MW00845527

Textbook of Palliative Care

Roderick Duncan MacLeod
Lieve Van den Block
Editors

Textbook of Palliative Care

Volume 2

With 194 Figures and 184 Tables

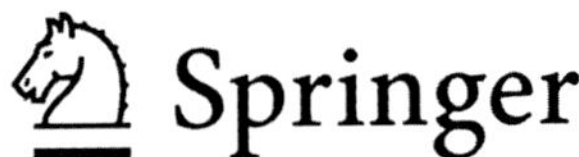

Editors
Roderick Duncan MacLeod
The University of Sydney
School of Medicine
Sydney, Australia

Palliative Care, HammondCare
University of Sydney
Sydney, NSW, Australia

Harbour Hospice
Auckland, New Zealand

Lieve Van den Block
VUB-UGhent End-of-Life Care Research Group
Department of Family Medicine and Chronic Care and Department of Clinical Sciences
Vrije Universiteit Brussel (VUB)
Brussels, Belgium

ISBN 978-3-319-77738-2 ISBN 978-3-319-77740-5 (eBook)
ISBN 978-3-319-77739-9 (print and electronic bundle)
https://doi.org/10.1007/978-3-319-77740-5

Library of Congress Control Number: 2019932976

This Springer imprint is published by the registered company Springer Nature Switzerland AG
The registered company address is: Gewerbestrasse 11, 6330 Cham, Switzerland

Foreword by Luc Deliens

We recently commemorated the 100th birth anniversary of Cicely Saunders, born in 1918. She began her education by studying philosophy, politics, and economics at the University of Oxford and then qualified as a nurse during the Second World War in the Nightingale Home and Training School in London; as a medical social worker, again at Oxford; and then as a medical doctor in the 1950s at King's College London. Her multidisciplinary educational background, combined with her personal experience (she twice fell in love with dying patients, both Polish refugees) which included a period of what she called "pathological grieving" after a series of bereavements, will have had an impact on her thinking and the development of the concept of palliative care, but also on her activism and her decades-long campaign against the terminal neglect of those who are dying and the medicalization of death. She wrote her first medical paper on care for dying people in 1957, and by the summer of 1967, she had initiated palliative care as an interdisciplinary concept at St. Christopher's Hospice in London, in the establishment of which she was involved. She is now acknowledged worldwide as one of the founders of the palliative care and hospice movement. Ever since, the field of palliative care has grown rapidly across the world, and the scientific evidence for its effectiveness is steadily growing, as is the list of countries with a national palliative care policy. The number of scientific journals covering death, dying, supportive care, palliative care, and end-of-life care is also rapidly growing, and about 20 of these have an impact factor indexed by the Web of Science, with around 5 being classified in the upper quartile of their domain. Hence, this textbook is timely and one of the indicators that palliative care as a clinical as well as a scientific domain has come to full growth.

"Palliative care" can be understood in several ways. It can be understood as a clinical specialism for medical doctors, as it is now recognized by the Royal College of Physicians as a specialty within the UK; it can also be understood as a specialist palliative care service, e.g., an inpatient hospice or palliative care unit, in which a multidisciplinary team delivers the care of people with serious illnesses, or, as a concept of care, a holistic philosophy of care taking into account more than just medical problems such as the burden of physical symptoms. This is reflected in the holistic definition of palliative care by the World Health Organization in which (apart from the medical aspects), nursing, social, psychological, and existential aspects are covered, or ideally should be covered. The latter suggests that there is a difference between what palliative care is in the real world and what it should be in the reality of our health-care systems; in most countries, the quality of palliative care in most care settings or contexts is suboptimal or can potentially be improved and further developed. This textbook can help clinicians, students, health-care providers, managers, researchers, and also policy-makers to improve their knowledge and skill in palliative care.

This textbook presents 101 chapters in 11 different parts: Palliative Care: Definitions, Development, Policies; Symptom Assessment and Management; Palliative Care Professionals and Provision; Organization of Palliative Care in Different Settings; Palliative Care in Specific Disease Groups; Palliative Care in Specific Populations; Palliative Care Emergencies; Ethics of Palliative Care and End-of-Life Decision-Making; Research in Palliative Care; Public Health Approach in Palliative and End-of-Life Care; and Financial Aspects and Cost-Effectiveness in Palliative Care. It offers a synthesis of the practice and knowledge base that has grown over the last 50 years. Since Cicely Saunders developed the concept of palliative care, focusing on preventing harm to people who are dying and promoting their quality of life, the field has evolved professionally and now covers a complex and wide range of aspects of care for all people with a serious illness, involving informal or family carers and volunteers as well as health-care professionals. Palliative care promotes life until death and should be understood as different from the narrow concept of terminal care. In order to challenge this narrow understanding, palliative care should also embrace the knowledge and skills of the disciplines of health promotion and public health, the latest developments of which are well covered in this textbook.

Cicely Saunders' multidisciplinary background is well reflected by the contents of the *Textbook of Palliative Care* and by its editors, a palliative care doctor, Professor Rod MacLeod from New Zealand, and a social scientist and clinical psychologist, Professor Lieve Van den Block from Belgium. The textbook, with over 100 chapters, covers the breadth of the domain, including clinical, health services, and public health-related aspects of palliative care. The editors should be congratulated on this impressive academic achievement and, more specifically because they have consulted a wide range of clinicians, far more social scientists, and public health experts than any other textbook on palliative care. I hope that this book, available online as well as in print, soon finds its way into the classrooms, universities, and vocational schools of all involved in the care of those who are dying or those with serious illness.

Professor of Palliative Care Research at Ghent University, Ghent, and VUB University Brussels, Belgium

Luc Deliens

Foreword by Sheila Payne

Palliative care has come of age. No longer can we claim, or make excuses, that palliative care is a young or novice discipline. This impressive *Textbook of Palliative Care* with over 100 chapters offers convincing evidence that palliative care is now a mature discipline. The textbook provides a comprehensive overview of numerous topics that form the core and substance of the discipline. The global reach of the chapter contributors and the distinguished section editors and the overall guidance from two remarkable editors have produced an outstanding testament to not only palliative care's place within medicine but also, importantly, within society.

However, let me caution you from any feelings of complacency and premature celebration. There are still many challenges ahead. We know from the work of the Lancet Commission on pain relief and palliative care that on a global scale, there remain very poor access to palliative care and woefully insufficient affordable and accessible pain relief (Knaul et al. 2017). According to the authors, in 20 health conditions where there were identifiable palliative care needs, 84% account for deaths in adults and 60% in children. Global projections indicate that between 40 and 80 million patients with advanced disease need access to palliative care, with 78–95% of them living in low- and middle-income countries (Knaul et al. 2017). Shockingly, infants and children have even less access to pain relief and palliative care than adults (Knaul et al. 2017).

One way forward is to ensure that the key principles of palliative care are taught as a fundamental part of all basic and post-basic health and social care education programmes. Let me draw a comparison here with the recognition of communication skills as a core element of all courses. When I trained as a nurse in the early 1970s in a well-respected London teaching hospital, my only communication skills education was the well-worn advice for nurses working in hospital wards, which was to *draw the curtains and reassure the patient.* Quite how I might provide that 'reassurance', when the poor patient was likely to be facing an uncomfortable, painful and/or embarrassing procedure, was never revealed. Fortunately, communication skills education is now a core topic in virtually all medical, nursing and other health professional programmes. In some countries, it is even mandatory. In my view, likewise, palliative care core competencies also need to be embedded in all health and social care programmes as essential aspects of professional education (Gamondi et al. 2013).

So what will be the future challenges facing palliative care? We need to be prepared to 'give it away' so that basic palliative care practices and knowledge move beyond the restricted domains of certain places such as specialist palliative care units, or disease groups such as those with cancer, or age groups, or professional disciplinary boundaries. I am not arguing that there is no future for specialist palliative care, as the people working in these settings, and with this expertise, are essential to drive the education of others; improve the quality of care, through research and reflective practice; and provide leadership. However, to ensure universal coverage and access to basic palliative care, more energy, resource and leadership need to be devoted to spreading the political and policy message that palliative care is not a luxury for the few but a fundamental human right.

Universal access to high-quality palliative care may not be quite within our grasp yet but should be a goal for everyone. Suffering, especially avoidable suffering, blights the lives of millions of people, creating a lasting impact on their families in terms of financial burden and emotional distress. Addressing the challenges of responding compassionately, while drawing on the best scientific evidence, to ameliorate suffering for those with complex, advanced and life-limiting conditions lies at the heart of palliative care. This textbook is a good example of this commitment to improve care for all in need.

This textbook is truly outstanding. I am not going to highlight specific chapters, as I am sure that all contributors will have fulfilled their brief under the guidance of the editorial team. It is a textbook to dip into, relishing the quality of the information contained in these pages. You, dear reader, will make your choices, but let me urge you to venture into new areas, perhaps reading those chapters that are outside your normal interest zone. Become a critical consumer of the material and resources presented in this textbook. How does it compare to your practice? What does it challenge you to think about in a new and different way? What do you agree with? This textbook, developed by an international team of experts, offers guidance on the development and establishment of all aspects of palliative care services, and it wonderfully captures the flourishing of a mature discipline.

Emeritus Professor
International Observatory on End of Life Care
Lancaster University
UK

Sheila Payne

References

Gamondi C, Larkin P, Payne S. Core competencies in palliative care: an EAPC White Paper on palliative care education – part 1. Eur J Palliat Care. 2013;20(2):140–5.

Knaul FM, Farmer PE, Krakauer EL, De Lima L, Bhadelia A, Jiang Kwete X, et al. Alleviating the access abyss in palliative care and pain relief-an imperative of universal health coverage: the Lancet Commission report. Lancet. 2017. https://doi.org/10.1016/S0140-6736(17)32513-8

Preface

Nothing in life is to be feared, it is only to be understood.

Attributed to Marie Curie. *On ne doit rien craindre dans la vie—il suffit de comprendre* in Université Laval, Faculté de médecine, Société medicale des hôpitaux universitaires de Québec, Laval médical (1951), 16, 569

Palliative care has been identified as a discrete part of healthcare for over 50 years, and yet we still find ourselves having to explain the nature and practice of palliative care to many of our professional colleagues and to the public in general. Healthcare education and training has been slow to recognize the vital importance of ensuring that *all* practitioners have a good understanding of what is involved in the care of people with serious or advanced illnesses and their families. Because of this limited exposure, many laypeople and professionals still have understandable fear and anxiety about death and dying.

However, the science of palliative care is advancing, and our understanding of the evidence concerning many aspects of palliative care is developing rapidly. There are now excellent research teams and facilities around the world exploring different characteristics of this essential aspect of healthcare from a wide range of disciplines.

There have been many authoritative books on various facets of palliative care produced over the last years. In planning this *Textbook of Palliative Care,* we hoped to produce a comprehensive, clinically relevant, and state-of-the-art book, aimed at advancing palliative care, as a science, a clinical practice, and an art.

For this major reference work, we have been able to draw on our own collective experience and the goodwill of many fine people from around the world. We have endeavored to produce a *Textbook* that showcases the multi- and interdisciplinarity of palliative care and is unique in bringing together authors from all fields of palliative care – physical, psychological, social, and existential or spiritual. The majority of them are internationally recognized experts in their chosen discipline. We have been helped by dozens of authors and the committed section editors, who have given their time, expertise, and wisdom to ensure that this work can be disseminated around the globe to assist in the understanding of all aspects of illness and disease near the end of life as well as death, dying, and into bereavement. Our authors have drawn not only on the evidence available but also on their own phronesis or practical wisdom. They have summarized and extended the state of the art in their field and challenge the reader with new insights, challenges, opportunities, and potential future evolutions. We are deeply indebted to all those who have been involved in the preparation, writing, and editing of this work. They all undertook their work with enthusiasm and commitment.

We expect this *textbook* will be of value to practitioners in all disciplines and professions where the care of people approaching death is important, specialists as well as nonspecialists, in any setting where people with serious advanced illnesses reside. It can also be an important resource for researchers, policy-makers, and decision-makers – national or regional – as well as for laypersons, patients, and/or families, seeking to learn more about palliative care. Neither the science nor the art of palliative care will stand still, so we hope to be able to keep this *textbook* updated as the authors find new evidence and approaches to care.

Our special appreciation goes to Vasowati Shome and Tina Shelton of Springer who have guided us expertly through the process of creating this reference work – we are deeply indebted to them.

March 2019

Roderick Duncan MacLeod
Lieve Van den Block

Contents

Volume 1

About the Editors

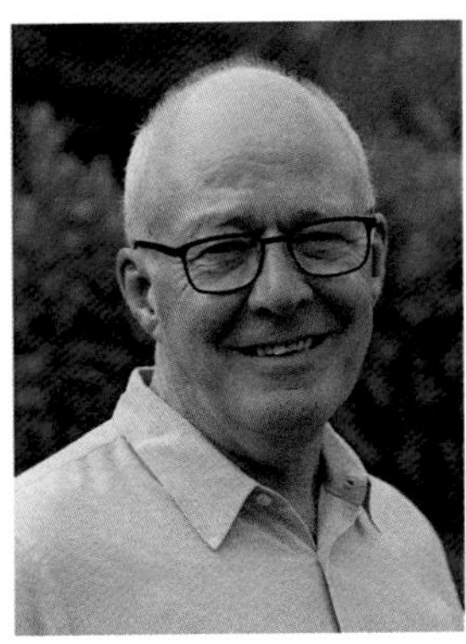

Roderick Duncan MacLeod is a Palliative Medicine Specialist at Harbour Hospice in Auckland, New Zealand, and Consultant to HammondCare in Sydney where he is also Honorary Professor in the University of Sydney School of Medicine.

He gained his primary medical degrees from the University of Dundee in 1976 and went on to train for general practice. He was a Principal in general practice for almost 10 years before moving to the discipline of palliative care. He was first appointed as Medical Director of the Dorothy House Foundation in Bath, England, in 1989 after having completed a period of prolonged study leave exploring palliative care in the community. In 1994, he was appointed Medical Director and subsequently Director of Palliative Care at the Mary Potter Hospice in Wellington, New Zealand. He was made a Fellow of the Royal College of General Practitioners (UK) in 1999. He was a Foundation Fellow of the Royal Australasian College of Physicians, Australasian Chapter of Palliative Medicine, in 2000. He received his Ph.D. in 2001 from the University of Glamorgan (Prifysgol De Cymru) for his work and publications on "Changing the Way that Doctors Learn to Care for People Who Are Dying."

In 2003, he was appointed to New Zealand's first Chair in Palliative Care as the inaugural South Link Health Professor in Palliative Care at the University of Otago Dunedin School of Medicine and in 2013 was appointed Conjoint Professor in Palliative Care at the University of Sydney and worked clinically as Senior Staff Specialist in Palliative Care for HammondCare in Sydney. He has been a Member of the Australasian Chapter of Palliative Medicine

Education Committee, the NZ National Health Committee – Working Party on Care of People Who Are Dying, the NZ Palliative Care Expert Working Group, and the Council of the Asia Pacific Hospice Network. He was appointed to the Expert Advisory Group (Physician Education) and the Chapter of Palliative Medicine Committee of the Royal Australasian College of Physicians and the NZ Ministry of Health Palliative Care Advisory Group. He has also held a number of roles within Hospice NZ.

He has published over 130 peer-reviewed articles in the field of palliative care in national and international journals and has written over 20 chapters for palliative care texts. In addition, he has been on editorial boards of international peer-reviewed journals in the field of palliative care and has reviewed manuscripts for over 25 different academic journals. He has also published two anthologies of poetry, exploring what it might be like to approach death and experience bereavement and loss.

He is one of the authors of *The Palliative Care Handbook*, which has become a freely available standard text for healthcare professionals in New Zealand and parts of Australia.

He was appointed a Member of the New Zealand Order of Merit by Her Majesty Queen Elizabeth II in the Queen's birthday honors in 2015.

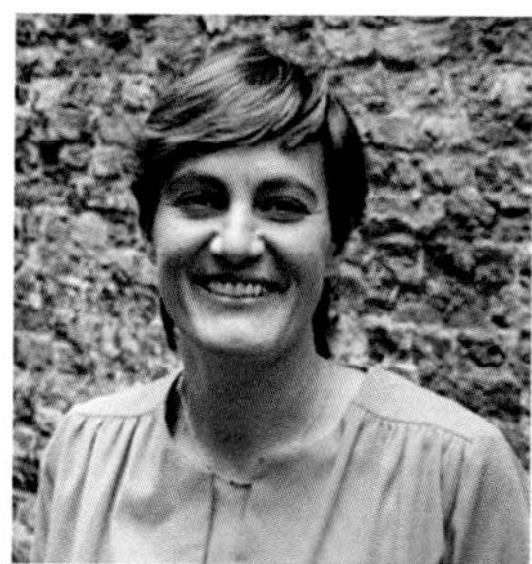

Lieve Van den Block is Professor of Ageing and Palliative Care at the Vrije Universiteit Brussel (VUB) and Chair of the Ageing and Palliative Care Research Programme at the End-of-Life Care Research Group of the VUB and Ghent University in Belgium. She holds a Ph.D. in Medical Social Sciences and a master's in Clinical Psychology. Professor Van den Block has been involved in palliative care research for over 15 years, focusing on national and international public health and interventional research aimed at monitoring and improving palliative and end-of-life care. She has received several scientific awards for her work, including the 2014 Early Researcher Award of the European Association for Palliative Care. She has published over 100 peer-reviewed articles on palliative care and is editor and author of several books and chapters. Her work has been supported by grants from the European Commission, national fundamental and applied research foundations, and leading medical and health charities.

Section Editors

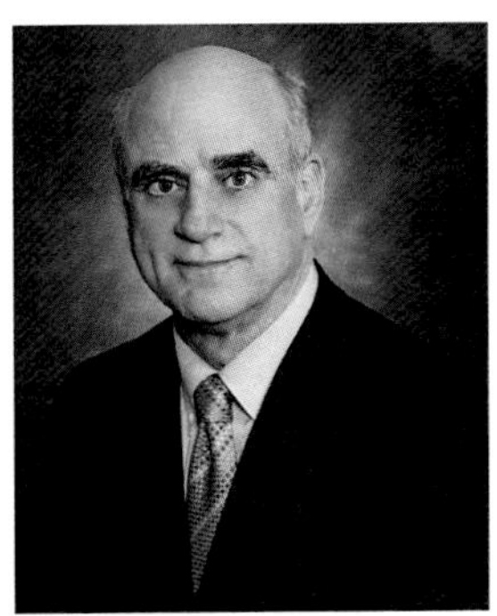

Stephen R. Connor Worldwide Hospice Palliative Care Alliance, London, UK

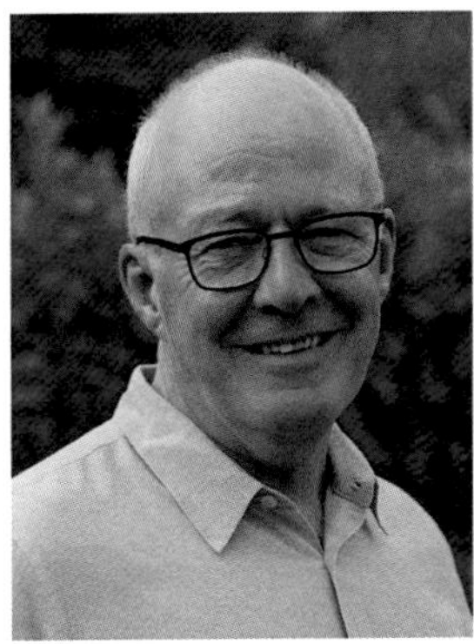

Roderick Duncan MacLeod The University of Sydney School of Medicine, Sydney, Australia

Palliative Care, HammondCare, University of Sydney, Sydney, NSW, Australia

Harbour Hospice, Auckland, New Zealand

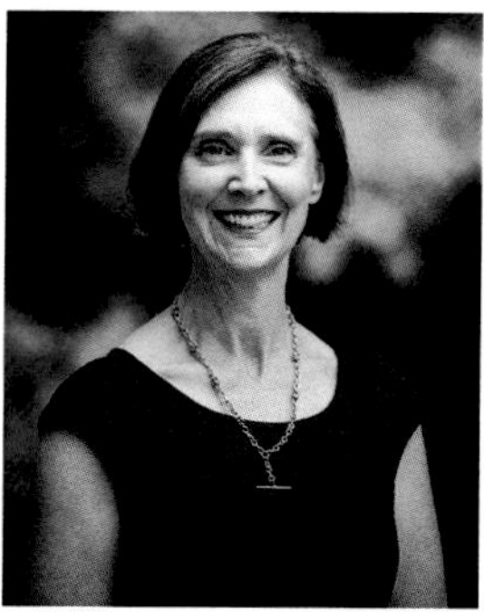

Melanie Lovell Centre for Learning and Research in Palliative Care, HammondCare, Sydney Medical School, Faculty of Health, University of Technology Sydney, Greenwich, NSW, Australia

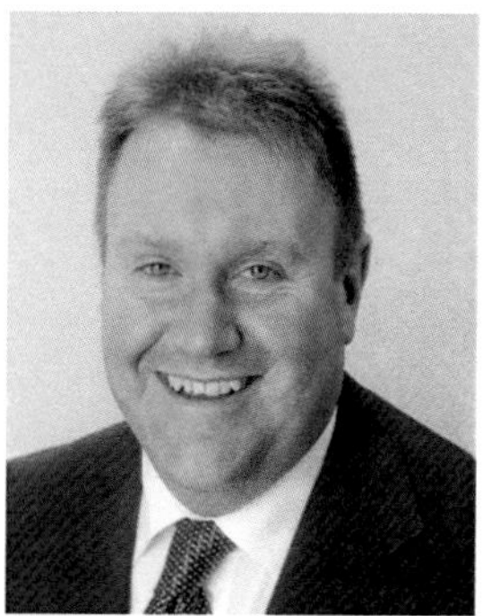

Philip Larkin University of Lausanne, Lausanne, Switzerland

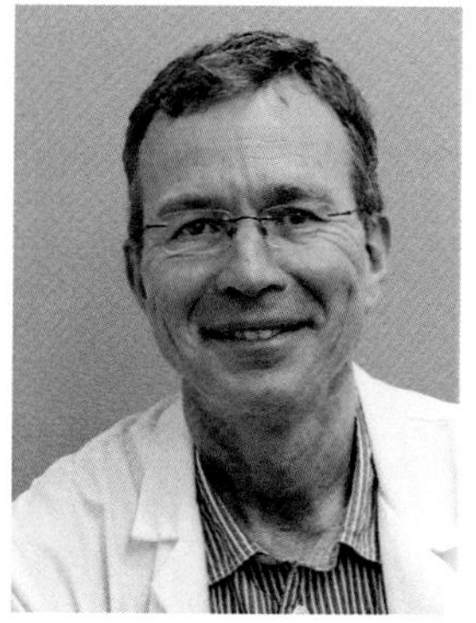

Steffen Eychmüller Universitäres Zentrum für Palliative Care, Bern, Switzerland

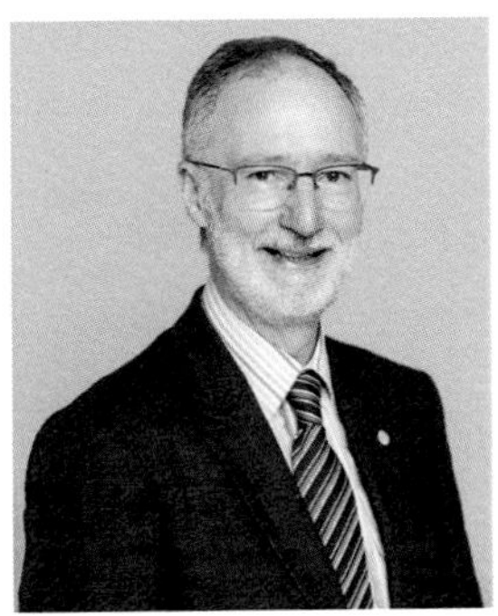

David Oliver Tizard Centre, University of Kent, Canterbury, Kent, UK

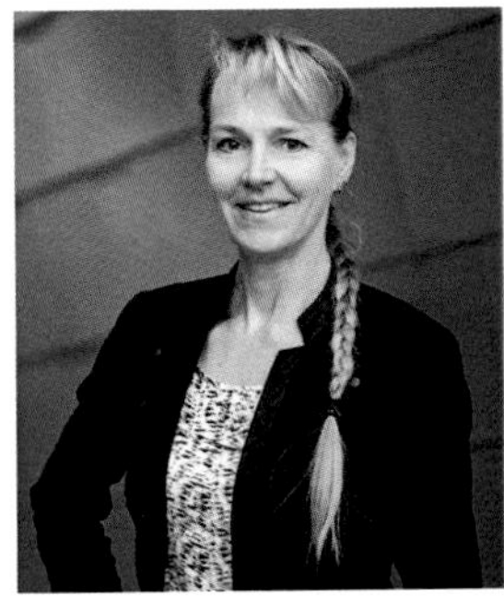

Jenny T. van der Steen Department of Public Health and Primary Care, Leiden University Medical Center, Leiden, The Netherlands

Radboud university medical center, Department of Primary and Community Care, Nijmegen, The Netherlands

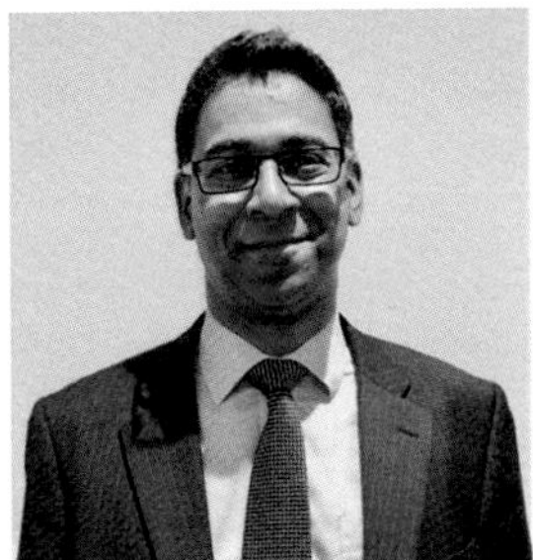

Leeroy William Palliative Medicine, Monash Health, Eastern Health, Monash University, Melbourne, VIC, Australia

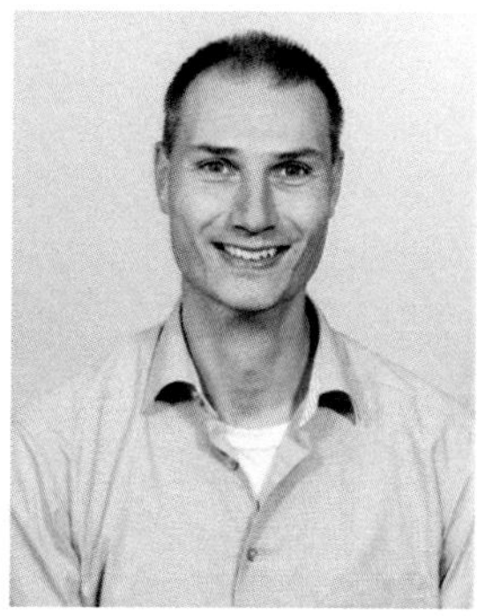

Jeroen Hasselaar Department of Anesthesiology, Pain and Palliative Medicine, Radboud University Medical Center, Nijmegen, The Netherlands

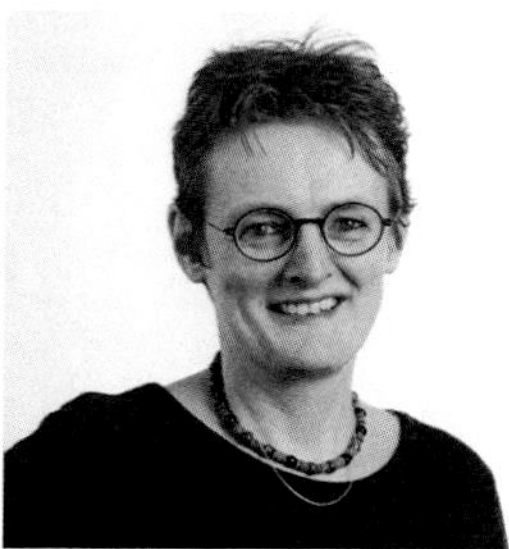

Agnes van der Heide Erasmus University Medical Center, Rotterdam, Netherlands

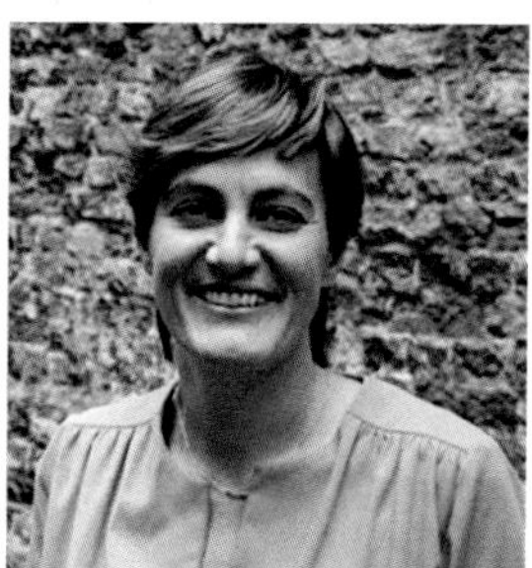

Lieve Van den Block VUB-UGhent End-of-Life Care Research Group, Department of Family Medicine and Chronic Care and Department of Clinical Sciences, Vrije Universiteit Brussel (VUB), Brussels, Belgium

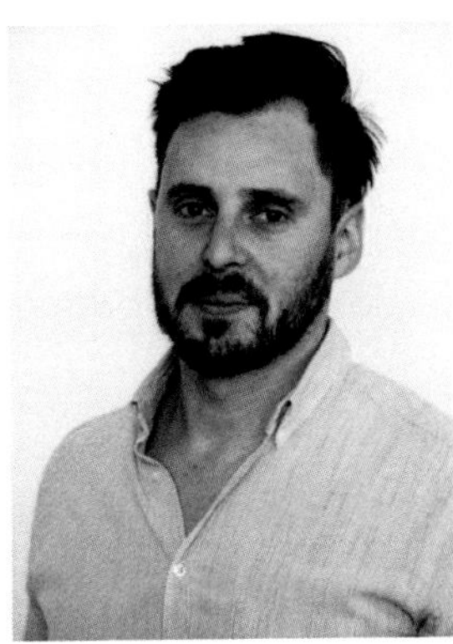

Joachim Cohen End-of-Life Care Research Group, Vrije Universiteit Brussel (VUB) and Ghent University, Brussels, Belgium

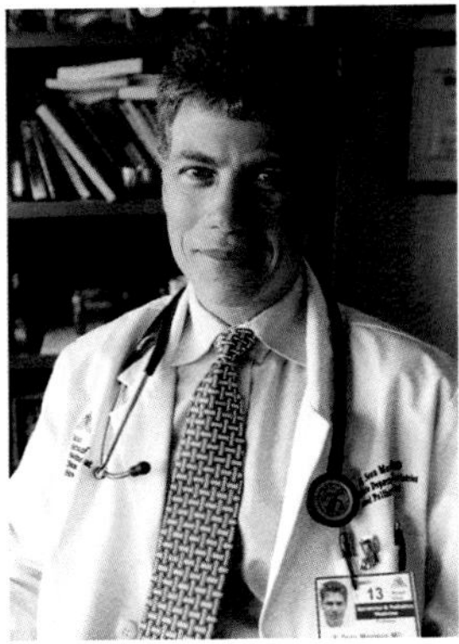

R. Sean Morrison Brookdale Department of Geriatrics and Palliative Medicine, Icahn School of Medicine at Mount Sinai, New York, NY, USA

Contributors

Meera Agar Faculty of Health, University of Technology Sydney, Ultimo, NSW, Australia

South Western Sydney Clinical School, School of Medicine, University of New South Wales (UNSW), Sydney, NSW, Australia

Ingham Institute for Applied Medical Research, Liverpool, NSW, Australia

Palliative Care Service, South Western Sydney Local Health District, Sydney, NSW, Australia

Jacqui Allen University of Auckland, Grafton, Auckland, New Zealand

Jordi Amblàs University of Vic-Central University of Catalonia, Barcelona, Spain

Ingrid Amgarth-Duff Faculty of Health, University of Technology Sydney, Ultimo, NSW, Australia

María Arantzamendi ICS. ATLANTES: Dignidad humana, enfermedad avanzada y cuidados paliativos, Universidad de Navarra, Pamplona, Spain

Rebecca A. Aslakson Department of Medicine and Division of Primary Care and Population Health, Section of Palliative Care; Department of Anesthesiology, Perioperative and Pain Medicine, Stanford University, Stanford, CA, USA

Emma Bateman Cancer Treatment Toxicities Group, School of Medicine, University of Adelaide, Adelaide, SA, Australia

Lesley S. Batten College of Health, Massey University, Palmerston North, New Zealand

James M. Beattie Cicely Saunders Institute, King's College, London, UK

Bertrand Behm Palliative Medicine, Geisinger Health System, Danville, PA, USA

Kirsty Beilharz Music Engagement, Palliative Care, HammondCare, University of New South Wales, Kolling Institute and University of Edinburgh Visiting Fellow, Sydney, NSW, Australia

Alazne Belar ICS. ATLANTES: Dignidad humana, enfermedad avanzada y cuidados paliativos, Universidad de Navarra, Pamplona, Spain

Jan Bernheim End-of-Life Care Research Group, Vrije Universiteit Brussel (VUB) and Ghent University, Brussels, Belgium

Megan Best University of Sydney, Sydney, NSW, Australia

University of Notre Dame Australia, Broadway, NSW, Australia

Priyanka Bhattarai Faculty of Health, Improving Palliative, Aged and Chronic Care Through Clinical Research and Translation, University of Technology Sydney, Ultimo, NSW, Australia

School of Nursing, University of Notre Dame Australia-Sydney, Darlinghurst, NSW, Australia

Carrie Bourassa Indigenous and Northern Health, Health Sciences North Research Institute, Sudbury, ON, Canada

Institute of Indigenous Peoples' Health, Canadian Institute of Health Research, Sudbury, ON, Canada

Frank Brennan Palliative Care Physician, St George and Calvary Hospitals, Sydney, Australia

Katherine Bristowe King's College London, Cicely Saunders institute of Palliative Care, Policy and Rehabilitation, London, UK

Ingrid Bullich Socio-Health Program, General Management of Health Planning, Government of Catalonia, Barcelona, Spain

Shirley H. Bush Department of Medicine, Division of Palliative Care, University of Ottawa, Ottawa, ON, Canada

Bruyère Research Institute, Ottawa, ON, Canada

Ottawa Hospital Research Institute, Ottawa, ON, Canada

Philippa Cahill School of Medicine, The University of Notre Dame Australia, Darlinghurst, NSW, Australia

Belinda A. Campbell Department of Radiation Oncology and Cancer Imaging, Peter MacCallum Cancer Centre, Melbourne, Australia

Rachel Campbell Northern Ireland Medical and Dental Agency, Belfast, UK

Bridget Candy Marie Curie Palliative Care Research Department, University College London, London, UK

Keryln Carville Silver Chain Group and Curtin University, Perth, WA, Australia

Carlos Centeno ATLANTES Research Program, Institute for Culture and Society, University of Navarra, Pamplona, Spain

Palliative Care Unit, Clínica Universidad de Navarra, University of Navarra, Pamplona, Spain

Kenneth Chambaere End-of-Life Care Research Group, Vrije Universiteit Brussel (VUB) and Ghent University, Brussels, Belgium

Emily Chang Starship specialist paediatric palliative care service, Auckland City Hospital, Auckland, New Zealand

Rebecca Chin Radiation Oncology, Sydney Adventist Hospital, The University of Sydney, Sydney, NSW, Australia

Katherine Clark Cancer and Palliative Care Network NSLHD, Northern Sydney Cancer Centre Royal North Shore Hospital, St Leonards, NSW, Australia

Northern Clinical School, The University of Sydney, Camperdown, NSW, Australia

Jean B. Clark Hospital Palliative Care Service Palmerston North Hospital, MidCentral Health, Palmerston North, New Zealand

School of Nursing, Massey University, Palmerston North, New Zealand

Josephine M. Clayton Centre for Learning and Research in Palliative Care, HammondCare; and Sydney Medical School, University of Sydney, Sydney, NSW, Australia

Dianne Clifton RANZCP, St Vincent's Hospital Melbourne, Cabrini Hospital, Albert Road Clinic, Hawthorn Road Consulting Suites, International Psycho-oncology Society, University of Melbourne, Fitzroy, VIC, Australia

Psychosocial Cancer Care, St Vincent's Hospital Melbourne, Fitzroy, VIC, Australia

Joachim Cohen End-of-Life Care Research Group, Vrije Universiteit Brussel (VUB) and Ghent University, Brussels, Belgium

Andrew Cole Rehabilitation, HammondCare and University of New South Wales, Sydney, NSW, Australia

Sarah Combes King's College London, Florence Nightingale Faculty of Nursing, Midwifery and Palliative Care, London, UK

St Christopher's Hospice, London, UK

Stephen R. Connor Worldwide Hospice Palliative Care Alliance, London, UK

Xavier Costa University of Vic-Central University of Catalonia, Barcelona, Spain

Gregory B. Crawford Northern Adelaide Palliative Service, Northern Adelaide Local Health Network, Adelaide, SA, Australia

Discipline of Medicine, University of Adelaide, Adelaide, SA, Australia

Agnes Csikos Department of Primary care, Pecs University, Pécs, Hungary

David Currow IMPACCT – Improving Palliative Aged Care through Clinical Research and Translation, Faculty of Health, University of Technology Sydney, Ultimo, NSW, Australia

Wolfson Palliative Care Research Centre, Hull York Medical School, University of Hull, Hull, UK

J. Randall Curtis Division of Pulmonary, Critical Care, and Sleep Medicine, Harborview Medical Center, Cambia Palliative Care Center of Excellence, University of Washington, Seattle, WA, USA

Nathan Davies Centre for Ageing Population Studies, Research Department of Primary Care and Population Health, University College London, London, UK

Mellar P. Davis Department of Palliative Care, Geisinger Medical Center, Danville, PA, USA

Aline de Vleminck End-of-life care research group, Department of Family Medicine and Chronic Care, Vrije Universiteit Brussel, Jette, Belgium

Karen Detering Advance Care Planning Australia, Austin Health, Melbourne, VIC, Australia

Rachel E. Diamond Palliative Care Division, Department of Medicine, University of Rochester Medical Center, Rochester, NY, USA

Michelle DiGiacomo Improving Palliative, Aged, and Chronic Care through Clinical Research and Translation (IMPACCT), Faculty of Health, University of Technology Sydney, Ultimo, NSW, Australia

Julia Downing International Children's Palliative Care Network, Durban, South Africa

Ross Drake Starship specialist paediatric palliative care service, Auckland City Hospital, Auckland, New Zealand

Jaimee Dudley University of Auckland, Auckland, New Zealand

Mathew Dutton Wound Management Clinical Nurse Consultant, St George Hospital, Sydney, Australia

Elizabeth S. Dylke Faculty of Health Sciences, University of Sydney, Sydney, NSW, Australia

Peter Eastman Department of Palliative Care, Barwon Health, North Geelong, VIC, Australia

Department of Palliative and Supportive Care, Royal Melbourne Hospital/ Melbourne Health, Parkville, VIC, Australia

Sara Ela World Health Organization Collaborating Center for Public Health Palliative Care Programs, Catalan Institute of Oncology, University of Vic-Central University of Catalonia, Barcelona, Spain

Prudence Ellis Speech Pathology, HammondCare, Greenwich, NSW, Australia

Catherine Evans King's College London, Cicely Saunders Institute of Palliative Care, Policy and Rehabilitation, London, UK

Sussex Community NHS Foundation Trust, Brighton General Hospital, Brighton, UK

Gail Ewing Centre for Family Research, Department of Psychology, University of Cambridge, Cambridge, UK

Carlos Fernandez Palliative Medicine, Geisinger Health System, Danville, PA, USA

Diana Ferreira Flinders University, Bedford Park, SA, Australia

Jane Fletcher Melbourne Psycho-oncology Service, Cabrini Health, Epworth Hospital, Monash University, Melbourne, VIC, Australia

Janette Fodera Arts on Prescription, HammondCare, Sydney, NSW, Australia

Abigail E. Franklin HammondCare Palliative and Supportive Care Service, Greenwich Hospital, Sydney, NSW, Australia

Claire Fraser Faculty of Health, Improving Palliative, Aged and Chronic Care Through Clinical Research and Translation, University of Technology Sydney, Ultimo, NSW, Australia

Xavier Gómez-Batiste World Health Organization Collaborating Center for Public Health Palliative Care Programs, Catalan Institute of Oncology, Barcelona, Spain

University of Vic-Central University of Catalonia, Barcelona, Spain

Wei Gao Cicely Saunders Institute of Palliative Care, Policy and Rehabilitation, King's College London, London, UK

Rachel Gibson Cancer Treatment Toxicities Group, School of Medicine, University of Adelaide, Adelaide, SA, Australia

Division of Health Sciences, University of South Australia, Adelaide, SA, Australia

Gunn Grande Division of Nursing, Midwifery and Social Work, School of Health Sciences, Faculty of Biology, Medicine and Health, University of Manchester, Manchester, UK

Gareth P. Gregory Monash Haematology, Monash Health, Clayton, VIC, Australia

School of Clinical Sciences at Monash Health, Monash University, Clayton, VIC, Australia

Stephanie Grimes Musgrave Park Hospital, Belfast, UK

Kate Grundy Christchurch Hospital Palliative Care Service, Christchurch, New Zealand

Liz Gwyther School of Public Health and Family Medicine, University of Cape Town and Hospice Palliative Care Association of South Africa, Cape Town, South Africa

Christopher Hall Australian Centre for Grief and Bereavement, Mulgrave, VIC, Australia

Richard Harding Cicely Saunders Institute, Department of Palliative Care Policy and Rehabilitation, Florence Nightingale Faculty of Nursing, Midwifery and Palliative care, King's College London, London, UK

Jeroen Hasselaar Department of Anesthesiology, Pain and Palliative Medicine, Radboud University Medical Center, Nijmegen, The Netherlands

Nilay Hepgul Cicely Saunders Institute of Palliative Care, Policy and Rehabilitation, King's College London, London, UK

Agnes Higgins School of Nursing and Midwifery, Trinity College Dublin, Dublin, Ireland

Irene J. Higginson Cicely Saunders Institute of Palliative Care, Policy and Rehabilitation, King's College London, London, UK

Jo Hockley Primary Palliative Care Research Group, Centre for Population Health Sciences, The Usher Institute of Population Health Sciences and Informatics, The University of Edinburgh, Edinburgh, Scotland

Russell Hogg Obstetrics and Gynaecology, Royal North Shore Hospital, The University of Sydney, Sydney, NSW, Australia

Annmarie Hosie Faculty of Health, University of Technology Sydney, Ultimo, NSW, Australia

Doris Howell Lawrence S. Bloomberg Faculty of Nursing, University of Toronto, Toronto, ON, Canada

Princess Margaret Cancer Center, University Health Network, Toronto, ON, Canada

Peter Huggard School of Population Health, Faculty of Medical and Health Sciences, University of Auckland, Auckland, New Zealand

Jayne Huggard School of Nursing, Faculty of Medical and Health Sciences, University of Auckland, Auckland, New Zealand

Geralyn Hynes School of Nursing and Midwifery, Trinity College Dublin, Dublin, Ireland

Akshay Ilango RANZCP, Melbourne, VIC, Australia

Monash Health, Melbourne, VIC, Australia

Austin Health, Melbourne, VIC, Australia

Sarina R. Isenberg Department of Health, Behavior and Society, Johns Hopkins Bloomberg School of Public Health, Baltimore, MD, USA

Temmy Latner Centre for Palliative Care and Lunenfeld-Tanenbaum Research Institute, Sinai Health System, Toronto, ON, Canada

Department of Family and Community Medicine, University of Toronto, Toronto, ON, Canada

Birgit Jaspers Department of Palliative Medicine, University Hospital Bonn, Bonn, Germany

Bridget Johnston Centre for Health Policy and Management, Trinity College Dublin, Dublin, Ireland

Marion Jones Auckland University of Technology, Auckland, New Zealand

Dorothy Keefe Cancer Treatment Toxicities Group, School of Medicine, University of Adelaide, Adelaide, SA, Australia

Puneeta Khurana Palliative Care Division, Department of Medicine, University of Rochester Medical Center, Rochester, NY, USA

Sharon L. Kilbreath Faculty of Health Sciences, University of Sydney, Sydney, NSW, Australia

Maartje S. Klapwijk Healthcare Organisation Marente, Voorhout, The Netherlands

Department of Public Health and Primary Care, Leiden University Medical Center, Leiden, The Netherlands

Slavica Kochovska Improving Palliative, Aged, and Chronic Care through Clinical Research and Translation (IMPACCT), Faculty of Health, University of Technology Sydney, Ultimo, NSW, Australia

Eric L. Krakauer Harvard Medical School, Boston, MA, USA

Center for Palliative Care, Harvard Medical School, Boston, MA, USA

Division of Palliative Care and Geriatrics, Massachusetts General Hospital, Boston, MA, USA

Department of Palliative Care, University of Medicine and Pharmacy, Ho Chi Minh City, Vietnam

Dmitrij Kravchenko Department of Palliative Medicine, Universitätsklinikum Bonn (AöR), Bonn, Germany

Sophia Lam Department of Medicine, Cairns and Hinterland Hospital and Health Service, Cairns, QLD, Australia

Jonathan Langton Department of Interventional and Diagnostic Imaging, Monash Health, Clayton, Australia

Anne M. Larson Department of Internal Medicine, Division of Gastroenterology, University of Washington, NW Hepatology/UW Medicine, Seattle, WA, USA

Cristina Lasmarías World Health Organization Collaborating Center for Public Health Palliative Care Programs, Catalan Institute of Oncology, University of Vic-Central University of Catalonia, Barcelona, Spain

Lis Latta Dunedin School of Medicine, University of Otago, Dunedin, New Zealand

Brian Le Department of Palliative and Supportive Care, Royal Melbourne Hospital/Melbourne Health, Parkville, VIC, Australia

Carlo Leget University of Humanistic Studies, Utrecht, The Netherlands

Richard Logan Cancer Treatment Toxicities Group, School of Medicine, University of Adelaide, Adelaide, SA, Australia

School of Dentistry, University of Adelaide, Adelaide, SA, Australia

Melanie R. Lovell HammondCare Palliative and Supportive Care Service, Greenwich Hospital, Sydney, NSW, Australia

Northern Clinical School and Kolling Institute, The University of Sydney, Sydney, NSW, Australia

Joe Low Marie Curie Palliative Care Research Department, University College London, London, UK

Tim Luckett Improving Palliative, Aged and Chronic Care through Clinical Research and Translation, Faculty of Health, University of Technology Sydney, Sydney, NSW, Australia

Emmanuel Luyirika African Palliative Care Association, Kampala, Uganda

Roderick Duncan MacLeod The University of Sydney School of Medicine, Sydney, Australia

Palliative Care, HammondCare, University of Sydney, Sydney, NSW, Australia

Harbour Hospice, Auckland, New Zealand

Matthew Maddocks Cicely Saunders Institute of Palliative Care, Policy and Rehabilitation, King's College London, London, UK

Arno Maetens End-of-Life Care Research Group, Vrije Universiteit Brussel (VUB) and Ghent University, Brussels, Belgium

Linda Magann Palliative Care Clinical Nurse Consultant, St George Hospital, Sydney, Australia

Catherine Mandel Swinburne Neuroimaging, Swinburne University of Technology, Melbourne, VIC, Australia

Kathleen Mason School of Nursing, University of Auckland, Auckland, New Zealand

Peter May Centre for Health Policy and Management, Trinity College Dublin, Dublin, Ireland

The Irish Longitudinal study on Ageing (TILDA), Trinity College Dublin, Dublin, Ireland

Janet McElhaney Health Sciences North Research Institute, Sudbury, ON, Canada

Michelle Meiring School of Public Health and Family Medicine, University of Cape Town and Hospice Palliative Care Association of South Africa, Cape Town, South Africa

Geoffrey Mitchell Primary Care Clinical Unit, Faculty of Medicine, University of Queensland, Brisbane, Australia

Martin Mücke Department of Palliative Medicine, Universitätsklinikum Bonn (AöR), Bonn, Germany

Tess Moeke-Maxwell School of Nursing, Faculty of Medical and Health Sciences, University of Auckland, Auckland, New Zealand

Anne Morgan Christchurch, New Zealand

R. Sean Morrison Brookdale Department of Geriatrics and Palliative Medicine, Icahn School of Medicine at Mount Sinai, New York, NY, USA

Fliss E. M. Murtagh Wolfson Palliative Care Research Centre, Hull York Medical School, University of Hull, Hull, UK

Caroline Nicholson King's College London, Florence Nightingale Faculty of Nursing, Midwifery and Palliative Care, London, UK

St Christopher's Hospice, London, UK

Supportive and End of Life Care (Nursing), St. Christopher's Hospice/King's College, London, UK

Simon Noble Marie Curie Palliative Care Research Centre, Division of Population Medicine, Cardiff University, Cardiff, UK

Charles Normand Centre for Health Policy and Management, Trinity College Dublin, Dublin, Ireland

Cicely Saunders Institute Of Palliative Care, Policy and Rehabilitation, King's College London, London, UK

Eric Oleson First Nations University of Canada, Regina, SK, Canada

David Oliver Tizard Centre, University of Kent, Canterbury, Kent, UK

Koen Pardon End-of-Life Care Research group, Vrije Universiteit Brussel and Ghent University, Brussels, Belgium

Faculty of Medicine and Life Science, Faculty of Business Economics, Hasselt University, Diepenbeek, Belgium

Sally Paul School of Social Work and Social Policy, University of Strathclyde, Glasgow, UK

Cathy Payne All Ireland Institute of Hospice and Palliative Care (AIIHPC), Dublin, Ireland

Institute of Nursing and Health Research, Ulster University, Newtownabbey, UK

Sheila Payne International Observatory on End of Life Care, Lancaster University, Lancaster, UK

Leena Pelttari EAPC Task Force on Volunteering in Hospice and Palliative Care in Europe, Hospice Austria, Vienna, Austria

Yolanda W. H. Penders Epidemiology, Biostatistics and Prevention Institute, University of Zürich, Zürich, Switzerland

Jane L. Phillips Faculty of Health, Improving Palliative, Aged and Chronic Care Through Clinical Research and Translation, University of Technology Sydney, Ultimo, NSW, Australia

School of Nursing, University of Notre Dame Australia-Sydney, Darlinghurst, NSW, Australia

Lara Pivodic End-of-Life Care Research Group, Vrije Universiteit Brussel (VUB) and Ghent University, Brussels, Belgium

Peter Poon Supportive and Palliative Medicine, Monash Health, Eastern Palliative Care, Monash University, Clayton, VIC, Australia

Kathy Pope Department of Radiation Oncology and Cancer Imaging, Peter MacCallum Cancer Centre, Melbourne, VIC, Australia

Christopher Poulos Centre for Positive Ageing, HammondCare and University of New South Wales, Hammondville, NSW, Australia

Roslyn Poulos The School of Public Health and Community Medicine, University of New South Wales, Sydney, NSW, Australia

K. M. Prasanna Kumar Centre for Diabetes and Endocrine Care, Bengaluru, India

Timothy E. Quill Palliative Care Division, Department of Medicine, University of Rochester Medical Center, Rochester, NY, USA

Mike Rabow General Internal Medicine, University of San Francisco, San Francisco, CA, USA

Lukas Radbruch Department of Palliative Medicine, University Hospital Bonn, Bonn, Germany

Centre of Palliative Care, Malteser Hospital Seliger Gerhard Bonn/Rhein-Sieg, Bonn, Germany

Suzanne Rainsford Medical School, Australian National University, Canberra, Australia

Calvary Healthcare Bruce, Clare Holland House Campus, Canberra, Australia

Sharp Street Surgery, Cooma, NSW, Australia

Pallavi D. Rao Centre for Diabetes and Endocrine Care, Bengaluru, India

Mpho Ratshikana-Moloko University of the Witswatersrand, Johannesburg, South Africa

Kasper Raus Ghent University Hospital, Ghent, Belgium

Valentina Razmovski-Naumovski South Western Sydney Clinical School, School of Medicine, University of New South Wales (UNSW), Sydney, Australia

Rab Razzak Outpatient Palliative Medicine, Johns Hopkins Medicine, Johns Hopkins School of Medicine, Baltimore, USA

Sally Regel Department of Palliative Care, Geisinger Medical Center, Danville, PA, USA

John Y. Rhee ATLANTES Research Program, Institute for Culture and Society, University of Navarra, Pamplona, Spain

Icahn School of Medicine at Mount Sinai, New York, NY, USA

Judith Rietjens Department of Public Health, Erasmus MC, Rotterdam, CA, The Netherlands

Jillian P. Riley National Heart and Lung Institute, Imperial College, London, UK

Rocio Rojí Departamento Medicina Paliativa, Clínica Universidad de Navarra, Pamplona, Spain

Margaret Ross Department of Psychosocial Cancer Care, St Vincent's Hospital, Melbourne, VIC, Australia

Karen Ryan Mater Misericordiae University Hospital and St Francis Hospice, Dublin, Ireland

University College Dublin, Belfield, Dublin 4, Ireland

Tony Ryan School of Nursing and Midwifery, The University of Sheffield, Sheffield, UK

Libby Sallnow Palliative Care Physician, University College London Hospital and Central and North West London NHS Trust, London, UK

Pau Sanchez Socio-Health Program, General Management of Health Planning, Government of Catalonia, Barcelona, Spain

Christine Sanderson Calvary Palliative and End of Life Care Research Institute, Calvary Health Care Kogarah, Sydney, NSW, Australia

Department of Medicine, University of Notre Dame Australia Darlingurst, Kogarah, NSW, Australia

Sebastià Santaeugènia Chronic Care Program, General Management of Health Planning, Government of Catalonia, Barcelona, Spain

Ros Scott Dundee University is School of Education and Social Work, Dundee, UK

Davinia S. E. Seah Sacred Heart Health Service, St Vincent's Hospital, NSW, Australia

School of Medicine, University of Notre Dame Australia, Darlinghurst, NSW, Australia

St Vincent's Clinical School, University of New South Wales, NSW, Australia

Jake Shortt Monash Haematology, Monash Health, Clayton, VIC, Australia

School of Clinical Sciences at Monash Health, Monash University, Clayton, VIC, Australia

Philip J. Siddall Department of Pain Management, HammondCare, Sydney, NSW, Australia

Sydney Medical School – Northern, University of Sydney, Sydney, NSW, Australia

Thomas J. Smith JHMI, The Johns Hopkins Hospital, Baltimore, MD, USA

Rosalie Stephen Cancer and Blood Services, Auckland City Hospital, Auckland, New Zealand

Sigrid Sterckx Department of Philosophy and Moral Sciences, Ghent University, Ghent, Belgium

Carol A. Stone Marie Curie Hospice, Belfast, UK

Geoff Sussman Faculty of Medicine, Nursing and Health Science, Monash University, Melbourne, Australia

Helena Talbot-Rice St Christopher's Hospice, London, UK

Damien Tange Department of Cancer Surgery, Peter MacCallum Cancer Centre, Melbourne, VIC, Australia

Kathryn A. Tham Royal Melbourne Hospital Palliative Care, Parkville, VIC, Australia

Jill Thistlethwaite University of Technology Sydney, Sydney, NSW, Australia

William Thompson Cancer and Blood Services, Auckland City Hospital, Auckland, New Zealand

Rebecca Tiberini St Michael's Hospice, Hastings, UK

Frances Toohey Faculty of Medical and Health Sciences, University of Auckland, Auckland, New Zealand

John M. Troupis Department of Diagnostic Imaging, Monash Health, Clayton, Australia

Irene Tuffrey-Wijne Faculty of Health, Social Care and Education, Kingston University and St George's, University of London, London, UK

Karen Turner Royal Free London NHS Foundation Trust and Marie Curie Hospice Hampstead, Florence Nightingale Scholar, London, UK

Lieve Van den Block VUB-UGhent End-of-Life Care Research Group, Department of Family Medicine and Chronic Care and Department of Clinical Sciences, Vrije Universiteit Brussel (VUB), Brussels, Belgium

Sophie van Dongen Department of Public Health, Erasmus MC, Rotterdam, CA, The Netherlands

Jelle van Gurp IQ healthcare/Ethics of healthcare, Radboud University Medical Center, Nijmegen, The Netherlands

Evert van Leeuwen Professor Emeritus of IQ healthcare/Ethics of healthcare, Radboud University Medical Center, Nijmegen, The Netherlands

Martine van Selm Amsterdam School of Communication Research, University of Amsterdam, Amsterdam, The Netherlands

Jenny T. van der Steen Department of Public Health and Primary Care, Leiden University Medical Center, Leiden, The Netherlands

Radboud university medical center, Department of Primary and Community Care, Nijmegen, The Netherlands

Gaëlle Vanbutsele End-of-Life Care Research group, Vrije Universiteit Brussel and Ghent University, Brussels, Belgium

Jan Vandevoorde Department of Family Medicine and Chronic Care, Vrije Universiteit Brussel (VUB), Brussels, Belgium

Simone Veronese Fondazione FARO, palliative care, Torino, Italy

Willem Vink Christchurch Hospital Palliative Care Service, Christchurch, New Zealand

Claudia Virdun Improving Palliative, Aged, and Chronic Care through Clinical Research and Translation (IMPACCT), Faculty of Health, University of Technology Sydney, Ultimo, NSW, Australia

Kris Vissers Department of Anesthesiology, Pain and Palliative Care, Radboud University Medical Center, Nijmegen, The Netherlands

Catherine Walshe International Observatory on End of Life Care, Lancaster University, Lancaster, UK

Eswaran Waran Royal Darwin Hospital, Tiwi, NT, Australia

Territory Palliative Care, Tiwi, NT, Australia

Renee Weller Department of Palliative Care, Geisinger Medical Center, Danville, PA, USA

Patrick White Primary Care Respiratory Medicine, School of Population Health and Environmental Science, King's College London, London, UK

Leeroy William Palliative Medicine, Monash Health, Eastern Health, Monash University, Melbourne, VIC, Australia

Michelle K. Wilson Cancer and Blood Services, Auckland City Hospital, Auckland, New Zealand

Rachel Wiseman Canterbury District Health Board, Christchurch, New Zealand

Erica Witkamp Faculty of Nursing and Research Centre Innovations in Care, Rotterdam University of Applied Sciences, Rotterdam, The Netherlands

Part IV

Organization of Palliative Care in Different Settings

Home Care, Primary Care

50

Geoffrey Mitchell

Contents

G. Mitchell (✉)
Primary Care Clinical Unit, Faculty of Medicine,
University of Queensland, Brisbane, Australia
e-mail: g.mitchell@uq.edu.au

R. D. MacLeod, L. Van den Block (eds.), *Textbook of Palliative Care*,
https://doi.org/10.1007/978-3-319-77740-5_48

Abstract
Care at the end of life has developed into a sophisticated specialty, historically modeled around the needs of incurable cancer in terms of complex, rapidly developing symptomatology and psychopathology in a predictable time frame. It is ill-equipped to manage people dying of other conditions, and the aging of the population will see the rise of multimorbidity, frailty, dementia, and organ failure as predominant causes of disability and death. The existing specialized, hospital-focused, and subspecialized health system that currently manages very ill people will not be able to cope with the complexity, multimorbidity, and unpredictability that characterize the future. Generalists, particularly community-based services, will inevitably have a very significant role to play.

This chapter examines the role of primary care, specifically general practice, in managing end-of-life care. It describes the similarities between the aims and objectives of general practice and palliative care, the scope of generalist end-of-life care, the past performance of general practice at the end of life, and models of care that can enhance both GP performance and integration between specialists and generalists. It concludes with initiatives that will facilitate national policy development to promote effective end-of-life care.

1 Introduction

The world has made spectacular advances in overcoming illnesses as diverse as cancer and sepsis. As a result, the average survival rate has increased dramatically, and the improvements in quality of life for most of those years have been impressive. Most of us can be confident that we will be living well into our 80s. While we celebrate "conquering cancer" (and other diseases), what is not discussed much at all is that there is a limit to the length of time we will live. The vast majority of people will die between the ages of 70 and 90 and virtually are all dead by about 100 years of age (World Health Organization 2015). Medical advances have simply delayed the inevitable.

As the population ages rapidly, so the absolute number of deaths per annum will rise. The absolute numbers who will die has to increase faster than the rate at which we are aging. Etkind et al. estimate that the number of people dying per annum in the UK will rise by 25.4% as a result of a higher proportion of older people (from 17.7% $\geq$ 65 in 2014 to 24.2% in 2040) (Etkind et al. 2017). Australian predictions suggest that the picture will continue to escalate beyond 2040. By 2016, the number of deaths was predicted to rise by over 250% from 2011 to 2061 (Australian Bureau of Statistics 2016) (Fig. 1). Moreover, the number whose dying can be anticipated and who will probably benefit from palliative care will escalate from approximately 75% in 2014 to up to 87% in 2040 (Etkind et al. 2017). The need for skilled end-of-life care will escalate.

In addition, the nature of the causes of death is changing. Gill et al. analyzed the cause of death of previously well 70-year-old people and found that the greatest cause of death was frailty (28%), followed by any organ failure (21%), cancer (19%), and dementia (14%) (Gill et al. 2010). Seventy-nine percent of this cohort had a predictable course to death, with the majority of people dying after a prolonged period of disability and ill health. Frailty, the most common cause, is caused by an accumulation of age-related illnesses, impacting on bodies with less capacity to maintain homeostasis. Older people will be taking more medicines than before, with the accompanying risks of expected and unexpected adverse events and drug interactions.

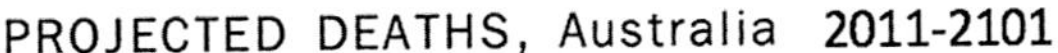

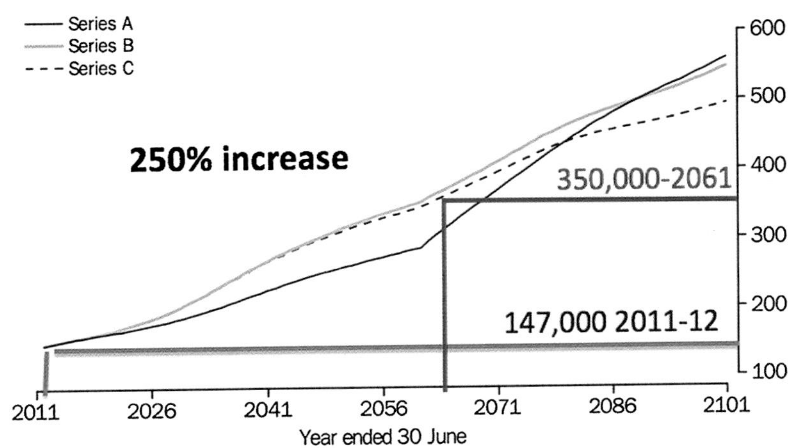

Fig. 1 Annual deaths from 2011 to 2101 in Australia

2 Society's Response: Palliative Care

Society's response to dying has changed dramatically since Cicely Saunders developed a systematic and deliberate response to the problems of distressing deaths from terminal cancer. The sustained study of pain and symptom management and a complete change in approach to death from a perceived medical failure to an expected part of the human experience have had profound effects on modern health care.

Better understanding of pain management and the development the specialized institutions to manage the end of life were the initial response. Better understanding of the management of other symptoms, the psychology of dying, vastly improved communication skills, and better organization of care have put very high quality of care in reach of most people with cancer in developed countries. Indeed, the proportion of people dying of cancer who access palliative care is around 68 percent (Rosenwax and McNamara 2006). Specialist palliative care has largely aligned with cancer care. Palliative care services are often co-located with oncology departments. There may be beds allocated to palliative care services, or the service may be a consultative service to other clinical units.

This model has served these patients well, particularly with timely referral. It is not perfect, particularly when patients are referred too late to have a demonstrable impact on the patient and family's well-being. There are two main reasons the majority of palliative care services manage cancer. The first is historical. The dramatic and tragic course of cancer for many patients makes improvement of the end of life an obvious backdrop for this sort of care. Secondly, with relatively predictable time courses and relatively predictable symptoms, it has been relatively easy to design service delivery to suit end-of-life cancer care.

However, the proportion of people without cancer who die without accessing specialist palliative care is disturbingly high (Rosenwax and McNamara 2006), in spite of the symptom burden of conditions like advanced heart failure being the equivalent of that of advanced lung cancer (Murray et al. 2002). There are several problems in providing specialist palliative care to this group. First, the illness trajectory of these conditions is variable (Fig. 2). A typical organ failure trajectory has multiple relapses and remissions, and the timing of these is unpredictable. Secondly, a person with organ failure may have a prognosis of years before death. The same applies to the person with advanced multimorbidity. They often have substantial care needs relating to mounting disability, but it might take years to recognize that the person is approaching death. Many will have dementia, which in the latter stages limits the ability to undertake more than

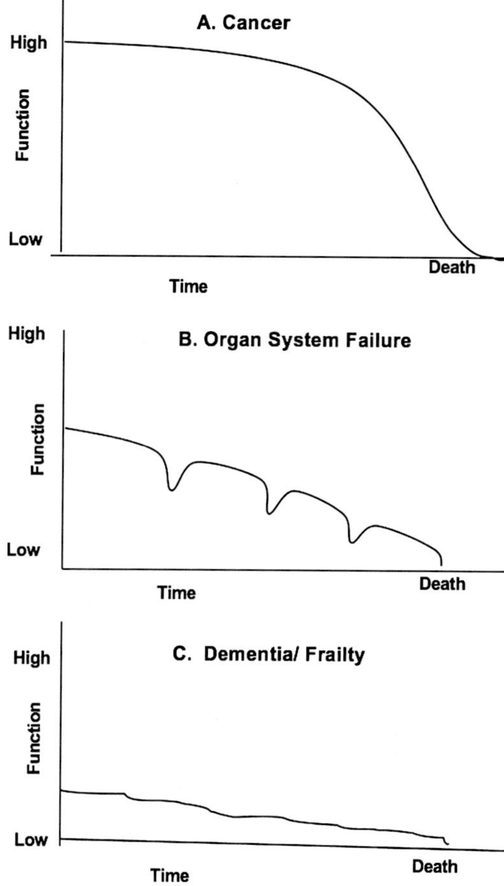

Fig. 2 Trajectories of illness at the end of life

the most basic of activities of daily living. In addition, people with dementia also suffer substantial symptom burden over and above the burden of the underlying condition. For example, approximately half of all people with advanced dementia are reported to suffer pain to some degree (van Kooten et al. 2016).

The end-of-life care model designed for the intense, accelerating need for care seen in cancer palliative patient is not going to work in most people with nonmalignant disease approaching end of life. Currently, about 80% of the patients of specialist palliative care units have a primary diagnosis of cancer (Australian Institute of Health and Welfare 2014). Who looks after the non-cancer deaths? Certainly not specialist palliative care – they are being stretched with the current illness mix. The number of referrals to Australian specialist palliative care services grew by 52% in the decade from 2002 to 2012 (Australian Institute of Health and Welfare 2014), and the services have little ability to take more on. More of the same is not going to work, and urgent attention needs to be paid to alternative models of care.

This chapter aims to describe the place of primary care in the care of people at the end of life, with a particular emphasis on primary care. It examines how ideal primary palliative care could work and the evidence in support of integrating primary care into the management of complex end-of-life conditions. In addition, it demonstrates the performance of general practice as reflected by a systematic review of the literature undertaken to 2014. Finally, it documents some of the major policy initiatives that seek to embed primary palliative care into routine end-of-life care.

3 General Practice, Primary Care and Palliative Care

There are major similarities between the definitions of general practice and of palliative care (Box 1). Both emphasize the importance of treating the whole person. Both emphasize the importance of high-quality assessment and management of people's problems. In addition, family practice emphasizes health promotion and prevention and understanding the context in which the patients live work. End-of-life care is a natural fit for primary care.

Box 1 Definitions of Palliative Care and General Practice

WHO Definition of Palliative Care

Palliative care is an approach that improves the quality of life of patients (adults and children) and their families who are facing the problems associated with life-threatening illness, through the prevention and relief of suffering by means of early identification and correct assessment and treatment of pain, and other

(*continued*)

Box 1 (continued)
problems, whether physical, psychosocial, or spiritual (World Health Organization 2004).

European Definition of General/ Family Practitioner

General practitioners/family doctors are specialist physicians trained in the principles of the discipline. They are personal doctors, primarily responsible for the provision of comprehensive and continuing care to every individual seeking medical care irrespective of age, sex, and illness. They care for individuals in the context of their family, their community, and their culture, always respecting the autonomy of their patients. They recognize they will also have a professional responsibility to their community. In negotiating management plans with their patients, they integrate physical, psychological, social, cultural, and existential factors, utilizing the knowledge and trust engendered by repeated contacts. General practitioners/family physicians exercise their professional role by promoting health, preventing disease, and providing cure, care, or palliation. This is done either directly or through the services of others according to health needs and the resources available within the community they serve, assisting patients where necessary in accessing these services. They must take the responsibility for developing and maintaining their skills, personal balance, and values as a basis for effective and safe patient care (WONCA Europe 2011).

In fact, as experts in multimorbid care, general practice is where most of end-of-life care should and probably already does take place. It is not clear whether GPs understand that they are already providing end-of-life care as they manage multimorbid and frail older people. There are different perceptions of what palliative care and end-of-life care actually comprise. The classic picture of palliative care involves intense care at the end of life: managing uncontrolled symptoms, rapidly changing and accumulating symptom burden, patient fears, and relatives who are frightened and distressed. And that is what a lot of end-of-life care is like. However, there is another form of end-of-life care which ideally takes place much earlier – months from death is ideal. Here there is a recognition of the inevitability of dying at some stage in the future. Together with the patient, future patient wishes are articulated. Clinicians anticipate future medical and situational problems and start to put into place strategies to manage these when they arise. These are both legitimate forms of end-of-life care but very different (Fig. 3).

4 Multidimensional Care

Murray et al. have gone further to describe the nature of palliative care, calling it a four-dimensional activity. These dimensions are physical, psychological, social, and spiritual dimensions of care (Murray et al. 2007). This framework is very useful in identifying and planning treatment. Different versions of this work have been done. For example, Eychmüller and colleagues (Eychmeuller 2012) have also undertaken work to identify the essential elements of palliative care, developing the SENS structure of palliative care planning and treatment: ***S****ymptoms* both current and anticipated; ***E****nd-of-life decisions* that have to be made; the ***N****etwork of care* required around the patient; and ***S****upport for the family* required to manage the situation. They go on to define the goals of comprehensive care: the so-called 4-S goals, improving ***Self-help*** capacities; promoting ***Self-determination***; ensuring ***Safety***; and assuring ***Support*** for the family.

5 Consumer Expectations of the Role of GPs and Primary Care at the End of Life

A systematic review by Johnson et al. (under review) identified the expectations of patients and their immediate carers of the role of GPs and primary care health professionals at the end of life.

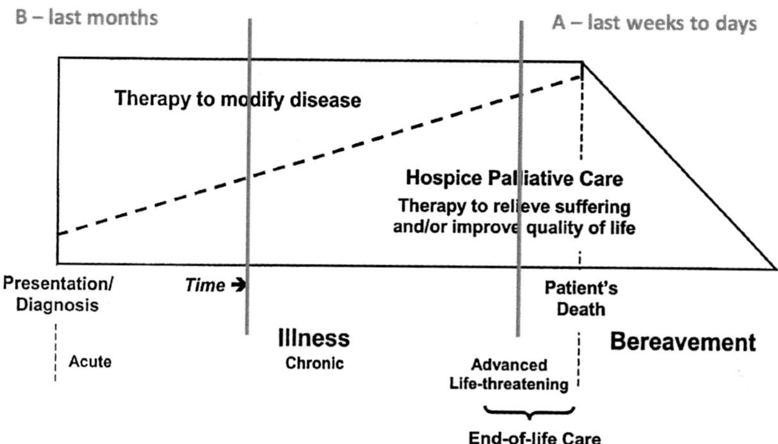

Fig. 3 Different aspects of palliative care dependent on time from death

Continuity of care was considered an important aspect of care (Borgsteede et al. 2006; Neergaard et al. 2008). Different elements were identified in the literature:

1) *Relational continuity of GP care.* Patients and their immediate carers prefer that care is provided by the same known GP (with backup from the same clinic when necessary), rather than different GPs (Borgsteede et al. 2006). Further, patients also preferred to continue their relationship with the GP across different care settings, thus requiring ongoing and close cooperation between the patient's GP and their specialists during the final illness. This relationship should ideally persist with the next of kin, even after the death of the patient.

2) *Informational consistency.* The patient's primary care providers should be the repository of the patients' clinical information. This information should be shared across all health providers to promote consistent care and reduce the need for patients to continually retell their story (Neergaard et al. 2008). Effective means of information sharing is an increasing theme for health care in general. Having a shared clinical record is already a reality in some jurisdictions (e.g., Spain, UK) but not others. Sharing information between specialists and carers is eventually being developed in other places (e.g., Australia). Until that is universal, some means of information sharing should be devised, and primary care practitioners are in a good position to enable that to happen.

3) *Consistency of information provision.* The role of caring is highly stressful, and most carers do not have a health-care background. They are being asked to care for the most unwell people and need good information to do this job. Minor differences in the information provided create anxiety and distress. Consistency of information provision minimizes this problem (Boyd et al. 2004). GPs can be the providers of information or the interpreters of information from others to allay concerns and ensure high-quality care provision.

Interprofessional communication. Patients and carers believe that high-quality interprofessional communication regarding diagnosis, treatment, and prognosis facilitates good end-of-life care (Borgsteede et al. 2006). While patients developed strong rapport and relationships with health professionals in the acute care setting (Aabom and Pfeiffer 2009), they needed to see overt collaboration between those health professionals and other agencies involved in palliative care provision and their GP to feel confident that all health professionals were working together (Neergaard et al. 2008). The GP could be a key carer if the GP-patient relationship was established and effective. Some patients suggested that GPs should be proactive in engaging with health professionals such as oncologists and palliative care services and that oncologists should inform patients of the important role of GPs in end-of-life care (Borgsteede et al. 2006; Neergaard et al. 2008).

Patients believe they benefit from a strong therapeutic relationship with their GP (Slort et al. 2011). Consistently seeing the same GP contributed to a greater knowledge of the personal needs and preferences of the individual, increasing trust and mutual understanding (Michiels et al. 2007). The GP in such a therapeutic relationship would take time to be engaged and "listen carefully," be able to deal with strong emotions, and be able to assist patients with advance care planning to improve patient, carer, and family outcomes (Slort et al. 2011).

Patients observed that they were often the subjects of a health professional-led approach to care, rather than a partnership between health professionals, the patient, and any relevant carers and family members (Boyd et al. 2004). They considered such a partnership a more effective approach, which would empower patients and their carers and facilitate patient-centered care. The limited palliative care experience of some GPs was perceived by some patients and carers to impact on their ability to provide more than basic psychosocial and carer support (Farber et al. 2003).

A ***GP's communication skills*** were particularly valued by both patients and carers (Borgsteede et al. 2006; Neergaard et al. 2008; Grande et al. 2004). Attributes such as trustworthiness, respect, kindness, caring, sympathy, honesty, and sensitivity fostered constructive and collaborative relationships between GPs, patients, and carers (Grande et al. 2004). Patients preferred GPs to be open and initiate discussions about end of life (Slort et al. 2011).

Ready access to and availability of GPs and other health professionals were considered fundamental to good end-of-life care (Borgsteede et al. 2006; Neergaard et al. 2008). Patients needed to be able to see their GP without protracted waiting times for appointments or having to wait for long periods on the day of appointments (Borgsteede et al. 2006). As a patient deteriorated, having a GP who was available out of hours and who conducted home visits was essential if the patient wished to remain at home (Borgsteede et al. 2006; Neergaard et al. 2008; Slort et al. 2011). A GP's lack of time was a barrier to continuity of care.

Patients expect GPs to be competent at diagnosing problems and in the management of their symptoms (Borgsteede et al. 2006), but this was not always the case (Grande et al. 2004). They wanted GPs to be well informed about their condition, how to manage symptoms, and to be aware of the side effects of treatment (Borgsteede et al. 2006; Slort et al. 2011). Patients wanted information about symptoms and their management to be shared with them (Grande et al. 2004).

Patients and carers expect GPs to facilitate or enlist help from other agencies to enhance EOL care. In particular, shared care between GPs, community services, and specialist services was appreciated by them, including engagement with palliative care services when required (Neergaard et al. 2008). Community support services can facilitate access to equipment and supplies.

While some patients and carers identified the importance of the psychological, social, and spiritual support which could be provided by GPs (Grande et al. 2004), others had not considered that they might use the GP for non-biomedical or nontreatment-related issues. They did not want to inconvenience or disturb a busy GP for what they considered "minor matters," despite increasing psychosocial concerns as the disease progressed. Some clinicians described their patient care largely in terms of treating the disease.

6 What Does End of Life Look like in the Community?

End-of-life care in primary care comprises escalating need for care starting months from death and some intense care at the end of life. There are three essential elements to this "early palliative care." First, in order for deliberate planning and management to take place, there has to be a conscious recognition that the end of life is approaching. When that decision is made, then some form of planning should take place. Finally, the health team needs to be ready to enact the plan when the time comes.

7 Essential Steps in Primary Palliative Care

7.1 Identifying Approaching End of Life

Identifying people approaching the end of life seems such a simple proposition, and yet it is not often deliberately done. The identification of patients for palliative care tends to rely on practitioners' subjective judgment (intuition and knowledge), rather than established guidelines (Harrison et al. 2012). Cancer patients had the greatest likelihood of being identified as being in need of palliative care. Patients with non-malignant but advanced and progressive illnesses were less likely to be formally identified for palliative care prior to death (Harrison et al. 2012). This may be because of a perception that palliative care is only the care at the end of life.

Our group has done recent work (under review) that shows that GPs' recognition of approaching end of life is tacit, and they will not often raise it with patients de novo, unless the patient raises the possibility first. If patients raise it, then proceeding to appropriate planning is relatively smooth. If they do not, then the GP is loathe to raise the possibility of impending death. However, the GPs reported that they did subtly, perhaps consciously, shift their care toward comfort care.

Burridge et al. (Burridge et al. 2011) describe "consultation etiquette" – where the patient is too polite to "bother the doctor" with their problems and doctor is too polite to raise issues like this one with the patient. Thus consideration of very important issues like this one is deferred and perhaps never addressed.

7.1.1 Attempts at Systematic Identification of Patients Nearing the End of Life in Primary Care

There have been concerted attempts to systematize the identification of patients approaching the end of life. Keri Thomas of England initiated this movement and developed a sophisticated process of identification through screening of GP patient lists, planning care, and enacting the plan – the so-called Gold Standards Framework (Thomas 2007). There have also been other tools or checklists to assist in the identification of people approaching the end of life. A systematic review has identified four main identification tools and assesses their practicality in the practice setting (Maas et al. 2013). What is clear is that any systematic identification process has to be compatible with the health systems in which they operate. The tools available very clearly illustrate this. Gomez-Batiste in Catalonia, Spain, developed a tool (NECPAL) that could interrogate electronic records and required smaller amounts of input from clinicians (Gomez-Batiste et al. 2013). Spain has a single electronic record that follows the patient through the entire health system. Thomas' Prognostic Indicator Guide (PIG) (Thomas 2011) works in the context of UK's system of capitation payments and rewards for meeting public health targets. This enables practice staff to spend time searching patient records for people suitable for a Palliative Care register and be rewarded for doing so. This will not work in a fee-for-service environment like the Netherlands or Australia, where practitioners only get paid for seeing patients.

Research into the implementation of screening tools has taught several lessons. In the Netherlands, a tool was developed that identified people with advanced cancer and end-stage lung and heart failure, but not those with non-specific frailty or multimorbidity (Thoonsen et al. 2015). The project trained GPs in its use – a good strategy in a fee-for-service environment. However, in an RCT, there was no difference in patient identification when all GPs who were randomized to training in the tool were considered, as half the intervention group did not use it (Thoonsen et al. 2015). However, there were significant improvements in patient identification and multifaceted care when analyzing those GPs who did use the tool (Thoonsen et al. 2015). The Supportive and Palliative Indicator Tool (SPICT) has been the one most used internationally (Highet et al. 2014). It is short (one page) and more inclusive than exclusive of patients through the use of broad categories of disability. It is also constantly being revised and upgraded through web page (www.spict.org), inviting commentary and registration of its use. It has been translated into several languages as well.

A literature review of the impact of the Gold Standards Framework (Shaw et al. 2010) showed that, in spite of financial incentives to maintain palliative care registers, many people who did die did not appear on the register, as it contained predominantly people with advanced cancer. Why this was the case is yet to be fully determined.

While the concept of screening patient lists is very logical on paper, it appears that converting the idea into practice is another issue. We learn from this literature that GPs recognize deterioration to death with cancer more easily than for end-stage nonmalignant disease. We also learn that relying on GPs to use a tool offered to them is no guarantee of use, even if use does achieve the desired result.

Our group wondered whether there was benefit in using screening tools at all and tested the ability of screening tools to predict death against GP intuition (Mitchell et al. 2018a). We showed that screening tools was more effective than intuition in predicting those who did die but only among those patients that a GP considered were at risk of death. There was no difference between the groups in identifying people who died when whole practice lists of patients over 70 were screened. There was also a very high false-positive rate of identification of risk of death with both techniques. We showed that deliberately screening for likely death was not a useful means of identifying the cohort of people with end-of-life needs, and recognition of escalating needs was a better approach to explore.

Taking identification out of the hands of GPs and making screening an automatic procedure, for example, through electronic records surveillance, may have promise (Mason et al. 2015). The problem will be to have a screening process to identify people at risk, but with appropriately modest false-positive rates. A positive test demands a response, and a high false-positive test will place an unreasonable burden on practitioners if developing a comprehensive care plan is the response. Either a graded response proportional to the level of risk is developed, or a less sensitive and more specific set of search criteria are generated.

Zheng et al. did elegant work in Scottish general practices to see if the problem of end-of-life recognition was the term "palliative" (Zheng et al. 2013). They showed that people with non-malignant diseases – organ failure and frailty/multimorbidity/dementia – were hardly ever placed on the practice palliative care register as at risk of dying compared with cancer, where three-quarters of cancer patients were identified on the register and in a timely manner. By changing the title of the register to a "supportive needs register," recognition of people who died from nonmalignant was 40% at the time of death, and much earlier recognition occurred.

One issue is that dying in primary care is a low prevalence event in primary care. As the population ages, patient deaths will become more prevalent. However, while patient death will never be a routine event, the incidence of frail and multimorbid patients will rise, all of whom will die. At what point should a doctor "change gears"? Should it be a sudden transition, or a gradual escalation of response to need? The answers to these questions are not yet clear.

In summary, identification of the patient is the essential first step to proactive end-of-life care. While appearing logical, it is in fact highly complex to enact it systematically in the community.

7.2 Planning Care

Once a person is identified as requiring palliative care, ideally some sort of plan needs to be generated. This again is not as easy as it sounds. There are two elements to proactive care planning – advance care planning and clinical care planning (Fig. 4).

7.2.1 Advance Care Planning

Much effort has been made to facilitate advance care decision-making. The rationale is that medical care needs to reflect the individual's goals and aspirations for the remainder of their life, along with preferences for the type of health care they want to have. This is very important in hospital practice, so that care which can be very expensive and which may not produce demonstrable

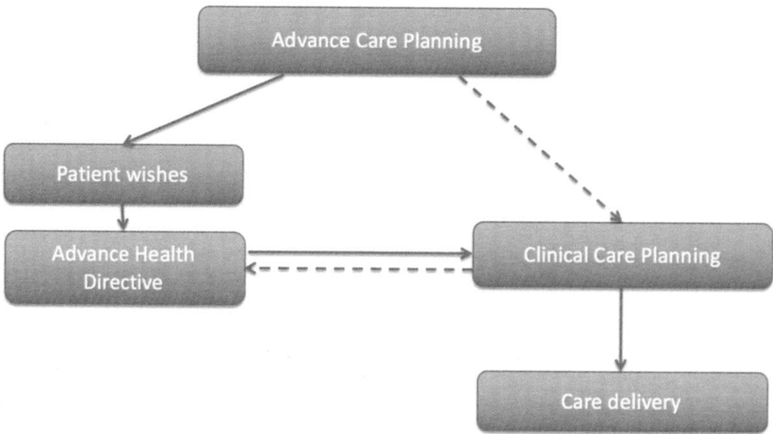

Fig. 4 A concept map of care planning for the end of life (Mitchell. 2014a)

benefits is only offered to those who really want it. The second element of advance care planning is to appoint substitute decision-makers in the event that the person cannot articulate decisions for themselves. These people are usually, but not always, next of kin.

7.2.2 Clinical Care Planning

A second form of care planning is also highly desirable but less considered. This is clinical care planning. Most people with serious illness have predictable complications. For example, a person who has severe heart failure will almost certainly wake up in the middle of the night breathless at some point in the future. What can be done to prevent that? What actions can minimize the breathlessness and facilitate the patient settling without an emergency admission to hospital when it does happen? It should be possible to anticipate these issues and prepare plans that can be enacted when the anticipated problems arise.

7.2.3 Integrating Specialist and Generalist Care

Being ill with multiple conditions can be problematic. Hillman describes a health system where the consequences of lack of integration include a lack of clear decision-making, deferral of critical decisions these often being made by intensive care specialists by default (Hillman and Cardona-Morrell 2015). Gawande describes multiple personal experiences of a loss of focus on the whole person, with decisions being made for reasons far removed from what the patient wants or will provide long-term benefit (Gawande 2014).

General practitioners manage multimorbidity as a matter of course. They are also usually very aware of the personality and social circumstances of the individual, which becomes important in anticipating the needs of people at the end of life.

Management of patients with multimorbid problems is not well coordinated between GP and the specialist team(s). A systematic review of integration programs that deliberately integrated general practitioners with specialists found only 14 such studies (Mitchell et al. 2015). By contrast, there are dozens of studies testing integration in a range of specialist settings. Here integration means integration of different specialist treatment modalities. Actual interventions aimed at bringing medical specialities together are unusual. For example, a Cochrane review of integration in COPD care involved 26 studies, only 2 of which aimed to improve interprofessional integration (Kruis et al. 2013).

Bringing together the contextual knowledge of GPs and the content knowledge of specialists should be of benefit to patients facing the end of life. A number of interventions supporting this form of care have been tested.

The one with the strongest evidence base is case conferences between specialists and GPs.

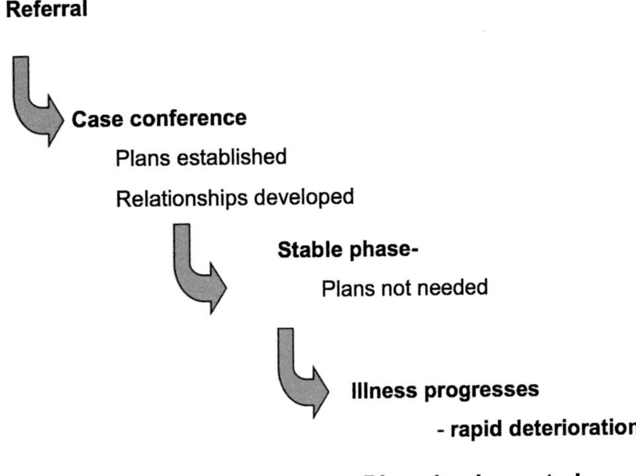

Fig. 5 Mechanism of action of GP specialist case conferences at the end of life

The rationale is that GPs know the context of the patient and their family, while specialist teams have the content expertise. The combination of these two things should be effective in improving patient outcomes. Australian general practice is funded through a blending of fee-for-service and outcomes based funding. In recognition of the importance of integrating GPs into the care of complex and chronic conditions, government rebates for participating in case conferences with other health professionals are available. Both trials used this opportunity to test the above hypothesis. Abernethy et al.'s study (the world's largest randomized controlled trial in palliative care) showed 30% reductions in admissions to hospitals and a mean 10% improvement in maintenance of functional capacity from diagnosis to death (Abernethy et al. 2013). Mitchell et al. showed improvements in the patient's quality of life in the last month of life (Mitchell et al. 2008b).

The assumed mechanism of action for this improvement was that the case conference took place and a joint plan of action was negotiated and the palliative care team members and the GP became acquainted with each other, creating communication channels. This plan was often not enacted immediately because there was often a latent period when the patient was stable. However, when deterioration did occur, the latent communication channels were activated, plans were in place and enacted promptly, and the patient's outcomes were better than those of normal care (Fig. 5).

It appears that a key element of successful GP specialist integration is buy-in from the GPs. Active negotiation of the plan between specialists and GPs appears to work better than passive receipt by a GP of a plan formulated by the specialists – someone else's plan (Mitchell et al. 2008a). Thus the major difference between the program impact was that the GP was an integral part of the planning process – he or she had buy-in – whereas in the geriatrics trial, the primary care practitioner was a passive recipient of someone else's care plan.

7.3 Implementing Care

Once patient and carer needs are identified and care planned, the plan has to be implemented. Recent work (under review) indicates that the GPs' understanding of the patient's willingness to accept their nearness to death determines how overtly a plan to implement end-of-life care is articulated. If the patient can articulate an awareness and acceptance of impending death, then the GP will discuss end-of-life care overtly. If not, then GPs instinctively and subtly changes care goals to include issues of importance at the end of life.

8 What Are the Outcomes for Primary Care-Delivered Palliative Care?

The following sections examine how well GPs perform palliative care from different perspectives. They arise from the series of systematic reviews mentioned in the acknowledgments at the commencement of the chapter.

8.1 Symptoms (Mitchell et al. 2018)

8.1.1 GP-Identified Symptoms

General practitioners (GPs) found symptoms associated with the terminal phase as the most distressing for the patient (Mitchell and Seamark 2016). Of those patients who were cared for at home in the terminal phase of their disease, the main symptom was fatigue, which was a documented symptom in almost all patients (Leemans et al. 2012). Other common symptoms included anorexia, drowsiness, pain, dyspnea, and psychological distress. Pain was perceived as causing less suffering than these in the terminal phase (Mitchell and Seamark 2016).

8.1.2 Did GPs Respond Adequately to Patient Symptoms?

Primary health-care professionals were well placed to recognize symptom issues in palliative care patients. A study comparing agreement on symptom assessments between patients at home with those of nurses and GPs demonstrated high levels of symptom identification (Ewing et al. 2006). Gastrointestinal problems such as nausea, vomiting, and constipation were recognized by GPs more than by the patients themselves. Nonmedical health professionals were more likely to note psychological issues and bestow greater significance to them than patients did themselves. Pain scores were comparable between all groups throughout.

In general, GPs expressed confidence responding to the symptoms identified by their palliative patients (Leemans et al. 2012; Blazekovic-Milakovic et al. 2006; Kuin et al. 2004; Canto et al. 2000). They felt most comfortable in responding to pain. They were least comfortable managing dyspnea, followed by fatigue. However, a study in Spain identified that the majority of GPs felt confident managing pain, dyspnea, and epilepsy by themselves (Canto et al. 2000).

General Psychological Care General practitioners perceived emotional support as being one of the most important aspects of palliative and terminal care they managed (Blazekovic-Milakovic et al. 2006; Ledeboer et al. 2006). They used supportive conversations, assistance with administration procedures, coordination of care, and management of carer and family distress to address patient distress (Canto et al. 2000; Demagny et al. 2009). While GPs felt they were predominantly comfortable providing this care, there were a number of challenges. GPs were often troubled by conversations about death and spirituality (Kelly et al. 2008). In one study, only half of GPs had involved patients in conversations regarding dying, viewing patient stoicism, and the presence of other family members as common barriers. Spirituality was seen as a difficult subject, often viewed by GPs as involving only religious beliefs, and thus rarely discussed. A common theme throughout all such studies was a lack of formal education and experience in this area, with GP eager to participate in further training (Canto et al. 2000).

8.1.3 Effectiveness of GP Symptom Control

(a) ***Pain***. While most general practitioners had adequate knowledge of general pain management, deficits in some GPs' knowledge of treating cancer pain may have resulted in ongoing pain at the end of life (Anquinet et al. 2011). They were also challenged by managing comorbid symptoms, such as neurological symptoms in patients with high-grade gliomas (Sizoo et al. 2010).

There was insufficient evidence available to assess whether GP management provided adequate relief: assessment of suffering, effective cancer pain management (Gott et al. 2010), patients' roles in end-of-life care and advance care planning, artificial nutrition and hydration, and the understanding of sedation versus euthanasia in relation to pain management (Anquinet et al. 2011).

(b) ***Breathlessness***. GPs were reluctant to prescribe opioids for breathlessness associated with severe COPD, even though they were aware of their proven benefit (Gott et al. 2010; Young et al. 2012). The main reasons for their hesitancy were the lack of education or knowledge of guidelines (Young et al. 2012), perceived scarce evidence supporting expert groups' recommendations for the long-term use of opioids for breathlessness (Young et al. 2012), and the fear of censure (Gott et al. 2010; Young et al. 2012). Some GPs would rather hospitalize patients than prescribe opioids for breathlessness (Gott et al. 2010).

8.1.4 Gastrointestinal Symptoms

One community-based audit showed that 30 of 88 patients were prescribed laxatives (Mitchell and Seamark 2016). Of these 11 were co-prescribed with opioids and 19 for non-opioid-related constipation. Thirty-six patients of the 88 patients had nausea. Most were treated with a single antiemetic, or two antiemetics tried sequentially, while only two had a combination of two antiemetics. In one study, gastrointestinal symptoms were reported as the most frequent symptoms identified by GPs (Borgsteede et al. 2007a). GPs identified nausea and vomiting as more prevalent and more severe than patients reported it, but under-recognized constipation as a problem (Ewing et al. 2006). In a 2002 survey of GPs prescribing an opioid, reported 57.6% would prescribe an antiemetic, only 33% a laxative (Oxenham et al. 2003; Borgsteede et al. 2009), and 20.7% both in the first few days (Barclay et al. 2002).

8.1.5 Depression

GPs experienced difficulties diagnosing and managing depression within the palliative care setting (Warmenhoven et al. 2012). GPs reported relying on clinical judgment, patient context, and the long-standing patient-doctor relationship to identify depression in palliative care patients, rather than making criterion-based diagnoses. The treatment of depression in palliative care was mainly supportive and non-specific, with antidepressants seldom prescribed.

8.1.6 Palliative Sedation

Palliative sedation is a recent phenomenon, performed when standard treatment is not able to control troubling symptoms. By sedating the patient to the point of unconsciousness, it removes awareness of the symptom and alleviates patient distress. The practice is only infrequently required (Donker et al. 2013) and should always be administered after close consultation with the patient and family. Continuous deep sedation until death does not always guarantee the dying process was free from symptoms (Anquinet et al. 2013). There was disagreement among practitioners about which symptoms actually necessitate palliative sedation (Sercu et al. 2014), as well as the potentially life-shortening intentions of sedation (Sercu et al. 2014). Reassuringly, a systematic review has showed palliative sedation does not shorten life expectancy (Beller et al. 2015).

A minority of GPs reported feeling pressure from patients, relatives, or colleagues to commence continuous sedation. This pressure was felt more strongly when patients experienced psychological symptoms (compared to physical symptoms) and when patients had greater estimated life expectancies (Blanker et al. 2012). Such pressure led to GPs seeking advice with respect to therapeutic options and/or specific information (Blanker et al. 2012; van Heest et al. 2009).

8.1.7 Barriers to Good Symptom Control

The need for more formal training in palliative care for GPs at both under- and postgraduate level was well documented (Farber et al. 2004; Hong et al. 2010; Walsh and Regan 2001; Groot et al. 2005). There was a particular need for education in the use of opioids (Hirooka et al. 2014; Gardiner et al. 2012; Todd et al. 2013; Salvato et al. 2003; Higginson and Gao 2012; Hawley et al. 2013) and referral for palliative radiotherapy (Vulto et al. 2009; Olson et al. 2012; Samant et al. 2006).

Another barrier identified by GPs was a lack of access to inpatient beds and home services support – often perceived as the result of bureaucracy – causing delay of essential symptom management or necessitating the patient to travel to hospital for simple procedures that could have been delivered in the home (Walsh and Regan 2001; Groot et al. 2007).

GP confidence in some settings providing palliative care was perceived as being low but increased with experience (Hirooka et al. 2014). The more frequently a GP performed palliative care activities, the more competent they felt (Farber et al. 2004; Gorlen et al. 2012). A death within a GP's population is a low prevalence event, which can exacerbates the GP's sense of inadequacy. However, those physicians who were more interested in palliative care did perform palliative care activities more frequently (Farber et al. 2004).

9 GP Understanding and Use of Opioid Therapy in Pain and Dyspnea Management

GPs were usually familiar with the management of common pain problems, the WHO guidelines on analgesics, and the use of oral opioids (Oxenham et al. 2003; Barclay et al. 2002). However, some gaps were identified: omission of rapid-release opioid use for breakthrough pain (Oxenham et al. 2003; Barclay et al. 2002), not prescribing laxatives and antiemetics when giving opioids (Oxenham et al. 2003; Barclay et al. 2002; Borgsteede et al. 2007b), and difficulty in converting oral opioids to subcutaneous forms (Oxenham et al. 2003; Barclay et al. 2002; Linklater 2008).

Older GPs (Young et al. 2012; Ben Diane et al. 2005), GPs with more experience in the treatment of terminally ill patients (Ben Diane et al. 2005), and those trained in palliative care and pain management (Ben Diane et al. 2005; Mas et al. 2010) were more likely to prescribe strong opioids. They were more comfortable prescribing opioids for cancer patients (Young et al. 2012; Borgsteede et al. 2007b) compared with other conditions and more particularly in the terminal phase (Harrison et al. 2012). Patient factors positively associated with GP opioid prescription included younger age (Harrison et al. 2012; Hirakawa et al. 2007) higher pain levels (higher pain associated with more opioid prescriptions) (Mas et al. 2010), repeated requests for pain medication (Mas et al. 2010), and the presence of relatives caring for the patient.

9.1 Advance Health Directives

9.1.1 Uncertainty about the Timing of ACP

Advance care planning (ACP) is done ad hoc in the terminal phase, is sometimes discussed but not documented, or is not done at all (Evans et al. 2013; Meeussen et al. 2011; Snyder et al. 2013; Vandervoort et al. 2012). Difficulties associated with the unpredictability of the end-of-life trajectory and the absence of a clear beginning of the final stages of non-cancer patient deaths created uncertainty among clinicians about when such a discussion should be initiated (Meeussen et al. 2011; De Vleminck et al. 2014; Evans et al. 2014). Consequently, for non-cancer patients, ACP often occurs in the last week of life (Meeussen et al. 2011; Snyder et al. 2013) despite patients' preference to have a discussion with their GP earlier (Robinson et al. 2012). Discharge from hospital was a common trigger for initiating ACP (Meeussen et al. 2011; Boyd et al. 2010). ACP is more likely to be completed if the patient was in hospital as opposed to the community, as the hospital-treating doctors were more likely to recognize changing clinical status (Boyd et al. 2010).

Several ***factors that influenced the completion of ACP by GPs*** were identified. In terms of provider characteristics, an advance care plan was more likely to be completed if the GP was older and had more clinical experience (Snyder et al. 2013); if the GP was comfortable discussing ACP (Farber et al. 2004; Snyder et al. 2013; Evans et al. 2014); if they had appropriate education and training in ACP (De Vleminck et al. 2014; Robinson et al. 2012; Boyd et al. 2010; Cartwright et al. 2014; Rhee et al. 2013); and if the GP was involved and trained in palliative care (Farber et al. 2004). There were also issues with the quality of ACP, as studies showed that where end-of-life discussions took place, not all holistic aspects were addressed such as spiritual and existential concerns, social issues, and cultural differences (Farber et al. 2004; Snyder et al. 2013; Evans et al. 2014). Lack of time was also described as a barrier to ACP (Brown 2002).

Patient characteristics and patient interest in ACP also influenced the GP's involvement. If patients lacked awareness of their diagnosis and prognosis or did not initiate such a discussion, ACP was often not raised by the GP (De Vleminck et al. 2014). GPs also found it difficult to introduce ACP to patients who are not already interested or informed about it (Brown 2002). Older patients with non-cancer diseases often had less detailed ACP discussions (Evans et al. 2014). Despite these influences, patients want to discuss ACP with their GP but at a much earlier phase (Robinson et al. 2012).

Other factors that influenced completion or implementation of ACP were identified as concerns about the legal standing (Rhee et al. 2013; Robinson et al. 2013) and currency of ACP documents (Bull and Mash 2012), confusion around the terminologies and systems particularly with substitute decision-making (Cartwright et al. 2014), uncertainty around validity of ACP forms given there are multiple available (Robinson et al. 2013), concerns about making binding decisions about the future given the uncertainties of disease trajectories, and lack of awareness that ACP can be modified (Boyd et al. 2010; Rhee et al. 2013; Robinson et al. 2013).

In addition, organizational and care setting factors were found to influence the completion of an advance care plan. Incorporating ACP as part of standard care and having organizational protocols and systems for ACP, especially in residential care facilities, were found to be important in increasing the use of advance care plans (De Vleminck et al. 2014; Mitchell et al. 2011). ACP was also more likely to be considered in the context of end-of-life care and in the provision of palliative care (Evans et al. 2014; Boyd et al. 2010).

10 Determinants of whether the Completed Advance Care Plans or Directives Are Implemented

These included advance care plan factors such as its availability, currency, and legality of the forms (Rhee et al. 2013; Robinson et al. 2013; Bull and Mash 2012), timing of ACP (Meeussen et al. 2011), patient illness factors (e.g., quality of life of patient, level of functionality, and prognostication), organization and care setting factors (e.g., prioritizing life-sustaining treatments, policies, and protocols to support use of advance care plans), awareness, and attitudes of health professionals and family to ACP (e.g., families' understanding of the disease progression, GPs' desire to avoid family dissent) (Rhee et al. 2013).

10.1 Caring for Carers

Ninety percent of patient care in the final year of life occurs at home (Hinton 1994), with many patients moving to an inpatient setting in the final days of life. Hence, much of the burden of caregiving is managed in the community, with the greatest burden falling on primary caregivers (Aoun 2004). Care may be equivalent to a full-time job, with 20% of caregivers providing full-time or constant care (Aoun 2004).

Caring for a patient with end-of-life needs carries a number of implications. It is often provided by people who are themselves elderly and/or ill, and caregiving may exacerbate the illness burden. Caregivers of patients receiving PC have lower quality of life (QoL-impairment in physical functioning, general health, and vitality) and worse overall physical health than caregivers of patients receiving curative or active treatment (Weitzner et al. 1999). As patients deteriorate physically, caregiver QoL worsens, suggesting a greater need for support at this time (Grunfeld et al. 2004). Furthermore, while many caregivers feel positively about caregiving and derive deep satisfaction in this role, caregivers may also experience a number of physical and psychosocial issues, including reduced social contact, significant financial burden, sadness, anger, or resentment which may increase the risk of psychiatric morbidity and complicated grief (Aoun et al. 2014). Additionally, caregivers report a number of unmet needs across a variety of areas, including information, communication, and support from services (Aoun et al. 2005). Family members whose own needs are not identified and addressed early have greater needs and less trust and confidence in the health-care system and cope more poorly in the later stages than families who have been informed and supported throughout the course of the illness (Kristjanson and White 2002).

However, despite the shift to include family members and primary caregivers as active participants in PC (Sepulveda et al. 2002), it is still common that the primary focus of the caregiver and of health professionals is on the needs and comfort of the patient, meaning that caregiver needs and distress may be considered secondary to the patient's and may be (Butler et al. 2005). For example, in 2003/2004, the patient was the client in 98.3% of referrals to Home and Community Care services, yet caregivers are a target group of that program. It has also been suggested that caregivers may be reluctant to raise their own needs with their health-care provider, as they do not wish to put their own issues before the patient's or bother the health-care professional (Hudson et al. 2004). On the other hand, health-care professionals are often working under tight time restraints, with the average Australian general practice consultation in lasting only 14.9 minutes (Britt et al. 2016), making it difficult to assess both the patient and caregivers needs in one appointment. Countering this short-time period is the fact that GPs frequently see patients several times to resolve a complex problem.

11 Does Primary Care Involvement Impact on the End-of-Life Outcomes?

Although international literature highlights GPs' variable levels of knowledge about PC and symptom control (Barclay et al. 2003) and their lower perceived levels of competence in these areas compared to specialist PC services, GPs are in an optimal position to evaluate and assess the needs of caregivers. GPs are usually the first point of contact for patients and their caregivers and generally have an established relationship with the patients with palliative care needs as well as having an important contextual knowledge of the family and of the illness. Canadian research indicates that palliative care patients with a regular GP are less likely to seek care from emergency departments (Burge et al. 2003a) and are less likely to die in hospital (Burge et al. 2003b).

Whether the effort of involving the patient in end-of-life care ultimately depends on whether patient and carers are better off with GP involvement. What is the evidence that patients and carers do better with the involvement of their GP, compared with those who have little or no GP involvement?

11.1 Integrated Primary-Secondary Care

We have already presented the controlled trial evidence of the impact of case conferences between GPs and specialist palliative teams managing mainly cancer patients (Abernethy et al. 2013; Mitchell et al. 2008b). An RCT of facilitated family meetings at which GPs were invited to attend for terminal dementia patients in aged care homes showed no group effect on quality of life but improvements in pharmacological and non-pharmacological management of symptoms (Agar et al. 2017).

There is lower level evidence in favor of integrated care specialists and GPs caring for people at the end of life for nonmalignant end-of-life disease as well. Case conferences in end-stage heart failure showed impressive reductions in hospitalization, emergency visits, emergency visits not requiring admission (Mitchell et al. 2014b), and costs (Hollingworth et al. 2016). A uniform pain control pathway reduced palliative patient's pain in rural settings (Tateno and Ishikawa 2012), while half of head and neck cancer patients whose GP used a telephone advice service died at home, but half also had some level of uncontrolled symptoms (Ledeboer et al. 2006).

It is important to observe that these initiatives were all initiated by specialist services and reached out to general practitioners. It is clear that the primary care and specialist care work in very different ways. GPs tend to react to problems, and their systems are often designed around reaction. By contrast, specialist services are organizations and are more used to working with multidisciplinary teams. They are in a far better situation to initiate collaborative models of care. Active collaboration between them improves outcomes but requires considerable effort to embed such initiatives. Stakeholders need to feel that the outcomes are worth the time and effort.

11.2 Advance Care Planning

There is some evidence that where an advance care plan is in place and implemented, patient preferences and wishes are more likely to be followed (Evans et al. 2013). Other patient outcomes of ACP include anticipated symptoms being identified earlier, greater control with symptom management, (Auerbach and Pantilat 2004) greater patient satisfaction with the GP, (Tierney et al. 2001) and increased support, contact, and visits by GPs in the last week of life (Evans et al. 2013; Meeussen et al. 2011). Moreover, when an advance care plan is completed, patients are more likely to die in their preferred place of death (Vandervoort et al. 2012).

11.3 Caring for Carers

There is one study of GP identification and management of the needs of carers of advanced cancer patients. Using a self-completed needs checklist to identify carer problems, the GP and carer addressed these issues in a carer-focused consultation. This found improvements in outcomes for carers who were anxious or depressed at baseline and who were caring for more ill people and enabled the identification of more needs than the normal care control group (Mitchell et al. 2013).

11.4 Place of Death

There is a significant association between home visits by GPs to patients with advanced cancer with the possibility of dying at home and not hospital (e.g., Burge et al. 2003b; Neergaard et al. 2009). Similar findings on the likelihood of home death were also found for home visits by community nurses to cancer patients (Neergaard et al. 2009).

12 Policy Initiatives

End-of-life care policy has largely focused on specialist palliative care and its role at the very end of life. By and large cancer care is its focus, and the principles and processes of specialist services are well established. Only now is it becoming clear that a far bigger issue is developing – the population is aging, most will die of diseases other than cancer, and the current way of caring for patients is simply not viable to manage massively increased numbers of frail, multimorbid people. In 2014, the World Health Organization passed a resolution declaring end-of-life care of fundamental importance (World Health Organization 2014), thus committing member countries to improving end-of-life care. A core part of this declaration was the central role primary care had to play in providing end-of-life care. Work done by Murray and colleagues through the European Association of Palliative Care Primary Care working group had underpinned that initiative. They developed a set of guidelines based on Stjernsward's work, to allow nations or regions to analyze their end-of-life policy in terms of four high level principles, policy settings, drug availability, education, and implementation (Stjernsward et al. 2007) (Fig. 6), and created a means of evaluating national health systems to show the extent of involvement of primary care in end-of-life care. They evaluated 29 European countries' responses to show a range of facilitators and barriers to primary care end-of-life care (Murray et al. 2015) (Table 1). From that work, national policy to address these issues can arise. The Toolkit has been translated into several languages.

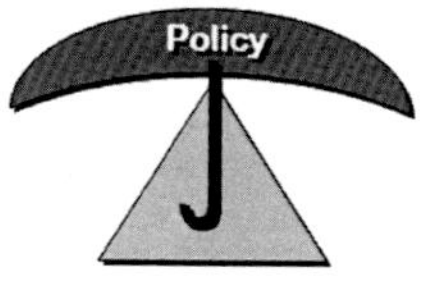

Fig. 6 Policy framework for developing palliative care services (Stjernsward et al. 2007)

Table 1 Barriers and opportunities to facilitate primary care involvement in end-of-life care provision (Murray et al. 2015)

Barriers	Opportunities
Lack of knowledge and skills among GPs and nurses	Training opportunities available in some countries
Financial systems not permitting reimbursements for palliative care	Examples of established primary care infrastructure
Issues hindering opiate prescribing	New national strategies supporting palliative care
Lack of professional or specialist support	Developing clinical networks in many countries
Poor identification of patients requiring palliative care	All patients have access to primary care
Limited public understanding and stigmatization of and palliative care	Increasing political support

Another international initiative has been led by Murray and Mitchell as co-Chairs – the International Primary Palliative Care Collaborative. This group was established in 2005 and has over 300 members from around the world. Its remit is to promote primary palliative care across the world through research, teaching, and local policy development. It has played an important part in developing the considerable momentum that has been evident in the last few years. Excellent work is currently happening in countries across the globe, bringing the critical role of primary care at the end of life to the attention of national governments.

13 Conclusion

Primary care and palliative care share a close affinity through an emphasis on the management of the whole person. In the age of specialist palliative care, a narrow view of end-of-life care has emerged which focuses on the last few weeks of life and largely relating to cancer and some particularly difficult degenerative diseases. The rapid aging of the population will lead to swelling numbers of deaths, with the major contributors being frailty, multimorbidity, organ failure, and dementia. These diseases, with their slowly accumulating needs and unpredictable illness course, are much more difficult to plan for, and a completely new approach to end-of-life care is warranted.

Further, the multidimensional nature of whole person care needs to be acknowledged and care arranged to meet these diverse needs.

Primary care has to take a major role in this. Complex medical problems will demand better integration of care between patients, carers, primary care practitioners, and specialists. This will be a difficult transition for health systems built on disease and system-focused, subspecialist care, but one that has to commence now.

References

Aabom B, Pfeiffer P. Why are some patients in treatment for advanced cancer reluctant to consult their GP? Scand J Prim Health Care. 2009;27(1):58–62.

Abernethy AP, Currow DC, Shelby-James T, Rowett D, May F, Samsa GP, et al. Delivery strategies to optimize resource utilization and performance status for patients with advanced life-limiting illness: results from the "palliative care trial" [ISRCTN 81117481]. J Pain Symptom Manag. 2013;45(3):488–505.

Agar M, Luckett T, Luscombe G, Phillips J, Beattie E, Pond D, Mitchell G, Davidson PM, Cook J, Brooks D, Houltram J, Goodall S, Chenoweth L, Quinn TJ. Effects of facilitated family case conferencing for advanced dementia: A cluster randomised clinical trial. PLOS ONE. 2017;12(8):e0181020

Anquinet L, Rietjens JAC, Van Den Block L, Bossuyt N, Deliens L. General practitioners' report of continuous deep sedation until death for patients dying at home: a descriptive study from Belgium. Eur J Gen Pract. 2011;17(1):5–13.

Anquinet L, Rietjens JAC, Vandervoort A, Van Der Steen JT, Vander Stichele R, Deliens L, et al. Continuous deep sedation until death in nursing home residents with dementia: a case series. J Am Geriatr Soc. 2013;61(10):1768–76.

Aoun S. The hardest thing we have ever done: full report of the national inquiry into the social impact of caring for terminally ill people. Canberra: Palliative Care Australia; 2004.

Aoun SM, Kristjanson LJ, Currow DC, Hudson PL. Caregiving for the terminally ill: at what cost? Palliat Med. 2005;19(7):551–5.

Aoun S, Breen L, Rumbold B, McNamara B, Hegney D. Findings of a community survey of bereavement experience: support for a public health approach. Palliat Med. 2014;28(6):581–2.

Auerbach AD, Pantilat SZ. End-of-life care in a voluntary hospitalist model: effects on communication, processes of care, and patient symptoms. Am J Med. 2004;116(10):669–75.

Australian Bureau of Statistics. 3303.0 – Causes of Death, Australia, 2015. Canberra: Australian Government; 2016.

Australian Institute of Health & Welfare. Palliative Care Services in Australia 2014. Canberra: AIHW; 2014. Report No.: Cat. no. HWI 128

Barclay S, Todd C, Grande G, Lipscombe J. Controlling cancer pain in primary care: the prescribing habits and knowledge base of general practitioners. J Pain Symptom Manag. 2002;23(5):383–92.

Barclay S, Wyatt P, Shore S, Finlay I, Grande G, Todd C. Caring for the dying: how well prepared are general practitioners? A questionnaire study in Wales. Palliat Med. 2003;17(1):27–39.

Beller EM, van Driel ML, McGregor L, Truong S, Mitchell G. Palliative pharmacological sedation for terminally ill adults. Cochrane Database Syst Rev. 2015;1:CD010206.

Ben Diane MK, Peretti-Watel P, Pegliasco H, Favre R, Galinier A, Lapiana JM, et al. Morphine prescription to terminally ill patients with lung cancer and dyspnea: French physicians' attitudes. J Opioid Manag. 2005;1(1):25–30.

Blanker MH, Koerhuis-Roessink M, Swart SJ, Zuurmond WW, van der Heide A, Perez RS, et al. Pressure during decision making of continuous sedation in end-of-life situations in Dutch general practice. BMC Fam Pract. 2012;13:68.

Blazekovic-Milakovic S, Matijasevic I, Stojanovic-Spehar S, Supe S. Family physicians' views on disclosure of a diagnosis of cancer and care of terminally ill patients in Croatia. Psychiatr Danub. 2006;18(1–2):19–29.

Borgsteede SD, Graafland-Riedstra C, Deliens L, Francke AL, van Eijk JTM, Willems DL. Good end-of-life care according to patients and their GPs. Br J Gen Pract. 2006;56(522):20–6.

Borgsteede S, Deliens L, Beentjes B, Schellevis F, Stalman WAB, Van Eijk JTM, et al. Symptoms in patients receiving palliative care: a study on patient-physician encounters in general practice. Palliat Med. 2007a;21(5):417–23.

Borgsteede SD, Deliens L, Van Der Wal G, Francke AL, Stalman WAB, Van Eijk JTM. Interdisciplinary cooperation of GPs in palliative care at home: a nationwide survey in the Netherlands. Scand J Prim Health Care. 2007b;25(4):226–31.

Borgsteede SD, Deliens L, Zuurmond WWA, Schellevis FG, Willems DL, Van der Wal G, et al. Prescribing of pain medication in palliative care. A survey in general practice. Pharmacoepidemiol Drug Saf. 2009;18(1):16–23.

Boyd KJ, Murray SA, Kendall M, Worth A, Frederick Benton T, Clausen H. Living with advanced heart failure: a prospective, community based study of patients and their carers. Eur J Heart Fail. 2004;6(5):585–91.

Boyd K, Mason B, Kendall M, Barclay S, Chinn D, Thomas K, et al. Advance care planning for cancer patients in primary care: a feasibility study. Br J Gen Pract. 2010;60(581):e449–e58.

Britt H, Miller G, Henderson J, Bayram C, Harrison C, Valenti L, et al. General practice activity in Australia 2015–16. Sydney: Sydney University Press; 2016. Contract No: 40.

Brown M. Participating in end of life decisions. The role of general practitioners. Aust Fam Physician. 2002;31(1):60–2.

Bull A, Mash B. Advance directives or living wills: reflections of general practitioners and frail care coordinators in a small town in KwaZulu-Natal. South African Family Practice. 2012;54(6):507–12.

Burge F, Lawson B, Johnston G. Family physician continuity of care and emergency department use in end-of-life cancer care. Med Care. 2003a;41(8):992–1001.

Burge F, Lawson B, Johnston G, Cummings I. Primary care continuity and location of death for those with Cancer. J Palliat Med. 2003b;6(6):911–8.

Burridge LH, Mitchell GK, Jiwa M, Girgis A. Consultation etiquette in general practice: a qualitative study of what makes it different for lay cancer caregivers. BMC Fam Pract. 2011;12:110.

Butler LD, Field NP, Busch AL, Seplaki JE, Hastings TA, Spiegel D. Anticipating loss and other temporal stressors predict traumatic stress symptoms among partners of metastatic/recurrent breast cancer patients. Psychooncology. 2005;14(6):492–502.

Canto ME, Canaves JL, Xamena JM. De Lluch Bauza Amengual M. Management of terminal cancer patients: attitudes and training needs of primary health care doctors and nurses. Support Care Cancer. 2000;8(6):464–71.

Cartwright C, Montgomery J, Rhee J, Zwar N, Banbury A. Medical practitioners' knowledge and self-reported practices of substitute decision making and implementation of advance care plans. Intern Med J. 2014; 44(3):234–9.

De Vleminck A, Pardon K, Beernaert K, Deschepper R, Houttekier D, Van Audenhove C, et al. Barriers to advance care planning in cancer, heart failure and dementia patients: a focus group study on general practitioners' views and experiences. PLoS One. 2014;9(1):e84905.

Demagny L, Holtedahl K, Bachimont J, Thorsen T, Letourmy A, Bungener M. General practitioners' role in cancer care: a French-Norwegian study. BMC Res Notes. 2009;2:200.

Donker GA, Slotman FG, Spreeuwenberg P, Francke AL. Palliative sedation in Dutch general practice from 2005 to 2011: a dynamic cohort study of trends and reasons. Br J Gen Pract. 2013;63(615):e669–e75.

Etkind SN, Bone AE, Gomes B, Lovell N, Evans CJ, Higginson IJ, et al. How many people will need palliative care in 2040? Past trends, future projections and implications for services. BMC Med. 2017;15(1):102.

Evans N, Pasman HR, Vega Alonso T, Van den Block L, Miccinesi G, Van Casteren V, et al. End-of-life decisions: a cross-national study of treatment preference discussions and surrogate decision-maker appointments. PLoS One. 2013;8(3):e57965.

Evans N, Costantini M, Pasman HR, Van Den Block L, Donker GA, Miccinesi G, et al. End-of-life communication: a retrospective survey of representative general practitioner networks in four countries. J Pain Symptom Manag. 2014;47(3):604–19.

Ewing G, Rogers M, Barclay S, McCabe J, Martin A, Campbell M, et al. Palliative care in primary care: a study to determine whether patients and professionals agree on symptoms. Br J Gen Pract. 2006;56(522): 27–34.

Eychmeuller S. SENS is making sense – on the way to an innovative approach to structure palliative care problems. Ther Umsch. 2012;69(2):87–90.

Farber SJ, Egnew TR, Herman-Bertsch JL, Taylor TR, Guldin GE. Issues in end-of-life care: patient, caregiver, and clinician perceptions. J Palliat Med. 2003;6(1):19–31.

Farber NJ, Urban SY, Collier VU, Metzger M, Weiner J, Boyer EG. Frequency and perceived competence in providing palliative care to terminally ill patients: a survey of primary care physicians. J Pain Symptom Manag. 2004;28(4):364–72.

Gardiner C, Gott M, Ingleton C, Hughes P, Winslow M, Bennett MI. Attitudes of health care professionals to opioid prescribing in end-of-life care: a qualitative focus group study. J Pain Symptom Manag. 2012; 44(2):206–14.

Gawande AA. Being mortal: medicine and what matters in the end London: profile books; 2014.

Gill TM, Gahbauer EA, Han L, Allore HG. Trajectories of disability in the last year of life. N Engl J Med. 2010;362(13):1173–80.

Gomez-Batiste X, Martinez-Munoz M, Blay C, Amblas J, Vila L, Costa X, et al. Identifying patients with chronic conditions in need of palliative care in the general population: development of the NECPAL tool and preliminary prevalence rates in Catalonia. BMJ Support Palliat Care. 2013;3(3):300–8.

Gorlen T, Gorlen TF, Vass M, Neergaard MA. Low confidence among general practitioners in end-of-life care and subcutaneous administration of medicine. Dan Med J. 2012;59(4):A4407.

Gott M, Gardiner C, Small N, Payne S, Seamark D, Halpin D, et al. The effect of the shipman murders on clinician attitudes to prescribing opiates for dyspnoea in end-stage chronic obstructive pulmonary disease in England. Prog Palliat Care. 2010;18(2):79–84.

Grande GE, Farquhar MC, Barclay SIG, Todd CJ. Valued aspects of primary palliative care: content analysis of bereaved carers' descriptions. Br J Gen Pract. 2004; 54(507):772–8.

Groot MM, Vernooij-Dassen MJFJ, Crul BJP, Grol RPTM. General practitioners (GPs) and palliative care: perceived tasks and barriers in daily practice. Palliat Med. 2005;19(2):111–8.

Groot MM, Vernooij-Dassen MJFJ, Verhagen SCA, Crul BJP, Grol RPTM. Obstacles to the delivery of primary palliative care as perceived by GPs. Palliat Med. 2007;21(8):697–703.

Grunfeld E, Coyle D, Whelan T, Clinch J, Reyno L, Earle CC, et al. Family caregiver burden: results of a longitudinal study of breast cancer patients and their principal caregivers. CMAJ. 2004;170(12): 1795–801.

Harrison N, Cavers D, Campbell C, Murray SA. Are UK primary care teams formally identifying patients for palliative care before they die? Br J Gen Pract. 2012;62(598):e344–e52.

Hawley P, Liebscher R, Wilford J. Continuing methadone for pain in palliative care. Pain Res Manage. 2013;18(2):83–6.

Higginson IJ, Gao W. Opioid prescribing for cancer pain during the last 3 months of life: associated factors and 9-year trends in a nationwide United Kingdom cohort study. J Clin Oncol. 2012;30(35):4373–9.

Highet G, Crawford D, Murray SA, Boyd K. Development and evaluation of the supportive and palliative care indicators tool (SPICT): a mixed-methods study. BMJ Support Palliat Care. 2014;4(3):285–90.

Hillman KM, Cardona-Morrell M. The ten barriers to appropriate management of patients at the end of their life. Intensive Care Med. 2015;41(9):1700–2.

Hinton J. Can home care maintain an acceptable quality of life for patients with terminal cancer and their relatives? Palliat Med. 1994;8:183–96.

Hirakawa Y, Masuda Y, Kuzuya M, Iguchi A, Uemura K. Age-related differences in care receipt and symptom experience of elderly cancer patients dying at home: lessons from the DEATH project. Geriatr Gerontol Int. 2007;7(1):34–40.

Hirooka K, Miyashita M, Morita T, Ichikawa T, Yoshida S, Akizuki N, et al. Regional medical professionals' confidence in providing palliative care, associated difficulties and availability of specialized palliative care services in Japan. Jpn J Clin Oncol. 2014;44(3):249–56.

Hollingworth S, Zhang J, Vaikuntam BP, Jackson C, Mitchell G. Case conference primary-secondary care planning at end of life can reduce the cost of hospitalisations. BMC Palliat Care. 2016;15(1):84.

Hong TC, Lam TP, Chao DVK. Barriers for primary care physicians in providing palliative care service in Hong Kong – qualitative study. Hong Kong Practitioner. 2010;32(1):3–9.

Hudson P, Aranda S, Kristjanson L. Meeting the supportive needs of family caregivers in palliative care: challenges for health professionals. J Palliat Med. 2004;7:19–25.

Kelly B, Varghese FT, Burnett P, Turner J, Robertson M, Kelly P, et al. General practitioners' experiences of the psychological aspects in the care of a dying patient. Palliat Support Care. 2008;6(2):125–31.

Kristjanson L, White K. Clinical support for families in the palliative care phase of hematologic or oncologic illness. Hematol Oncol Clin North Am. 2002;16:745–62.

Kruis AL, Smidt N, Assendelft WJ, Gussekloo J, Boland MR, Rutten-van Molken M, et al. Integrated disease management interventions for patients with chronic obstructive pulmonary disease. Cochrane Database Syst Rev. 2013;10:CD009437.

Kuin A, Courtens AM, Deliens L, Vernooij-Dassen MJFJ, Van Zuylen L, Van Der Linden B, et al. Palliative care consultation in the Netherlands: a nationwide evaluation study. J Pain Symptom Manag. 2004;27(1):53–60.

Ledeboer QC, Van der Velden LA, De Boer MF, Feenstra L, Pruyn JF. Palliative care for head and neck cancer patients in general practice. Acta Otolaryngol. 2006;126(9):975–80.

Leemans K, Van den Block L, Bilsen J, Cohen J, Boffin N, Deliens L. Dying at home in Belgium: a descriptive GP interview study. BMC Fam Pract. 2012;13:4.

Linklater GT. Promoting patient-centredness in undergraduate palliative care education. Med Educ. 2008;42(11):1126–7.

Maas EA, Murray SA, Engels Y, Campbell C. What tools are available to identify patients with palliative care needs in primary care: a systematic literature review and survey of European practice. BMJ Support Palliat Care. 2013;3(4):444–51.

Mas C, Albaret MC, Sorum PC, Mullet E. French general practitioners vary in their attitudes toward treating terminally ill patients. Palliat Med. 2010;24(1):60–7.

Mason B, Boyd K, Murray SA, Steyn J, Cormie P, Kendall M, et al. Developing a computerised search to help UK general practices identify more patients for palliative care planning: a feasibility study. BMC Fam Pract. 2015;16:99.

Meeussen K, Van Den Block L, Echteld M, Bossuyt N, Bilsen J, Van Casteren V, et al. Advance care planning in Belgium and the Netherlands: a nationwide retrospective study via sentinel networks of general practitioners. J Pain Symptom Manag. 2011;42(4):565–77.

Michiels E, Deschepper R, Van Der Kelen G, Bernheim JL, Mortier F, Vander Stichele R, et al. The role of general practitioners in continuity of care at the end of life: a qualitative study of terminally ill patients and their next of kin. Palliat Med. 2007;21(5):409–15.

Mitchell G. The effect of case conferences between general practitioners and palliative care specialist teams on the quality of life of dying people [PhD]. Brisbane: University of Queensland; 2005.

Mitchell G, Seamark D. Dying in the community: general practitioner treatment of community-based patients analysed by chart audit. Palliat Med. 2016;17(3):289–92.

Mitchell GK, Brown RM, Erikssen L, Tieman JJ. Multidisciplinary care planning in the primary care management of completed stroke: a systematic review. BMC Fam Pract. 2008a;9:44.

Mitchell GK, Del Mar CB, O'Rourke PK, Clavarino AM. Do case conferences between general practitioners and specialist palliative care services improve quality of life? A randomised controlled trial (ISRCTN 52269003). Palliat Med. 2008b;22(8):904–12.

Mitchell G, Nicholson C, McDonald K, Bucetti A. Enhancing palliative care in rural Australia: the residential aged care setting. Aust J Prim Health. 2011;17(1):95–101.

Mitchell GK, Girgis A, Jiwa M, Sibbritt D, Burridge LH, Senior HE. Providing general practice needs-based care for carers of people with advanced cancer: a randomised controlled trial. Br J Gen Pract. 2013;63(615):e683–e90.

Mitchell G. End of life care for patients with cancer. Aust Fam Physician. 2014a;43(8):356–361.

Mitchell G, Zhang J, Burridge L, Senior H, Miller E, Young S, Donald M, Jackson C. Case conferences between general practitioners and specialist teams to plan end of life care of people with end stage heart failure and lung disease: an exploratory pilot study. BMC Palliat Care. 2014b;13:24.

Mitchell GK, Burridge L, Zhang J, Donald M, Scott IA, Dart J, et al. Systematic review of integrated models of health care delivered at the primary-secondary interface: how effective is it and what determines effectiveness? Aust J Prim Health. 2015;21(4):391–408.

Mitchell GK, Senior HE, Rhee JJ, Ware RS, Young S, Teo PC, Murray S, Boyd K, Clayton JM. Using intuition or a formal palliative care needs assessment screening process in general practice to predict death within 12 months: A randomised controlled trial. Palliat Med. 2018a;32(2):384–394. https://doi.org/10.1177/0269216317698621

Mitchell G, Senior H, Johnson C, Fallon-Ferguson J, Williams B, Monterosso L, Rhee J, McVey P, Grant M, Aubin M, Nwachukwu H, Yates P. Systematic review of general practice end-of-life symptom control. BMJ Support Palliat Care. 2018b. https://doi.org/10.1136/bmjspcare-2017-001374.

Murray SA, Boyd K, Kendall M, Worth A, Benton TF, Clausen H. Dying of lung cancer or cardiac failure: prospective qualitative interview study of patients and their carers in the community. BMJ. 2002; 325(7370):929.

Murray SA, Kendall M, Grant E, Boyd K, Barclay S, Sheikh A. Patterns of social, psychological, and spiritual decline toward the end of life in lung cancer and heart failure. J Pain Symptom Manag. 2007;34(4): 393–402.

Murray SA, Firth A, Schneider N, Van den Eynden B, Gomez-Batiste X, Brogaard T, et al. Promoting palliative care in the community: production of the primary palliative care toolkit by the European Association of Palliative Care Taskforce in primary palliative care. Palliat Med. 2015;29(2):101–11.

Neergaard MA, Olesen F, Jensen AB, Sondergaard J. Palliative care for cancer patients in a primary health care setting: bereaved relatives' experience, a qualitative group interview study. BMC Palliat Care. 2008;7:1.

Neergaard MA, Vedsted P, Olesen F, Sokolowski I, Jensen AB, Sondergaard J. Associations between successful palliative cancer pathways and community nurse involvement. BMC Palliat Care. 2009;8:18.

Olson RA, Lengoc S, Tyldesley S, French J, McGahan C, Soo J. Relationships between family physicians' referral for palliative radiotherapy, knowledge of indications for radiotherapy, and prior training: a survey of rural and urban family physicians. Radiat Oncol. 2012;7(1):73.

Oxenham D, Duncan R, Fischbacher M. Cancer pain management in Lanarkshire: a community-based audit. Palliat Med. 2003;17(8):708–13.

Rhee JJ, Zwar NA, Kemp LA. Why are advance care planning decisions not implemented? Insights from interviews with Australian general practitioners. J Palliat Med. 2013;16(10):1197–204.

Robinson C, Kolesar S, Boyko M, Berkowitz J, Calam B, Collins M. Awareness of do-not-resuscitate orders: what do patients know and want? Can Fam Physician. 2012;58(4):e229–33.

Robinson L, Dickinson C, Bamford C, Clark A, Hughes J, Exley C. A qualitative study: Professionals' experiences of advance care planning in dementia and palliative care, 'a good idea in theory but'. Palliat Med. 2013;27(5):401–8.

Rosenwax LK, McNamara BA. Who receives specialist palliative care in Western Australia – and who misses out. Palliat Med. 2006;20(4):439–45.

Salvato C, Aretini G, Serraglia D, Terrazzani G, Debetto P, Giusti P, et al. Opioid prescription for terminally ill outpatients in a district of northern Italy: a retrospective survey. Pharmacol Res. 2003;48(1):75–82.

Samant RS, Fitzgibbon E, Meng J, Graham ID. Family physicians' perspectives regarding palliative radiotherapy. Radiother Oncol. 2006;78(1):101–6.

Sepulveda C, Marlin A, Yoshida T, Ullrich A. Palliative care; the World Health Organization's global perspective. Journal of Pain Management. 2002; 24:91–6.

Sercu M, Pype P, Christiaens T, Derese A, Deveugele M. Belgian general Practitioners' perspectives on the use of palliative sedation in end-of-life home care: a qualitative study. J Pain Symptom Manag. 2014;47(6): 1054–63.

Shaw KL, Clifford C, Thomas K, Meehan H. Improving end-of-life care: a critical review of the gold standards framework in primary care. Palliat Med. 2010; 24(3):317–29.

Sizoo EM, Braam L, Postma TJ, Pasman HRW, Heimans JJ, Klein M, et al. Symptoms and problems in the end-of-life phase of high-grade glioma patients. Neuro-Oncology. 2010;12(11):1162–6.

Slort W, Schweitzer BPM, Blankenstein AH, Abarshi EA, Riphagen I, Echteld MA, et al. Perceived barriers and facilitators for general practitioner-patient communication in palliative care: a systematic review. Palliat Med. 2011;25(6):613–29.

Snyder S, Hazelett S, Allen K, Radwany S. Physician knowledge, attitude, and experience with advance care planning, palliative care, and hospice: results of a primary care survey. Am J Hosp Palliat Med. 2013; 30(5):419–24.

Stjernsward J, Foley KM, Ferris FD. The public health strategy for palliative care. J Pain Symptom Manag. 2007;33(5):486–93.

Tateno Y, Ishikawa S. Clinical pathways can improve the quality of pain management in home palliative care in remote locations: retrospective study on Kozu Island, Japan. Rural Remote Health. 2012;12(4):1992.

Thomas K, editor. Improving community palliative care in the UK using the gold standards framework. Ninth Australian palliative care conference. Melbourne: Palliative Care Australia; 2007.

Thomas K. The gold standards framework prognostic Indicator guidance (PIG). 4th ed. Shrewsbury: Gold Standards Framework; 2011.

Thoonsen B, Vissers K, Verhagen S, Prins J, Bor H, van Weel C, et al. Training general practitioners in early identification and anticipatory palliative care planning: a randomized controlled trial. BMC Fam Pract. 2015;16(1):126.

Tierney WM, Dexter PR, Gramelspacher GP, Perkins AJ, Zhou XH, Wolinsky FD. The effect of discussions about advance directives on patients' satisfaction with primary care. J Gen Intern Med. 2001;16(1):32–40.

Todd A, Husband A, Richardson R, Jassal N, Robson P, Andrew I. Are we using oxycodone appropriately? A utilisation review in a UK tertiary care Centre. Eur J Hosp Pharm: Sci Pract. 2013;20(2):125–8.

van Heest F, Finlay I, Kramer J, Otter R, Meyboom-de Jong B. Telephone consultations on palliative sedation therapy and euthanasia in general practice in the Netherlands in 2003: a report from inside. Fam Pract. 2009;26(6):481–7.

van Kooten J, Binnekade TT, van der Wouden JC, Stek ML, Scherder EJ, Husebo BS, et al. A review of pain prevalence in Alzheimer's, vascular, frontotemporal and Lewy body dementias. Dement Geriatr Cogn Disord. 2016;41(3–4):220–32.

Vandervoort A, van den Block L, van der Steen JT, Stichele RV, Bilsen J, Deliens L. Advance directives and physicians' orders in nursing home residents with dementia in Flanders, Belgium: prevalence and associated outcomes. Int Psychogeriatr. 2012;24(7):1133–43.

Vulto A, van Bommel M, Poortmans P, Lybeert M, Louwman M, Baart R, et al. General practitioners and referral for palliative radiotherapy: a population-based survey. Radiother Oncol. 2009;91(2):267–70.

Walsh D, Regan J. Terminal care in the home–the general practice perspective. Ir Med J. 2001;94(1):9–11.

Warmenhoven F, van Rijswijk E, van Hoogstraten E, van Spaendonck K, Lucassen P, Prins J, Vissers K, van Weel C. How family physicians address diagnosis and management of depression in palliative care patients. Ann Family Med 2012;10(4):330–336.

Weitzner MA, McMillan SC, Jacobsen PB. Family caregiver quality of life: differences between curative and palliative cancer treatment settings. J Pain Symptom Manage. 1999;17(6):418–28.

WONCA Europe. The European definintion of general practice/ family medicine. WONCA Europe: 2011 edition. Munich, 2011. Accessed 31/3/2018.

World Health Organization. Definition of Palliative Care. WHO Geneva, 2004. www.who.int/cancer/palliative/definition/en/. Accessed 28/6/18.

World Health Organization. Strengthening of palliative care as a component of integrated treatment throughout the life course. 2014. Contract No.: http://apps.who.int/gb/ebwha/pdf_files/WHA67/A67_R19-en.pdf.

World Health Organization. World health report on ageing and health. Geneva: WHO; 2015.

Young J, Donahue M, Farquhar M, Simpson C, Rocker G. Using opioids to treat dyspnea in advanced COPD: attitudes and experiences of family physicians and respiratory therapists. Can Fam Physician. 2012;58(7):e401–e7.

Zheng L, Finucane A, Oxenham D, McLoughlin P, McCutcheon H, Murray S. How good is primary care at identifying patients who need palliative care? A mixed methods study. Eur J Palliat Care. 2013;20(5):216–22.

Palliative Care in Residential Settings 51

Jo Hockley

Contents

Abstract

Many residential care settings for older people have been established on a culture of rehabilitation. However, this is changing. In many Western countries, recent policy is encouraging frail older people to stay longer in their own homes before going into 24-h care. As a result, on admission to these settings, older people are often considerably more dependent and frail than 10 years ago.

The palliative care needs of frail older people with multiple comorbidities admitted to residential care settings are significant. Palliative care is core to their work; such settings are now being compared to the former hospices that founded the hospice movement some 50 years ago. Hospices have an important role to play in reaching out to staff in

J. Hockley (✉)
Primary Palliative Care Research Group, Centre for Population Health Sciences, The Usher Institute of Population Health Sciences and Informatics, The University of Edinburgh, Edinburgh, Scotland
e-mail: Jo.hockley@ed.ac.uk

R. D. MacLeod, L. Van den Block (eds.), *Textbook of Palliative Care*,
https://doi.org/10.1007/978-3-319-77740-5_49

residential care settings and the frail older people they care for in order to support and enhance a palliative care approach.

This chapter describes some of the differences between palliative care for people with advanced cancer (often dying in mid-life) and those dying as a frail older person at the end of their lives with multiple comorbidities. It highlights a number of different quality improvement initiatives through which staff in residential care settings can be supported to adopt a greater palliative care approach.

Currently, nearly a quarter of the population in the UK, in Canada, and the USA die in care homes. In other countries, such as The Netherlands and Norway where there is greater on-site healthcare provision including physicians, it is nearer 50% of the country's population.

1 Introduction

This chapter aims to bring: greater awareness to the important place that residential care settings increasingly play in the care of frail older people at the end of life; highlight differences between the populations in these facilities compared to that of hospices; suggest opportunities and initiatives where a palliative care approach might be enhanced; and, finally, use narratives to bring alive important aspects.

For many years, residential care settings have been seen as places for rehabilitation where older people were admitted for companionship and to maintain independence for as long as possible. So much so that, in the UK prior to 2000, while a few frail older people died in the care home they were living in, most residents were admitted to the local hospital to die. Increasingly, however, countries across the world are concerned about how to meet the cost of institutional elderly care and are encouraging the provision of more care for older people in their own homes. Consequently, on admission to a place providing 24-h care, older people are now considerably frailer.

The result of such a policy has meant that there is not only greater frailty in people living in their own homes, which in itself needs to be proactively managed, but the majority of residents living/dying in residential care settings now have advanced, progressive, incurable diseases (IAHPC 2017) – ranging from Parkinson's disease and stroke to a number of different dementias. Gone are the places where the majority of residents would survive more than 3 or 4 years. The average length of stay in UK care homes is now 15 months with the majority of people dying within a year of admission to a care home with on-site nurses (Kinley et al. 2014a). Currently, nearly a quarter of the population in the UK, Canada, and the USA die in care homes; in other countries (i.e., The Netherlands and Norway) where there is greater on-site healthcare provision including physicians, it is nearer 50% of the population.

Staff working in residential care settings are being encouraged to develop their palliative care skills; however, palliative care is still not part of statutory training for residential care settings in many countries. This rise in both the complexity and number of comorbidities of frail older people requiring 24-h care at a later stage demands a higher level of skill and communication within facilities especially facilities where there is no on-site nursing (Handley et al. 2014).

Different terms associated with residential settings globally are now outlined before considering the following: the population of those who live and work in these settings; geriatrics and palliative care and the differing dying trajectories of frail older people; different models and initiatives to enhance palliative care in these settings; components of successful implementation of initiatives and their sustainability; and, innovations for the future.

2 Residential Care Settings Giving 24-H Care to Frail Older People

Froggatt and colleagues undertook a comprehensive mapping and classification of European care homes (with and without nursing) and their palliative care provision collecting data from 29 European countries (Froggatt et al. 2017a).

Their aim was to develop a typology of palliative care activity with respect to the implementation of various palliative care initiatives. They identified three types of facility: Type 1 ("on-site" physicians and nurses and care assistants), Type 2 ("on-site" nurses and care assistants but "off-site" physicians), and Type 3 ("on-site" care assistants with "off-site" physicians and nurses) (Froggatt et al. 2017b). Although the distinction over the years between Type 2 and Type 3 care homes with the regard to the professionals working there remains much the same, the distinction between the people living in these types of facilities is diminishing as the general residential setting population becomes distinctly frailer. Many countries worldwide are now merging the distinction between "low" and "high" care or "residential" and "nursing" care in institutions.

There are different terms used to describe the 24-h residential care given to frail older people and often more than one in the same country (see Table 1). For the purpose of this chapter, residential care settings for people requiring 24-h care will be called "long-term care facilities" (LTCFs) unless talking specifically about a certain country when the name relevant to that country will be used.

Every country has different ways of funding the 24-h care of frail older people. However, there are three broad categories of facilities: independent private ("for profit"), independent charitable foundations ("not for profit"), and government (health/local authority) in most countries. How care is funded for frail older people is gaining increasing attention by researchers and politicians in light of the aging population.

Globally, the development of palliative care services in residential care settings has, in the main, been less well developed than in other settings such as hospitals or hospices with their home care teams. An exception is The Netherlands. Here, in the 1980s, following a 5-year research project at Antonius IJsselmonde, Rotterdam (a 230-bedded nursing home), specific palliative care wards were created in large nursing home organizations in recognition of the needs of frail older people at the end of life (Baar 1999; Baar and van der Kloot Meijburg 2002).

In contrast, in the UK, where palliative care was first developed through hospices and their home care teams, it was not until the turn of the twenty-first century that palliative care services reached out to care homes. Many long-stay geriatric wards were closed down in 1990s, and the money was given to social care who then paid independent care homes to care for older people. While the social care needs of frail older people were considerably advanced, because care homes were now placed outside the NHS, they became isolated from palliative care developments occurring in the NHS and more difficult to reach.

3 The LTCF Population

3.1 Residents and Their Families

Those over 85 years are the fastest growing segment of the population in many western countries. In the UK, this group is projected to more than double by 2039 and is associated with increasing incidence of dementia (ONS 2014). In the UK, those requiring 24-h care in 2030 are projected to increase by 82% with an increasing demand from 400,000 to 630,000 care home places (Jagger et al. 2011).

As has already been mentioned, the LTCF population globally are increasingly frail with multiple comorbidities. In the UK, as many as 80% of residents in care homes have dementia or severe cognitive impairments (Alzheimers Society 2013). It is well documented that people with advanced dementia living in LTCFs can experience "social death" where they are passive recipients or objects of care being robbed of a meaningful interaction in the last months/years of life (Watson 2016). Holistic care and the importance of recognizing that the mind is not separate from the body but intricately made up of mind, body, and soul cannot be over emphasized especially in relation to someone with advanced dementia.

A white paper on the palliative care needs for people with dementia (van der Steen et al. 2014) details complete consensus from experts across 23 European countries in relation to the following:

Table 1 Type of 24-h residential care facility according to country

Country	Name given to facility	Staff employed in facilities	How funded
Australia (type 2 and 3)	Aged Care Facilities (ACFs)	RNs: Registered nurses ENs: Enrolled nurses PCAs: Personal care attendants AHPs: Allied health professionals	Health and social care Privately funded
USA (type 1 and 2)	Skilled Nursing Facilities (SNFs) or Long-term care facilities (LTCFs) or Continuing Care Retirement Communities (CCRCs)	RNs: Registered nurses LVNs: Licensed vocational nurses CNAs: Certified nurse aides CMAs: Certified medication aides APRNs: Advanced practice registered nurses	Medicare Medicaid Private insurance
Canada (type 2 and 3)	Long-term residential care facilities (LTC) or Nursing homes or Homes for the aged	RNs: Registered nurses LPNs: Licensed practical nurses or registered qualified nursing assistants PSW: Personal support worker Type 2 will have the above + physiotherapists + occupational therapists	Variation across the country – currently debating a universal public insurance scheme for long-term care (Grignon and Bernier 2012)
Europe (type 1, 2 and 3) Norway, Finland, Italy, and the Netherlands have elderly care physicians in their nursing homes	Long-term care facilities (LTCFs) or Nursing homes (NHs) or Care homes and care homes with on-site nurses (CHs; CHs-N)	RNs: Registered nurses NAs: Nursing assistants SCW: Social care workers	Different funding models across the different countries – mixture between "health and social care" funding, insurance, privately funded. Care of older people in the Netherlands, for example, is nearly completely covered by a national health insurance plan

Type 1: "On-site" nurses + care assistants + elderly care physicians
Type 2: "On-site" nurses + care assistants; "off-site" physician/s
Type 3: "On-site" care assistants only; "off-site" nurse/s + physician/s
Froggatt et al. (2017b)

- Person-centered care, communication, and shared decision-making
- Optimal treatment of symptoms and providing comfort
- Setting care goals and advance planning
- Continuity of care
- Psychosocial and spiritual support
- Family care and involvement
- Education of the healthcare team
- Societal and ethical issues

The domains provide a framework to guide important aspects of LTCF palliative care development in clinical practice, policy, and research.

3.2 Management and Staffing

Leadership of LTCFs is one of the single most important aspects for high-quality care for frail older people and its continuity in such settings. If staff are valued and supported by management in helping them progress and develop, then this generally cascades down into good care of residents and families. When one sees defensive care and/or poor communication especially in relation to palliative and end-of-life care, then this is often a result of poor leadership and poor role models where staff do not feel supported.

There is a wide variation between countries and even within different LTCF organizations in the same country in relation to staff development. The majority of staff have little healthcare training. Many young people choose to work in these facilities because they want to help frail older people; they come to help dress, feed, and chat to older people. Unfortunately, they are often not prepared with the demands of the work and the fact that many frail older people, who they have got to know very well over the months/year, will die in the LTCF.

In the UK, the majority of formal carers will be encouraged to have some vocational training –50% of staff in a care home should have Level 2 NVQ/SVQ (National/Scottish Vocational Qualification). Such a qualification is based around personal care, moving and handling, nutrition, oral care, etc. for frail older people but does not often include knowledge about different comorbidities and how to communicate about life/death issues. However, despite this, LTC staff are not unskilled. Often they have considerable insight into situations but are not given the opportunity or support to voice their opinions.

In most countries, there are little or no nurses working in LTCFs and no on-site medical support with some exceptions like The Netherlands and Norway. In the UK, only a quarter of care homes have on-site nurses. Where there are nurses, the ratio is in the region of 1 nurse to 30 residents with the rest of the staff being formal care workers. With increasing pressure on workloads and the "risk" that some LTCF staff feel when not having the knowledge and competencies in the care they are being increasingly asked to give, it is not surprising there is a high turnover of staff. In the UK, this has now reached worryingly high proportions. It could be argued that because of the lack of distinction is diminishing between older people residing in the different LTCF/care home settings and because managers are being encouraged not to transfer frail older people in the last months of life, that all LTCFs/care homes should provide "high" care and employ nurses and even care home doctors.

4 Geriatrics and Palliative Care

In 2017, both geriatric and palliative care specialists celebrate important milestones in their development as a speciality – geriatrics celebrate 70 years and palliative care celebrate 50 years. Dame Cicely gained huge insights from well-known physicians in the care of older people to underpin the hospice movement. It was Professor Worcester's seminal work, The Care of the Aged, the Dying and the Dead (1935), which had prominence both in Dame Cicely's writing and on her bookshelf.

In 1989, at the First International Conference on Palliative Care of the Elderly, Balfour Mount (1989, p. 7) also drew interesting analogies between geriatric practice and palliative care:

> Both make the whole person and his or her family the focus of care, while seeking to enhance quality of life and maintain the dignity and autonomy of the individual. Judicious use of investigations are advocated and both eschew unwarranted treatment while providing symptom control and relief of suffering. Both are necessarily multi-disciplinary and both are areas which prompt phobic reactions from society at large. . ..

However, despite the similarities drawn above, there are also differences not only between the settings but also within the care practices (see Table 2).

Respecting the choices of frail older people toward the end of life is extremely important. In 2012, a global initiative called "choosing wisely" was set up to help clinicians and patients engage in conversations about unnecessary tests/treatments and make wise and effective care choices. This initiative now involves professionals from

Table 2 Differences between cancer palliative care and end-of-life care in the elderly dying (Hockley 2002). (Reproduced with kind permission from Open University Press, Buckingham MK18 1XW)

Cancer palliative care	End-of-life care in the elderly dying
Focus in one disease process	Multiple disease processes
Emphasis on dying in mid-age or younger when life is generally seen as being "cut short"	Natural ending of life often understood by both the resident and those caring within the context of care homes
Clearer concept of "prognosis" so terminal care can be planned	Less predictable dying trajectory following a more dependent, lengthier disease process
Professional holistic relationship between patient and staff	Often a much closer/ emotional relationship between resident and care home staff as resident becomes "part of the family" and may have lived in the care home months/ year
More support from family/friends	Less support from family/ friends – often care home staff and other residents seen as family
Both patient and family often want life extended	Elderly, frail people in nursing homes frequently speak about dying and that it would be nice "to go to bed one night and not wake up"
Morphine and other medication frequently used to control symptoms	Pain requiring strong opioids less common
Multidisciplinary model of care	Nurses and care workers having the greatest input of care
Patients more often cognitively intact	Greater percentage of residents in nursing homes are cognitively impaired

across 20 countries. As a result of this initiative, the Long-term Care Medical Directors Association of Canada have come up with six recommendations (see Table 3) that are all evidence-based with their relevant resources (https://choosingwiselycanada.org/long-term-care/). Such recommendations emphasize the importance of palliative care and geriatricians working together for the best care of frail older people.

Table 3 Recommendations from choosing wisely (Jones 2017)

1.	*Don't send the frail resident of a nursing home to the hospital unless their urgent comfort and medical needs cannot be met in their care home.* Transfers to hospital for assessment and treatment of a change in condition have become customary; however, they are of uncertain benefit and may result in increased morbidity
2.	*Don't use antipsychotics as a first choice to treat behavioral and psychological symptoms of dementia.* People with dementia can sometimes be disruptive, behave aggressively, and resist personal care. There is often a reason for this behavior, and identifying and addressing the causes can make drug treatment unnecessary
3.	*Don't do a urine dip or urine culture unless there are clear signs and symptoms of a urinary tract infection (UTI).* Unless there are UTI symptoms, such as urinary discomfort, abdominal/back pain, frequency, urgency, or fever, testing should not be done. Testing often shows bacteria in the urine, with as many as 50% of those tested showing bacteria present in the absence of localizing symptoms to the genitourinary tract
4.	*Don't insert a feeding tube in individuals with advanced dementia. Instead, assist the resident to eat.* Inserting a feeding tube does not prolong or improve quality of life in patients with advanced dementia. If the resident has been declining in health with recurrent and progressive illnesses, they may be nearing the end of their life and will not benefit from feeding tube placement
5.	*Don't continue or add long-term medications unless there is an appropriate indication and a reasonable expectation of benefit in the individual patient.* Long-term medications should be discontinued if they are no longer needed (e.g., heartburn drugs, antihypertensives), as they can reduce the resident's quality of life while having little value for a frail elder with limited life expectancy
6.	*Don't order screening or routine chronic disease testing just because a blood draw is being done.* Unless treatment can be given that would add to quality of life, don't do these tests. What is considered routine testing may lead to harmful overtreatment in frail residents nearing the end of their life

4.1 Different Dying Trajectory

When reaching out to LTCFs with quality improvement initiatives or supporting end-of-life care, it is important not to impose the more familiar model of palliative care developed for

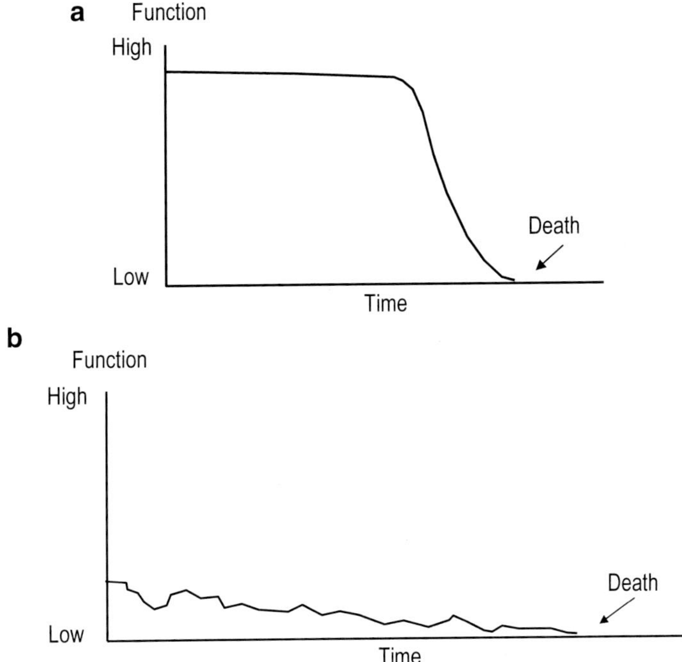

Fig. 1 (**a**) Different dying trajectories – cancer (Lynn and Adamson 2003). (**b**) Dwindling trajectory of frail older people – especially those with advanced dementia (Lynn and Adamson 2003)

people with advanced cancer. There is a difference between palliative care that has been developed for people with advanced cancer, typically from within specialist palliative care and the hospice movement, and palliative care for frail older people dying at the end of life from multiple comorbidities.

The dwindling dying trajectory, so well described by Lynn and Adamson (2003), is very different from the well-known, fairly predictable cancer trajectory – see Fig. 1a, b.

The phrase "bounce back" is an unknown phenomenon when caring for people dying in a hospice or a hospital and is uniquely tied to the dwindling trajectory of frail older people. A frail older person is seen to deteriorate, their medication is reviewed and discontinued, a greater attention to fluid intake is taken, and as a result the person "bounces back."

The danger of imposing a specialist palliative care model in the last days of life, where often opiates and hyoscine are used routinely, onto a frail older person who is dying with advanced dementia is vividly highlighted in the following case study (see Case Study A).

Case Study A: Mrs. A: 89 Years: Advanced Dementia (2012)

The Care Home Project Team at St Christopher's Hospice, London, (https://www.stchristophers.org.uk/education/training-and-research/care-homes/) was involved in development and training in a local care home without on-site nurses. The care home manager had contacted the local community palliative care team to come and review Mrs. A with advanced dementia who was dying. Mrs. A was in her late 80s and had been in the care home for a number of years; with her advancing dementia, she was pleasantly confused. However, she was now very frail and not drinking and clearly had days/week to live.

The community palliative care team were used to putting up syringe drivers when a person at home or in a care home without on-site nurses was dying. Because Mrs. A was slightly agitated, they decided

(*continued*)

to put up a syringe driver with a small dose of diamorphine 10 mg and Buscopan 20 mg/24 h. Within 3 days, Mrs. A had changed from her pleasant confusion to being increasingly agitated, shouting out, and unmanageable.

The Care Home Project Team were contacted and advised the immediate discontinuation of the syringe driver – the opiates had clearly accumulated because of Mrs. A's "old kidneys," and appropriate dehydration at the end-of-life. She was clearly dying but had no pain. It took the administration of s/c fluids and phenobarbitone to help reduce Mrs. A's distress, and she died peacefully 3 days later.

A different scenario (see Case Study B) highlights the benefits of "working alongside" staff in LTCFs – listening to what they would normally do, being open to learn from them in relation to the last day/s of life, and not imposing a specialist palliative care knowledge.

Case Study B: Miss B: 91 Years: Advanced Dementia (2004)

During research into death and dying in care homes with on-site nurses, staff were being supported to implement the "integrated care plan for the last days of life" (Hockley et al. 2005). Miss B, who had worked for many years as pharmacist, was now dying. She had been a "feisty" lady and had lived in the care home several years. If she didn't like your approach when you were helping her with her medication, you were in danger of the tablets being thrown back in your face. However, she now was very frail, reasonably calm, and just able to sip the fluids offered to her. The staff nurse asked for advice, and a typical response from a nurse specialist in palliative care was given: s/c diamorphine 2.5 mg and s/c Buscopan 10 mg. Importantly, the staff nurse offered her thoughts – she had worked in the care home sector for many years and had had some training in palliative care. She queried why opiates were being considered when Miss B had no pain. She also queried the use of Buscopan as it would only increase the dryness in Miss B's already dry mouth and suggested: "What about giving a small dose of diazepam rectally to calm her?" Immediately the importance of what the staff nurse was saying was recognized. Following the rectal diazepam, Miss B was still able to take sips of fluid – the care assistants took it in turns to sit with her reading some favorite poetry. Miss B died 12 h later – peacefully and comfortable.

As can be seen from Case Study B, the dying process of frail older people is often a natural process requiring little extra medication. William Osler (1849–1919) is well known for saying "pneumonia is the old man's friend," and although written over 150 years ago before the invention of antibiotics, it is as relevant today as it was in the nineteenth century.

Dying itself is not painful (Worcester 1935) – it is only painful in situations where there is unrelieved pain prior to the last days of life. An appropriate assessment of the situation taking into account the frailty, natural dehydration of frail older people, and any specific distressing symptoms must be made and a syringe driver only used if symptoms are severe. Often occasional s/c medication is all that is necessary in frail older people.

A small percentage of deaths in LTCFs can be quite sudden and, despite the person being in their 90s, is seen as "unexpected." An "acute" event like a silent pneumonia can often prompt admission to an acute hospital and sadly the person's dies in unfamiliar surroundings. The dwindling dying trajectory however is the most common type of dying in LTCFs, and generally speaking if properly acknowledged, the death will occur in the LTCF.

5 Different Models and Initiatives to Enhance Palliative Care in LTCFs

It is well documented that palliative care education on its own does not change practice in the often hierarchical structures of LTCFs (Froggatt 2001) that have for many years adopted a rehabilitation culture. However, we know that when education is done alongside implementing a specific tool, for example, advance care planning documentation, there is a greater chance of developing a palliative care approach to care.

Many LTCFs eagerly respond to new initiatives in relation to improving palliative and end-of-life care especially when supported by an outside agency such as a local university or hospice. Effectiveness of a project depends not only on the enthusiasm of the LTCF staff to develop their practice but also the support given by manager/management. Projects benefit when there is both a "top-down" and "bottom-up" approach. However, the current trend of short-term funding of programs is unlikely to bring about long-lasting change unless a funded sustainability initiative has been proposed at the beginning of the project (Hockley and Kinley 2016).

A number of tools, quality improvement initiatives, and models have been developed. These are now described, firstly, from a focus on the implementation of individual aspects of palliative care such as advance care planning or pain assessment in advanced dementia and, secondly, the implementation of a system that addresses multiple aspects of palliative care.

5.1 Individual Tools

If given the task to choose what might be the "key" developments of a palliative care approach in care homes, it would be impossible to list all such initiatives. Nonetheless, there are a number of tools that are gathering evidence of their effectiveness and are described below.

5.1.1 Advance/Anticipatory Care Planning and DNACPR Decisions

Advance/anticipatory care planning (ACP) is reported to decrease inappropriate hospital admissions of frail elderly residents with palliative care needs (Hockley and Kinley 2016). Documentation may take the form of an advance statement of wishes and preferences, an advance decision to refuse treatment (a legal document refusing specific treatment), and/or a surrogate decision-maker in the appointment of a Lasting Power of Attorney for Health and Welfare. These documents are then available to guide care if the individual loses the ability to make decisions or communicate their wishes. However, there are multiple preconditions related to successful ACP in LTCFs which occur at different levels of the organization (Gilissen et al. 2017).

Who in the LTCF Should Undertake These Conversations?

Until recently, the dominant culture in LTCFs has been a "striving to keep alive," and it is not always straightforward for staff to embrace discussions around ACP – especially when they have limited healthcare knowledge.

Most frail older people know they are facing the last year/s of their life. The very fact that they have now been admitted for 24-h care because they can no longer manage to care for themselves at home is every indication to them that this is likely to be their last move; to deny this is to discredit their autonomy and their ability to know their own body. Many residents are very open to discussions in relation to their wishes at the end of life (Stone et al. 2013). However, for many LTCF staff, often young with little healthcare training, conversations about care at the end of life can be extremely daunting.

Learning how to undertake such conversations is really important, and considerable support and education is often required. Learning can be very effective when seeing other people undertaking such a conversation (either through role modeling by an experienced clinician or through watching videos) and/or through role play alongside some communication skills training such as Sage and

Thyme (http://www.sageandthymetraining.org.uk/about). Sitting in with an experienced professional is probably the most useful.

In the UK, discussions about what a resident might want to achieve before becoming very frail, and whether they have thought about who they might want close-by at the end, can be undertaken by experienced social care workers. However, any detailed health-related discussions such as an event that might result in an action like going to hospital must be undertaken by properly qualified healthcare professionals.

With the increasing likelihood that many frail older people are likely to die within months of admission to a LTCF, conversations in relation to wishes toward the end of their life are most important. Such conversations are very individual (often requiring at more than one conversation) and must be documented accordingly.

Relatives are key to these conversations, and while they might like to think they know what their family member wants, sometimes they can be misguided. It is important to include where possible both resident and family in such conversations.

When Should Such Conversations Take Place?

The timing of conversations about the care in the last weeks of life including discussions regarding "do not attempt cardio-resuscitation" (DNACPR) needs to be adopted into routine practice of the facility. Most LTCFs will review residents' care plans on a monthly and 6-month basis; these therefore become the ideal times. For residents who have been in the LTCF a number of months/year/s, then the 6-month review (unless there is a sudden deterioration) is perfectly acceptable opportunity for such a conversation to be added to the end of the general discussion. For someone being admitted to a LTCF, especially if they are frail and ill, the timing is likely to be different.

It is important that the doctor/nurse establishes within a week of admission whether a DNACPR decision is to be signed. More detailed conversations about care at the end of life need to be undertaken once the resident and family have settled into the care home – and likely not to take place until the end of the 1st month in the care home.

There are a considerable number of forms and pamphlets that have been developed and are widely available. However, it is the importance of the conversation that is paramount – and the process should not be a "tick box" exercise. It is really important that such conversations are undertaken by staff who feel competent, having had the opportunity of sitting in with doctors/senior nurses to witness how it is done; such role modeling is very important if care home staff are to become competent.

5.1.2 Monthly Multidisciplinary Meetings

Good coordination of care especially in the last year of life is vital if the needs of frail older people in care homes are to be identified and managed appropriately. Monthly multidisciplinary meetings in the care home bring together all those who not only know the person but also those who have expertise to advise and ensure that care is properly coordinated.

In the UK, the Gold Standards Framework (http://www.goldstandardsframework.org.uk), promoting the development of a palliative care approach both in peoples' own homes and care homes, has advocated the importance of monthly multidisciplinary meetings for over 10 years now.

A simple palliative care register completed at a monthly multidisciplinary meeting in the LTCF prompts staff about different aspects of care, i.e., advance care planning/DNACPR, symptom control issues, and family communication. One of three triggers indicating that a resident is nearing the end of life is the "surprise question" (Thomas 2011):

> would I be surprised if [Mrs B] died in the next. . .three months, six months, year?

This question is asked at the meeting in conjunction with two other triggers: deterioration over the previous month/s and specific clinical indicators related to certain conditions. As a result of this questioning, the resident is categorized as likely having day/s, week/s, or month/s to live. Importantly, it is often the formal care workers in daily contact with the frail older person who are best able to answer this "surprise" question despite often having little advanced health education. It is important that they are present to discuss their specific residents. Once it is considered likely that the LTCF staff believe the person to be nearing the end of life – even though that might still be month/s away – it is important that there is open communication with the rest of the staff, to the resident (as appropriate), and family.

Such a monthly multidisciplinary meeting not only helps to build teamwork and trust across the different professions as well as good coordination of palliative care. Working with services provided during the day, at night, and at weekends is key to providing seamless quality palliative care in LTCFs.

5.1.3 Pain Assessment/Management Tools

Some diseases and conditions create varying degrees of pain for individuals. Older people often suffer in silence with their pain as they believe arthritis and other musculoskeletal conditions are part of growing old and therefore to be endured. LTCF residents have been found to have considerably more pain compared to the same population living in their own homes (Husebo et al. 2012).

Systematic pain assessment on admission and the use of relevant documentation can contribute to effective pain assessment and management. We know that pain has a combination of physical, emotional, social, and spiritual elements which Dame Cicely Saunders called "total pain." However, with 80% of frail older people in LTCFs having dementia or severe cognitive impairment, pain in these people needs to be assessed differently to that of people with cancer pain. It is often more complex to assess/manage pain in people with advanced dementia than it is in people with cancer (see Case Study C).

Case Study C: Pain Assessment in a Person with Advanced Dementia Unable to Verbalize Her Pain

During a year's study in a particular LTCF, I had got to know the majority of the 40 residents very well indeed. Mrs. C and her husband had been residents for a couple of years – she was a charming but muddled lady in her mid-80s with advanced dementia, while Mr. C had recently been diagnosed with advanced prostate cancer. One day when coming into the LTCF, instead of Mrs. C being up and about dusting the staircase, I noticed her sitting by the front door rubbing her knees. This was a change to Mrs. C's normal activity of walking around the house making sure that everything was spick and span.

At the time, although this was not the focus of the study, I had become interested in the difference between assessing pain in people with advanced dementia and assessing pain in people with advanced cancer in a hospice/community. I had read about the importance of assessing the nonverbal response to pain in people with advanced dementia and in particular the Doloplus2-scale (Lefebvre-Chapiro and the Doloplus Group 2001). The rubbing of the knees was new, and I was interested to find out her level of pain.

The manager happily told me who Mrs. C's carer was, and we proceeded to Mrs. C's room in order to undertake a pain assessment. Using a scale of 0–10, I asked Mrs. C "if '0' is no pain at all and '10' is the most excruciating pain you have ever had in all your life, what score would you give the pain in your knees?" Almost immediately Mrs. C told me 8/10. Ashamedly, because she didn't look as though she was in that much pain, I wondered whether she had become muddled and had really meant 2/10. To confirm my musings, the carer and I

(*continued*)

went away and completed the Doloplus2-scale together.

The Doloplus2-scale pain assessment tool (see Table 4) checks ten reactions at four levels (0–3) divided into three domains: somatic reactions, behavioral reactions, and psychosocial. A total score of 5 or more is likely to represent pain. When the carer added up our scoring of Mrs. C's pain, it came to 15. We realized together that Mrs. C had very real pain. We slowly titrated the analgesics that included starting oral morphine. Gradually over 3 weeks, the morphine was increased until Mrs. C was up and doing her dusting again. She remained stable on MST 30 mg bd alongside paracetamol for a number of months walking around and doing her dusting. She died reasonably suddenly in the LTCF about 4 months later.

There are many different pain assessment scales for use with people with advanced dementia unable to express their pain verbally (Lichtner et al. 2014). There are probably four that have had repeated scrutiny in relation to validity and reliability testing:

- *PAINAD*: This tool (http://geriatrictoolkit.missouri.edu/cog/painad.pdf) has five domains and is a relatively simple tool for nurses/care staff to use (Warden et al. 2003). Tool reliability is good for interrater reliability, but internal consistency is only moderate, and stability has not been demonstrated. http://prc.coh.org/Review%20of%20Tools%20for%20Pain%20Assessment/Review%20of%20Tools%202004/PAINAD/PAINAD_Indepth.pdf
- *ABBEY*: The ABBEY (Abbey et al. 2004) scale is similar to the PAINAD in that it is easy to complete. However, reliability and validity have been shown not to be strong. http://prc.coh.org/PainNOA/ABBEY_D.pdf
- *PACSLAC*: the Pain Assessment Checklist for Seniors with Limited Ability to Communicate (Fuchs-Lacelle and Hadjistavropoulos 2004) has been developed in Canada. It covers four domains: facial expressions × 13, activity/body movement × 20, social/personality/mood × 12, and others × 15. Prospective evaluation has added to the tool's reliability and validity. http://prc.coh.org/PainNOA/PACSLAC_D.pdf
- *Doloplus2-scale*: The Doloplus2-scale (Lefebvre-Chapiro and the Doloplus Group 2001) was specifically developed by geriatricians in France for people with advanced dementia who were no longer able to verbalize their pain. Although more complex to use, its reliability and validity are strong. http://prc.coh.org/PainNOA/Doloplus%202_Tool.pdf (Torvik et al. 2010).

Further studies evaluating the above tools and their efficacy and ease of use in the assessment/management of pain in frail older people with dementia by LTCF staff would be useful.

5.1.4 Documentation for the Last Days of Life

Dame Cicely Saunders (1918–2005) is well known for saying, "How someone dies remains in the memory of those who live on." This is extremely important in LTCF settings where often the majority of staff have little healthcare training. Some sort of documentation to help guide these last days is of vital importance.

Developed and adapted from the Liverpool Care Pathway (Ellershaw and Wilkinson 2003) for specific use in care homes, the *Integrated Care Plan for the Last Days of Life* (Hockley et al. 2005; Watson et al. 2006), further developed to more recent documentation called the *Integrated Personalised Plan for the last days of life* (http://www.stchristophers.org.uk/care-homes/research/ipp) (IPP), has managed to ride the storms of controversy in relation to the Liverpool Care Pathway. A recent audit report outlines the first 50 completed IPPs and the success of its use in care homes in south London (Coleman et al. 2017).

The importance of at least 90% staff in a setting where such documentation is being used was highlighted by Ellershaw and Wilkinson (2003)

Table 4 Doloplus2-scale (http://prc.coh.org/PainNOA/Doloplus%202_Tool.pdf)

DOLOPLUS-2 SCALE BEHAVIOURAL PAIN ASSESSMENT IN THE ELDERLY

NAME : Christian Name : Unit :

Behavioural Records

		DATES			
SOMATIC REACTIONS					
1• Somatic complaints	• no complaints	0	0	0	0
	• complaints expressed upon inquiry only	1	1	1	1
	• occasionnal involuntary complaints	2	2	2	2
	• continuous involontary complaints	3	3	3	3
2• Protective body postures adopted at rest	• no protective body posture	0	0	0	0
	• the patient occasionally avoids certain positions.	1	1	1	1
	• protective postures continuously and effectively sought.	2	2	2	2
	• protective postures continuously sought, without success.	3	3	3	3
3• Protection of sore areas	• no protective action taken	0	0	0	0
	• protective actions attempted without interfering against any investigation or nursing	1	1	1	1
	• protective actions against any investigation or nursing	2	2	2	2
	• protective actions taken at rest, even when not approached	3	3	3	3
4• Expression	• usual expression	0	0	0	0
	• expression showing pain when approached	1	1	1	1
	• expression showing pain even without being approached	2	2	2	2
	• permanent and unusually blank look (voiceless, staring, looking blank)	3	3	3	3
5• Sleep pattern	• normal sleep	0	0	0	0
	• difficult to go to sleep	1	1	1	1
	• frequent waking (restlessness)	2	2	2	2
	• insomnia affecting waking times.	3	3	3	3
PSYCHOMOTOR REACTIONS					
6• washing &/or dressing	• usual abilities unaffected	0	0	0	0
	• usual abilities slightly affected (careful but thorough)	1	1	1	1
	• usual abilities highly impaired, washing &/or dressing is laborious and incomplete	2	2	2	2
	• washing &/or dressing rendered impossible as the patient resists any attempt	3	3	3	3
7• Mobility	• usual abilities & activities remain unaffected	0	0	0	0
	• usual activities are reduced (the patient avoids certain movements and reduces his/her walking distance	1	1	1	1
	• usual activities and abilities reduced (even with help,the patient cuts down on his/her movements)	2	2	2	2
	• any movement is impossible, the patient resists all persuasion	3	3	3	3
PSYCHOSOCIAL REACTIONS					
8• Communication	• unchanged	0	0	0	0
	• heightened (the patient demands attention in an unusual manner)	1	1	1	1
	• lessened (the patient cuts him/herself off)	2	2	2	2
	• absence or refusal of any from of communication	3	3	3	3
9• Social life	• participates normally in every activity (meals, entertainment, therapy workshop)	0	0	0	0
	• participates in activities when asked to do so only	1	1	1	1
	• sometimes refuses to participate in any activity	2	2	2	2
	• refuses to participate in anything	3	3	3	3
10• Problems of behaviour	• normal behaviour	0	0	0	0
	• problems of repetitive reactive behaviour	1	1	1	1
	• problems of permanent reactive bahaviour	2	2	2	2
	• permanent behaviour problems (without any external stimulus)	3	3	3	3
	SCORE				

COPYRIGHT

in their original book and has underpinned the work of Coleman et al. (2017). The individual care home setting has managed to be more rigorous in achieving such training than in the acute hospital setting with the myriad of staff to be taught. Training should include the use of a "case scenario" alongside the documentation so that training isn't being taught via a PowerPoint presentation in isolation of real-life situations. It is important to note that any care given is only as good as the person giving the care, and while "using the IPP does not in itself assure quality of care, the use of such a plan can provide homes with evidence that their care is consistent" (Coleman et al. 2017, p. 41).

5.1.5 Valuing and Supporting Staff Support After Death: Reflective Debriefing Sessions – UK

For many young untrained staff, talking about and caring for people who are dying are frightening and the powerful triggers to any of their own unresolved grief (Holman et al. 2011). With the increasing number of frail older people dying in LTCFs, meaningful support through reflective debriefing sessions has been found to be helpful (Hockley 2014).

Staff often become very close to residents – especially if the resident has been in the LTCF for a number of months or even years. Reflecting on the death in a structured way is a useful support for staff and an innovative way of learning from practice – a tool has been developed (Hockley 2014). The aim of a reflective debriefing sessions is:

- To use the experience of caring for a resident who has died as a basis for learning about end-of-life care
- To be a place where "death and dying" can be safely and openly discussed and where support can be actively shown
- To construct knowledge about end-of-life care of frail older people dying in LTCFs in order to develop a palliative care culture in these settings
- To increase team cohesion between different shifts and across different roles that include not only nurses and carers but different ancillary staff who have known the resident and/or family

Sessions are held monthly with an emphasis on a "no blame" culture. The deaths of residents who have died during the previous weeks are formerly discussed. Such a session lasts about 45 min (a maximum of an hour). If there is no death during the month, then these sessions can be used for informal teaching on any subject that the LTCF manager thinks will be helpful. The essential point is for the sessions to be planned in the diary at a specific point each month of the year so it becomes routine practice and not just something that might happen if there is a significantly bad death. It is important that the LTCF manager be present wherever possible at the reflective debriefing sessions.

The outline of a session is as follows:

- For someone within the group to give a short portrait (no more than a couple of minutes) of the person who has died and the knowledge they had of the family
- What led up to the death – was it sudden or anticipated, etc.
- How did staff fell things went – What went well? What didn't go so well?
- What could have been done differently?
- What needs to change in the LTCF as a result of the reflection?

Each reflection can inform practice and should be used not only as a building block to learning but as a celebration of good practice. Reflection is not a passive contemplation but an active, deliberate process that requires commitment, energy, and a willingness to learn as a team.

5.2 Tools Incorporating Whole System Change to Create a Palliative Care Approach

Not surprisingly, the "individual initiatives" that have been highlighted above do in time promote a palliative care culture to emerge. However, there are initiatives that champion a "whole system" development in one project. Establishing a system which addresses a number of different aspects of palliative/end-of-life care alongside an educational initiative is probably one of the most effective ways to encourage a greater palliative care approach in LTCFs. However, it is sustaining such initiatives that is of vital importance and will be discussed in Sect. 6.

5.2.1 The Gold Standards Framework for Care Homes: UK/Europe

The most notable whole system change in relation to palliative care/care homes in the UK has been the Gold Standards Framework in Care Homes (GSFCH) (http://www.goldstandardsframework.org.uk/care-homes-training-programme). Professor Keri Thomas, founder of the GSF program, saw the need in the early 2000s for better collaboration and communication in relation to palliative and end-of-life care in the community (Thomas 2003), furthered the vision to encompass a program for care homes (GSFCH) (Badger et al. 2009; Thomas 2016).

The GSFCH program is a 2-year accredited program divided into three parts: a *preparatory phase, an implementation phase, and a consolidation phase*. The *preparatory phase (6 months)* is extremely important phase encouraging not only the staff, residents, and families to take part but also the local GP/s and specialist palliative care team/s external to the care home.

Care homes from a regional area are encouraged to sign up for the course and as part of the payment will be given all the documentation/folders/videos, etc. Each care home manager appoints GSFCH "champions" who will attend 4 training days during the *implementation period (9–12 months)* and be responsible for disseminating the information to the rest of the care home staff in between each of the 4 days. The number of "champions" is never less than two and will vary depending on the size of the care home. The *consolidation period (6 months)* helps care home staff to work on aspects that they are unsure about and at the same time prepare a portfolio for accreditation. An "after-death analysis" audit is undertaken on a number of residents' deaths before commencing the course and compared to those during/after the completion of the GSFCH program.

The GSFCH provides care home organizations with a number of key aspects of documentation in relation to advance care planning "Thinking Ahead"; prognostic indicator guide; the monthly multidisciplinary supportive care register; the PACA, a summary of resident and carer needs and concerns; the PEPSI COLA Aide Memoire, an holistic assessment tool; and significant event analysis that is completed following a death and helps staff reflect and feel supported.

In 2008, St Christopher's Hospice developed a Care Home Project Team to "reach out" to local care homes (http://www.stchristophers.org.uk/education/training-and-research/care-homes/). It became the first GSFCH regional center in the UK and over a 5-year period reached out to all the 71 care homes with on-site nurses in the area, encouraging them to take part. By the end of 5 years, the percentage of care home residents dying in hospital had reduced from 44% to 22% (Hockley and Kinley 2016).

As a result of GSFCH program, the UK National Health Service developed documentation "Route to Success" to encourage local regions to develop the palliative care needs of their residents in care homes (http://www.nwcscnsenate.nhs.uk/files/7714/3040/1087/Route_To_Success_Care_Homes_updated_Apr2015.pdf?PDFPATHWAY=PDF/). Different localities then developed different tools such as the "Six Steps to Success" and "Steps to Success" programs. While making it locally relevant, some programs have lacked resources when it comes to accreditation, ongoing support, and sustainability.

5.2.2 The PACE Program: Europe

The PACE program (www.eupace.eu) is a randomized controlled trial looking at whole system change in the adoption of a palliative care approach in LTCFs across six European countries (Van den Block et al. 2016; Smets et al. 2018). The PACE program was developed following a number of quality improvement initiatives in care homes and is framed around six steps: advance care planning, mapping changes in a resident's condition, monthly multidisciplinary meetings, pain and symptom assessment, care in the last days of life, and reflective debriefing sessions for staff following a death. The intervention is complete, and outcomes from the PACE program are awaited.

5.2.3 Palliative Approach Toolkit for Residential Aged Care Facilities: Australia

Deborah Parker and colleagues from Blue Care Research and Development Unit and the University of Queensland developed the "Palliative Approach Toolkit for Residential Aged Care Facilities" – an evidence-based knowledge translation product for staff in aged care facilities in Australia (https://www.caresearch.com.au/caresearch/tabid/3629/Default.aspx). The Toolkit is a set of clinical care, educational and management resources, and a "comprehensive 'how to' guide featuring a step by step approach to implementing a new model of palliative care. It includes policies and procedures, education and training for staff" (Parker 2013). The success of the project was realized when the Australian Government Department of Health funded a national rollout of the Toolkit under the Encouraging Better Practice in Aged Care (EBPAC) initiative between October 2013 and December 2014 (https://www.caresearch.com.au/Caresearch/Portals/0/PA-Tookit/Training%20Support%20Materials/PowerPoint%20Presentation.pdf).

5.2.4 Namaste Care Program: Improving the Quality of Life for Residents with Advanced Dementia: USA and UK

The Namaste Care program was developed by Joyce Simard in the early 2000s in the USA (Simard 2013). Joyce had worked as a social worker in LTCFs and was interested in the importance of meaningful activity to improve the quality of life for people with advanced dementia. She had set up innovative meaningful activity for those with mild to moderate dementia ("The Club") but noticed that many people with advanced dementia just sat on the edges of such activity with little engagements or otherwise didn't attend, remaining alone in their bedrooms.

Namaste is an Indian greeting which means "to honor the spirit within." Namaste Care is a multidimensional program that includes physical, sensory, and emotional elements. The purpose of Namaste is to give comfort and pleasure to people with advanced dementia through sensory stimulation, especially the use of touch. It aims to restructure the care for people with advanced dementia who are often immobile/confined to a wheelchair and incontinent failing in their speech.

Namaste runs for 2-h in the morning and 2-h in the afternoon, 7 days a week, and aims to increase engagement through the five senses (hearing, sight, touch, taste, and smell). It requires no additional staffing. The Namaste Care worker assigned to run the program for that day will work with all those in the facility with advanced dementia as defined above. It is likely that there will be 6–8 such residents within a facility of 60 people. Once they have been helped with breakfast, instead of remaining in their room, these residents are brought to the Namaste Care "space" (whether an adapted dining area or a dedicated space). Here they will be greeted by name, made very welcome and checked for discomfort and pain. The Namaste Care worker will engage with each as appropriate during the next 2 h – doing a hand massage, helping with a drink, combing a resident's hair, applying cream to the face, giving a footbath, and offering cut-up fruit and tasty titbits.

When it is felt a resident would benefit from being part of program, a family meeting is held to understand from them things that will bring pleasure and trigger memories for their family member. This meeting is also an opportunity to acknowledge the resident's deterioration from dementia in the positive context of offering more appropriate care. Finally, the meeting is an opportunity to establish the overarching goal of a peaceful, dignified death in familiar surroundings in the care home.

Namaste Care has now been implemented in LTCFs in a number of countries including the USA, Japan, Australia, and the UK. A toolkit is freely available from the St Christopher's Hospice website (http://www.stchristophers.org.uk/education/resources). There are several core elements of the program (see Table 5).

A recent study evaluating Namaste Care in six care homes found that, where there is strong

Table 5 Core elements of the Namaste Care program (Stacpoole et al. 2016)

1	"Honoring the spirit within"	The guiding principle of Namaste Care is a respectful and compassionate approach to individuals with advanced dementia
2	The presence of others	Namaste residents are brought together as a social group with a dedicated Namaste Care worker, so each resident feels "included" in their community
3	Comfort and pain management	Comfortable seating and pain assessment/management are the essential first step toward enabling Namaste residents to relax, engage, and express how they feel
4	Sensory stimulation	The program incorporates stimulation of the five senses (touch, hearing, sight, smell, taste). Music, color, therapeutic touch and massage, aromatherapy oils, and food treats are all part of the multisensory environment created in the Namaste room
5	Meaningful activity	In Namaste, personal care is provided as a meaningful activity, even though the Namaste residents will usually have had their morning wash. The focus is on pleasure rather than personal hygiene. Hands and face are gently washed with a warm flannel and patted dry with a soft towel. Moisturizing creams are applied, and the Namaste Care worker uses this opportunity to make eye contact and talk affirmatively with the resident. Hand and face washing is part of everyone's life experience and usually results in a sense of well-being. The Namaste Care worker will explore individual wishes and preferences and adapt activities to meet people's needs
6	Life story	Knowledge of the resident's life story is key to adapting the program of activities and interventions so that they are meaningful for each person
7	Food treats and hydration	The Namaste Care worker offers drinks and food throughout the session (being mindful of any swallowing difficulties). This creates extra opportunities to improve hydration and nutrition and contribute to the residents' health and well-being
8	Care worker education	Care workers involved in Namaste require education about dementia and all aspects of the care program. The care workers need support to feel confident
9	Family meetings	Holding a family meeting when a resident is going to start the Namaste Care program creates a further bond between the family/friends and the care staff, opening up the conversation about end-of-life care. Families are encouraged to take part in the Namaste sessions when they visit
10	Care of the dying and after-death care	The care that residents enjoy in the Namaste Care program can be transferred to the bedroom when the person is unwell and when they are dying
11	After-death reflection	Dedicating time to remembering a resident after their death supports the care staff emotionally. Reflecting on what went well, and any difficulties, provides an opportunity for care staff to learn from the experience and improve the care they give to residents when they are dying

leadership, adequate staffing, and good nursing and medical care, the Namaste Care program can improve quality of life for people with advanced dementia in care homes by decreasing behavioral symptoms (Stacpoole et al. 2015).

Implementing such a program actively demonstrates a person-centered relationship-based holistic culture for people with advanced dementia. Those with advanced dementia are not isolated but included in a program that is set to bring them enjoyment through the senses focusing on the palliative care needs including pain and agitation in the end stages of dementia. The Namaste Care worker reports any distress and lack of engagement of those at a session – people cannot engage if they are uncomfortable. The beneficial effect of Namaste Care on the family and staff has also been shown to be significant (Stacpoole et al. 2017).

6 Components of Successful Implementation of Initiatives

Implementing quality improvement initiatives is an interplay of three elements (Kitson et al. 1998, 2008):

- The "context" where the development is to take place (McCormack et al. 2002)

- The quality of the "evidence" that backs up what is being implemented (Rycroft-Malone et al. 2004)
- The level of "facilitation" required based on the "context" and "evidence" (Harvey et al. 2002)

For each of the above elements, different "situations" prevail (Kitson et al. 1998) which makes the element "not so effective" ("low") or "very effective" ("high"). In their model, Kitson and colleagues suggest that for successful implementation of a quality improvement initiative, there has to be a minimum of two "highs" associated with the three elements. For example, in the *context* of many LTCFs, there is no on-site multidisciplinary team, the majority of staff have little healthcare education, and many lack a learning culture. It can therefore be deduced that many LTCFs have a "low" *context* and any LTCF quality improvement initiative therefore needs to have a "high" evidence base + "high" facilitation.

The importance of understanding the multidimensional aspects of implementing quality improvement initiatives in LTCFs cannot be emphasized enough. A recent quality improvement initiative implementing the GSFCH framework ("high" evidence) using "high" facilitation showed four times the number of LTCFs gaining GSFCH accreditation compared to normal facilitation (Kinley et al. 2014b).

The importance of how an initiative is facilitated is often vital to its success. Just giving a LTCF a certain toolkit with little information on how to implement the change will be likely to fail. Where there is no effective facilitation, then any outcome will rely heavily on the care facility ability to "take hold" of the project and its ability to implement it.

Facilitation of 'whole system change' tools discussed in the previous section (such as GSFCH, PACE, Namaste) when supported well by specialist palliative care can be extremely beneficial – not only do colleagues in specialist palliative care increase their understanding of the chronic illness trajectory of frail older people in LTCFs, but such collaboration enables LTCFs to be connected and supported while they develop their own palliative care approach.

6.1 Sustainability When Undertaking Quality Improvement

Evaluations of many quality improvement initiatives in LTCFs have been encouraging. However, the importance of sustaining what has been implemented cannot be emphasized enough especially in light of the current high turnover of staff in LTCFs.

Whether it is just a simple tool or whole systems change, the importance of building in some sustainability initiative into the wider project is extremely important. Sustainability is not without cost but sustainability can be cost effective. Many initiatives, even when LTCF staff and management are keen to develop a palliative care approach, can fail because of lack of sustainability and support of the LTCF once the project is over. This raises a debate about the value of funding short-term initiatives/projects without a long-term vision (Hockley and Kinley 2016).

Little evidence exists regarding sustaining interventions in practice in LTCFs, but where these organizations have contributed financially toward to a sustainability initiative once the implementation has been completed, it has continued to empower, support, and develop staff (Kinley et al. 2017).

7 Future Issues and the Need for Innovation

By 2050 there will be more people in the world over the age of 60 than under the age of 15 years old (UNFPA 2012). It is important to start thinking differently about LTCFs if we are to improve the palliative care needs of frail older people. It is vital that LTCFs are seen as places where frail older people can live out the remaining months/year/s in the knowledge that their end can be in the place where they have got to know and trust the staff.

Increasingly, LTCFs are innovating how they care; whether it is developing a more homely atmosphere for frail older people with advanced dementia (http://hogeweyk.dementiavillage.com/en/) or encouraging greater emphasis on student involvement and training in order to attract and retain staff (Kirkvold 2008).

Further innovation in relation to palliative care and LTCFs involves technology. Countries, especially those with large rural areas, have developed videoteleconferencing technology (VTC) to support the palliative care needs of LTCF residents' alongside staff training. The need to evaluate such services is important.

Finally, here in Scotland, development is underway to build a teaching/research-based care centre (The Vision for a Teaching/Research-based Care Centre). Based on the "hospice model" of holistic person-centered relationship-based care for people with advanced progressive incurable diseases, it will provide a centre of clinical excellence alongside being a resource for training and coordination of research across the region. With the majority of frail older people requiring 24-h care having a diagnosed dementia or severe cognitive impairment, the emphasis will be on advanced dementia with plans to innovate in relation to proactive respite care and support of families.

It would appear that developing palliative care in LTCFs is now very much on the political agenda. There is a danger however that LTCFs become overwhelmed by all the different education courses, quality improvement initiatives, and research. It is important for there to be a coordinated approach to work with LTCFs in a locality so that they are not inundated with different projects but that a "homely" atmosphere be maintained.

8 Conclusion

William Osler's quote "pneumonia is the old man's friend" was written prior to the considerable developments that have occurred in medicine over the last 70 years within which time geriatrics/gerontology and palliative care have both created their own specialties. The coming together of these specialties in the care of frail older people in residential care facilities is a vital area requiring expansion while recognizing Osler's wise words.

Mutual learning between those passionate with the care of frail older people in residential care settings and those experienced in the palliative care needs of people facing the end of life, while bearing in mind not to impose what has been learned from a cancer "model of palliative care" onto residential care settings, will bring remarkable elegance to the care of frail older people.

This chapter has described a number of initiatives – "stand-alone" as well as "whole system" change initiatives. The emphasis must be on sustainability of such initiatives and the support of staff in residential care settings. An important "white paper" details the areas for practice development and research for people with advanced dementia being cared for in residential care settings. This alone if acted upon will break the isolation that staff caring for the 24-h needs of frail older people often feel.

Competent multidisciplinary working to support the palliative care needs of people in residential care settings will not only reduce inappropriate hospital admissions but is likely to enhance staff support, reduce turnover, respect what really matters to frail older people and their wishes at the end of life, and improve their quality of death.

References

Abbey JA, Piller N, DeBellis A, Esterman A, Parker D, Giles L, Lowcay B. The Abbey pain scale. A 1-minute numerical indicator for people with late-stage dementia. Int J Palliat Nurs. 2004;10(1):6–13.

Alzheimer's Society. Low expectations. Attitudes on choice, care and community for people with dementia in care homes. 2013. Available at https://www.alzheimers.org.uk/download/downloads/id/1705_alzheimers_society_low_expectations_executive_summary.pdf. Accessed 7 July 2017.

Baar F. Palliative care for the terminally ill in the Netherlands: the unique role of the nursing homes. Eur J Palliat Care. 1999;6(5):169–72.

Baar F, van der Kloot Meijburg H. The role of the physician in nursing home care in The Netherlands. In: Hockley J, Clark D, editors. Palliative care for older people in care homes. Buckingham: Open University Press; 2002. p. 104–19.

Badger F, Clifford C, Hewison A, Thomas K. An evaluation of the implementation of a programme to improve end of life care in nursing homes. Palliat Med. 2009;23:502.

Coleman J, Levy J, Wiggins S, Kinley J. Using a new end-of-life care plan in nursing homes. Nurs Resid Care. 2017;19(1):38–41.

Ellershaw J, Wilkinson S. Care of the dying: a pathway to excellence. Oxford: Oxford University Press; 2003.

Froggatt K. Palliative care and nursing homes: where next? Palliat Med. 2001;15(1):42–8.

Froggatt K, Payne S, Morbey H, Edwards M, Finne-Soveri H, Gambassi G, Pasman RH, Szczerbińska K, Van Den Block L, on behalf of PACE. Palliative care development in European care homes and nursing homes: application of a typology of implementation. JAMDA. 2017a. https://doi.org/10.1016/j.jamda.2017.02.016. Published online: April 13, 2017. Accessed 13 June 2017.

Froggatt K, Arrue B, Edwards M, Finne-Soveri H, Morbey H, Payne S, Szczerbinska K, van den Noortgate, N, van den Block L. Palliative care systems and current practices in long term care facilities in Europe. 2017b. Available from http://www.eapcnet.eu/Portals/0/Policy/EU%20sup_proj_/PACE/EAPC_PACE_WP1_Deliverable_January_26_2017_final_amended%20typos.pdf. Accessed 5 May 2017.

Fuchs-Lacelle S, Hadjistavropoulos T. Development and preliminary validation of the pain assessment checklist for seniors with limited ability to communicate (PACSLAC). Pain Manag Nurs. 2004;5(2):37–49.

Gilissen J, Pivodic L, Smets T, Gastmans C, Stichele RV, Deliens L, Van den Block L. Preconditions for successful advance care planning in nursing homes: a systematic review. Int J Nurs Stud. 2017;66:47–59.

Grignon M, Bernier NF. Financing long-term care in Canada. Montreal: Institute for Research on Public Policy; 2012. http://irpp.org/research-studies/study-no33/. Accessed 5 July 2017.

Handley M, Goodman C, Froggatt K, Mathie E, Manthorpe J, Barclay S, Crnag C, Iliffe S. Living and dying: responsibility for end-of-life care in care homes without on-site nursing provision – a prospective study. Health Soc Care Community. 2014;22(1):22–9.

Harvey G, Loftus-Hills A, Rycroft-Malone J, Titchen A, Kitson A, McCormack B, Seers K. Getting evidence into practice: the role of function of facilitation. J Adv Nurs. 2002;37(6):577–88.

Hockley J. Organizational structures for enhancing standards of palliative care. In: Hockley J, Clark D, editors. Palliative Care for Older People in Care Homes. p165–181. Open University Press: Buckingham; 2002.

Hockley J. Learning, support and communication for staff in care homes: outcomes of reflective debriefing groups in two care homes to enhance end-of-life care. Int J Older People Nurs. 2014;9(2):118–30.

Hockley J, Kinley J. A practice development initiative supporting care home staff deliver high quality end-of-life care. Int J Palliat Nurs. 2016;22(10):474–81.

Hockley J, Dewar B, Watson J. Promoting end-of-life care in nursing homes using an 'integrated care pathway for the last days of life'. J Res Nurs. 2005; 10(2):135–52.

Holman D, Sawkins N, Hockley J. Experience of use of advance care planning in care homes. In: Thomas K, Lobo B, editors. Advance care planning in end of life care. Oxford: Oxford University Press; 2011.

Husebo BS, Wilco P, Achterberg WP, Lobbezoo F, Kunz M, Lautenbacher S, Kappesser J, Tudose C, Strand LI. Pain in patients with dementia: a review of pain assessment and treatment challenges. Nor Epidemiol. 2012;22(2):243–51.

IAHPC. Definition of palliative care. International Association of Hospice and Palliative Care Manual on Palliative Care; 2017. https://hospicecare.com/resources/publications/getting-started/5-what-is-palliative-care. Accessed 17 June 2017, Houston, Texas: USA.

Jagger C, Collerton JC, Davies K, Kingston A, Robinson L, Eccles MP, von Zglinicki T, Martin-Ruiz C, James OF, Kirkwood TB, Bond J. Capability and dependency in the Newcastle 85+ cohort study: projections of future care needs. BMC Geriatr. 2011;11:21. https://bmcgeriatr.biomedcentral.com/articles/10.1186/1471-2318-11-21. Last Accessed 17 June 2017.

Jones R. Choosing wisely for frail residents of long-term care homes: six recommendations. BCMJ. 2017; 59(6):300–1. http://www.bcmj.org/council-health-promotion/choosing-wisely-frail-residents-long-term-care-homes-six-recommendations

Kinley J, Hockley J, Stone L, Dewey M, Hansford P, Stewart R, McCrone P, Behum A, Sykes N. The provision of care for residents dying in UK nursing care homes. Age Ageing. 2014a;43:375–9.

Kinley J, Stone L, Dewey M, Levy J, Stewart R, McCrone P, Sykes N, Hansford P, Begum A, Hockley J. The effect of using high facilitation when implementing the Gold Standards Framework in Care Homes programme: a cluster randomised controlled trial. Palliat Med. 2014b;28(9):1099–109.

Kinley J, Stone L, Butt A, Kenyon B, Santos Lopes N. Developing, implementing and sustaining an end-of-life care programme in residential care homes. Int J Palliat Nurs. 2017;23(4):186–93.

Kirkvold M. The Norwegian teaching home program: developing a model for systematic practice development in the nursing home sector. Int J Older People Nurs. 2008;3:282–6.

Kitson A, Harvey G, McCormack B. Enabling the implementation of evidence based practice: a conceptual framework. Qual Health Care. 1998;7:149–58.

Kitson A, Rycroft-Malone J, Harvey G, McCormack B, Seers K, Titchen A. Evaluating the successful implementation of evidence into practice using the PARiHS framework: theoretical and practical challenges. Implement Sci. 2008;3:1. https://implementationscience.biomedcentral.com/articles/10.1186/1748-5908-3-1. Last Accessed 1 July 2017.

Lefebvre-Chapiro S, the Doloplus Group. The Doloplus-2 scale – evaluating pain in the elderly. Eur J Palliat Care. 2001;8:191–4.

Lichtner V, Dowding D, Esterhuizen P, Closs J, Long AF, Corbett A, Briggs M. Pain assessment for people with dementia: a systematic review of systematic reviews of pain assessment tools. BMC Geriatr. 2014;14:138. https://bmcgeriatr.biomedcentral.com/articles/10.1186/1471-2318-14-138. Last Accessed 17 June 2017.

Lynn J, Adamson DM. Living well at the end of life. Adapting healthcare to serious chronic illness in old age. Washington, DC: Rand Health; 2003.

McCormack B, Kitson A, Harvey G, Rycroft-Malone J, Titchen A, Seers K. Getting evidence into practice: the meaning of 'context'. J Adv Nurs. 2002;38(1):94–104.

Mount B. First international conference on palliative care of the elderly. In: Hockley J, Clark D, editors. Palliative care for older people in care homes. Buckingham: Open University Press; 1989. p. 166. 2002.

ONS. National population projections: 2014-based statistical bulletin. London: UK: Office of National Statistics; 2014. https://www.ons.gov.uk/peoplepopulationandcommunity/populationandmigration/populationprojections/bulletins/nationalpopulationprojections/2015-10-29

Parker D. National rollout of the palliative approach toolkit for residential aged care facilities supporting residential aged care facility management and staff to deliver high quality palliative care for residents. 2013. Available from https://www.caresearch.com.au/Caresearch/portals/0/documents/whatispalliativecare/pa-toolkit/1-pa_toolkit_brochure-dl_websafe.pdf. Accessed 11 June 2017.

Rycroft-Malone J, Seers K, Titchen A, Harvey G, Kitson A, McCormack B. What counts as evidence in evidence-based practice? J Adv Nurs. 2004;47(1):81–90.

Simard J. The end-of-life Namaste care program for people with dementia. 2nd ed. Baltimore: Health Professions Press; 2013.

Smets T, Onwuteaka-Philipsen B, Miranda R, Pivodic L, Tanghe M et al. Integrating palliative care in long-term care facilities across Europe (PAC): protocol of a cluster randomized controlled trial of the 'PACE Steps to Success' intervention in seven countries. BMC Palliative Care. 2018;17(47). Open Access https://doi.org/10.1186/s12904-018-0297-1.

Stacpoole M, Hockley J, Thompsell A, Simard J, Volicer L. The Namaste care programme can reduce behavioural symptoms in care home residents with advanced dementia. Int J Geriatr Psychopharmacol. 2015;7:702–9.

Stacpoole M, Thompsell A, Hockley J. Toolkit for implementing the Namaste care programme for people with advanced dementia living in care homes. 2016. Available from http://www.stchristophers.org.uk/wp-content/uploads/2016/03/Namaste-Care-Programme-Toolkit-06.04.2016.pdf. Accessed 13 June 2017.

Stacpoole M, Hockley J, Thompsell M, Simard J, Volicer L. Implementing the Namaste Care Programme for residents with advanced dementia: exploring the perceptions of family and staff in UK care homes. Ann Palliat Med. 2017;6(4):327–339.

Stone L, Kinley J, Hockley J. Advance care planning in care homes: the experience of staff, residents and family members. Int J Palliat Nurs. 2013;19(11):550–557.

Thomas K. Caring for the dying at home: companions on the journey. Oxford: Radcliffe Publishing; 2003.

Thomas K. The GSF prognostic indicator. The Gold Standards Framework Centre in End of Life Care CIC. UK: The Royal College of General Practitioners; 2011. http://www.goldstandardsframework.org.uk/cd-content/uploads/files/General%20Files/Prognostic%20Indicator%20Guidance%20October%202011.pdf. Accessed 24 June 2017.

Thomas K. Summary of evidence: Gold Standards Framework in Care Homes (GSFCH) training programme. 2016. Available from http://www.goldstandardsframework.org.uk/cd-content/uploads/files/GSF%20Care%20Home%20Evidence%20Summary%20Updated%20Oct%202016%20MSR%281%29.pdf. Accessed 11 June 2017.

Torvik K, Kaasa S, Kirkevold O, Saltvedt I, Holen J, Fayers P, Rustoen T. Validation of Doloplus-2 among nonverbal nursing home patients – an evaluation of Doloplus-2 in a clinical setting. BMC Geriatr. 2010;10(9). https://doi.org/10.1186/1471-2318-10-9. Accessed 17 June 2017.

UNFPA. Ageing in the twenty-first century: a celebration and a challenge. New York: United Nations Population Fund; 2012. http://www.unfpa.org/sites/default/files/pub-pdf/Ageing%20report.pdf. Accessed 17 June 2017.

van den Block L, Smets T, van Dop N, Adang E, Andreasen P, Collingridge Moore D, Engels Y, Finne-Soveri H. Comparing palliative care in care homes across Europe (PACE): protocol of a cross-sectional study of deceased residents in 6 EU countries. JAMA. 2016;17(6):566. https://doi.org/10.1016/j.jamda.2016.03.008. Accessed 7 July 2017.

Van der Steen J, Radbruch L, Hertogh C, de Boer ME, Hughes J, Larkin P, Franke AL, Junger S, Gove D, Firth P, Koopmans R, Volicer L, on behalf of the EAPC. White paper defining optimal palliative care in older people with dementia: a Delphi study and recommendations from the European Association for Palliative Care. Palliat Med. 2014;28(3):197–209.

Warden V, Hurley AC, Volicer L. Development and psychometric evaluation of the Pain Assessment in Advanced Dementia (PAINAD) Scale. J Am Med Dir. 2003;4:9–15.

Watson J, Hockley J, Dewar B. Barriers to implementing an integrated care pathway for the last days of life in nursing homes. Int J Palliat Nurs. 2006;12(15):234–240.

Watson J. Developing the senses framework to support relationship-centred care for people with advanced dementia until the end of life in care homes. Dementia. 2016; December 6. https://doi.org/10.1177/1471301216682880.

Worcester A. The care of the aged, the dying and the dead. 2nd ed. Springfield: Charles C Thomas; 1935.

Hospital Care

52

Kate Grundy and Willem Vink

Contents

K. Grundy (✉) · W. Vink
Christchurch Hospital Palliative Care Service,
Christchurch, New Zealand
e-mail: kate.grundy@cdhb.health.nz; willem.vink@cdhb.health.nz

R. D. MacLeod, L. Van den Block (eds.), *Textbook of Palliative Care*,
https://doi.org/10.1007/978-3-319-77740-5_50

Abstract
Hospitals are where we find the most seriously ill people in our society. Patients go there to receive lifesaving and life-prolonging treatment, but they are also where many will deteriorate and die. Care for these people and their families is therefore core business for hospitals, and this is being increasingly recognized internationally. Hospitals are also facing the challenge of how best to meet the needs of a population that is becoming ever older and frailer. When in an acute care facility, patients with advanced disease require palliative care in its broadest sense, and when their needs are complex, they deserve reliable and timely access to specialist support.

This chapter will look at the provision of palliative care in the acute setting, from the perspective of a dedicated team, working in a small provincial city in the South Island of New Zealand. It will explore how this service has developed and how it operates and thrives within its unique healthcare setting. A broad range of challenges and opportunities are discussed as well as issues such as information technology, team sustainability, and education provision. Ultimately the aim is to promote a culture change in health that promotes universal access to holistic care at the end of life.

1 Introduction

Specialist palliative care is well recognized internationally as a core component of health service delivery. People with palliative care needs often move from one care setting to another, and the skills and expertise that are provided and supported by those with specialist training need to be readily available. The ideal system is supported and configured to ensure that quality and compassionate care at the end of life is available in a timely way to everyone who needs it, wherever they are located.

The reality is however that in the minds of many (including healthcare professionals, administrators, and funders), palliative care is what happens in hospices and in people's homes, not in acute hospitals. It is often assumed that palliative care is delivered only by nurses who have a calling to provide an alternative option for care when death is inevitable. Grateful and generous communities donate money and provide time as volunteers to supplement government funding. It is viewed as separate and different to the multidisciplinary, quality-driven, holistic, and supportive services that are needed across the wider health system, including in hospitals.

Hospitals are where people who are living with and ultimately dying from chronic progressive illnesses and conditions seek treatment for (usually) short periods during an acute episode or exacerbation (Clark et al. 2014). This is certainly the case in New Zealand, as it is in many other developed countries. Community care has expanded and developed to encompass those who are very unwell and disabled and many acute problems are able to be managed very comprehensively without admission. However, hospitals are where people often look to in times of crisis, and staff should be able to recognize when a person is at risk of dying and respond accordingly. This is achieved best when their department or service recognizes the importance of this issue and is configured appropriately with access to all the necessary resources, policies, and guidelines.

Expectations vary as to what hospitals can provide, but most patients will be hoping that treatment will work and that they will be returned to health. Supporting this belief are the ever-expanding array of specialties and subspecialties which flourish as medicine evolves and more treatment options become available. Hospitals are often where it becomes apparent that cure is not possible, that the person's future is far from certain, and that the priority now is the relief of suffering.

Hospitals are also where a large proportion of our population die. In the period 2000–2013 in New Zealand, 33.9% of all deaths occurred in publicly funded hospitals. This figure is closer to

50% for Australian hospitals (Ireland 2017). The majority of these deaths are able to be anticipated given the progressive nature of the person's medical condition or conditions.

Studies conducted in Australia, the UK, and Belgium have concluded that at any one time, 13–36% of hospital inpatients meet the criteria for palliative care need. A New Zealand estimate from 2013 using the Gold Standards Framework criteria is entirely consistent at 19.8% (Gott et al. 2013). The proportion of in-hospital deaths with a palliative care status identified in hospital databases (from that same Australian study) sits at 44% in 2013–2014 which is up from 37% in 2009–2010. Looking more broadly, it is apparent that the majority of deaths are preceded by a period of deterioration over weeks to months where there was the opportunity to instigate a palliative approach and involve specialist services if required. This issue was cited in a 2008 paper by Project Muse where it was stated that 75–80% of decedents have a dying process that typically occurs over a few weeks to many months (Wilson et al. 2008). Despite these statistics, many are still surprised that such a large proportion of the care provided in hospitals is for patients nearing the end of their lives. Such information should be used to inform end-of-life care policy in hospitals (Clark et al. 2016).

Acceptance of the need for a palliative philosophy in acute care is far from the norm. As far back as 2001, it was stated that "the hospital environment reflects the business of life in society, which still denies the naturalness and inevitability of death. The culture of practice in the acute care setting is inherently related to life supporting and life prolonging activities" (Middlewood et al. 2001). The inclusion of palliative care can be an uneasy fit, but it "has presented an alternative philosophy to guide the care for dying patients... there is a need to integrate palliative care services into the acute care setting to assist the transition of goals from investigative and treatment orientated care to improving quality of life" (Middlewood et al. 2001). This issue of integration has become one of the central functions of palliative care services and will be covered later.

2 Normalizing Death and Dying

The overriding focus for doctors continues to be on returning patients to health using the diagnostic and treatment skills in which they were trained. However, essential to ensuring that palliative care is both available and of high quality is the recognition that dying is inevitable for each and every patient and agreeing that expert and timely care should be delivered with compassion. When it is apparent that a patient is not responding to active treatment or they do not want life-prolonging measures, doctors "step onto the threshold" of a new place, the place of realizing that this person is not improving, not taking the normal path, and perhaps preparing for the end of life and/or even imminent death. Dying brings health professionals face to face with their own mortality. For most this is a frightening landscape. It can be a place of discomfort on many spheres, not just physical. Palliative care operates right on this threshold. Dying often brings everyone into a liminal space, uncharted territory. In hospitals enabling this acceptance to occur is particularly challenging.

The rapid pace of hospital diagnostics and treatments now needs a reduced pace and a slow and listening presence. Assessing where the discomfort is, helping patients and families navigate this landscape and all the uncertainty it brings. Uncovering where the fear lies and transitioning people to a place of understanding and hope, through confident care and management of symptoms, are the essence of the palliative care approach.

The wider nursing and multidisciplinary team in hospitals is strongly influenced by the medical paradigm. This medically oriented hierarchy within hospitals tends to give weight to the narrative set by doctors, and it can be hard for nurses or others to break into this with their own observations and assertions or to give voice to the person's unique concerns and priorities regarding their future care.

The acknowledgement of palliative care brings a fresh perspective to any acutely unwell patient's care. It makes available a different way of thinking particularly with regard to goals of treatment and the role of the carer and wider family/whānau. (**Whānau**: extended family, family group, or a familiar term of address to a number of people. In the modern context, the term is sometimes used to include friends who may not have any kinship ties to other members (Moorfield 2015) (ISBN 978-0-947491-36-9 (online)).). Hospital palliative care teams can assist with difficult decisions, weighing up the risks and burdens versus benefits of treatment options in real time. They can assist with the transition from active treatment to a palliative approach, uncovering what is most important to the person. This is the unique set of skills that those with specialist training in palliative care and palliative medicine bring to the acute care setting.

In New Zealand, five recurring themes regarding the provision of care to palliative patients in the acute setting have been identified. These are as follows: symptom control and burden, communication with health professionals, decision-making related to patient care and management, inadequate hospital environment, and interpersonal relationships with health professionals (Robinson et al. 2015). These are areas of care provision that can be deliberately addressed by hospital palliative care teams. Ideally, palliative care should be "at the table" when vulnerable patients are discussed. This may go some way to ensuring that a palliative approach is actively considered and that teams are reminded to glean the person's wishes in the light of any clinical concerns or worsening prognosis.

3 New Zealand Context

In New Zealand, hospitals are operated and funded by district health boards who are also responsible for delivering a full range of services in community settings. This is overseen by the New Zealand Ministry of Health (MOH) (Cumming et al. 2013). There is a strong imperative to provide a seamless care experience for consumers, and this is made more achievable given that there is no competition for patient numbers and no conflicting interests across care settings.

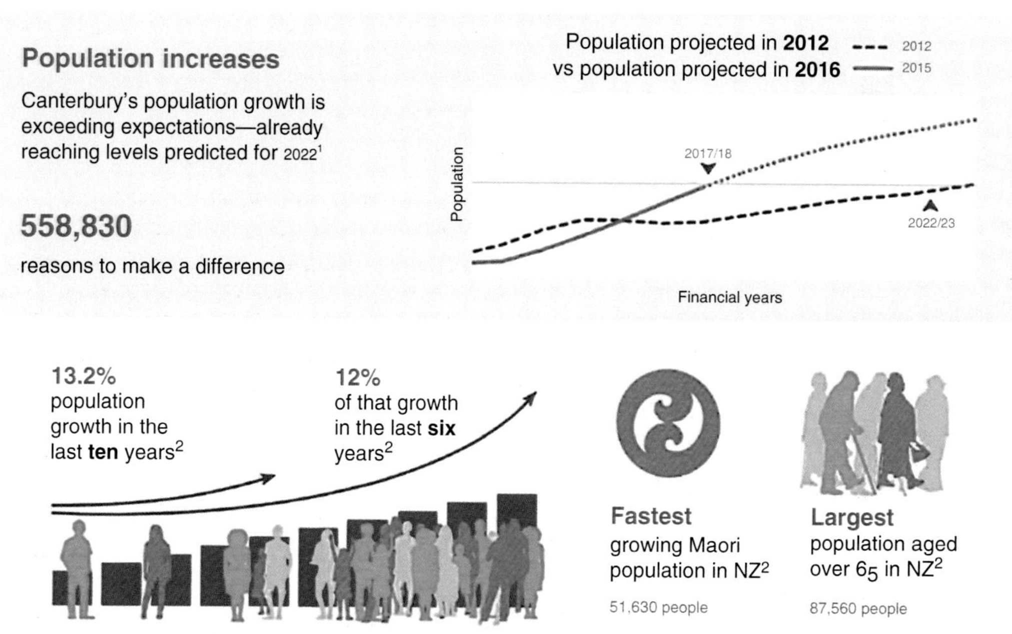

Fig. 1 Challenges of population growth in Canterbury

The insights detailed in this chapter are based on the experience of establishing a hospital palliative care service in Christchurch, Canterbury. Canterbury is located on the east coast of the South Island of New Zealand. The total population of NZ is 4.8 million. The Canterbury District Health Board (CDHB) encompasses one major population group with an overall population of 558,830. The following graphic is taken from the CDHB Annual Report 2016/2017 and illustrates current population challenges, including the high proportion of residents aged over the age of 65 years (http://www.cdhb.health.nz/About-CDHB/corporate-publications/Documents/Canterbury%20DHB%20Annual%20Report%20year%20ended%2030%20June%202017%20%28PDF%2C%202MB%29.pdf).

The Christchurch Hospital is a tertiary-level teaching hospital with approximately 650 beds. There is a second hospital in the north of the city with approximately 300 beds. The hospital palliative care team accepts referrals from both hospitals and consults on a regular basis. There is also a rural hospital with approximately 70 beds in Ashburton in the south of the region. There is a close relationship with the much smaller DHB on the West Coast (WCDHB) which has a highly dispersed mainly rural population of approximately 32,600. A large range of specialist services on the West Coast are provided by the CDHB, and some, including palliative care, are enhanced and supported by the CDHB through agreements and alliances.

Projections of the need for palliative care in all settings in New Zealand were published in 2016 (McLeod 2016). These are based on historic patterns from 2000 to 2013 and demonstrated that palliative care was needed for 73.5% of all deaths in public hospitals. Deaths in acute hospitals are often sudden and unexpected, but there are also a large number where the death can be anticipated and prepared for (Gott et al. 2013). It is anticipated that the South Island will experience an increase in total deaths of 44% over the period 2016–2038, as the population ages and the "baby boomers" begin to reach the end of their lives. As a consequence, it is projected that the need for palliative care will increase by 47% – an increase of 35% in public hospitals and a much bigger increase of 75% in aged residential care.

When considering the need for palliative care services, it is noted that this analysis is done on the basis of place of **death** and not place of **care**. The need for hospital palliative care at older ages is therefore dependent on the extent to which people are hospitalized. It is also a concern that aged residential care facilities will not be expanded as extensively as the predictions suggest, putting additional pressure on home care. Hospitals may also see an increase in admissions for the elderly as a result.

The introduction and sustainability of specialist palliative care in New Zealand hospitals have been very challenging, despite it being a clear recommendation in the palliative care strategy for over 15 years (Minister of Health 2001). In the analysis from 2016 (http://www.cdhb.health.nz/About-CDHB/corporate-publications/Documents/Canterbury%20DHB%20Annual%20Report%20year%20ended%2030%20June%202017%20%28PDF%2C%202MB%29.pdf), the need for palliative care in different settings was assessed, and it is interesting to note that a high proportion of deaths occur outside of hospitals, relative to other countries (Broad et al. 2013). Contributing to this might be the fact that only 25.8% of cancer patients died in public hospitals, in contrast to approximately 56% of cancer patient deaths in England and Wales. It is interesting to note that the largest increase in place of death for cancer patients in New Zealand has been in residential care (Palliative Care Council 2014). In addition to this, an overarching priority of the New Zealand MOH is to provide care "close to home," drawing attention away from acute care as the default option (http://www.health.govt.nz/publication/better-sooner-more-convenient-health-care-community). These factors combined may be contributing to a lack of focus on allocating sufficient resources to hospitals for end-of-life care.

3.1 Definitions

All health systems are complex, and navigating them can be challenging, both as health professionals and as consumers. Talking about death and dying is also not easy, and confusion can occur when the phrase *palliative care* is used both for the type of care provided to people with a life-limiting or life-threatening condition and for some, **but not all**, of the health professionals tasked with delivering that care. Palliative care organizations are well placed to be involved in developing local models of care and promoting integration across care settings.

Definitions can be confusing, and in order to clarify the situation, the New Zealand Palliative Care Glossary was developed (2nd edition, MOH 2015) to assist with promoting the Framework. Terms such as a "palliative care approach," "primary palliative care," and the "palliative care system" are included, and socializing these concepts has been occurring incrementally.

Palliative Care Approach: an approach to care which embraces the definition of palliative care. It incorporates a positive and open attitude toward death and dying by all service providers working with the person and their family and respects the wishes of the person in relation to their treatment and care.

Primary Palliative Care: is provided by all individuals and organizations who deliver palliative care as a component of their service and who are not part of a specialist palliative care team.

Specialist Palliative Care: palliative care provided by those who have undergone specific training and/or accreditation in palliative care/ medicine, working in the context of an expert interdisciplinary team of palliative care health professionals. It may be provided by hospice- or hospital-based palliative care services where people have access to at least medical and nursing palliative care specialists.

Specialist Palliative Care Service: a team or organization whose core work focuses on delivering palliative care, for example, a hospice or hospital palliative care team.

Palliative Care System: comprises specialist palliative care services, primary palliative care providers, and the other factors that enable them to deliver palliative care, such as communication and coordination between providers. It is not simply the existence of primary palliative care providers and palliative care services that comprises the palliative care system; it is the links between them that tie together "a system."

Supporting the delivery of primary palliative care are specialist services. These include

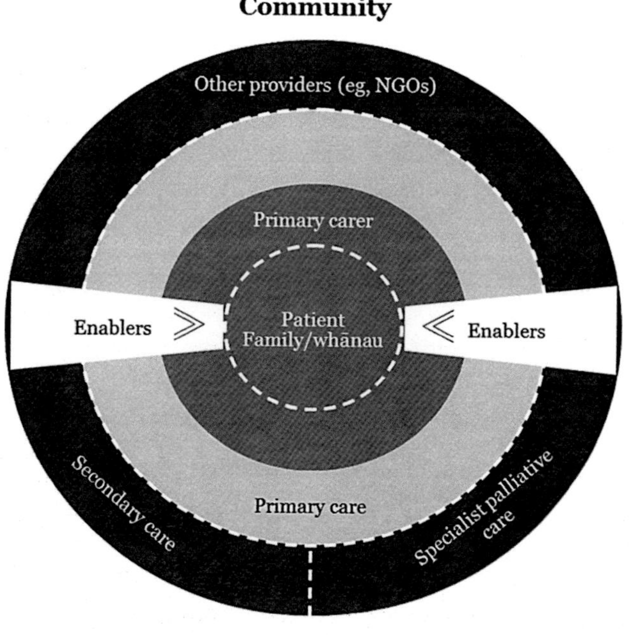

Fig. 2 Support for the patient and family/whanau https://www.health.govt.nz/system/files/documents/publications/resource-capability-framework-adult-palliative-care-services-v2.pdf

hospices and community palliative care teams AND hospital palliative care teams. Hospice inpatient and community services are very well embedded across New Zealand, and they are still considered the face of palliative care in society.

3.2 Models of Care

In 2012, the Resource and Capability Framework for Integrated Adult Palliative Care Services in New Zealand (the Framework) (Ministry of Health 2012) was developed. This outlines a model of care which explicitly recognizes that the majority of palliative care in New Zealand is delivered and coordinated by those without specialist training in palliative care, working outside a hospice or palliative care service/team, i.e., primary palliative care. The current arrangement across both the CDHB and the WCDHB is aligned with this Framework. The following graphic is taken from the Framework document.

The delivery of specialist palliative care in the acute care environment has grown organically in New Zealand, as has been the case around the world. It is contingent on supportive and sympathetic organizational leadership and a shared vision for integration of care across settings. This was fortunate to happen in CDHB leading to the creation of the Christchurch Hospital Palliative Care Service in 1999. The same cannot be said across the country with the establishment of hospital services proving very hard to realize in some DHBs.

The service in Canterbury started with a part-time physician and the recruitment of a full-time specialist nurse a few months later. Now the service employs two physicians, a nurse practitioner, two nurse specialists, registered nursing cover for planned leave, and a full-time registrar training position. The team is located within the Canterbury Regional Cancer and Haematology Service and is funded as a component of the medical and surgical division of the Hospital.

It remains the case that some hospitals in New Zealand still have **no** specialist palliative care presence at all. This is problematic and disappointing and has been allowed to happen because of the lack of a clear MOH directive for DHBs in this regard. Some hospital services are limited to in-reach nurses from hospices, with or without DHB input and often with restricted medical oversight.

Although the interdisciplinary consult liaison team is the usual model of care in hospitals, there are other models utilized in other countries. For example, there are dedicated palliative care units within some hospitals in the UK funded by the National Health Service (NHS). These units have led directly to an increase in home death rate, a reduction in deaths in the acute care hospital setting, and better integration of community, hospital, and palliative care unit team facilitating admissions and discharges and have raised the profile of palliative care within the trust (Grogan et al. 2016). (Trusts are organizations within the National Health Service which serve either a geographical area or a specialized function (such as an ambulance service). In any particular location, there may be several trusts involved in the different aspects of healthcare for a resident.).

Regardless of model, the key aspect of hospital palliative care is providing a higher level of expertise in complex symptom management, psychosocial support, communication, grief, and bereavement. Ideally, this process involves a full multidisciplinary approach and requires negotiation, coordination, communication, and collaboration as well as clinical knowledge and expertise.

The overarching goal is integration across the "whole of system" (Ministry of Health 2017a, b). This is increasingly necessary given the growing burden of chronic conditions. Ensuring that care at the end of life and following bereavement is equitable, of high quality, and available to everyone, **wherever they are located**, can only be achievable by empowering, teaching, and supporting "primary palliative care" providers in all settings, including hospitals. The issue of integration will be covered later in this chapter, but it is worth noting that following the release of the Framework (Ministry of Health 2012), momentum to configure specialist services with improved integration as a focus has indeed increased across New Zealand.

In the South Island, this imperative of integration is led by the South Island Alliance, covering all five DHBs. Since 2014, palliative care has been represented on the Alliance by the Palliative Care Workstream (https://www.sialliance.health.nz/our-priorities/palliative-care/).

The graphic below illustrates the functions of the SIA with "population health" and "experience of care" being two of its core principles. Of particular relevance to those working in and promoting universal access to palliative care is that "people die with dignity" is one of the eight key priorities (https://www.sialliance.health.nz/UserFiles/SouthIslandAlliance/Image/Outcomes%20Framework_020715.jpg).

4 Hospital Palliative Care Services

As noted earlier, approximately one third of all deaths occur in hospital in New Zealand. Recent trajectories predict this will remain steady over time (http://www.cdhb.health.nz/About-CDHB/corporate-publications/Documents/Canterbury%20DHB%20Annual%20Report%20year%20ended%2030%20June%202017%20%28PDF%2C%202MB%29.pdf; Palliative Care Council 2011). Regardless of whether the risk of dying has been acknowledged, consumers quite rightly expect that alongside active treatment of an advanced progressive condition, attention is paid to pain and any other distressing symptoms and that communication around diagnosis, prognosis, and options for care and treatment is conducted sensitively and with compassion and respect.

While there is an expectation that all health professionals provide supportive and palliative care, it would be fair to say that many do not have sufficient knowledge or understanding to do so effectively, or they feel out of their depth with initiating a palliative approach, particularly in complex situations. Hospital palliative care as a specialist area developed in response to a recognition that many people were dying in acute hospitals without ready access to expert symptom control and a timely referral to palliative care is increasingly recognized as an essential service within the hospital system.

The symptom burden of hospitalized patients is high. "Many patients in hospital with uncontrolled symptoms including pain, nausea, vomiting, constipation, anorexia and dyspnoea" (Jack et al. 2003). The impact of hospital palliative care team has been studied with positive results. "Analysis of the data showed statistically significant improvements in the symptoms of pain, nausea, insomnia, anorexia and constipation following interventions by the team. Discussion regarding diagnosis significantly change the insight of both patients and relatives, and appropriate placement was facilitated. This study has demonstrated the significant contribution that could be made to patient care by a hospital palliative care team" (Ellershaw et al. 1995).

Within hospitals, the primary model of care delivery is the interdisciplinary consultation team (Kelly and Morrison 2015). This is generally referred to as a "consult liaison service." The palliative care team needs to work alongside the treating team and respond to the prevailing discomfort around death and dying, offering clinical support, reassurance, and education. Teams build on the care provided by the primary clinical team to enhance the capability and capacity and quality of the overall service provided while emphasizing the normality of dying. Ideally, teams need not only to be competent but also accessible and nonjudgmental. Within the palliative care team, experience levels and areas of expertise will differ requiring collaboration and support. It is preferable at times for two team members to see an individual patient.

Where hospital services are present, thought needs to be given to two aspects which may extend the "consultation liaison model." The first is "admitting rights" which is the ability to admit patients under a palliative care specialist. The other is about "prescribing rights" which is the acceptance that palliative care team members (doctors or nurse practitioners) can prescribe and amend medications. The situation in the CDHB has not changed since the service was established with the team being able to prescribe freely, in consultation with the treating team, but all patients are admitted under another specialist with palliative care providing advice and support. This model has served us well but has been challenged a few times over the years.

4.1 Clinical Roles and Functions of Hospital Teams

It is our observation that hospital teams vary considerably in size and personnel depending on available resources. Appendix B of the Framework has outlined the essential composition and clinical functions in the New Zealand context, and teams have used these as a guide and as a vehicle for discussions with funders and managers (Ministry of Health 2012).

The constitution of a hospital-based palliative care team also varies depending on the will and influence of clinical leaders within the individual organization. Many hospital palliative care services began with one nurse or one doctor, sometime in-reaching from a local hospice. One person does not make a team, and successful services depend on their being a team structure for mutual support, sustainability, and professional safety. It is generally recognized that medical and nursing involvement is required **at a minimum**, ideally supported by some administration hours, sufficient to assist the team with the typing, data collection, and general administration.

The hospital team functions are as follows:

- Five days a week on-site service (with after-hours telephone cover)
- Consultation, advice, and liaison with referring multidisciplinary team (MDT)
- Advanced assessment (initial and ongoing) and care planning – medical, nursing, psychosocial, and spiritual
- Liaison – community (primary care) aged care, hospital teams, hospice (inpatient and community services), and pain services
- Input into family meetings
- Input into discharge planning
- Input into advance care planning
- Input into end-of-life care pathway implementation

Nonclinical functions were also included in the framework. These were considered critical to enhance the knowledge and skills of primary palliative care providers and to ensure leadership and strategic direction for palliative care:

- Clinical education – both formal/structured and informal
- Supervision/training (medical and nursing)
- Leadership and strategic planning
- Quality improvement
- Research/audit
- Clinical data collection
- Access to clinical supervision
- Appropriate networks and engagement (local, regional, and national)

An ideal service would be able to offer consultation liaison services 7 days a week and the option of in-person specialist review after-hours for complex or emergency cases. To date this comprehensive coverage has not been possible in any New Zealand hospital, and even providing after-hours telephone cover is proving difficult for most hospital teams. Provision of after-hours telephone advice has been achieved recently in Christchurch and involves the sharing of senior staff across the hospital and the hospice/community services. This arrangement is based on a close working collaboration that has developed over years.

It is apparent that hospital palliative care teams often demonstrate the benefits of a flat hierarchy. This is where the views of the whole team are equally valuable and decisions are made after attending to members' views and ensuring that there has been open and honest dialogue. As a minimum, this requires hospital teams to consist of nurses AND doctors as members and a strong alignment with allied health in the wider hospital to include social, cultural, and spiritual care. Some teams include social worker and/or counselor/psychologist as members of the specialist team, and this can compensate for when there is inexperience in these areas in the wider hospital.

It is important to emphasize that there is a need for hospital teams to operate in a time-constrained environment which can be challenging. Trust and rapport with patients and families must be established very quickly, in what is a busy and fast-paced environment. The median time from referral to discharge or death for the Christchurch service is 4 days, and this is inclusive of weekends where the team are not on site.

Anecdotally, the case mix for hospital palliative care is somewhat different to hospice and community services, with acute deaths and non-malignant conditions more strongly represented. In Christchurch Hospital, the proportion of new referrals who have a non-cancer diagnosis sits at approximately 40%, a number that has been consistent over the last 5 years. The proportion of new referrals who die during an episode of care has also been stable over time at 25%. Three quarters of referrals therefore are discharged from hospital to community settings, making it an imperative that the process of transfer of care is robust and well-planned (Unpublished data from Christchurch Hospital Palliative Care Database, New Zealand).

Further analysis of the Christchurch data has confirmed the impression that a higher proportion of patients seen by our service die in hospital if they have a nonmalignant condition. Eighteen percent of cancer new referrals to the palliative care team died during that first episode, compared to 49% of non-cancer new referrals. This difference is striking. These patients (and their families) may not be aware of the seriousness of the situation at the time of admission or the possibility that they might be close to death. This raises many issues in regard to community and health system preparedness that is likely to become more important as the general population ages (Unpublished data from Christchurch Hospital Palliative Care Database, New Zealand).

Ward-based referrals are not the only activity undertaken by hospital palliative care teams. Across all disciplines, clinics are a core component of specialist services in acute hospitals. Increasingly these are not led by doctors but by specialist nurses conducting clinics in areas such as oncology, diabetes, wound care, and infectious diseases. Hospital-based palliative care clinics are variably utilized, and this is often a reflection of capacity. It also depends on whether ambulatory care is provided by the local community-based/hospice service. It can be confusing for patients and referrers if there are multiple options for outpatient intervention in palliative care (particularly in a publically funded health system like New Zealand), and it is important not to have unnecessary duplication of resources.

In Christchurch, palliative care services work collaboratively with a number of other specialty areas with clinics and multidisciplinary support processes that complement each other and promote integration. Having combined clinics to address particular areas can work very well and include but are not limited to nephrology (for end-stage kidney disease), motor neurone disease, and heart failure.

Pediatric palliative care is a specialty area on its own, and most adult specialists (medical and nursing) do not feel it is appropriate to be offering advice to their pediatric colleagues. However, the volume of patients in pediatric practice is low, and it takes much longer to accumulate a broad experience base. There is enormous value in some situations for providing collaboration and support. It is an issue that is very worthwhile considering.

Access to bereavement support including formal counseling is ad hoc and often absent. Hospices generally have well-developed services and link very effectively with other community providers. Some hospital-based services such as intensive care and pediatric oncology have policies that include bereavement support, but it is the exception rather than rule. This is the subject of a current project in our DHB.

4.2 Nonclinical Roles

The knowledge and wisdom of individuals within the hospital palliative care team are often utilized by other teams around the hospital to discuss complex patients and debrief over difficult issues, especially in cases where there is particular sensitivity or emotion. This is perhaps because of having expertise in communication skills but also because as a discipline palliative care sits slightly outside the traditional medical model and therefore brings a different perspective and a sense of neutrality. This listening ear can be highly valued in the stressful environment of acute medical care.

The influence of hospital palliative care extends beyond the patients and the clinical teams caring for them. Ideally the reach should be directly into the realm of quality and patient safety as this is at the heart of what we do. Hospitals receive regular feedback on their services, and criticism is often leveled at issues around poor end-of-life care and communication. Building a profile in the organization where the service is valued for providing guidance and advice is invaluable. This can involve assisting with the processing of complaints in a constructive and meaningful, driving institutional change around policy and priority setting for dying patients.

The requirement for "noncontact time" (the time spent on issues not relating directly to patient care) is specifically identified within the employment contract of doctors in New Zealand. This is very relevant for palliative care where education, service development, research, and continuing professional development must be undertaken. Other staff, most specifically nurses, also require noncontact time for these endeavors. For everyone the ability to prioritize this above clinical work is extremely challenging.

4.3 Staff Training

Advanced medical training to specialist level across Australia and New Zealand is delivered through the Royal Australasian College of Physicians (RACP). New Zealand has a nationally funded program, and palliative medicine registrars work in hospital palliative care for a minimum of 6 months to develop their palliative care skills in an acute setting. This is a mandatory requirement for training. All palliative medicine specialists employed by the CDHB have a role in undergraduate medical student teaching both in the hospital and in the hospice.

Nursing students have little exposure in most undergraduate programs to opportunities to improve generic symptom assessment and treatment skills as well as communication skills. Allied health staff have even less. Palliative care forums worldwide continue to advocate for increased training in all undergraduate programs.

Postgraduate university posts for palliative medicine and palliative care nursing are gradually becoming more common but are still inadequate for the research that is required and for providing sound evidence for clinical decision-making. This is particularly the case in New Zealand. The CDHB is fortunate to have a specialist in post who is also employed as a Senior Clinical Lecturer for the University of Otago.

While numbers are still small, the introduction of nurse practitioners (NP) approximately 15 years ago in New Zealand has assisted in increasing advanced assessment skills and increased pharmacology knowledge among palliative care nurses. This has been valuable in the acute hospital environment as well as rural and community settings and has raised the bar regarding clinical reasoning, knowledge, and prescribing of medications by nurses. The NP role supports the philosophical stance of palliative care in many hospital teams – that nursing, allied health, and doctors consult on the same group of patients. Allowance is made for the clinical experience of the individual practitioner in relation to the complexity of the case, but otherwise there is no differentiation.

Hospital palliative care teams need to prioritize their own ongoing learning which may include journal clubs, hospital grand rounds, complex case management reviews, mortality meetings, cancer multidisciplinary meetings (MDMs), etc. Combined continuing medical education (CME) with other disciplines such as oncology are also highly beneficial and usually easily accessible in the hospital environment. Such meetings also provide opportunity to discuss patients with complex symptoms. Within the hospital system, specific meetings can be set up to review imaging and discuss patients with complex pain issues. This has happened in Christchurch and is proving invaluable in the treatment of patients with pain who require a broader team discussion. Appropriate patients may then be selected for palliative procedures such as cementoplasty/

vertebroplasty, ablation techniques, and nerve blocks as well as palliative surgery and radiotherapy. These meetings provide opportunity for specific ongoing learning as procedures are refined or new innovations become available.

As hospital teams grow, the risk emerges of referring teams getting conflicting advice, depending on who from palliative care responds on each occasion. This needs to be managed proactively as it can erode trust in the wider team. Having agreed symptom management guidelines that the whole team adheres to sets a platform for the main problems that are encountered. Complex cases, where creative thinking may be required, need to come back to the team so that a consensus is developed. Every effort should be made to ensure that each team member does not work independently, with synergy of practice being of paramount importance, while still valuing each other's unique skills and ideas.

Another issue that causes concern is when the advice of palliative care is in conflict with the treatment plan of the referring team. This is not an uncommon situation and requires diplomacy and care to minimize confusion and polarization. Ultimately a consensus is usually reached as long as the needs and preferences of the patient are put at the center. The palliative care perspective is not always correct of course, so mutual respect and humility are very useful attributes.

4.4 Prompt Response to Clinical Need

As hospital palliative care services have been established, so have referral criteria to manage the flow of referrals and to guide referrers. In New Zealand the Framework identifies three main criteria for specialist referral. These are as follows:

1. The patient has active progressive and advanced disease or life-limiting illness.
2. The patient has a level of need that exceeds the resources of the primary palliative care provider. The Framework states that palliative care services "should provide direct management support of patients their families and whānau where more complex palliative care needs exceeds the resources of the primary care provider."

   There has also been agreement that the level of input is "needs based" rather than based on diagnosis or prognosis and in some cases where that level of need becomes extraordinary examples include:

   "Uncontrolled or complicated symptoms, specialised nursing requirements related to mobility functioning or self-care, emotional behavioural difficulties related to the illness such as uncontrolled anxiety or depression."
3. The patient agrees to the referral if competent to do so (or an advocate agrees on their behalf).

On the basis of these criteria, a referral for a specialist palliative care assessment can be activated. The referral is made according to **patient need**. Sometimes patients with a longer or unknown prognosis are referred, and this is entirely consistent with the model of care. It has been recommended that individual service referral criteria in New Zealand are based on the national guidelines. As noted in the Framework, "the subsequent level of involvement/intervention, treatment plan and care package be negotiated with the patient, carer and referring team" (Ministry of Health 2012).

Patients can also be discharged from palliative care services either through patient choice or because their needs have been met and ongoing care can be effectively managed without regular input from specialist services. Discussion with and referral back can be made at any time.

Another recommendation is that teams articulate a target response time for new referrals to be seen once the referral has been received. Not infrequently, referred patients will be in acute pain or close to death. These are sometimes referred to as "late" referrals and to a certain extent are inevitable. Teams should make themselves as approachable as possible to help mitigate this issue, and responding quickly with advice and support is essential. Local policy is that patients are seen the same day if at all possible. While this may not always be achievable, it should be the ideal as responding to acute need/demand for acutely unwell patients is core business for hospital palliative care. In many cases, the issues affecting the person and/or their family have been present for some time before the referral is generated, so waiting any longer only compounds distress for patients, families, and staff.

Triaging of referrals is a complex and fraught issue. The task of making a referral is often delegated to junior staff who may not appreciate the full picture and struggle to articulate the purpose or urgency. Speaking to the most appropriate member of the referring team (which may be a senior) is often required. To complicate things further, there are often additional concerns that have not been identified by the referring team. Wherever possible, patients should be prepared for a palliative care referral and have agreed for it to occur. The presence of a specific support person may be required. Working alongside referrers on a daily basis is essential to improve their capacity to identify and respond to palliative and end-of-life issues. Over time, referral practices improve and true teamwork emerges.

4.5 Complex Decision-Making and Ethical Challenges

Palliative care skills are generic and required in all locations; however, working in the acute hospital environment allows clinicians to be involved at the coalface for active treatment decisions as they are unfolding during an acute admission. The availability of specialist palliative care support when a patient is in the emergency department or being admitted to intensive care as well as for acute assessment teams such as in general medicine, general surgery, oncology, cardiology, hematology, and older person's health is highly beneficial. Being accepted as part of the wider team requires mutual trust and respect; benefits are significant, and they can work both ways. Palliative care as a specialty needs to stay current with practice trends and developments for the benefit of all patients and also improves interdepartmental communication and collaboration.

Patients with palliative care needs derive many benefits from hospital admissions. Robinson et al. reported that "families felt relieved when they were admitted to hospital. This was seen as relief from the responsibility of decision making associated with caring for someone with a serious illness" (Robinson et al. 2015). Primary teams defer to the hospital palliative care service particularly when patients with complex symptoms or psychosocial issues are admitted when they lack the confidence to manage the case alone (Ireland 2017). Access to specialist palliative care in the hospital environment has a demonstrated effectiveness in reducing the symptom burdens of dying person, whether these be physical or psychosocial (Le and Watt 2010). There are also established benefits for carers (Higginson and Evans 2010). This occurs despite that fact that a member of the hospital palliative care team cannot be at every ward-based multidisciplinary meeting or mortality meeting, just like they cannot be present at every cancer MDM, but the profile of palliative care within the acute hospital should ideally be such that teams can call on a team member to provide a palliative care viewpoint or option in most situations where that is needed.

A regular reason for referral is when ethical challenges arise or where there is conflict between the wishes of the treating team and those of the patient and/or family unit. These cases are distressing for health professionals, and the palliative care team can act as a "sounding board" or "wise ear." This is a form of collegial support which is increasingly important in the acute environment.

It should also be routine that a health professional with advanced knowledge in end-of-life care will assist in the development and socialization of policies and processes linked to complex decision-making. This can be achieved by contributing to initiatives such as the transition from active treatment to a palliative approach, determining and documenting goals/ceiling of care, advance care planning, medical guidance plans for incompetent patients, and policies regarding resuscitation decisions and documentation. It also requires an understanding of how to discuss these delicate issues with consumers.

4.6 Education, Mentoring

The training and education of healthcare professionals who work in acute hospitals are paramount and linked closely to the issues of transitioning patients from active treatment to a palliative approach and end-of-life care. Medical staff trained in the biomedical model with curative intent should be introduced to the basic concepts of palliative care early in their training and be given the opportunity to think about their own mortality and the importance of compassion, empathy, person-centered care, communication, and self-care.

Face-to-face education sessions for ward-based staff are expensive to deliver for resource-constrained hospitals, and this has led an increasing demand for online learning packages. These are also more easily accessible for healthcare professionals working across 24-h shifts, but such programs are time-consuming to produce. Even once implemented, these tools cannot completely eliminate the need for personal contact with experts in the field, especially when teaching sensitive and challenging content that may trigger deeply personal responses that need to be carefully managed.

It is important to maximize informal teaching opportunities and to mentor ward nursing and medical staff and students. This is part of the day-to-day work of hospital palliative care teams. This ongoing requirement can be a heavy workload for inherently numerically small hospital teams but is absolutely necessary.

An excellent opportunity for palliative care education is as part of any communication skills training that happens within the hospital. Teaching and role-playing of breaking bad news/end-of-life care consultations with patients and families are also required. The introduction of advance care planning programs in acute care in recent years has also provided the opportunity for healthcare professionals to improve their communication skills and to encourage them to better acknowledge that people have unique preferences, goals, priorities, and fears when it comes to care at the end of life. Both of these should be taught in the hospital setting, and opportunities for collaboration should be sought with other specialty groups to give weight to the importance of the topic in the eyes of the learners and the organization. Collaborating on teaching also spreads the load which is important for small services with stretched resources.

There is a very high turnover of clinical staff in acute hospitals, not limited to just doctors and nurses, so keeping everyone familiar with the place of palliative care, the role of the service, the availability of resources, and opportunities for education needs to be constantly refreshed. Part of the challenge is to empower staff without de-skilling them. This requires resisting the temptation to do everything ourselves!

New Zealand is an increasingly multicultural society with significant numbers of the registered and unregistered workforce having trained overseas. English may also not be their first language. This may lead to cultural, clinical, and ethical challenges regarding care at the end of life that require targeted education and support.

4.7 Guideline and Pathway Development

Throughout the world, various palliative care guidelines have been developed (e.g., NICE Guidelines in the NHS (https://www.nice.org.uk/guidance/qs13)) to assist in one of the most important purposes of palliative care – the education and support of healthcare professionals. Developing guidelines based on best practice and research is challenging with the relative paucity of robust studies in palliative care. The Christchurch Hospital Palliative Care Guidelines were developed approximately 15 years ago. They were initially only available for hospital-based staff on the intranet, but in more recent times, they have been refined and made available to all health professionals on the CDHB Internet site (http://cdhb.palliativecare.org.nz/). They have been widely accessed and referenced by individuals and services both across NZ and internationally.

Another platform for improving access to localized and relevant information has been HealthPathways (https://www.healthpathwayscommunity.org/About.aspx). In the CDHB there

1. Baseline assessment

A health practitioner undertakes a baseline assessment when they think a person may be entering their last days for life. This change in condition acts as a prompt to ensure conversations occur with the person and with their family/whānau.

If a person in their last days of life has a level of need that exceeds the resources of the primary palliative care provider, that provider should refer them to specialist palliative care.

Table 1: Baseline assessment summary

Te taha tinana: *Physical health*		Te taha hinengaro: *Mental health*	
1.1	Recognition the person is dying or is approaching the last days of life	1.5	Assessment of the person's preferences for care
1.2	Identification of the lead health practitioner	**Te taha whānau: *Extended family health***	
1.3	Assessment of physical needs	1.6	Identification of communication barriers
1.4	Review of current management and initiation of prescribing of anticipatory medication	1.8	The family/whānau's awareness of the person's changing condition
1.7	The person's awareness of their changing condition	1.9	Discussion of cultural needs
1.11	Provision of food and fluids	1.15	Provision of information to the family/whānau about support and facilities
1.12	Availability of equipment to support the person's care needs	**Te taha wairua: *Spiritual health***	
1.13	Consideration of cardiac devices	1.10	Provision of opportunity for the person and family/whānau to discuss what is important to them
1.14	Advice to relevant agencies of the person's deterioration		

Fig. 3 Baseline assessment at last days of life

is a version for general practice teams and community care and another version for the hospital. HealthPathways have been adopted in many other areas in New Zealand and localized as needed but based on the same principle of a shared platform of information across all settings of care.

A number of location-specific pathways have been developed by the palliative care team. The most notable ones are in the emergency department and the intensive care unit. Both of these areas are highly experienced at dealing with serious life-threatening illness and death but wanted to appreciate and understand the nature and benefits of palliative care in order to improve their services and ensure that transfers were safer and more in line with ward- or community-based care. It has been a mutually beneficial process and is an ongoing work in progress.

New Zealand has also recently released Te Ara Whakapiri: principles and guidance for care at the end of life and the Te Ara Whakapiri Toolkit (April 2017) (Ministry of Health 2017c). The two documents are suitable for all healthcare settings, including acute care, and a process of implementation is currently underway. The program was developed in response to the withdrawal of the Liverpool Care Pathway for the Dying Patient in 2015. The following graphic is taken from the section of the guidance that covers the baseline assessment that is conducted on all people identified as dying, regardless of their location. Te Reo Maori, the language of New Zealand's indigenous peoples, is used throughout the document as a recognition of the need for culurally appropriate care at the end of life.

4.8 Liaison with Community Services

A key aspect of providing seamless palliative care is being able to transfer patients to community-based services upon discharge from hospital. This requires knowledge of what they can provide and their level of expertise. It also requires close links with specialist palliative care service(s). This interface is improved if there is good sharing of electronic patient data to ensure all information is accurate and up to date and shared in a timely fashion. Ideally this should be inclusive of patients in their own homes, those residents in aged residential care facilities (care homes) as well as any other locations such as supported care homes for those with intellectual disability, and those in prisons or other facilities.

Effective liaison also requires a relationship of trust so that when setting up discharge arrangements from hospital, there is confidence in what follow-up services will be there to for each patient and family. This may be as simple as ascertaining whether the patient can be seen promptly by the community palliative care team and/or district nurse. Hospital teams can act as a "bridge" with the community, and fully understanding the capacity and capability of the local providers is essential to avoid inflated expectations.

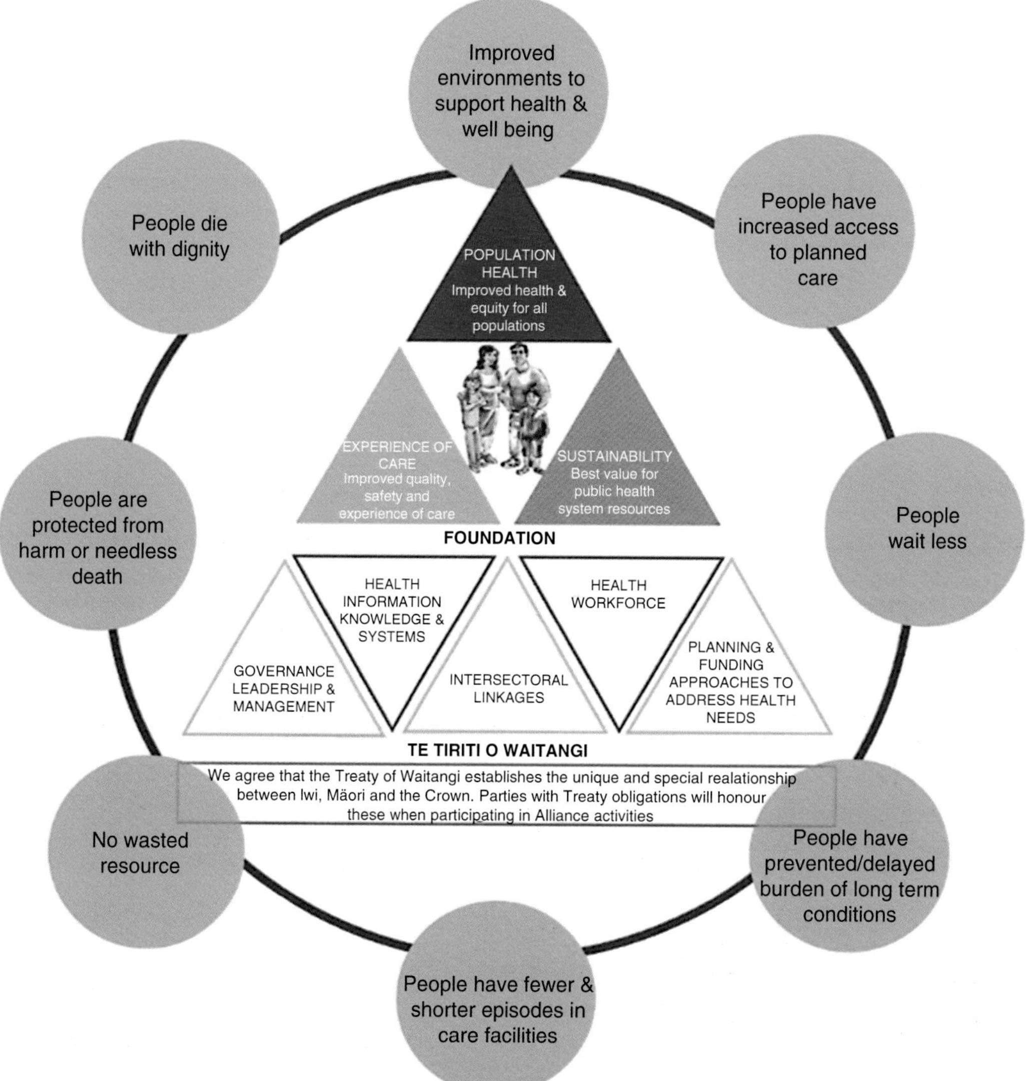

Fig. 4 Best for people, best for system outcomes framework https://www.sialliance.health.nz/system-outcomes-framework-graphic/

Sometimes patients cope better than expected, and sometimes they need to fail in order to understand the extent of their limitations. All of these issues need to be communicated effectively with our community colleagues.

It is imperative in the New Zealand system that the general practice team (also known as the primary healthcare team) is considered at all times. Having a general practitioner (GP) who is supportive is critical to the functioning of the primary palliative care team as the model of care. This is because specialist palliative care in the community is contingent on a collaborative GP relationship.

Models of community care and the organization of palliative care services will vary from country to country and within regions. As part of the model of care in Canterbury, the DHB has an agreement between the hospital and the community (Nurse Maude (https://www.nursemaude.org.nz/)) to work as a single specialist unit – *Canterbury Integrated Palliative Care Services*. Even though the two arms are funded separately, the vision, planning, and operational goals are aligned to eliminate gaps and waste and to enhance the consumer and health professional experience.

Even within a small country such as New Zealand, models of care vary; however, organizations such as the South Island Alliance (SIA) are promoting a more uniform approach. The SIA is funded and supported by the five South Island DHBs which has enabled the region to work collaboratively to develop more innovative and efficient health services than could be achieved independently. The SIA has been a driving factor in improving access, quality, and service development in a wide range of clinical areas.

In order to ensure a connected community of care, access to real-time information such as current medications, results, specialist assessments and letters, acute care plans, advance care plans, goals of care documents, etc. is becoming a universal expectation internationally. Making this happen with diverse IT systems, privacy concerns, and IT logistics is a significant barrier to providing comprehensive integrated palliative care. Improving IT systems and software programs are bridging these gaps; however, having information accessible to all the relevant health professionals in real time is proving to be an ongoing challenge. The SIA is helping spearhead IT integration across the South Island within the limitations of the systems available. Change can be difficult for staff, but benefits are steadily being realized.

4.9 Information Technology

As mentioned above, data sharing and transfer of patient information across healthcare settings is of paramount importance and is an increasingly complex endeavor. Hospital palliative care teams can usually access all the same information as colleagues from other areas within the acute environment, but this does not always translate to the same access for specialist doctors, nurses, and allied health staff working in community settings. This inevitably leads to delays, errors, and frustrations. Working collaboratively with IT services is essential in ensuring that the care of dying patients is seen as just as important as those being treated actively.

In 2013, the Health Information Standards Organisation in NZ developed a suite of national data definitions for specialist palliative care (Health Information Standards Organisation 2013a, b). These have helped drive consistency in hospice services, but as yet there have been no resources available to standardize, measure, and report on activity, demographics, and trends in hospital practice. This issue has been much more proactively addressed in other countries but will not be reported here.

An important way of maximizing productivity for small services is to invest in IT innovations such as Telehealth (videoconferencing). This has been a very successful vehicle in the CDHB especially for rural consultations, for complex case meetings which are conducted regionally, and for staff support.

4.10 Building and Sustaining the Team

New Zealand as well as most other countries has a shortage of skilled palliative care medical and nursing staff let alone allied health staff. "Growing your own" where possible appears to be the best option available. As mentioned earlier, the RACP has a training program to specialist and diploma level, and these are well utilized. Many New Zealand hospitals are accredited for palliative medicine training, but the number of funded positions is insufficient to meet current and future needs. This issue will no doubt be familiar internationally. In regard to nursing staff, a trust fund is available in New Zealand for two placements per year where a registered nurse can train in palliative care for a 2-year period. Working in the hospital setting is part of the training program, but places and funding are limited, and efforts to improve the situation have not yet been forthcoming.

The recruitment of a "team" is dependent on many factors not least the availability of skilled personnel with appropriate qualifications and experience. Growing the specialty within nursing and succession planning for services is an ongoing challenge. More creative ways to upskill registered nurses in palliative care are required. Working in hospitals is different to hospices, and although many of the necessary skills can be gleaned in hospice or community care, the swift-moving and highly pressured environment in acute care can make it hard for nurses in particular to feel that their input is having any influence.

Leadership in the team is also important to consider and foster. One of the benefits of having a flat structure within hospital teams is being able to share leadership responsibilities, to cover personnel when others are away, and to take collective responsibility for accepting challenging cases. Leadership in any team sets the direction, philosophy, and culture of the service, but the entire team must "share the vision."

Formal orientation to a new position within a hospital team is critical, with clear directions and guidance as to how referrals are managed, how workload is contained, how to seek help, and how to keep skills and knowledge current. Even small teams need orientation packs for new or visiting team members. Teams develop very intricate patterns of behavior that can be mystifying to the outsider; therefore, writing down what your team does helps new personnel to integrate more smoothly and operate effectively.

Maintaining a team in the acute hospital environment requires close professional working relationships and high levels of trust in each other's work as well as the checks and balances of paper ward rounds, patient review meetings, audits, and ongoing research projects. It also requires each individual team member to take responsibility for the emotional, psychological, and spiritual demands inherent in a busy hospital palliative care practice. Reflective professional supervision should be encouraged and funded (as is the case in the CDHB) as well as informal debriefing among the team members as needed. It is a forum where the complexities of the interpersonal interactions that underpin the provision of healthcare can be explored in a supportive and confidential setting (https://www.nzma.org.nz/journal/read-the-journal/all-issues/2010-2019/2016/vol-129-no-1434-6-may-2016/6884). Regular team business meetings can also be helpful and occasional team-building activities. These are essential to create sustainability.

Ideally team members should be supported to utilize their individual strengths and strong enough to tolerate their differences. This is particularly challenging at times of growth and when managing change such as a new manager or leader.

There is no doubt that small teams can fall into the trap of spreading themselves too thinly. An example of this might include the common request for a palliative care physician to be present at every cancer MDM. There are more than 12 individual meetings in the CDHB, each lasting at least an hour and run sometimes every week. Meeting this request is impossible, and each case must be looked at individually to maximize the resource.

Small teams are very vulnerable – both in regard to the myriad of unrealistic expectations placed on them by others but also to the teams' own internal dynamics. Palliative care attracts health professionals with a strong vocation and a desire to venture where others are unable or unwilling to tread, and this can make team members overly sensitive to a fear of failure to meet their own high standards.

It is important to foster relationships with management that are attuned to these pressures, expectations, and dynamics so that they can empower and support hospital teams to develop and thrive, despite the pressure placed upon them. This can make the difference between a team that is able to adapt and change successfully and one that is only able to "tread water" and survive.

5 Raising the Profile and Promoting Culture Change

Having a clear and visible profile within the hospital requires individual commitment and managerial support. Some examples of how this might be achieved include making and taking the opportunity to present at departmental meetings and hospital grand rounds, contributing to hospital newsletters, developing policies and pathways, and participating in strategic projects and hospital-wide meetings. The function of hospital palliative care is not only to provide excellent clinical advice and support but also to be politically astute and active. Being seen to be involved in the workings of the wider hospital system is critically important.

Hospital palliative care teams, when working well, influence and change the culture within the organization around care of the dying. They legitimize dying as being "OK" even within a curative model, and they allow other health professionals to ask for help in both an end-of-life situation and to assist in managing difficult symptom management and complex social needs. They also advocate for patients especially those who are vulnerable. Hospital palliative care teams promote a way of thinking that turns around the notion prevalent in acute care of "what can we do to the patient" to "what is best for the person." Having a palliative care presence in hospitals challenges a model of care that may no longer be appropriate.

There are many examples of patients having more than one team or multiple teams involved in their care and no one team taking the lead. The patient who is left languishing without any direction or plan lost in the complex world of acute hospital care. These are the situations in which patients or family members feel they have little choice other than to lodge complaints against "the system." Added to these are the environmental factors of acute care hospitals. Due to pragmatism and cost, multi-bedded rooms with few, if any, alternative spaces make it extremely difficult for any personal or reflection time let alone private conversations with family members or other healthcare professionals. Discussing spiritual care or fears around dying is extremely challenging in the acute care environment for patients, family, chaplains, pastoral care, and palliative care team members. Therefore, hospital palliative care teams need to use their position within the healthcare system to advocate for patients and to influence change.

6 Palliative Care and Hospital Costs

Despite the fact that death and dying are ubiquitous in hospitals, acceptance of the value of a palliative care presence is far from universal. This may be, in part, due to the reticence of hospices to venture into the acute environment, wishing to preserve the identity and separateness of the hospice philosophy of care. It may also be due to an assumed lack of evidence that they are of benefit. This, however, is not actually the case. Palliative care teams have been shown to improve quality of life for patients with advanced cancer and in a recent study to extend survival (Temel et al. 2010). "Furthermore, palliative care programs can reduce hospital costs by ameliorating pain and other distressing symptoms that increase hospital lengths of stay and cause medical complications; can reduce overuse of unnecessary, ineffective or marginally effective services; and can develop transition plans that result in safe hospital discharges with lower likelihood of readmission" (Morrison et al. 2011).

Cost savings attributable to palliative care services in hospitals have been extensively reported in international studies (Kelly and Morrison 2015; Morrison et al. 2008; Simoens et al. 2010). The paper by Ireland in 2017 examined access to palliative care services during a terminal hospital admission and concluded that intervention rates and hospital costs were reduced. Involvement from palliative care was associated with significantly lower hospital costs in the order of $5000–8000 (Australian dollars) for all patient groups, but most particularly for those with non-cancer diagnoses. Shorter terminal episodes and greater palliative care-related cost reductions have been identified for patients with diagnoses other than cancer. The paper states that the total costs of these episodes were reduced by 28% for cancer patients and 36% for other patients with much lower rates of ICU admissions and operative procedures being the chief drivers of cost reductions. A prospective multisite cohort study published in 2017 noted that reduced length of stay is the biggest driver of cost saving from early consultation for patients with advanced cancer. Patient- and family-centered discussions on goals of care and transition planning initiated by palliative care consultation teams were felt to be at least as important in driving cost savings as the reduction of unnecessary test and pharmaceuticals identified in other studies (May et al. 2017).

It is worthy to include a note of caution when extrapolating such specific findings to individual situations. "Funding models are a very important consideration and they need to be well understood to ensure best practice and minimise perverse incentives. Before we can conduct cross-national comparisons of costs and impact of palliative care, we need to understand the funding and policy context for palliative care in each country of interest" (Groeneveld et al. 2017).

7 Integrated Palliative Care

Integration is required to ensure that palliative care is available and effective for all who need it. This needs to occur across all settings of care and is dependent on collaboration, trust, respect, and mutual support.

A definition of integration is included in a recent systematic review in Europe. "Integrated palliative care involves bringing together administrative, organisational, clinical and service aspects in order to realise continuity of care between all factors involved in the care network of patients receiving palliative care. It aims to achieve quality of life and a well-supported dying process for the patient and the family in collaboration with all the caregivers, paid and unpaid" (Garralda et al. 2016).

The recommendations from this project are well worth reflecting on, and they address the issue from three levels.

At a policy (macro) level, the focus is on:

1. National policy development
2. Earmarked funding
3. Measurable outcomes
4. Public engagement

At an organizational (meso) level, the following requirements are emphasized:

1. Identify gaps (often communication).
2. Include the multidisciplinary team.
3. Ensure seamless working across systems.
4. Acknowledge that **one size does not fit all.**
5. Promote formal structures specifically targeting integrated care.

At an individual patient/family (micro) level, the report also emphasizes the following;

1. Personalized communication to enable patients to express their preferences for their care, e.g., via formal advance care planning
2. Identification of patients before crises occur, e.g., goals of care
3. Involvement of family/whānau
4. Integration of care across agencies
5. Established communication systems

Many of these points resonate with work that has been occurring in New Zealand, but there is still a long way to go. The work of agencies such as the Health Quality and Safety Commission (https://www.hqsc.govt.nz/our-programmes/patient-deterioration/), the Advance Care Planning Cooperative (http://www.advancecareplanning.org.nz/), the Canterbury Initiative (http://www.canterburyinitiative.org.nz/) (including

HealthInfo and HealthPathways), and the South Island Alliance (https://www.sialliance.health.nz/UserFiles/SouthIslandAlliance/Image/Outcomes%20Framework_020715.jpg) are helping palliative care organizations with promoting integrated care at the end of life and service development.

8 Conclusion

An important indicator of how effectively a health system is operating is how well it cares for the most vulnerable members of society. The dying are extremely vulnerable, and it is pleasing to see that New Zealand features highly in a global context with a ranking of third in the 2010 report by the Economist Intelligence Unit (http://graphics.eiu.com/upload/eb/qualityofdeath.pdf). Despite this, coverage and integration are incomplete, and hospitals remain a major area for improvement.

Within Christchurch Hospital, in addition to medical and nursing partners, it has been beneficial to identify champions in areas such as pharmacy, social work, occupational therapy, acute pain management, counseling, and mental health. These have helped to support the wider interdisciplinary team with their care of routine and complex cases, and collectively they serve to raise the bar in regard to interdisciplinary team commitment to quality palliative and end-of-life care. This is part of creating a shared vision for care of the dying across the whole health system.

Back in 1994, it was recognized that having "palliative care in a hospital. . ..is an issue of justice and equity, and gives structure to compassion" (Lickiss et al. 1994). As indicated throughout this chapter, more recent studies have validated this over and over, providing a clear and welcome message for providers, commissioners, and funders of health services. It is summarized very eloquently in this final paper. "In the intense pressure for health services to do things differently and more cost effectively, specialist palliative care teams may have a central role in delivering better care and outcomes while reducing acute care use in last weeks of life, and should be resourced and commissioned to do so" (Murtagh 2014).

Given the aging population and the ongoing expectation that hospitals will remain central to the delivery of care at the end of life, hospital palliative care must not be forgotten. The relatively poor profile of palliative care in acute settings and in society in general, the observation that high proportions of nonmalignant patients are only being recognized as dying in the final stages, and the vulnerability of small teams are just some of the challenges that need to be faced. Palliative care is not an optional extra. Targeted effort is required to drive improvements in outcomes for patients and families and to ensure that **all** health professions are equipped to look after palliative patients in their care.

References

Broad JB, Gott M, Kim H, Boyd M, Chen H, Connolly MJ. Where do people die? An international comparison of the percentage of deaths occurring in hospital and residential aged care settings in 45 populations, using published and available statistics. Int J Publ Health. 2013;58(2):257–67. Available at http://www.ncbi.nlm.nih.gov/pubmed/22892713

Clark D, Armstrong M, Allan A, Graham F, Carnon A, Isles C. Imminence of death among hospital inpatients: prevalent cohort study. Palliat Med. 2014;28(6):474–9. Available at http://www.ncbi.nlm.nih.gov/pubmed/24637342

Clark D, Schofield L, Graham FM, Isles C, Gott M, Jarlbaek L. Likelihood of death within one year among a national cohort of hospital inpatients in Scotland. J Pain Symptom Manag. 2016;52:e2–4. Available at http://www.ncbi.nlm.nih.gov/pubmed/27262261

Cumming J, McDonald J, Barr C, Martin G, Gerring Z, Daubé J, Gericke C. New Zealand health system review. In: Health systems in transition, vol 3, no 4, p 272. Asia Pacific Observatory on Health Systems and Policies; 2013. Available at http://www.wpro.who.int/asia_pacific_observatory/hits/series/nez/en/

Ellershaw JE, Peat SJ, Boys LC. Assessing the effectiveness of a hospital palliative care team. Palliat Med. 1995;9:145. Available at https://www.ncbi.nlm.nih.gov/pubmed/7541684

Garralda E, Hasselaar J, Carrasco JM, Van Beek K, Siouta N, Csikos A, Menten J, Centeno C. Integrated palliative care in the Spanish context: a systematic review of the literature. BMC Palliat Care. 2016;15(1):1. https://doi.org/10.1186/s12904-016-0120-9. Available at https://bmcpalliatcare.biomedcentral.com/articles/10.1186/s12904-016-0120-9

Gott M, Frey R, Raphael D, O'Callaghan A, Robinson J, Boyd M. Palliative care need and management in the acute hospital setting: a census of one New Zealand hospital. BMC Palliat Care. 2013;12:15. Available at http://www.ncbi.nlm.nih.gov/pubmed/23537092

Groeneveld EI, Cassel JB, Bausewein C, Csikós Á, Krajnik M, Ryan K, Haugen DF, Eychmueller S, Gudat Keller H, Allan S, Hasselaar J, García-Baquero Merino T, Swetenham K, Piper K, Fürst CJ, Murtagh FE. Funding models in palliative care: lessons from international experience. Palliat Med. 2017;31(4): 296–305. https://doi.org/10.1177/0269216316689015. Epub 2017 Feb. Available at https://www.ncbi.nlm.nih.gov/pubmed/28156188

Grogan E, Paes P, Peel T. Excellence in cost-effective impatient specialist palliative care in the NHS a new model. Clin Med. 2016;16:7. Available at https://www.ncbi.nlm.nih.gov/pubmed/26833508

Health Information Standards Organisation. National specialist palliative care data definitions standard, HISO 10039.2. Wellington: Health Information Standards Organisation, Ministry of Health; 2013a. Retrieved from http://www.ithealthboard.health.nz/who-we-work/hiso

Health Information Standards Organisation. National specialist palliative care data business process standard, HISO 10039.1. Wellington: Health Information Standards Organisation, Ministry of Health; 2013b. Retrieved from http://www.ithealthboard.health.nz/who-we-work/hiso

Higginson IJ, Evans CJ. What is the evidence that palliative care teams improve outcomes for cancer patients and their families? Cancer J. 2010;16:423–34.

http://cdhb.palliativecare.org.nz/

http://graphics.eiu.com/upload/eb/qualityofdeath.pdf

http://www.advancecareplanning.org.nz/

http://www.canterburyinitiative.org.nz/

http://www.cdhb.health.nz/About-CDHB/corporate-publications/Documents/Canterbury%20DHB%20Annual%20Report%20year%20ended%2030%20June%202017%20%28PDF%2C%202MB%29.pdf

http://www.health.govt.nz/publication/better-sooner-more-convenient-health-care-community

https://www.healthpathwayscommunity.org/About.aspx

https://www.hqsc.govt.nz/our-programmes/patient-deterioration/

https://www.nice.org.uk/guidance/qs13

https://www.nursemaude.org.nz/

https://www.nzma.org.nz/journal/read-the-journal/all-issues/2010-2019/2016/vol-129-no-1434-6-may-2016/6884

https://www.sialliance.health.nz/our-priorities/palliative-care/

https://www.sialliance.health.nz/UserFiles/SouthIslandAlliance/Image/Outcomes%20Framework_020715.jpg

Ireland AW. Access to palliative care services during a terminal hospital episode reduces intervention rates and hospital costs. Intern Med J. 2017;47:549. Available at https://www.ncbi.nlm.nih.gov/pubmed/28195682

Jack B, Hillier V, Williams A, Oldham. Hospital-based palliative care teams improve the symptoms of cancer patients. Palliat Med. 2003;17:498–502. Available at https://www.ncbi.nlm.nih.gov/pubmed/14526882

Kelly AS, Morrison RS. Palliative care for the seriously ill. N Engl J Med. 2015;373(8):747–55. Available at www.nejm.org/doi/full/10.1056/NEJMra1404684

Le B, Watt J. Care of the dying in Australia's busiest hospital: benefits of palliative care consultations and methods to enhance access. J Palliat Med. 2010;168:855–60.

Lickiss JN, Wiltshire J, Glare PA, Chye RW. Central Sydney Palliative Care Service: potential and limitations of an integrated palliative care service based in a metropolitan teaching hospital. Ann Acad Med Singap. 1994;23(2):264–70. Available at https://www.ncbi.nlm.nih.gov/pubmed/7521620

May P, Garrido MM, Cassel JB, Kelley AS, Meier DE, Normand C, Smith TJ, Morrison RS. Cost analysis of a prospective multi-site cohort study of palliative care consultation teams for adults with advanced cancer: where do cost-savings come from? Palliat Med. 2017;31(4):378–86. https://doi.org/10.1177/0269216317690098. Epub 2017 Feb 3. Available at https://www.ncbi.nlm.nih.gov/pubmed/28156192

McLeod H. The need for palliative care in New Zealand. Technical Report prepared for the Ministry of Health, June 2016. 2016. Available at http://centraltas.co.nz/health-of-older-people/tools-and-guidance/

Middlewood S, Gardner G, Gardner A. Dying in hospital: medical failure or natural outcome. J Pain Symptom Manag. 2001;22(6):1035–41. Available at https://www.ncbi.nlm.nih.gov/pubmed/11738166

Minister of Health. The New Zealand palliative care strategy. Wellington: Ministry of Health; 2001. Available at http://www.health.govt.nz/publication/new-zealand-palliative-care-strategy

Ministry of Health. Resource and capability framework for integrated adult palliative care services in New Zealand. Wellington: Ministry of Health Manatū Hauora; 2012. Available at http://www.health.govt.nz/publication/resource-and-capability-framework-integrated-adult-palliative-care-services-new-zealand

Ministry of Health. New Zealand palliative care glossary. Wellington: Ministry of Health; 2015. Available at http://www.health.govt.nz/publication/new-zealand-palliative-care-glossary

Ministry of Health. Palliative care action plan. Wellington: Ministry of Health; 2017a. Available at http://www.health.govt.nz/publication/palliative-care-action-plan/

Ministry of Health. Review of adult palliative care services in New Zealand. Wellington: Ministry of Health; 2017b. Available at http://www.health.govt.nz/publication/review-adult-palliative-care-services-new-zealand

Ministry of Health. Te Ara Whakapiri: principles and guidance for the last days of life. Wellington: Ministry of Health; 2017c. Available at http://www.health.govt.nz/publication/te-ara-whakapiri-principles-and-guidance-last-days-life

Morrison RS, Penrod JD, Cassel JB, Caust-Ellenbogen M, Litke A, Spragens L, Meier DE. Cost savings associated with US hospital palliative care consultation programs. Arch Intern Med. 2008;168(16):1783–90. https://doi.org/10.1001/archinte.168.16.1783. Available at https://www.ncbi.nlm.nih.gov/pubmed/18779466

Morrison SR, Dietret J, Ladwig S, Quill T, Sacco J, Tangeman J, Meier D. Palliative care consultation teams cut hospital costs for Medicaid beneficiaries. Health Aff. 2011;30:454–63. Available at http://jamanetwork.com/. On 22 July 2017

Moorfield JC. 2015. Te Aka Online Māori-English, English-Māori Dictionary and Index 2015. Available at http://www.maoridictionary.co.nz

Murtagh F. Can palliative care teams relieve some of the pressure on acute services. BMJ. 2014;348:g3693. https://doi.org/10.1136/bmj.g3693. (Published 6 June 2014). Available at https://www.ncbi.nlm.nih.gov/pubmed/24906714

Palliative Care Council. National health needs assessment for palliative care phase 1 report: assessment of palliative care need. Wellington: Palliative Care Council of New Zealand; 2011. Available at http://www.health.govt.nz/publication/national-health-needs-assessment-palliative-care-phase-1-report-assessment-palliative-care-need

Palliative Care Council. Cancer deaths in New Zealand, 2000 to 2010. Working paper No. 6, October 2014. Wellington: Cancer Control New Zealand; 2014.

Robinson J, Gott M, Gardiner C, Ingleton C. A qualitative study exploring the benefits of hospital admissions from the perspectives of patients with palliative care needs. Palliat Med. 2015;29(8):703–10. Available at https://www.ncbi.nlm.nih.gov/pubmed/25769983

Simoens S, Kutten B, Keirse E, Berghe PV, Beguin C, Desmedt M, Deveugele M, Léonard C, Paulus D, Menten J. The costs of treating terminal patients. J Pain Symptom Manag. 2010;40(3):436–48. https://doi.org/10.1016/j.jpainsymman.2009.12.022. Epub 2010 Jun 25. Available at https://www.ncbi.nlm.nih.gov/pubmed/20579838

Temel JS, Greer JA, Muzikanski A, Gallagher ER, Adamane S, Jackson VA, et al. Early palliative care for patients with metastatic non-small-cell lung cancer. N Engl J Med. 2010;363(8):733–42.

Unpublished data from Christchurch Hospital Palliative Care Database, New Zealand.

Wilson DM, Birch S, Sheps S, Thomas R, Justice C, MacLeod R. Researching a best-practice end-of-life care model for Canada. Can J Aging. 2008;27(4):319–30. Available at https://www.ncbi.nlm.nih.gov/pubmed/19606565

Palliative Care in the Intensive Care Unit (ICU)

53

Rebecca A. Aslakson and J. Randall Curtis

Contents

R. A. Aslakson
Department of Medicine and Division of Primary Care and Population Health, Section of Palliative Care; Department of Anesthesiology, Perioperative and Pain Medicine, Stanford University, Stanford, CA, USA
e-mail: aslakson@stanford.edu

J. R. Curtis (✉)
Division of Pulmonary, Critical Care, and Sleep Medicine, Harborview Medical Center, Cambia Palliative Care Center of Excellence, University of Washington, Seattle, WA, USA
e-mail: jrc@uw.edu; jrc@u.washington.edu

Abstract

Palliative care is a medical specialty and philosophy of care that focuses on reducing suffering among patients with serious illness and their family members, regardless of disease diagnosis or prognosis. As critical illness is often life-threatening and confers significant disease-related symptom burdens, palliative care and palliative care specialists can aid in identifying goals of care, reducing symptom burden, and improving quality of life among intensive care unit (ICU) patients and their

R. D. MacLeod, L. Van den Block (eds.), *Textbook of Palliative Care*,
https://doi.org/10.1007/978-3-319-77740-5_51

family members. Palliative care in the ICU can be delivered by the ICU team itself, specialist-trained palliative care consultants, or a combination of both. Though initial reports describing end-of-life care practices in the ICU were published in 1976, the modern era of palliative care research in the ICU began in the early 2000s. Since 2010, the Improving Palliative Care in the ICU (IPAL-ICU) Advisory Board has published a series of articles exploring opportunities and barriers to palliative care delivery in the ICU, particularly across different ICU types, ICU providers, and ICU patient populations. Furthermore, initiatives to improve delivery of "family-centered care" in the ICU frequently also correlate with palliative care practices. To date, over 40 palliative care and palliative care-related interventions targeting ICU patients and families have been trialed and published with results showing mixed effectiveness on outcomes such as ICU length of stay, patient and family symptoms, and family member satisfaction; several randomized trials provide important insights into interventions that improve patient and family outcomes as well as those that do not.

1 Introduction

The chapter aim is to discuss the history, delivery models, evidence base, opportunities for, and barriers to palliative care delivery in the intensive care unit.

Critically ill patients often require the most sophisticated technological treatments that modern medicine can offer and are at significant risk of death during or after the intensive care unit (ICU). In addition, ICU patients are at risk for significant morbidity with physical and psychological suffering that can occur both during and after ICU care (Angus et al. 2004; Teno et al. 2013; Wunsch et al. 2010; Cox et al. 2007, 2009; Choi et al. 2014; Puntillo et al. 2010; Herridge et al. 2011; Dowdy et al. 2005; Iwashyna et al. 2010; Davydow et al. 2008, 2009; Nelson et al. 2006a; Needham et al. 2012). Family members and caregivers of ICU patients are also at risk of increased morbidity, especially psychological morbidity (Needham et al. 2012; de Miranda et al. 2011; Swoboda and Lipsett 2002; Van Pelt et al. 2007; Anderson et al. 2008; Siegel et al. 2008; Cameron et al. 2016). The ICU is also a frequent place of patient death, often following a decision to withhold or withdraw life-sustaining treatments when those treatments no longer meet the patient's goals of care as identified by the patient, family member, and/or clinicians (Angus et al. 2004; Teno et al. 2013; Prendergast and Luce 1997). Finally, due to the burdens of critical illness, many ICU patients are unable to make medical decisions (Nelson et al. 2006a; Prendergast and Luce 1997; Silveira et al. 2010). Consequently, family members, caregivers, or other surrogate decision-makers must often work with the ICU team to make complicated, nuanced decisions that ideally attempt to balance a patient's previously expressed wishes with an evolving and often repetitive and cumulative barrage of critical illness-related insults to patient mortality, morbidity, and short- and long-term quality of life (Schenker et al. 2013; Scheunemann et al. 2015; White et al. 2007, 2012; White and Curtis 2006; Zier et al. 2012; Nelson et al. 2017). As critical illness confers significant disease-related symptom burdens, complex values-based decision-making and surrogate decision-making, and nontrivial risk of death, palliative care provided by ICU clinicians and palliative care specialists can aid in reducing symptom burden, facilitating decision-making, and improving quality of life among ICU patients and their family members (Kelley and Morrison 2015; Aslakson et al. 2014a).

2 Recent History of Palliative Care and Ethical Controversies in the ICU

By the late 1960s, the advent of life-supporting technologies – particularly ventilators – and the recognition of a survival benefit conferred through close physiological monitoring and intense nursing for critically ill patients led to the inception of ICUs (Luce 2010). ICUs rapidly became not only a physical care location but also a nexus for a progressively multidisciplinary team with expertise in selection and delivery of the complex treatments required to optimize patient survival despite severe, life-threatening illness. Indeed, the ICU with its combination of cutting-edge technologies and specialized care teams enabled patient survival through many previously fatal medical conditions. Yet, since inception, ICUs inherently illuminate the boundaries of modern medical care and consequently compel patients, family members, clinicians, and the medical community as a whole to confront and debate if and when aggressive medical treatments are personally, pragmatically, and ethically acceptable.

The advent of ICUs and ICU care has spurred multiple decisional, ethical, and legal conundrums, often involving palliative and end-of-life care-related issues and frequently surrounding the withdrawal or withholding of medical technologies (Luce 2010). By the mid-1960s, ethicists and ICU clinicians began to question the value of sustaining a patient's physiologic life when that patient had sustained a severe, irreversible neurologic insult; by 1968, the Harvard Commission published criteria for brain death and from those criteria evolved treatment pathways for when and how brain dead patients could or should be separated from physiologically supportive technologies, such as ventilators (School, A.H.C.o.t.H.M. 1968). By 1976, a prominent *New England Journal of Medicine* article acknowledged that ICUs are a frequent place of patient death and that ICU clinicians "promulgate and discuss publicly explicit policies about the deliberate withdrawal or non-application of life-prolonging measures" and that it is an "open secret" that "such measures are in fact regularly withheld or withdrawn" (Fried 1976; Optimum care for hopelessly ill patients, 1976). From the 1970s through the early 2000s, life-supporting technologies inherent to the ICU also instigated a series of legal cases in the United States to explore and define whether and when life-supportive technologies could be withdrawn or withheld; the legal cases involving the care of Karen Quinlan and Nancy Cruzan underlie modern ICU practices about if and when life-sustaining treatments can be withheld or withdrawn based on a patient's previously expressed wishes (In re Quinlan 1976; Cruzan v. Director, Missouri Department of Health 1990). Even in modern critical care practice, ethical, legal, and professional debates continue about what ICU-based technologies – such as extracorporeal membranous oxygenation (ECMO) – constitute the boundary of acceptable medical care and in what circumstances those technologies could or should be deployed (Fan et al. 2016).

There has been important regional variation in how decisions have been made regarding withholding and withdrawing life support. For example, a study across Europe conducted in the early 2000s found that much higher proportion of deaths were preceded by withdrawing life support in Northern Europe compared to Southern Europe, while withholding life support was more common in Southern Europe (Sprung et al. 2003). Withdrawal of life support is also less common in many countries in Asia, Africa, and South America. Some of these differences are undoubtedly driven by religious influences (Sprung et al. 2007). However, it is important to note that there is also considerable variability within countries or even among physicians in a single ICU suggesting that lack of consensus and limited education play an important role in this variability (Mark et al. 2015). A recent study suggests that differences are decreasing across Europe, which may be the result of increased consensus and education.

Given these tensions surrounding if and when medical technologies are medically feasible, ethically acceptable, and pragmatically likely to facilitate patient and family medical goals, it is not surprising that early palliative and end-of-life care-related interventions and trials have involved ICUs and ICU patients, family members, and clinicians (Aslakson et al. 2014b). By the late 1980s, a hospital in the state of Michigan in the United States began to evaluate whether a "comprehensive supportive team" for "hopelessly ill" ICU patients, primarily those with hypoxic encephalopathy and advanced dementia, could improve the quality of care and end-of-life care through focused provision of physical comfort, psychosocial support, and family support (Field et al. 1989; Carlson et al. 1988). Through the early to mid-1990s, further ICU-based, palliative care-related interventions, often led by nurses, trialed whether enhanced communication strategies – informational booklets, daily phone calls to family members, and/or goal-related communication between ICU clinicians and family members – could improve family member-related outcomes such as satisfaction, anxiety, and/or informational awareness. By the late 1990s and early 2000s, the modern era and definitions of palliative care and palliative care practices commenced and consequently spurred a cohort of trials attempting to integrate palliative care principles, and sometimes palliative care specialists providers, into routine ICU care.

3 Defining Palliative Care in the ICU for the Coming Decade

Palliative care is a rapidly growing interprofessional specialty as well as an approach to care by all clinicians who care for patients with serious illness. The key domains of palliative care in the adult ICU, which have been defined by patients and families (Nelson et al. 2010a) as well as by expert consensus (National Consensus Project for Quality Palliative Care 2013; Clarke et al. 2003), include effective management of distress from physical, psychological, and spiritual symptoms; timely and sensitive communication about appropriate goals of intensive care in relation to the patient's condition, prognosis, and values; alignment of treatment with patient values; attention to families' needs and concerns; planning for care transitions; and support for clinicians. Palliative care is often optimally provided together with life-prolonging care, a coordinated approach that has been supported by major societies representing critical care professionals (Lanken et al. 2008; Selecky et al. 2005; Truog et al. 2008; Carlet et al. 2004; Cox et al. 2007, 2009; Choi et al. 2014; Puntillo et al. 2010) and by the World Health Organization (2018) and that is embraced by patients and families (Nelson et al. 2010a). Therefore, palliative care is not a mutually exclusive alternative, nor simply a sequel to failed attempts at life-prolonging care, but rather an integral component of comprehensive care for critically ill patients from the time of ICU admission.

4 Delivery Models of Palliative Care

Palliative care can be in many different clinical settings and can be provided by the following (Nelson et al. 2010b; Quill and Abernethy 2013; Committee on Approaching Death: Addressing Key End of Life Issues; Institute of Medicine 2015):

- Frontline, nonspecialist providers (termed primary or generalist palliative care)
- A specialist, interdisciplinary team with advanced training and skills in symptom management and communication about goals of care, prognosis, and treatment options (termed specialty or consultative palliative care)
- Some combination of both (termed mixed)

This conceptualization is particularly relevant for delivery of palliative care in the ICU (Fig. 1). The ICU team itself is inherently interdisciplinary

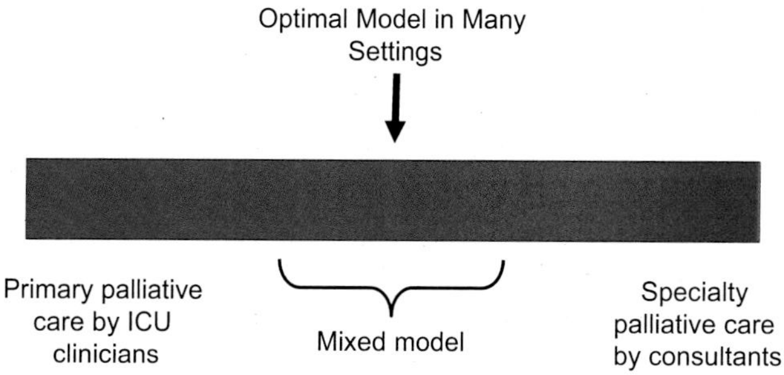

Fig. 1 Conceptualization of palliative care delivery model spectrum – optimal model is based on availability of specialty palliative care and on ICU primary palliative care expertise

and often includes doctors, nurses, social workers, chaplains, respiratory therapists, and pharmacists who are trained and specially skilled to address the unique needs of critically ill patients and their families (Nelson et al. 2010b). In mixed palliative care in the ICU, the primary palliative care provided by this ICU team is further supplemented by care provided by the specialty palliative care interdisciplinary team (Nelson et al. 2010b).

Core elements of palliative care, such as basic symptom management and discussion of goals of care in relation to the patient's prognosis and preferences, should be part of routine critical care practice and within the competency of all ICU clinicians. However, sometimes the optimal care of a critically ill patient may call for more advanced palliative care skills and specialist expert input. Goal setting with a family experiencing unusual distress or internal conflict, symptom management for patients with refractory symptomatology, supporting a bereaved family, or providing continuity of care after the patient is discharged from the ICU are examples of clinical challenges for which a critical care clinician may wish to obtain expert consultation from a palliative care specialist team (Quill and Abernethy 2013). In addition, sometimes a palliative care specialist can serve as a "third party" to help mediate conflict between the ICU team and the patient or family.

After more than a decade of rapid expansion, expert palliative care through a palliative care consultation is now available at the majority of US hospitals, although smaller and/or for-profit hospitals are less likely to have palliative care consult services. Availability of hospital-based palliative care consult services is much more variable in Europe, Asia, and South America although developing in many areas, and where they are developed, they often have less interaction with the ICU than in the United States. Specialty palliative care services have often developed from within oncology, geriatrics, or primary care and may consequently have less experience and integration in the ICU setting. However, as interest in improving palliative care in the ICU increases, this setting can offer an opportunity for palliative care specialists to increase their presence, both in supporting better primary palliative care through ICU clinician education and provision of supportive tools and also in providing specialty palliative care consultation for patients and family members with unmet palliative needs after primary palliative care.

Workforce shortages for palliative care specialists may limit availability of palliative care consultations, at least in the near term (Goldsmith et al. 2008). In addition, excessive reliance on specialty palliative care could fragment care, potentially complicate therapeutic relationships between patients and ICU care clinicians, as well as diminish impetus for ICU clinicians to cultivate and maintain primary palliative care skills (Accreditation Council for Graduate Medical Education 2018). Indeed, a key issue for palliative care in the ICU is to determine how best to utilize existing specialist palliative care resources as well as how to optimally integrate those resources into existing primary palliative care practices and pathways.

Previous palliative care trials in the ICU have frequently used triggers to identify which patients should receive specialist palliative care (Aslakson et al. 2014b). In past trials, triggers have included both diagnoses, such as hypoxic encephalopathy, multiple organ failure for multiple days, or advanced dementia, as well as non-specific assessments such as ICU clinician belief that a patient is "likely to die" and/or intra-ICU team conflicts regarding a patient's likely survival and/or quality of life following critical illness. Ultimately, the provision of primary versus specialist palliative care should be fluid over time, unique to each ICU, and based on multiple factors including unit culture toward palliative and end-of-life care, ICU clinician primary palliative care competence and capacity, the availability of palliative care specialist resources, ICU patient and family desire for specialist palliative care, and/or systematic triggers or goals championed by ICU and/or hospital clinicians and leadership.

When specialty palliative care clinicians are interested in increasing their impact in the ICU setting, either through supporting primary palliative care or providing specialty palliative care consultation, it is very important that the palliative care clinicians become familiar with the functioning and culture of the ICU. In our experience, two key barriers to effective palliative care consultation in the ICU setting include ICU clinician suspicion that palliative care clinicians will advance an agenda of withholding or withdrawing life support and belief among some ICU clinicians that they already provide high-quality primary palliative care. Understanding such barriers is essential to overcoming them. For example, in the ICU where ICU clinicians are suspicious of the agenda of palliative care clinicians, reassuring ICU clinicians about the lack of such an agenda is essential. However, in the ICU where ICU clinicians believe they provide high-quality primary palliative care, the key to overcoming this barrier is to highlight areas of palliative care that the ICU clinicians are less focused on, such as anticipatory bereavement support and supporting palliative care needs after ICU discharge.

5 Palliative Care Needs Both Within and After the ICU

In this chapter, we focus on studies conducted in adult ICUs in North America and Europe, where existing data demonstrate important opportunities to improve all core components of palliative care in the ICU. For example, multiple studies confirm that symptom distress is prevalent at high levels of severity among critically ill patients (Puntillo et al. 2010, 2014; Puntillo 1990). Communication between clinicians and families is often delayed and fragmented (White et al. 2007; Azoulay et al. 2000; McDonagh et al. 2004). When families meet with ICU physicians, they frequently have insufficient time to share their perspectives on the patient's goals and values or express their own concerns (McDonagh et al. 2004). ICU physicians may miss opportunities for empathic response to emotions, leaving families too distressed to absorb or integrate information they need for surrogate decision-making (Curtis et al. 2005; Selph et al. 2008). Some patients spend their last days in the ICU because planning for care in a more suitable or preferred setting is inadequate. In addition, transitions from one setting to another (e.g., acute care, critical care, long-term care, and home care) are increasingly frequent but often without adequate support for patients and families (Teno et al. 2013). Among those who require prolonged mechanical ventilation, data show that during the year following ICU discharge, patients will make multiple transitions across a variety of facilities, spending an average of 74% of all days in a hospital or post-acute care facility or dependent on a high level of home healthcare (Unroe et al. 2010). Finally, the need to support ICU clinicians more effectively for the emotional strain of ICU practice is evident from the widespread problems of burnout, depression, moral distress, and conflict across disciplines on the critical care team (Azoulay et al. 2009; Studdert et al. 2003a, b; Breen et al. 2001).

The burden of critical illness for patients and family members continues after the ICU. Decreases in hospital mortality from critical illnesses, such as sepsis, acute respiratory distress syndrome (ARDS), and major cardiac or neurologic events, have not diminished the relevance of palliative care in the ICU but rather underscored the importance of anticipating and attending to the palliative care needs of those who survive intensive care as well as those who succumb. As ICU survivors increase in number and investigators examine the experience of these patients and their families more fully, the burdens of survivorship are coming into clearer view (Needham et al. 2012). A broad array of physical and psychological symptoms along with impairments of function and cognition continue to impair the quality of patients' lives (Cox et al. 2009; Choi et al. 2014; Herridge et al. 2003, 2011; Iwashyna et al. 2010; Davydow et al. 2008, 2009; Adhikari et al. 2011; Dowdy et al. 2006; Pandharipande et al. 2013; Boyle et al. 2004). During the 1st year after ICU discharge, ARDS survivors commonly report debilitating insomnia, fatigue, and pain along with emotional lability, depression, and anxiety (Cox et al. 2009). In addition to ongoing functional limitations and decrements in physical quality of life, these survivors have psychological sequelae for as long as 5 years (Herridge et al. 2011). A systematic review of depression in general ICU survivors found that the median point prevalence of clinically significant depressive symptoms within 14 months of ICU discharge was 28%, and depression in the early post-ICU period predicted longer-term depressive symptoms (Davydow et al. 2009). ICU survivors also struggle with chronic pain that is associated with decrements in health-related quality of life (Boyle et al. 2004). New and clinically significant cognitive impairment follows critical illness for a broad range of survivors (Pandharipande et al. 2013). Some ICU patients surviving acute critical illness remain critically ill on a chronic basis, with protracted or permanent dependence on mechanical ventilation and other intensive care therapies (Nelson et al. 2010c). For this "chronically critically ill" patient group, symptom burden is heavy, functional and cognitive outcomes are very poor, and 1-year mortality is over 50%, exceeding that for many malignancies (Nelson et al. 2004, 2006a; Jubran et al. 2010). Families struggle with their own symptoms and with strains of caregiving (Cox et al. 2009; Needham et al. 2012; de Miranda et al. 2011; Swoboda and Lipsett 2002; Van Pelt et al. 2007; Choi et al. 2011; Pochard et al. 2005). Among family members of critically ill patients, anxiety and depression are common and may persist long after the ICU, along with post-traumatic stress disorder and complicated grief (Anderson et al. 2008; Siegel et al. 2008; Pochard et al. 2005). Thus, a distinctive "postintensive care syndrome" is now recognized not only in patients but also in families (Needham et al. 2012). Effective integration of palliative care during the treatment of acute and chronic critical illness may help patients and families prepare more fully for challenges to come in the days, months, and years after discharge from intensive care.

In addition, the use of intensive care for patients approaching the end of life continues. Approximately one in five deaths in the United States occurs during or shortly after intensive care, with more deaths occurring in the ICU than in any other setting in the hospital (Angus et al. 2004). In the United States, patients over age 65 with severe chronic illness are less likely to die in the hospital and more likely to receive hospice care than they were a decade ago, but ICU treatment during the last month of life has concurrently increased (Teno et al. 2013; Goodman et al. 2011). For patients over age 65 receiving ICU treatment, particularly among those who are mechanically ventilated, the risk of death within 3 years of discharge is nearly three times that of matched controls in the general population (Wunsch et al. 2010). These trends are likely to continue as aggressive medical and surgical treatments are offered to a growing population of older adults with multiple comorbid conditions. For now and the foreseeable future, palliative care will thus remain an essential element of critical care practice, both during and after ICU admission.

6 The Modern Era of Palliative Care in the ICU: Evaluating the Evidence Base

Data for this chapter were drawn from systematic and comprehensive narrative reviews as well as a recent research agenda on palliative care in the ICU (Aslakson et al. 2014a, b, 2017; Khandelwal et al. 2015; Scheunemann et al. 2011). Interventions can be grouped into broad domains based on the intervention target – ICU patient, family members, ICU clinician team, system, and/or multilevel (Table 1) – although some interventions are "bundled" with multiple targets. Interventions can also be organized based on content and goals. It is important for palliative care specialists interested in supporting patients and families in the ICU to understand this evidence base for both primary and specialty palliative care in the ICU.

Structured approaches to communication. Interventional research to date has focused mainly on testing proactive, structured approaches to clinician communication with families, implemented either by the interdisciplinary ICU team or by consultants specializing in palliative care or biomedical ethics (Aslakson et al. 2014b; Curtis et al. 2016; Andereck et al. 2014; Carson et al. 2016). This research has been summarized in several comprehensive reviews (Aslakson et al. 2014b; Khandelwal et al. 2015; Scheunemann et al. 2011). Most studies were conducted in a single center using a pre-post design. In those studies, the communication

Table 1 Examples of ICU-based palliative care interventions and representative studies

Primary target	Examples	Summary of findings	Sample of references
Patient	NONE		
Family	Intervention booklet for family; intensive nurse-, social worker-, or physician-led communication; standardized or structured family meetings; family support coordinator or navigator; family presence during ICU rounds	Mixed – no effect or change in family satisfaction or depression scores, reduced ICU length-of-stay, reduced nonconsensus between ICU clinicians and families; increased DNR and comfort care orders; increased order choosing "aggressive" interventions; improved frequency of communication with ICU providers; decreased ICU costs	Daly et al. 1994; Lilly et al. 2000; Lilly et al. 2003; Azoulay et al. 2002; Burns et al. 2003; Curtis et al. 2016
Clinician team	Education about ethics; education about communication skills; Palliative care team rounds with ICU team	Increased proportion of ICU patients receiving palliative care consultation; reduced ICU length-of-stay	Holloran et al. 1995; Villarreal et al. 2011
System	Palliative care or comfort care order set	No change; increased pastoral care involvement; reduced hospital length-of-stay	Treece et al. 2004; Hall et al. 2004
Multi-level	Palliative care consultation; ethics team consultation; transition of patient out from ICU team to "comprehensive support care team"; ICU clinician education about communication and more frequent and intensive communication with family; clinician education about palliative care communication with designation of local champions and standardized comfort care order sets; communication facilitator	No change; reduced ICU and hospital length-of-stay; reduced treatment intensity; reduced depression, anxiety, and PTSD prevalence among family members; improved nurse quality of death and dying scores; increased frequency of family conferences; increased frequency of prognosis being discussed in family conferences; increased DNR status designation	Carlson et al. 1988; Field et al. 1989; Schneiderman et al. 2000; Campbell and Guzman 2003; Schneiderman et al. 2003; Campbell and Guzman 2004; Lautrette et al. 2007; Norton et al. 2007; Curtis et al. 2008; Curtis et al. 2011

interventions were associated with significant reductions in resource utilization (e.g., shorter ICU length of stay) without increases in mortality, as well as with decreases in discord among decision-makers for ICU patients. However, in one of the largest pre-post studies conducted in five ICUs in two academic medical centers which tested the effect of regular, structured family meetings for patients in the ICU for 5 days or more, there was no significant reduction in ICU length of stay or other utilization outcomes (Daly et al. 2010). Importantly, a multicenter, randomized trial testing a protocol-based strategy for family meetings together with a brochure addressing bereavement found that family members had significant decreases in depression, anxiety, and post-traumatic stress disorder at 3 months after the death of a loved one in the ICU (Cox et al. 2012). Informational brochures have also been independently evaluated and shown in a multicenter, prospective randomized trial to improve family comprehension and satisfaction with information provided by ICU clinicians (Azoulay et al. 2002). These studies suggest that a structured approach to communication with patients and family members in the ICU is one of the most important targets for primary and specialty palliative care interventions.

Support for families and surrogate decision-making. A number of interventions have been designed to support families of ICU patients through increased involvement of the families or more explicit support for surrogate decision-making (Aslakson et al. 2014b; Scheunemann et al. 2011; Curtis et al. 2016; Carson et al. 2016). Examples include an intervention promoting greater involvement of family members in patient care rounds, a critical care family assistance program, a social worker specifically counseling and supporting ICU families, an ICU family clinic, a communicator facilitator to support ICU families, and a palliative care specialty-trained communicator to convene prognosis-related meetings for family meetings of chronically critically ill patients. Although results vary across studies, these studies suggest such interventions are promising and require further evaluation.

Decision support tools. Several tools have been developed to support surrogate decision-making in the ICU. For example, a short video to support decision-making about resuscitation increased surrogates' knowledge of CPR and the proportion of patients with DNR directives at the time of ICU discharge or death (McCannon et al. 2012). An ICU admission assessment tool to help identify surrogate decision-makers and clarify decision-making standards was associated with shorter LOS and lower total hospital charges for patients requiring mechanical ventilation for 4 days or more (Hatler et al. 2012). A decision aid for surrogates of patients on prolonged mechanical ventilation was associated with less discordance between physicians and surrogates as well as with improved quality of communication as perceived by families and lower hospital costs (Cox et al. 2012). Decision support tools are likely an important area for future research.

ICU diaries, order sets, and "death rounds." Some additional tools have been evaluated to support patients, families, and clinicians. A randomized, controlled multicenter study in Europe evaluated an intervention in which healthcare staff and family contributed to a handwritten diary including photographs that recorded events and experiences on a daily basis during the patient's ICU stay and was provided to the patient 1 month after ICU discharge (Jones et al. 2010). As measured at 3 months after the ICU, this intervention significantly reduced the incidence of new-onset post-traumatic stress disorder among survivors of critical illness when compared to usual care. Another tool included the development of standardized order sets to support clinicians, prepare families, and ensure patient comfort during limitation of life support (Treece et al. 2004). Regular sessions for ICU clinician debriefing after patient deaths have been evaluated for supporting clinicians (Hough et al. 2005). Evidence supports use of these types of tools to support patients, family members, and ICU clinicians.

Multifaceted quality improvement. Multifaceted quality improvement approaches have also been used to improve palliative care in the ICU. The largest and most rigorous study to date was a multicenter, cluster randomized controlled trial that tested a multicomponent intervention comprising education of ICU clinicians, identification of local palliative care "champions" in the ICU, standardization of palliative care order sets, and feedback to ICU clinicians about palliative care-related outcomes. Although this intervention was initially successful at the investigators' own center (Curtis et al. 2008), the multicenter cluster randomized trial found no differences in outcomes including quality of dying as assessed by families or nurses, family satisfaction, ICU length of stay before death, or time from ICU admission to withdrawal of life-sustaining therapies (Curtis et al. 2011). These studies suggest that such interventions may be more successful when generated by and targeted for the needs of each institution.

Tailoring of palliative care interventions for sub-specialty ICUs. A few studies and expert opinion-informed guidelines have addressed further unique palliative care barriers and needs in sub-specialty types of ICUs. Existing data describe cultural tension surrounding palliative and end-of-life care among surgical providers and in surgical intensive care units (Buchman 2010; Buchman et al. 2002, 2003; Cassell et al. 2003a; Olson et al. 2013; Schwarze et al. 2010, 2013). Not surprisingly, studies demonstrate lower utilization of specialist palliative care providers among surgical patient populations (Rodriguez et al. 2015), and a systematic review of palliative care in surgical populations notes relatively few trials and that most existing trials are small and of low to moderate quality (Lilley et al. 2016). Nonetheless, expert opinion supports thoughtful tailoring of palliative care interventions to surgical intensive care units (Lilley et al. 2017; Mosenthal et al. 2012). In addition, existing data regarding specialist palliative care interventions in surgical intensive care units is promising. A single center, before-after study tested a multifaceted interdisciplinary intervention to integrate palliative care into standard care in a trauma ICU. After the intervention, symptom management and goals of care were discussed more frequently on rounds, and while ICU mortality was unchanged, the intervention was associated with shorter length of stay in the ICU and hospital for patients who died. A similar intervention in the same institution for liver transplant surgical ICU patients was associated with earlier consensus around goals of care, earlier and more frequent use of DNR and withdrawal of life-sustaining treatment order, and shorter surgical ICU length of stay, with unchanged mortality. Further expert statements address tailoring of palliative care in both neurocritical care units and burn critical care units (Frontera et al. 2015; Ray et al. 2017).

7 Opportunities and Challenges for ICU Palliative Care Improvement

Ongoing challenges for optimal integration of palliative care in ICU settings have been identified and it is important that palliative care specialists interested in supporting critically ill patients, family members, and clinicians understand these challenges (Kirchhoff and Beckstrand 2000; Nelson 2006; Fassier et al. 2005). In a survey of a large, nationally representative sample of nurse and physician directors of US adult ICUs, respondents reported on perceived barriers at the level of the patient/family, clinician, and institution (Nelson 2006). Important barriers included unrealistic expectations on the part of patients, families, and clinicians about patient prognosis or effectiveness of ICU treatment, inability of patients to participate in treatment discussions, insufficient training of physicians in relevant communication skills, and competing demands for clinicians' time. Similar perspectives have been articulated by critical care professionals in Europe, along with distinct issues facing these clinicians including cultural variations across different European countries as well as a history of more decision-making by clinicians, and less involvement of families, as compared to North American settings (Fassier et al. 2005).

Special challenges for efforts to integrate palliative care in surgical ICU settings care have been noted. These include surgeons' strong sense of personal responsibility for patient outcomes (Buchman et al. 2002; Cassell et al. 2003b), disparate surgical provider opinions about the adequacy of communication regarding prognosis (Aslakson et al. 2010), and what has been described as a "covenantal" relationship in which the surgeon commits to protect the patient and the patient commits to endure the operation and sequelae (Buchman 2010; Cassell et al. 2003b). In a national survey of surgeons, more than 40% reported conflict with intensive care physicians and nurses with respect to appropriate goals of postoperative care (Olson et al. 2013). In addition, many responding surgeons described difficulties in managing clinical aspects of poor outcomes, communicating with the family and patient about such outcomes, and coping with their own discomfort about these outcomes (Olson et al. 2013).

8 Surrogate Decision-Making

The vast majority of ICU patients are incapacitated and dependent on family or other surrogates for medical decision-making (Nelson et al. 2006a; Prendergast and Luce 1997). Qualitative studies are increasingly illuminating the perspectives, concerns, and needs of these surrogates (Schenker et al. 2013; Boyd 2010; Evans et al. 2009; Apatira et al. 2008; Schenker et al. 2012). Most surrogates favor timely discussion of prognosis by ICU clinicians as necessary for decision-making as well as for emotional and practical preparation for the possibility that the patient could die (Apatira et al.

2008). Surrogates appear to recognize and accept that uncertainty about prognosis is unavoidable yet still wish to discuss expected outcomes (Herridge et al. 2003). At the same time, they experience intrapersonal tensions, acknowledging that information about an unfavorable prognosis may be painful as well as helpful (Schenker et al. 2012, 2013). Surrogate behaviors in response to these tensions include focusing on details rather than the larger picture, relying on personal instincts or beliefs, and, at times, rejecting prognostic information (Schenker et al. 2013; Nelson et al. 2017). Awareness of surrogates' perspectives may help ICU and palliative care clinicians more fully address their concerns and needs, thereby facilitating effective shared decision-making. Palliative care specialists can play an important role in helping ICU clinicians understand and address these concerns and needs.

ICU clinician approaches that maximize family-centered communication, provide support for families, and incorporate active listening are associated with increased family satisfaction, improved surrogate decision-making, and psychological well-being of surrogates (McDonagh et al. 2004; Curtis et al. 2005; West et al. 2005; Stapleton et al. 2006). Palliative care specialists can play a key role in supporting these approaches. Based on qualitative research and expert opinion, clinicians are encouraged to help surrogates "plan for the worst" while "hoping for the best" (Back et al. 2003). Other communication strategies suggested by existing evidence include explicit expression of empathy (Selph et al. 2008; Pollak et al. 2007); affirmative exploration of family concerns and comprehension with adequate time for listening by clinicians (White et al. 2007; Azoulay et al. 2000; McDonagh et al. 2004); assurance that the patient will not be abandoned or allowed to suffer should life-sustaining treatments be withdrawn (West et al. 2005; Stapleton et al. 2006); support for critical decisions made by family members, such as whether the patient would want to limit or continue life-sustaining therapies (Stapleton et al. 2006; Back et al. 2005); and, when possible, advance care planning discussions between surrogates and high-risk patients prior to the need for ICU care or the next episode of critical illness (Majesko et al. 2012).

9 Operationalizing Core Palliative Care Components as Measures of ICU Quality

As interest in value-based care rises, ICU and palliative care clinicians are increasingly working together to implement palliative care quality measures in the ICU. Key domains of ICU palliative care quality have been identified and made operational as specific measures that focus on care processes and outcomes (Mularski et al. 2006; Aslakson and Bridges 2013). Focusing primarily on processes, the "Care and Communication Bundle" was developed and tested as part of a national performance improvement initiative by the Voluntary Hospital Association (VHA), Inc. (Nelson et al. 2006b). The measures in this bundle are triggered by time periods in the ICU, with emphasis on proactive, early performance of key processes (e.g., identify medical decision-maker and resuscitation status before Day 2 in the ICU, offer social work and spiritual care support before Day 4, and conduct an interdisciplinary family meeting no later than Day 5). Specifications are precise (e.g., the family meeting measure defines "interdisciplinary" as including at least the attending physician; a member of another discipline such as a nurse, social worker, or chaplain; and the patient and/or his or her family, as documented in the medical record, and must include discussion of prognosis, goals of care, and the patient's and family's needs and preferences) (Nelson et al. 2006b). Similar Day 1 and Day 3 communication measures were tested in a statewide ICU collaborative project in Rhode Island (Black et al. 2013). Significant increases were seen in compliance with these measures, while improvements in compliance varied across ICU type with less improvement in open, nonteaching, and mixed medical-surgical ICUs. Most patient-specific outcome measures were unchanged, although there was an increase in patients discharged from ICU to inpatient hospice. Additional studies evaluating performance on ICU palliative care quality measures show wide variation both within and across hospitals and even within individual intensive care units, as well as low performance levels overall on most items and little improvement over recent years (Penrod et al. 2011, 2012; De Cato et al. 2013).

The quality of ICU palliative care should also be evaluated by structure and outcome measures in addition to process measures (Curtis et al. 2006; Pronovost et al. 2001). The relationship of ICU palliative care process measures to desired patient and family outcomes requires further investigation.

10 Resources Available to Support Integrating Palliative Care and Critical Care

Training opportunities for ICU clinicians. Several interventions have focused on training ICU clinicians to deliver palliative care more effectively. Some approaches include communication skills training (Lilly et al. 2000, 2003; Lautrette et al. 2007; Norton et al. 2007) and education on ethics and conflict resolution (Schneiderman et al. 2003; Browning et al. 2007). These training programs are often conducted or supported by palliative care specialists. For intensivists and hospitalists in the United States, the Harvard Medical School Center for Palliative Care offers an annual two-and-half-day course that provides clinicians with information and skills needed to offer high-quality palliative care to critically ill patients and their families. "Critical Care Communication" (C3), another intensive course focusing specifically on communication skills, was offered to physicians training in critical care at the University of Pittsburgh. In workshops for pediatric critical care providers, the "Program to Enhance Relational and Communication Skills" used "parent-actors" to simulate pediatric, values-based, and/or end-of-life conversations (Browning et al. 2007; Meyer et al. 2009). The VitalTalk program offers specific communication training on palliative care and communication skills and also offers a smartphone-based supplemental application. A 1-day workshop was developed specifically to train bedside critical care nurses in skills they need for active and effective participation along with physicians in interdisciplinary meetings with ICU families (Krimshtein et al. 2011). Of nurses receiving this training and surveyed before and after it ($n = 74$), the average proportion self-rating skills as "very good/excellent" rose significantly, and almost all nurses reported that, after training, they had an increased awareness of special contributions they could make and felt more able to initiate interdisciplinary family meetings. The End-of-Life Nursing Education Consortium (ELNEC), an international education initiative to improve palliative care, has developed a critical care-specific course for nurses. A before-after study in three medical and surgical ICUs in a single community hospital tested a 90-min program of interdisciplinary team training to enhance communication with ICU families (Curtis et al. 2013). Along with clinicians' confidence in communication with families, family satisfaction with ICU communication improved significantly. Yet, this randomized trial of a communication skills building workshop for residents and nurse practitioners did not show an improvement in the patient- and family-level outcomes. These studies identify questions and challenges with showing improvements in patient and family outcomes with educational interventions. One-day communication training programs for ICU clinicians have also been offered at some European intensive care congresses over the past decade including the European Society of Intensive Care Medicine, although such training programs seem less common in Europe and other parts of the world than the United States.

Web-based resources. Extensive resources for use in ICU palliative care improvement efforts are readily accessible, and palliative care specialists could consider offering these resources to their ICU colleagues. Many of these are available on the Website of The IPAL-ICU Project, which is sponsored by the National Institutes of Health and the Center to Advance Palliative Care (CAPC). This Website is password-protected and requires an institutional or individual membership to CAPC to be able to access the materials. Yet, once accessed, those materials are extensive and include a library of relevant references, a variety of practical improvement tools (e.g., family meeting planner and documentation template, data collection instrument for quality monitoring, pocket cards for guidance on symptom management and communication), materials for patients and families (e.g., family meeting brochure), and links to curricula for professional education. In addition, the IPAL-ICU Advisory Board has published an expanding series of articles addressing key issues for efforts to improve palliative care in different types of critical care settings (Nelson et al. 2010b, 2011, 2013, 2015; Puntillo et al. 2014; Mosenthal et al. 2012; Ray et al. 2017; Lustbader et al. 2012).

Professional practice recommendations. Multiple societies representing critical care professionals have published practice recommendations and/or guidelines related to important aspects of ICU palliative care, and these are evidence-based and extensively referenced (Lanken et al. 2008; Selecky et al. 2005; Truog et al. 2008; Carlet et al. 2004; Davidson et al. 2017; Mularski et al. 2013; Mahler et al. 2010; Barr et al. 2013; Yancy et al. 2017; Holloway et al. 2014). Palliative care specialists may be able to use these practice recommendations and guidelines to support improved primary and specialty palliative care in the ICU. For example, the American College of Critical Care Medicine has published consensus recommendations for end-of-life care in the intensive care unit (Truog et al. 2008), as well as clinical practice guidelines for support of the family in the patient-centered intensive care unit (Davidson et al. 2017) and for management of pain, agitation, and delirium (Barr et al. 2013). Similarly, the American Thoracic Society (ATS) published a clinical policy statement on palliative care for patients with respiratory diseases and critical illnesses (Lanken et al. 2008). The American College of Chest Physicians (ACCP) published a position statement on palliative and end-of-life care for patients with cardiopulmonary diseases (Griffin et al. 2007). In addition, both ATS and ACCP have specifically addressed the management of dyspnea (Mularski et al. 2013; Mahler et al. 2010). The American Heart Association (AHA) and American College of Cardiology Foundation included palliative care in their management plan for patients with severe heart failure (Yancy et al. 2017), and the AHA and American Stroke Association have published a statement advocating for palliative care for stroke patients (Holloway et al. 2014). Finally, among five recommendations published as part of the 2014 "Choosing Wisely" campaign, the Critical Care Societies Collaborative recommends that clinicians not "continue life support for patients at high risk for death or severely impaired functional recovery without offering patients and their families the alternative of care focused entirely on comfort" (Halpern et al. 2014). These and other resources can help ICU and palliative care clinicians to strengthen their knowledge and skills and support integration of primary and specialty palliative care as a routine part of critical care practice.

Synergy with family-centered care interventions. Over the past decade, efforts to improve family-centered care in the ICU have burgeoned concurrent to those to improve delivery of palliative care in the ICU (Davidson et al. 2017). Indeed, as psychosocial support of family members is a key component of palliative care, so the two are different facets of the same entity, and interventions to improve family-centered ICU care cannot help but to advance palliative care – often primarily palliative care – content and to improve integration of palliative care practices and providers into ICU care practices.

11 Conclusion and Summary

Palliative care evaluates and treats patient symptoms, provides psychosocial support for patients and families, and identifies and integrates a patient's personal goals into medical treatment. Over the last two decades, intervention studies have explored how to better provide palliative care together with critical care, including incorporating palliative care specialists and supporting critical care clinicians in the delivery of primary palliative care. Moreover, efforts to improve family-centered care in the ICU are synergistic with those to improve palliative care. Evidence supports the benefits of palliative care in the critical care setting, although the most effective and efficient ways to achieve these benefits are not yet clear. Critical care professional society statements call for delivery of primary palliative care by ICU clinicians as well as provision of specialist palliative care, when needed. Existing educational tools and resources enable ICU clinicians to improve their palliative care knowledge and skills and to help palliative care clinicians identify opportunities to support critically ill patients, their families, and their ICU clinicians. Future research is needed to better determine how best to provide palliative care to critically ill patients and their families both in the ICU and beyond.

References

Accreditation Council for Graduate Medical Education. Program requirements for graduate medical education in hospice and palliative medicine. 2018. Available from http://www.acgme.org/Portals/0/PFAssets/ProgramRequirements/540_hospice_and_palliative_medicine_2017-07-01.pdf?ver=2017-05-03-135824-423. Accessed 15 April 2018.

Adhikari NKJ, et al. Self-reported depressive symptoms and memory complaints in survivors five years after ARDS. Chest. 2011;140(6):1484–93.

Andereck WS, et al. Seeking to reduce nonbeneficial treatment in the ICU: an exploratory trial of proactive ethics intervention*. Crit Care Med. 2014;42(4):824–30.

Anderson WG, et al. Posttraumatic stress and complicated grief in family members of patients in the intensive care unit. J Gen Intern Med. 2008;23(11):1871–6.

Angus DC, et al. Use of intensive care at the end of life in the United States: an epidemiologic study. Crit Care Med. 2004;32(3):638–43.

Apatira L, et al. Hope, truth, and preparing for death: perspectives of surrogate decision makers. Ann Intern Med. 2008;149(12):861–8.

Aslakson RA, Bridges JF. Assessing the impact of palliative care in the intensive care unit through the lens of patient-centered outcomes research. Curr Opin Crit Care. 2013;19(5):504–10.

Aslakson RA, et al. Surgical intensive care unit clinician estimates of the adequacy of communication regarding patient prognosis. Crit Care. 2010;14(6):R218.

Aslakson RA, Curtis JR, Nelson JE. The changing role of palliative care in the ICU. Crit Care Med. 2014a;42(11):2418–28.

Aslakson R, et al. Evidence-based palliative care in the intensive care unit: a systematic review of interventions. J Palliat Med. 2014b;17(2):219–35.

Aslakson RA, et al. Developing a research agenda for integrating palliative care into critical care and pulmonary practice to improve patient and family outcomes. J Palliat Med. 2017;20(4):329–43.

Azoulay E, et al. Half the families of intensive care unit patients experience inadequate communication with physicians. Crit Care Med. 2000;28(8):3044–9.

Azoulay E, et al. Impact of a family information leaflet on effectiveness of information provided to family members of intensive care unit patients: a multicenter, prospective, randomized, controlled trial. Am J Respir Crit Care Med. 2002;165(4):438–42.

Azoulay E, et al. Prevalence and factors of intensive care unit conflicts: the conflicus study. Am J Respir Crit Care Med. 2009;180(9):853–60.

Back AL, Arnold RM, Quill TE. Hope for the best, and prepare for the worst. Ann Intern Med. 2003;138(5):439–43.

Back AL, et al. Approaching difficult communication tasks in oncology. CA Cancer J Clin. 2005;55(3):164–77.

Barr J, et al. Clinical practice guidelines for the management of pain, agitation, and delirium in adult patients in the intensive care unit. Crit Care Med. 2013;41(1):263–306.

Black MD, et al. A multifaceted intervention to improve compliance with process measures for ICU clinician communication with ICU patients and families. Crit Care Med. 2013;41(10):2275–83.

Boyd EA, et al. "It's not just what the doctor tells me:" factors that influence surrogate decision-makers' perceptions of prognosis. Crit Care Med. 2010;38(5):1270–5.

Boyle M, et al. The effect of chronic pain on health related quality of life amongst intensive care survivors. Aust Crit Care. 2004;17(3):104–6. 108-13

Breen CM, et al. Conflict associated with decisions to limit life-sustaining treatment in intensive care units. J Gen Intern Med. 2001;16(5):283–9.

Browning DM, et al. Difficult conversations in health care: cultivating relational learning to address the hidden curriculum. Acad Med. 2007;82(9):905–13.

Buchman TG. Surgeons and their patients near the end of life. Crit Care Med. 2010;38(3):995–6.

Buchman TG, et al. Who should manage the dying patient?: rescue, shame, and the surgical ICU dilemma. J Am Coll Surg. 2002;194(5):665–73.

Buchman TG, et al. Families' perceptions of surgical intensive care. J Am Coll Surg. 2003;196(6):977–83.

Burns JP, et al. Results of a clinical trial on care improvement for the critically ill. Crit Care Med. 2003;31(8):2107–17.

Cameron JI, et al. One-year outcomes in caregivers of critically ill patients. N Engl J Med. 2016;374(19):1831–41.

Campbell ML, Guzman JA. Impact of a proactive approach to improve end-of-life care in a medical ICU. Chest. 2003;123(1):266–71.

Campbell ML, Guzman JA. A proactive approach to improve end-of-life care in a medical intensive care unit for patients with terminal dementia. Crit Care Med. 2004;32(9):1839–43.

Carlet J, et al. Challenges in end-of-life care in the ICU. Statement of the 5th international consensus conference in critical care: Brussels, Belgium, April 2003. Intensive Care Med. 2004;30(5):770–84.

Carlson RW, Devich L, Frank RR. Development of a comprehensive supportive care team for the hopelessly ill on a university hospital medical service. JAMA. 1988;259(3):378–83.

Carson SS, et al. Effect of palliative care-led meetings for families of patients with chronic critical illness: a randomized clinical trial. JAMA. 2016;316(1):51–62.

Cassell J, et al. Surgeons, intensivists, and the covenant of care: administrative models and values affecting care at the end of life- updated...including commentary by Buchman TG and Stewart RM. Crit Care Med. 2003a;31(5):1551–9.

Cassell J, et al. Surgeons, intensivists, and the covenant of care: administrative models and values affecting care at the end of life – updated. Crit Care Med. 2003b;31 (5):1551–7. Discussion 1557-9.

Choi J, et al. Caregivers of the chronically critically ill after discharge from the intensive care unit: six months' experience. Am J Crit Care. 2011;20(1):12–22. Quiz 23.

Choi J, et al. Self-reported physical symptoms in intensive care unit (ICU) survivors: pilot exploration over four months post-ICU discharge. J Pain Symptom Manag. 2014;47(2):257–70.

Clarke EB, et al. Quality indicators for end-of-life care in the intensive care unit. Crit Care Med. 2003;31(9):2255–62.

Committee on Approaching Death: Addressing Key End of Life Issues; Institute of Medicine. Dying in America: improving quality and honoring individual preferences near the end of life. Washington, DC. Copyright 2015 by the National Academy of Sciences. All rights reserved: National Academies Press; 2015.

Cox CE, et al. Differences in one-year health outcomes and resource utilization by definition of prolonged mechanical ventilation: a prospective cohort study. Crit Care. 2007;11(1):R9.

Cox CE, et al. Surviving critical illness: acute respiratory distress syndrome as experienced by patients and their caregivers. Crit Care Med. 2009;37(10):2702–8.

Cox CE, et al. Development and pilot testing of a decision aid for surrogates of patients with prolonged mechanical ventilation. Crit Care Med. 2012;40(8):2327–34.

Cruzan v. Director, Missouri Department of Health, in 110 S Ct 2841; 1990.

Curtis JR, et al. Missed opportunities during family conferences about end-of-life care in the intensive care unit. Am J Respir Crit Care Med. 2005;171(8):844–9.

Curtis JR, et al. Intensive care unit quality improvement: a "how-to" guide for the interdisciplinary team. Crit Care Med. 2006;34(1):211–8.

Curtis JR, et al. Integrating palliative and critical care: evaluation of a quality-improvement intervention. Am J Respir Crit Care Med. 2008;178(3):269–75.

Curtis JR, et al. Effect of a quality-improvement intervention on end-of-life care in the intensive care unit: a randomized trial. Am J Respir Crit Care Med. 2011;183(3):348–55.

Curtis JR, et al. Effect of communication skills training for residents and nurse practitioners on quality of communication with patients with serious illness: a randomized trial. JAMA. 2013;310(21):2271–81.

Curtis JR, et al. Randomized trial of communication facilitators to reduce family distress and intensity of end-of-life care. Am J Respir Crit Care Med. 2016;193 (2):154–62.

Daly K, et al. The effect of two nursing interventions on families of ICU patients. Clin Nurs Res. 1994;3 (4):414–22.

Daly BJ, et al. Effectiveness trial of an intensive communication structure for families of long-stay ICU patients. Chest. 2010;138(6):1340–8.

Davidson JE, et al. Guidelines for family-centered care in the neonatal, pediatric, and adult ICU. Crit Care Med. 2017;45(1):103–28.

Davydow DS, et al. Posttraumatic stress disorder in general intensive care unit survivors: a systematic review. Gen Hosp Psychiatry. 2008;30(5):421–34.

Davydow DS, et al. Depression in general intensive care unit survivors: a systematic review. Intensive Care Med. 2009;35(5):796–809.

de Miranda S, et al. Postintensive care unit psychological burden in patients with chronic obstructive pulmonary disease and informal caregivers: a multicenter study. Crit Care Med. 2011;39(1):112–8.

DeCato TW, et al. Hospital variation and temporal trends in palliative and end-of-life care in the ICU. Crit Care Med. 2013;41(6):1405–11.

Dowdy DW, et al. Quality of life in adult survivors of critical illness: a systematic review of the literature. Intensive Care Med. 2005;31(5):611–20.

Dowdy DW, et al. Quality of life after acute respiratory distress syndrome: a meta-analysis. Intensive Care Med. 2006;32(8):1115–24.

Evans LR, et al. Surrogate decision-makers' perspectives on discussing prognosis in the face of uncertainty. Am J Respir Crit Care Med. 2009;179(1):48–53.

Fan E, et al. Venovenous extracorporeal membrane oxygenation for acute respiratory failure: a clinical review from an international group of experts. Intensive Care Med. 2016;42(5):712–24.

Fassier T, et al. Care at the end of life in critically ill patients: the European perspective. Curr Opin Crit Care. 2005;11(6):616–23.

Field BE, Devich LE, Carlson RW. Impact of a comprehensive supportive care team on management of hopelessly ill patients with multiple organ failure. Chest. 1989;96(2):353–6.

Fried C. Editorial: terminating life support: out of the closet. N Engl J Med. 1976;295(7):390–1.

Frontera JA, et al. Integrating palliative care into the care of neurocritically ill patients: a report from the improving palliative care in the ICU project advisory board and the center to advance palliative care. Crit Care Med. 2015;43(9):1964–77.

Goldsmith B, et al. Variability in access to hospital palliative care in the United States. J Palliat Med. 2008;11(8):1094–102.

Goodman DC, Esty AR, Fisher ES, et al. Trends and variation in end-of-life care for medicare beneficiaries with severe chronic illness. Hanover: The Dartmouth Institute for Health Policy and Clinical Practice; 2011.

Griffin JP, et al. Palliative care consultation, quality-of-life measurements, and bereavement for end-of-life care in patients with lung cancer: ACCP evidence-based clinical practice guidelines (2nd edition). Chest. 2007;132 (3 Suppl):404s–22s.

Hall RI, Rocker GM, Murray D. Simple changes can improve conduct of end-of-life care in the intensive care unit. Can J Anaesth. 2004;51(6):631–6.

Halpern SD, et al. An official American Thoracic Society/ American Association of Critical-Care Nurses/American College of Chest Physicians/Society of Critical Care Medicine policy statement: the choosing wisely (r) top 5 list in critical care medicine. Am J Respir Crit Care Med. 2014;190(7):818–26.

Hatler CW, et al. The effect of completing a surrogacy information and decision-making tool upon admission to an intensive care unit on length of stay and charges. J Clin Ethics. 2012;23(2):129–38.

Herridge MS, et al. One-year outcomes in survivors of the acute respiratory distress syndrome. N Engl J Med. 2003;348(8):683–93.

Herridge MS, et al. Functional disability 5 years after acute respiratory distress syndrome. N Engl J Med. 2011;364 (14):1293–304.

Holloran SD, et al. An educational intervention in the surgical intensive care unit to improve ethical decisions. Surgery. 1995;118(2):294–8. discussion 298-9.

Holloway RG, et al. Palliative and end-of-life care in stroke: a statement for healthcare professionals from the American Heart Association/American Stroke Association. Stroke. 2014;45(6):1887–916.

Hough CL, et al. Death rounds: end-of-life discussions among medical residents in the intensive care unit. J Crit Care. 2005;20(1):20–5.

In re Quinlan, in 755 A2A 647. 1976, cert denied: NJ.

Iwashyna TJ, et al. Long-term cognitive impairment and functional disability among survivors of severe sepsis. JAMA. 2010;304(16):1787–94.

Jones C, et al. Intensive care diaries reduce new onset post traumatic stress disorder following critical illness: a randomised, controlled trial. Crit Care. 2010;14(5): R168.

Jubran A, et al. Depressive disorders during weaning from prolonged mechanical ventilation. Intensive Care Med. 2010;36(5):828–35.

Kelley AS, Morrison RS. Palliative care for the seriously ill. N Engl J Med. 2015;373(8):747–55.

Khandelwal N, et al. Estimating the effect of palliative care interventions and advance care planning on ICU utilization: a systematic review. Crit Care Med. 2015;43 (5):1102–11.

Kirchhoff KT, Beckstrand RL. Critical care nurses' perceptions of obstacles and helpful behaviors in providing end-of-life care to dying patients. Am J Crit Care. 2000;9(2):96–105.

Krimshtein NS, et al. Training nurses for interdisciplinary communication with families in the intensive care unit: an intervention. J Palliat Med. 2011;14(12):1325–32.

Lanken PN, et al. An official American Thoracic Society clinical policy statement: palliative care for patients with respiratory diseases and critical illnesses. Am J Respir Crit Care Med. 2008;177(8):912–27.

Lautrette A, et al. A communication strategy and brochure for relatives of patients dying in the ICU. N Engl J Med. 2007;356(5):469–78.

Lilley EJ, et al. Palliative care interventions for surgical patients: a systematic review. JAMA Surg. 2016;151 (2):172–83.

Lilley EJ, et al. Palliative care in surgery: defining the research priorities. J Palliat Med. 2017;20:702–9.

Lilly CM, et al. An intensive communication intervention for the critically ill. Am J Med. 2000;109(6):469–75.

Lilly CM, et al. Intensive communication: four-year follow-up from a clinical practice study. Crit Care Med. 2003;31(5 Suppl):S394–9.

Luce JM. A history of resolving conflicts over end-of-life care in intensive care units in the United States. Crit Care Med. 2010;38(8):1623–9.

Lustbader DR, et al. Physician reimbursement for critical care services integrating palliative care for patients who are critically ill. Chest. 2012;141(3):787–92.

Mahler DA, et al. American College of Chest Physicians consensus statement on the management of dyspnea in patients with advanced lung or heart disease. Chest. 2010;137(3):674–91.

Majesko A, et al. Identifying family members who may struggle in the role of surrogate decision maker. Crit Care Med. 2012;40(8):2281–6.

Mark NM, et al. Global variability in withholding and withdrawal of life-sustaining treatment in the intensive care unit: a systematic review. Intensive Care Med. 2015;41(9):1572–85.

McCannon JB, et al. Augmenting communication and decision making in the intensive care unit with a cardiopulmonary resuscitation video decision support tool: a temporal intervention study. J Palliat Med. 2012;15(12):1382–7.

McDonagh JR, et al. Family satisfaction with family conferences about end-of-life care in the intensive care unit: increased proportion of family speech is associated with increased satisfaction. Crit Care Med. 2004;32(7):1484–8.

Meyer EC, et al. Difficult conversations: improving communication skills and relational abilities in health care. Pediatr Crit Care Med. 2009;10(3):352–9.

Mosenthal AC, et al. Integrating palliative care in the surgical and trauma intensive care unit: a report from the Improving Palliative Care in the Intensive Care Unit (IPAL-ICU) Project Advisory Board and the Center to Advance Palliative Care. Crit Care Med. 2012;40 (4):1199–206.

Mularski RA, et al. Proposed quality measures for palliative care in the critically ill: a consensus from the Robert Wood Johnson Foundation Critical Care Workgroup. Crit Care Med. 2006;34(11 Suppl): S404–11.

Mularski RA, et al. An official American Thoracic Society workshop report: assessment and palliative management of dyspnea crisis. Ann Am Thorac Soc. 2013;10 (5):S98–106.

National Consensus Project for Quality Palliative Care, editor. Clinical practice guidelines for quality palliative care. 3rd ed. Pittsburgh: National Consensus Project for Quality Palliative Care; 2013.

Needham DM, et al. Improving long-term outcomes after discharge from intensive care unit: report from a stakeholders' conference. Crit Care Med. 2012;40(2):502–9.

Nelson JE. Identifying and overcoming the barriers to high-quality palliative care in the intensive care unit. Crit Care Med. 2006;34(11 Suppl):S324–31.

Nelson JE, et al. The symptom burden of chronic critical illness. Crit Care Med. 2004;32(7):1527–34.

Nelson JE, et al. Brain dysfunction – another burden for the chronically critically ill. Arch Intern Med. 2006a;166 (18):1993–9.

Nelson JE, et al. Improving comfort and communication in the ICU: a practical new tool for palliative care performance measurement and feedback. Qual Saf Health Care. 2006b;15(4):264–71.

Nelson JE, et al. In their own words: patients and families define high-quality palliative care in the intensive care unit. Crit Care Med. 2010a;38(3):808–18.

Nelson JE, et al. Models for structuring a clinical initiative to enhance palliative care in the intensive care unit: a report from the IPAL-ICU Project (Improving Palliative Care in the ICU). Crit Care Med. 2010b;38(9):1765–72.

Nelson JE, et al. Chronic critical illness. Am J Respir Crit Care Med. 2010c;182(4):446–54.

Nelson JE, et al. Integrating palliative care in the ICU: the nurse in a leading role. J Hosp Palliat Nurs. 2011;13 (2):89–94.

Nelson JE, et al. Choosing and using screening criteria for palliative care consultation in the ICU: a report from the Improving Palliative Care in the ICU (IPAL-ICU) Advisory Board. Crit Care Med. 2013;41(10):2318–27.

Nelson JE, et al. Integration of palliative care in the context of rapid response: a report from the Improving Palliative Care in the ICU advisory board. Chest. 2015;147 (2):560–9.

Nelson JE, et al. The voice of surrogate decision-makers. Family responses to prognostic information in chronic critical illness. Am J Respir Crit Care Med. 2017;196 (7):864–72.

Norton SA, et al. Proactive palliative care in the medical intensive care unit: effects on length of stay for selected high-risk patients. Crit Care Med. 2007;35(6):1530–5.

Olson TJP, et al. Surgeon-reported conflict with intensivists about postoperative goals of care. JAMA Surg. 2013;148(1):29–35.

Optimum care for hopelessly ill patients. A report of the clinical care committee of the Massachusetts General Hospital. N Engl J Med. 1976;295(7):362–4.

Pandharipande PP, et al. Long-term cognitive impairment after critical illness. N Engl J Med. 2013;369 (14):1306–16.

Penrod JD, et al. Implementation and evaluation of a network-based pilot program to improve palliative care in the intensive care unit. J Pain Symptom Manag. 2011;42(5):668–71.

Penrod JD, et al. Meeting standards of high-quality intensive care unit palliative care: clinical performance and predictors. Crit Care Med. 2012;40(4):1105–12.

Pochard F, et al. Symptoms of anxiety and depression in family members of intensive care unit patients before discharge or death. A prospective multicenter study. J Crit Care. 2005;20(1):90–6.

Pollak KI, et al. Oncologist communication about emotion during visits with patients with advanced cancer. J Clin Oncol. 2007;25(36):5748–52.

Prendergast TJ, Luce JM. Increasing incidence of withholding and withdrawal of life support from the critically ill. Am J Respir Crit Care Med. 1997;155 (1):15–20.

Pronovost PJ, et al. Developing and implementing measures of quality of care in the intensive care unit. Curr Opin Crit Care. 2001;7(4):297–303.

Puntillo KA. Pain experiences of intensive care unit patients. Heart Lung. 1990;19(5 Pt 1):526–33.

Puntillo KA, et al. Symptoms experienced by intensive care unit patients at high risk of dying. Crit Care Med. 2010;38(11):2155–60.

Puntillo K, et al. Palliative care in the ICU: relief of pain, dyspnea, and thirst – a report from the IPAL-ICU Advisory Board. Intensive Care Med. 2014;40(2):235–48.

Quill TE, Abernethy AP. Generalist plus specialist palliative care – creating a more sustainable model. N Engl J Med. 2013;368(13):1173–5.

Ray DE, et al. Care of the critically ill burn patient. An overview from the perspective of optimizing palliative care. Ann Am Thorac Soc. 2017;14(7):1094–102.

Rodriguez R, et al. Utilization of palliative care consultation service by surgical services. Ann Palliat Med. 2015;4(4):194–9.

Schenker Y, et al. I don't want to be the one saying 'we should just let him die': intrapersonal tensions experienced by surrogate decision makers in the ICU. J Gen Intern Med. 2012;27(12):1657–65.

Schenker Y, et al. "It hurts to know... and it helps": exploring how surrogates in the ICU cope with prognostic information. J Palliat Med. 2013;16(3):243–9.

Scheunemann LP, et al. Randomized, controlled trials of interventions to improve communication in intensive care: a systematic review. Chest. 2011;139(3):543–54.

Scheunemann LP, et al. How clinicians discuss critically ill patients' preferences and values with surrogates: an empirical analysis. Crit Care Med. 2015;43(4):757–64.

Schneiderman LJ, Gilmer T, Teetzel HD. Impact of ethics consultations in the intensive care setting: a randomized, controlled trial. Crit Care Med. 2000;28(12):3920–4.

Schneiderman LJ, et al. Effect of ethics consultations on nonbeneficial life-sustaining treatments in the intensive care setting: a randomized controlled trial. JAMA. 2003;290(9):1166–72.

School, A.H.C.o.t.H.M. A definition of irreversible coma, report of the Ad Hoc Committee of the Harvard Medical School to examine the definition of brain death. JAMA. 1968;205:337–40.

Schwarze ML, Bradley CT, Brasel KJ. Surgical "buy-in": the contractual relationship between surgeons and patients that influences decisions regarding life-supporting therapy. Crit Care Med. 2010;38(3):843–8.

Schwarze ML, et al. Surgeons expect patients to buy-in to postoperative life support preoperatively: results of a national survey. Crit Care Med. 2013;41(1):1–8.

Selecky PA, et al. Palliative and end-of-life care for patients with cardiopulmonary diseases: American College of Chest Physicians position statement. Chest. 2005;128 (5):3599–610.

Selph RB, et al. Empathy and life support decisions in intensive care units. J Gen Intern Med. 2008;23 (9):1311–7.

Siegel MD, et al. Psychiatric illness in the next of kin of patients who die in the intensive care unit. Crit Care Med. 2008;36(6):1722–8.

Silveira MJ, Kim SY, Langa KM. Advance directives and outcomes of surrogate decision making before death. N Engl J Med. 2010;362(13):1211–8.

Sprung CL, et al. End-of-life practices in European intensive care units: the Ethicus study. JAMA. 2003;290 (6):790–7.

Sprung CL, et al. The importance of religious affiliation and culture on end-of-life decisions in European intensive care units. Intensive Care Med. 2007;33(10): 1732–9.

Stapleton RD, et al. Clinician statements and family satisfaction with family conferences in the intensive care unit. Crit Care Med. 2006;34(6):1679–85.

Studdert DM, et al. Nature of conflict in the care of pediatric intensive care patients with prolonged stay. Pediatrics. 2003a;112(3 Pt 1):553–8.

Studdert DM, et al. Conflict in the care of patients with prolonged stay in the ICU: types, sources, and predictors. Intensive Care Med. 2003b;29(9):1489–97.

Swoboda SM, Lipsett PA. Impact of a prolonged surgical critical illness on patients' families. Am J Crit Care. 2002;11(5):459–66.

Teno JM, et al. Change in end-of-life care for Medicare beneficiaries: site of death, place of care, and health care transitions in 2000, 2005, and 2009. JAMA. 2013;309(5):470–7.

Treece PD, et al. Evaluation of a standardized order form for the withdrawal of life support in the intensive care unit. Crit Care Med. 2004;32(5):1141–8.

Truog RD, et al. Recommendations for end-of-life care in the intensive care unit: a consensus statement by the American College [corrected] of Critical Care Medicine. Crit Care Med. 2008;36(3):953–63.

Unroe M, et al. One-year trajectories of care and resource utilization for recipients of prolonged mechanical ventilation: a cohort study. Ann Intern Med. 2010;153 (3):167–75.

Van Pelt DC, et al. Informal caregiver burden among survivors of prolonged mechanical ventilation. Am J Respir Crit Care Med. 2007;175(2):167–73.

Villarreal D, et al. A model for increasing palliative care in the intensive care unit: enhancing interprofessional consultation rates and communication. J Pain Symptom Manag. 2011;42(5):676–9.

West HF, et al. Expressions of nonabandonment during the intensive care unit family conference. J Palliat Med. 2005;8(4):797–807.

White DB, Curtis JR. Establishing an evidence base for physician-family communication and shared decision making in the intensive care unit. Crit Care Med. 2006;34(9):2500–1.

White DB, et al. Toward shared decision making at the end of life in intensive care units: opportunities for improvement. Arch Intern Med. 2007;167(5):461–7.

White DB, et al. Nurse-led intervention to improve surrogate decision making for patients with advanced critical illness. Am J Crit Care. 2012;21(6):396–409.

World Health Organization. 2018. WHO definition of palliative care. Available from: http://www.who.int/cancer/palliative/definition/en/. Accessed 15 April 2018.

Wunsch H, et al. Three-year outcomes for Medicare beneficiaries who survive intensive care. JAMA. 2010;303 (9):849–56.

Yancy CW, et al. 2017 ACC/AHA/HFSA focused update of the 2013 ACCF/AHA guideline for the management of heart failure: a report of the American College of Cardiology/American Heart Association task force on clinical practice guidelines and the Heart Failure Society of America. J Card Fail. 2017;23(8):628–51.

Zier LS, et al. Surrogate decision makers' interpretation of prognostic information: a mixed-methods study. Ann Intern Med. 2012;156(5):360–6.

Palliative Care in Rural Settings

54

Suzanne Rainsford

Contents

S. Rainsford (✉)
Medical School, Australian National University,
Canberra, Australia

Calvary Healthcare Bruce, Clare Holland House Campus,
Canberra, Australia

Sharp Street Surgery, Cooma, NSW, Australia
e-mail: suzanne.rainsford@anu.edu.au

R. D. MacLeod, L. Van den Block (eds.), *Textbook of Palliative Care*,
https://doi.org/10.1007/978-3-319-77740-5_47

Abstract
To ensure the provision of end-of-life care is relevant to individual communities, it must not only reflect the needs of the dying person and their family but also the diverse geography and cultures in which they live. Studies consistently report that rural residents perceive themselves as different to their urban counterparts and clearly hold distinct views on what it means to die well. Currently there is no international consensus on the definition of rurality and remoteness. Rural settings are not homogeneous, and there is considerable individual, cultural, and ethnic diversity both within and between rural locations. Rural communities are close-knit, and known for their social solidarity, community commitment, and loose support networks. While there are many benefits of rural residency, significant challenges exist in the provision of quality end-of-life care. The needs of rural residents are shaped by decreased access and availability of services. While this potentially has a negative influence on outcomes, it is offset by local support networks. Rural palliative care is mostly primary care, with limited access to specialist multidisciplinary palliative care services. Home is the initial preferred place of death for most rural residents; however, when home is not possible, rural hospitals and residential aged care are considered appropriate alternatives, providing they are within ones' community. The universal rural theme is that if rural residents are unable to die at home, then it is essential that their place of death is within their local community.

1 Introduction

To ensure the provision of end-of-life care is relevant to individual communities, it must not only reflect the needs of the dying person and their family but also the diverse geography and cultures in which they live (Bakitas et al. 2015; Cottrell and Duggleby 2016). In general, populations are becoming more urbanized, with the estimated proportion of rural dwellers falling from 70.5% in 1950 to 46% in 2015 (WHO 2014). The highest proportion of rural populations remains in the developing regions, such as sub-Saharan Africa. For example, 84% of Uganda's population is considered rural, compared to 30% in Canada (World Bank 2016). While the size of many individual rural populations is decreasing, they are also aging, often at a faster rate than urban populations. In developed nations, the phenomenon of "sea-change" and "tree-change," adds to the graying of some rural populations, as older urban dwellers leave the cities in search of the more relaxed rural lifestyle (Castleden et al. 2010). Between 2000 and 2030, the growth rate in Australia's population aged 65-years or older is expected to rise by 139%, with a 180% increase anticipated in rural areas (Australian Government Department of Health 2008).

Studies consistently report that rural residents perceive themselves as different to their urban counterparts and clearly hold distinct views on what it means to die well (Wilson et al. 2009a, b; Robinson et al. 2010). In relation to palliative and end-of-life care, rural areas typically have fewer health and social services, as compared to urban areas resulting in substantial differences in the provision of care. As a consequence, some people must move away from their rural community to receive the care required.

Most rural end-of-life research has been focused on healthcare services (intervention studies, needs assessment, program planning and evaluation, education and finances) and professional attitudes, education, and practices (Bakitas et al. 2015). There is also a focus on determining the urban/rural differences, rather than finding ways to explore the unique factors associated with rural health and in particular rural palliative care (Boarders 2017). Currently, there is a paucity of studies documenting rural end-of-life care experiences and perspectives from the recipients of such care – the patients and their family caregivers (Robinson et al. 2009).

The objective of this chapter is to describe palliative care in rural settings. This is a challenge due to the significant heterogeneity between rural settings. While the rural literature contains a number of excellent rural studies undertaken in sub-Saharan Africa and Asia, overall it is biased toward developed nations, especially Canada, the United Kingdom, Australia, and the United States of America. While attempting to remain inclusive, this chapter is written from the perspective of one Australian rural palliative medicine specialist.

This chapter begins by defining "rural" and exploring the challenges of developing a universal consensus on definition. This is followed by a description of rural residents and the nature of palliative healthcare services in rural settings. The challenges and benefits of receiving and delivering palliative care in rural locations are explored. Place of death in rural settings is described. The chapter concludes with a discussion on the concept of the "good" rural death.

2 The Challenges of Defining "Rural"

Currently, there is no international consensus on rural definition or universal rurality or remoteness index. In the absence of homogeneity within health services and cultural context, it is difficult to compare rural areas, not only between countries but also within countries. "Rural" is a multifaceted concept and can be interpreted in a number of ways. Rural settings encompass large towns with services, smaller towns with limited services, villages, hamlets, and farms of varying degrees of isolation, with some locations metro-adjacent or easily accessible to services, and others isolated by geography or weather; some locations are inland and others coastal. Policy-makers and service providers base definitions on population size, population density or demographics, or distance from urban centers and services. For example, since the early 1990s, four different geographic classifications have been developed in Australia (AIHW 2004): Rural, Remote and Metropolitan Areas classification [RRMA, 1994], in which the index of remoteness is based on the straight line distance to service centers and the distance from other people based on population density; Accessibility/Remoteness Index of Australia [ARIA, 1997], based on the road distance from the closest service center; Australian Standard Geographical Classification [ASGC, 2001], which uses the average distance from each populated locality to the closest service center (population 1000–4999 persons), as well as the larger urban service centers; and Modified Monash Model [MMM, 2015], based on ASGS with the additional subdivision of regional Australia into four categories based on the population size. The classification applied has significant implications on funding, service provision, and financial incentives to attract general practitioners to areas of need.

The definition of rural is complex and cannot be limited to geography based on distances from urban service centers or population densities. The provision of palliative care in rural settings is not only influenced by geographical borders and boundaries. In a rural study conducted by Giesbrecht et al. (2016), formal and informal caregivers in rural Canada identified five forms of borders and boundaries that impact on the delivery, and receiving, of palliative care: political (national/federal and state/provincial borders), jurisdictional (formal borders within states/provinces created by different health authorities), geographical (especially in terms of distances and isolation), professional (boundaries between organizations and specialities that determined specific roles of service providers), and cultural (differences in cultural norms, practices, behaviors, and communications, especially those that distinguished differences between rural and urban dwellers and between Aboriginal and non-Aboriginal peoples).

"Rurality" is a term increasingly used to differentiate rural people as a distinct cultural group consisting of "small human communities, whose values of mutual aid and shared history still focus on pride and a sense of belonging to a community, a territory, or family. Rural areas are characterised by dynamic and social, cultural and economic practices centred on proximity, conviviality, mutual aid and cooperation" (Ministere des affaires municipales et des regions du Quebec 2007). While urban dwellers may not acknowledge or appreciate rurality as a separate entity, rural people openly state "that there are important differences between dying in a rural community and dying in a large city" (Wilson et al. 2009b, p. 316).

3 The Characteristics of Rural Residents

Despite significant cultural and ethnic diversity between rural communities, rural people are united by the fact they live in rural areas and believe they have some unique perspectives on, and concerns about, dying well and end-of-life care. Rural and urban residents share the desire for autonomy, a pain-free death, and quality end-of-life care; rural residents frequently have an openness and awareness of death and dying (Wilson et al. 2009a) and have been described as "more accepting of death and less likely to intervene to delay death" (Kirby et al. 2016, p. 1).

Some rural residents perceive differences between those living on farms and those residing in rural towns. Those residents living on farms have been described as more independent, resilient, and adept at problem-solving than rural town dwellers. This resilience (flexibility and the capacity to recover quickly from adversity) and self-reliance (the ability to problem solve rather than relying on others) is not necessarily a personality trait but, more out of necessity, born out of personal experiences and expectations with farmers adept to multitasking and finding novel ways to solve multiple problems.

Rural people are also identified by their deep concern for their community and its members (Kirby et al. 2016). Strong relationships and informal community services are important factors that facilitate end-of-life care within rural communities. The high level of community support fosters a strong sense of belonging and attachment to the community (physical, social, and autobiographical). While "country" has special cultural significance for Aboriginal and Indigenous peoples, many rural dwellers prefer to receive care and die in their community as "being at home is like a brick being in the right place: this is my land and these are my people" (Devik et al. 2015, p. 7). While the rural environment can quickly become unsafe and one of isolation, it has the capacity to be a source of great comfort, security, reassurance, and identity, while for many rural people, the urban environment is viewed negatively (e.g., noisy, unfamiliar, and impersonal).

4 Nature of Rural Palliative Healthcare Services

Quality palliative care is considered the right of every dying person, regardless of where they live (WHO 2015). In 2011, 44.6% of all deaths in the United States of America occurred under hospice (palliative) care (NHPCO 2012). In sub-Saharan Africa, the estimated proportion is less than 5% (Grant et al. 2011). The proportion of rural residents receiving specialist palliative care is significantly lower than for urban residents. The palliative care needs of rural and remote residents "are related to context [. . ..] and are shaped by reduced access and availability of services" (Kirby et al. 2016, p. 1). Access to palliative care services differs widely across rural locations – both within countries and between countries, with the commonality being "gaps" in service provision.

As in any location, primary healthcare providers are pivotal to the provision of rural palliative care. While many of the needs of patients and family caregivers are universal, priorities differ between rural and urban dwellers and between developed and developing nations. The nature of service gaps is dependent on context, with many rural areas, especially in developing countries, lacking the basics of healthcare such as trained primary care health workers, basic medicines (such as morphine), and equipment. In Australia, and other developed countries, increased costs associated with healthcare delivery, decreasing numbers of rural healthcare providers, and centralization of services have all impacted negatively on access to rural and remote healthcare services.

In a number of developed countries, such as Australia, Britain, and Canada, extensive work is being undertaken to address these problems and to ensure palliative care services are provided locally (AIHW 2014).

5 Challenges of Rural Residency

Much of the current rural literature emphasizes the unique challenges associated with rural residency. The obvious challenges relate to isolation and distance from specialist services in major urban centers; however, rural residents face other barriers to receiving quality end-of-life care, as outlined below.

5.1 Distance and Travel

For many rural residents, distance is the greatest negative influence on rural end-of-life care. Many rural patients travel for investigations, diagnosis, and treatment. Commuting can be stressful, exhausting, inconvenient, expensive (Lockie et al. 2010; Pesut et al. 2010; Duggleby et al. 2011; Grant et al. 2011; Devik et al. 2013), and even dangerous or impossible, depending on the weather (Castleden et al. 2010). Despite this, some regard travel for treatment a price for living in a beautiful place, and a compromise they have to make for living at home, that is, "to live in a place that contributes to their overall health" (Wiik 2011, p. 12). While the time taken to reach certain services may be comparable to some urban areas, the actual distances can be considerably more and often at higher speeds. One patient receiving palliative care in rural Australia compared the time taken to travel from her farm to the local hospital, with that of her children who live in the city: "Here you're 20-kilometres but it translates to 15-minutes. In [the city], five-kilometres translates into 15-minutes" (Rainsford 2017, p. 192). While traveling can be acceptable in the early stages of disease, with some residents treating it as "a day out" (Devik et al. 2015), distance and travel become more problematic as patients become more ill and fatigued, when symptoms become more troublesome and when patients enter the terminal phase. Traveling becomes not just an inconvenience but can be associated with physical distress.

Once patients can no longer travel, they often report being disconnected from their specialists (medical, nursing, and allied health), who have been a source of valued support. A time of grieving sometimes follows, for both the patient and their family.

The issues of distance and travel are not just about seeking healthcare support. Distance and travel also impact on family caregivers, regardless of whether they live locally or away. Family caregivers are faced with a number of scenarios while caring for their family member: the out-of-town family having to travel to visit their family member, often leaving their own children and responsibilities for extended periods of time, the local family traveling to the distant tertiary hospital or out-of-region hospice to visit their family member, the anguish of family members trying to decide whether to seek medical help locally or in more distant specialist facilities, and the costs of travel and accommodation when there is no family home to stay in when visiting or supporting family members in hospital or residential aged care. Traveling has been reported to impact negatively on the health of some family caregivers (Lockie et al. 2010).

Most families hope to be present at the time their family member dies. The fear of not being present can be significant and is compounded by the sense of geographical separation (Castleden et al. 2010). When family caregivers have to travel to out-of-region hospitals or hospices to be with their family member, the travel distances become more problematic. While rural family caregivers have a strong desire to be present at the time of death, they have to balance fulfilling their responsibilities at home or the farm with maintaining a bedside vigil away from home.

Traveling out of region, to access services not available locally, increases the risk of fragmented care (Duggleby et al. 2011). Without impeccable clinical handover and coordination of care, the quality of care can be compromised. The greatest support need of many rural patients with a terminal illness, and their family caregivers, especially in developed countries, is informational. Effective communication between healthcare professionals and patients/family caregivers reduces pain and distress, empowers carers to fulfill their responsibilities, facilitates smooth transitions of care, and allows patients and families to prepare for death (Rainsford et al. 2017). When surveyed, most patients and family caregivers report to be satisfied with the standard of communication by rural healthcare professionals (Devik et al. 2013); however, a number of communication difficulties are commonly reported. These include receiving conflicting or untimely information and uncertainty in identifying the lead physician.

However, opinions regarding the effect of distance on the quality of care are divided, with some rural residents seeing it as a major barrier to receiving home-based palliative care, and therefore achieving a home death (Dembinsky 2014), and others not viewing distance and rural residency a disadvantage (Devik et al. 2015). With advanced illness, the patients and family caregivers' sense of solitude (previously seen as an advantage of rural life) can become one of isolation (Duggleby et al. 2011). Geographic isolation can also contribute to the greater unmet emotional needs of rural caregivers, as they often lack the support of others going through similar experiences (Brazil et al. 2014).

5.2 Accessibility to In-Home Services

The availability of rural healthcare professionals to support patients dying at home becomes problematic the greater the travel distance and the more protracted the terminal phase. The most isolated rural locations are the least likely to have access to in-home care and support. Geographical distance limits accessibility to home-based services, especially for patients living outside the home visit boundary. Home visits become less frequent, especially in bad weather, and are often not available at short notice or after hours. Daily home visits to adjust medications, often required during the last days of life, are less likely to be available the further one lives from the service town. Some rural GPs provide on-call medical cover for rural hospitals. As rural generalists, this on-call cover can be in the emergency department, general wards, maternity, anesthetics, and/or operating theatres. In small towns, the on-call doctor is often the only doctor in town after hours and on weekends. While some doctors may be able to leave the hospital briefly to home visit a patient in close proximity to the hospital, they cannot leave town to visit patients living in surrounding villages or farms. In other rural locations, the service provided by GPs is on a part-time basis, with no daily access to medical support.

Mobile phones, computers, and internet access can help reduce the sense of rural isolation by maintaining contact with distant family and improving access to healthcare professionals; however, these technologies are often unreliable or not available in more remote areas (Lockie et al. 2010; Pesut et al. 2010). For some patients, a phone call is not sufficient and does not replace the physical presence of the nurse or doctor (Pesut et al. 2010; Hansen et al. 2012). In an Australian study, one husband living on a farm, felt "unsupported and alone" when the face-to-face presence of "qualified medical advice" was not available the night before his wife died (Rainsford 2017). Robinson et al. (2010) reported that some rural residents familiar with telehealth were not impressed with the service and found it unreliable and expensive. It cannot be presumed that all rural residents have sufficient literacy to use the technology and that phone and internet connections are available in all houses or in all communities.

Consistent with their urban counterparts, rural family caregivers often feel responsible for ensuring the dignity and comfort of their loved ones during their final days and experience distress, guilt, and anger when circumstances prevent them fulfilling this role (Revier et al. 2012).

While rural family caregivers take on the responsibility of providing direct care, many also take on the role of managing and coordinating care while being an advocate for their family member (Pesut et al. 2014); however, "few [are] physically, emotionally, or educationally prepared for the tasks and responsibilities of caregiving" (Revier et al. 2012, p. 5), especially as the illness progresses.

5.3 Lack of Local Specialist Services and Expertise

While travel distances restrict patients from visiting their specialists, the lack of local specialized personnel and facilities offering life-prolonging interventions is often considered a disadvantage of rural residency. However, as patients become more unwell, they and their family caregivers often acknowledge that the need for further complex interventions is no longer necessary, and in-fact, helps ensure a better quality of dying. During a bereavement interview, one rural family caregiver commented that "not [being] hooked up to machines" facilitated a more dignified death for his father who achieved a home death on their farm (Rainsford 2017, p. 203).

Unlike metropolitan and some regional areas, most rural and remote locations do not have specialist palliative care services and are reliant on primary healthcare providers. In some locations, GPs and community nurses may be supported by a specialist palliative care nurse. The lack of a specialist service could be viewed as a limitation of the quality of palliative care for rural residents. While GPs often struggle with managing complex issues, such as complex pain and high dose opiates, they do deliver sound and effective palliative care, and rural patients and their family caregivers appreciate the care provided by their primary care professionals (Mitchell 2002). Rural primary care physicians are frequently highly praised for their honesty and presence at the time of death.

The benefits of primary care-led palliative care must not be overlooked. These benefits include increased continuity of care, which often continues when patients are transferred from home to hospital or residential aged care, being cared for by health professionals who have a long standing professional relationship and knowledge of the individual and their family (sometimes intergenerational), and access to continuing care and bereavement support for family members. As a member of the rural community, rural health professionals are also familiar with the broader issues and the unique rural culture within rural communities.

Compared to their urban colleagues, rural primary healthcare professions face additional challenges in providing quality evidenced based end-of-life care. Rural healthcare professionals often find themselves in the dual role of healthcare provider and community member. As members of the community they are not anonymous and are often faced with planning and providing end-of-life care for close friends, neighbors, and colleagues (Beckstrand et al. 2012). Added to this is the difficulty of taking study leave to attend educational programs to up-date knowledge and maintain competencies and skills. Travel distances are compounded by the difficulty of recruiting locums to fill in during periods of absence. Travel distances also limit opportunities for team meetings, which can compound the emotional and physical isolation of independent healthcare professionals. Many rural locations have a single "unofficial" palliative care champion, and in their absence the whole system may stagnate or even disintegrate.

Rural patients are more likely than urban patients to visit their primary care physician (or GP) and the hospital emergency room and less likely to be admitted to an inpatient hospice or make use of respite services (Brazil et al. 2013). For rural patients and their family caregivers, being cared for in their community and by people they know is often more important that receiving specialist care (Veillette et al. 2010).

5.4 Lack of Allied Health Support

A multidisciplinary team is central to the provision of quality palliative care. While medical, nursing, and informal family care are the backbone of rural palliative care, limitations in accessing allied health support are often cited as a disadvantage of rural residency. In some circumstances, the lack of services and choice of commodities is just an inconvenience, for others the limitations, for example, home nursing, reduce the chance of patients dying at home.

Access to physiotherapy, occupational therapy, social work, counselors, and pastoral care varies depending on location and population. In some rural locations, when these services are available, they are often restricted to inpatient settings in the local rural hospital or are limited by the cost of private fees. Ongoing bereavement counseling is limited in most rural and remote communities. Community pharmacists are valued members of the multidisciplinary team; however, they are not present in all rural locations, and when available, after-hour services are either limited or nonexistent. Specific medications for symptom management are frequently not available at short notice.

6 Benefits of Rural Residency

Despite the challenges faced by rural communities, quality palliative care can be, and is, provided locally. In many ways, the benefits of rural living outweigh the disadvantages. The great sense of community is one benefit of rural living and a major contributor to quality end-of-life care. Another positive of rural living, voiced by many rural residents, is the beauty and tranquility of the rural lifestyle. Despite limited health services, many believe rural living has positive health benefits, and many could not contemplate living in a more urbanized location. Rural residents often speak of feeling "safe" in their isolation; however, when they, and especially those on isolated farms, are diagnosed with a terminal illness, due to the limited availability of medical, nursing and community support, the isolation can contribute to home becoming an unsafe place (Rainsford 2017).

6.1 Personalized Care

Features of care that facilitate quality rural end-of-life care include personalized care (Hansen et al. 2012), "knowing," and "being known" by the healthcare workforce (Pesut et al. 2011), and a willingness of healthcare workers to go beyond their professional duty. The concept of "being known" and "knowing others" is a unique feature of rural communities and extends into rural hospitals and residential aged care. Unlike many large urban institutions, there is often a small turnover of rural staff, within rural institutions, that facilitates personalized care. "Being known" promotes a sense of acceptance, where patients are known for who they are rather than being known for their illness. The workforce within rural community health, hospital, and residential aged care is usually members of the community and known to the patients and their families. This familiarity can assist patients and their families to have confidence in the care provided and can often ease the distress of transferring from home to hospital or residential aged care, for end-of-life care.

However, loss of privacy and anonymity and an expectation that friends will always be available are perceived as barriers (Pesut et al. 2011). Often the quality of care provided is dependent on the personality of the healthcare provider, with difficulties arising if personality conflicts arise, as often no alternative provider is available (Devik et al. 2013). Loss of anonymity can also be problematic if patients are self-conscious of their deteriorating state. Issues of confidentiality can also arise when family caregivers are forced into the dual relationship of family protector and community member. This can result in a spirit of independence as patients and their family caregivers may restrict both formal and informal support in an attempt to keep their personal circumstances private.

6.2 Informal Community Support

The informal support provided by family, friends, neighbors, and the community is significant, with some considering that family is the "most important" factor (Devik et al. 2013, 2015) and essential for culturally congruent care (Mixer et al. 2014). In many rural areas, the profile of informal rural caregivers reflects the social change in family structure. As previously noted, many rural populations are graying and decreasing in size due to internal migration, as younger family members move to more urbanized areas in search of education and employment. Compared to urban areas, rural caregivers are now more likely to be younger and a non-first-degree relative (Burns et al. 2015).

Rural communities are often described as "very close knit with incredible volunteer bases, and very generous people... who are genuinely concerned about the community" (Castleden et al. 2010, p. 287). Informal community support is highly valued by rural residents and is perceived to be unique to rural communities and a significant advantage of rural residency. It is reported to have a positive influence on rural end-of-life care as it contributes to a sense of solidarity, as people take care of each other (Devik et al. 2015). Community support cannot be taken for granted and is highly reciprocal, with those who have contributed most to their rural community often receiving the highest amount of support from that community (Pesut et al. 2011).

Informal support is mostly direct and practical, such as food, transport, sitting with a patient, and domestic help; however, some support is indirect, with many community members unaware of the significance of a friendly smile or "hello."

There is an assumption that, due to reduced access and availability of services and support, rural caregivers would have higher levels of needs and greater unmet needs than their urban counterparts. However, rural communities are often resourceful when no specialist services are available. Local support networks are created in response to the unspoken responsibility and commitment to care for community members when one identifies as a member of the community. Compared to urban caregivers, rural caregivers perceive the same low level of carer burden and good level of support (Kirby et al. 2016). Rural caregivers are more positive about the caregiving experience than their urban counterparts, with most reporting the experience to be as expected or better than expected. Rural caregivers are also more likely to perceive their deceased family member to have been comfortable during the last 2 weeks of life (Burns et al. 2015). Despite the great sense of community support, the greatest unmet needs identified by rural family caregivers, in both developed and developing countries, remain the tangible or practical needs (Brazil et al. 2013, 2014; Grant et al. 2011).

For some patients receiving treatment in small rural health facilities, a special "subcommunity" can develop, where patients and their family caregivers find mutual support in other patients. For other rural patients and family caregivers, despite the strong sense of community, as disease progresses and patients lose mobility and independence, a sense of isolation can develop as often there is no one in the community who has experienced the same situation, "I am part of my community but I feel alone. Family and friends come to visit me, but I feel isolated as they are unable to understand what is happening to me and my wife" (Duggleby et al. 2011, p. 2).

Despite the perceived willingness to volunteer, it has been suggested that rural community members may volunteer out of obligation, rather than a true desire to be involved. Likewise, formal care providers may also feel pressured to provide services above and beyond that expected of their urban counterparts, because there is often no alternative (Castleden et al. 2010).

6.3 Formal Support

Depending on the locality, formal support can be readily available, limited, or nonexistent. Most rural patients, especially in developed countries, have access to primary palliative care through their general practitioners and community nurses. With the exception of those living in regional towns, most, if not all, rural patients are required to travel to receive specialist care. In contrast to the majority of urban medical practices, most rural GPs and community nurses live in the community where they work, with friendships commonly developing between healthcare professionals and their patients. Healthcare providers' obligations often extend far beyond the professional role with some providers going to extraordinary lengths to be available, and take great "pride in being able to make it work – through responsive, creative, highly individualized care" (Robinson et al. 2010, p. 81).

In many rural areas, it is not unusual for residents to have their "own" GP. Some rural residents are supported by the same GP and community nurse over a prolonged period, often from the time of diagnosis. The advantages of "being known" and continuity of care enhance the sense of trust in the healthcare providers. The concept of "knowing" also extends to the healthcare providers, who are often known by, and know of, other service providers.

6.4 Convenience of Rural Residency

Despite the travel distances, once in town, there are conveniences often not found in cities. When family caregivers are "time poor," the lack of traffic congestion is a commonly reported benefit of rural residency. Parking at rural hospitals and medical centers is usually free and in close proximity to the front door.

7 Place of Death in Rural Palliative Care

In rural settings, relationships between place and one's self are often stronger than for urban residents, so one would expect that rural people would view dying at home an essential feature of the "good" rural death. Place of death is often considered in terms of geographical location (community) and physical space (home, hospital, residential aged care). Consistent with urban dwellers, surveyed rural residents do indicate that, if faced with a life-limiting illness, home is their preferred place of death, surrounded by family and friends (Veillette et al. 2010), and, in the case of Aboriginal and Indigenous peoples, connected to their land and family (McGrath 2007). However, inconsistencies exist in the current rural literature due to limited and small studies, heterogeneous rural definitions, and rural data embedded in mixed geographical studies (Rainsford et al. 2016a). Also, most rural studies are either population surveys reporting hypothetical preferences of healthy people or retrospective bereavement interviews/questionnaires of families and carers. Few studies report preferences directly from patients, i.e., those facing an end-of-life situation. Therefore, rural preferences for place of death are not clearly understood.

In contemporary rural studies, more than half of rural participants expressed a preference for dying at home; however, this is not a universal finding. Locations with stronger traditional cultures and values exhibit the strongest preferences for, and the highest numbers of, home deaths; however, these locations often have less access to hospitals, hospices, and residential aged care (Rainsford et al. 2016a). Rural residents are often considered disadvantaged by the lack of rural inpatient hospice facilities, with rural hospitals and residential aged care acting as substitutes for inpatient hospice (Menec et al. 2010). While wishing to remain home, studies indicate that many rural residents and their family caregivers accept the need to alternate between home and hospital, providing the length of hospital stay is kept to the minimum.

Currently, there is great variation in the rate of home deaths between rural settings. Rates range from just over 10% to 80%, with a large cluster around 25% (Rainsford et al. 2016a). Compared to urban residents, the chance of dying at home in rural areas is often dependent on the specific rural setting and cause of death. Rural residents who die of cancer in South Australia have been reported to have a greater chance of dying at home than urban residents (Hunt et al. 2001). Likewise, people living in rural England with COPD (Higginson et al. 2017) and living in parts of rural Europe with cancer (Cohen et al. 2010) are less likely to die in hospital than patients residing in urban locations. However, a Canadian study by Lavergne et al. (2015) reported no significant difference in the odds of dying in hospital for urban and rural residents with a terminal illness, organ failure, or frailty.

The most frequently cited reasons for leaving home are symptom control and carer distress. Factors influencing place of care/place of death in rural settings are not clearly identified in the literature but, when reported, include patients' functional status and clinical condition, carer and social networks, and health-system facilities. With limited medical and nursing support at home to respond to changes in patients' conditions, the influence of rural residency has the potential to render rural homes, especially farms and outliers, more susceptible to become unsafe, earlier, and more frequently than most urban homes.

Deciding on place of death is a complex process, in which wishes and preferences are not necessarily the same. Rural patients change their preferences as illness progresses, with most accepting that a home death may not be possible. For many rural patients, hospital becomes their preference, and an acceptable alternative to home, especially in the last 48-hours and providing they are located within the patients' community (Robinson et al. 2010). Rural hospitals are often a substitute for inpatient hospice care.

Rural hospitals could be perceived as less safe than urban hospitals, due to the lack of specialist palliative care and expertise; however, this is often not the perception of rural patients. The familiarity and personal attention provided by rural hospitals, and the benefit of being known, creates a safe place within rural hospitals. At end of life, the inability of small rural hospitals to provide aggressive and often futile interventions is often perceived as an enabler to maintaining dignity. However, this experience is not universal. When local hospitals are perceived as unsafe, or under-resourced for "active" treatment, some rural residents choose to move away from their community, to specialist palliative care facilities or larger hospitals. Safety is not simply following procedures and policies. Safety is aligned with trust. Trust is based on prior knowledge of the hospital, and dependent on the moment-to-moment experience of care, not only for the patient but also their family. The biggest barriers to using hospital-based palliative care services for Indigenous peoples are the lack of cultural awareness by healthcare professionals and not being able to die "in country" (Kelly et al. 2009; Grant et al. 2011; Dembinsky 2014).

When available, residential aged care is a significant provider of rural palliative and end-of-life care for those aged 65 years and older; however, this option is not available in all rural regions. Availability of residential aged care varies significantly, not only within countries but between countries. In some Australian rural locations, it is not uncommon for patients who are unable to return home from hospital to be transferred to residential aged care for end-of-life care. Consistent with urban residential aged care, current workloads and staff shortages create challenges for registered nurses to be available, in a timely fashion, to attend to the acute palliative care needs of residents.

The congruence between preferred and actual place of care and place of death has been mooted as a quality outcome for palliative care, with health policies aimed at enabling people to die in their preferred place. Based on the current literature, the assumption is that for most people, the preferred place of care and place of death is home, being in a familiar place, surrounded by family and/or friends. With limited studies reporting the actual and preferred place of death, there is currently insufficient data to draw any conclusions as to the degree of congruence within rural settings.

Robinson et al. (2010) suggest that a death at home is not necessarily the most appropriate or desirable place in rural settings, due to often limited palliative care resources, especially after hours. The significant burden and cost (financial, physical, and emotional) to family caregivers, caring for a family member at home, is often overlooked. Patients may only be able to die well and have a "good death" if they leave their home or farm to die in the rural hospital. Therefore, it remains unclear if the "push" to increase the rate of home deaths in rural settings is justified.

If rural residents are unable to die at home, then most consider it important that they die within their community. Many rural residents will sacrifice access to specialist palliative care to ensure they are not displaced from their rural community. Dying within community is one factor contributing to the "good" rural death.

8 The Concept of the "Good" Rural Death

The "good death" is a difficult concept to define and is dependent on individual interpretations, perspectives, and priorities formulated by cultural, religious, and political values and beliefs.

There is significant overlap between urban and rural views, highlighting that all people, regardless of where they live, have some common needs and desire a "good death." The elements considered essential for a "good" rural death go beyond culture and ethnicity; however, the context and priority placed on each factor differ from the urban perspective (Kirby et al. 2016). The essential elements include those that maintain quality of life for the patient and their family and address the physical, emotional, social, spiritual, and cultural needs of the dying person and their family caregivers.

The dominant theme, from both developed and developing countries, is that a rural "good death" is one that is peaceful, free of pain, and without suffering (Rainsford et al. 2016b). The themes describing the "good" rural death parallel the urban view and include a "controlled" death, with control over symptoms, place of death, decision-making, manner of death, and independence (Wilson et al. 2009a, b; Veillette et al. 2010); a "timely" death, which is a death coming "naturally and after a long and well-spent life" (van der Geest 2004, p. 899) after having had opportunity to say goodbye to family; a "dignified" death by maintaining identity, self-worth, integrity, and control (Wilson et al. 2009a; Devik et al. 2013); a "social" death, such as to die within the community with family present (Wilson et al. 2009a, b); and a "noble" death such as through enduring the situation (Grant et al. 2003; Devik et al. 2013).

Rural residents consider family and community important, especially at end of life, because "the togetherness of the family members makes you feel they love you and are not abandoning you" (Grant et al. 2003, p. 163). In some cultures, the family and community play an important role after the death of a family member, by ensuring specific rituals are carried out.

The strong connection to one's rural/remote community means that dying within one's rural locality is frequently identified as a critical element in achieving a "good death." If it is not possible to die at home surrounded by family, then it is important to die within the rural community, as "home or home community… [is] the only place where the dying person [can] be close to the many people who have meaning for them" (Wilson et al. 2009b, p. 316). In Ghana, dying away from home is considered "bad" and disgraceful; however, partial restoration can be achieved by "bringing the dead body home" (van der Geest 2004, p. 909).

8.1 Physical Support (Pain and Symptom Management)

Good pain and symptom control is the overriding factor reported to ensure a "good death." Pain relief is central to maintaining quality of life through the dying journey, not just for the patient but also the family caregiver. Most dying people and families fear pain. While inadequate pain control is reported in developed countries, moderate to severe pain often dominates the lives of patients in rural sub-Saharan Africa, due to the shortage or absence of pain medication and healthcare workers (Grant et al. 2011). Anticipating medication requirements, when commuting long distances, is an important consideration for some rural patients (Pesut et al. 2010; Lockie et al. 2010).

8.2 Emotional Support

Strong emotional support is a facilitator of quality rural end-of-life care. Faith and hope are central to emotional well-being. Hope is often maintained through connection with family, friends, and being linked to something outside the illness. The serenity and peacefulness of many rural settings are an advantage of rural residency.

8.3 Social Support

As previously indicated, rural communities provide significant social support (both formally and informally) for patients and family caregivers. This support is an enabler of the "good death" and is dependent on good communication, information, the presence of healthcare professionals, and the support of other patients. The solidarity of rural communities and mutual support of neighbors is unique to rural settings (Wilson et al. 2009a; Robinson et al. 2010).

8.4 Spiritual Support

Spiritual connection and faith foster hope, with faith seen as an enabler to persevering in life as death draws near. Faith is fundamental to rural Appalachians and their transition through end-of-life care (Mixer et al. 2014). In many rural communities, church support is not limited to spiritual issues, as congregations often also provide physical and financial support.

8.5 Cultural Influences on the "Good" Rural Death

In addition to the influence of rural residency, cultural beliefs and values influence how individuals view end-of-life care and preferences for management, interventions, conversations, and place of care and death. This chapter is written mostly from a western point of view, where there is an emphasis on individualism, autonomy, quality of life, privacy, science, and the nuclear family. Other cultures may place greater emphasis on interdependence, extended family, village community, and respect for elders and traditional healers. In more traditional rural settings, for example, Kenya, "powerful cultural traditions [make] it difficult for social needs to be met" (Grant et al. 2003, p. 163). In many developing countries, while Christianity has influenced the concept of the "good" and "bad" death, it has not replaced, but instead has been interpreted and applied to, traditional beliefs. These beliefs can significantly impact on the health and well-being of the community, descendants, and ancestors (Grant et al. 2003, 2011). The "good death" is often regarded as one that does not disrupt the life and health of the community (van der Geest 2004). In contrast, rural residents in developed countries often view the "good death" in light of a biomedical model, placing greater emphasis on autonomy, the process of dying, and minimizing any sense of struggle. Stoicism and the culture of "not complaining" are a feature of rural residents in both developed (Devik et al. 2013) and developing countries (Grant et al. 2003).

9 Summary

Regardless of place of residency, all people desire a "good death." The goal of palliative care is to ensure the dying person and their family is free of suffering and distress. However, the provision of palliative care in rural settings is variable and dependent on the degree of rurality. Currently there is no international consensus on the definition of rurality and remoteness. There is considerable individual, cultural, and ethnic diversity with regard to preferences for end-of-life care. Rural culture is distinct from urban culture, with rural residents holding unique perspectives on what it means to die well. Rural communities are close-knit and known for their social solidarity, community commitment, and loose support networks. While there are many benefits of rural residency, significant challenges exist. The needs of rural residents are shaped by decreased access and availability of services. While this potentially has a negative influence on outcomes, it is offset by local support networks. Rural palliative care is mostly primary care, with limited access to specialist multidisciplinary palliative care services. Home is the preferred place of death for most rural residents; however, when home is not possible, rural hospitals and residential aged care are considered appropriate alternatives, providing they are within ones' community.

10 Conclusion

To ensure palliative care is relevant to individual communities, it must reflect the needs of the dying person and their family, and the diverse geography and cultures of the community in which they live. While there are many similarities between urban and rural end-of-life care, there are many significant differences. Rural settings are not homogeneous. While studies indicate that rural residents are mostly satisfied with the level of palliative care provided, there are huge, and often unacceptable, variations, especially in remote and developing regions. The universal rural theme is that if rural residents are unable to die at home, then it is essential that their place of death is within their local community.

References

Australian Government Department of Health. Report on the audit of health workforce in rural and regional Australia; 2.5.2 Trends in population ageing. 2008. http://www.health.gov.au/internet/publications/publishing.nsf/Content/work-res-ruraud-toc~work-res-ruraud-2~work-res-ruraud-2-5~work-res-ruraud-2-5-2. Accessed 15 Jul 2016.

Australian Institute of Health and Welfare (AIHW). Rural, regional and remote health: a guide to remoteness classifications. Rural health series no. 4. Cat. no. PHE 53. Canberra: AIHW; 2004. http://www.aihw.gov.au/publication-detail/?id=6442467589. Accessed 19 Aug 2017.

Australian Institute of Health and Welfare (AIHW). Palliative care services in Australia 2014, Cat. No. HWI 128. Canberra: AIHW; 2014.

Bakitas MA, Elk R, Astin M, Ceronsky C, Clifford KN, Dionne-Odom JN, et al. Systematic review of palliative care in the rural setting. Cancer Control. 2015;22(4): 450–64.

Beckstrand RL, Giles VC, Luthy KE, Callister LC, Heaston S. The last frontier: rural emergency nurses' perceptions of end-of-life care obstacles. J Emerg Nurs. 2012;38(5):E15–25.

Boarders T. Advancing the field of rural health research (ed). J Rural Health. 2017;33:3–4.

Brazil K, Kaasalainen S, Williams A, Rodriguez C. Comparing the experiences of rural and urban family caregivers of the terminally ill. Rural Remote Health. 2013;13:2250.

Brazil K, Kaasalainen S, Williams A, Dumont S. A comparison of support needs between rural and urban family caregivers providing palliative care. Am J Hosp Palliat Care. 2014;31(1):13–9.

Burns C, Dal Grande E, Tieman J, Abernethy AP, Currow D. Who provides care for people dying of cancer? A comparison of a rural and metropolitan cohort in a south Australian bereaved population study. Aust J Rural Health. 2015;23:24–31.

Castleden H, Crooks VA, Schuurman N, Hanlon N. "Its not necessarily the distance on the map…": using place as an analytical tool to elucidate geographical issues central to rural palliative care. Health Place. 2010;16:284–90.

Cohen J, Houtter D, Onwuteaka-Philipsen B, Miccinesi G, Addington-Hall J, Kaasa S, et al. Which patients with cancer die at home? A study of six European countries using death certificate data. J Clin Oncol. 2010;28(13):2267–73.

Cottrell L, Duggleby C. The "good death": an integrative literature review. Palliat Support Care. 2016:1–27. https://doi.org/10.1017/S1478951515001285.

Dembinsky M. Exploring Yamatji perceptions and use of palliative care: an ethnographic study. Int J Palliat Nurs. 2014;20(8):387–93.

Devik SA, Enmarker I, Wiik GB, Hellzen O. Meanings of being old, living on one's own and suffering from incurable cancer in rural Norway. Eur J Oncol Nurs. 2013;17(6):781–7.

Devik SA, Helizen O, Enmarker I. "Picking up the pieces" – meanings of receiving home nursing care when being old and living with advanced cancer in a rural area. Int J Qual Stud Health Well-Being. 2015;10:28382.

Duggleby WD, Penz K, Leipert BD, Wilson DM, Goodridge D, Williams A. 'I am part of the community but...' the changing context of rural living for persons with advanced cancer and their families. Rural Remote Health. 2011;11(3):1733.

Giesbrecht M, Crooks VA, Castleden H, Schuurman N, Skinner M, Williams A. Palliating inside the lines: the effects of borders and boundaries on palliative care in rural Canada. Soc Sci Med. 2016;168:273–82.

Grant E, Murray SA, Grant A, Brown J. A good death in rural Kenya? – listening to Meru patients and their families talk about care needs at the end of life. J Palliat Care. 2003;19(3):159–67.

Grant L, Brown J, Leng M, Bettega N, Murray SA. Palliative care making a difference in rural Uganda, Kenya and Malawi: three rapid evaluation field studies. BMC Palliat Care. 2011;10(8):1–10.

Hansen L, Cartwright JC, Craig CE. End-of-life care for rural-dwelling older adults and their primary family caregivers. Res Gerontol Nurs. 2012;5(1):6–15.

Higginson IJ, Reilly CC, Bajwah S, Maddocks M, et al. Which patients with advanced respiratory disease die in hospital? A 14-year population-based study of trends and associated factors. BMC Med. 2017;15(19):1–12.

Hunt RW, Fazekas BS, Luke CG, Roder DM. Where patients with cancer die in South Australia, 1990–1999: a population-based review. Med J Aust. 2001;175 (10):526–9.

Kelly L, Linkewich B, Cromarty H, Pierre-Hansen NS, Antone I, Gilles C. Palliative care of first nations people: a qualitative study of bereaved family members. Can Fam Physician. 2009;55(4):394–5.

Kirby S, Barlow V, Saurman E, Lyle D, Passey M, Currow D. Are rural and remote patients, families and caregivers needs in life-limiting illness different from those of urban dwellers? A narrative synthesis of the evidence. Aust J Rural Health. 2016;24:289–99.

Lavergne MR, Lethbridge L, Johnston G, Henderson D, D'Intino AF, McIntyre P. Examining palliative care program use and place of death in rural and urban contexts: a Canadian population-based study using linked data. Rural Remote Health. 2015; 15:3134.

Lockie SJ, Bottorff JL, Robinson CA, Pesut B. Experiences of rural family caregivers who assist with commuting for palliative care. Can J Nurs Res. 2010;42 (1):74–91.

McGrath P. 'I don't want to be in that big city; this is my country here': research findings on aboriginal peoples' preference to die at home. Aust J Rural Health. 2007; 15(4):264–8.

Menec V, Nowicki S, Kalischuk A. Transfers to acute care hospital at the end of life: do rural/remote regions differ from urban regions? Rural Remote Health. 2010;10:1281.

Ministere des affaires municipales et des regions du Quebec. Texte complet de la Politique nationale de la ruralite 2007–2014. 2007. Translated and cited in Wilson et al. 2009a. p. 316.

Mitchell GK. How well do general practitioners deliver palliative care? A systematic review. Palliat Med. 2002;16:457–64.

Mixer S, Fornehed ML, Varney J, Lindley LC. Culturally congruent end-of-life care for rural Appalachian people and their families. J Hosp Palliat Nurs. 2014;16 (8):526–35.

NHPCO. Facts and figures: hospice care in America. Alexandria: National Hospice and Palliative Care Organization; 2012.

Pesut B, Robinson CA, Bottorff JL, Fyles G, Broughton S. On the road again: patient perspectives on commuting for palliative care. Palliat Support Care. 2010;8(2):187–95.

Pesut B, Bottorff JL, Robinson CA. Be known, be available, be mutual: a qualitative ethical analysis of social values in rural palliative care. BMC Med Ethics. 2011;12:19.

Pesut B, Robinson CA, Bottorff JL. Among neighbors: an ethnographic account of responsibilities in rural palliative care. Palliat Support Care. 2014;12(2):127–38.

Rainsford S. The influence of place of death and rural residency on the 'good death'. A doctoral thesis. The Australian National University, Canberra; 2017. https://openresearch-repository.anu.edu.au/handle/1885/140950

Rainsford S, MacLeod RD, Glasgow NJ. Place of death in rural palliative care: a systematic review. Palliat Med. 2016a;30(8):745–63.

Rainsford S, MacLeod RD, Glasgow NJ, Wilson DM, Phillips CB, Wiles RB. Rural residents' perspectives on the rural 'good death': a scoping review. Health Soc Care Commun. 2016b. https://doi.org/10.1111/hsc.12385.

Rainsford S, MacLeod RD, Glasgow NJ, Phillips CB, Wiles RB, Wilson DM. Rural end-of-life care from the experiences and perspectives of patients and family caregivers: a systematic literature review. Palliat Med. 2017;31:895–912.

Revier SS, Meiers SJ, Herth KA. The lived experience of hope in family caregivers caring for a terminally ill loved one. J Hosp Palliat Nurs. 2012;14(6):438–46.

Robinson CA, Pesut B, Bottorff JL, Mowry A, Broughton S, Fyles G. Rural palliative care: a comprehensive review. J Palliat Med. 2009;12(3):253–8.

Robinson CA, Pesut B, Bottorff JL. Issues in rural palliative care: views from the countryside. J Rural Health. 2010;26(1):78–84.

van der Geest S. Dying peacefully: considering good death and bad death in Kwahu-Tafo. Ghana Soc Sci Med. 2004;58:899–911.

Veillette A, Fillion L, Wilson DM, Thomas R, Dumont S. La belle mort en milieu rural: a report of an ethnographic study of the good death for Quebec rural francophones. J Palliat Care. 2010;26(3):159–66. 158p

Wiik GB. Don't become a burden and don't complain: a case study of older persons suffering from incurable cancer and living alone in rural areas. Nurs Rep. 2011;1(e3):7–14.

Wilson DM, Fillion L, Thomas R, Justice C, Bhardwaj PP, Veillette AM. The "good" rural death: a report of an ethnographic study in Alberta, Canada. J Palliat Care. 2009a;25(1):21–9.

Wilson DM, Fillion L, Thomas R, Justice C, Veillette AM, Bhardwaj P. Planning and providing for a good death using rural French-Canadian and English-Canadian insights. Rev Neurosci. 2009b;20(3–4):313–9.

World Bank. Rural populations. 2016. http://data.worldbank.org/indicator/SP.RUR.TOTL.ZS. Accessed 3 Sept 2017.

World Health Organisation (WHO). Global health observatory data. 2014. Accessed 3 Sept 2017. http://www.who.int/gho/urban_health/situation_trends/urban_population_growth/en/.

World Health Organisation (WHO). Palliative care, Fact sheet N°402 2015. http://www.who.int/mediacentre/factsheets/fs402/en/. Accessed 3 Sept 2017.

Informal/Family Caregivers

55

Gunn Grande and Gail Ewing

Contents

Abstract

This chapter considers the importance of informal carers in enabling patients to remain at home towards the end of life, providing extensive hours of care and covering a range of caregiving tasks, including physical, emotional, and social care and monitoring. It highlights the considerable impact that caregiving has mainly on carers' psychological health, but also their general wellbeing, and it reviews the evidence on factors that predict worse impact, key elements of which are carers' own appraisal of their situation and their preparedness. The chapter describes how carers occupy two main roles: that of a co-worker and of being a client themselves, and the main areas with which they need support to enable them to support the patient as co-workers, and to look after their own health

G. Grande (✉)
Division of Nursing, Midwifery and Social Work, School of Health Sciences, Faculty of Biology, Medicine and Health, University of Manchester, Manchester, UK
e-mail: Gunn.grande@manchester.ac.uk

G. Ewing
Centre for Family Research, Department of Psychology, University of Cambridge, Cambridge, UK
e-mail: ge200@cam.ac.uk

R. D. MacLeod, L. Van den Block (eds.), *Textbook of Palliative Care*,
https://doi.org/10.1007/978-3-319-77740-5_52

and wellbeing as clients. It reviews the limited success interventions for carers have had to date, some of the challenges that need to be overcome, the importance of individualized, person-centered interventions, and some of the assessment tools that may help facilitate tailored support. It also highlights that assessment in itself is unlikely to be of benefit without clear procedures for discussion of and response to identified problems. Finally, it considers factors required for implementation of carer support within palliative care practice, including procedures for identifying carers, recording carer data and for intervention delivery, as well as organizational level support to sustain implementation including leadership, staff training, protected time, and carer champions. However, fundamental to achieving consistent carer support is the question of whether carers are true clients of palliative care services.

1 Introduction: The Importance of Carers

Informal carers make a substantial contribution to patient care. In the UK, it is estimated that informal carers of people of all conditions provide care to the value of £132 billion per year, close to the annual healthcare spending of £134 billion (Buckner and Yeandle 2015). In Australia, the cost of replacing the hours of informal caregiving with formal care would be equivalent to 60% of the spending on the health and social care work industry (Carers Australia 2015), while in Canada carers have been estimated to provide 80–90% of home care (Romanow 2002).

The size of the contribution of informal carers in palliative and end of life care is less clear. Caregiving hours are in this situation likely to be considerably higher compared to caregiving in general, thus representing a sizable input, but input from formal services is also likely to increase. A recent study from England found that informal caregiving amounted to more than twice the cost of formal healthcare among patients with advanced chronic disease and refractory breathlessness (Dzingina et al. 2017). Conversely, an Irish study found that informal caregiving accounted for 22% of total costs in the last year of life among patients receiving specialist palliative care (Brick et al. 2017). These estimates will depend on the caregiving context and what tasks are considered. Formal care input is likely to have been different in the two above studies. Further, Brick et al. (2017) only focused on carers' assistance with activities of daily living and out of pocket expenditure. Dzingina et al. (2017) considered hours "on call" in addition to more practical or physical caregiving tasks. Arguably, to gain a true picture of the value of caregiving (and impact on the carer), we need to consider caregiving in the broader sense, not just practical and physical elements but also their constant vigilance: a lot of carer time at home involves monitoring of the patient's condition and being on call. This in one sense mirrors the situation in inpatient care, where monitoring and being able to call on assistance when needed is an important aspect of care. Time spent looking after patients' psychological and social needs is also important in maintaining patients' psychological wellbeing and personhood, which arguably are important elements of holistic care.

Not surprisingly, the efforts of informal carers are crucial in enabling care to take place at home towards the end of life. The vast majority of patients prefer to be looked after at home towards the end of life, and although the percentage who actually wants to die at home may be smaller, these may still form the majority (Gomes et al. 2013a). Studies consistently show that the availability of carers is a major and consistent predictor of likelihood of dying at home: patients who have a primary carer, are married, live with relatives, have an extended family or carer network are more likely to achieve a home death than their counterparts (Gomes and Higginson 2006; Grande and Ewing 2008; Burns et al. 2013). Similarly, a substantial proportion of "inappropriate" hospital admissions may be carer initiated or due to carers' inability to cope (Reyniers et al. 2017; Gott et al. 2013, respectively).

Current healthcare policies often promote care in the community over inpatient care towards end of life based on patient preferences and costs, where hospital inpatient care accounts for the majority of healthcare costs (Gardiner et al. 2017). However, sustaining care in the community is heavily dependent on carers' efforts, and this policy normally does not take into account the impact on carers and the size and economic value of their contribution (Gardiner et al. 2017). For instance, The National End of Life Care Programme (NEoLCP 2012) in England estimated that end of life community care was likely to be cheaper than acute hospital care, but this calculation only considered the costs of health and social care provision, not the costs of carers' contribution. Literature reviews indicate that the costs of palliative care is lower than standard care, but economic evaluations consistently fail to consider carers' time and out-of-pocket costs (Smith et al. 2013; Gomes et al. 2013b; Penders et al. 2017). Support for carers was explicitly excluded from the NHS Palliative Care Tariff recommended by the Palliative Care Funding Review (DH 2011) for England, despite the PCFR's emphasis on enabling patient death at home.

Proper recognition of carers' input, consideration of the impact on carers, and how we support them will be of increasing importance in the future. In the UK, the number of carers in the population increased by 16.5% from 2001 to 2015. More importantly, there was an increase of nearly 43% in carers providing 20–49 h and 33% in those providing >50 h per week (Buckner and Yeandle 2015). Our reliance on carers is likely to continue to increase in years to come, particularly for end of life care. Projections in the UK indicate there will be increases in people over 85, those with life limiting illness (Buckner and Yeandle 2015), in dependency in the final years of life (Kingston et al. 2017) and in the number deaths (ONS 2013). These demographic changes are likely to be mirrored at least across the developed world. Health and social care services are likely to struggle to meet these future demands, and carers are likely to have to make up much of the shortfall.

This chapter will give an overview of who carers are, what they do, what impact caregiving has on them and who may be worst affected, what support they need, what may help carers in terms of interventions, and how we embed carer support within palliative care.

2 Who Are the Carers?

Carers have been defined as "lay people in a close supportive role who share in the illness experience of the patient and who undertake vital care work and emotion management" (NICE 2004). They are usually first degree relatives, most often a spouse or adult child of the patient (Abernethy et al. 2009), but can also be more distant relatives, friends, or neighbors. In fact, the wider network of carers may have a more prominent role than is often realized. For instance, a population based study in Australia by Burns et al. (2013) found that of those reported providing "hands on care" for someone at end of life, only 44% were first degree relatives (a spouse, child, parent, or sibling) and 56% were extended family, friends, and others. Nevertheless, first degree relatives were more likely to do daily care and to care for a longer period. Therefore, the main burden of care is still likely to fall on the closest relatives.

Other characteristics are likely to define those who provide the most care. Abernethy et al. (2009) found that carers who provided more frequent care (daily or several times a week) were more likely to be women. Those providing more intermittent care compared to daily care were more likely to be younger (<60 years), have higher education, be in paid work and to be wealthier, as well as being more likely to be children, parents, other relatives, or friends of the patient.

3 What Do Carers Do?

Carers in general provide substantial hours of care per week. National data from England indicate that the majority of carers (62%) provide up to 19 h per week, although 24% provide 50 h or more (Buckner and Yeandle 2015). Carers of people with cancer have been estimated to provide

15–24.5 h per week (Van Houtven et al. 2010; Round et al. 2015, respectively). However, this is unlikely to reflect the intensity of caregiving towards the end of life.

To gain an overview of carer hours and tasks in the patient's final months of life, we conducted a national census post-bereavement survey of everyone who had reported the death of a relative from cancer in England during a two-week period in 2015 (Rowland et al. 2017). Respondents were asked to estimate how many hours they spent on a range of caregiving tasks in a typical week during the patient's last 3 months of life. A total of 1504 (28.5%) of 5270 relatives completed the survey and 91% provided information on hours of care. These carers reported spending a median of 69 h and 30 min on caregiving per week (interquartile range 28:37–115:15 h). Carers of people with cancer may therefore on average spend nearly 10 h per day 7 days per week on caregiving during the patient's final months. This may still not provide the full picture of informal care contributions: 60% of respondents reported receiving additional informal help in the patient's last 3 months, mostly from family, but also friends and neighbors, and the extent of this help was a median of 20 h per week (Interquartile range 7.3–50 h). While we do not have similar data for carers of people dying from other conditions, their contribution is also likely to be substantial.

Carers carried out a broad range of support tasks within their caregiving hours (Rowland et al. 2017). Most spent time on social and emotional support for the patient (83%), followed by shopping (79%), cleaning, preparing food/drink, general administration, organizing/attending appointments and helping with symptoms (all between 70–73%), personal care (64%), travelling with the patient (58%), and maintenance/miscellaneous jobs (55%).

Carers can also have considerable out of pocket expenditure in relation to caregiving. In a study of 13 European countries, Penders et al. (2017) found such expenditure in the last year of life to amount to 2–25% of median household income. In our national survey for England (Rowland et al. 2017), carers were asked to report total out of pocket expenditure during the deceased person's last 3 months. Seventy one percent reported such expenditure, with a median total expenditure of £370 among those reporting figures, including spending on travel, meals, medical equipment, and care supplies. Additionally, 17% reported "one off" expenses during the total time of caregiving with a median expense of £2000, including mobility equipment, furniture, or house adaptations. These expenditures relate to a country with public health service coverage and are likely to be considerably higher where people pay for private medical and nursing care.

4 Impact of Caregiving on Carers

Caregiving has considerable impact on carers' own psychological and physical health (Stajduhar et al. 2010). Studies have found carers to have worse psychological health compared with the general population (Dumont et al. 2006; Grov et al. 2005; Gotze et al. 2014; Kenny et al. 2010; Zapart et al. 2007), although some studies show them to have similar or better physical health than the norm (Grov et al. 2005; Zapart et al. 2007; Kenny et al. 2010). Compared with carers of people with non-terminal conditions, carers of palliative and end of life patients have worse emotional health and physical health (Williams et al. 2014; Wolff et al. 2007). They have even been found to have greater prevalence of anxiety and depression than patients themselves (Braun et al. 2007; Gotze et al. 2014; Grunfeld et al. 2004). In general, research seems to show that caregiving has the greatest and most consistent impact on carers' psychological health, and patterns seem to be similar at least across English-speaking countries and Europe (Dumont et al. 2006; Stajduhar et al. 2010; Wolff et al. 2007; Williams et al. 2014; Grov et al. 2005; Zapart et al. 2007; Kenny et al. 2010; Gotze et al. 2014).

The level of impact on the mental health among carers of palliative and end of life patients gives cause for concern. Studies using standard measures that enable identification of clinically significant levels of distress have found a prevalence of anxiety ranging from 34% to 47% among these carers during caregiving (Grov et al. 2005; Gotze et al. 2014; Grunfeld et al. 2004; Rumpold et al. 2016) and a prevalence of depression of 39%

(Braun et al. 2007). However, results may not be fully generalizable. These studies mainly have recruited carers for oncology/tertiary care (Grov et al. 2005; Grunfeld et al. 2004; Braun et al. 2007; Rumpold et al. 2016) or palliative care services (Zapart et al. 2007; Kenny et al. 2010; Gotze et al. 2014), and specialist services may produce better outcomes than generalist services. Conversely, patients referred to these services may also have more complex needs. Only Dumont et al. (2006) recruited carers both through generalist and specialist care, and found significant levels psychological morbidity to be between 41% and 62%. Only two studies have considered population data (Wolff et al. 2007; Williams et al. 2014). However, these used single item, non-standard scales of emotional impact which do not allow us to ascertain levels of clinical significance. Furthermore, most studies have included large proportions of carers of patients who are not yet in the final months of life and who may still be relatively well (Wolff et al. 2007; Grov et al. 2005; Zapart et al. 2007; Kenny et al. 2010; Gotze et al. 2014; Grunfeld et al. 2004; Braun et al. 2007; Rumpold et al. 2016), thus not indicating the full impact of caregiving on carers during the course of the patients' illness.

To gain insights into psychological morbidity and general health during end of life caregiving for a broader population of carers we investigated psychological and general health in our 2015 national census post-bereavement survey of carers of people who died from cancer in England (Grande et al. 2018). We asked for carers' retrospective reports of how they felt during the patient's last 3 months of life using the GHQ-12, a standard measure of psychological morbidity, and the EQ-VAS, an established single item scale for general health. We compared carers' reports with scores from the general population using the Health Survey for England 2014. Survey responses indicated that 83% of carers had clinically significant psychological morbidity compared with 15% in the general population, and their psychological morbidity scores were 5–7 times higher than population scores across all age groups. Carers also overall had worse general health than the general population, but differences were less marked than for psychological morbidity, and carer and population scores converged towards older age with carers age 75 and over in fact scoring better than the population. Given that these are retrospective carer reports, we have to treat the absolute scores with some caution. However, carers were surveyed 4 months post-bereavement to enhance accuracy of recall. Further, the GHQ-12 mainly focuses on psychological functioning, e.g., ability to concentrate or to make decisions, rather than more subjective general feelings. We can therefore probably conclude with some certainty that levels of psychological morbidity among carers during end of life care are very high relative to the general population.

However, it is important to recognize that many carers also can see caregiving as positive and rewarding alongside the challenges and problems experienced. We therefore must understand these positive aspects and how we can help preserve these, while seeking to ameliorate some of the negative impacts from caregiving. Reviews of caregiving (Funk et al. 2010; Li and Loke 2013) report that positive aspects of caregiving include gaining a sense of reward, personal growth, growing closer to the patient and demonstrating love, gaining a feeling of self-esteem and accomplishment, and finding life enriching and meaningful features within the experience. However, the Funk et al. (2010) review notes that these findings may reflect carer coping processes that use positive interpretation and identification of rewards as part of meaning-based ways of coping. Nevertheless, this should not invalidate these processes in any way or indicate that we should not seek to support these ways of coping.

5 When Are Carers More Likely to Suffer Negative Impacts from Caregiving?

Not surprisingly, the patient's disease burden (i.e., level of functioning and symptoms) appears to have negative impact on carers' psychological health, quality of life, and perceived burden (Stajduhar et al. 2010; Hirdes et al. 2012; Lee et al. 2013; Tang et al. 2013). Similarly carers have greater psychological morbidity (Burridge et al. 2009; Tang et al. 2013; Grant et al. 2013; Hirdes et al. 2012) and worse health (Lee et al. 2013) as patients' approach death, where closeness to death is again likely to be associated with greater patient disease burden.

Hours of caregiving may also matter. A national survey of carers in general (Hirst 2005) found that increased hours were related to worse carer psychological health. Results are less clear for palliative care, however. Whilst some studies have found that longer hours of caregiving are associated with worse carer psychological health (Hirdes et al. 2012) and physical health (Kenny et al. 2010; Yoon et al. 2014), other hospice care studies have found no relationship (Washington et al. 2015).

Several demographic and contextual variables also affect impact of caregiving. A closer relationship with the patient may relate to more negative impact. Research indicates that spouses and/or (adult) children suffer greater psychological morbidity (Gotze et al. 2014; Hirdes et al. 2012; Tang et al. 2013) than less close relations. Spouses also report worse physical health (Park et al. 2012; Yoon et al. 2014) than other carers, but spouses may often also be older carers and therefore have worse physical health due to age. Good social network support is associated with reduced carer psychological morbidity (Gotze et al. 2014; Tang et al. 2013), health problems (Park et al. 2012), and perceived burden (Lee et al. 2013). Conversely, competing carer commitments may make caregiving more demanding. Stajduhar (2013) highlights that a growing number of carers, termed the "sandwich" generation, may be juggling caregiving for older parents with care for younger children and work which may be detrimental to their own health. However, more research is probably required into how the sum total of carers' commitments impact on carer health. Women generally report greater psychological morbidity during caregiving than men (Burridge et al. 2009; Stajduhar et al. 2010) and may also have worse physical health than male carers (Kenny et al. 2010; Park et al. 2012; Washington et al. 2015). Younger carers may suffer more psychological impact than older carers (Stajduhar et al. 2010), although Given et al. (2004) found middle aged carers to be more affected than younger and older carers, possibly representing the "sandwich generation." In contrast, older carers report worse physical health than younger carers (Kenny et al. 2010; Park et al. 2012; Yoon et al. 2014), but this may simply reflect the link between physical health and age. Carers with lower education on the whole seem to have worse psychological and physical health (Stadjuhar et al. 2010; Park et al. 2012) compared with those with higher education. Financial burden may be related to worse carer psychological morbidity (Gotze et al. 2014), and higher income or better financial support to better physical health and less perceived carer burden (Lee et al. 2013; Park et al. 2012; Yoon et al. 2014).

However, carers' own personal reactions and subjective appraisals of burden are probably more important in determining the impact of caregiving on their health and wellbeing than the actual, "objective" demands of caregiving or demographic and contextual variables. Review of the quantitative literature indicates that better outcomes are, for instance, associated with carers' perception of benefits of caregiving, as well as better preparation for caregiving and lower difficulty with tasks, a greater sense of meaning and comfort with caregiving tasks; and the feeling of greater role esteem, self-efficacy, and confidence in relation to caregiving (Stajduhar et al. 2010; Li and Loke 2013). "Reframing" coping strategies, including acceptance and redefinition, and positive religious coping also relate to better outcomes (Stajduhar et al. 2010; Li and Loke 2013). Reviews of the qualitative literature also indicates that carers often lack preparation, knowledge, and ability for caregiving and that lack of preparedness is associated with negative psychological outcomes (Funk et al. 2010). This clearly provides pointers for interventions with carers.

6 What Do Carers Say They Need Help with?

Given that carers' own appraisal of their caregiving situation is likely to be of prime importance in determining the impact of caregiving on them, it is crucial to understand how individual carers appraise their situation, what they struggle to manage, and where they feel they need additional support. To help with this, we investigated what carers normally need support with when looking after someone during palliative or end of life care, in order to help improve individualized carer assessment and support and highlight what areas we may generally need to address to support them. We conducted a large-scale qualitative study involving 75 bereaved carers in focus groups and interviews (Ewing and Grande 2013). Participants were carers of patients who had been referred to one of five hospice home care services across the UK.

Findings showed that carers' support needs fell into two broad groups: carers needed support to enable them to support the patient in their role as a key "co-worker." They also needed support to look after their own wellbeing in their role as a "client" in their own right. Responses indicated that carers felt a deep sense of responsibility for the patient's care and may be more willing to talk about their needs as "co-workers," and more reluctant to talk about their own needs (see Sect. 8). However, we have to recognize that to fully support carers, we must address their support needs both in their roles as co-worker and client. Within each role, carers' needs for support encompassed seven broad domains (see Box 1).

Box 1 Support needs of carers as co-workers or clients during end of life caregiving

Enabling carers to care (co-worker role)	Direct support for carers (client role)
Knowing who to contact when concerned	Own physical health concerns
Understanding the patient's illness	Dealing with their own feelings and worries
Knowing what to expect in the future	Beliefs or spiritual concerns
Managing symptoms and giving medicine	Practical help in the home
Talking to the patient about their illness	Financial, legal, or work issues
Equipment to help care for the patient	Having time for themselves in the day
Providing personal care for the patient	Overnight break from caring

The 14 domains were incorporated into a Carer Support Needs Assessment Tool (CSNAT). To ensure the 14 domains captured, the support needed by carers during palliative and end of life care, we conducted a validation study with 225 carers who were currently supporting a patient who had been referred to one of six UK hospice home care services (Ewing et al. 2013). Carers completed a postal survey indicating if they needed more support with any of the 14 support need domains or with "anything else," and completed standard measures of strain, distress, preparedness, global health, and positive appraisals of caregiving. Survey results showed that all the 14 domains were used by somebody to indicate further need for support. Further, only five of 225 carers wrote that they needed help with "anything else" that was not already fully covered by the existing domains, and what they added was nevertheless very closely related to existing domains, e.g., information on services available in the area. Need for further support with the domains was significantly correlated with increased carer strain and distress, worse global health, and reduced preparedness for caregiving, but not to positive appraisals (Ewing et al. 2013). Further linear regression analysis showed that a need for more support explained the greatest variance in strain (47%), followed by global health (35%), distress (29%), and preparedness (27%), but explained very little variance in positive appraisals (9%) (Grande et al. 2012). In terms of direction of these relationships, it is probably more likely that insufficient support predicts worse carer health and wellbeing, and that a lack of carer preparedness predicts a need for more support, but the nature of these relationships requires further investigation.

The validation study results indicate that the 14 domains were both comprehensive and sufficient in capturing carers' support needs and that they related to important measures of health and wellbeing. This study and subsequent research (Aoun et al. 2015a) show that the main domain carers need more support with are "knowing what to expect in the future," "dealing with your feelings and worries," "having time for yourself in the day" and "understanding your relative's illness." However, carers' support needs will differ and all the domains will be important to someone.

It is furthermore important to recognize that carers will differ in the individual support needs they have within any given domain and correspondingly the supportive input that they will require to meet those needs (Ewing and Grande 2013). Needing more support with symptom and medication management, for instance, will encompass a range of different support needs. These may include a need to understand the medicine regimen; what side effects to expect; being involved in discussions about symptom control; knowing at what point there is cause for alarm so that further help should be sought; or something else specific to the individual. Each of these scenarios requires different input and only the carer can define what supportive input is helpful in their case. While the 14 domains therefore comprehensively capture the broad areas that need to be considered when supporting carers, it is important that carers have the opportunity to express their individual support needs and to define what input would actually help with these needs.

7 How Well Have We Done in Supporting Carers to Date?

There is limited evidence to date that interventions have been effective in improving carer outcomes. An early systematic review by Lorenz et al. (2008) found that in general there was moderate evidence that palliative, supportive, and end of life care interventions increased carer satisfaction, but only weak evidence that such care actually improved carer outcomes This review did, however, find moderate evidence that interventions for carers of people with dementia were beneficial, but these may not necessarily be relevant to other palliative and end of life carers (e.g., they may focus on dealing with behavior problems or personality change). A Cochrane review (Candy et al. 2011) of supportive interventions, mainly to improve the psychological health of carers of patients in the terminal phase of their illness, found that interventions reduced carer distress short-term, but the effect was small (effect size $d = 0.15$). Further, there were no significant improvements in coping and quality of life. A more recent Cochrane review of home palliative care interventions by Gomes et al. (2013b) concluded that the overall evidence for improvement was nonsignificant, inconclusive, or conflicting with only some individual studies indicating shorter term improvement in burden, sense of reward, or reduced distress.

Part of the problem in assessing the effect of palliative and end of life interventions on carers is the wide range of interventions considered, so that it is difficult to draw clear and consistent conclusions and establish the "active components" of an intervention that may make a difference. Lorenz et al.'s (2008) review included regular palliative care and enhanced palliative care, group interventions and individual interventions. Gomes et al. (2013b) considered both regular and enhanced home palliative care, which again comes in many forms. Candy et al.'s (2011) review was more focused but still encompassed a considerable range of supportive interventions. Another problem is that many of the above interventions were mainly aimed at the patient, e.g., home palliative care, so it is perhaps unsurprising that they did not show a clear impact on carers, although there was a hope that carers would benefit. Further, even when interventions are targeted at carers, there may be a lack of effect because the intervention that is offered does not fit with what carers actually need (Buck et al. 2013; Levesque et al. 2010). Conclusions from Lorenz et al.'s review (2008) were that interventions were more likely to be effective when they were individually targeted and when they had multiple components (not just focused on one aspect).

To achieve meaningful improvements in carer outcomes, we therefore probably need to design interventions that are specifically focused on carers, more responsive to their individual needs and that address the range of needs or problems they may have. This means we need to understand the perspective of carers themselves; look at the whole individual; and let carers define what they need and let that drive the intervention. This comes back to asking carers themselves what it is they need support with, and sits squarely within the person-centered, holistic approach to support and care which is normally seen as core to palliative and end of life care.

8 Fitting Interventions to Carers' Considerations, Situation, and Individual Needs

There are several challenges that have to be overcome to ensure a fit between intervention (or support offered) and carers: negotiating carers' dual role and ambivalence at receiving help; restraints of location, time, and energy; and ensuring support fits the needs of individual carers.

As we have seen, carers have a dual role as both co-worker and client. Norms and expectations (held by carers themselves, but also sometimes by patients, family, and services) mean that carers often do not see themselves as legitimate care recipients and are ambivalent about receiving help or taking a break from caregiving. Carers may only accept support if they feel this will help them care and does not take resources and attention away from the patient (Harding and Higginson 2001). To provide effective support, we need to recognize these dynamics, help legitimize the expression of need for help and support, and ensure that help is on carers' own terms. This is likely to require a proactive approach as carers themselves are often reluctant to express what they themselves need help with, may not know what aspects of support are available or what it is legitimate to ask for support with. While volunteering that they need help is often difficult for carers, being asked about needs and/or offered help as part of an established, formal process may help overcome barriers. It may also help if this is done in such a way that carers do not have to express their needs in front of the patient (Ewing and Grande 2018).

Any standardized interventions need to be sensitive to the dilemmas and constraints of the carer role. They need to recognize the potential conflict between carers' desire to sustain caregiving and looking after their own needs. Respite may for instance be easier for carers to accept in the form of briefer daytime breaks or overnight sitting, rather than inpatient admission. Help with the patient's personal care may be more acceptable if the carer can still be present and involved. In each case, it is important to know what carers want; some may want a complete break from caregiving, but for others this can be hard to accept, although they need a rest and some support. Interventions that depend on carers leaving the patient, e.g., to attend group activities or therapies, are often also practically difficult for carers, unless formal care for the patient forms part of the intervention, and even then carers need to feel this is an acceptable solution for the patient. Carer interventions that can be delivered at home or during delivery of day care, outpatient or inpatient care for the patient may therefore prove more feasible. Joint patient/carer interventions may provide a solution and be desirable where the aim of the intervention for instance is to foster communication or joint problem solving. However, this may inhibit expression of carers' own needs and concerns. Interventions that to some extent can be tailored are also likely to be of more use to carers who will have limited time and energy. For instance, one can hypothesize that access to bitesize, individualized information is likely to be more helpful than bigger, standardized chunks. Any standard intervention needs to be developed from carers' perspective to ensure they actually fit carers' situation and address what they need. It is therefore essential that we engage carers in the design of general interventions or support services for carers.

If we are to provide more individualized support, however, this normally requires individual assessment of need for support. There are two broad approaches that can be taken to assessing carers' need for support: assessment of adverse effects of caregiving or more direct assessment of the problems that carers need support with.

Assessment of adverse effects of caregiving enables identification of carers that are suffering particularly high impacts from caregiving, which enables us to focus intervention resources on those most in need of help and most likely to benefit from intervention. Numerous tools exist that may be used for assessment of adverse effects during caregiving (Hudson et al. 2010). The main groups of adverse outcomes that have been considered include psychological morbidity, subjective burden, and quality of life. Measures of psychological morbidity have not been developed specifically for carers, but general measures have successfully been used with the carer population. These include the Hospital Anxiety and Depression Scale (HADS), the Beck Depression Inventory (BDI) (Hudson et al. 2010), and the General Health Questionnaire (GHQ-12) (Grande et al. 2018), all of which are relatively short (12–21 items) with good reliability. The single item Distress Thermometer has also been used as a brief screening tool for anxiety and depression in carers to identify those who may require further follow up (Zwahlen et al. 2008). Measures of subjective burden, or strain, have been specifically developed for carers to capture burdens related to the caregiver situation. These include the Zarit Burden Interview (ZBI), the Caregiver's Burden Scale in End-of-Life Care (CBS-EOLC), and the Caregiver Strain Index (CSI) (Hudson et al. 2010). Again these are relatively short (13–22 items) with good reliability. The Family Appraisal of Caregiving Questionnaire for Palliative Care (FACQ-PC; 25 items) seeks to capture both strain and distress, as well as positive appraisals (Hudson et al. 2010). Questionnaires that have been used to measure carers' quality of life include both generic questionnaires and questionnaires specifically developed or adapted for carers. The former include the SF-36 and the Quality of Life Scale (QOLS) (16 items). The latter include the Quality of Life in Life-Threatening Illness – Family carer version (QOLTTI-F) and the Caregiver Quality of Life Index – Cancer (CQOLC) scale (Hudson et al. 2010) with 16 and 35 items, respectively, all again with good reliability.

These measures can give an indication that a carer is experiencing adverse effects from caregiving likely to need further intervention. However, these measures still require us to then identify the individual areas of difficulty or needs the carer has as well as appropriate courses of action to help ameliorate the psychological morbidity, burden or poor Quality of Life. Appropriate action may for instance be to target carers' psychological appraisals of caregiving burden and improve coping, resilience, and capabilities, or more direct intervention with the day to day problems they experience with caregiving. In any case, actions should involve discussion with carers regarding what may help. Further, one would ideally want to try to intervene before burden, psychological morbidity and deteriorating quality of life reach critical levels, where possible.

Here more direct assessment of the issues that carers need support with or that give rise to distress can help by providing practical pointers for meaningful action or earlier intervention to prevent adverse impacts reaching critical levels. Tools that may help with this include The Needs Assessment Tool – Caregivers (NAT-C), Carer Support Needs Assessment Tool (CSNAT), Carers' Alert Thermometer (CAT), and The Family Inventory of Needs (FIN). The NAT-C (Mitchell et al. 2010) is a 32 item tool developed from the literature and 25 interviews with practitioners and carers. It can be self-completed by carers or together with a practitioner and enables carers to indicate their levels of concern on a range of issues including physical and psychological wellbeing, spiritual, existential, social, financial and legal concerns, and whether they would like to discuss them with their GP or other practitioner. The CSNAT (Ewing and Grande 2013), as previously noted, contains 14 items or domains and was developed from focus groups with 75 bereaved carers. It is intended to be self-completed by carers and enables them to indicate whether they need more support with looking after the patient or with preserving their own wellbeing (Box 1). The Carers' Alert Thermometer (CAT) (Knighting et al. 2016) contains 10 items about the carers' caring situation and their health and wellbeing. It is designed for practitioners to complete to identify any alerts that require further intervention. The Family Inventory of Needs (FIN) (Kristjanson et al. 1995) identifies areas of importance to the carer where services "fall short." Its

20 items represent a range of needs, mainly in relation to information including having questions answered honestly, knowing what treatment the patient is receiving, and what to do for the patient. It enables carers to rate how important each item is to them and indicate the extent to which these are met by practitioners.

However, assessment tools in and of themselves are unlikely to improve carer outcomes. If used as a questionnaire or form without subsequent discussion of, and response to, identified problems, none of these tools are likely to have beneficial impact on carer outcomes. Both the NAT-C and CSNAT are examples of tools that have been designed to be used as part of a defined intervention process, and whose impact has subsequently been tested through trials. In the NAT-C intervention, the completion of the tool by the carer is intended to be followed by a discussion of the NAT-C with their GP or other practitioner. As part of the process, the GP is supported by resource folder outlining potential carer problems and suggested resources and strategies that may help (Mitchell et al. 2010). A randomized controlled trial of this intervention with GPs indicated that for carers with clinical anxiety at baseline, the intervention improved mental wellbeing, and for those with clinical depression at baseline, the intervention slowed the worsening of depression (Mitchell et al. 2013).

The CSNAT is explicitly designed be part of a person-centered process that is led by the carer, although facilitated by practitioners. Early CSNAT feasibility work with practitioners highlighted the important features of this process to ensure it has meaningful impact and represents a truly person-centered comprehensive approach (the CSNAT Approach; Ewing et al. 2015). The CSNAT Approach is encapsulated in five stages, which also have relevance for other assessments: (1) Introduction: It is important to ensure the carer understands that the tool is part of a process of assessment that gives them the opportunity to consider their own support needs as distinct from the patient not just another leaflet or form. (2) Carer consideration of needs: The carer needs time to consider what areas they need support with, in privacy if required. Whatever time they require, carers need to know they will then have opportunity to discuss identified support needs with a practitioner. (3) Assessment conversation: In completing the CSNAT, the carer will have highlighted domains where they need more support and then prioritized those most pressing for them at the moment. The focus of the conversation is on the carers' individual needs within the domain(s) they have prioritized, to establish the particular issue they need help with and what supportive input they feel would help in relation to this. As highlighted earlier, carers will differ in the supportive input that they need within each domain, so it is important not to work from set assumptions by the practitioner as to the problem and its solution. (4) Shared action plan: Supportive input is based on the assessment conversation; it summarizes and documents actions put in place. This can take different forms: actions carers themselves take to access support (self-help or help from family); support directly delivered by practitioners such as "active listening," reassurance, advice giving, provision of information (which may be accomplished within the visit/contact); signposting the carer to other sources of support or referral to other agencies. Not all support needs have to be met by the practitioner or their organization. (5) Shared review: Carers' support needs change and so review of their situation needs to be ongoing. The prompt for a review can come from either the carer or the practitioner. It is important that carers are aware that they may raise their support needs at any time.

Further feasibility studies and trials showed that use of the CSNAT to support carers was seen as valuable both by practitioners and carers. Practitioners felt that use of such an assessment tool opened up different conversations with carers, challenged their assumptions regarding what carers needed help with, and improved expression, visibility and "legitimacy" of support needs (Ewing et al. 2016). The carers themselves felt that this helped them identify and express support needs that would otherwise not be possible; that it enabled necessary reflection, although this could at times be challenging; and that it provided them with validation, reassurance, and empowerment (Aoun et al. 2015b). Cluster trials of the impact of the CSNAT intervention on carer outcomes found that the intervention group had significantly lower levels of strain during caregiving from baseline to follow up (effect size, d = 0.35) (Aoun et al. 2015a) and that they had significantly lower early grief and better psychological and physical health post-bereavement (Grande et al. 2017).

9 How Do We Implement Carer Support in Practice?

Successful development and trialing of interventions will not be of broader benefit unless evidence-based practice can be implemented and integrated into mainstream care. This normally entails a change in practice, which requires change not only at the level of individual practitioners but also at organization level to provide the structures and processes needed to support implementation and sustain it longer term, beyond a research project or practice initiative. The challenges of implementing change can be overlooked within policy, practice, and research. The MORECare Guidance for palliative care research recommends that implementation should be considered from the outset, within development, piloting and testing stages (Higginson et al. 2013).

In England, the Government's strategy for palliative care has for a long time highlighted that there should be assessment and support for carers as well as patients (DH End of Life Care (EOLC) Strategy 2008; NPEoLP Ambitions for Palliative and End of life Care 2015). Yet within this strategy, there has been no consideration of how this will be implemented in practice for carers. It was largely in response to this gap in the Government's 2008 strategy that the CSNAT was developed. However, our feasibility testing, trial, and implementation work with the CSNAT intervention helped us begin to identify the factors that need to be in place for successful implementation of change in practice in general and the assessment and support for carers in particular.

These lessons were consolidated and extended in a UK project to develop key recommendations for implementation of comprehensive, person-centered carer assessment, and support in end of life care. The project involved research review and stakeholder consultation through three interlinked stages: (1) secondary analysis of rich data from pragmatic implementation of person-centered carer assessment and support within 36 palliative care services using the CSNAT intervention; (2) new focus groups with hospice practitioners/leads, and (3) wide consultation with stakeholders from hospice, hospital, community, policy, and academia as well as carer groups to confirm and validate the set of recommendations. Box 2 lists the resulting ten recommendations, all of which were identified as key issues for implementation of carer assessment and support in practice and not consistently met by current provision in end of life care. Broadly, the first four recommendations indicate what needs to be

Box 2 Ten recommendations for achieving organizational change to enable provision of comprehensive, person-centered assessment and support for family carers towards the end of life

1. Consistent identification of carers within the care setting.
2. Demographic and contextual data on who the carer is and their situation.
3. A protocol for assessing carers and responding to the assessment.
4. A recording system for carer information, separate from patient data.
5. A process for training practitioners about carer assessment and support.
6. Available time/workload capacity for carer assessment and support.
7. Support from senior managers for carer assessment and support.
8. Role models/champions for carer assessment and support.
9. Pathways for communication about carer assessment and support.
10. Procedures for monitoring/auditing processes and outcomes of carer assessment and support.

embedded in organizations to provide person-centered support for carers and the remaining six are the structures and processes needed to successfully implement and sustain this approach in practice. Together they illustrate the whole-systems approach that need to be taken to implementation (Ewing and Grande 2018).

While developed for carer assessment and support, these principles are likely to have general applicability for implementation of interventions to support carers. The context for each recommendation is described in more detail below.

Underpinning any carer interventions is the need to know who the patient's main carer or carers are. Current practice of carer identification can be quite ad hoc, allowing many carers to slip through the net. A more systematic and proactive approach is necessary for **Consistent identification of carers within the care setting** as many carers do not self-identify and can miss out on much needed support. This is particularly the case where they see themselves in relationship terms, as a wife/husband or son/daughter of the patient and do not recognize themselves as a "carer." In these circumstances, a questions such as "who provides the patient with most support" (who is not a healthcare professional) can be helpful in carer identification.

Closely linked to carer identification is the recommendation for **Demographic and contextual data on who the carer is and their situation**, to aid communication with carers and awareness of their circumstances. Even where carers are known to palliative care services, there can be a lack of documentation about them. Our project found this was particularly the case in hospital settings where the primary focus is on the patient but was also true in hospices. There was a lack of basic information such as number of carers known to the organization, and even for identified carers contact information and basic details about their situation or needs were often not recorded. This again makes it difficult to sustain meaningful intervention.

The project's third recommendation – **A protocol for assessing carers and responding to the assessment** is a principle that translates to implementation in general, in that there has to be a clear protocol for how any new intervention is to be delivered in practice. In terms of delivering consistent carer assessment and support, this normally represents a considerable practice change: identification of carers' needs may currently be missed altogether, and when it does take place, is often an informal, practitioner-led approach conducted as part of the patient assessment or takes the form of "doorstep conversations" (Ewing et al. 2015) when carers don't want to talk in front of the patient. Further, solutions are often based on practitioners' assumptions rather than identified by carers. A clear protocol is a prerequisite for implementing consistent, comprehensive, person-centered carer assessment and support. This puts carers on a more equal footing to patients and helps legitimize their support in palliative and end of life care.

A recording system for carer information, separate from patient data, is to ensure that information on carers is recorded in a defined location for record keeping and future reference. This is an issue linked to consistent carer identification and data gathering. If this information cannot be easily accessed and utilized, it is unlikely to aid effective interventions. Current health record systems focus on patients: any information that is recorded about carers is usually done within the patient record, often under family support. However, a systems change in recording processes is needed if carers are to be consistently identified and supported. Flexibility to develop separate carer records will vary across settings with particular challenges for hospital-based palliative care teams, but many hospices are already developing separate carer record systems.

Fundamental to achieving consistency in practice with carers is putting in place **a process for training practitioners about carer assessment and support**. Training is core to ensure everyone is on board with the purpose and procedures of the intervention and how it is different from existing practice, otherwise what may be a beneficial intervention at conception, may change to become ineffective or even detrimental in its implementation (Neuberger et al. 2013). It is, for instance, important to identify the differences between a comprehensive, person-centered approach and current practice for those already working to support carers in everyday practice. Training about carer assessment and support also has resonance across all settings and at all stages: from broader carer awareness raising early in nurse education to understand the key role of carers in end of life care; to assist more junior frontline staff who are unfamiliar with identifying carer needs; through to more experienced practitioners who feel they "already do" carer assessment and support, providing an opportunity to "up their game."

Available time/workload capacity for carer assessment and support: For implementation of any intervention, organizations need to consider how to make sufficient time to plan, implement, and sustain a change in practice. For carer assessment and support the leadership in organizations needs to decide whether this is part of their "core" business, rather than an "add-on" to patient care, only when time allows. If core, organizations need to consider how to make sufficient time for meaningful implementation. Investment of time on carers in the short-term can achieve longer-term gains in averting crises. However achieving capacity at practitioner level for this new way of working not only requires a mind-shift away from a focus solely on patients but also time and resources for its practical implementation by frontline staff.

Support from senior managers for carer assessment and support: This is crucial to provide a wider strategic overview and the authority for implementation of new interventions across all settings. This includes (1) initiating the change from current practice and (2) driving forward the new way of working through facilitating training and ensuring workforce capacity for implementation. Input from senior managers is vital to sustaining the change to comprehensive, person-centered assessment and support in the longer term, through review, improving processes and providing evidence to commissioners to support palliative care delivery for carers, not just patients.

Role models/champions for carer assessment and support: This highlights the need for organizational support at several levels for implementation. Rather than managers, champions need to be credible practitioners committed to the new intervention and able to promote its implementation in practice. Champions provide essential facilitation through creating a positive culture around the new way of working, cascading training and support to practitioners working with carers as well as acting as a source of advice. Organizational investment in the role is crucial to ensure champions are supported and have the necessary resources but also that the role continues even if the original post-holder moved on.

Pathways for communication about carer assessment and support: Different communication processes are important to embed and sustain new ways of working. This needs to operate both between and within different organizational levels. Two-way processes are required: (top down) from service leads and champions to communicate what is expected of practitioners and to provide help and advice, but also (bottom up) feedback by practitioners who are implementing a new intervention about what is helping or hindering its use in practice. Putting in place peer discussions for problem solving and sharing of good practice provides further opportunities to support a different way of working.

Procedures for monitoring/auditing processes and outcomes of carer assessment and support: This is not always well done within palliative care services; yet these are key organizational activities for internal purposes to measure progress towards targets and review work done by the services in supporting carers. Crucially, these processes can communicate impact of service delivery on carer outcomes, demonstrating achievements in carer assessment and support to external agencies such as commissioners of palliative care services and other funding bodies.

Overall, achieving comprehensive, person-centered assessment and support for carers is not without challenges for palliative care delivery. The first main challenge is that this way of working with carers is not commonplace: It represents a substantial change in practice for end of life care, not just for practitioners directly supporting carers but for organizations in terms of the structures and process that need to be in place. The ten recommendations identify the building blocks to achieving the necessary organizational changes. There is, however, a second and perhaps more difficult challenge of addressing the question of where carers "fit" within palliative care provision. Since its beginnings, palliative care has had an ethos of services being there for the carer and family, not just the patient. While this is a strong philosophy, its translation into practice is hindered by the many issues underpinning the ten recommendations. If carers are to be identified, assessed, and supported in end of life care, the fundamental question of whether or not they are to be viewed as true clients of services (and therefore their care and support can become legitimized through commissioning and funding processes) has to be addressed.

10 Conclusion and Summary

This chapter has shown that family carers provide vital support for patients towards the end of life. Formal services clearly have an essential part to play, but resource constraints mean that the time and support they can provide will always remain limited. Family carers therefore undertake the main bulk of patient care and support and make care at home viable. Our dependence on carers is likely to increase in light of a projected increase in the older population and number of deaths.

Carers suffer adverse consequences from caregiving, particularly in terms of their mental health. The prevalence of clinically significant psychological morbidity among carers during end of life care may indeed be so high that it can be deemed a public health problem. However, there is considerable individual variation in who is most affected. While the patient's disease burden and hours of caregiving have some impact on carers' health, impact also depends on carers' demographic characteristics and context, and in particular on carers' own subjective appraisals and preparedness for caregiving. This indicates that there is considerable scope for intervention.

In terms of what may help, carers support needs fall into two broad areas: firstly, they need support to enable them to support the patient, in their role as "co-workers"; secondly, they need support to look after their own health and wellbeing, as "clients" in their own right. Both areas need to be addressed if we are to fully support carers. It is important to realize that the type of supportive input carers need in each case varies greatly from individual to individual, and that "one size does not fit all." This implies that it is important to take an individualized approach to carer support and to ensure that the assessment of carers' support needs and identification of what supportive input would help, is carer-led.

Reviews indicate that interventions to support carers so far have had fairly limited success. Part of the problem may be that interventions have not been specifically designed to support carers or that what is provided has not matched what carers actually need. Again more individualized interventions that encompass a broader range of needs appear to be more successful. Further, any intervention should be designed with carers' situation and concerns in mind and include meaningful carer involvement in its development.

Individualized, tailored intervention is difficult to achieve without some form of assessment of need. This may be in the form of assessing which carers are suffering critically high levels of adverse impact on their health and wellbeing and focusing efforts on these carers. However, this still requires identification of what intervention is appropriate. Assessment may also be in the form of directly assessing what carers say they need more support with, to enable more direct and potentially more preventative interventions with carers. However, assessment in itself is not likely to be beneficial without subsequent discussion and follow up.

If we are to implement carer support within mainstream palliative care practice, this is likely to require a considerable change in practice which entails a whole-systems approach to implementation. Such a whole-system implementation would need to encompass organizational procedures for identifying carers and recording carer information, as well as protocols for how to support carers. To implement and sustain such a change, wider organizational support is also required in terms of leadership, staff training, champions for driving change forward, protected time for supporting carers, communication pathways, and procedures for auditing and monitoring change.

However, the fundamental, underlying question that needs to be addressed if we are to provide consistent, meaningful carer support within palliative care is where carers fit within palliative care provision. We have to decide whether supporting carers is simply an add-on which only is covered on a more intermittent basis or whether it is part of "core" business which is consequently funded and has protected time.

References

Abernethy A, Burns C, Wheeler J, Currow D. Defining distinct caregiver subpopulations by intensity of end-of-life care provided. Palliat Med. 2009;23(1):66–79.

Aoun SM, Grande G, Howting D, Deas K, Toye C, Troeung L, et al. The impact of the Carer Support Needs Assessment Tool (CSNAT) in community palliative care using a stepped wedge cluster trial. PLoS One. 2015a;10(4):e0123012. https://doi.org/10.1371/journal.pone.0123012.

Aoun S, Deas K, Toye C, Ewing E, Grande G, Stajduhar K. Supporting family caregivers to identify their own needs in end-of-life care: qualitative findings from a stepped wedge cluster trial. Palliat Med. 2015b;29(6):508–17. https://doi.org/10.1177/0269216314566061.

Braun M, Mikulincer M, Rydall A, Walsh A, Rodin G. Hidden morbidity in cancer: spouse caregivers. J Clin Oncol. 2007;25(30):4829–34.

Brick A, Smith S, Normand C, O'Hara S, Droog E, Tyrrell E, Cunningham N, Johnston B. Costs of formal and informal care in the last year of life for patients in receipt of specialist palliative care. Palliat Med. 2017;31:356–68.

Buck HG, Zambroski CH, Garrison C, McMillan SC. Everything they were discussing, we were already doing: hospice heart failure caregivers reflect on a palliative caregiving intervention. J Hosp Palliat Nurs. 2013;15(4):218–24.

Buckner L, Yeandle S. Valuing Carers 2015 – the rising value of carers' support. Carers UK. 2015. https://www.carersuk.org/for-professionals/policy/policy-library/valuing-carers-2015.

Burns CM, Abernethy AP, Dal Grande E, Currow DC. Uncovering an invisible network of direct caregivers at the end of life: a population study. Palliat Med. 2013;27(7):608–15.

Burridge LH, Barnett AG, Clavarino AM. The impact of perceived stage of cancer on carers' anxiety and depression during the patients' final year of life. Psycho-Oncology. 2009;18(6):615–23.

Candy B, Jones L, Drake R, et al. Interventions for supporting informal caregivers of patients in the terminal phase of a disease. Cochrane Database Syst Rev. 2011;15(6):CD007617. https://doi.org/10.1002/14651858.CD007617.pub2.

Carers Australia. The economic value of informal care in Australia in 2015. 2015. http://www.carersaustralia.com.au/storage/Access%20Economics%20Report.pdf. Last accessed 25 June 2018.

Department of Health. End of life care strategy: promoting high quality care for all adults at the end of life. London: Department of Health; 2008.

Department of Health. Palliative care funding review: funding the right care and support for everyone. 2011. https://www.gov.uk/government/uploads/system/uploads/attachment_data/file/215107/dh_133105.pdf.

Dumont S, Turgeon J, Allard P, Gagnon P, Charbonneau C, Vezina L. Caring for a loved one with advanced cancer: determinants of psychological distress in family caregivers. J Palliat Med. 2006;9(4):912–21.

Dzingina MD, Reilly CC, Bausewein C, Jolley CJ, Moxham J, McCrone P, Higginson IJ, Yi D. Variations in the cost of formal and informal health care for patients with advanced chronic disease and refractory breathlessness: a cross-sectional secondary analysis. Palliat Med. 2017;31:369–77.

Ewing G, Grande GE. Development of a Carer Support Needs Assessment Tool (CSNAT) for end of life care practice at home: a qualitative study. Palliat Med. 2013;27(3):244–56. https://doi.org/10.1177/0269216312440607.

Ewing G, Grande GE. Providing comprehensive, person-centred assessment and support for family carers towards the end of life: 10 recommendations for achieving organisational change. London: Hospice UK; 2018.

Ewing G, Brundle C, Payne S, Grande G. The Carer Support Needs Assessment Tool (CSNAT) for use in palliative and end of life care at home: a validation study. J Pain Symptom Manag. 2013;46(3):395–405. https://doi.org/10.1016/j.jpainsymman.2012.09.008.

Ewing G, Austin L, Diffin J, Grande G. Developing a person-centred approach to carer assessment and support. Br J Community Nurs. 2015;20(12):580–4.

Ewing G, Austin L, Grande G. The role of the Carer Support Needs Assessment Tool in palliative home care: a qualitative study of practitioners' perspectives of its impact and mechanisms of action. Palliat Med. 2016;30(4):392–400.

Funk L, Stajduhar KI, Toye C, Aoun S, Grande G, Todd C. Part 2: home-based family caregiving at the end of life: a comprehensive review of published qualitative research (1998–2008). Palliat Med. 2010;24:594–607.

Gardiner C, Ingleton C, Ryan T, Ward S, Gott M. What cost components are relevant for economic evaluations of palliative care, and what approaches are used to measure these costs? A systematic review. Palliat Med. 2017;31(4):323–37.

Given B, Wyatt G, Given C, et al. Burden and depression among caregivers of patients with cancer at the end of life. Oncol Nurs Forum. 2004;31:1105–17.

Gomes B, Higginson IJ. Factors influencing death at home in terminally ill patients with cancer: systematic review. BMJ. 2006;332(7540):515–21.

Gomes B, Calanzani N, Gysels M, Hall S, Higginson IJ. Heterogeneity and changes in preferences for dying at home: a systematic review. BMC Palliat Care. 2013a;12:7. https://doi.org/10.1186/1472-684X-12-7.

Gomes B, Calanzani N, Curiale V, McCrone P, Higginson IJ. Effectiveness and cost-effectiveness of home palliative care services for adults with advanced illness and their caregivers. Cochrane Database Syst Rev. 2013b;6(6):CD007760. https://doi.org/10.1002/14651858.CD007760.pub2.

Gott M, Frey R, Robinson J, Boyd M, O'Callaghan A, Richards N, et al. The nature of, and reasons for, 'inappropriate' hospitalisations among patients with palliative care needs: a qualitative exploration of the views of generalist palliative care providers. Palliat Med. 2013;27(8):747–56.

Gotze H, Brahler E, Gansera L, Polze N, Kohler N. Psychological distress and quality of life of palliative cancer patients and their caring relatives during home care. Support Care Cancer. 2014;22(10):775–8.

Grande GE, Ewing G. Death at home unlikely if informal carers prefer otherwise: implications for policy. Palliat Med. 2008;22:971–2.

Grande G, Ewing G, Sawatzky R. Supporting family carers: the relative importance of different support domains in explaining negative and positive impacts from caregiving. In: Palliative medicine: Abstracts of the 7th World Research Congress of the European Association for Palliative Care (EAPC). 2012; 26:408.

Grande G, Austin L, Ewing G, O'Leary N, Roberts C. Assessing the impact of a Carer Support Needs Assessment (CSNAT) intervention in palliative home care: a stepped wedge cluster trial. BMJ Support Palliat Care. 2017;7:326–34.

Grande G, Rowland R, van den Berg B, Hanratty B. Psychological morbidity and general health among family caregivers during end of life cancer care: a retrospective census survey. Palliat Med online first. 2018. https://doi.org/10.1177/0269216318793286.

Grant M, Sun V, Fujinami R, Sidhu R, Otis-Green S, Juarez G, et al. Family caregiver burden, skills preparedness, and quality of life in non-small cell lung cancer. Oncol Nurs Forum. 2013;40(4):337–46.

Grov EK, Dahl AA, Moum T, Fossa SD. Anxiety, depression, and quality of life in caregivers of patients with cancer in late palliative phase. Ann Oncol. 2005;16(7):1185–91.

Grunfeld E, Coyle D, Whelan T, et al. Family caregiver burden: results of a longitudinal study of breast cancer patients and their principal caregivers. Can Med Assoc J. 2004;170(12):1795–801.

Harding R, Higginson I. Working with ambivalence: informal caregivers of patients at the end of life. Support Care Cancer. 2001;9(8):642–5.

Higginson IJ, Evans CJ, Grande G, Preston N, Morgan M, McCrone P, Lewis P, Fayers P, Harding R, Hotopf M, Murray SA, Benalia H, Gysels M, Farquhar M, Todd C. Evaluating complex interventions in end of life care: the MORECare statement on good practice generated by a synthesis of transparent expert consultations and systematic reviews. BMC Med. 2013;11:111. https://doi.org/10.1186/1741-7015-11-111.

Hirdes JP, Freeman S, Smith TF, Stolee P. Predictors of caregiver distress among palliative home care clients in Ontario: evidence based on the interRAI palliative care. Palliat Support Care. 2012;10(3):155–63.

Hirst M. Carer distress: a prospective, population-based study. Soc Sci Med. 2005;61:697–708.

Hudson PL, Trauer T, Graham S, Grande G, Ewing G, Payne S, Stajduhar KI, Thomas K. A systematic review of instruments related to family caregivers of palliative care patients. Palliat Med. 2010;24:656–68.

Kenny PM, Hall JP, Zapart S, Davis PR. Informal care and home-based palliative care: the health-related quality of life of carers. J Pain Symptom Manag. 2010;40(1):35–48.

Kingston A, Wohland P, Wittenberg R, Robinson L, Brayne C, Matthews F, Jagger C on behalf of Cognitive Function and Ageing Studies Collaboration. Is late-life dependency increasing or not? A comparison of the Cognitive Function and Ageing Studies (CFAS). Lancet. 2017;390(10103):1676–84.

Knighting K, O'Brien MR, Roe B, Gandy R, Lloyd-Williams M, Nolan M, et al. Gaining consensus on family carer needs when caring for someone dying at home to develop the Carers' Alert Thermometer (CAT): a modified Delphi study. J Adv Nurs. 2016;72(1):227–39.

Kristjanson LJ, Atwood J, Degner LF. Validity and reliability of the family inventory of needs (FIN): measuring the care needs of families of advanced cancer patients. J Nurs Meas. 1995;3:109–26.

Lee KC, Chang W-C, Chou W-C, Su P-J, Hsieh C-H, Chen J-S, et al. Longitudinal changes and predictors of caregiving burden while providing end-of-life care for terminally ill cancer patients. J Palliat Med. 2013;16(6):632–7.

Levesque L, Ducharme F, Caron C, Hanson E, Magnusson L, Nolan J, Nolan M. A partnership approach to service needs assessment with family-caregivers of an aging relative living at home: a qualitative analysis of the experiences of caregivers and practitioners. Int J Nurs Stud. 2010;47:876–87.

Li Q, Loke AY. The positive aspects of caregiving for cancer patients: a critical review of the literature and directions for future research. Psycho-Oncology. 2013;22(11):2399–407.

Lorenz KA, Lynn J, Dy SM, et al. Evidence for improving palliative care at the end of life: a systematic review. Ann Intern Med. 2008;148:147–59.

Mitchell G, Girgis A, Jiwa M, Sibbritt D, Burridge L. A GP caregiver needs toolkit versus usual care in the management of the needs of caregivers of patients with advanced cancer: a randomized controlled trial. Trials. 2010;11:115. http://www.trialsjournal.com/content/11/1/115.

Mitchell GK, Girgis A, Jiwa M, Sibbritt D, Burridge LH, Senior HE. Providing general practice needs-based care for carers of people with advanced cancer: a randomised controlled trial. Br J Gen Pract. 2013;63:e683.

National End of Life Care Programme. Reviewing end of life care costing information to inform the QIPP End of Life Care Workstream. Whole systems partnership. 2012. http://www.thewholesystem.co.uk/docs/EoLC_QIPP_Costings_Report.pdf.

National Institute for Clinical Excellence. Guidance on Cancer Services. Improving supportive and palliative care for adults with cancer. The manual. London: NICE; 2004.

National Palliative and End of Life Care Partnership. Ambitions for Palliative and End of Life Care: a national framework for local action 2015–2020. 2015. NHS England. London.

Neuberger J, Guthrie C, Aaronvitch D. More care, less pathway: a review of the Liverpool Care Pathway. London: Department of Health; 2013. https://assets.publishing.service.gov.uk/government/uploads/system/uploads/attachment_data/file/212450/Liverpool_Care_Pathway.pdf. Last accessed 22 June 2018.

Office of National Statistics. 2012-based National Population Projections (Released: 6 November 2013). London: ONS; 2013. [Online] Available from: http://www.ons.gov.uk/ons/rel/npp/national-population-projections/2012-based-projections/stb-2012-based-npp-principal-and-key-variants.html.

Park C-H, Shin DW, Choi JY, Kang J, Baek YJ, Mo HN, et al. Determinants of the burden and positivity of family caregivers of terminally ill cancer patients in Korea. Psycho-Oncology. 2012;21(3):282–90.

Penders YWH, Rietjens J, Albers G, Croezen S, Van den Block L. Differences in out-of-pocket costs of healthcare in the last year of life of older people in 13 European countries. Palliat Med. 2017;31(1):42–52.

Reyniers T, Deliens L, Pasman HR, Vander Stichele R, Sijnave B, Houttekier D, et al. Appropriateness and avoidability of terminal hospital admissions: results of a survey among family physicians. Palliat Med. 2017;31(5):456–64.

Romanow RJ. Building on values: the future of healthcare in Canada. Commission on the Future of Health Care in Canada. 2002. http://publications.gc.ca/site/eng/237274/publication.html. Last accessed 25 May 2018.

Round J, Jones L, Morris S. Estimating the cost of caring for people with cancer at the end of life: a modelling study. Palliat Med. 2015;29:899–907.

Rowland C, Hanratty B, Pilling M, van den Berg B, Grande G. The contributions of family care-giving at end-of-life: a national post-bereavement census survey of cancer carers' hours of care and expenditures. Palliat Med. 2017;31(4):346–55.

Rumpold T, Schur S, Amering M, et al. Informal caregivers of advanced-stage cancer patients: every second is at risk for psychiatric morbidity. Support Care Cancer. 2016;24(5):1975–82.

Smith S, Brick A, O'Hara S, Normand C. Evidence on the cost and cost-effectiveness of palliative care: a literature review. Palliat Med. 2013;28(2):130–50.

Stajduhar KI. Burdens of family caregiving at the end of life. Clin Invest Med – Medecine Clinique et Experimentale. 2013;36(3):E121–6.

Stajduhar KI, Funk L, Toye C, Grande G, Aoun S, Todd C. Part 1: home-based family caregiving at the end of life: a comprehensive review of published quantitative research (1998–2008). Palliat Med. 2010;24:573–93.

Tang ST, Chang W-C, Chen J-S, Wang H-M, Shen WC, Li C-Y, et al. Course and predictors of depressive symptoms among family caregivers of terminally ill cancer patients until their death. Psycho-Oncology. 2013;22(6):1312–8.

Van Houtven CH, Ramsey SD, Hornbrook MC, Atienza AA, van Ryn M. Economic burden for informal caregivers of lung and colorectal cancer patients. Oncologist. 2010;15:883–93.

Washington KT, Pike KC, Demiris G, Parker Oliver D, Albright DL, Lewis AM. Gender differences in caregiving at end of life: implications for hospice teams. J Palliat Med. 2015;18(12):1048–53.

Williams AM, Wang L, Kitchen P. Differential impacts of care-giving across three caregiver groups in Canada: end-of-life care, long-term care and short-term care. Health Soc Care Community. 2014;22(2):187–96.

Wolff JL, Dy SM, Frick KD, Kasper JD. End-of-life care: findings from a national survey of informal caregivers. Arch Intern Med. 2007;167(1):40–6.

Yoon S-J, Kim J-S, Jung J-G, Kim S-S, Kim S. Modifiable factors associated with caregiver burden among family caregivers of terminally ill Korean cancer patients. Support Care Cancer. 2014;22(5):1243–50.

Zapart S, Kenny P, Hall J, Servis B, Wiley S. Home-based palliative care in Sydney, Australia: the carer's perspective on the provision of informal care. Health Soc Care Community. 2007;15(2):97–107.

Zwahlen D, Hagenbuch N, Carley MI, Recklitis CJ, Buchi S. Screening cancer patients' families with the distress thermometer (DT): a validation study. Psycho-Oncology. 2008;17(10):959–66.

Volunteers in Palliative Care

56

Bridget Candy, Joe Low, Ros Scott, and Leena Pelttari

Contents

B. Candy (✉) · J. Low
Marie Curie Palliative Care Research Department, University College London, London, UK
e-mail: b.candy@ucl.ac.uk; joseph.low@ucl.ac.uk

R. Scott
Dundee University is School of Education and Social Work, Dundee, UK
e-mail: r.z.scott@dundee.ac.uk

L. Pelttari
EAPC Task Force on Volunteering in Hospice and Palliative Care in Europe, Hospice Austria, Vienna, Austria
e-mail: leena.pelttari@hospiz.at

R. D. MacLeod, L. Van den Block (eds.), *Textbook of Palliative Care*,
https://doi.org/10.1007/978-3-319-77740-5_120

Abstract

Volunteers are key members of the hospice and palliative care team. In some countries, they are the only source of care provision for a person at a palliative stage of a disease. This chapter highlights both the importance of volunteers in these settings and the impact their contribution makes to care. The chapter covers the definitions of volunteering, the historical development of volunteering in hospice and palliative care, as well as research evaluation to document volunteer practice, an understanding of their distinct role in patient and family care, and assessment of their impact on patients and their families experience. The chapter also provides five case studies from volunteers across the world on their experiences in volunteering.

1 Introduction and Aim of the Chapter

Like the concepts of hospice and palliative care, volunteering can be described variously. For volunteering what is distinctive and important in these settings is that volunteering is inextricably linked to the development of the modern hospice and palliative care movement. Volunteering is also distinctive and important in hospice and palliative care because of the breadth and depth of volunteer involvement not only in directly supporting the provision of care but in leading some services, in administrative roles, in fundraising, and in influencing organization and the care it provides. Volunteers may also have a special and unique role in direct patient and family care. This has been described as "being there," which may involve a social or quiet presence, and a link between the patient and their family and health professionals. Reliance in hospice and palliative care on the work of volunteers is likely to increase with the aging global population and increased recognition of the need to provide access to hospice and palliative care to all irrespective of disease.

Research evaluation in hospice and palliative care is needed to both evaluate what interventions work and what work best and where. Evaluation is also needed to help understand how an intervention may work. Such research evaluation includes the contribution of volunteers. With finite resources in hospice and palliative care and a growing demand for these services, it is important to know how best to involve and support volunteers, to recognize their distinct contribution, and to sustain the large contribution they make in these settings.

The aim of this chapter is to provide an overview of both the importance of and evidence on understanding the role and impact of the contribution of volunteers in hospice and palliative care.

2 What Do We Mean by Volunteering in Hospice and Palliative Care?

Before focusing on volunteering in hospice and palliative care, it is worth considering volunteering more generally in order to gain an understanding of its breadth, diversity, and complexity. Volunteering means many things to many people. For some, it can be seen as a force for good in making a difference, yet for others it can be a reminder of difficult times, for example, under some communist regimes, where volunteering was compulsory for children and adults. As a result, volunteering is often less prevalent in former communist countries. The word "volunteering" in reality encapsulates a diverse range of people of all ages, motivations, skills, activities, and contexts. We will, therefore, explore a number of volunteering constructs before narrowing these down to be clear about what we mean by volunteering in hospice and palliative care in this chapter. The United Nations (UN) describes volunteering as happening at all levels: individual, community, national, and global (United Nations 2015). They consider that volunteering encompasses "traditional forms of mutual aid and self-help, as well as formal service delivery" in addition to "enabling and promoting participation and engaging through advocacy, campaigning and or activism" (p. xiv). The UN defines volunteering as "activities ... undertaken of free will, for the general public good and where monetary reward is not the principal motivating factor" (United Nations 2015, p. xiv). In seeking to apply more generic volunteering definitions to hospice and palliative care, the European Association of Palliative Care (EAPC) Task Force on Volunteering in Hospice and Palliative Care arrived at a specific definition following consultation across a number of countries. They propose the following definition in their EAPC White Paper "...the time freely given by individuals, with no expectation of financial gain, within some form of organised structure other than the already existing social relations or familial ties, with the intention of improving the quality of life of adults and children with life-limiting conditions and those close to them (family and others)" (Goossensen et al. 2016).

Within such a broad definition, there are necessarily many different volunteering models and structures ranging from informal to formal. Informal volunteering may be defined as individuals giving help without payment to others outwith their family (Rochester et al. 2016). This type of volunteering often operates outwith any recognized organization and often within local communities (United Nations 2015). One example of this might be the person motivated by the plight of refugees who travels overseas to provide help as an independent individual, unrelated to any organization. In contrast, Rochester et al. (2010) describe formal volunteering as help for which no remuneration is given, which benefits people or the environment and is undertaken through organizations (Rochester et al. 2016). An example of this would be the person who offers specific help regularly on a voluntary basis within an statutory, not-for-profit, or private organization.

Volunteering in hospice and palliative care is often only understood solely in terms of formal volunteering traditionally seen in many well-resourced countries, and that is provided within a dedicated hospice, at home, or in specialist units within a general hospital. This is typified by a hierarchical structure within which volunteers are managed by paid staff, work regularly in specified roles within limited and boundaried activities. This structure, however, does not include all possible ways of volunteering in hospice and palliative care in different countries. For instance, the community (and volunteer) led approach to volunteering in hospice and palliative care as seen in countries such as India or Africa and the "almost-at-home-houses" well established within the Netherlands (Kiange 2018) in addition to those within the UK such as Hospice Neighbours and Compassionate Neighbours. In reality, therefore, within hospice and palliative care volunteering in the same way as in the wider context of volunteering, there is a spectrum of volunteering.

What we mean by volunteering in this chapter, therefore, draws upon the definition from the EAPC Task Force on Volunteering White Paper, recognizing that hospice and palliative care volunteering encompasses a broad spectrum of activities and structures ranging from more informal volunteer-led approaches to formal service delivery models (Goossensen et al. 2016). Having arrived at a working definition, the next section will now go on to consider some of the origins of hospice and palliative care volunteering.

3 History of Hospice and Palliative Care Volunteering

Hospice and palliative care has evolved in diverse ways in different countries, often influenced by culture, society, and available resources (Morris et al. 2013). This can also be seen in the development of volunteering. It is beyond the scope of this chapter to consider this in detail, and so this section will give a brief overview giving examples from a number of countries.

In many countries throughout the world, volunteering is inextricably linked to the development of hospice and palliative care services and the support that the services offer to patients and families. Scott (2015) suggests that volunteers were instrumental in establishing many palliative care services particularly hospices (Scott 2015), while Radbruch and Payne (2010) describe the development of hospice care in general as "a civil rights movement based on volunteering" (Radbruch and Payne 2010) (p. 26). The work of Dame Cicely Saunders, considered by many to be the founder of the modern hospice movement, has been influential in the development of palliative care in many countries. Having worked as a volunteer herself, she was committed to the involvement of volunteers as a fundamental part of St Christopher's Hospice in London, UK, from its inception in 1967 (Howlett and Scott 2018).

A Volunteer in Australia Describes Her Experiences

My journey volunteering began in 2013 when I decided to apply to Concord Palliative Care Unit. I went to the orientation with no idea of what was actually involved but just knew that I wanted to "put back" something into the community. I was excited to be part of the team in palliative care that could make just the smallest amount of difference at a time when both the patients and family were under duress. For 12 months, I did the weekend "jolly trolley," taking around an array of sweets and beverages. It was almost like the naughty trolley and many of the patients loved the fact that even though they were desperately ill, they could sort of cheat a bit and eat and drink things perceived "not allowed." Many times they just loved to chat and pass some time before loved ones arrived. Others shared intimate life experiences and confided their most inner thoughts and frailties. I felt so privileged to not only get a firsthand account of their lives but also to feel like I was in the inner circle. To them they reached out to a stranger and for just a small amount of time felt connected to the outside world, not the new world they had become accustomed to, and had some sort of normality. In turn, each week I would walk away knowing that in some shape or form I had given them just a little respite from their stresses and made them feel like they were important and valued. Many did not have family and friends, and even though it saddened me to think that they were going it alone, they weren't totally alone, because as a volunteer I was there to ensure that they had a helping hand and I was there to listen and also support them in the little time they had. I felt like I was part of one of the most important, intimate part of a patients' life, and it humbled me.

In Austria and Poland, it was volunteers in conjunction with catholic and protestant churches who were influential in establishing hospice and palliative care services (Krakowiak and Pawłowski 2018; Pelttari and Pissarek 2018). In Poland, it is interesting to note that this development took place in the face of significant political opposition (Krakowiak and Pawłowski 2018). In Germany, hospice and palliative care volunteering developed "in parallel" with palliative medicine. Hesse and Radbruch (2018) describe this as a "citizen's movement" motivated by poor societal attitudes to death and dying (Hesse and Radbruch 2018) (ibid.). Volunteering emerged somewhat differently in Australia where UK hospice models (involving dedicated hospice units within the community) were less common with palliative care considered as a clinical rather than community issue (Huntir 2018). Volunteers, therefore, became involved in hospitals and community health centers or separate not-for-profit organizations with close links to hospital networks (ibid.). In the Netherlands, having considered the UK hospice model, there was a move toward more community-led hospice care (Goossensen and Somsen 2018). While in many countries hospice and palliative care development was a reaction to poor care of the dying, in Africa, the involvement of volunteers was in response to the overwhelming challenge of communicable diseases such as HIV and TB (Kiange 2018).

So far the focus has been on adult services, and it is worth taking a moment to consider what is known about volunteers within pediatric hospice and palliative care. Children's services developed at a later date than adult, when the first children's hospice, Helen House opened in Oxford in the UK in 1982. In the UK, however, the children's hospice and palliative care sector was slower to embrace volunteering than their adult equivalents. Burbeck et al. (2013) suggest this may be due to stakeholder anxiety about the complexity of the children's conditions and the number of professionals already involved in the lives of families caring for a child with a life-threatening and life-limiting condition and issues involved in safeguarding children and young people (Burbeck et al. 2013). Volunteering in this sector has evolved to a stage where currently in the UK most not-for-profit children's hospices and some voluntary and statutory community pediatric palliative care teams now involve volunteers. Likewise in Austria, volunteers often take care of siblings, and there is a special curriculum for volunteers in pediatric hospice and palliative care.

What seems to emerge from this history is the strong influence that people from local communities can have in responding to the palliative and end of life care needs of others.

4 Influences of and on Volunteering in Palliative Care

As we have seen in the last section, volunteers made a significant contribution to the development of hospice and palliative care in many countries. The involvement of volunteers, however, necessarily has significant influence on organizations. As members of the local community offering their time and skills with no expectation of financial reward, volunteers bring a wide range of skills, individual values, and perspectives that affects organizational culture and values. Indeed Scott (2013) identifies a number of key organizational areas which are influenced by volunteers including (1) diversification of available skills, such as professionals providing their skills as volunteers, and service quality, (2) leadership and governance, (3) financial sustainability, and (4) support of local communities and general public (Scott 2013).

This section, therefore, focuses briefly on the role of volunteers (discussed in more depth in further sections) in order to explore how different volunteering activities influence both the care of patients and families and the organization more widely. It is important to recognize that volunteering in turn is also affected by a range of external factors, and this section also explores the ways in which volunteering can be affected by societal and demographic factors.

In considering the diversity of volunteering roles in hospice and palliative care, the EAPC Task Force in Volunteering White paper, as earlier mentioned groups these under three distinct headings: (1) volunteers from local communities who provide direct practical or social support to patients and their families, or who provide other skills to the organization which may include fundraising, administration, catering, and gardening; (2) governance volunteers, trustees, and board members of hospices and other not-for-profit services; and (3) professionals using their professional skills in a voluntary capacity, for example, doctors, nurses, and chaplains (Goossensen et al. 2016). These roles may take place in many different settings including inpatient hospices, day hospices, in the community in patients' homes, hospitals, specialized units and elsewhere, and care homes (Goossensen et al. 2016).

Volunteers enable hospice and palliative care services to increase the range and enhance the quality of services offered (Scott 2015). A brief scoping of the research literature indicates that volunteers can have a beneficial influence on the care of patients and families; this includes that they can help to make care more person centered and less medicalized (Morris et al. 2015; Claxton-Oldfield 2015a; Block et al. 2010; Wilson et al. 2005; Pesut et al. 2014), while Luijkx and Schols (2009) highlight that volunteers make life less stressful for families caring for a loved one at end of life (Luijkx and Schols 2009). Indeed Herbst-Damm and Kulik's (2005) study found that volunteer support can extend survival time in terminally ill patients (Herbst-Damm and Kulik 2005). A more in-depth discussion of the research evidence on the impact of volunteers in hospice and palliative care can be found in Sect. 6 of this chapter.

The role of volunteers in the leadership and governance of not-for-profit organizations is often little recognized. As trustees (or non-executive board directors), these volunteers carry strategic and legal accountability for ensuring that organizations in particular hospices are effectively run and meet regulatory requirements. Volunteer trustees, therefore, have significant influence on the culture, leadership, and future direction of hospice and palliative care services. It is somewhat perplexing, however, that this voluntary strategic leadership is often responsible for the restrictions and boundaries imposed on other volunteering roles, influencing the activities that volunteers can and cannot undertake.

Morris et al. (2015) suggest that volunteers play a key role in bringing the local community into hospices and in extending the reach of the hospice and palliative care services in supporting patients and families at home (Morris et al. 2015). McKee et al. (2010) suggest that volunteers "inhabit a unique third culture of care" (p. 103) and play a vital role within community networks that enable high-quality hospice and palliative care (McKee et al. 2010). These themes are further explored in Sect. 5.3.

The influence of volunteers extends as already documented beyond patient care, and in some countries, volunteers are also involved in raising awareness of hospice and palliative care and in generating income to support the delivery of services (Scott 2015). Wilson et al. (2005), while recognizing a lack of evidence, suggest that volunteers may be important to the viability of organizations (Wilson et al. 2005). A later research study by Scott (2015) in the UK supports this hypothesis and found that volunteers were essential to the sustainability of not-for-profit hospices, with a number of respondents indicating that without volunteer support, their services would close (Scott 2015).

It is possible, however, that the influence of volunteers may be felt beyond hospice and palliative care organizations. Scott (2015) highlights the role of volunteers in educating the public about hospice and palliative care and including to "dispel myths and taboos" (p. 81) (Scott 2015). For example, in Austria, in common with a number of other countries, this includes hospice and palliative care volunteers going in to schools to talk to children about death, dying, and hospice and palliative care. The Council of Europe (2003) suggests that the role of volunteers in hospice and palliative care "is often underestimated" and contends that volunteers help to normalize dying and contextualize death as a societal rather than solely a medical issue (Council of Europe 2003) (ibid. p. 67).

While volunteering may influence a number of aspects of hospice and palliative care, there are a number of external influences which can impact on volunteering itself including culture, society, politics, legislation, or regulation. Culture affects not only how volunteering is perceived but can also encourage or inhibit the development of volunteering. As noted earlier, the level of volunteering may be affected by political influences, but this is not always the case. Globisch (2005) suggests that there is little tradition in Denmark of volunteering in healthcare settings (Globisch 2005). The reasons cited are the high level of female employment (who at least traditionally volunteered more than their male counterparts) and resistance from staff in the hospice and palliative care sector (ibid.).

Changes in volunteering are also evident in a number of countries as a result of societal changes. Howlett and Scott (2018) highlight that volunteers in many countries today have less time available and want their time to be utilized wisely (Howlett and Scott 2018). Today's hospice and palliative care volunteers may demand more from their experience than earlier generations. They may be motivated by personal and professional development, seeking responsibility and meaningful activities (ibid.). This poses challenges for hospice and other palliative care organizations which may see the increased involvement of the community as volunteers as key in helping to address the current and future growing demand as populations age.

In the light of these changes in and effects on volunteering, there is perhaps one further influence that is worth considering before leaving this section. The EAPC launched "Voice for Volunteering," the EAPC Madrid Charter on Volunteering in Hospice and Palliative Care in May 2017 (European Association of Palliative Care 2017). The purpose of this Charter is to emphasize the importance of and embed volunteering within hospice and palliative care. The aims of the Charter are:

- Promote the successful development of volunteering for the benefit of patients, families and the wider hospice and palliative care community.
- Recognise volunteering as a third resource alongside professional care and family care, with its own identity, position and value.
- Promote research and best practice models in the recruitment, management, support, integration, training and resourcing of volunteers. (ibid.)

The Charter calls for organizations to recognize the role of volunteers in direct patient care as one of "being there" which is described as focusing on the "human connection on 'being with' the person, that is the basis for sensing what kind of support the volunteer can provide to this particular person at this particular time." Actions outlined in the Charter are targeted at individual, organizational, local, and national levels and encompass areas such as recognizing the role of volunteers, effective management, training, and support, and identify volunteering as a key area for evaluation and research (ibid.).

5 Using Research to Understanding the Volunteers Role in Hospice and Palliative Care

5.1 Why Use Research to Understand the Volunteers Role in Hospice and Palliative Care?

The previous sections have highlighted many aspects of the volunteering in the context of hospice and palliative care such as definitions and the development of the modern hospice movement. They have also raised discussions about the complexity of the volunteering role and the many influences which mold this role, both on a personal (e.g., expectations) and on a wider societal and organizational level. At the same time, little is currently known from a population viewpoint about how volunteers deliver care in hospice and palliative care, in particular the level of activities provided within hospice and palliative care and in what settings do these activities occur? What are volunteers' own experiences? Are they overall good or bad? How do volunteers perceive their role and do they feel adequately prepared to perform it?

It is obviously important to understand these issues. Volunteers are as already stated often a vital resource in the delivery of care. To ensure that they continue to play an active role and do not suffer from burnt-out, research is needed to inform best practice. Although volunteers work has historically been linked closely to the development of the hospice movement (Goossensen et al. 2016), it is important to ensure that volunteers help provide good quality care, especially in an age where there is a growing emphasis on accountability. Within this context and to help plan services for the future at a population, it is necessary to quantify the types of care delivered by volunteers and in what settings. To help answer these questions robustly, research provides a range of tools.

Firstly, to recap what is research? It is the systematic and rigorous progress of inquiry that aims to describe processes and develop explanatory concepts in order to contribute to the scientific body of knowledge. Conducting good quality research facilitates the production of reliable and valid data from which effective and acceptable decisions can be applied to the broadest set of phenomena. This chapter section explores the research looking at volunteers in patient- and family-facing roles in hospice and palliative care to:

1. Quantify the activities of volunteers
2. Explore the role of volunteers
3. Discuss limitations in current research and to explore potential ways forward in future research

There are, as discussed earlier in this chapter, Sect. 2, different types of roles and settings that volunteers may work in within hospice and palliative care. These differences can be grouped in various ways: (1) community volunteering both in direct patient and family care-facing contact and in indirect facilitative roles, (2) voluntary board membership, and (3) professionals working within their discipline without receiving payment (Goossensen et al. 2016). The focus in this chapter section (and subsequent sections on research) is on research evidence in regard to patient- and family care-facing volunteers in hospice and palliative care settings. This focus is chosen as it is important to understand in what way volunteers have a direct impact on patient and family experience. At the same time, volunteers have unique concerns and challenges that exist in the role of providing care to patients and family in these settings. These include involvement in caring for very vulnerable patients of persons with non-professional training. Research evaluating their role in such care could also help combat any element of resistance and difficulty volunteers may suffer in establishing a link with some paid staff within the palliative care sector. The focus on research in this area is also needed as the number of volunteers is likely to increase greatly due to insufficient numbers of available professional staff to care for the growing demand for hospice and palliative care. Moreover there is now increasingly global interest in understanding the extent and best practice of volunteer involvement in providing this support (Morris et al. 2013) as demonstrated by the EAPC charter for volunteering in hospice and palliative care (see Sect. 4).

It is important to highlight that the focus of this section and subsequent research sections in this chapter aims to provide an international context to research looking at volunteers in hospice and palliative care. However, we acknowledge that most of the studies conducted in these settings have been conducted in Europe, North America, and Australia and may not be relevant to all volunteer hospice and palliative care services in other areas of the world.

5.2 What Activities Do Volunteers in Hospice and Palliative Care Engage in?

Previous studies have grouped the main roles of volunteers in hospice and palliative care in patient- and family-facing roles into five areas: emotional, social, practical, informational, and spiritual (Wilson et al. 2005; Claxton-Oldfield 2015b). Large surveys, e.g., national or international, are important tools in helping to illuminate the broader picture and quantify the breadth and depth of the role of volunteer involvement in patient- and family-facing care, as they illustrate both the settings where volunteers work within hospice and palliative care and the types of activities they engage in within these settings. Several large national surveys have been conducted across different European countries such as the UK, Poland, and Belgium or the various countries involved in the recent EAPC Taskforce initiative on volunteers. These surveys have both confirmed and quantified that most volunteers are involved in a wide range of patient-facing roles, meeting and greeting patients (Burbeck et al. 2014a), providing emotional support/psychosocial care to patients (Burbeck et al. 2013, 2014a; Pabst et al. 2017; Pawłowski et al. 2016; Vanderstichelen et al. 2017) and bereavement support, feeding patients or cleaning rooms (Burbeck et al. 2013; Pawłowski et al. 2016), and providing a range of complementary and diversional therapies, pastoral/faith-based services, and beauty/hairdressing (Burbeck et al. 2014a).

Two published surveys have looked at where volunteers work by care setting. One within the Flemish healthcare system found that volunteers based in palliative care units were more likely to be involved in direct patient care compared with those based in medical oncology unit. These volunteers were also more likely to be providing psychological, spiritual, and existential care (Vanderstichelen et al. 2017). The other, a UK-based survey of volunteers in adult hospice and palliative care services, found that volunteers were more likely to be involved in day care, bereavement services, and with in-patients, but less likely to be involved in home care (Burbeck et al. 2014a). In looking at volunteer involvement in patient and family-facing care delivery, those working in the voluntary sector (when compared to those working in the statutory sector) were more likely to be involved in the range of specific activities such as creative/diversional therapies, complementary/alternative therapies, counseling, pastoral/faith-based activities, and hair dressing/beauty, and where in many cases, volunteers were entirely responsible for the running of these services (Burbeck et al. 2014a).

A Volunteer in India Describes His Experiences

I head the creative wing to improve the ambience of Institute of Palliative Medicine. Late one evening, while walking to my room passing by the patients' wards, I saw her sitting by the window waving at me with a bright smile. Rishna was suffering from brain tumor. A bright chirpy 12-year-old girl with a sparkle in her eyes who was interested in Art. I had told Rishna that I'd get her art supplies the last time she was here. Now that she was back. I had the art supplies in my room and planned to give it to her on the way back. Something came up and it was too late to visit her. So I kept the supplies in my bag and decided to visit her first thing in the morning.

Next morning I went by her room but she was sleeping. Little did I know that her condition was bad and she was on heavy medication. I went by her room later that afternoon, she was still sleeping. My heart sank a little, but I hoped that next morning she would be better and I would be able to keep my word. Things just got from bad to worse and soon she was terminal. A few days later, she deteriorated progressively never recovering to her former state. I knew that with her condition, there was no coming back, but I never thought, the day I walked past her room would be the last time I would see her smile – her death posed a lot of questions to me – why didn't I give her the art supplies at the moment itself? Why did I put it off? How granted did I take that moment, thinking I would get a chance the next day – that incident taught me the value of a moment – the moment I had lost. It was a learning lesson for me to cherish every moment then on. In our daily life, there are those little moments we take for granted but only realize the value of that moment once it's gone. Later that week I got a call from my friend saying another girl has been admitted in the same room as Rishna was and she is interested in coloring. I went back with coloring supplies!

Most surveys have investigated the involvement of volunteers in adult services, but it is important not to forget the role of the volunteer in hospice and palliative pediatric care where additional potential ethical issues exist in how volunteers are involved given the relatively young age of the population and societal attitudes to caring for this group. Moreover, there are often general structural differences between children's and adult hospice and palliative care services. For example, in the UK, this care may be delivered to an individual child over a number of years, which in many cases may additionally involve the provision of education and play. Despite the complexities of providing pediatric palliative care, surveys in this area though are extremely limited, with only one study looking specifically at the involvement of volunteers in the delivery of pediatric palliative care (Burbeck et al. 2013). Although this study was conducted in the UK, some limited comparisons can be made with countries which have a similar service provision. In comparing the activities of volunteers between adult and children services, there were common aspects in their roles. In both cases, volunteers' most common activities included greeting visitors to the service, serving meals and drinks in the hospice, and assisting with social activities. In both settings, many of their services provided by the hospices, such as complementary therapies and pastoral care services, were dependent on volunteers running these services. Nevertheless, clear differences existed between volunteers in both settings. The number of volunteers in this UK survey in pediatric services (median 25 volunteers per service such as a dedicated hospice) is small compared to a UK survey in adult services (median 85 volunteers per service) (Burbeck et al. 2014a). Volunteers in pediatric hospice and palliative care were also found to be less likely to have direct patient care contact with children, but more likely to be involved in music and arts-based activities, befriending, and complementary therapies provision for the whole family. They were also not involved in any aspect of home care (Burbeck et al. 2013). In addition to structural differences with adult service, these findings may reflect that pediatric hospice and palliative care is compared to adult care a relatively recent development with potentially few beds available and a volunteer's role which is less well-defined. However, it should be noted that this survey in pediatric services was undertaken over 5 years ago and services have evolved since then. For instance, some community teams in the UK now involve volunteers.

There are difficulties underlying the current published literature in this area. There are as demonstrated few published surveys. The focus of the research questions of some of these surveys do not specifically address the role of volunteers per se but have their focus on topics such as specific training issues for volunteers (Pawłowski et al. 2016) or the role of motivation in volunteers (Pabst et al. 2017). Some surveys are "in progress," published in abstract only thereby lack sufficient detail (Vanderstichelen et al. 2017). Another difficulty, in generalizing these findings on how volunteers deliver patient-facing care in hospice and palliative care, is that different countries have different structural systems and cultural values in how they run their hospice and palliative care services and what is permissible for volunteers to do. It is also important to highlight that the focus in this section is on surveys published in peer-reviewed journals. There will be other surveys documented elsewhere such as "in-house" yearly service surveys. Only surveys published in peer-reviewed journals were discussed in this section because such papers are in general (across all types of research) likely to be of higher quality or reliability than non-peer reviewed as they are published based on approval of a board of professional experts. There may also be other surveys not noted in this section published in peer-reviewed journals, this is as they were not published in English. These restrictions may have limited the findings in this section.

5.3 What Volunteers in Patient- and Family-Facing Roles Within Hospice and Palliative Care Settings Understand About Their Role

The previous section explored the role of volunteers in the context of the activities that they performed in different settings within hospice and palliative care. It is equally important to understand how volunteers see their role. In this section, the perspectives of volunteers in patient- and family-facing roles in hospice and palliative care are explored using the findings of qualitative designed studies. Although we acknowledge that quantitative designed studies (those that predominantly provide numerical data), particularly large surveys, may be useful in identifying general trends, qualitative research are more valuable in exploring a phenomenon from the perspective of the individuals experiencing it, in this case what volunteers understand about their role, and there are now numerous qualitative studies available exploring this.

In the first part of this current section, the review of qualitative studies by Burbeck et al. (2014b) is critiqued and presented on how volunteers perceive their role and also how other key stakeholders (such as patient and their families and professional staff) perceive the role of the volunteer in hospice and palliative care. In the second part, the results of this review are compared with qualitative studies published since the review.

The Burbeck et al. review uses a qualitative evidence synthesis approach in its interpretation of how volunteers understand their role. The synthesis explores the qualitative analysis from all known qualitative studies (Burbeck et al. 2014b). It takes a thematic approach in the synthesis of the individual studies analysis; in doing so it considers connections, similarities, and differences between the findings of each study. This may identify "higher-order" key themes not identified in any study but only apparent in the pooling of their findings. This can produce a deeper and potentially new understanding of what the volunteers may understand of their role. This review identified 12 studies, mainly from North America (7/12) or Europe (4/12), but with 1 study originating from Uganda. The total sample comprises of 294 participants who were mostly volunteers but also other stakeholders relevant to understanding the role of the volunteer including a patient and their family and hospice and palliative care staff. Most participants were female.

The review identified three theme clusters in the studies. Theme 1 highlights the *distinctness of the volunteers' role*, in which the volunteer saw their role as having an identity separate from paid staff. This distinct role was often described in terms of recognized work boundaries. Volunteers felt they were not restricted in either the tasks or the time they could offer to patients or families in the same way that paid staff were. Volunteers saw their roles characterized by two factors: independence in that the task that they would perform would not be done by a paid member of staff and surrogacy which was possible due to the blurred relationship between volunteers and patients. Within these role characterizations, volunteers act either as "go-between" between the patients and their family and members of staff or as advocates for patients and families in representing the interests of these people. These roles highlight the surrogate nature of the volunteer role, where volunteers potentially become an "additional" members of the family due the person time at the hospice.

Theme 2: characteristics of the role. This theme highlights *the social nature of the volunteer role*, as opposed to being task-orientated. This aspect of the volunteers' role is further illustrated by the value that volunteers feel that they provide patients and family in terms of social support, notably in providing emotional support and "being there" for them. The perceived social aspect was seen as a motivating factor for volunteering in a hospice setting.

Theme 3: volunteers experience of the role, defined in terms of its ambiguity, flexibility, and informality and their relationship with paid members of staff. The synthesis identified *ambiguity in how volunteers understood the role*. Volunteers viewed the flexibility and informality of their role positively, but at the same time, they found it stressful when there was uncertainty around the tasks that they should be doing. The relationship between volunteers and paid staff was central in shaping the volunteers' experience of their role, in particular the way that staff controlled their role by restricting the availability of patient information or treating volunteers as subordinates. The synthesis highlighted tensions between the perceptions of informality of the volunteers' role with the growing formalization of their roles, through the need to be increasingly professionalized, often due to the increased need to work within a legal framework.

This review provides a distinct understanding of how volunteers perceive their role in patient and family-facing settings. It also highlights many issues that planners and managers of hospice and palliative care services may need to be aware of to facilitate the best of volunteers' contributions, namely, that it can be perceived as social in nature and it may also be about dealing with the ambiguous nature of the volunteers' role. This review by including 12 studies of different populations of volunteers, as well as some other key stakeholders such as family members, enabled the role of the volunteer to be constructed from a range of different perspectives. The studies reviewed came from a variety of North American and European countries, which increased the generalizability of the findings to a wide range of healthcare settings. Furthermore, the review explored differences in care settings, with volunteers working in inpatients services adopting a quasi-professional approach to their role while those volunteering in home-based care tended to act more as surrogate family members. Nevertheless, there are some methodological issues that need to be considered when interpreting the findings from this review, in particular the range of questions asked by the researchers from the 12 studies in collecting their primary data where not all directly asking about the role of the volunteer.

Since the publication of the Burbeck et al. (2014) review (Burbeck et al. 2014b), four relevant qualitative studies on volunteers perspectives in hospice and palliative care have been published (Brighton et al. 2017; Dean and Willis 2017; Gale 2015; Söderhamn et al. 2017). The studies are European, three from the UK and one from Norway. Unlike the studies analyzed in the Burbeck review where the volunteers were all from dedicated hospices and palliative care units, the volunteers from two of these studies came from community palliative care (Gale 2015; Söderhamn et al. 2017). These studies have explored the volunteer experience to varying degrees. One study focused on the impact of how working with patients near the end of life influenced volunteers own experience and attitudes toward death and dying (Gale 2015). The second looks at how the experience of volunteers are affected by the training and support provided by a palliative care coordinator (Söderhamn et al. 2017). The remaining two have used the volunteer experience as a means of identifying how to improve training for volunteers working with people with palliative care needs (Brighton et al. 2017; Dean and Willis 2017).

The main findings from these studies chime closely with the three themes identified from the Burbeck et al. review. These include dilemmas around the development of close relationships, friendships, between volunteers and patients (Gale 2015; Söderhamn et al. 2017) and doing tasks not performed by health care professionals (Brighton et al. 2017), "being there" (Söderhamn et al. 2017), and providing emotional and social support to family members (Söderhamn et al. 2017). Nevertheless, the theme of increasingly professionalism and regulation (Gale 2015; Söderhamn et al. 2017) is reflected in the later studies, particularly the importance of volunteers having a clarified role and provided with sufficient knowledge to carry out the task (Söderhamn et al. 2017). Likewise, it is equally important for health professionals to be aware of the volunteers' role (Söderhamn et al. 2017).

A Volunteer in Canada Describes Her Experiences

On a practical level, I have, over the years, been involved with fundraising, for example, the Christmas "Angel's Remembered" campaign, the annual "Hike for Hospice," and giving presentations in the community to bring awareness to the topic and services available. I also teach the "communication with the dying and their loved ones" component of the volunteer training program for a local hospice organization once every year or so. However, mostly I have offered emotional, social, and practical support to patients/clients, for example, accompanying people to medical appointments, taking them for drives, and walking them around

(*continued*)

hospital grounds or their own gardens or homes. I have given hand massages and sometimes used a relaxation technique known as Reiki when requested. I have spent time with the dying person's loved ones listening and talking and listening again to their stories, fears, and concerns for their loved ones and sometimes their concerns for their own future when thinking about their inevitable and impending aloneness. And, last but not least and, by far what I mostly enjoy is the countless hours I have spent just sitting with or at the bedside of the dying person – many of those hours were spent in silence as they lay sleeping or were semicomatose/comatose due to the disease (or more often, due to the drugs used for symptom control of the disease). On these occasions, I will often just touch a hand or a shoulder periodically to remind them that they are not alone. If it is expected to be a long stretch of time with someone who is unconscious, I will take a book with me and during breaks from reading I often find myself watching the breathing patterns and will imagine the person in their life before they entered the final stages. Since we don't currently have any freestanding hospices in our area, I visit people in their homes and the hospitals.

My role as a hospice palliative care volunteer over the last 25 plus years has offered me the opportunity to meet some wonderful people that I likely otherwise would not have met, at a time in their life when they were often the most vulnerable – whether they were the patient/client or the loved one (s). Front-line volunteering has, at times, offered me experiences that have stretched me out of my comfort zone whether through dealing with uncomfortable situations due to stressful family dynamics or because sometimes witnessing the suffering of an individual is just simply almost too much to bare. Then there have been the times when I have felt a bit like a fraud because I've been sure that I have been getting more out of the relationship than I was giving. No matter the situation, every person I have met has taught me something about myself and about life. It has always been a great privilege to be involved – as cliché as that sounds, it's the truth, as anyone who has journeyed with a dying person will tell you. Volunteering in this field has had a profound impact in shaping my life – for the better!

In palliative care, feeling unprepared to perform certain tasks related to their role is a challenge facing many volunteers in direct contact with patients and their families; this includes dealing with imminently dying patients or subsequent bereavement issues with family members (Dean and Willis 2017). Likewise, similar challenges also apply to volunteers working in hospital settings, who, through their roles of acting as hospital guides, chaplain volunteers, and ward visitors and assisting with patient discharge to home, work with patients with palliative and end of life care needs, involving difficult and emotionally intensive encounters (Brighton et al. 2017). These studies emphasize the importance of providing good support to its volunteers (Gale 2015), potentially through a mentor (Söderhamn et al. 2017). There is recognition that tailor-made training is an important element to support volunteers carry out their role (Brighton et al. 2017; Dean and Willis 2017).

5.4 Limitations of Research on the Volunteers' Role in Patient and Family-Facing Support in Hospice and Palliative Care

Studies in this area confirm the broad range of activities that volunteers are involved in and have provided a greater understanding of how volunteers understand their role and how they experience it. Nevertheless, current studies, particularly looking at the volunteer experience, are limited. The majority of studies have originated from North America, Australia, or Europe (mainly the UK or the Scandinavian countries), with the main findings limited in their generalizability. More studies need to be conducted and published from other European countries and from countries outside North America and Europe. The samples used in these studies have mainly been volunteers, apart from three studies from the Burbeck et al. (2014) review (Burbeck et al. 2014b) which identified three studies exploring either the patient or family members' perspectives of the volunteer role. Although these studies provide a relevant basis to understanding the experience of volunteers, it is equally important to understand the perspectives of all stakeholders, including those who receive care from these volunteers, namely, the patients or their family members as well as those who work closely with volunteers such as nurses. More studies are needed to explore the perspectives of these groups as findings from these groups will enable us to see how they compare with those from volunteer only studies and so build up a wider picture about the role of volunteers in hospice and palliative care. Such an approach has been used in a qualitative study looking at the collaboration between volunteers and staff in a pediatric palliative care unit, which identified communication, particularly good information flow as a key factor in successful collaboration between volunteers and staff (Meyer et al. 2018).

The qualitative studies identified have all used interviews or focus groups to collect their data. While these methods can allow a wide range of topics to be discussed, there are several limitations. Although the interviewees have some flexibility in responding to interviewers' questions, the interviewers/researchers exert control in determining what topics are covered during the interviews or focus groups and how they are discussed. There is also an assumption in conducting interviews and focus groups that what participants say is what they actually do, but this may not be the case in many situations. Interviews and focus groups, by their very nature, do not look at the interaction between how participants interact with their social environment. Within the field of volunteer research, other alternative methods may be more appropriate in teasing out the social interactions between volunteers and other potential stakeholders such as patients, family members, and health professionals working in hospice and palliative care institutions. One such method is ethnography, where the researcher participates openly in the field they are studying and immerses themselves in that social environment, observing the interactions of the topic being explored and recording detailed field notes. This methodology is useful in examining health beliefs and the organization of health care. Although time-consuming, such studies would provide a deeper and richer understanding of how volunteers in hospice and palliative care interact with other agencies.

6 Using Research to Understand the Impact of Patient- and Family-Facing Volunteers in Hospice and Palliative Care

In this section, the focus is on research to assess the impact of patient- and family-facing volunteers in hospice and palliative care settings. The section opens with a discussion on what is the value of evaluating volunteers' involvement in patient care within hospice and palliative care settings. By this, what is meant is on whether the contribution of the volunteer has an influence on the patient or their family, such as in their well-being or care satisfaction. This is followed with an outline on how we may evaluate impact. Presentation and a critique are then made of the findings of studies that have evaluated the impact of patient- and family-facing volunteers in hospice and palliative care. Considering the limitations in this evidence base, the next subsection highlights the challenges in evaluation. The section concludes with discussion on the way forward in assessing impact.

A Volunteer in Austria Describes Her Experiences

Here we are, sitting in a small cafe in the 16th district of Vienna. Mrs. M. sits in her wheelchair, drinks a black coffee, and smokes a cigarette. She starts talking about her uncle's suicide. "You know, he had colon cancer, just like I do. He couldn't bear the pain, the physical limitations and the fear anymore. He had two children and he was Catholic, very religious. I don't know how he could possibly...". Tears are flooding her eyes. It's been a year now that I am with her and her family, and it's the first time this strong, brave, and self-reflective woman is crying in my presence. When saying goodbye this day, she shakes my hand longer and more firmly than she usually does. "Thank you," she says, looking deeply into my eyes. This moment makes me realize that I am where I'm supposed to be, doing what matters to me.

During my work as a hospice volunteer, I am honored to experience many situations like this. I feel blessed how much trust, openness, and gratefulness I receive and that I can be there for someone, simply by listening with an open mind and heart. These intimate encounters also allow me to experience myself in a unique way: Being fully present and compassionate, I feel very connected to others, and my experiences and relationships seem more meaningful.

Some other day, I am sitting with Mrs. M. and her husband in their living room. They hardly ever talk about her illness and the impact it has on their lives. During the conversation, Mr. M. looks at me and speaks about how he admires his wife and her strength, what a loving mother she is and how proud he is to be her husband. Mrs. M. sits right next to him and tries to establish eye contact with him. He doesn't react and keeps looking at me, as if he couldn't look at her while saying those words. It feels like magic and I wonder if my presence made this possible. And I am overwhelmingly grateful to witness it.

6.1 Do We Need to Evaluate the Impact of Patient- and Family-Facing Hospice and Palliative Care Volunteers?

In answer to the question on why do we need to evaluate the impact of hospice and palliative care volunteers, let us first take this as a health or social care intervention that involves the contribution of volunteers. If we look broadly at health and social care evaluations, we find that many, be they drug treatments, non-drug, or services, in hospice and palliative care and elsewhere have been implemented without rigorous research to assess their impact. This includes the exploration on the barriers and facilitators to the best implementation in practice of an intervention. In other words, there are interventions that lack sufficient evidence to either recommend or not recommend. In hospice and palliative care because of historic underfunding in research, and because of the complexities in undertaking research in these settings, under-evaluation may be more extensive than in many other areas of healthcare. On the other hand, it may seem intuitive that many healthcare, palliative or otherwise, interventions help and indeed for some evaluation are unnecessary, inappropriate, or even unethical. Many of the most effective treatments have not been the subject of evaluation by controlled trial, including external defibrillation, which is used to start a stopped heart (Howick 2011). In hospice and palliative care, there are clear ethical issues to consider in conducting research that involves withholding from a proportion of the study participants (those in the control or comparison arm of a trial) additional care, which while not of established benefit may be unlikely to cause harm (Casarett 2009). However, without rigorous evaluation, the impact of interventions on important outcomes is not fully known nor is it known what is the better approach to care. This is not to challenge the value of clinical experience in the provision of good quality healthcare. In the evaluation of care interventions though, clinical judgment does not provide an adequate basis for detecting at population level modest beneficial or adverse effects (Howick 2011). For instance, a review of all published trials on a particular drug or of a new supportive therapy or service perhaps involving a volunteer or a nurse may find a higher rate of adverse events in patients taking the drug or having the supportive therapy compared to those receiving usual care. Unaided by comparative studies, a clinician (who is likely to have seen fewer patients needing the drug or supportive therapy than those participating in trial evaluations) will be less likely to detect this.

The provision of hospice and palliative care varies across countries as does, as demonstrated earlier in this chapter, the role of the volunteer. However, what is consistent is the extensive depth and breadth of volunteer involvement in these settings particularly in the community, in home care, and in dedicated hospice and palliative care facilities. In many countries, the volunteers' contribution was critical to the development and to the sustainability of hospice and palliative care services. In other countries, volunteering is the workforce providing hospice and palliative care. Moreover, alongside the growing global number of older people, there is growing demand for hospice and palliative care. There are insufficient numbers of professional staff to respond to this need, and there may need to be an even greater reliance in many countries on volunteers to help provide care and support. In recognition of this, some governments have endorsed policies that may directly or indirectly promote informal caregivers like volunteers to assume a greater share of care provision at the end of life (Alcock 2010). In parallel, a recent development within hospice and palliative care has been called to adopt the principles of public health to further promote community volunteering to fill the growing gaps in professional support services (Abel and Kellehear 2016). Thereby to identify and accelerate best practice, there has never been a more pressing time for the need to have robust and relevant evaluation of the impact of volunteers in hospice and palliative care.

6.2 How Do We Evaluate the Impact of Patient- and Family-Facing Volunteers in Hospice and Palliative Care?

In answer to the how do we evaluate, firstly we should consider what we should evaluate. A starting point is to consider why patient- and family-facing volunteers are needed in hospice and palliative care. The reasons include as noted earlier, but are not limited to, to enable services to be provided, to allow finite resources to go further, to involve the community, and to provide more holistic care. It is also worth considering to whom patient- and family-facing volunteers make a difference. This could be as already noted the difference made to patients and their families experience. It could also be the difference made to volunteers, the difference made to the local community, and difference made to the organization (e.g., organizational capacity, staff able to focus on specialist roles, reaching more people, and in providing a wider range of services). Exploring all these points though is beyond the scope of this chapter. They are noted here to highlight some of the broad scope of what could be evaluated.

There are various study designs that can be used to measure volunteers' impact on patient and family experience. Randomized controlled trials (RCTs) are considered the gold standard to evaluate the effects of an intervention. This study design more than any other reduces the risk of biased results. However, for various reasons including ethical, there are limited numbers of RCTs in hospice and palliative care. These reasons will be discussed further later in this section. There are though other designed studies that allow, although to a lesser extent, the evaluation of the impact of an intervention to be measured. This is by comparing, like a RCT, one group that experienced the intervention of interest, here volunteers, with another group who do not experience the "volunteer intervention." These include a range of different designed studies such as quasi-randomized controlled trials, controlled before-and-after studies, and interrupted time series.

The work of Methods Of Researching End of life Care (MORECARE) project aimed to provide evidence-based guidance on research methods in end of life and palliative care (Higginson et al. 2013). One of their recommendations, it is important to note here, is for the use of research exploring patient and family experience in intervention development. These experiences can be gathered via qualitative research methods which are extremely useful in understanding the mechanisms behind what any intervention may achieve.

6.3 Differences Made to Patients and Families in Hospice and Palliative Care: Choice of Outcomes

Comparative studies, such as trials, can tell us a lot about a whether a treatment works, whether it is cost-effective, and whether it causes no serious harm. What such a study can tell is dependent on the outcomes selected. The impact assessment of many care interventions in hospice and palliative settings is characterized as involving a range of different measures. For instance, in a Cochrane systematic review on the effectiveness of home palliative care services, there were eight items of interest in regard to whether the service made a difference to the patient and their family. These items were satisfaction with care, symptom controlled, physical functioning, quality of life, time spent at home, death at home, and caregiver pre- and post-bereavement outcomes (Gomes et al. 2009). Multiple outcome assessments may be undertaken in a study in part as it may be unclear what outcomes an intervention may impact on. It is also because in hospice and palliative care, the impact of many interventions is known to be broad, and one outcome measure is insufficient to assess this. Take, for instance, how palliative care is defined by the World Health Organization (WHO). This is as an "approach that improves the quality of life (QOL) of patients and their families facing the problem associated with life-threatening illness, through the prevention and relief of suffering by means of early identification and impeccable assessment and treatment of pain and other problems, physical, psychosocial and spiritual" (World Health Organization 2018). Since it is a goal of palliative care, it would seem appropriate that a key outcome to evaluate the impact of the involvement of patient- and family-facing volunteer is patient and family QOL. But assessment may also include other measures to assess prevention and relief of suffering on varied domains (e.g., pain, other symptoms, emotional, social, and spiritual). This broadness, though, is not the only thing that is not straightforward in hospice and palliative care research. Outcome assessments are complex because of the changing nature of the patients' condition and its impact on symptoms and physical, emotional, social, and spiritual needs. Moreover, in hospice and palliative care where a person's health is deteriorating, in regard to the assessment of QOL, for example, you may not necessarily be focusing in measuring whether the intervention leads to an improvement or not. Evaluation of an intervention may be on measuring whether it limits decline or halts decline in QOL.

The role of a patient and family-facing volunteer can be considered, as discussed in Sect. 5, as distinct from those of healthcare professionals and families role in caring and support. If we follow an overarching theme in the qualitative literature of "being there," then perhaps we have another way we should evaluate the impact of volunteers, namely, on outcomes relating to the social nature of the role of the volunteer. Another complementary way to identify relevant outcomes to assess what the benefit of patient- and family-facing volunteers in hospice and palliative care is what patients and families value in the involvement of volunteers? However, there a few qualitative studies specifically exploring the experiences of patients and their families on receiving support from a volunteer. One qualitative study conducted individual interviews with ten bereaved women

(Weeks et al. 2008). The overarching theme that emerged in their analysis was that volunteers had a unique social role in care:

> And I think, for [my husband], the fact of having somebody from outside, not just staff, is important. I think the staff that deal with you all the time, there is some humiliation in your situation that staff has to deal with at another level, his physical needs, so this is strictly someone to talk and be there, a friendly face, a kind face. (Bereaved wife Weeks et al. 2008)

6.4 What Is the Best Evidence on the Impact of Volunteers in Hospice and Palliative Care?

There are few comparative studies that have evaluated the impact of patient- and family-facing volunteers in hospice and palliative care (Candy et al. 2015). Of these, there is only one known RCT (Walshe et al. 2016). Other comparative studies include retrospective studies of datasets (Block et al. 2010; Herbst-Damm and Kulik 2005). In two of these three studies, the volunteers who delivered the intervention provided weekly social home visits, of up to 3 h (Block et al. 2010; Walshe et al. 2016). In the other, it is not reported what volunteers did or how often they provided support (Herbst-Damm and Kulik 2005).

The ELSA study was a UK-based pragmatic RCT, a prospective wait-list trial that assessed the impact of volunteer-delivered support services at the end of life (Walshe et al. 2016). The intervention involved volunteers providing tailored face-to-face support to people who were anticipated to be in their last year of life. Support was deemed to be supplementary to usual forms of health and social care. It commonly involved befriending weekly visits of between 1 and 3 h, but it could also involve signposting the recipient to relevant services. The setting was in the community, most commonly this was the patient's home. The intervention was compared to usual care. The primary outcome of interest was the impact on change in QOL at 4 weeks after the start of the intervention. Other outcomes assessed were whether the intervention reduced loneliness, affected the perception of social support, or impacted on the use of health and social care services. The study enrolled 196 patients. It was found that there was no statistically significant difference in impact on change in QOL between volunteer-provided support and those in the treatment as usual trial arm. Overall the trial authors noted that "there were trends in the data in favour of the intervention, but the effect is small, and related to reducing the rate of decline rather than improving outcomes." However, the study was underpowered, and the authors had questions about their choice of outcome measures, in that the one they used may not have addressed QOL appropriately within the context of end of life. Therefore, they concluded the effectiveness of these volunteer services remains unknown.

The Herbst-Damm and Kilik (2005) comparative study undertook secondary analysis of a dataset of survival rates of 290 US hospice patients comparing those who received volunteer home visits with those who did not. Volunteers who provided the home visits were trained to listen, to provide conversation, and to provide if requested personal grooming needs such as trimming nails or combing hair. They found that those who received volunteers' visits ($n = 94$) lived longer than those who did not, on average of an 80-day increase in survival. Specifically, and controlling in their survival analysis for patients' physical status (Karnofsky score at study entry), they demonstrated (using Cox's proportional Hazard Model) that neither marital status nor gender independently predicted survival, but the survival rate for those receiving visits was almost three times that of those who were not visited by a volunteer (likelihood ratio, 2.9; p value <0.001).

The third comparative study was by Block and colleagues. It compared satisfaction with care of (United Nations 2015) families whose relative received care from hospices that involved greater volunteer involvement in direct care with (Goossensen et al. 2016) those who received care in hospices with less volunteer involvement (Block et al. 2010). The study using the US National Hospice and Palliative Care Organization National Data Set (NDS) undertook a secondary analysis of hospice programs using the number of direct patient care volunteer hours.

These programs provide support in the home, freestanding hospices, hospitals, nursing homes, and other long-term facilities. The data did not provide detail on what the volunteer involvement in care entailed. Obtained using information from 57,353 individuals from 32% ($n = 305$) of hospice organizations that provided data for the NDS were families' perception of the quality of care. They analyzed "excellent" ratings of care by the number of volunteer hours reported by hospices using a multivariate analysis model that adjusted for hospice characteristics, such as the number of care staff (full-time equivalents) and patient characteristics (diagnosis and hospice length of stay). They found statistically significantly more relatives rated care as "excellent" in those hospices reporting the highest number of volunteer hours per patient week (3.3 h), compared with those reporting the lowest number of hours (0.245 h); coefficient, 6%; and 95% confidence interval, 4–9%.

In conclusion while the RCT found limited evidence of benefit, the other two studies of weaker design report statistically significant positive outcomes in the involvement of patient- and family-facing volunteers in hospice and palliative care. There are limited conclusions to be drawn as the evidence base to date is of low quality. This is as the studies were few, the studies differed in setting and evaluation, and for two the research design was at a higher risk of biased results. While there remains as there is for volunteer-delivered service elsewhere limited evidence on their efficacy (Jenkinson et al. 2013), there are some relevant comparative studies underway. This includes, for instance, in Ireland a pilot randomized trial of a volunteer-led community social and practical support intervention for adults with life-limiting illness.

6.5 Challenges and Way Forward in Evaluation of the Impact of Volunteers in Hospice and Palliative Care

There is a paucity of well-designed evaluations on the impact of hospice and palliative care, not just in services involving volunteers in these settings. There are many methodological and ethical challenges in evaluation in hospice and palliative care (Krouse et al. 2004). The ethical issues, while not unique to these settings, may be more compounded in these settings. The population is vulnerable, and for which inviting and seeking consent to be part of research is complicated because of emotional distress, potential decline in mental capacity, invasiveness of treatment, and physical and mental burden of taking part in an evaluation. In trials, there is also the issue of the "no treatment arm." This is the risk that those allocated to this arm of the trial will receive suboptimal support and care. Although one could argue the other way around, those in the intervention may receive suboptimal support and care. There are other methodological issues that while may not be unique to hospice and palliative care, they may be more extensive in these settings. This includes heterogeneity in population; patients may be dying from a broad range of diseases which have different rates of progression. This if not considered in planning and analysis may lead to bias results. In a trial, for example, this is when in one arm there are a higher proportion of the participants despite randomization have a disease with a shorter prognosis (Hoerger 2017). Results are also at a risk of biases as in these settings as there are often high attrition rates due to declining physical or mental incapacity or death. Other issues include the need for surrogate respondents and difficulty as already noted in selection of outcomes.

This is not to suggest there are no trials. For instance, although disappointingly, a recent systematic review on the association of palliative care and patient and family caregiver outcomes was unable to draw strong conclusions on impact even though it included many trials (Kavalieratos et al. 2016). It included several combined analyses (meta-analyses) of data from up to 13 RCTs. Its conclusion was limited because of issues in the trial evidence including heterogeneity of outcome measures and poorly conducted trials.

So are these challenges insurmountable for research on impact of patient- and family-facing volunteers in hospice and palliative care? It is worth remembering that hospice and palliative care research is a relatively new endeavor, but at the same time, there is a growing body of researchers and hospice and palliative care research groups around the world who are successful in attracting competitive research funding (Johnson et al. 2017). While there is a need for more focused research attention to better understand how to maximize their contribution while providing better support for volunteers' (Pesut et al. 2014), there are groups exploring how to improve research methods in palliative care (Higginson et al. 2013). This includes the authors of the one RCT of a volunteer intervention in palliative care, they highlight the use of wait-list controls to overcome issues of withholding a potentially beneficial intervention to people who have shorten lives, and they also recommend to enhance completion and reduce attrition and ease of ethical approval short and easy to complete measures (Walshe et al. 2016).

7 Training of Volunteers in Hospice Palliative Care

This section focuses on the training of volunteers in hospice and palliative care. It begins with a discursive section which poses questions on the need to train volunteers. This is followed by a brief exploration of the tensions that exist between training volunteers to be effective in their roles while nurturing the humanity and freedom that characterizes volunteering. This section concludes by examining the limited evidence base on volunteer training in hospice and palliative care and considers the way forward.

7.1 Why Do We Need to Train Volunteers in Hospice and Palliative Care?

There is limited research evidence in the field of hospice and palliative care on the effectiveness and value of volunteer training (Dean and Willis 2017; Horey et al. 2015). Despite this, it is accepted in many countries that training volunteers in hospice and palliative care is good practice, and it is likely that there are few instances where volunteers receive no preparation or training whatsoever. At a minimum, volunteers are likely to receive an introduction to the organization and guidance on the boundaries of their role (Brighton et al. 2017; Dean and Willis 2017). So why is it that training volunteers seems to be so embedded in practice? Is it to enable volunteers to be effective and have confidence in their role; to enable paid staff, patients, and families to trust that volunteers have the right skills; or to satisfy legislative or regulatory requirements? Does the training take a theoretical approach or is the focus on helping volunteers to reflect on and develop their natural skills in responding to the needs those they support? In taking a theoretical approach, do we risk volunteers becoming more like professionals and losing their unique role as community "friend" or "neighbor"; what is the role that we need them to play?

In reality, it may be a mixture of some or all of these reasons and approaches to training depending on the volunteer activity, the organizational philosophy and wider influences as outlined in Sect. 4. The Council of Europe (2003) states that volunteers in hospice and palliative care must receive appropriate training and that "willingness to help not enough" (Council of Europe 2003) (p. 67). Radbruch and Payne (2010) take this a step further stating that such volunteers should receive "an accredited instruction course" and receive ongoing training along with supervision and support (Radbruch and Payne 2010). As highlighted in Sect. 5, training has an important role to play in supporting volunteers to carry out their role (Brighton et al. 2017; Dean and Willis 2017), in which effective training programs are important in mitigating stress for volunteers (Claxton-Oldfield 2015b). Volunteers sought flexibility in deciding what topics they wanted to be trained on, according to their interest and need at the time. Volunteers wanted to be taught by highly respected staff working in the field, which was particularly important for those volunteers working in acute hospitals (Brighton et al. 2017). Volunteers did not think online teaching would be suitable as part of their training (Brighton et al. 2017; Dean and Willis 2017). As part of their training package, volunteers benefitted from shadowing "experienced" volunteers (Dean and Willis 2017) or being followed up by a highly skilled mentor on a regular basis, who would be able to monitor the volunteer's progress or clarify their role (Söderhamn et al. 2017).

The EAPC Madrid Charter on Volunteering in Hospice and Palliative Care considers that the aim of training is to prepare volunteers for the hospice and palliative care environment and to help them to develop their own natural human ability to reach out others (European Association of Palliative Care 2017).

Before moving on to explore volunteer training in different countries, there remains a question about training for the volunteer professional who offers their skill as a doctor, nurse, chaplain, or complementary therapist without payment. What training do these volunteers require? Are there limits to their role enforced either by their professional body legislation/regulation or by the organization? Does the professional need to learn to become a volunteer?

7.2 What Is Happening Across Countries?

In considering some of these questions, it is helpful to explore what is happening in different countries. A study undertaken in Belgium found that 91% of hospice and palliative care volunteers received training, with only 33% of organizations providing mandatory training (Vanderstichelen et al. 2017). Austria, the Netherlands, and Germany have national curricula for volunteering. In Austria, for example, the required basic volunteer training is 120 h, comprising 80 h of theory and 40 h of practice (Pelttari and Pissarek 2018). All volunteers must undertake the basic training with additional training of 80 h (40 theory and 40 practice) for children's palliative care volunteers. Bereavement volunteers must undertake a separate training of 110 h or may add an additional 80 h to the basic training. In the Netherlands, volunteer training is provided over seven sessions and includes online learning (ibid) (Goossensen and Somsen 2018). In Germany, 100–120 h of training is proposed, and funding for volunteer coordinator roles is dependent on volunteers being trained (Hesse and Radbruch 2018).

Canada has a national volunteer training program of approximately 30 h available to hospice and palliative services. Claxton-Oldfield suggests that a typical hospice volunteer training program would include an overview of hospice palliative care, the roles of the multidisciplinary team, volunteer roles, multicultural faith and spiritual perspectives, clinical care, death, dying and bereavement, and communication and coping skills in addition to volunteer policies and procedures (Claxton-Oldfield 2015b).

A Volunteer in Scotland Describes Her Experiences

I have been a volunteer massage therapist within a Marie Curie Hospice for 3 years now. In an earlier life, I was a career civil servant working for the Scottish Government. At age 54, I was given the opportunity of early retirement and that is when my second, and more satisfying, working life began. A few years previously, I had studied in my spare time for a Diploma in Swedish Massage so I decided to build on this by qualifying in sports and remedial massage therapy. I was fortunate to be offered two part-time jobs, one in a private swimming club and the other in a health clinic which is where I gained real experience and honed my skills. For reasons I will explain, I had wanted to be able to offer treatments to patients coping with a cancer diagnosis, and, when I felt I had sufficient basic skills, I was lucky enough to study massage for people living with cancer. I now volunteer 1 day a week at the Edinburgh hospice and treat inpatients, day patients, outpatients, and also carers and bereaved carers.

The first time I had personal experience of the beneficial effects of massage was, sadly, 20 years ago when my late husband

(*continued*)

was receiving palliative care in hospital. His back was often uncomfortable and I used to climb up behind him in his hospital bed and, with no training – and questionable skills! – would knead his muscles and stroke his back to give him relief. In the latter stages of his illness, he loved me gently massaging his feet. When you are in despair and would do anything to help ease your loved one's pain, being able to do even these small personal things for him helped me cope too. I think, even then, I had made up my mind that this was something I'd like to do for others although it was many years before I felt emotionally able to do so. Although my husband had no hospice care, members of my family and two close friends did, and I had seen firsthand how wonderfully caring the whole environment is and, particularly, how special the staff are who work there. When I got the opportunity to join them, I was delighted. I had not expected it to be easy, but, initially, I struggled quite badly with my sadness for both the patients and their loved ones and my mind and dreams were full of some of these people for days after my weekly session and sometimes longer. Fortunately, I was well supported by both staff within Marie Curie and fellow therapists and began to realize that these were common emotions and that being able to discuss coping mechanisms with others was invaluable. As time passed, while still very moved by particular people and their situations, I found myself able to put my emotions in perspective and just feeling glad that I can help in some small way. Being invited into patients' lives at this poignant stage and knowing that the gentle touch massage gives some pleasure and relief from pain and discomfort in their final days feels such a privilege.

I have also found that my role extends beyond that of massage therapist particularly when treating carers and people who have been bereaved. It may be the safe, warm, and welcoming environment in which we see people or just that they feel able to talk freely to someone outwith their family, but I find that a significant part of my job is listening to their troubles and fears and empathizing and supporting them where I can. I love working with the patients at Marie Curie. There are some tears but lots of laughter and lightheartedness too, and I gain so much more from being there than I give.

Without a national volunteer education program in the UK, it falls to individual hospice and palliative care organizations develop their own training courses for volunteers. However, anecdotal evidence suggests that training topics are common to many organizations and are very similar to those delivered in Canada as outlined above. In addition organizations may require volunteers to undertake some core mandatory training relevant to their role such as infection control, health and safety, moving and handling, and food safety. Resources have recently been launched for community children's palliative care volunteering in the UK entitled "Together We Can"; these online materials from Together for Short Lives include a six-module training program of approximately 21–24 h.

Australia offers a Palliative Care Training Resource Kit in addition to a handbook for Palliative Care Volunteers. The length of training is determined by the needs of the service and varies from 2 to 8 days in length (Huntir 2018). The context in the USA is somewhat different as volunteers are a mandatory part of hospice and palliative care for any hospice that receives payment from Medicare (Brock and Herndon 2017). Under this provision, the training of volunteers is required but not prescribed. However, a 16 h training program is suggested by the National Hospice and Palliative Care Organization. They suggest that this should include hospice ethos, services and aims, confidentiality, protecting the rights of patients and families, family dynamics, understanding the impact of dying, death and bereavement, and coping strategies. In addition, volunteers should be clear about their role, accountability and reporting structure.

It might be considered, therefore, that the training is firmly embedded within the concept of hospice and palliative care volunteering. It is interesting to note that this extends to community-driven hospice and palliative care services. For example in Neighbourhood Network in Palliative Care in Kerala in India those interested in helping receive 16 h of training (Kumar and Numpeli 2005).

7.3 What Do We Know About the Impact of Training

A review published in 2005 sought to describe the dominant topics in research literature on volunteering in hospice and palliative care. The review focused on publication years 1988–2004 (Wilson et al. 2005). Of the three overarching themes identified in the literature, one was on descriptions of volunteer training programs and training needs. Ten years later, a Cochrane systematic review sought to evaluate the effect of training programs for volunteers in patient- and family-facing roles in hospice and palliative care (Horey et al. 2015). This review focused on comparative prospective studies, such as RCTs. They sought evaluations of training programs according to any stated or implied purpose: of whether the program was intended to build skills for the volunteer's role, to enhance volunteers coping, or to maintain service standards. No relevant well-designed studies were identified. In their conclusions, they highlight that they excluded some comparative prospective trials on volunteer training in this setting (this is because of limitations in the trial design prevented meaningful comparison between those who received volunteer training and those who did not). This they suggest indicates that rigorous research in this area is possible. Although since this publication to our knowledge there have been no new trials published.

8 Conclusion

This chapter has explored volunteering from both practice and research perspectives in both adult and children's hospice and palliative care. While countries and cultures may approach hospice and palliative care differently, there is a surprising similarity in the roles and involvement of volunteers. Research suggests that their roles are distinct from those of paid staff; they are perceived by volunteers as less task oriented and more social in nature. Their activities are diverse, and volunteer presence in hospice and palliative care spans many different contexts in which care is delivered. Volunteering is not without its challenges, however. Research shows that volunteers themselves sometimes feel unprepared for what they face highlighting the importance of good support and training. There is much anecdotal evidence but a paucity of empirical evidence on the impact of volunteering in hospice and palliative care and of the content and effectiveness of training. This chapter has also explored the ethical and research challenges of identifying and measuring outcomes for volunteering and concluded that these are not insurmountable.

Clearly embedded in the history and development of hospice and palliative care across many countries, volunteering plays an essential role in contributing to leadership, fundraising and governance, patient and family experience, and public education. Volunteers, as community members, play an important part in helping to normalize death and dying as a social issue. If we are serious about delivering truly holistic hospice and palliative care to patients and families, we need to recognize and address the vital role played by volunteers.

References

Abel J, Kellehear A. Palliative care reimagined: a needed shift. BMJ Support Palliat Care. 2016;6:21–6. https://doi.org/10.1136/bmjspcare-2015-001009.

Alcock P. A strategic unity: defining the third sector in the UK. Voluntary Sect Rev. 2010;1(1):5–24.

Block EM, Casarett DJ, Spence C, Gozalo P, Connor SR, Teno JM. Got volunteers? Association of hospice use of volunteers with bereaved family members' overall rating of the quality of end-of-life care. J Pain Symptom Manag. 2010;39(3):502–6.

Brighton LJ, Koffman J, Robinson V, Khan SA, George R, Burman R, et al. 'End of life could be on any ward really': a qualitative study of hospital volunteers' end-of-life care training needs and learning preferences. Palliat Med. 2017;31(9):842–52.

Brock CM, Herndon CM. A survey of hospice volunteer coordinators: training methods and objectives of current hospice volunteer training programs. Am J Hosp Palliat Med. 2017;34(5):412–6.

Burbeck R, Low J, Sampson EL, Scott R, Bravery R, Candy B. Volunteer activity in specialist paediatric palliative care: a national survey. BMJ Support Palliat Care. 2013. https://doi.org/10.1136/bmjspcare-2012-000355.

Burbeck R, Low J, Sampson EL, Bravery R, Hill M, Morris S, et al. Volunteers in specialist palliative care: a survey of adult services in the United Kingdom. J Palliat Med. 2014a;17(5):568–74.

Burbeck R, Candy B, Low J, Rees R. Understanding the role of the volunteer in specialist palliative care: a systematic review and thematic synthesis of qualitative studies. BMC Palliat Care. 2014b;13(1):3.

Candy B, France R, Low J, Sampson L. Does involving volunteers in the provision of palliative care make a difference to patient and family wellbeing? A systematic review of quantitative and qualitative evidence. Int J Nurs Stud. 2015;52(3):756–68.

Casarett D. Ethical issues in palliative care research. In: Oxford textbook of palliative medicine. Oxford: Oxford University Press; 2009.

Claxton-Oldfield S. Hospice palliative care volunteers: the benefits for patients, family caregivers, and the volunteers. Palliat Support Care. 2015a;13(3):809–13.

Claxton-Oldfield S. Got volunteers? The selection, training, roles, and impact of hospice palliative care volunteers in Canada's community-based volunteer programs. Home Health Care Manag Pract. 2015b;27(1):36–40.

Council of Europe. Recommendation of the Committee of Ministers to member states on the organisation of palliative care. Stockholm: Ipisisim Vulpute ver Ii ese; 2003.

Dean A, Willis S. 'A strange kind of balance': inpatient hospice volunteers' views on role preparation and training. Prog Palliat Care. 2017;25(6):1–7.

European Association of Palliative Care. Voice for volunteering. The EAPC Madrid Charter on volunteering in hospice and palliative care. Available from: http://www.eapcnet.eu/Themes/Resources/VolunteeringCharter.aspx (accessed 12th June 2018); 2017.

Gale B. O-26 Making a difference – stories from community hospice volunteers. BMJ Supportive & Palliative Care. 2015;5:A82.

Globisch MD. Denmark. In: Gronemeyer R, Fink M, Globisch M, Schumann F, editors. Helping people at the end of their lives hospice and palliative care in Europe. Berlin: Lit Verlag; 2005.

Gomes B, Calanzani N, Curiale V, McCrone P, Higginson IJ. Effectiveness and cost-effectiveness of home palliative care services for adults with advanced illness and their caregivers. Cochrane Database Syst Rev. 2009;(6):CD007760.

Goossensen A, Somsen J. Volunteering in hospice and palliative care in the Netherlands. In: Scott R, Howlett S, editors. The changing face of volunteering in hospice and palliative care: an international perspective. Oxford: Oxford University Press; 2018.

Goossensen M, Somsen J, Scott R, Pelltari L. Defining volunteering in hospice and palliative care in Europe: an EAPC white paper. Eur J Palliat Care. 2016;23(4):184–191.

Herbst-Damm KL, Kulik JA. Volunteer support, marital status, and the survival times of terminally ill patients. Health Psychol. 2005;24(2):225.

Hesse M, Radbruch L. Volunteering in hospice and palliative care in Germany. In: Scott R, Howlett S, editors. The changing face of volunteering in hospice and palliative care: an international perspective. Oxford: Oxford University Press; 2018.

Higginson IJ, Evans CJ, Grande G, Preston N, Morgan M, McCrone P, et al. Evaluating complex interventions in end of life care: the MORECare statement on good practice generated by a synthesis of transparent expert consultations and systematic reviews. BMC Med. 2013;11(1):111.

Hoerger M. Randomization failure in palliative care RCTs. Palliat Med. 2017;32:533–4. https://doi.org/10.1177/0269216317727159.

Horey D, Street A, O'Connor M, Peters L, Lee S. Training and supportive programs for palliative care volunteers in community settings. Cochrane Database Syst Rev. 2015;(7):CD009500.

Howick JH. The philosophy of evidence-based medicine. Oxford: Wiley; 2011.

Howlett S, Scott R. Pulling it all together. In: Scott R, Howlett S, editors. The changing face of volunteering in hospice and palliative care: an international perspective. Oxford: Oxford University Press; 2018.

Huntir A. Volunteering in hospice and palliative care in Australia. In: Scott R, Howlett S, editors. The changing face of volunteering in hospice and palliative care: an international perspective. Oxford: Oxford University Press; 2018.

Jenkinson CE, Dickens AP, Jones K, Thompson-Coon J, Taylor RS, Rogers M, et al. Is volunteering a public health intervention? A systematic review and meta-analysis of the health and survival of volunteers. BMC Public Health. 2013;13(1):773.

Johnson MJ, Ekstrom M, Currow DC. In response to C Walshe,'The state of play'. Palliat Med. 2017;31(8):772–3.

Kavalieratos D, Corbelli J, Zhang D, Dionne-Odom JN, Ernecoff NC, Hanmer J, et al. Association between palliative care and patient and caregiver outcomes: a systematic review and meta-analysis. JAMA. 2016;316(20):2104–14.

Kiange K. Volunteering in hospice and palliative care in Africa. In: Scott R, Howlett S, editors. The changing face of volunteering in hospice and palliative care: an international perspective. Oxford: Oxford University Press; 2018.

Krakowiak P, Pawłowski L. Volunteering in hospice and palliative care in Poland and Eastern Europe. In: Scott R, Howlett S, editors. The changing face of volunteering in hospice and palliative care: an international perspective. Oxford: Oxford University Press; 2018.

Krouse RS, Rosenfeld KE, Grant M, Aziz N, Byock I, Sloan J, et al. Palliative care research: issues and opportunities. Cancer Epidem Biomar Prevent. 2004;13(3): 337–9.

Kumar S, Numpeli M. Neighborhood network in palliative care. Indian J Palliat Care. 2005;11(1):6.

Luijkx KG, Schols JM. Volunteers in palliative care make a difference. J Palliat Care. 2009;25(1):30.

McKee M, Kelley ML, Guirguis-Younger M, MacLean M, Nadin S. It takes a whole community: the contribution of rural hospice volunteers to whole-person palliative care. J Palliat Care. 2010;26(2):103.

Meyer D, Schmidt P, Zernikow B, Wager J. It's all about communication: a mixed-methods approach to collaboration between volunteers and staff in pediatric palliative care. Am J Hosp Palliat Med. 2018. https://doi.org/10.1177/1049909117751419.

Morris S, Wilmot A, Hill M, Ockenden N, Payne S. A narrative literature review of the contribution of volunteers in end-of-life care services. Palliat Med. 2013;27(5):428–36.

Morris SM, Payne S, Ockenden N, Hill M. Hospice volunteers: bridging the gap to the community? Health Soc Care Community. 2015;25:1704–13.

Pabst K, Pelttari L, Scott R, Jaspers B, Loth C, Radbruch L. The role and motivation of volunteers in hospice and palliative care in Europe. 15th World Congress of the European Association for Palliative Care, Madrid, Spain; 2017.

Pawłowski L, Lichodziejewska-Niemierko M, Pawłowska I, Leppert W, Mróz P. Nationwide survey on volunteers' training in hospice and palliative care in Poland. BMJ Support Palliat Care. 2016. https://doi.org/10.1136/bmjspcare-2015-000984.

Pelttari L, Pissarek A. Volunteering in hospice and palliative care in Austria. In: Scott R, Howlett S, editors. The changing face of volunteering in hospice and palliative care: an international perspective. Oxford: Oxford University Press; 2018.

Pesut B, Hooper B, Lehbauer S, Dalhuisen M. Promoting volunteer capacity in hospice palliative care: a narrative review. Am J Hosp Palliat Med. 2014;31(1):69–78.

Radbruch L, Payne S. White paper on standards and norms for hospice and palliative care in Europe: part 2. Eur J Palliat Care. 2010;17(1):22–33.

Rochester C, Paine AE, Howlett S, Zimmeck M, Paine AE. Volunteering and Society in the 21st Century. Basingstoke: Pallgrave Macmillan; 2010.

Rochester C, Paine AE, Howlett S, Zimmeck M, Paine AE. Volunteering and society in the 21st century. Springer; 2016.

Scott R. Strategic asset or optional extra: the impact of volunteers on hospice sustainability. Unpublished doctoral thesis, University of Dundee. Available from http://ethos.bl.uk/OrderDetails.do?uin=uk.bl.ethos.585509; 2013.

Scott R. "We cannot do it without you"- the impact of volunteers in UK hospices. Eur J Palliat Care. 2015;22 (2):80–3.

Söderhamn U, Flateland S, Fensli M, Skaar R. To be a trained and supported volunteer in palliative care–a phenomenological study. BMC Palliat Care. 2017; 16(1):18.

United Nations. State of the world's volunteeerism report: Transforming Governance. United Nations Volunteer Programme. Available from: https://www.unv.org/sites/default/files/2015%20State%20of%20the%20World%27s%20Volunteerism%20Report%20-%20Transforming%20Governance.pdf; 2015.

Vanderstichelen S, Houttekier D, Cohen J, Van Wesemael Y, Deliens L, K Chambaere. Describing the size and type of care tasks of the volunteer workforce in palliative care: a nation-wide survey. 15th world congress of the European association for palliative care, Madrid, Spain; 2017.

Walshe C, Algorta GP, Dodd S, Hill M, Ockenden N, Payne S, et al. Protocol for the End-of-Life Social Action Study (ELSA): a randomised wait-list controlled trial and embedded qualitative case study evaluation assessing the causal impact of social action befriending services on end of life experience. BMC Palliat Care. 2016;15(1):60.

Weeks LE, Macquarrie C, Bryanton O. Hospice palliative care volunteers: a unique care link. J Palliat Care. 2008;24(2):85.

Wilson DM, Justice C, Thomas R, Sheps S, MacAdam M, Brown M. End-of-life care volunteers: a systematic review of the literature. Health Serv Manag Res. 2005;18(4):244–57.

World Health Organization. WHO definition of palliative care. 2018. Available from: http://www.who.int/cancer/palliative/definition/en/.

Part V

Palliative Care in Specific Disease Groups

Palliative Care and Cancer

57

Koen Pardon and Gaëlle Vanbutsele

Contents

K. Pardon (✉)
End-of-Life Care Research group, Vrije Universiteit Brussel and Ghent University, Brussels, Belgium

Faculty of Medicine and Life Science, Faculty of Business Economics, Hasselt University, Diepenbeek, Belgium
e-mail: koen.pardon@vub.ac.be

G. Vanbutsele
End-of-Life Care Research group, Vrije Universiteit Brussel and Ghent University, Brussels, Belgium
e-mail: gaelle.vanbutsele@vub.ac.be

R. D. MacLeod, L. Van den Block (eds.), *Textbook of Palliative Care*,
https://doi.org/10.1007/978-3-319-77740-5_56

Abstract

There is a growing trend in oncology, both in research and in clinical practice, toward the early integration of palliative care into regular oncology treatment, from diagnosis of advanced cancer onward. This new care approach has been developed to tackle two major problems insufficiently addressed by traditional methods which seriously affect the quality of life of advanced cancer patients – the undertreatment of symptoms and the overtreatment of the cancer itself. Although these problems can also be observed in other life-threatening diseases such as heart failure and dementia, the early integration of palliative care is gaining ground particularly in oncology, as the specific, more recognizable symptoms of advanced cancer and the relative predictability of time of death make it more suitable for early palliative care.

Recently, several models of the early integration of palliative care into regular oncological health services have been developed. In some of these models, the oncologists themselves are responsible for the palliative care of the patient during the illness trajectory, and in others specialist palliative care teams are integrated into regular oncology care. There is accumulating evidence that supports the value of early integration of specialist palliative care teams both in outpatient and inpatient settings. However, despite this evidence, palliative care is still largely seen, and applied, only in the later stages. In this chapter, several barriers to the early integration of palliative care related to healthcare professionals, to patients and family, and to the healthcare system itself are identified and discussed.

1 Introduction

There is a growing trend in oncology, both in research and in clinical practice, toward the early integration of palliative care into regular oncology treatment, from diagnosis of advanced cancer onward. This trend is in accordance with the 2002 definition of palliative care by the World Health Organization (WHO) which clearly states that palliative care is applicable early in the course of a life-threatening illness, in conjunction with disease-modifying and life-prolonging therapies, and is not limited to end of life or terminal care when death is likely to occur within a few days or weeks (WHO 2002). According to the WHO, the goals of palliative care, such as improving quality of life through comprehensive symptom management and patient and family support, are ideally applied throughout the trajectory of a serious illness like an advanced cancer. More recently, in 2016, on the basis of accumulating evidence, the American Society of Clinical Oncology (ASCO) issued an official guideline stating that inpatients and outpatients with advanced cancer should receive dedicated palliative care services, early in the disease course, concurrent with active treatment (Ferrell et al. 2017). With this, an important step has been taken toward actual integration into clinical practice.

Figure 1 describes the new model of early integrated palliative care; this differs from the old but still much used model in which palliative care is seen as an attachment to the curative and life-extending phase. This figure is an adaptation of the figure that was developed by Lynne and Adamson in 2003 (with permission of RAND Health) (Lynn and Adamson 2003). In the old model, palliative care is only initiated when there are no options left. In the new model, palliative care starts at diagnosis by evaluating whether the patient has palliative care needs. As the disease progresses, palliative care becomes increasingly important, though in a varying way, according to the patient's needs; additionally, it also focuses on those close to the person who is dying, both before and after death.

This chapter discusses (1) which problems in traditional oncology care have led to the development of this new approach, (2) what models of early integration of palliative care in oncology are being developed and proposed, (3) why the integration of palliative care is gaining ground particularly in oncology rather than in other diseases such as heart disease and dementia, (4) what the research evidence says about the early integration of palliative care into oncology, and (5) what the current state of affairs is with regard to the actual integration of palliative care into clinical practice and which barriers have to be overcome in order to improve it.

2 Problems Insufficiently Addressed by Traditional Oncology Care

There are several problems that seriously affect the quality of life of people with advanced cancer which are insufficiently addressed by traditional

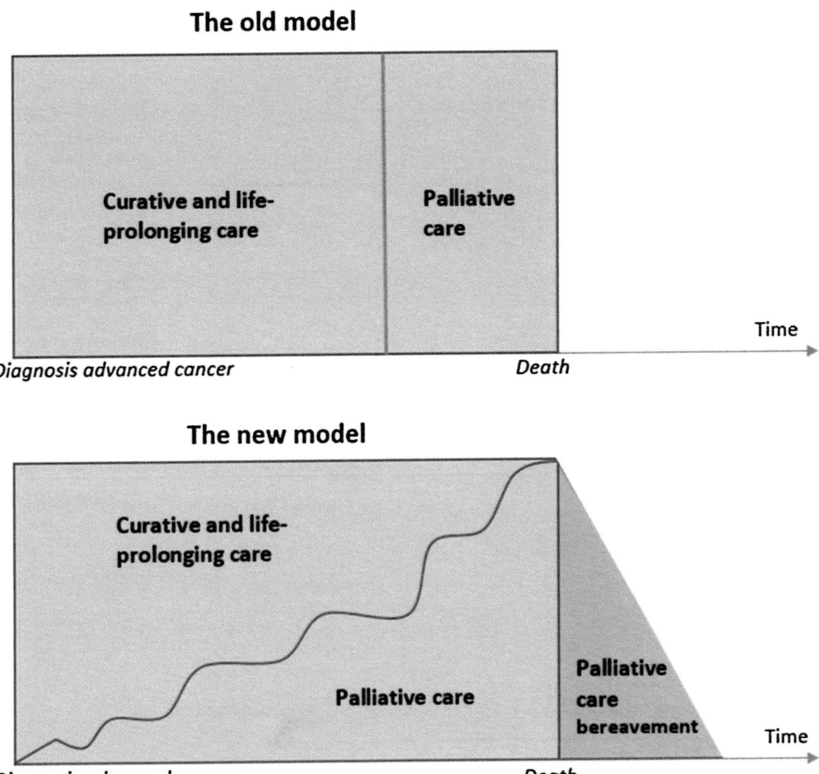

Fig. 1 The old and new model of early integrated palliative care in oncology care

oncology care, a situation that has led to the development of the new approach of early integration of palliative care into oncology care. Perhaps the most obvious of these is that people with advanced cancer with limited life expectancy often suffer from multiple symptoms – on the physical, psychological, social, and existential levels – that appear to be undertreated. A recent study of pain from the USA, one of the most frequent and debilitating of symptoms, shows that of 3123 ambulatory patients with invasive breast, gastrointestinal, or lung cancer, 33% of those who were suffering from pain were receiving inadequate analgesic prescribing, a problem that persisted even after a 1-month follow-up (Fisch et al. 2012). A study in a teaching hospital in Australia examined the treatment of nausea in hospitalized cancer patients and concluded that nausea is often inadequately treated, with more than one third of nauseated patients either not being prescribed an antiemetic or not having taken prescribed medication (Greaves et al. 2009). Studies with regard to other common symptoms in advanced cancer, such as dyspnea, constipation, loss of appetite, and depression, show similar results.

One of the reasons for undertreatment of symptoms is their underdiagnosis; according to a European multicenter study, healthcare providers underestimate symptom intensity in one out of ten patients, with variations between cancer diagnoses (Laugsand et al. 2010). Other related reasons include the strong orientation of healthcare providers toward cure or life prolongation rather than quality of life, a lack of expert knowledge of symptom management, and limited time to spend with patients.

A second problem is that people with advanced and incurable cancer run the risk of overtreatment, of receiving continued burdensome treatment with only marginal positive effect, if any, but with many adverse effects. This has been demonstrated in several studies; a population-based retrospective study in Ontario, Canada, for instance, used administrative data to examine aggressiveness of end-of-life cancer care. The care was deemed aggressive if there was at least one of the following indicators: the last dose of chemotherapy received within 14 days of death, more than one emergency department visit within 30 days of death, more than one hospitalization within 30 days of death, or at least one intensive care unit admission within 30 days of death. It was observed that almost 25% of patients experienced at least one occurrence of potentially aggressive end-of-life care, and this was most likely in breast, lung, or hematological malignancies (Ho et al. 2011). The researchers also remarked that chemotherapy and intensive care unit utilization was higher in the USA than in Ontario.

This tendency to overtreat can be ascribed to oncologists whose orientation is naturally toward cure and life prolongation, but it might also be related to the wishes of the person who is dying, who may prefer to receive aggressive treatment for as long as possible. However, research shows that the treatment approach has often not been thoroughly discussed with the patient and thus does not always correspond with their fully informed preferences. There is ample empirical evidence that most patients with serious life-threatening illness prefer to avoid hospitalizations and aggressive care when their illness is advanced.

Both problems, the undertreatment of the symptoms and the overtreatment of the cancer, can be tackled by the early integration of palliative care into regular oncological care. The WHO defines palliative care as an approach that improves the quality of life of patients and their families facing the problems associated with life-threatening illness, through the prevention and relief of suffering by means of early identification and impeccable assessment and treatment of pain and other problems, physical, psychosocial, and spiritual (WHO 2002). In palliative care the expertise exists to diagnose and treat the many symptoms that advanced cancer patients experience. The focus of palliative care on the quality rather than quantity of life acts as a good counterbalance to the use of possibly futile aggressive treatments. The integration of the two care systems, i.e., oncology with its focus on disease-oriented treatment and palliative care with its focus on symptom reduction and quality of life, can ensure that people who are dying and those close to them receive the best possible care, tailored to their wishes and their needs.

3 Early Palliative Care Is Gaining Ground More in Oncology than in Other Medical Specialties

The early integration of the palliative care model is gaining ground in oncology more than in other medical specialties. This is unexpected because the problems of cancer patients that, as described above, originally led to integrated palliative care do not only affect oncology patients but also others with life-limiting diseases such as heart failure and dementia. Considering heart failure, for instance, a US study compared the symptom burden, depression, and lack of existential well-being of heart failure patients with that of advanced cancer patients and found that both groups had a similar number of physical symptoms, depression scores, and scores for spiritual well-being, after adjustment for age, gender, marital status, education, and income. The authors concluded that heart failure patients, particularly those with more severe heart failure, need the option of palliative care just as much as advanced cancer patients do (Bekelman et al. 2009). Another study in Belgium, Europe, interviewed people with cancer, chronic obstructive lung disease, heart failure, or dementia at different phases of the illness trajectory. They were asked how they experienced the care needs related to their disease from diagnosis onward. The results revealed that various problems and care needs, i. e., physical, practical, psychological, social, existential, and financial, as well as needs for information and communication, were present in every disease group (Beernaert et al. 2016). The needs occurred both in the earlier phases, from diagnosis onward, and in the later phases in the illness trajectory of every disease group.

One explanation for the leading role of oncology in the early integration of palliative care can be found in the specific disease pathway of cancer compared with other diseases such as heart failure and dementia (Lynn and Adamson 2003). The cancer pathway is characterized by the presence of various symptoms that are highly recognizable and by a relatively predictable time of death. As a result, the match with palliative care is possibly much greater than it is with other diseases. Heart failure usually results in a slow deterioration of the state of health, interspersed with more acute phases of deterioration. Any of these acute phases can result in a more or less "sudden" death. In such patients, there is much less clarity about the imminence of death. The third pathway, dementia, is characterized by a steady period of decline in functional and mental capacity; death itself is usually the result of the occurrence of an acute infection.

The different pathways of cancer, heart failure, and dementia are described in Fig. 2 (with

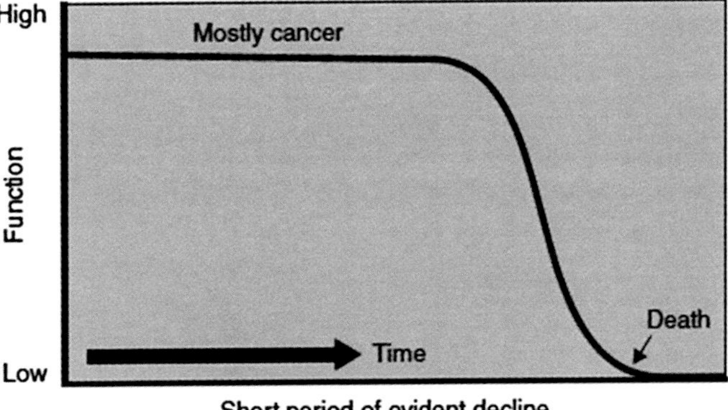

High
Mostly heart and lung failure
Function
Death
Time
Low
Long-term limitations with intermittent serious episodes

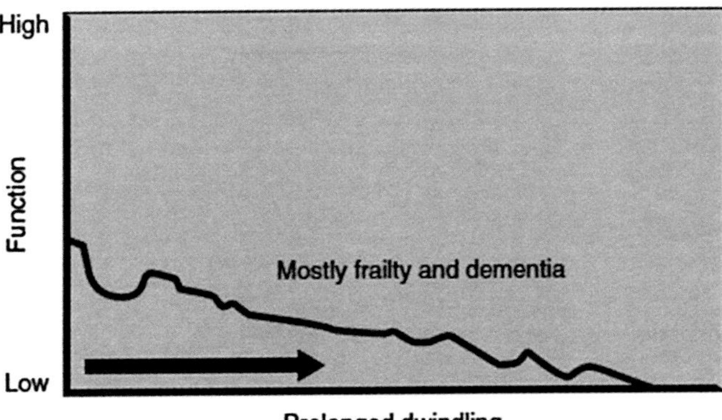

Fig. 2 The typical disease pathway of cancer, heart failure, and dementia

permission of RAND Health). It has to be noted that these disease pathways describe an overall trajectory that is not always applicable to individual patients. This means that even in cancer patients the disease trajectory cannot always be predicted, even with the best prognostic tools and skills. The predictability of the disease trajectory can also depend on the specific cancer diagnosis. The pathway of hematological cancer, for example, is characterized by acute exacerbations and a rapid dying trajectory, resulting in difficulties for hematologists in assessing the right time to refer to palliative care. For some cancer types such as breast and colorectal cancers, there is an evolution toward chronic disease, and the differences with nonmalignant disease have become less. Moreover, the development of new immunotherapies that are effective for some people can add years to a life, further complicating the prognostic estimations of physicians. However, the limited predictability of life-threatening diseases, whether cancer or other conditions, does not need to be a barrier to the early integration of palliative care. Palliative care is in its essence a holistic approach that is focused on the person and not on the disease. This means that it is important in palliative care to evaluate every person separately to assess whether they have palliative care needs and to offer palliative care if indicated, rather than to start from a specific diagnosis.

4 Models of Early Integration of Palliative Care into Oncological Care

Models of early integration of palliative care within regular oncological health services have only recently begun to be developed. Bruera et al., for instance, described three possible models and levels of integration of palliative care services within oncology care: a solo practice model, a congress practice model, and a fully integrated palliative care model (Bruera and Hui 2012). The first, the solo practice model, requires the oncologist to manage all aspects of cancer care, i.e., the treatment of the cancer as well as supportive and palliative care. To be able to achieve this, the oncologist has to fully integrate palliative care knowledge and skills into their daily practice. The second, the "congress" practice model, is one in which the oncologist does not provide palliative care but refers patients to multiple consultants for the management of pain, distress, fatigue, and other symptoms. This requires some knowledge and skills in palliative care by the oncologist as it is important to be able to diagnose the palliative care symptoms of the patient and to assess the need for professional help with these symptoms. The third, the fully integrated palliative care model, is one in which the oncologist focuses on cancer-specific treatments while the palliative care team systematically attends to the patient's physical symptoms and psychosocial concerns. In this model, the oncologist and palliative care physicians comanage care in a complementary manner, thereby reducing the need for the extensive use of outside consultants.

These three models each have their advantages and disadvantages. The solo practice model, for example, has the advantage that both medical disease-oriented care and palliative care are provided by one person, requiring fewer visits for the patient and less coordination between specialists. The disadvantage is that oncologists are often not trained in palliative care and may not always have the time to take on this task. The congress practice model has the advantage that the oncologist can refer to experts and does not need to have all the expertise, but the disadvantage is that there is often limited communication and coordination of care. On the other hand, good coordination and close cooperation are possible in the fully integrated care model, but this coordination can only be effective if good care pathways or protocols are established and followed.

Bruera's three models, however, conceal something that is often mentioned in the literature – the distinction between general and specialist palliative care (Quill and Abernethy 2013). General palliative care is care that is provided by regular healthcare professionals who have basic palliative care knowledge and skills.

In concrete terms, general palliative care would mean that the oncologist engages in systematic basic symptom assessment and management, in discussions about prognosis and goals of care, in shared decision-making, and in timely care planning.

Specialist palliative care involves the separate discipline of palliative care as provided by multidisciplinary teams in hospitals, in outpatient clinics, and in palliative home care. In this case, the palliative care is provided by physicians, nurses, and other specialists who have received special training and whose main activity is to provide palliative care. This form of palliative care is what most people understand as palliative care. Specialized palliative care has become increasingly available in recent years. Researchers at the University of Lancaster, UK, for instance, have identified the existence of 16,000 hospices and/or palliative care units worldwide – standalone units or those attached to a hospital – that treat patients in the final phase of life through the provision of adequate symptom relief (Lynch et al. 2013). The countries in the top category for such provision are Austria, Australia, Belgium, Canada, France, Germany, Hong Kong, Iceland, Ireland, Italy, Japan, Norway, Poland, Romania, Singapore, Uganda, and the UK. According to this WHO-recognized classification, these countries have developed a critical mass in the field of palliative care, spread across various locations within the country. This means there is a complete range of various forms of palliative care from multiple service providers. In these countries both professional caregivers and society and government as a whole are aware of the need and importance of palliative care; there is widespread though heavily regulated availability of morphine and other analgesics. In addition, the specialist healthcare providers are organized into one or more palliative care associations (WPCA and WHO 2014). Unfortunately, there is still a large group of countries, 75 in total, where no center for palliative care exists. These are mainly countries with a low gross national income.

The question arises of which model of early integration of palliative care into oncology is preferable. Much research has been undertaken looking at the third model of full and early integration of specialist palliative care in oncology care, and strong evidence for the effectiveness of this model has been found. However, one clear disadvantage of this model is that it is time intensive and expensive, which raises the question of whether the full integration of specialist palliative care is actually feasible in times of increased aging and increased numbers of chronically ill people. For this reason it has been suggested and argued that the support of a fully integrated model throughout the disease course is not necessary but is only required when the patient develops complex palliative care needs. At other times general palliative care, i.e., that provided by an oncologist who has had a basic training in palliative care, will suffice. In other words, in this scenario the best overall model would be one in which integrated specialist palliative care is being interchanged with general palliative care provided by the oncologist, depending on the complexity and the severity of the palliative care needs of the patient.

5 Research Evidence for the Value of Early Integration of Palliative Care into Oncology

There is accumulating scientific evidence that demonstrates the added value of models of early integration of specialist palliative care provided by an interdisciplinary palliative care team both in outpatient and inpatient settings. Other models of early palliative care in oncology, such as the model of general palliative care in oncology, have not been studied thoroughly, and therefore no definitive statements can be made regarding their effectiveness.

The randomized controlled trial (RCT) studies that have tested the early and fully integrated specialist palliative care model are discussed below. These trials were strongly based on others that studied palliative care in the home or hospital setting but have the specific feature that the palliative care was provided early in the disease trajectory to maximize the beneficial effects on quality of life and symptom burden of the person who is dying and those close to them.

5.1 Temel et al. (USA): Study 1

Temel et al. undertook an RCT with 151 outpatients with metastatic non-small cell lung cancer (NSCLC) who were treated in the thoracic oncology clinic of Massachusetts General Hospital in the USA (Temel et al. 2010). They compared early specialist palliative care integrated into standard oncology care versus standard oncology care alone with no palliative care provision or care provided only late in the disease course. The researchers chose to study newly diagnosed metastatic lung cancer patients because they have a median life expectancy of less than 1 year and experience a high symptom burden.

The early palliative care intervention consisted of consultations with the patient by a member of the hospital palliative care team shortly after diagnosis and at least monthly thereafter. The palliative care team of the hospital consisted of six palliative care physicians and an advanced practice nurse. The consultations were guided by newly developed palliative care guidelines that differed from the existing guidelines for standard palliative care in that the clinicians were specifically encouraged to assess physical and psychosocial symptoms throughout the disease trajectory, to establish goals of care and to assist with treatment decision-making and coordination of care. Table 1 gives an overview of the early palliative care guidelines.

Table 1 Ambulatory palliative care guidelines in the study of Temel et al.

1. Illness understanding/education
Inquire about illness and prognostic understanding
Offer clarification of treatment goals
2. Symptom management – inquire about uncontrolled symptoms with a focus on:
Pain
Pulmonary symptoms (cough, dyspnea)
Fatigue and sleep disturbance
Mood (depression and anxiety)
Gastrointestinal (anorexia and weight loss, nausea and vomiting, constipation)
3. Decision-making
Inquire about mode of decision-making
Assist with treatment decision-making, if necessary
4. Coping with life-threatening illness
Patient
Family/family caregivers
5. Referrals/prescriptions
Identify care plan for future appointments
Indicate referrals to other care providers
Note new medications prescribed

The researchers found that the people in the early palliative care group had a significantly higher quality of life compared with those in the standard care group alone at 12 weeks after baseline. The percentage of patients with depression at 12 weeks was significantly lower in the palliative care group than in the standard care group, but there was no difference between groups in scores for symptoms of anxiety. With regard to end-of-life care, 33% of those who were assigned to early palliative care compared with 54% of the standard oncology group had received aggressive end-of-life care. Another important finding that drew the attention of the medical community was that patients receiving early palliative care had a longer median survival rate than those in the standard care group (11.6 versus 8.9 months since diagnosis). It is not yet clear what precisely causes the increased survival time in the early palliative care group. The researchers concluded that early integration of palliative care for patients with metastatic non-small cell lung cancer is a clinically meaningful and feasible care model that has effects on quality of life and survival that are similar to the effects of first-line chemotherapy.

5.2 Temel et al. (USA): Study 2

Temel et al. then conducted a further RCT with 350 patients with newly diagnosed incurable lung cancer (NSCLC, small cell, or mesothelioma) or non-colorectal gastrointestinal cancer (pancreatic, esophageal, gastric, or hepatobiliary) recruited from the Massachusetts General Hospital (Temel et al. 2017). Patients were randomly assigned to the intervention group providing at least monthly consultations with a palliative care clinician plus usual care or the control group providing usual care alone.

There was no significant improvement in quality of life in the early integration group at

12 weeks after baseline, but there was at the 24-week time point. People in the intervention group also had lower depression at week 24, controlling for baseline scores. At 24 weeks there were also significantly more in the intervention group who had discussed their end-of-life wishes with their oncologist than in the control group. Exploratory analyses of the study outcomes by cancer type revealed important differences in both cancer groups. Lung cancer patients in the intervention group improved in quality of life from baseline to 12 weeks, while those lung cancer patients in the control group reported worsened quality of life. On the other hand, the non-colorectal gastrointestinal cancer patients improved in quality of life in both groups with no differences between groups. Thus, there seems to be a difference in the effect of the intervention depending on cancer type.

5.3 Bakitas et al. (USA): Study 1

Bakitas et al. studied 322 patients with different types of newly diagnosed advanced cancer in a rural comprehensive cancer center, affiliated outreach clinics, and a Veterans Affairs Medical Center (USA). In this study, people were randomly assigned to early palliative care and usual care (intervention group) versus usual care alone (control group) (Bakitas et al. 2009). The intervention consisted of a multicomponent psycho-educational intervention (the ENABLE study: Educate, Nurture, Advise, Before Life Ends) that was given shortly after diagnosis of advanced or recurrent cancer. Trained palliative care advanced practice nurses undertook four weekly educational sessions with the patient and monthly telephone sessions thereafter for follow-up. The sessions focused on patient activation, empowerment, and self-management; patients learned important palliative care principles and crisis prevention through the practice of problem solving, symptom management, communication, and advance care planning. The nurses also had a referring role to other healthcare professionals when this was indicated in order to improve quality of life. Patient-reported outcomes were measured on baseline, at 1 month and every 3 months until death or study completion.

Patients in the palliative care group had significant higher quality of life scores compared with control group patients, better mood, a trend toward lower symptom intensity, but no different resource use (i.e., days in hospital, days in intensive care unit, number of emergency department visits). The survival time in the intervention group was not significantly higher compared with the control group.

5.4 Bakitas et al. (USA): Study 2

Bakitas et al. conducted another RCT later on in the same centers with a similar intervention to determine at what time in the illness trajectory it is best to begin early palliative care; they compared two early palliative care groups, one in which palliative care was begun after enrollment, within 30–60 days (early palliative oncology care), and one in which palliative care was started 3 months after enrollment (still early but delayed palliative oncology care compared with the other group) (Bakitas et al. 2015). The researchers found no significant differences in the patient-reported outcomes of quality of life and symptom impact at 3, 6, and 12 months after enrollment. However at 1 year, a 15% survival advantage was found in the early palliative oncology care group. The precise mechanism of the prolonged survival is not clear yet and can have many possible causes according to the researchers.

5.5 Zimmerman et al. (Canada)

Zimmerman et al. undertook a cluster RCT in the Princess Margaret Cancer Centre in Toronto, Canada, in which 24 medical oncology clinics were randomized to early palliative care integrated in standard cancer care or standard cancer care alone (Zimmermann et al. 2014). A total of 461 advanced cancer patients with solid tumors with a clinical prognosis of 6–24 months participated. The core intervention of early palliative care comprised a consultation and follow-up in

Table 2 Components of the intervention of early palliative care in the study of Zimmerman et al.

1. Within 1 month of recruitment: a multidisciplinary assessment of symptoms, psychological distress, and social support. The duration of this consultation was approximately 60–90 min
2. One week after the first consultation and thereafter as needed: routine telephone contact from a palliative care nurse
3. On a monthly basis: outpatient palliative care follow-up. The duration of these follow-up consultations was 20–50 min
4. 24/7: an on-call service for telephone management of urgent issues

the oncology palliative care clinic by a palliative care physician and nurse. The components of the intervention are described in more detail in Table 2.

The results of the study showed that there was no significant improvement in the early palliative care group compared with the control group at 3 months after enrollment, but there was at 4 months. Their satisfaction with care was significantly better both at 3 and 4 months, and the symptom scores were significantly better at 4 months. There were no significant differences in the specific problems of patients in their interactions with nurses and doctors. Looking at the effects of early palliative care on the caregivers, a significant improvement in their satisfaction with care was observed, while the results regarding their quality of life were inconclusive (McDonald et al. 2017).

5.6 Maltoni et al. (Italy)

Maltoni et al. conducted a multicenter RCT study in Italy of 207 outpatients with metastatic or locally advanced inoperable pancreatic cancer (Maltoni et al. 2016b). The goal was to compare the impact of standard cancer care with systematic early palliative care on the one hand with that of standard cancer care with on-demand palliative care on the other hand. The difference between the two groups was that in the first group all participants received palliative care as a standard, whereas in the second group it was only provided if there was an explicit request from a doctor or patient.

The intervention and trial were very similar to Temel's study. Patients in the intervention arm were given an appointment with a palliative care specialist who used a checklist of topics that were the same as those used by Temel. They were seen every 2–4 weeks until death by a member of the palliative care team. Palliative care appointments and interventions initiated by the palliative care specialist were shared with the oncologist.

Systematic early palliative care significantly improved quality of life 3 months after baseline compared with on-demand palliative care. There were fewer people with depression and anxiety in the intervention group, but the difference was not significant. There was no difference in overall survival between the two groups. With regard to the aggressiveness of end-of-life care, there were differences in favor of the intervention group on some indicators, in particular the use of hospice services and chemotherapy provided in the last 30 days of life (Maltoni et al. 2016a).

5.7 Overall Assessment of Research

When we compare the six trials, there are a number of similarities and differences. Looking at the intervention that was being evaluated, in all studies it involved early integration of specialist palliative care into standard oncological care and consisted of at least monthly patient consultations by a member of the specialist palliative care team. In the studies of Bakitas et al., the first consultations were highly educational, which was not the case in the other studies, and the subsequent monthly consultations were conducted by telephone because of the rural setting in which the study took place. The palliative care guidelines on which the consultations were based were most clearly described in Temel and Maltoni's study. According to these guidelines, the following topics were required to be discussed in the consultations with the person and those close to them: illness perception, symptom management, medical decision-making, coping with the illness, and referral to other healthcare professionals. In the study of Zimmerman et al., the description of the intervention explicitly mentioned – besides the monthly consultations – the possibility of telephone contact with a palliative care nurse if needed and 24/7 on-call service for the telephone management of urgent issues.

Different patient populations were studied in the six studies. The first study of Temel and the study of Maltoni examined one type of cancer, i.e., non-small cell lung cancer and pancreatic cancer, respectively, both being very deadly cancers with a high symptom burden. In the second study of Temel, two types of cancers were studied, incurable lung cancer and non-colorectal gastrointestinal cancer. In the studies of Zimmerman and Bakitas, a heterogeneous group of patients with different types of advanced cancer were studied. In all studies, quality of life was the primary factor investigated, and an effect was found in all studies. However, this effect was not observed in Temel's second study and in Zimmerman's study at the intended 3 months after baseline, but only at 6 and 4 months after baseline, respectively. It seems that the palliative care intervention may require longer than 3 months before having a noticeable effect on quality of life. The other outcomes that were often investigated in the studies were depression, anxiety, symptom burden, use of resources, and survival time. These outcome measures were sometimes significantly improved in the intervention group compared with the control group, and sometimes they were not, depending on the study. Increased survival time in the intervention group was only significant in the first study of Temel and in the second study of Bakitas.

6 Actual Integration into Clinical Practice: Barriers to Overcome

Despite the established principle of early integration of palliative care in oncology and evidence of its benefits, research evaluating the use and timing of both general and specialist palliative care shows that, overall, it is still both seen and applied as terminal care (Quill and Abernethy 2013; Beernaert et al. 2013; Van den Block et al. 2008). A survey to determine the availability and degree of integration of palliative care services in the USA showed that the median duration from referral to specialist palliative care was 90 days before death for outpatient clinics, 7 days for inpatient consultation teams, and 7 days for palliative care units (Hui et al. 2010). A study on referral practices of oncologists to specialized palliative care conducted in Canada also showed that referral was late in the disease trajectory for patients with uncontrolled symptoms (Wentlandt et al. 2012). In Belgium, about 60% of patients who did not die suddenly of cancer were referred to a palliative care service, and for about half of those, this was less than 20 days before death (Beernaert et al. 2013).

Using specialist palliative care does not, of course, necessarily reflect whether or not palliative care was being provided, as regular care could also have been aimed at improving the quality of life of patients and those close to them by addressing their palliative care needs. There are however several studies that indicate that this is not the case. Mortality follow-back studies in Belgium, for instance, have looked at the type of care delivered in the final 3 months of life and demonstrated that, in a majority of cases, the aim of care shifted to comfort or palliation only in the final weeks of life (Beernaert et al. 2013; Van den Block et al. 2008).

Several studies have been done to examine why palliative care is often offered only very late in the disease trajectory when death is imminent, if at all. Three types of barriers have been identified that play a role in the lack of early integration of palliative care in oncology – barriers related to the healthcare professionals, barriers related to the person who is dying and those close to them, and barriers related to the healthcare system.

6.1 Barriers Relating to Healthcare Providers

At the level of healthcare providers, one of the main barriers is the fact that many oncologists still have the idea that palliative care equals terminal care and that palliative care thus only needs to be initiated at the end of life. In order to address this barrier, it is important that healthcare providers become well-informed about the benefits of early palliative care, both through scientific literature and textbooks such as this one and through their own professional organizations. A good and important step was taken by the American Society of Clinical Oncology (ASCO), which established a provisional clinical opinion in 2012 based on the first RCT study of Temel stating that patients with metastatic NSCLC should be offered concurrent palliative care and standard oncologic care at initial diagnosis (Smith et al. 2012). By 2016, ASCO updated this provisional clinical opinion reflecting changes in evidence since the Temel study and recommending that all patients with advanced cancer should receive palliative care early in the disease course, concurrent with active treatment (Ferrell et al. 2017).

Even if oncologists are convinced of the benefits of early palliative care, they are still sometimes hesitant to discuss and initiate it because of fear that the use of the term palliative care will take away hope from their patient. Research has indeed shown that oncologists tend to avoid discussing more difficult topics such as prognosis, life expectancy, and palliative care, even if the patient wants this information (Pardon et al. 2011). Some investigators have suggested using the term supportive care instead of palliative care, in order to address this problem. There are studies that have demonstrated that renaming palliative care as supportive care effectively led to more referrals to palliative care. A study by the MD Anderson Cancer Center in Texas, for example, observed a 41% increase in palliative care consultations and a quicker referral to palliative care after a name change (Dalal et al. 2011).

Another barrier at the level of oncologists is that very often they have not received any training at all in palliative care and thus lack basic palliative care knowledge, skills, and attitudes (Aldridge et al. 2016). A basic training in palliative care is fundamental in enabling oncologists and other regular health professionals to recognize palliative care needs. It would also facilitate oncologists in providing general palliative care themselves whenever necessary and in referring to and working with specialist palliative care teams in the case of complex problems. Training in palliative care is also important because it may contribute to the elimination of other barriers such as the idea that it is the duty of the oncologist to provide palliative care themselves or the negative image of palliative care they may have as a result of negative experiences in their clinical practice. For the integration of palliative care in oncology, it is additionally important that oncologists have specific knowledge of how palliative care is organized in their country, to what degree palliative care services are accessible and available, and what the legal and financial framework is for the cooperation between oncology and palliative care.

Besides barriers at the level of the oncologist, there are also barriers at the level of palliative care professionals. One barrier is that early integration of palliative care into oncology leads to a greater workload for palliative care specialists, who are already underrepresented and often overburdened (Kain and Eisenhauer 2016). Another barrier for successful integration might be that the palliative care experts are insufficiently informed about the therapies the patient is receiving from diagnosis on, the side effects of these therapies, and the overall expertise and modus operandi of oncologists in relation to their patients.

6.2 Barriers Relating to the Person Who Is Dying and Those Close to Them

One barrier relating to the person who is dying and those close to them is that they often think of palliative care as terminal care, as many regular healthcare professionals do, although terminal care is only part of what palliative care provides. Patients who participated in the RCT of Zimmerman were asked after the study how they had viewed palliative care before the study had started (CAPC 2015; Zimmermann et al. 2016). In their answers it became clear that most patients associated palliative care with death, dependence, and end-of-life comfort care in inpatient settings. This perception changed for those who received the intervention of early palliative care, even though they still thought that the term itself was very much associated with stigma and that it needed to be better explained by healthcare professionals. An important step toward eliminating this barrier is to educate the public about palliative care through awareness campaigns and through more accurate information provision by healthcare professionals. Another way is to change the name as discussed above.

6.3 Barriers Relating to the Healthcare System

The early integration of palliative care into oncology is challenging because it questions the adequacy and efficacy of the current structure and organization of the healthcare system as it exists in many countries. The current healthcare system is primarily organization-centered, with limited communication and cooperation between the different specialties that are involved in care and between the different healthcare settings (hospital, nursing home, home). The aim of the integration of services however is to enhance cooperation and communication and organize healthcare around the person who is dying and his or her needs. To be able to let healthcare services cooperate more and to make the patient central is another way of working that is not financially and structurally endorsed in the current system. In many countries, for instance, the financing of healthcare is such that technical performance may be rewarded, while the quality of care and the time spent on communication and coordination is less highly regarded.

The current system thus needs to a certain extent to be changed from an organization-centered to a patient-centered system, and one way of doing this is to develop pathways or protocols (Kaasa et al. 2017). These are structured, multidisciplinary care plans that clearly identify who is responsible for care in the various disciplines and how communication will be achieved. Care pathways also make clear what resources are needed to make optimal integrated care possible during the disease trajectory. Researchers have stressed the importance of such care pathways and have clarified that they should reflect different needs, different goals, and different forms of expertise and that therefore different pathways need to be developed for different subgroups of patients. Information and communication technology (ICT) can be very helpful in developing integrated palliative care models. ICT can, for example, facilitate communication between healthcare providers, carers, and the patient through shared digital medical records, interdisciplinary meetings using video communication, and digital educational or informational programs for the patient, helping them to understand and to cope with their condition. ICT can also be used to enable systematic and automatic monitoring of symptoms, allowing professional and informal carers and the patient to respond rapidly to clinical changes, symptoms, and other care needs in a population where time is of the essence. However in order for care pathways and ICT to be successful, the input and support of all stakeholders – e.g., healthcare professionals, patients, hospital administrators, and health policymakers – in the development, evaluation, and implementation of these tools is of crucial importance.

The WHO captures the use of protocols, care pathways, and ICT to improve the care of patients with chronic or life-threatening disease under the heading "Health Technology" which it defines as "the application of organized knowledge and skills in the form of devices, medicines/vaccines, procedures and systems developed to solve a health problem and improve quality of lives" (WHO 2007). Although health technology is a fast-moving field that offers huge possibilities, it has yet to be developed and evaluated thoroughly in the domain of the early integration of palliative care in oncology.

Another barrier on the level of the healthcare system that hinders the widespread integration of palliative care in oncology is that of costs. Palliative care services in most countries are too understaffed to be able to take on the extra workload of the early integration of palliative care and thus require new investment and incentives. In the USA, for instance, a study found that there is only one palliative medicine physician for every 1200 people with a life-threatening disease. In comparison, for every 141 newly diagnosed cancer patients, there is one oncologist (CAPC 2015). Several studies point out that investing in palliative care has a cost neutral or even a cost-saving effect. Palliative care interventions, for instance, limit the number of hospitalizations at the end of life, and such hospitalizations make up 5% of the healthcare costs of a dying patient. Two studies in US hospitals revealed that the implementation of specific palliative care consultation programs helped to bring down overall healthcare costs in the last months of life (Ciemins et al. 2007; Penrod et al. 2006). The early integration of palliative care might typically involve the withholding and withdrawal of expensive surgery as well as of life-prolonging therapies such as chemotherapy, hormone therapy, or radiotherapy, which can compensate for the costs of the new palliative care interventions.

7 Conclusion and Summary

The severity and multiplicity of symptoms of advanced cancer warrant a comprehensive care approach, integrating adequate oncology treatment with general and specialist palliative care options. Evidence for the benefits of the early integration of palliative care into oncological care is very promising but has not yet been widely translated into implementation in clinical practice. For this to happen in the future, it will be necessary to disseminate information about the beneficial effects of the early integration of palliative care into oncology and confront the misapprehension that palliative care is only terminal care. Moreover, organizational and structural changes in healthcare systems will be necessary in order to support the efforts of healthcare professionals to collaborate intensively and effectively with each other and with the person who is dying and those close to them, for the benefit of all involved.

References

Aldridge MD, Hasselaar J, Garralda E, van der Eerden M, Stevenson D, McKendrick K, Centeno C, Meier DE. Education, implementation, and policy barriers to greater integration of palliative care: a literature review. Palliat Med. 2016;30(3):224–39. https://doi.org/10.1177/0269216315606645.

Bakitas M, Lyons KD, Hegel MT, Balan S, Brokaw FC, Seville J, Hull JG, Li Z, Tosteson TD, Byock IR, Ahles TA. Effects of a palliative care intervention on clinical outcomes in patients with advanced cancer: the project ENABLE II randomized controlled trial. JAMA. 2009;302(7):741–9. https://doi.org/10.1001/jama.2009.1198.

Bakitas MA, Tosteson TD, Li Z, Lyons KD, Hull JG, Li Z, Dionne-Odom JN, Frost J, Dragnev KH, Hegel MT, Azuero A, Ahles TA. Early versus delayed initiation of concurrent palliative oncology care: patient outcomes in the ENABLE III randomized controlled trial. J Clin Oncol. 2015;33(13):1438–45. https://doi.org/10.1200/jco.2014.58.6362.

Beernaert K, Cohen J, Deliens L, Devroey D, Vanthomme K, Pardon K, Van den Block L. Referral to palliative care in COPD and other chronic diseases: a population-based study. Respir Med. 2013;107(11):1731–9. https://doi.org/10.1016/j.rmed.2013.06.003.

Beernaert K, Deliens L, De Vleminck A, Devroey D, Pardon K, Block LV, Cohen J. Is there a need for early palliative care in patients with life-limiting illnesses? Interview study with patients about experienced care needs from diagnosis onward. Am J Hosp Palliat Care. 2016;33(5):489–97. https://doi.org/10.1177/1049909115577352.

Bekelman DB, Rumsfeld JS, Havranek EP, Yamashita TE, Hutt E, Gottlieb SH, Dy SM, Kutner JS. Symptom burden, depression, and spiritual well-being: a comparison of heart failure and advanced cancer patients. J Gen Intern Med. 2009;24(5):592–8. https://doi.org/10.1007/s11606-009-0931-y.

Bruera E, Hui D. Conceptual models for integrating palliative care at cancer centers. J Palliat Med. 2012;15(11):1261–9. https://doi.org/10.1089/jpm.2012.0147.

CAPC. Report card Center to Advance Palliative Care (CAPC): America's care of serious illness—a state-by-state report card on access to palliative care in our nation's hospitals. http://reportcard.capc.org/pdf/state-by-state-report-card.pdf. edited by Center to Advance Palliative Care (CAPC). 2015.

Ciemins EL, Blum L, Nunley M, Lasher A, Newman JM. The economic and clinical impact of an inpatient palliative care consultation service: a multifaceted approach. J Palliat Med. 2007;10(6):1347–55. https://doi.org/10.1089/jpm.2007.0065.

Dalal S, Palla S, Hui D, Nguyen L, Chacko R, Li Z, Fadul N, Scott C, Thornton V, Coldman B, Amin Y, Bruera E. Association between a name change from palliative to supportive care and the timing of patient referrals at a comprehensive cancer center. Oncologist. 2011;16(1):105–11. https://doi.org/10.1634/theoncologist.2010-0161.

Ferrell BR, Temel JS, Temin S, Alesi ER, Balboni TA, Basch EM, Firn JI, Paice JA, Peppercorn JM, Phillips T, Stovall EL, Zimmermann C, Smith TJ. Integration of palliative care into standard oncology care: American society of clinical oncology clinical practice guideline update. J Clin Oncol. 2017;35(1):96–112. https://doi.org/10.1200/jco.2016.70.1474.

Fisch MJ, Lee JW, Weiss M, Wagner LI, Chang VT, Cella D, Manola JB, Minasian LM, McCaskill-Stevens W, Mendoza TR, Cleeland CS. Prospective, observational study of pain and analgesic prescribing in medical oncology outpatients with breast, colorectal, lung, or prostate cancer. J Clin Oncol. 2012;30(16):1980–8. https://doi.org/10.1200/jco.2011.39.2381.

Greaves J, Glare P, Kristjanson LJ, Stockler M, Tattersall MH. Undertreatment of nausea and other symptoms in hospitalized cancer patients. Support Care Cancer. 2009;17(4):461–4. https://doi.org/10.1007/s00520-008-0511-4.

Ho TH, Barbera L, Saskin R, Lu H, Neville BA, Earle CC. Trends in the aggressiveness of end-of-life cancer care in the universal health care system of Ontario, Canada. J Clin Oncol. 2011;29(12):1587–91. https://doi.org/10.1200/jco.2010.31.9897.

Hui D, Elsayem A, De la Cruz M, Berger A, Zhukovsky DS, Palla S, Evans A, Fadul N, Palmer JL, Bruera E. Availability and integration of palliative care at US cancer centers. JAMA. 2010;303(11):1054–61. https://doi.org/10.1001/jama.2010.258.

Kaasa S, Knudsen AK, Lundeby T, Loge JH. Integration between oncology and palliative care: a plan for the next decade? Tumori. 2017;103(1):1–8. https://doi.org/10.5301/tj.5000602.

Kain DA, Eisenhauer EA. Early integration of palliative care into standard oncology care: evidence and overcoming barriers to implementation. Curr Oncol. 2016;23(6):374–7. https://doi.org/10.3747/co.23.3404.

Laugsand EA, Sprangers MA, Bjordal K, Skorpen F, Kaasa S, Klepstad P. Health care providers underestimate symptom intensities of cancer patients: a multicenter European study. Health Qual Life Outcomes. 2010;8:104. https://doi.org/10.1186/1477-7525-8-104.

Lynch T, Connor S, Clark D. Mapping levels of palliative care development: a global update. J Pain Symptom Manag. 2013;45(6):1094–106. https://doi.org/10.1016/j.jpainsymman.2012.05.011.

Lynn J, Adamson D. Living well at the end of life. Adapting health care to serious chronic illness in old age. Santa Monica: RAND; 2003.

Maltoni M, Scarpi E, Dall'Agata M, Schiavon S, Biasini C, Codeca C, Broglia CM, Sansoni E, Bortolussi R, Garetto F, Fioretto L, Cattaneo MT, Giacobino A, Luzzani M, Luchena G, Alquati S, Quadrini S, Zagonel V, Cavanna L, Ferrari D, Pedrazzoli P, Frassineti GL, Galiano A, Casadei Gardini A, Monti M, Nanni O. Systematic versus on-demand early palliative care: a randomised clinical trial assessing quality of care and treatment aggressiveness near the end of life. Eur J Cancer. 2016a;69:110–8. https://doi.org/10.1016/j.ejca.2016.10.004.

Maltoni M, Scarpi E, Dall'Agata M, Zagonel V, Berte R, Ferrari D, Broglia CM, Bortolussi R, Trentin L, Valgiusti M, Pini S, Farolfi A, Casadei Gardini A, Nanni O, Amadori D. Systematic versus on-demand early palliative care: results from a multicentre, randomised clinical trial. Eur J Cancer. 2016b;65:61–8. https://doi.org/10.1016/j.ejca.2016.06.007.

McDonald J, Swami N, Hannon B, Lo C, Pope A, Oza A, Leighl N, Krzyzanowska MK, Rodin G, Le LW, Zimmermann C. Impact of early palliative care on caregivers of patients with advanced cancer: cluster randomised trial. Ann Oncol. 2017;28(1):163–8. https://doi.org/10.1093/annonc/mdw438.

Pardon K, Deschepper R, Vander Stichele R, Bernheim J, Mortier F, Schallier D, Germonpre P, Galdermans D, Van Kerckhoven W, Deliens L. Are patients' preferences for information and participation in medical decision-making being met? Interview study with lung cancer patients. Palliat Med. 2011;25(1):62–70. https://doi.org/10.1177/0269216310373169.

Penrod JD, Deb P, Luhrs C, Dellenbaugh C, Zhu CW, Hochman T, Maciejewski ML, Granieri E, Morrison RS. Cost and utilization outcomes of patients receiving hospital-based palliative care consultation. J Palliat Med. 2006;9(4):855–60. https://doi.org/10.1089/jpm.2006.9.855.

Quill TE, Abernethy AP. Generalist plus specialist palliative care–creating a more sustainable model. N Engl J Med. 2013;368(13):1173–5. https://doi.org/10.1056/NEJMp1215620.

Smith TJ, Temin S, Alesi ER, Abernethy AP, Balboni TA, Basch EM, Ferrell BR, Loscalzo M, Meier DE, Paice JA, Peppercorn JM, Somerfield M, Stovall E, Von Roenn JH. American society of clinical oncology provisional clinical opinion: the integration of palliative care into standard oncology care. J Clin Oncol. 2012;30(8):880–7. https://doi.org/10.1200/jco.2011.38.5161.

Temel JS, Greer JA, Muzikansky A, Gallagher ER, Admane S, Jackson VA, Dahlin CM, Blinderman CD, Jacobsen J, Pirl WF, Billings JA, Lynch TJ. Early palliative care for patients with metastatic non-small-cell lung cancer. N Engl J Med. 2010;363(8):733–42. https://doi.org/10.1056/NEJMoa1000678.

Temel JS, Greer JA, El-Jawahri A, Pirl WF, Park ER, Jackson VA, Back AL, Kamdar M, Jacobsen J, Chittenden EH, Rinaldi SP, Gallagher ER, Eusebio JR, Li Z, Muzikansky A, Ryan DP. Effects of early integrated palliative care in patients with lung and GI cancer: a randomized clinical trial. J Clin Oncol. 2017;35(8):834–41. https://doi.org/10.1200/jco.2016.70.5046.

Van den Block L, Deschepper R, Bossuyt N, Drieskens K, Bauwens S, Van Casteren V, Deliens L. Care for patients in the last months of life: the Belgian sentinel network monitoring end-of-life care study. Arch Intern Med. 2008;168(16):1747–54. https://doi.org/10.1001/archinte.168.16.1747.

Wentlandt K, Krzyzanowska MK, Swami N, Rodin GM, Le LW, Zimmermann C. Referral practices of oncologists to specialized palliative care. J Clin Oncol. 2012;30(35):4380–6. https://doi.org/10.1200/jco.2012.44.0248.

WHO. Definition of palliative care. 2002. www.who.int/cancer/palliative/definition/en

WHO. Definition:Health Technology. 2007. www.who.int/health-technology-assessment/about/healthtechnology/en/

WPCA, and WHO. Global atlas of palliative care at the end of life. 2014.

Zimmermann C, Swami N, Krzyzanowska M, Hannon B, Leighl N, Oza A, Moore M, Rydall A, Rodin G, Tannock I, Donner A, Lo C. Early palliative care for patients with advanced cancer: a cluster-randomised controlled trial. Lancet. 2014;383(9930):1721–30. https://doi.org/10.1016/s0140-6736(13)62416-2.

Zimmermann C, Swami N, Krzyzanowska M, Leighl N, Rydall A, Rodin G, Tannock I, Hannon B. Perceptions of palliative care among patients with advanced cancer and their caregivers. CMAJ. 2016;188(10):E217–27. https://doi.org/10.1503/cmaj.151171.

Palliative Care and Neurodegenerative Diseases

58

David Oliver and Simone Veronese

Contents

Abstract

Neurological disease is a major cause of disability and death across the world. There is increasing evidence that palliative care is effective in managing symptoms, maintaining and improving quality of life, and helping patients

D. Oliver (✉)
Tizard Centre, University of Kent, Canterbury, Kent, UK

S. Veronese
Fondazione FARO, palliative care, Torino, Italy
e-mail: simone.veronese@fondazionefaro.it

R. D. MacLeod, L. Van den Block (eds.), *Textbook of Palliative Care*,
https://doi.org/10.1007/978-3-319-77740-5_58

and families cope with the deterioration. As the disease progression varies, both between diseases and for individuals, palliative care may be involved for varying periods of time, and may need to be involved episodically throughout the disease progression. Careful assessment of all the issues – physical, psychosocial, and spiritual – will allow appropriate management and support for patients and families. Carer support is very important as families face all the issues of coping with a progressive disease. Recognition of the later stages of life is helpful in enabling patients, families, and professionals to be able to prepare for the dying phase and manage all the issues appropriately.

1 Introduction

1.1 Extent of the Problem

Neurological disease is a major cause of ill health, disability, and death across the world. In 2015 it was estimated that 12% of all deaths worldwide were due to neurological disease – this included progressive disease, stroke (10% of all deaths), and infections (WHO 2006). These disease groups vary greatly, and there is individuality for each patient – as the symptoms, progression, and prognosis can vary from person to person.

The commonest causes of death from neurological disease are cerebrovascular disease (10.2%), dementias (0.81%), epilepsy (0.21%), Parkinson's disease (PD) (0.20%), and multiple sclerosis (MS) (0.03%) (OFNS 2012). Infections are common – with tetanus and meningitis causing 0.4% of deaths worldwide. The distribution varies greatly across the world, and neurological disease accounts for a higher percentage of deaths (16.8%) in lower middle-income countries, compared to 13.2% in high-income and 8.2% in low-income countries (WHO 2006). There is the expectation that these figures will increase over the coming decades, as the majority of neurological diseases develop with increasing age, and by 2030 it has been estimated that 12.22% of all deaths will be due to neurological disease (WHO 2006).

Palliative care may be appropriate for many of these disease groups. In some instances, there may be a sudden deterioration and death may be unexpected – such as in epilepsy or cerebrovascular disease. The principles of holistic care within palliative care may be appropriate for all these people as they face a sudden deterioration in their functional state and quality of life. However with many progressive diseases, there is a slow and gradual progression, and there is no curative treatment, with the best that treatment can offer being the slowing of progression or the management of symptoms.

Although progressive neurological diseases are relatively rare individually, as a group they do cause both morbidity and mortality. The common progressive diseases are motor neurone disease/amyotrophic lateral sclerosis (MND/ALS) with a prevalence of 7/100,000, Parkinson's disease (PD) 180/100,000 but with a prevalence of 1750/100,000 for people over 80 years, dementias 700/100,000, multiple systems atrophy 5/100,000, progressive supranuclear palsy 7/100,000, Huntington's disease 6/100,000, and multiple sclerosis 80–140/100,000 but with higher rates in higher-income and northerly areas compared to lower-income or lower-latitude countries (WHO 2006; OFNS 2012; Alzheimer's Society 2015).

Thus neurological disease does lead to morbidity, disability, and death, and with the aging of the population on many countries, there will be increasing numbers of people affected and increasing palliative care needs.

2 Role of Palliative Care

Palliative care may be seen as appropriate for many neurological diseases which have no curative treatment and progress over time – such as MND/ALS, PD, MS, MSA, PSP, HD – and the World Health Organization definition of palliative care defines palliative care as helpful for "life-threatening illness" (WHO 2002). Moreover for other diseases which may have a more sudden onset, such as cerebrovascular disease (stroke), there may be an uncertainty of the prognosis and future progression with many people left with severe disability and/or the risk of further deterioration and death.

Even for the progressive diseases, the prognosis and progression can be very variable, and patients have to cope with uncertainty of the future – both in terms of quality of life and prognosis. The prognosis of MND/ALS is usually 2–3 years from diagnosis, which may only be made after a year of symptoms, but 25% of people are alive at 5 years from diagnosis and 5–10% at 10 years (Shaw et al. 2014). PD has an average prognosis of 14 years but many people live 20–30 years, and as they are elderly there may be only a small reduction in life expectancy.

Palliative care has been increasingly recommended for neurological disease, and a consensus document from the European Association for Palliative Care (EAPC) and the European Academy of Neurology (EAN) has recommended that "palliative care should be considered early in the disease trajectory, depending on the underlying prognosis" (Oliver et al. 2016). Moreover there have been many guidelines recommending palliative care for different diseases, such as MND/ALS (Andersen et al. 2012) and PD (NICE 2006), and for neurology in general (Boersma et al. 2014).

However it is often considered that palliative care is only appropriate at the end of life, and referral for care may be very late in the disease progression. Within cancer there has been increased awareness of the effectiveness of early palliative care involvement, and a study of lung cancer patients showed that not only did early palliative care involvement improve quality of life and reduce depressive symptoms, but the prognosis was extended from 8.9 months to 11.6 months (Temel et al. 2010). Other studies have suggested early integration of palliative care within oncological services, so that patients' problems can be identified and managed appropriately (Gaertner et al. 2011).

As the prognosis of progressive neurological diseases varies – average prognoses are MND/ALS 2–3 years, PD 14 years, MSA 9 years, PSP 7 years, MS 30 years, and Alzheimer's disease 8–10 years – the involvement of early palliative care can be complex. However earlier involvement, according to the person's particular needs, can be very helpful in improving quality of life and managing symptoms, and also establishing a relationship with a multidisciplinary team so that the care can be easily accessed and accepted as the disease progresses (Oliver 2014). This approach, considering all aspects of care – physical, psychosocial, and spiritual – and considering family as well as patient, is the basis of palliative care. Although this approach may be helpful over a long period of time, the involvement of palliative care may be episodic, responding to particular issues (Bede et al. 2009). For instance, for a person with ALS, there may be particular concerns and issues at diagnosis, consideration of a gastrostomy, development of respiratory problems, and consideration of ventilatory support as the person deteriorates at the end of life (Oliver 2014).

3 Palliative Care in Neurological Disease: Evidence of Effectiveness

From the WHO definition of palliative care, it is clear that the measurement of the effectiveness of palliative care should be focused on the improvement of the individual quality of life (IQoL) of both patients and families and on the other physical, psychosocial, and spiritual issues that can be caused by the advanced disease.

Effectiveness can also be gauged by the evaluation of the complex services provided by palliative care, considering the wide range of these facilities. These vary in different countries and health services, and palliative care can be considered as a "simple approach" adopted by any health-care provider to severely ill patients or provided by primary medicine operators for patients with a low burden of palliative care needs (often known as generalist palliative care) or the specialist palliative care, provided by multidisciplinary services, with training and ongoing involvement in the care of people with complex needs in specific settings like hospice inpatient facilities, home specialist palliative care, or hospital teams.

The role of palliative care services in terms of impact of care, outcome measurement, and effectiveness has been increasingly studied. In 2003 the first study reporting the positive impact of palliative care was released (Higginson et al. 2003). A later review showed that the evidence for benefit from specialized palliative care is sparse and limited by methodological shortcomings (Zimmermann et al. 2008). More recently other researchers highlighted how palliative care can have a moderate positive effect on the main palliative care outcome (IQoL) (Catania et al. 2015), the integration of early palliative care can improve QoL and mood (Bakitas et al. 2009), and, even though not being a primary outcome, survival increased in patients with advanced lung cancer (Temel et al. 2010). Palliative care has been shown to have cost savings (Smith and Wasner 2014).

In patients affected by long-term neurodegenerative conditions, palliative care provision and integration with neurological services remains heterogeneous. There is a need for an improved model of integration that should be rigorously tested for effectiveness. Nevertheless the impact of palliative care services on the specific outcomes of patients severely affected by neurological disorders was studied for the first time by the King's College London palliative and supportive group for people with multiple sclerosis (MS) (Higginson et al. 2008). A phase 2 randomized controlled study was performed comparing a fast track group of patients who received immediately the palliative care service versus a control group who had a waiting list of 3 months before being cared for. This study showed how the involvement with the palliative care service appeared to positively affect some key symptoms and reduced informal caregiver burden and is cost effective (Higginson et al. 2009; Edmonds et al. 2010).

Using the same methodology, a similar RCT was repeated widening the service to a mix of neurological disorders (ALS, MS, PD, and related disorders). Fifty patients were randomized to receive immediate specialist palliative care (SPC) versus standard care (SC). This study showed how patients who received SPC input reported a significant clinical and statistical improvement in IQoL and in important physical symptoms like pain, dyspnea, quality of sleep, and bowel symptoms versus those who had SC (Veronese et al. 2015). Patients in the fast track group received home care multidisciplinary visits and were seen by palliative care physicians, nurses, physiotherapist, and psychologist if required. The team was in contact with the neurological service if specific issues emerged. On average, patients received weekly visits for all the duration of the study (16 weeks), and the service was not discontinued at the end of the follow-up.

An Italian multicenter, phase 3 RCT studied the impact of a home based palliative care approach (HPA) on the needs of patients with severe MS and their informal carers (Solari et al. 2015). The preliminary findings indicate that HPA reduced symptom burden, but there was no evidence of HPA efficacy on patient QoL or secondary patient and carer outcomes. The difference in the intensity of the service provision may explain the lack of effectiveness as the team were less experienced, and it may show that a specialist palliative care approach is necessary to really affect patient experience.

This available evidence shows that there is strong interest in elucidating the appropriate role of palliative care for people with neurological conditions. At present there is data showing a positive impact of palliative care on patients and their carers, even though the intensity of care or specific service that is ideal for such a heterogeneous group of disorders is not exactly clear. The model suggested by Bede (Bede et al. 2009) and adopted in a NHS document in the UK (NELCP 2010) represents the optimal option for the challenge of providing the correct amount of care at the right times during the disease trajectory. This approach creates useful links with the specialist palliative care services for significant moments where palliative care issues emerge and to better identify the end-of-life phase which is obviously inherent to palliative care.

4 Physical Symptom Management

Patients affected by advanced neurological conditions suffer a high burden of physical symptoms, often not adequately assessed and treated (Veronese et al. 2017). In the consensus review on the development of palliative care for patients with chronic and progressive neurological disease (Oliver et al. 2016), three recommendations focus on the importance of assessing and treating physical symptoms:

- Proactive assessment of physical and psychosocial issues is recommended to reduce the intensity, frequency, and need for crisis intervention.
- Physical symptoms require thorough differential diagnosis, pharmacological and non-pharmacological management, and regular review.
- The principles of symptom management, as part of the wider palliative care assessment, should be applied to neurological care.

Studies showed that many symptoms in people severely affected by multiple sclerosis (MS) are as highly prevalent and severe as those experienced by patients with advanced cancer and that increased disability is associated with increased severity for some symptoms (Higginson et al. 2006). Patients with late-stage PD, MSA, and PSP experience a complex mix of non-motor and motor symptoms. In a 1-year follow-up, symptoms are not resolved and half of the patients deteriorate. Palliative problems are predictive of future symptoms, suggesting that an early palliative assessment might help screen for those in need of earlier intervention (van Vliet et al. 2016). In ALS the impact of unmet physical issues is also very high (O'Brien et al. 1992), and the fear of choking to death, related to the shortness of breath, can be a leading cause for requests of hastening death (Veldink et al. 2002).

4.1 Motor Symptoms

In general, advanced neurological conditions cause motor complications and physical disability that impact deeply in the IQoL of patients and cause high burden of care to the informal carers (Veronese et al. 2015). Clinically, motor impairment can appear as muscular flaccidity, typical when the second motor neurone is involved such as in traumatic paralysis, in some forms of ALS, or in spinal cord metastasis. In other conditions, the patient can suffer from muscular rigidity or spasticity, like in stroke, MS, movement disorders, and ALS forms with prevalent first motor neurone involvement. Other muscular symptoms can be spasms, cramps, fasciculation, or myoclonus.

Some of these symptoms can be treated by modulating the specific drugs for the primary disorder; for example, in IPD rigidity can be improved by increasing L-DOPA or dopaminergic drugs. Since most of these conditions do not respond to specific treatments, in the advanced stages motor symptoms are treated with a symptomatic approach. A combination of physical therapy and muscle relaxant and muscle relaxant drugs can be used for stiffness and rigidity, for example, in advanced MS or ALS. Even in the very advanced stages, when the patient is restricted to a wheelchair or bedbound, adequate stretching programs can be adopted and useful to control the pain related to stiffness, maintain joint elasticity, and prevent bedsores. Occupational therapists play a role in prescribing aids to compensate for the disability and can be useful for transferring, writing, and other activities of daily living. The use of medications like baclofen, tizanidine, or dantrolene can be effective as muscle relaxant, but doses must be individually titrated and re-evaluated on regular bases. Benzodiazepines have also a role in treating stiffness, taking into account the possible central side effects. Botulinum toxin injections are used for those patients whose rigidity does not respond to symptomatic treatments. This option can help in hygienic procedures like allowing the movement of thighs in MS of very rigid patients and facilitating personal care. In specific cases advanced treatments can be effective for motor symptoms and complications. Intrathecal continuous injection of baclofen is used in advanced MS for general rigidity, using a pump often positioned in the patients' abdomen (Otero-Romero et al. 2016). In IPD, selected patients' motor symptoms can be approached with specific options like apomorphine subcutaneous infusion, deep brain stimulation, and continuous intrajejunal infusion of levodopa-carbidopa intestinal gel (Worth 2013).

In most cases, however, motor complications cannot be effectively resolved, and patients and carers are exposed to the restless progression of disability. A role of palliative care is to help their assisted patient to accept the condition trying to enhance resilience and adaptation strategies. Disability is challenging, but feeling abandoned can be worse. One of the most touching quotes from the founder of modern palliative care, Dame Cicely Saunders, says: "You matter because you are you, and you matter to the end of your life. We will do all we can not only to help you die peacefully, but also to live until you die." According to this mandate, palliative care must face patients even when they cannot solve their problems, but continue providing help and promoting the residual quality of life.

Pain is a common and often unrecognized symptom in patients affected by neurodegenerative conditions (see Table 1).

Table 1 Prevalence of pain in neurologic conditions

Neurological disorder	Prevalence of pain	References
Parkinson's disease	40–86%	(Simuni and Sethi 2008)
Multisystem atrophy – MSA	88%	(Higginson 2012)
Progressive supranuclear palsy – PSP	60%	(Higginson 2012)
Multiple sclerosis	50–86%	(O'Connor et al. 2008; Bermejo et al. 2010)
ALS/MND	40–73%	(Miller et al. 1999)
Alzheimer's disease	57%	(Pautex et al. 2006)
Post stroke	14–85%	(Kumar et al. 2009; (Klit et al. 2009)
Spinal cord injury	64.9%	(Modirian et al. 2010)
Guillain-Barré syndrome	89%	(Moulin et al. 1997)

Chronic pain in patients with neurologic disorders has some challenging features to be considered. Chronic pain causes significant changes in function, anatomy, and chemistry of the brain (Borsook 2012); these changes are "brain-wide" including areas like the cerebellum, not normally involved in the pain system (Moulton et al. 2010). For many diseases the pathophysiology of pain remains unclear, but patients can suffer more than one pain at a time, and the symptom can be related or not related to the underlying disorder, in the latter case being due to comorbidity, but always painful (Lee et al. 2007). Finally the association of pain with depression and mood disorders is very common. This dangerous loop can worsen the intensity and the impact of both symptoms and makes difficult to understand and treat both. Furthermore, it is known how depression, hopelessness, and pain can drive the request for hastened death (Breitbart et al. 2000).

There are peculiar painful syndromes in different neurological conditions that should be tackled with specific approaches. In PDs and related disorders, pain can be musculoskeletal 70%, dystonic 40%, radicular neuropathic 20%, or central neuropathic 10% (Lee et al. 2007; Borsook 2012). Pain can increase and decrease with dopaminergic fluctuations or may be related to a central dopaminergic deficit and in both cases can be alleviated by adjusting L-DOPA medications (dystonic and central pain). Botulinum toxin may help involuntary muscular contractions related to dystonia, and neuropathic pain can benefit from anticonvulsants and other drugs used for this type of pain. NSAIDs may reduce local irritation and work on musculoskeletal pains, and opioids modulate pain pathways and can be useful in all pain syndromes.

4.2 Respiratory Symptoms

Patients affected by advanced neurodegenerative disorders frequently experience respiratory distress including dyspnea, weak cough, trouble in management of secretions, respiratory infections, neurogenic pulmonary edema, and noisy secretions at the end of life (death rattle).

Respiratory complications represent a frequent cause of death in advanced neurological patients since the muscular impairment can lead to dysfunction like choking, ineffective cough, and susceptibility to atelectasis and aspiration pneumonia (Aboussouan 2005).

In neuromuscular disorders, the main cause of respiratory symptoms is the muscular impairment directly caused by the neurological disease. In ALS respiratory impairment is caused by the lack of innervation, caused by the death of the motor neurones, and the following development of respiratory insufficiency with hypoventilation on the basis of diaphragmatic and intercostal muscle weakness (Mangera et al. 2012). In MS the nervous denervation and spasticity above all of the expiratory muscles can lead to the development of voluntary or autonomic respiration, diaphragmatic paralysis, paroxysmal hyperventilation, apneustic breathing, and neurogenic edema; the pattern depends on the location of the lesions in the brain, which follows both axonal and neuronal death. Muscular weakness and lack of coordination, worsening with the course of the disease, are involved in PD. In other disorders like HD or Alzheimer's disease, a combination of neurologic damage in the brain is responsible for the respiratory impairment and consequent symptoms.

Shortness of breath (dyspnea) is a personal unpleasant experience that can cause the fear of choking to death. It has been defined as "a subjective experience of breathing discomfort that consists of qualitatively distinct sensations that vary in intensity." This experience is the combined effect of multiple physiological, psychological, social, and environmental factors and can itself induce both physiological and behavioral reactions. It can be associated to an objective respiratory insufficiency or just being a subjective feeling. It is strongly related to anxiety and often it creates a dangerous loop in which both symptoms are enhanced and worsened. The prevalence of breathlessness and respiratory distress varies with the disease: Dementia 12–52%, PD 22–35%, ALS 81–88%, and MS 26% (Moens 2014; Lee et al. 2007).

Symptoms of respiratory insufficiency in ALS include dyspnea on exertion, supine dyspnea, marked fatigue, disturbed sleep (frequent nocturnal awakenings, excessive daytime sleepiness), cough, and morning headaches (Miller et al. 2009). Weak coughing may be tolerable for patients who have an intact swallowing mechanism and minimal airway secretions, but the onset of complications like acute bronchitis or bulbar dysfunction may precipitate a life-threatening crisis.

Patients with neurological disorders should be monitored in the course of the disease for the possible onset of respiratory problems. In ALS specific guidelines provide indications on the timing and the clinical decisions to be undertaken. In other conditions, however, the pulmonary function should be assessed since its earlier detection can lead to the improvement of patients' outcome (Aboussouan 2005).

Treatment of respiratory symptoms should start from the recognition and treatment of possible underlying causes (e.g., respiratory infections), toward a more palliative approach when there is not a treatable cause. In the latter case, both pharmacological and non-pharmacological options can be effective, often combined. Physical therapy can help in correct positioning of the patients, and help in clearing secretions with techniques including manually assisted coughing, and others such as oscillation or percussion use of aids such as the assisted cough machine. Speech and language therapy can help when there are problems of coordination or vocal cord adduction. Noninvasive ventilation (NIV) via external mask is often effective for the support of inspiratory muscle function (Aboussouan 2005), though it may be contraindicated in some patients such as ALS with bulbar impairment or patients with cognitive decline or agitation. It can improve QoL of patients and data suggest an increase in survival in ALS (Radunovic 2013).

Invasive ventilation (IV) via tracheostomy remains a debated issue. There are differences in the adoption of this treatment in different countries. Although IV may increase survival, the disease continues to progress to the extent that the person becomes "locked in," with no form of communication, or it becomes a burdensome therapy. There are also ethical issues as it is an expensive treatment and may lead to the request of withdrawal from the ventilator, which will usually lead to the person's death within a short time. There is strong consensus that NIV should be preferred to IV for many reasons, including ease of administration, less strain on caregivers, lower cost, greater portability, fewer infections, the virtual elimination of airway complications, and reduced need for hospitalization (Radunovic 2013). The impact on survival of ALS patients is not very clear since the literature shows a range of life protraction from less than 1 year to more than 40 months after tracheostomy. The role of family carers is very important in the constant care (24 h/ 7 days) required by patients in need of frequent tracheal aspiration. There are studies showing that the carers' QoL can be seriously affected by these tasks (Kaub-Wittemer et al. 2003).

Palliative and hospice care represent an alternative choice which can effectively impact on respiratory symptoms (Veronese et al. 2015), through the accurate use of drugs, like opioids, found useful in respiratory distress (Jennings et al. 2001) and recommended in specific guidelines and consensus reviews (Andersen et al. 2012; Miller et al. 2009).

4.3 Dysphagia and Swallowing Problems

Difficulties in coordination of the processes of contraction and relaxation of the various muscles involved in mastication, deglutition, and the progression of the bolus toward the stomach are common in neurodegenerative disorders causing difficulty with swallowing food, liquid, or saliva. The characteristics of the swallowing disorder can vary according to the neurological condition, the severity of the neurological disease, and other comorbidities. Dysphagia is considered as a general indicator of decline in any neurological disorder having a negative impact on survival above all if associated to weight loss (Thomas and Armstrong Wilson 2016). In late-stage PD, it occurs in up to 95% of patients and is associated with aspiration pneumonia. It is also very common in Parkinson's plus syndromes, and studies show that its onset has a negative prognostic meaning (Walshe 2014).

In advanced MS dysphagia affects 33% to 50% of patients, possibly because of uncoordinated respiration during swallowing.

Many people with ALS will experience problems with dysphagia (swallowing problems), which can make eating and drinking difficult. Dysphagia is reported to be prevalent in 30–100% of individuals depending on the type of ALS and the stage of disease affecting all individuals in the later stages of the disease. This can cause anxiety for people with ALS and their carers/family, who may have concerns about choking on food and liquids.

Dysphagia in advanced stages of dementia is associated with malnutrition and aspiration pneumonia which is a significant cause of death in this population. It is also prevalent in Huntington's disease and Prion diseases.

Managing swallowing issues can be really challenging for both patients and carers. Food and liquids are essential for living and are often associated to ethical and existential aspects. Help can be provided by an accurate assessment of the cause of dysphagia, treatment of underlying secondary causes, and advice on dietary modifications. Intervention can be focused on compensatory (changes in posture, modification of food and/or fluid, and adaptation of methods of eating and drinking) or rehabilitation techniques depending on the specific disorder.

Some treatments showed benefits for dysphagia in selected populations. Electrical stimulation and botulinum toxin treatment have been shown to be helpful in reducing the swallowing impairment in MS. In PD, speech and language therapy and dopaminergic drug adjustment are suggested to improve deglutition. Rotigotine patches can play a role in advanced PD when swallowing is impaired, but deep brain stimulation (DBS) did not show positive effects on dysphagia.

When swallowing becomes very difficult, distressing, very slow, or impossible, the tube feeding option can be considered. This is very often offered to ALS patients, even earlier stages, when first signs of swallowing impairment appear. This is due to the positive impact on QoL with improved dietary intake, and the patient may be able to continue to eat and taste his or her favorite food in small amounts. Furthermore, PEG placement should be done before a decrease in pulmonary function becomes clinically significant, to avoid surgical and postsurgical risks of respiratory complication. In terminal dementia or in other neurological diseases with significant cognitive impairment, there is no evidence of positive effect of tube feeding in terms of QoL, survival, or other patients' outcomes, and the placement and later care may cause distress and even mortality (Sampson et al. 2009).

Even when clinically appropriate, patients can refuse tube feeding for many personal reasons – for instance, they may not want any further treatment to prolong their life. In this case the decision should be respected, and the involvement of palliative and end-of-life care becomes very important. Advance care planning should involve these decisions that are to be reassessed frequently, because as problems progress, they may change their mind.

5 Psychosocial/Spiritual Care

Facing a neurological disease may lead to many psychological and emotional issues. These may depend on the physical issues that affect the person; for instance, a person with PD who has severe mobility issues may become more anxious and concerned about how they cope with day-to-day activities and become disturbed. The response will also be affected by the previous experiences and issues faced by the person and their family – for instance, if there have been difficulties within a relationship, these may be heightened when there are stresses associated with a progressive disabling illness. Moreover changes in cognition and communication may also affect the person's coping mechanisms and lead to increased distress.

There are many psychological issues that may be faced:

- Concerns about the diagnosis – this may be a disease which is unknown to the person, or they may have experience, such as someone with HD who often has memories and experiences from a family member who has suffered and died of HD.
- Concerns about increasing disability and dependency.
- Feelings of depression or anxiety as they face the various symptoms and disability due to the disease progression.
- Fears of the process of dying. Many neurological diseases are associated with a distressing death, which may have been highlighted in discussions and debates about dying or assisted dying. For instance, people with MND/ALS have talked publically of their fears when discussing and advocating assisted dying, talking of choking to death and their fears of distress.
- Fears of losing control, especially as they may fear losing mobility, communication, and cognition. These are possibilities for many neurological diseases and needed to be discussed and ways of minimizing the effects on the person and their family considered (Goldstein 2014).

There may be no easy answers for these fears and concerns, but it is important to allow patients and their families to discuss and express their feelings. An openness of professional carers allows this, and this again emphasizes the need for longer-term involvement with teams, so that trust is engendered and discussions can more easily occur.

Most people are part of a wider family or caring network and those close to them may have similar issues. They may have the same fears about deterioration, dependency, disability, dying, and death, and depending on the previous relationship, they may or may not be able to discuss these openly with the person. If communication and discussion is limited, this may in turn lead to more difficulties as trust is lost, and the issues increase for both parties if there is not the opportunity to discuss and resolve these issues. Moreover if the spouse or carers are elderly, they may be facing their own illnesses and comorbidities, including psychological or cognitive change, and they will thus find the issues very difficult to cope with (Smith and Wasner 2014). If the person has cognitive change or dementia, there may be great stresses within a household, and it may become increasingly difficult to cope at home, or extra care may be needed that further disrupts the previous normality.

There may be very practical issues faced by someone with a neurological disease as they become more disabled that may lead to fear, anxiety, and family conflicts – the roles within a family may become disrupted as the person becomes more disabled and is unable to perform their normal roles within the family and conflicts may arise; care within the housing may become more difficult, and consideration of changing the housing such as the installation of lifts or planning to move to more suitable accommodation may be needed, with ensuing stress and the potential for conflict.

There may also be spiritual issues faced by both the person and family. The experiences, beliefs, and values of any person will affect how they cope and manage with illness and disability. This may be particularly so for a person with a neurological disease who is facing increasing deterioration and dependency and death. These issues may be very important for their family as well. The beliefs may be manifested in a religious belief or practice, and the involvement of others from their religious group, such as a faith leader, may be helpful. However many people do not espouse such belief but still search for meaning and value in their life – their own individual spiritual values. All may find coping with these deeper questions, such as the meaning of life and death, very difficult. These issues may not have any easy answers but should be heard and acknowledged (Lambert 2014).

With all these areas of care, there is the need for listening and awareness of the possibility of concerns by all the professional carers involved. Sharing of concerns and encouraging families to share their concerns together are often helpful. Specialized counselling may be helpful for some, and access to this service is essential if we are to help patients cope with their disease.

6 Communication Issues

The need for careful communication with both the patient and family has been emphasized in the EAPC/EAN consensus document (Oliver et al. 2016) and may be especially important in neurological disease, due to the complexity and variability of the disease progression and the risks of both communication ability and the cognitive ability of the patients as the disease progresses (Oliver et al. 2016). The areas that may need particular attention are the following.

6.1 Diagnosis

The giving of the diagnosis of a progressive neurological disease will set the agenda for future care, and may influence the patient and their family's response and coping with the disease as it progresses. There is evidence from the telling of the diagnosis in cancer that the use of a protocol, such as the SPIKES protocol, allows an open and clear discussion and aids in the telling of bad news (Baile et al. 2000). Such a protocol suggests that consideration is given to **S**etting up the interview, with preparing the setting and ensuring all the information is available; assessing the patient's **P**erception by asking for their thoughts and views; obtaining the patient's **I**nvitation by ascertaining their wishes on the information they would wish; giving **K**nowledge and information, by giving clear information in small chunks and without bluntness or over negative views; addressing the patient's **E**motions with empathic responses; and setting a **S**trategy and **S**ummary at the end of the discussion so that the patient has a clear plan of the next steps to be taken (Baile et al. 2000).

It has been shown that the SPIKES protocol can be helpful in enabling neurologists to tell the diagnosis of MND/ALS. In Australia it was found that 36% of patients were dissatisfied with the telling of the diagnosis and patients were more satisfied if the neurologists spent longer time, responded empathetically, shared information and suggested realistic goals, explored the expectations of patient and family, and made a clear plan with follow-up (Aoun et al. 2015). Moreover 70% of neurologists in this same study found telling the diagnosis somewhat to very difficult, and 65% were stressed and anxious when delivering this news (Aoun et al. 2015, 2016). Families also were concerned when communication was not satisfactory and commented on long-term emotional stress in these circumstances (Aoun 2017). There is evidence that these skills can be acquired through training in a specific program (Lienard et al. 2010).

Throughout the disease progression, there is the need for good communication and discussion of the disease, its effects, and the future prognosis. This may need to be repeated many times, and patients and families may take this information on board in different ways at different times. Time is needed to ensure that they have the information they wish and to facilitate communication within families, so that they are able to be open together. It has also been suggested that two appointments allow patients and families more time to understand and discuss the news and then ask more questions at the second appointment (Seeber et al. 2016).

However there may be family situations when communication is not open and conflicts arise. The aim should be to allow the patient to discuss what they wish, within their abilities of communication and understanding. Families may need extra support, as they are facing the issues of loss and change in the same way as the patient, but with their own particular concerns and experiences that may color their reactions. This may be compounded when there are communication issues, due to dysarthria or dysphasia and cognitive change – as one family described: "He received a death sentence and it felt like I had received a life sentence."

6.2 Advance Care Planning

As communication and cognition may deteriorate with disease progression, knowing the wishes of the patient while they are able to communicate with them is important. Advance care planning (ACP) is "a voluntary process of discussion and review to help an individual who has capacity to anticipate how their condition may affect them in the future and, if they wish, set on record choices or decisions relating to their care and treatment so that these can be referred to by their carers – whether professional or family – in the event that they lose capacity to decide once their illness progresses" (Chapman 2012). It is a voluntary act, without coercion, and should be offered appropriately and over time and may need to be repeated and reviewed (Chapman 2012).

A person can give their wishes for many aspects of care and treatment including the place of care and death, foods they may like/dislike, how they would like to be cared for, their values, and the treatment options they may wish/may not wish to receive. They may be able, according to the country's legislation, to refuse certain treatments if they define these clearly and show that they realize that these decisions could lead to their death (Chapman 2012).

ACP may be as:

- An advance directive – where the patient defines treatments they do not wish to receive – such as admission to hospital, cardiopulmonary resuscitation, tracheostomy ventilation, antibiotics for a urinary or chest infection.
- Appointment of a proxy to make decisions when they are not able to do so – this proxy would be asked by the professional team for a decision in the same way as they would have asked the patient, if he had been able to make the decision.
- An expression of their general views on care and treatment – in the UK this is known as an advance statement and is not legally binding, but should be taken into consideration in the decision-making.

In the care of neurological patients, ACP has been found to be helpful (Voltz et al. 1998), and it has been shown that patients do wish their ACP to be adhered to (Jox et al. 2008). Moreover patients with MS did want to express their views, and if doctors avoided these discussions, patients felt that they were less empathetic (Buecken et al. 2012).

Thus ACP is helpful and should be considered for patients, particularly when loss of communication or cognition is a possibility. However this may not be easy as patients and families often do not want to consider the future, due to fears of what may happen and concerns that these considerations may precipitate a decline. Professionals may also be reluctant to discuss the issues, as they find it difficult and stressful and time consuming. Thus careful discussion early in the disease progression may be necessary if the patient is able to express their wishes easily, and ACP may need to be discussed on several occasions – the completion of ACP is "a process" over time, and careful explanation of the benefits for the person and their family needs to be stressed.

6.3 Wish for Hastened Death

There is evidence that people with neurological disease and their families may wish to discuss hastened death – euthanasia and assisted suicide (Stutzki et al. 2014) – even if this is not an option within the specific country. There is a debate as to whether hastened death is part of palliative care, and in Belgium the services often work together (Bernheim and Raus 2017), but the European Association for Palliative Care White Paper on euthanasia has stated clearly that there is a clear separation and palliative care does not include hastened death (Radbruch et al. 2015).

However there is a need to allow patients and their families to discuss these issues. The request may come from the fear of symptoms, and a distressing death, of dependency, or of maintaining control over their life and death. For instance, although many patients with ALS fear a distressing death, there is increasing evidence that with good palliative care, this is unlikely and choking to death, a common fear, is rare (Neudert et al. 2001). These issues should be discussed, and with clear explanation, planning for possible crises, and ACP, the wish may lessen. There will be a number of patients who will still wish to retain control, and in areas without any legislation, there will need to be ongoing support for the patient, their family, and all the professional teams involved (Ganzini et al. 1998).

6.4 Communication Issues

Communication may become complex for people with neurological disease because of loss of speech and/or cognition. Speech may be affected due to bulbar changes (affecting the mouth, tongue, and lips), the respiratory muscles/diaphragm (causing weakness of respiration and reducing the ability to articulate), the central neurological control of speech or damage to the speech centers of the brain. Careful assessment is necessary, involving speech and language therapy, to help patients communicate. This may involve relatively low-tech equipment, such as pad and paper or a communication board, to high-tech computer-based systems, and even systems based on eye gaze or electroencephalograms. Extra time is often necessary to allow the person to communicate, as even the most sophisticated computer communication system is much slower than normal speech. It is essential to allow people to communicate their wishes and allow them to complete the communication (Scott and McPhee 2014).

There may also be a loss of cognition, which may be complex and not immediately obvious. Subtle changes in understanding or language may not be understood by families or carers but cause distress to all as communication becomes confusing and the behavior affected. For instance, frontal lobe changes, which may be found in up to 50% of people with ALS, may affect decision-making, cause subtle language difficulties including word and sentence comprehension and word finding, increase distractibility, lead to impulsivity, and lead to difficulty in planning activities, forgetfulness, difficulty in judging the emotions of others, and loss of empathy (Goldstein 2014). These changes may be subtle but may affect the person's ability to function and carers, both family and professional, need to be aware of the possibility of needing to provide extra support in helping the person with decisions or activities. Reduction of the "cognitive load" when making decisions can be helpful, so that the information provided is limited and the decision is reduced to a small number of options, which may be possible for the person to understand (Goldstein 2014). Awareness of the possibility of cognitive change is essential when communicating with people with neurological disease so that they can be involved in discussions and decisions, within the limits of their abilities.

7 Support of Carers

Family or informal carers are persons who take care of patients affected by chronic illnesses, disability, or other care need, outside a professional or formal employment framework. They are considered as beneficiaries of palliative care according to the WHO definition (WHO 2002), but, above all in a home setting, they are often viewed as a co-worker or even a member of the caring team but as such may not be identified as having care needs in their own right (Grande and Ewing 2009). They are the ones who spend most of their time with patients and, therefore, can provide essential information on minimal changes in needs and health status. Family carers should be educated and trained in medication management and symptom control (Bede et al. 2009).

Early education on the practical, technical, and emotional aspects of providing end-of-life care may be required for those caring for people with nonmalignant disease when the trajectory of dying is more uncertain (Funk et al. 2010). Professionals need to "think family" and consider how support for family carers can affect the care of the patient, above all when they tend to have problems related to aging. Understanding the complexities of end-of-life care in the home and the support needs for family carers can improve services, and among the main areas of need identified by lay carers are social and psychological support, financial concerns, and the need for choice and information (McIlfatrick 2007). Assessment of carers of patients with severe MS has shown a need for qualified personnel and care coordination in day-to-day home care, in particular identifying personal hygiene, a supportive network, and the preservation of patient/carer roles within the family and community (Borreani et al. 2014).

As many family or lay carers have never seen a person deteriorate or die, they can be worried about the future: uncertainty about the disease progression; physical dependency; mental deterioration; and the need to take decisions on behalf of their loved ones can cause anxiety and have a negative impact on their daily life.

Considering informal carers of people affected by neurological disorders, some aspects are to be taken into account:

- Carers, as well as patients, are often very frightened of the dying process and may be more fearful of the process of dying than of death itself.
- Appropriate information on further support is essential as well as opportunities to share their concerns and fears.
- Some carers (e.g., those caring for MS patients) will have been told that their condition is not one people die from and therefore may be unprepared, especially where there has been a slow and severe progression and death occurs suddenly.
- Carers could be the first to recognize and interpret subtle changes in reduced energy, engagement, and mood as the neurological condition worsens. They may experience patients' acute crises that may require hospital admission (infections, trauma, agitation).
- They need information about significant changes in care management, for example, in oral feeding and hydration.
- They may feel they have already "lost" the person and experience episodes of grieving during the care management.
- They may need specialist palliative care for unmet needs requiring psychosocial or spiritual input from the services to prevent severe psychiatric illness and even suicide among carers.
- Cultural and religious differences around the end of life deserve respect.
- Support for carers should continue into bereavement.

The needs of carers should be assessed on a regular basis, and the support of carers – before and after death – is an indispensable part of palliative care, reducing complicated bereavement and improve patients' quality of life (Oliver et al. 2016).

The care needs of carers of patients with neurodegenerative conditions are extensive and when unmet may be related to negative changes in their quality of life. Issues can range from significant anxiety and insomnia, related to their role, to depression related to caregiver burden and social dysfunction. Family suffering increases when the neurological disorder reaches advanced stages, and also financial problems are to be taken into account (Whetten-Goldstein et al. 2000). As the disease progresses and end of life approaches, the primary caregivers and also the wider family of persons with progressive neurological conditions need more supportive interaction and information.

8 End-of-Life Care

The General Medical Council in the UK defines end of life (EoL) as patients who are "approaching the end of life" when they are likely to die within the next 12 months. This includes those patients whose death is expected within hours or days; those who have advanced, progressive incurable conditions; those with general frailty and coexisting conditions that mean they are expected to die within 12 months; those at risk of dying from a sudden acute crisis in an existing condition; and those with life-threatening acute conditions caused by sudden catastrophic events. The term "approaching the end of life" can also apply to extremely premature neonates whose prospects for survival are known to be very poor, and patients who are diagnosed as being in a persistent vegetative state (PVS) for whom a decision to withdraw treatment and care may lead to their death. The "end stage" of life may be considered as the final period or phase in the course of a progressive disease leading to a patient's death (GMC 2017).

The identification of when someone with an advanced neurological condition may be approaching the EoL phase of their illness is important, because it enables the appropriate action to be taken. The consensus review on the development of palliative care for patients with chronic and progressive neurological disease states that the recognition of deterioration in disease progression near the end of life is essential in enabling the provision of appropriate care and support for patients and their families. Once recognized it must be considered how a regular reassessment is important, with careful continued discussion to enable the changes to be recognized (Oliver et al. 2016).

Unfortunately there are challenges in recognizing EoL in many neurological disorders because of many factors:

- The long duration of disease with the involvement of complex multidisciplinary care (e.g., MS).
- Sudden death (e.g., ALS, MSA).
- The lack of a predictable or fluctuating course (e.g., PD).
- The involvement of specialist treatments (e.g., deep brain stimulation, continuous intrajejunal infusion of levodopa-carbidopa, or continuous apomorphine subcutaneous infusion).
- Neuropsychiatric problems (e.g., behavioral and cognitive changes) can appear throughout the course of the disease creating confusion between terminal delirium and treatable complications.

Rapidly progressive diseases may need palliative care early on in the disease trajectory, in some conditions even from diagnosis (Oliver 2014). The role of comorbidities needs to be considered as many people (in particular the elderly) die with, but not from, their neurological condition. Nevertheless the neurological disease may play a role in the dying process, often causing difficulties in medical decisions and the priorities of care.

Palliative care can play a role at different times in the progression of a neurological disease. Figure 1 shows how this has changed over the decades – in the past palliative care was often only considered at the end of life, and more recently there has been a gradual transition with both neurological and palliative care services collaborating in care. However palliative care may have a role throughout the disease progression and in an episodic way, according to the patient and family's needs. Early involvement will enable a relationship to be developed between the patient and family and the multidisciplinary team which will facilitate care and may also make it easier for professionals to recognize the deterioration at the end of life.

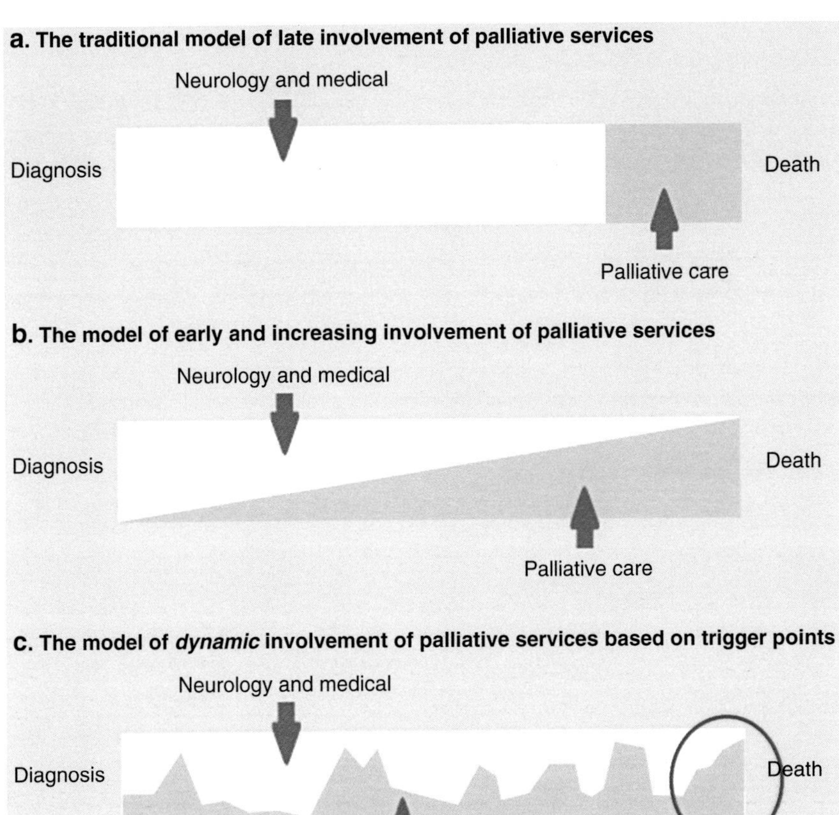

Fig. 1 Possible model of palliative care involvement in neurological disorders (Adapted from Bede et al.)

There are various instruments that can guide the clinician in the process of identification of an EoL trajectory. The Gold Standard Framework provides a multi-step decisional approach to identify patients approaching EoL Proactive Identification Guidance 2016 (GSF 2017). This toolkit is aimed at helping the primary medicine professional to screen the patients that they see and enter into the palliative care register those who are at risk of death and starts from the surprise question: "Would you be surprised if this patient were to die in the next 6–12 months?". If the answer is no, then the patient with advanced disease is further investigated in order to understand the desired choices of care and the presence and intensity of special need of supportive/palliative care. There is also the assessment of specific clinical indicators related to the main diagnosis that can indicate that the disorder is end stage. These indicators are also listed for neurological conditions like ALS, MS, PDs, stroke, and dementia. This approach helps to identify, assess, and plan for living well and dying well.

General triggers for EoL in neurological disorders were found to be rapid physical decline; significant complex symptoms, including pain; infection in combination with cognitive impairment; and risk of aspiration (NEOLCP 2010). Research has shown that the number of triggers increases as death approaches and the terminal phase was recognized for 72.6% of patients (Hussain et al. 2014).

The Supportive & Palliative Care Indicators Tool (SPICT™) is used to help identify people at risk of deteriorating and dying with one or multiple advanced illnesses for holistic, palliative care needs assessment and care planning (http://www.spict.org.uk/).

In the care planning of patients at the EoL, it is essential to assess important issues:

- The preferred place of care
  Including the desirability and feasibility of care for this person at home.
- The preferred place of death
  The person may feel better in his/her home or may feel more secure better in a more protective environment (such as a hospice or a nursing home).
- The family coping systems to deal with a death in their house
- The presence of other frail people at home who may need some protection – children, other seriously disabled family members, drug abuser, or alcohol addicted

In order to achieve a good quality of death, physical symptoms and psychosocial and spiritual issues are to be accurately addressed and reviewed any time the phase of illness changes, and the care plan has to be adapted.

Patients with ALS fear choking to death, even though there is good evidence that for those receiving good palliative care, most deaths are peaceful (Neudert et al. 2001). However, if they are not addressed, these worries can lead to desperation, and some patients are more likely to wish hastened death (Albert et al. 2005). The provision of appropriate medication "in case of need" may be appropriate – the Breathing Space Programme in the UK suggests the provision of morphine, midazolam, and glycopyrronium bromide injections in case of a sudden deterioration or distressing symptoms (Oliver 1996). For other conditions prevention of possible crises and careful planning of the EoL can be possible. The adopting of the principles of symptom management, as part of the wider palliative care assessment, should be applied to neurological care, allowing open discussion about the dying process and explanation that most patients will die peacefully with appropriate care.

9 Education

There is a need for information for all involved in the care of a person with a neurological disease. The diseases are relatively rare and may not have been encountered at all by patients and families and may be rarely seen by health and social care professionals. Thus there is the need for information to be available if the person is to attain the best quality of life and activity.

9.1 Patient and Family

At the time of diagnosis, patients and families may have limited information about what they face. However with some disease, which has a genetic component, they may be only too aware, having seen family members with the disease, such as in Huntington's disease. All need good and reliable information, but how this is provided is often difficult as some people may want limited information, whereas others feel let down if they develop new problems and feel that they have not been prepared beforehand. There is evidence that patients may seek information in different ways – "active seekers" who look for information, "selective seekers" who often rely on family members or friends to prescreen information and pass it on if they feel it is suitable, and "avoiders" who would rely on others to "buffer" and check any information (O'Brien 2004). Care is needed in allowing these people to receive information in the most effective way for them.

There are also issues if people look for information on the Internet, for although there are many excellent sites, often provided by specialist support societies, there are many misleading and erroneous sites and some which try to extort money for "cures" which are unsubstantiated or completely dishonest.

In the provision of information, awareness of the understanding of those involved is essential – many people may not be able to use written information due to literacy or language issues, and cultural differences may affect how information is perceived. However good information from reliable sources can be very positive, providing support and understanding and enabling care – for instance, awareness of behavioral changes in ALS when there is cognitive change enables family to understand why the person is acting in different ways and develop ways of coping and minimizing the difficult behavior (Goldstein 2014).

Specialist support groups and associations are very helpful in providing reliable information for people. They are able to provide specialist information for patients/families and professionals. They also help to facilitate general awareness of the issues facing people with the particular illness and help to raise funds for further research.

9.2 Professionals

There is increasing awareness of the need for professionals to be more aware of the needs of both patients with neurological disease and their carers/families. This may be for increased awareness of the role of palliative care for neurological/rehabilitation services and for increased knowledge of neurological disease for palliative care services (Creutzfelt et al. 2016). This is part of the ongoing development of health-care professionals in awareness of holistic care and the need for improved communication skills (Aoun et al. 2016).

10 Conclusions

The care of people with neurological disease can be complex and involves a wide multidisciplinary approach. There is a need for careful assessment and care needs to be individualized for every patient and family. This complexity is a challenge for palliative care services, as there is variable involvement over a variable period of time and collaboration and interaction with other professional teams. However with a careful collaborative approach, much can be done to improve the quality of life of this patient group.

To improve care further, it is hoped that there will be increased awareness of palliative care within neurology – including within guidelines on care. This will enable patients and families to receive the care they need. The numbers will increase over the coming years and decades as the population ages and all professionals will need to become more familiar with the palliative care of this population, who may also have multiple comorbidities.

The education of all professionals in the principles of palliative care will enable the approach to become more usual with a clearer understanding of the aims of management – often to minimize symptoms and allow people to live their lives as effectively as possible. As Dame Cicely Saunders, founder of St Christopher's Hospice where neurological patients were cared for from the opening in 1967, our aim should be "to help people live, live until they die."

References

Aboussouan LS. Respiratory disorders in neurologic diseases. Cleve Clin J Med. 2005;72(6):511–20.

Albert SM, et al. Wish to die in end-stage ALS. Neurology. 2005;65(1):68–74.

Alzheimer's Society. http://www.alzheimers.org.uk/site/scripts/documents_info.php?documentID=412. Accessed 26 July 2015.

Andersen PM, Abrahams S, Borasio GD, de Carvalho M, Chio A, Van Damme P, Hardiman O, Kollewe K, Morrison KE, Petri S, Pradat PF, Silani V, Tomik B, Wasner M, Weber M, The EFNS Task Force on Diagnosis and Management of Amyotrophic Lateral Sclerosis. EFNS guidelines on the clinical management of amyotrophic lateral sclerosis (MALS) – revised report of an EFNS task force. Eur J Neurol. 2012;19:360–75.

Aoun SM, Breen LJ, Howting D, Edis R, Oliver D, Henderson R, O'Connor M, Harris R, Birks C. Receiving the news of a diagnosis of motor neuron disease: what does it take to make it better? Amyotroph Lat Scler FTD. 2015;17:168–78.

Aoun SM, Breen LJ, Edis R, Henderson RD, Oliver D, Harris R, Howting D, O'Connor M, Birks C. Breaking the news of a diagnosis of motor neurone disease: a national survey of neurologists' perspectives. J Neurol Sci. 2016;367:368–74.

Aoun SM, Breen LJ, Oliver D et al. Family carers' experiences of receiving the news of a diagnosis of Motor Neurone Disease: A national survey. J Neurol Sci 2017; 372: 144–151.

Baile WF, Buckman R, Lenzi R, et al. SPIKES – a six step protocol for delivering bad news: application to the patient with cancer. Oncologist. 2000;5:302–11.

Bakitas M, Lyons KD, et al. Effects of a palliative care intervention on clinical outcomes in patients with advanced cancer: the project ENABLE II randomized controlled trial. JAMA. 2009;302(7):741–9.

Bede P, Hardiman O, O'Brannagain D. An integrated framework of early intervention palliative care in motor neurone disease as a model to progressive neurodegenerative disease. Poster at European ALS congress, Turin; 2009.

Bermejo PE, Oreja-Guevara C, Diez-Tejedor E. Pain in multiple sclerosis: prevalence, mechanisms, types and treatment. Rev Neurol. 2010;50:101–8.

Bernheim JL, Raus K. Euthanasia embedded in palliative care. Responses to essentialistic criticisms of the Belgian model of integral end-of-life care. J Med Ethics. 2017;43:489–494.

Boersma I, Miyasaki J, Kutner J, Kluger B. Palliative care and neurology: time for a paradigm shift. Neurology. 2014;83(6):561–7.

Borreani C, et al. Unmet needs of people with severe multiple sclerosis and their carers: qualitative findings for a home-based intervention. PLoS One. 2014;9: e109679.

Borsook D. Neurological diseases and pain. Brain. 2012;135:320–44.

Breitbart W, Rosenfeld B, et al. Depression, hopelessness, and desire for hastened death in terminally ill patients with cancer. JAMA. 2000;284:2907–11.

Buecken R, Galushko M, Golla H, Strupp J, Hahn M, Ernstmann N, Pfaff H, Voltz R. Patients feeling severely affected by multiple sclerosis: how do patients want to communicate about end-of-life issues? Patient Educ Couns. 2012;88:318–24.

Catania G, Beccaro M, et al. Effectiveness of complex interventions focused on quality-of life assessment to improve palliative care patients' outcomes: a systematic review. Palliat Med. 2015;29(1):5–21.

Chapman S. Advance care planning. In: Oliver D, editor. End of life care in neurological disease. London: Springer; 2012.

Creutzfelt CJ, Robinson MT, Holloway RG. Neurologists as primary palliative care providers. Communication and practice approaches. Neurol Clin Pract. 2016;6: 1–9.

Edmonds P, Hart S, Gao W, Vivat B, Burman R, Silber E, Higginson I. Palliative care for people severely affected by multiple sclerosis: evaluation of a novel palliative care service. Mult Scler. 2010;16:627–36.

Funk L, et al. Part 2: home-based family caregiving at the end of life: a comprehensive review of published qualitative research (1998-2008). Palliat Med. 2010;24:594–607.

Gaertner J, Wolf J, Hallek M, Glossmann J-P, Voltz R. Standardising integration of palliative care into comprehensive cancer therapy – a disease specific approach. Support Care Cancer. 2011;19:1037–43.

Ganzini L, Johnston WS, McFarland BH, Tolle SW, Lee MA. Attitudes of patients with amyotrophic lateral sclerosis and their care givers toward assisted suicide. N Engl J Med. 1998;339(14):967–73.

General Medical Council. End of life care: glossary of terms. Available from: http://www.gmc-uk.org/guidance/ethical_guidance/end_of_life_glossary_of_terms.asp. Accessed 8 Feb 2017.

Goldstein LH. Control of symptoms: cognitive dysfunction. In: Oliver D, Borasio GD, Johnston W, editors. Palliative care in amyotrophic lateral sclerosis- from diagnosis to bereavement. 3rd ed. Oxford: Oxford University Press; 2014. p. 107–25.

Grande GE, Ewing G. National Forum for hospice at home. Informal carer bereavement outcome: relation to quality of end of life support and achievement of preferred place of death. Palliat Med. 2009;23:248–56.

GSF, G.-S.-F. Proactive identification guidance. 2016. Available from: http://www.goldstandardsframework.org.uk/library-tools-amp-resources. Accessed 8 Feb 2017.

Higginson IJ, Finlay IG, et al. Is there evidence that palliative care teams alter end-of-life experiences of patients and their caregivers? J Pain Symptom Manag. 2003;25 (2):150–68.

Higginson IJ, Hart S, et al. Symptom prevalence and severity in people severely affected by multiple sclerosis. J Palliat Care. 2006;22:158–65.

Higginson IJ, Hart S, et al. Randomised controlled trial of a new palliative care service: compliance, recruitment and completeness of follow-up. BMC Palliat Care. 2008;7(1):7.

Higginson IJ, McCrone P, et al. Is short-term palliative care cost-effective in multiple sclerosis? A randomized phase II trial. J Pain Symptom Manag. 2009;38(6):816–26.

Hussain J, Adams D, Allgar V, Campbell C. Triggers in advanced neurological conditions: prediction and management of the terminal phase. BMJ Support Palliat Care. 2014;4:30–7.

Jennings AL, et al. Opioids for the palliation of breathlessness in terminal illness. Cochrane Database Syst Rev. 2001;(4). https://doi.org/10.1002/14651858.CD00266

Jox RJ, Krebs M, Bickhardt J, et al. How strictly should advance decisions be followed? The patients' opinion. Palliat Med. 2008;22:675–6.

Kaub-Wittemer D, et al. Quality of life and psychosocial issues in ventilated patients with amyotrophic lateral sclerosis and their caregivers. J Pain Symptom Manag. 2003;26(4):890–6.

Klit H, Finnerup NB, Jensen TS. Central post-stroke pain: clinical characteristics, pathophysiology, and management. Lancet Neurol. 2009;8:857–68.

Kumar B, et al. Central poststroke pain: a review of pathophysiology and treatment. Anesth Analg. 2009;108: 1645–57.

Lambert R. Spiritual care. In: Oliver D, Borasio GD, Johnston W, editors. Palliative care in amyotrophic lateral sclerosis – from diagnosis to bereavement. 3rd ed. Oxford: Oxford University Press; 2014.

Lee MA, et al. Measuring symptom load in idiopathic Parkinson's disease. Parkinsonism Relat Disord. 2007; 13(5):284–9.

Lienard A, Merckaert I, Libert Y, et al. Is it possible to improve residents breaking bad news skills? A randomised study assessing the efficacy of a communication skills training programme. Br J Cancer. 2010;103:171–7.

Mangera Z, Panesar G, Makker H. Practical approach to management of respiratory complications in neurological disorders. Int J Gen Med. 2012;5:255–63.

McIlfatrick S. Assessing palliative care needs: views of patients, informal carers and healthcare professionals. J Adv Nurs. 2007;57:77–86.

Miller RG, et al. Practice parameter: the care of the patient with amyotrophic lateral sclerosis (an evidence-based review): report of the Quality Standards Subcommittee of the American Academy of Neurology: ALS practice parameters task force. Neurology. 1999;52: 1311–23.

Miller RG, Jackson CE, Karsarkis EJ, England JD, Forshew D, Johnston W, et al. Practice parameter update: the care of the patient with amyotrophic lateral sclerosis: multidisciplinary care, symptom management, and cognitive/behavioural impairment (an evidence-based review). Neurology. 2009;73:1227–33.

Modirian E, et al. Chronic pain after spinal cord injury: results of a long-term study. Pain Med. 2010;11:1037–43.

Moens K, et al. Are there differences in the prevalence of palliative care-related problems in people living with advanced cancer and eight non-cancer conditions? A systematic review. J Pain Symptom Manag. 2014;48: 660–77.

Moulin DE, et al. Pain in Guillain-Barre syndrome. Neurology. 1997;48:328–31.

Moulton EA, Schmahmann JD, et al. The cerebellum and pain: passive integrator or active participator? Brain Res Rev. 2010;65:14–27.

National End of Life Care Programme. End of life care in long term neurological conditions: a framework for implementation: National End of Life Care Programme; 2010. www.mssociety.org.uk/sites/default/files/Documents/Professionals/End%20life%20care%20long%20term%20neuro%20conditions.pdf

Neudert C, Oliver D, Wasner M, Borasio GD. The course of the terminal phase in patients with amyotrophic lateral sclerosis. J Neurol. 2001;248:612–6.

NICE. Parkinson's disease in over 20s: diagnosis and management. 2006. Available from: https://www.nice.org.uk/guidance/cg35.

O'Brien MR. Information-seeking behaviour among people with motor neurone disease. Br J Nurs. 2004;13: 964–8.

O'Brien T, Kelly M, Saunders C. Motor neurone disease: a hospice perspective. Br Med J. 1992;304:471–3.

O'Connor AB, et al. Pain associated with multiple sclerosis: systematic review and proposed classification. Pain. 2008;137:96–111.

Office for National Statistics. 2012. www.ons.gov.uk/ons/rel/vsob1/mortality-statistics-deaths-registered-in-england-and-wales-dr/2012/dr-tables-2012-xls. Accessed 21 July 2015.

Oliver D. The quality of care and symptom control – the effects on the terminal phase of ALS/MND. J Neurol Sci. 1996;139(Suppl):134–6.

Oliver D. Palliative care. In: Oliver D, Borasio G, Johnston W, editors. Palliative care in amyotrophic lateral sclerosis- from diagnosis to bereavement. 3rd ed. Oxford: Oxford University Press; 2014.

Oliver DJ, Borasio GD, Caraceni A, de Visser M, Grisold W, Lorenzl S, Veronese S, Voltz R. A consensus review on the development of palliative care for patients with chronic and progressive neurological disease. Eur J Neurol. 2016;23:30–8. https://doi.org/10.1111/ene.12889.

Otero-Romero S, Sastre-Garriga J, et al. Pharmacological management of spasticity in multiple sclerosis: systematic review and consensus paper. Mult Scler. 2016;22: 1386–96.

Pautex S, et al. Pain in severe dementia: self-assessment or observational scales? J Am Geriatr Soc. 2006;54: 1040–5.

Radbruch L, Leget C, Müller-Busch C, Ellershaw F, de Conno F, Vanden BP. Euthanasia and physician-assisted suicide: a white paper from the European Association for Palliative Care. Palliat Med. 2015;30: 104–16.

Radunovic A, et al. Mechanical ventilation for amyotrophic lateral sclerosis/motor neuron disease. Cochrane Database Syst Rev. 2013;28(3):CD004427.

Sampson EL, Candy B, Jones L. Enteral tube feeding for older people with advanced dementia. Cochrane Database Syst Rev. 2009;15(2):CD007209.

Scott A, McPhee M. Multidisciplinary care: speech and language therapy. In: Oliver D, Borasio GD, Johnston W, editors. Palliative care in amyotrophic lateral sclerosis – from diagnosis to bereavement. 3rd ed. Oxford: Oxford University Press; 2014. p. 215–32.

Seeber AA, Pols AJ, Hijdra A, Grupstra HF, Willems DL, de Visser M. Experiences and reflections of patients with motor neuro disease on breaking the news in a two-tiered appointment : a qualitative study. BMJ Support Palliat Care. 2016;(1-9). https://doi.org/10.1136/bmjspcare-2015-000977.

Shaw C, Quinn A, Daniel E. Amyotrophic lateral sclerosis / motor neurone disease. In: Oliver D, Borasio G, Johnston W, editors. Palliative care in amyotrophic lateral sclerosis- from diagnosis to bereavement. 3rd ed. Oxford: Oxford University Press; 2014.

Simuni T, Sethi K. Nonmotor manifestations of Parkinson's disease. Ann Neurol. 2008;64(S2):S65–80.

Smith S, Wasner M. Psychosocial care. In: Oliver D, Borasio GD, Johnston W, editors. Palliative care in amyotrophic lateral sclerosis- from diagnosis to bereavement. 3rd ed. Oxford: Oxford University Press; 2014.

Solari A, Giordano A, et al. Home-based palliative approach for people with severe multiple sclerosis and their carers: study protocol for a randomized controlled trial. Trials. 2015;16(1):184.

Stutzki R, Weber M, Reiter-Theil S, Simmen U, Borasio GD, Jox RJ. Attitudes towards hastened death in ALS: a prospective study of patients and family caregivers. Amyotroph Lateral Scler Frontotemporal Degener. 2014;15(1–2):68–76.

Temel JS, Greer JA, Muzikansky A, et al. Early palliative care for patients with metastatic non-small-cell lung cancer. N Engl J Med. 2010;19:733–42.

Thomas, K. and J. Armstrong Wilson. The Gold Standards Framework Proactive Identification Guidance (PIG). 2016. Available from: www.goldstandardsframework.nhs.uk. Accessed 8 Feb 2017.

Veldink JH, Wokke JH, et al. Euthanasia and physician-assisted suicide among patients with amyotrophic lateral sclerosis in the Netherlands. N Engl J Med. 2002;346(21):1638–44.

Veronese S, Gallo G, et al. Specialist palliative care improves the quality of life in advanced neurodegenerative disorders: NE-PAL, a pilot randomised controlled study. BMJ Support Palliat Care. 2015. https://doi.org/10.1136/bmjspcare-2014-000788.

Veronese S, Gallo G, et al. The palliative care needs of people severely affected by neurodegenerative disorders: a qualitative study. Prog Palliat Care. 2017;25:11–6. https://doi.org/10.1080/09699260.2016.1193968.

van Vliet LM, Gao W, et al. How integrated are neurology and palliative care services? Results of a multicentre mapping exercise. BMC Neurol. 2016;16:63.

Voltz R, Akabayashi A, Reese C, Ohi G, Sass HM. End-of-life decisions and advance directives in palliative care: a cross cultural survey of patients and health-care professionals. J Pain Symptom Manag. 1998;16:153–62.

Walshe M. Oropharyngeal dysphagia in neurodegenerative disease. J Gastroenterol Hepatol Res. 2014;3(10):1265–71.

Whetten-Goldstein K, et al. Financial burden of chronic neurological disorders to patients and their families: what providers need to know. J Neurol Phys Ther. 2000;24:140–4.

World Health Organisation. Global burden of neurological disorders: estimates and projections. In: Neurological disorders- public health challenges. Geneva: World Health Organisation; 2006.

World Health Organization. Palliative care. 2002. www.who.int/cancer/palliative/definition/en/. Accessed 26 July 2015.

Worth PF. When the going gets tough: how to select patients with Parkinson's disease for advanced therapies. Pract Neurol. 2013;13:140–52.

Zimmermann C, Riechelmann R, et al. Effectiveness of specialized palliative care: a systematic review. JAMA. 2008;299(14):1698–709.

Palliative Care in Dementia

59

Nathan Davies, Maartje S. Klapwijk, and
Jenny T. van der Steen

Contents

N. Davies (✉)
Centre for Ageing Population Studies, Research
Department of Primary Care and Population Health,
University College London, London, UK
e-mail: n.m.davies@ucl.ac.uk

M. S. Klapwijk
Healthcare Organisation Marente, Voorhout,
The Netherlands

Department of Public Health and Primary Care, Leiden
University Medical Center, Leiden, The Netherlands
e-mail: M.S.Klapwijk@lumc.nl

J. T. van der Steen
Department of Public Health and Primary Care, Leiden
University Medical Center, Leiden, The Netherlands

Radboud university medical center, Department of Primary
and Community Care, Nijmegen, The Netherlands
e-mail: jtvandersteen@lumc.nl

R. D. MacLeod, L. Van den Block (eds.), *Textbook of Palliative Care*,
https://doi.org/10.1007/978-3-319-77740-5_113

Abstract

An optimal approach to palliative care for people with dementia has been defined by the European Association for Palliative Care with 11 domains including applicability of palliative care; person-centered care, communication, and shared decision-making; and setting care goals and advance care planning. Not all people with dementia will require specialist palliative care, and all involved in dementia care should be able to provide palliative care focusing on care and treatment which aims to increase the comfort and quality of life of the individual and supporting their family. There are many complications and symptoms which may arise for someone with dementia including increased infections, shortness of breath, swallowing difficulties, and pain which the individual may not be able to clearly express. These complications can lead to difficult decisions which need to be made by not only practitioners but also family caregivers as proxy. There should be a shared decision-making approach to these complications and symptoms, with advance care planning performed where possible. Caring for someone with dementia is one of the most difficult caring roles; support for family caregivers as part of a palliative approach is essential. Each person with dementia is different, and needs should be assessed on an individual basis, adopting a person-centered approach to care.

1 Introduction

With aging populations across the world, the numbers of people with dementia continuing to increase and with no known disease-modifying treatment, the delivery of high-quality palliative care is becoming a high priority for health and social care services. Dementia is often not recognized or understood as a terminal illness which will ultimately lead to death; however, research over the last decade has increased, and attention paid to palliative care for people with dementia continues to be recognized. Through the use of a case study/vignette (Mrs. S) in this chapter, we provide a definition of optimal palliative care for older people with dementia through the domains of the European Association for Palliative Care (EAPC) (van der Steen et al. 2014b). Drawing on a case study, we discuss common issues and symptoms for those with dementia including symptoms which may be experienced in the dying phase, and their associated treatments, considering the controversy of some of these treatments, such as artificial nutrition. The chapter considers the role of family caregivers in decision-making and the difficult decisions which are often left to them to make as proxy. The importance of family caregivers in dementia palliative care is highlighted including their health and psychological needs. Throughout this chapter we highlight the person-centered approach which should be adopted and needs and support should be considered on an individual basis.

2 Defining Palliative Care for People with Dementia

Palliative care has a great deal to offer for people with dementia. The trajectory of dementia usually involves multiple changes in condition and in the situation of people with dementia. What is needed is a care approach that is highly responsive to such changes, and which therefore explicitly incorporates and anticipates the future, to promote a feeling of being in control in a situation where people often feel loss of control. This does not mean that all people with dementia need specialist palliative care. Rather, with no cure of the disease available, the palliative approach may help as a reminder to focus care and treatment on maintaining or improving quality of life of the patient and supporting the family caregiver in changing and often difficult roles. As the course of the disease is much less predictable than, for example, with cancer, it is more problematic to limit palliative care in dementia to the end of life: when should that be? In order to integrate a palliative approach in dementia care, and for specialist palliative care to appreciate what is specific about dementia, a common understanding of what is needed from palliative care in dementia is needed.

A single sentence to define palliative care in dementia would not suffice. Therefore, in a Delphi study based on evidence and consensus among palliative care and dementia care experts, the European Association for Palliative Care (EAPC) sought to identify the important domains in palliative care in dementia to serve as a framework for development of practice, policy, and research (van der Steen et al. 2014b). This Delphi study focused on older people with dementia, as little is known about the specific issues of young-onset dementia at the end of life. Within each domain, the most important recommendations were provided to optimize palliative care in dementia, backed up by an explanation and evidence where available.

Box 1. Domains of Palliative Care in Older People with Dementia European Association for Palliative Care (EAPC) (van der Steen et al. 2014b)

1. Applicability of palliative care
2. Person-centered care, communication, and shared decision-making
3. Setting care goals and advance care planning
4. Continuity of care
5. Prognostication and timely recognition of dying
6. Avoiding overly aggressive, burdensome, or futile treatment
7. Optimal treatment of symptoms and providing comfort
8. Psychosocial and spiritual support
9. Family care and involvement
10. Education of the health-care team
11. Societal and ethical issues

The first domain is applicability of palliative care, because dementia is not always considered a terminal disease. It does shorten life expectancy (Rait et al. 2010), but perhaps more important is that dementia is a progressive disease and there needs to be continuous assessment of the needs of the individual, whether resulting in death with or from the dementia. Palliative care asserts that knowledge of and acceptance of the course of a disease, with no cure, is essential, even though this may be an emotionally charged area. In dementia there are indications that (on average) people die more comfortably and with better quality care when family and professional caregivers recognize dementia as a terminal disease before the dying phase (van der Steen et al. 2013). Also physicians perceived that patients suffered more in the final hours of life if their physician felt unprepared with an unexpected death (van der Steen et al. 2017a). Studies of advance care planning also speak to a general benefit of conceptualizing dementia as a terminal disease and preparation for declining health.

The important question then arises when palliative care should begin. In principle, when diagnosed with a terminal illness, one may wish to start and prepare. However, and especially with an early diagnosis, the end of life may still be far away. The exclusive focus on advance dementia seen in research suggests that moderate dementia is not yet a terminal disease (Mitchell et al. 2009). This is, however, difficult to maintain if half of people with dementia die before ever reaching the advanced stage, and after having experiencing a number of complications, with pneumonia and dehydration of cachexia occurring in moderate dementia as well (Hendriks et al. 2016). Moreover, people with advanced dementia may survive for many years (Gill et al. 2010), often referred to as dwindling; with good care, they may even form a selected subgroup of "survivors." The domain of prognostication and timely recognition of dying (Box 1) acknowledges difficulties in prognostication and is therefore typical for palliative care in dementia, where it is not usually a domain in itself in palliative care more generally or for other diseases.

The EAPC work also acknowledges that it is not possible to state a uniform and good starting point for palliative care for all people with dementia. Instead, palliative care is conceptualized as most compatible with two of three major care goals: maintenance of function and maximization of comfort (Fig. 1), which both relate strongly to quality of life. There may be a mixture of care goals, which can shift over time, with progressive dementia. Also, because this is a model, how exactly care goals may shift differs between individuals. In principle, however, palliative care can start at diagnosis (such as with naming of a proxy decision-maker; see advance care planning discussion Sect. 3 in this chapter), even though the care goal that overwhelmingly takes priority at that point may be life prolongation (Fig. 1).

Understanding the applicability and mainstays of palliative care in dementia is not only important for practice but also for policy making, given the benefits and slow uptake in, for example, national dementia strategies where, if included, palliative care is often regarded as care for the dying. Two other domains are relevant especially for policy makers, which are the final two domains (education of the health-care team and societal and ethical issues); however, these are beyond the scope of this chapter and as such not discussed.

The most important of the 11 domains (Box 1) of palliative care in people with dementia according to the experts – and perhaps for all patients with no dementia or palliative care needs – are optimal

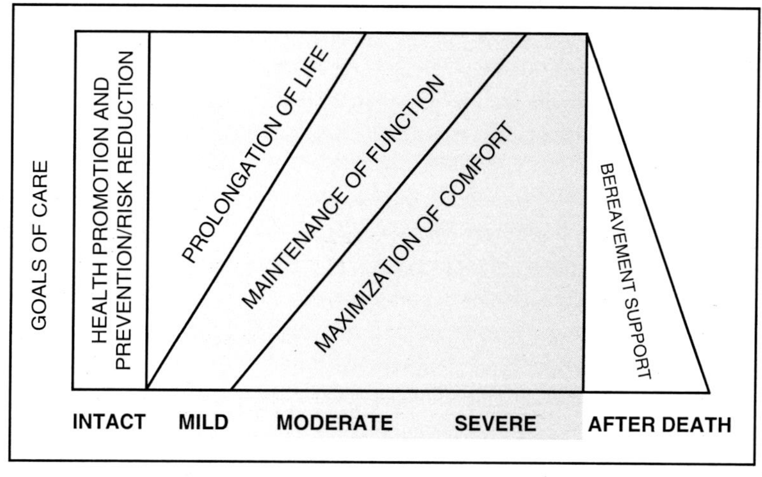

Fig. 1 Dementia progression and suggested prioritizing of care goals. The goals of maintenance of function and maximization of comfort are compatible with palliative care which aims to improve quality of life (van der Steen et al. 2014b. Copyright © 2014 by the Authors. Reprinted by permission of SAGE Publications, Ltd.)

treatment of symptoms and providing comfort and person-centered care, communication, and shared decision-making. Nevertheless, how this is being achieved is different with dementia than with several other terminal diseases; this is discussed in Sects. 4, 6, and 7. Several of the domains listed in Box 1 are emphasized more in palliative care in dementia than with palliative care in other diseases. These are the domains of setting care goals and advance care planning, because of missed opportunities when waiting for the patient to decline in cognitive functioning, and family care and involvement because of the great burden placed on families through both the physical and cognitive decline of the person with dementia. It may be argued that in advanced dementia or at the end of life, continuity of care, avoiding transfer and change or adding of new staff in the last phase, is also of special importance in people with dementia. The same may be true for the two domains that relate to a historical development of palliative care in response to an overly aggressive unilateral medical approach until (almost) dying: avoiding overly aggressive, burdensome, or futile treatment and psychosocial and spiritual support. Explicit attending to needs for spiritual care may fill a gap in dementia care practice, as spiritual care is nearly absent in most dementia guidelines and national dementia strategies (Durepos et al. 2017; Nakanishi et al. 2015).

Palliative care issues, however, may not be raised at all in the absence of a timely diagnosis of dementia which is shown in the case below.

Patient Case/Vignette Part 1 Mrs. S is an 82-year-old lady who lives at home. She has two children, a daughter and a son; her husband died 6 years ago. Her daughter visits her at home as much as possible. Her son lives abroad.

She has a history of a hypertension and has had a hysterectomy. She visits the GP regularly to check her blood pressure. Over the past year, she has visited her GP a few more times due to two urinary tract infections. She calls her daughter and son a couple of times a day and never remembers she has just called. Her daughter often finds moldy food in the fridge, and Mrs. S has got lost on her way home several times.

One day Mrs. S does not answer the phone; her daughter is worried and goes over to her mother. Mrs. S is lying next to the toilet; she does not know how long she has been on the floor. She can't use her right leg because she is in too much pain. Her daughter calls an ambulance, and in the hospital, a hip fracture is diagnosed.

During her stay in the hospital, Mrs. S gets very disoriented and hallucinates and is diagnosed with delirium. The possibility of dementia is mentioned, but at this point, it is not possible to run tests. Mrs. S's daughter agrees that her mother cannot go back home, and they decide to transfer Mrs. S to a rehabilitation unit.

3 Advance Care Planning

As can be seen in the case of Mrs. S, there has been little planning for her future care or treatment as her cognitive decline progresses and as her ability and capacity to make her own health, care, and welfare (including financial) diminishes. This stresses the importance of advance care planning.

3.1 Definition

Advance care planning (ACP) has been defined as "process of discussion that usually takes place in anticipation of a future deterioration of a person's condition, between that person and a care worker" (Henry and Seymour 2007). Advance care planning can include advance statements about wishes to inform subsequent treatment, for example, how one's religious beliefs should be reflected in care, or an advance decision to refuse treatment such as antibiotics to treat an infection. Included in the advance care plan are nonmedical decisions such as decisions about who should manage the individual's finances. An advance decision may sometimes be referred to as a living will, advance directive, advance policy making, or advance physician orders. It is important to highlight that ACP is a process of communication. It does not necessarily lead to a living will or nomination of a proxy decision-maker, it may also simply be conversations which are not documented; however, this is not recommended and documentation of decisions should be made when possible.

3.2 Why Is ACP Important in Dementia?

A timely diagnosis of dementia can be vital to encourage the process of ACP. As discussed above as cognitive decline progresses, an individual's ability to consider their own health and care needs deteriorates, along with their ability to make informed decisions. At this point many decisions are left to families to make in a shared decision-making process with practitioners, leaving families often unsure about their status and feeling guilty. ACP has demonstrated improved outcomes for both people with dementia and their caregivers (Dixon and Knapp 2018), including reduced depression, stress, and anxiety in family caregivers (Dixon and Knapp 2018). As is in the case of Mrs. S in patient case/vignette part 5, ongoing discussions around the future and complications may have reduced the surprise for the family when she deteriorated. There is little evidence, however, if there are subgroups of people who benefit more or less than others – for example, if there are people who would rather benefit from support in living one day at a time.

Patient Case/Vignette Part 2 Mrs. S in the rehabilitation unit is dependent on nurses' care, and she becomes more disoriented in time and place as her cognitive decline progresses. She has more difficulty finding words to express herself. After a while Mrs. S is diagnosed with dementia of Alzheimer type. Her children and the multidisciplinary team do not think Mrs. S can go back home, and they want to transfer her to a nursing home with a special dementia care unit. Her children feel quite guilty about this even more so since Mrs. S wants to go home.

3.3 What Should They Discuss and the Approaches: Who, How, and When?

The EAPC recommendations on optimal palliative care for people with dementia recognize ACP as a core domain (Box 1, domain 3) (van der Steen et al. 2014b). According to the EAPC, ACP should be considered early in the disease process shortly after diagnosis, continually reviewed as an ongoing process with the patient and family on a regular basis and following any significant change in health condition. As can be seen in Fig. 1, the care goals will change, and priorities may alter over time from life prolongation and maintenance of function in early dementia through to maximizing comfort in the severe/advanced stages of dementia.

However, there is ambiguity about when to start advance care planning. Starting shortly after diagnosis may not be appropriate for everyone and is currently not necessarily a common practice in many countries. In recognition that the optimal timing of initiating the process is highly individual, the EAPC recommends a minimum as to what should be done at diagnosis, which is to name a (future) substitute decision-maker. The health-care team may also just "plant the seed." Introducing planning and decision-making as early as possible is encouraged in many countries. Decisions about when to start ACP should be considered on an individual patient by patient level and should include both the person with dementia and those close to them.

There are many national guidelines across many countries which provide example templates for ACP, including how to begin discussions and what the discussions should include. Initial discussions may include identifying the wishes and preferences of an individual, including preference of where they would like to be cared for (e.g., hospital, nursing home, or at home), but this often depends on the care that is needed and how they may like their religious and spiritual beliefs incorporated in their care. Although an individual with dementia may express their preference of place of care throughout their dementia, for example, in the case of Mrs. S in patient case/vignette part 2. Often people with dementia want to remain at home, being a familiar environment and close to their relatives. Often, like in the case of Mrs. S, people are admitted to a hospital and are

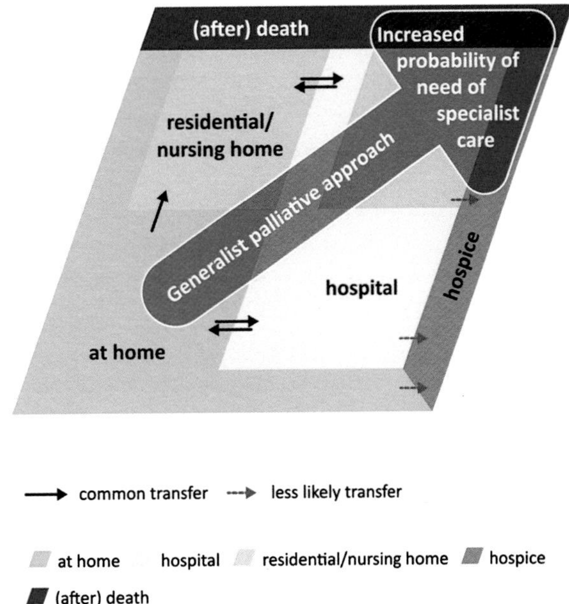

Fig. 2 Possible journey for person with dementia and health-care service transitions (Published with kind permission of © JT van der Steen, MS Klapwijk and N Davies 2018. All Rights Reserved)

afterward transferred to a nursing home because they need more care and staying at home is not safe anymore or the partner or relatives can't deliver the amount of care or guidance that is needed.

Figure 2 shows the different journeys for people with dementia; many live at home, but with the increase in care dependency, people are transferred to a hospital or a nursing home. Sometimes people are also admitted from home to a hospice or from a hospital or nursing home to a hospice. The discussions may then gradually move on to consider more specific decisions, such as treatment and scenarios of future health. These may include treatment such as artificial nutrition and hydration, the use of antibiotics for recurrent infections, and cardiopulmonary resuscitation. As with patients and families, physicians also differ in whether they feel comfortable with discussing future scenarios or rather focus on care goals and values with specific decisions postponed to when the situation occurs (van Soest-Poortvliet et al. 2015). There is a growing amount of literature surrounding planning with some placing high importance on what they regard as the necessity for people with dementia to complete advance care plans (Dixon and Knapp 2018).

3.4 Barriers

Despite many efforts internationally to encourage ACP for people with dementia, they are often not consulted about their wishes. ACP is less well developed across Europe, with much more work in Australia, Canada, and the USA. Several studies have identified a number of barriers why ACP does not occur including a lack of knowledge of ACP, difficulty of talking about such sensitive topics, fear of facing one's own mortality, organizational context, discontinuity of care, lack of a relationship with practitioners as well as within families, lack of time, as well as being made more complex in dementia by it often not being acknowledged as a terminal illness (van der Steen et al. 2014c). Many health and social care professionals are reported to lack the confidence, feel inexperienced, and need additional training and support in this area (Sampson et al. 2012). Health and social care staff in some countries believe that if they do not call emergency services in a crisis, there will be repercussions for them (Harrison Dening et al. 2012). This issue highlights the legal ambiguity that is often seen across countries of ACP (Jones et al. 2016). For example, in the UK, the legal document as part of ACP is the advance decision. The advance decision, however, is only legally binding if it complies with the Mental Capacity Act (2005), is valid (e.g., it is signed by the individual and a witness, and it specifies clearly the treatments the individual wishes to refuse), and applies to the situation. It is important to check the legal framework of decisions at the end of life in your country or region as this does differ.

3.5 Facilitators and Benefits

ACP potentially gives patients and families an opportunity to think about what is important for them and plan to try to ensure these wishes are met. However, it may not always be possible for the individual's wishes to be met, for example, as in the case of Mrs. S's wish to go home in patient case/vignette part 2. To facilitate ACP, practitioners should be available to educate families, and in particular, there should be a dedicated key facilitator to educate both practitioner and family. ACP can lead to reduced hospital admissions, unnecessary interventions, reduced costs (Robinson et al. 2012), and even reduced stress among family caregivers as discussed in Sect. 8.2 of this chapter.

Patient Case/Vignette Part 3 Finally Mrs. S has been moved from the rehabilitation unit to a unit (wing) for people with dementia in a nursing home. At first she seems to experience problems with her new environment; later she seems to feel better in her new rhythm of the unit.

At one point she starts to frown sometimes and to behave in an agitated manner. She cannot verbally express what she is feeling at those moments. At first nothing is found which could explain this. One day a nurse hears Mrs. S moaning and sees her frowning. Physical examination and a urine test lead to a diagnosis of a urinary tract infection, which is then treated with antibiotics.

4 Symptom Management

At the beginning of the disease, people with dementia live at home and are often still capable of expressing their feelings, for instance, pain. But with the progression of the disease, people often lose this ability to communicate verbally due to neuropathological changes. This is also reflected in functional and physical impairment and behavioral and psychological symptoms, for which people often have to be admitted to a nursing home. As the dementia progresses, the need for help rises, and the last year of living with dementia is known for a high level of disability with a high need for assistance in activities for daily living. Symptoms that are often described in studies of people with dementia include pain, shortness of breath, and agitation or other neuropsychiatric symptoms.

The clinical course of dementia shows that family or medical staff working with people with dementia should pay particular attention for symptoms of pain, shortness of breath, or anxiety (Hendriks et al. 2015; Hendriks et al. 2016). Often with the progression of the disease, people get urinary incontinence and later bowel incontinence and are at high risk for swallowing problems and aspiration, weight loss, pressure ulcers, infections (pneumonia and urinary tract infections), and febrile episodes, as can be seen in the case of Mrs. S (patient case/vignette part 3) (Mitchell et al. 2009).

4.1 Pain

The gold standard for the assessment of pain is self-report. This is often not possible in a later stage of dementia when people are often not capable of verbally expressing the experience of pain or lose the capacity of pain memory. Pain can result in behavior that challenges, for example, agitation or aggression if left untreated. In the case of Mrs. S, she can be seen to frown at times, and this is often coupled with agitation; this may be an indication that she is in pain. Pain can be experienced differently in people with different kinds of dementia or at different stages, related to the different neuropathological changes. Pain is however very common, 12–76%, in people with dementia, in all stages (van der Steen 2010).

Previous studies had suggested that people with dementia in nursing homes receive less pain medication compared to people without dementia; however, newer evidence suggests that there is no difference in people with or without dementia (Haasum et al. 2011) or it is even higher among people with dementia in some studies (Lövheim et al. 2008). Studies have also expressed concern about the overuse of opioids in people with dementia. It is therefore vital to ensure pain is a central component of continual assessment with a person with dementia, and an approach to maximizing comfort and quality of life is taken.

There are a number of instruments (pain scales) which can be used to assist staff identify pain in people with dementia if they are not able to verbally express this pain, such as the case with Mrs. S The team is alerted by the moaning and frowning suggesting she is in pain. The involvement of family and caregivers may be a very good way of assessing the patient, especially at home or just after admission in a nursing home, as they are familiar with changes in behavior or expression that may indicate distress. There are a large number of available instruments which have shown different reliability and validity, currently over 30, but for clinical practice, the Pain Assessment in Advanced Dementia (PAINAD) and Pain Assessment Checklist for Seniors with Limited Ability to Communicate (PACSLAC) are often recommended (Ellis-Smith et al. 2016). Research continues to look for an instrument that is reliable and valid and which can identify expressions specifically indicative for pain. In clinical settings it is important to evaluate the possibility of pain regularly and sometimes try the effect of analgesics, as well as assessment of current pain medication being received; is it still adequate and is it still necessary?

4.2 Shortness of Breath

Shortness of breath is often reported in studies of people with dementia with a range of 16–26% (Hendriks et al. 2015; Mitchell et al. 2009). Shortness of breath can be caused by different problems; common causes include pulmonary infection such as pneumonia or cardiac problems. Pneumonia may also be related to aspiration. Angina and pulmonary embolism are very difficult to recognize in people with dementia in cases where there are difficulties verbally expressing pain (chest) or shortness of breath.

4.3 Unmet Need/Challenging Behavior

Many feelings, for instance, pain as mentioned above, are the result of a sensation that is unpleasant, and they can lead to a change in the individual's behavior, which may be considered challenging. Many neuropsychiatric symptoms are seen in people with dementia and can have a great impact on the quality of life of that person and those surrounding them: family and caregivers.

Neuropsychiatric symptoms (NPS) (or behavioral and psychological symptoms of dementia (BPSD)) include delusions, hallucinations, depressive mood, anxiety, irritability/lability, apathy, euphoria, disinhibition, agitation/aggression, aberrant motor activity, and sleep or appetite changes (Cerejeira et al. 2012). The range of NPS prevalence in community-dwelling people with dementia is generally more than half of people (Borsje et al. 2015). These different types of behavior, often called challenging behavior, can also be frequently seen in nursing homes. Family or a regular staff member that know the person with dementia can often provide extra information on the cause of the behavior or have useful information on how to diminish this.

Infections such as a urinary tract infection are known to be a frequent cause of challenging behavior or even cause an episode of delirium; this is often the cause of admission to hospital for many people with dementia. The prevalence and incidence of delirium can be high in people with dementia, ranging from 8% in nursing homes to 89% in hospital and community populations (Boorsma et al. 2012; Fick et al. 2002). Many tools have been developed to assess delirium, including tools that are also used for people with dementia to ensure early recognition (Morandi et al. 2012), including the Richmond Agitation and Sedation Scale (RASS) and modified-RASS (m-RASS) (Morandi et al. 2016).

Agitation is often reported as one of the biggest behavioral challenges in people with dementia, and numbers ranging from 57% to 71% were found (Hendriks et al. 2015). However, for many, families are more concerned with pain, breathing problems, and memory problems than agitation (Shega et al. 2008). Pain and agitation are often reported simultaneously but a strong association was not found (van Dalen-Kok et al. 2015). Anxiety is also frequently reported in people with dementia, but this is also complex and difficult to test, due to an overlap with depression (Seignourel et al. 2008).

As can be seen in the case of Mrs. S, these symptoms and challenges often result in family caregivers acting as proxy, making decisions about the person with dementia's care when there is no advance care plan or in case of an advance care plan to check if the decision is in accordance with the ideas/wishes of the person with dementia. These are very difficult decisions for families as discussed in Sect. 6. One of the most difficult decisions is whether to move the person with dementia into a nursing home; in the case of Mrs. S, the family believe this is in the best interest of Mrs. S; however, they feel guilty about this decision as Mrs. S would like to return home (patient case/vignette part 2).

Patient Case/Vignette Part 4 After a few months in the nursing home, Mrs. S gets a fever, is short of breath, and coughs, and the amounts of fluids and food she takes are less than normal according to the nursing staff. The visiting physician diagnoses pneumonia and wants to talk to the family to discuss if Mrs. S should be sent to a hospital or not.

Mrs. S recovers from pneumonia, but she eats and drinks less every week. She can still walk but she is less stable and has a high risk of falling. She sometimes coughs during the meals. Her son asks if his mother should receive artificial hydration and feeding.

5 Treatment Options of Common Complications

In this section we refer to pharmacological and non-pharmacological treatment options for a variety of complications/symptoms which may arise before the person with dementia is in the dying phase. Later in this chapter (Sect. 9.2), we will discuss treatment in the dying phase.

5.1 Non-pharmacological Treatment Options (Including Spiritual Care)

In recent years person-centered care has been introduced in the care for people with dementia, and more evidence is showing the benefits of nondrug treatment, particularly for behavioral and psychological symptoms in relation to pain. Person-centered care is discussed in more detail later in this chapter in Sect. 7. The care for people with dementia should be multidisciplinary and include spiritual care. Studies show an effect of therapies like music therapy, massage, and aromatherapy, and these should be considered and need to be prioritized in clinical and research settings (Winblad et al. 2016). For example, music therapy has shown a reduction in the short term of depressive symptoms following at least five sessions, but there was little to no effect on agitation or aggression, and the long-term effects are yet to be studied (van der Steen et al. 2017b).

Every time when behavior changes, one has to pay attention to the possibility of medical conditions causing this change, for instance, infections, constipation, bladder retention, pressure sores, pressure sores or infections in the mouth, and side effects of medication, but also, for instance, changes in environment. Regular evaluation in a multidisciplinary team including the nursing staff, psychologist, physiotherapist, social care practitioner, occupational therapist, spiritual care counselor, dietitian, and a physician with evaluation on, among others, behavior, pain, medication, mobility, swallowing, weight change, and incontinence can help improve the quality of care for a person with dementia.

There are several environmental factors which should be considered when caring for someone with dementia. These may range from consideration about the aesthetics of the individuals' room and environment through to consistency of staff. In the home or nursing home, small alterations may help with orientation such as using different colored doors or pictures to help identify different rooms. It is important to ensure continuity of care when delivering palliative care for someone with dementia (van der Steen et al. 2014b). Continuity encompasses, ensuring the individual is able to remain in their preferred place of care with minimal disruption and minimizing the need for transfers between settings, continuity of the provision of care even if there is a transfer, and continuity of staff caring for the individual.

5.2 Pharmacological Treatment Options

Infections in persons with dementia are usually treated following national or regional antibiotic guidelines, like Mrs. S in the patient case/vignette part 3. As the dementia progresses, there should be a process of ongoing discussions as to what to expect from treatment (this may be part of ACP), for instance, antibiotics, and the likelihood of response to treatment. In some cases, a patient may not respond to treatment when they are too sick and are not capable of drinking and eating anymore. The use of antibiotics should be discussed with the family or advocate including the person with dementia if possible; it is viewed differently in different countries. In some countries the families have more influence on treatment decisions, and the practitioner may simply provide choices, whereas in others this may be a medical decision, in discussion with the wider multidisciplinary team and family. Antibiotics can prolong life but sometimes just for several days (van der Steen et al. 2012). See Sect. 6 on controversies and decision-making in this chapter.

When people with dementia are transferred to a hospital, they often receive intravenous treatment with antibiotics or fluid or even tube feeding. This treatment increases at the end of life but practice in different countries varies (Klapwijk et al. 2014; Mitchell et al. 2009), and they also vary over time; for example, there is a decline in feeding tubes used in the USA (Mitchell et al. 2016).

As pain medication, acetaminophen (paracetamol) is often used as a first-line treatment (Hendriks et al. 2015; Sandvik et al. 2016a), followed by the use of opioids to treat more severe pain which is nonreactive to acetaminophen (commonly used, up to 24%) (Hendriks et al. 2015; Pieper et al. 2017; Sandvik et al. 2016a; Griffioen et al. 2017). Antipsychotic drugs are frequently used to treat challenging behavior in dementia, often with no positive result and many adverse effects, like extrapyramidal symptoms, stroke, or death. Research and the EAPC white paper recommend that non-pharmacological treatment (see above) should be tried first for behavior which challenges (van der Steen et al. 2014b). Several other types of medication besides (typical and atypical) antipsychotic drugs are also used to treat neuropsychiatric symptoms: anxiolytics, sedatives, antidepressants, and anti-dementia drugs. More research is needed to gain a better understanding of how and when to start and stop these pharmacological treatments to optimize prescription in people with dementia, including for cases of delirium (Agar et al. 2017). Bronchodilators are often used in the treatment of shortness of breath; studies show different prevalence, ranging from 29% to 67% (Hendriks et al. 2015).

6 Controversies and Decisions

6.1 End-of-Life Decisions

The decisions which need to be made toward the end of life are often medically focused, relating to the complex symptoms which pose a dilemma for practitioners. However, many other nonmedical factors are also important and need to be considered, for example, spiritual care. As discussed in the previous section, difficult decisions both medical and nonmedical can include spiritual care, place of care, cardiopulmonary resuscitation, treatment of infections, management of eating and drinking problems, pain, shortness of breath, behavioral problems and hospitalization, as well as any comorbid conditions. In the case of Mrs. S, as she begins to eat and drink less, the son wishes to discuss the potential use of artificial hydration and feeding (patient case/vignette part 4).

In some countries, many are raising the option of euthanasia for people with dementia. This is legal in a small number of countries including the Netherlands when strict criteria are met, but many physicians are reluctant to fulfill such a preference in the absence of clear communication with the patient.

6.2 Who Should Make the Decisions?

Ultimately, health- and care-based decisions should be made by the individual/patient themselves. However, in many cases, by the time dilemmas such as difficulty with eating and swallowing arise, it is not possible due to a diminished capacity. Hence, the individual does not have the ability to make informed decisions. Despite efforts to increase advance care planning (ACP) with people with dementia, many people reach the end of life without one (see Sect. 3 earlier in this chapter). Some are not ready to have conversations about death and face their own mortality, and decision-making is left to families (Davies et al. 2014). Practitioners rely on families to know the wishes of the individual and to relay these with confidence and accuracy when making end-of-life decisions. However, caution should be taken by practitioners as family caregivers/proxies have been shown to have a low to moderate agreement with the person with dementia about preferences for end-of-life treatments (Harrison Dening et al. 2016). Practitioners should engage closely with families to understand the individuals' previous wishes and work with the family through a shared decision-making process.

6.3 What Gets in the Way of Making Decisions?

Many barriers have been identified by family caregivers/proxies which prevent them from making decisions about end-of-life care, including a lack of information, poor communication, difficult dynamics/conflict within families, limited emotional and practical support, and dynamic care systems (Davies et al. 2014; Lamahewa et al. 2018). Practitioners should provide clear information which is communicated in a sensitive and supportive manner, helping to facilitate the decision-making process. Social care practitioners can also act as mediators in family conflict to encourage supportive family relationships and aid decision-making.

It is not just family caregivers/proxies who have difficulties in making decisions; many practitioners lack the confidence to hold such difficult conversations and shy away from these discussions (Davies et al. 2013; Lamahewa et al. 2018). These difficult conversations require a high level of skill and a vast amount of experience to be conducted sensitively; many practitioners, and even experienced practitioners, dread such conversations. This leaves family caregivers often not knowing how to approach such conversations, being left to make difficult decisions and care plans, with many feeling doubts about their status.

6.4 Approaching Challenging Decisions/Dilemmas

There are relatively few professional guidelines which address end-of-life care for people with dementia. Until recently, many palliative care guidelines have focused on cancer such as the National Institute for Health and Care Excellence (NICE) (England and Wales). Practitioners should consult their national guidelines for both dementia and palliative care (see EAPC Atlas of Palliative Care in Europe), Alzheimer Europe, and consult the EAPC white paper on optimal palliative care for people with dementia (van der Steen et al. 2014b) as discussed in the symptom management, Sect. 4.

A recent practical toolkit for making decisions specific for end-of-life care of people with dementia used in conjunction with available guidance (Davies et al. 2016) consists of a series of heuristics (schematic patterns that can be applied in complex situations and function as prompts to initiate thinking and action) which offer a clinically familiar approach, are brief, are easy to remember, and lead to action. The toolkit covers key decisions including eating and swallowing difficulties, agitation/restlessness, reviewing treatment and interventions at the end of life (e.g., routine medication), and providing routine care at the end of life (e.g., changing dry bedsheets in the final days to hours of life). Examples of the heuristics are given in Figs. 3 and 4 and are discussed below with reference to common dilemmas and controversies.

6.5 Common Decision-Making Dilemmas and Controversies

A number of challenges and controversies around providing end-of-life care for people with dementia have been identified.

6.5.1 Hospitalization

In the process of attempting to manage symptoms and maintain quality of life, many people at the end of life often experience what are termed as avoidable hospital admissions (van der Steen 2010). This description of "avoidable" may be for a number of reasons including the nature and consequences of the condition, such as an infection (van der Steen 2010). These admissions often cause more pain and distress to both the individual and their family than remaining in their normal place of care. It is important, as in the example of Mrs. S (patient case/vignette part 4), to discuss the possibility of hospitalization with the relatives, discuss expectations, and make this decision together. Individuals can go to hospitals which have a focus on cure as opposed to care and may receive what is described as unnecessary tests or aggressive and invasive procedures. Cardiopulmonary resuscitation should be avoided in people with dementia, as it is less likely to be successful in people with dementia compared to those without. CPR can be very distressing for all those involved including both the person with dementia and the families, with those who are successfully resuscitated often being transferred to intensive care and dying a short while later.

6.5.2 Artificial Nutrition and Hydration

A common medical decision toward the end of life (like in the patient case/vignette part 4) is the introduction of artificial feeding when the individual is no longer able to swallow food, liquid, or medication. Many people, families and

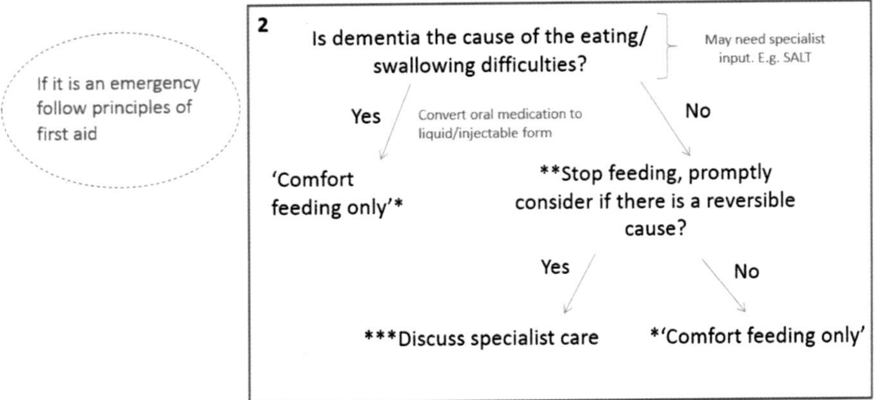

Fig. 3 Heuristic for eating/swallowing difficulties. *Comfort feeding may carry associated risks of aspiration; **Closely observe all intake particularly if changes to swallow function are suspected; ***Consider appropriateness on individual basis (Published with kind permission of © Nathan Davies and Steve Iliffe 2016. All Rights Reserved)

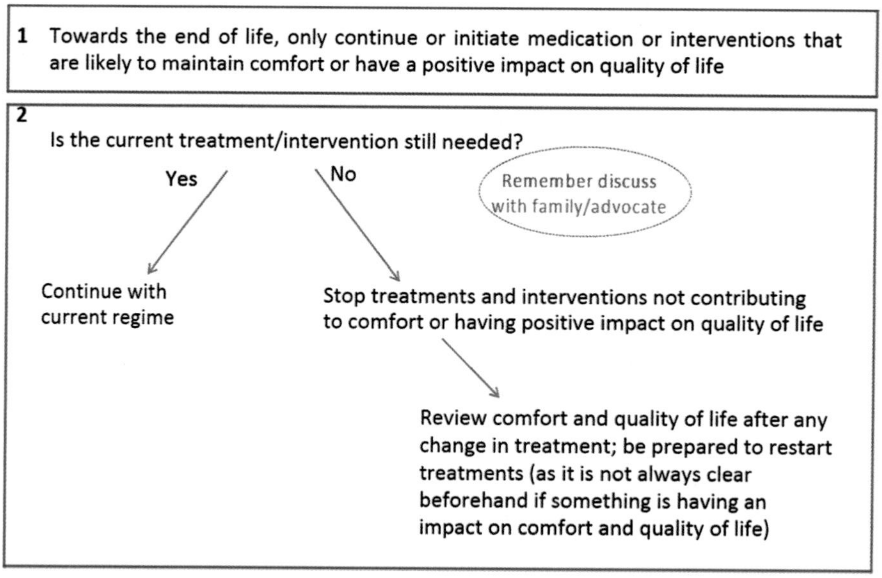

1 Towards the end of life, only continue or initiate medication or interventions that are likely to maintain comfort or have a positive impact on quality of life

2

Is the current treatment/intervention still needed?

Yes → Continue with current regime

No → Stop treatments and interventions not contributing to comfort or having positive impact on quality of life

Remember discuss with family/advocate

→ Review comfort and quality of life after any change in treatment; be prepared to restart treatments (as it is not always clear beforehand if something is having an impact on comfort and quality of life)

Fig. 4 Heuristic for initiating medication and interventions (Published with kind permission of © Nathan Davies and Steve Iliffe 2016. All Rights Reserved)

professional caring teams, believe that they cannot allow the individual to "starve to death," and they feel that the use of artificial feeding will extend life and prevent discomfort or further complications such as aspiration, potentially leading to an improvement in quality of life (Mitchell and Lawson 1999). In the UK, the Netherlands, and many other countries, the adoption of artificial nutrition and hydration has been a controversial topic for some time and remains so. The EAPC recommends that hydration (preferably subcutaneous) should only be provided if appropriate in the management of potentially reversible causes, such as infection, but should not be used in the dying phase when an individual loses their ability to swallow (van der Steen et al. 2014b). However, the EAPC white paper was unable to reach a consensus on this topic with the professionals they consulted, acting only to further highlight the controversy within this topic. It is unclear if rehydration therapy affects discomfort or indeed survival. A study of Italian nursing home patients with advanced dementia demonstrated that for almost all patients treated with intravenous rehydration therapy, the goal of treatment was to reduce symptoms and suffering. Despite this goal, discomfort was high overall, but symptom relief may be improved (van der Steen et al. 2018). More work to explore the effects of rehydration therapy and discomfort is needed.

The EAPC also recommends that permanent artificial feeding, using a gastrostomy or a nasogastric tube, should be avoided (van der Steen et al. 2014b). Careful and skillful hand feeding or comfort feeding should be provided. Comfort feeding refers to the process of eating for pleasure, providing small amounts of food, even though there may be associated risks such as aspiration. Practitioners together with families must balance the risks of feeding with the potential comfort and pleasure that eating may provide for the individual – Fig. 3 illustrates a heuristic which conveys a practical approach to how these decisions can be considered in the case of Mrs. S.

Currently there are no studies which show an association that artificial feeding offers benefits to the individual. On the contrary some studies have demonstrated they increase the chance of infection, aspiration, further complications (Palecek et al. 2010), and potentially mortality (Ticinesi et al. 2016). As with the limited understanding of pain in dementia, we similarly have a limited understanding around feelings of hunger and thirst in people with dementia. Data in the USA indicates a reduction in the use of feeding tubes in people with dementia (Mitchell et al. 2016).

6.5.3 Medication: Antimicrobial Treatment

The ability of antimicrobial treatment for recurrent infections in people with dementia to extend life or improve comfort is not well understood; however, some studies have demonstrated increased survival following antimicrobial treatment compared to no treatment or a palliative approach (van der Steen et al. 2012). The use of antimicrobials including oral, intramuscular, and intravenous for pneumonia has increased survival but was also associated with more symptoms reported in retrospect in the period from before to after the pneumonia in a nursing home population with advanced dementia (Givens et al. 2010). However, this was in the USA, where people with dementia and pneumonia with fewer symptoms were more likely not to be treated with antibiotics (van der Steen 2011). Another study used discomfort observed by independent, blinded observers measured with validated tools after antibiotic treatment, and discomfort levels were lower after antibiotic treatment (van der Steen 2011). A more recent study with the same strong methods showed that, with more symptom-relieving treatment provided, antibiotics were no longer associated with discomfort (van der Maaden et al. 2016). Antimicrobial use might be more beneficial for people in the earlier stages of dementia compared to the later stages, with no difference in mortality at in more advanced dementia between those receiving antimicrobial treatment and palliation and those not (Fabiszewski et al. 1990). Some studies have shown that increased survival after antibiotic treatment, but this may only last for a few days in some cases (van der Steen et al. 2012), which may be simply prolonging the dying process (van der Steen et al. 2012). Antimicrobial treatment is associated with renal failure, diarrhea, the use of intravenous lines, and skin rashes. After nearly 25 years of research investigating the effectiveness of antimicrobial treatment for people with dementia, the effects (benefits and adverse effects) are still unclear.

It is important to identify the source of the infection which may be causing symptoms such as fever and balance the benefits of treatment with the potential side effects and consequences. The EAPC recommends that antibiotics are appropriate for treating infections which have a goal of increasing comfort, but life-prolonging effects should be considered carefully (van der Steen et al. 2014b). This can be demonstrated through the heuristic in Fig. 4.

6.5.4 Other Medications

Treatments with other medications for preventive or symptomatic use can cause dilemmas too. Acetylcholinesterase inhibitors, HMG-CoA reductase inhibitors (statins), antihypertensive drugs, antihyperglycemic drugs, and anticoagulants are prescribed often in people with advanced dementia, but many medical guidelines provide an understanding of initiating such treatments but often do not include when and how to stop them. Discontinuation should be considered, but it can be difficult to determine what the effect can be and if stopping will contribute to a better quality of life (see Fig. 4); however, it can reduce the risks of side effects and drug interaction. Multidisciplinary meetings, medication review, and educational programs can help to improve appropriate medication use for people with advanced dementia in nursing homes.

7 Person-Centered Care

For many, being viewed as a person and treated with respect and dignity is, in addition to good symptom management, fundamental to a good death. This is consistent with what experts regard as the most important domains in palliative care with dementia: optimal treatment of symptoms and providing comfort and person-centered care, communication, and shared decision-making (van der Steen et al. 2014b). It can be argued that person-centered care is always important, but it may help to emphasize its importance in patients at risk of not being seen as a person anymore, which is the case with advanced dementia or when patients are not very responsive due to illness or at the end of life. Indeed, with admission to a nursing home, for example, as is the case with Mrs. S, family caregivers may be concerned that staff do not know the patient well enough to provide person-centered care, and as they live in a nursing home, they continue to lose their identity and may struggle to maintain this identity which is so important to person-centered care (Davies et al. 2017).

8 Family Caregivers of People with Dementia

8.1 Importance of Family Caregivers

An estimated 46.8 million people are living with dementia worldwide (Alzheimer's Disease International 2015), many of whom will be cared for by family caregivers and can be referred to as lay carers, untrained carers, informal carers, caregivers, or proxies. In the UK the Alzheimer's Society has insisted that without the help and support of family caregivers, the formal care system would collapse. Traditionally there are distinct boundaries between caregivers and the cared for. Caring in palliative care however may differ from caring for someone with a nonterminal physical or intellectual impairment. The boundary between the "caregiver" and the "cared for" is said to be somewhat blurred, because of the increasing need for support for the individual from the caregiver in palliative care. The caregiving career involves a variety of tasks in addition to meeting the physical and mental needs of the person with dementia. These include interaction with health and social care professionals, doing daily household chores, and escorting the person with dementia to various medical, dental, optical, and hairdressing appointments.

8.2 Effects of Caring for Someone with Dementia

It is well known that caring in general can be a stressful role and that the burden placed on the individual caregiver is often great, with limited opportunity to have breaks, socialize, and have whatever one may classify as a "normal" life. However, caring for an older person or a relative with dementia is thought to be one of the most stressful and difficult forms of caring. Caregivers as described in the portraits by Sanders and colleagues face the difficulty of coming to terms with the diagnosis and the loss of the person they once knew (Sanders et al. 2009). They may find difficulties with the individual's behavioral and cognitive decline, the loss of their own "normal" life, the role of caring, and finally the eventual death of the person. Uncertainty of death and the treatment options for people with dementia can lead to feelings of guilt among family caregivers; this is illustrated in patient case/vignette part 2. Caregivers of people with dementia have higher rates of various health problems, both physical and psychological, including depression and cardiovascular problems, resulting in increased doctor visits and an economical burden on health-care services, with a higher risk of mortality (Brodaty and Donkin 2009).

8.3 Supporting Caregivers

The lack of definitive split between the person with dementia and the caregiver can be conceptualized as what Twigg termed as carers as co-clients (Twigg 1989). Despite caregivers being seen as having a caring "career," the experience is not the same for all. Something which is often forgotten or not considered is that not all caregivers are loved by their relatives and conversely can be mistakenly labeled as "loved ones." The caregiver may endure a trajectory of caring from the encounter stage, where they are coming to terms with both the diagnosis of dementia and also their new role, moving onto an enduring stage at which point the caring intensity increases, through to the exit stage where they face the death of the individual and adapting to their new life (Lindgren 1993). As we discussed in Sect. 2 of this chapter, palliative care may cover all stages of this "caregiving career," and each individual caregiver may require more or less support at various stages

(Davies et al. 2014). A thorough caregiver's assessment should be completed with the family caregiver of the person with dementia, to identify their needs and levels of support required. This should be a holistic assessment considering medical as well as psychosocial aspects of care and support.

8.4 Grief, Loss, and Bereavement

Grief and loss when someone dies is to be expected with most people and is considered a normal response to death. Grief has been defined as "the reaction to the perception of loss with symptoms including yearning, sadness, anger, guilt, regret, anxiety, loneliness, fatigue, shock, numbness, positive feelings and a variety of physical symptoms unique to the individual" (Rando 2000).

Throughout the course of dementia, family caregivers may be experiencing a series of multiple losses, for example, loss of intimacy, companionship, control, personal freedom, and well-being among them (Chan et al. 2013). These losses can be described as part of anticipatory grief, that is, grief which occurs before the death of the individual (Rando 2000). Anticipatory grief occurs in 47–71% of family caregivers of people with dementia (Chan et al. 2013). The sometimes long projected course of dementia means that anticipating the death of the individual and ambiguity of what the future holds can be common among family caregivers. Anticipatory grief has been shown to have an association with depression, and depression is increased with anticipatory grief (Sanders and Adams 2005). However, some studies have suggested that what appears as clinical depression may actually be a grief reaction (Sanders and Adams 2005). Other factors which appear positively associated with increasing anticipatory grief include burden, non-English primary language in English-speaking countries, living with the person with dementia prior to being placed in a care home, and less satisfaction with care (Chan et al. 2013).

Grief appears to be more severe during the moderate to severe stages of dementia (Chan et al. 2013). However, as suggested, the needs of individual caregivers may differ, and this may also relate to their response to grief and loss. Individual caregivers may experience grief at different stages, and this should be carefully considered when supporting family caregivers. In particular, there may be a marked difference between spouses and adult children responding differently at different stages. Adult children appear to experience minimal grief in the early stages of dementia, most intense at the moderate stage, and the grief lessens toward the advanced stages with feelings of relief when the individual moves into a nursing home, for example. For spouses, grief appears to reflect a linear pattern increasing as dementia progresses; however, another work has suggested grief remains stable in advanced dementia and therefore may not continue to increase for all (Givens et al. 2011). It is important to reassure caregivers that relief after death is common and they should not feel guilty about this feeling; it can be part of the post-death grieving process (Chan et al. 2013). For some, grief may continue for some time after death, termed complicated grief if more than 6 months; this is termed as *persistent complex bereavement disorder* in the DSM-5, marked by an individual "incapacitated" by grief affecting their daily life.

Particular consideration and attention may be needed toward male caregivers who can find it difficult to openly accept their feelings of grief, strain, and distress (Sanders et al. 2003). Grief in some may be expressed in different ways or using different language, for example, portraying emotional dissociation from the person with dementia (Sanders et al. 2003). Males often have less stable social support networks and are less likely to seek assistance in dealing with their grief than females. This may be particularly pertinent in spouse male caregivers, who may be older and for whom grief may be particularly challenging, as they come to deal with the emotions associated with being alone at a time when their own social networks will be dwindling (Sanders et al. 2003).

In addition to regular caregiver assessments and reviews as mentioned, post-bereavement support should be offered to families (van der Steen et al. 2014b), including helping them adjust to a life of post-caring when much of this previous world will have disappeared. This may include as in the case of Mrs. S patient case/vignette part 5 a meeting at the nursing home with the family after their relative has died. Practitioners should identify caregivers who are at increased risk of grief (anticipatory, normal, and complicated grief), such as those with high levels of burden and depression, offering caregiver support at an early stage.

8.5 What Do Caregivers Want from Care?

The individuality of caregivers is not only reflected in the needs of them as a caregiver but also in their views of how palliative and end-of-life care should be provided for someone with dementia. Caregivers' views regarding the appropriate treatment in particular referring to the dilemmas discussed in Sect. 6 of this chapter lie on a spectrum of beliefs from provision of care purely aimed at comfort by relieving symptoms through to active/invasive/aggressive treatment which is aimed at "cure" (Davies et al. 2014). It is important to reflect on the stage of the dementia and provide information and education to family caregivers as to the progression of dementia (see Fig. 1) and appropriate treatment options (van der Steen et al. 2014b). However, it is also important to acknowledge that there is a great deal of diversity when families want to receive the information (individual and between countries). When considering families' views, there should be a recognition that they may not have the complex medical knowledge that many practitioners have and this may be their first experience caring for someone who is dying. Caregivers may focus on the psychosocial aspects of care as their main priorities (Davies et al. 2017). This is important to emphasize as we discussed previously that not all decisions are medically focused.

Patient Case/Vignette Part 5 Mrs. S gets weaker and is not able to walk anymore. She has lost a lot of weight in the past few months. She gets another case of pneumonia, is in bed all day, and doesn't eat or drink anything anymore; the nurses think that Mrs. S is going to die this time. For the daughter of Mrs. S, this comes as a surprise. The physician and the nursing staff make all sorts of arrangements, for example, on pain relief, treatment in case of shortness of breath, and prevention of pressure ulcers and constipation. A spiritual counselor is asked by the nursing home to visit Mrs. S. Mrs. S's daughter stays with her mother all the time. She frequently asks when her mother is going to die. After 3 days and nights, Mrs. S dies in the presence of her daughter.

A few weeks after the death of Mrs. S, the family is invited to attend a meeting with the nursing staff and the physician. They talk about the stay of their mother in the nursing home and the final days to death.

9 Dying with Dementia

A prognosis is very difficult to provide to a person with dementia (Brown et al. 2013). With the disease comes a decline in cognitive functioning, but it is very difficult to predict if a person with dementia is in the last months of life, whereas with cancer patients, end of life seems more predictable. People do not always reach the last phase of dementia, and about half of people with dementia may die before the advanced stages (Hendriks et al. 2016). In people with cancer and dementia, a high number of symptoms are found while dying in various settings, such as a hospice and nursing home. In the USA hospice generally refers to hospice care as a service. In many other countries across the world, such as the UK, a hospice is a physical building which delivers palliative care (see Fig. 2); however, few people with dementia will receive care here (Reyniers et al. 2015).

The 6-month mortality rate in nursing homes is high and often higher than anticipated (van der Steen et al. 2007). The most frequent causes of death are respiratory infections or cardiovascular disorders, and in later stages, people are often more dehydrated and cachectic due to eating/swallowing difficulties like Mrs. S in the patient case/vignette part 5 (Hendriks et al. 2014). Also in the earlier stages of dementia, there is an association between eating and drinking less and mortality (Hendriks et al. 2016).

Many people with dementia die in a nursing home, but the numbers differ between countries related to the available system of care for people with dementia. In some countries a large proportion of people will still die in a hospital (Reyniers et al. 2015). The different journeys from home to sometimes hospital, nursing home or hospice to death, and the increased need for palliative specialist care are shown in Fig. 2.

Prognosis for someone with dementia is difficult; however, the prediction of short-term mortality, for example, 1 week, is much more accurate (Casarett et al. 2012; Klapwijk et al. 2014). Even when death is expected within days, it is not possible to predict when exactly someone is going to die such as in the case of Mrs. S (patient case/vignette part 5).

Many studies on the last days of life of dementia show often burdensome symptoms like pain or shortness of breath, and this is also indicated by relatives, who in many cases experience death as a struggle. Only 50% of the relatives perceive death as peaceful in a Dutch study (De Roo et al. 2014).

In the literature a minority of nursing home residents with advanced dementia enter or are transferred to a hospice (Reyniers et al. 2015), but this also depends on available care system and the care that is required; not all people with dementia will require a hospice placement (see Fig. 2). Hospice care is often more for symptomatic treatment, often scheduled treatment of pain and shortness of breath. All people with dementia should get good quality of care at the end of life, not only in a hospice.

9.1 Symptoms in the Dying Phase

Several studies on the last days of life with dementia show high percentages of pain in the days before death, ranging from 15% to 78%; however, there are differences among studies, possibly also due to different measurement scales or methods (Hendriks et al. 2014, 2015; Klapwijk et al. 2014; Sandvik et al. 2016b). There is a high prevalence of shortness of breath in people with dementia increasing in the period to death sometimes even to 80% of people (Hendriks et al. 2015; Klapwijk et al. 2014; van der Steen 2010). Different behaviors are seen in the days before death. People are often in bed and can be unconscious. Restless behavior, anxiety, and agitation are seen in several studies, and also delirium has been reported (Hendriks et al. 2014, 2015; Vandervoort et al. 2013; Mitchell et al. 2009).

9.2 Treatment Options

9.2.1 Non-pharmacological Treatment Options (Including Spiritual Care)

Many of the non-pharmacological treatment options as described in Sect. 5.2 can also be used in the last days before death. The Namaste Care program, offering meaningful activities by a trained nursing assistant in nursing homes for people with advanced dementia, specifically describes the use of the program for the dying phase (Volicer and Simard 2015).

When a person with dementia reaches the dying phase, nursing staff and medical team should pay close attention to prevent constipation, bladder retention, and pressure sores. Regular mouth care should be started. People should be offered drinks and food, but it should not be forced upon them. The medication should be evaluated, and if oral medication can't be swallowed, it should be stopped. Regular evaluation of pain, shortness of breath, or discomfort is needed; observational instruments for pain or discomfort can be used in this phase, for example, the Discomfort Scale-Dementia of Alzheimer Type (DS-DAT) (Hurley et al. 1992). The presence of a pacemaker or implantable cardioverter defibrillator (ICD) should be checked, and in case one of these is present, it should be explained what to do to nursing staff and family.

It is important to highlight the needs of people are individual and some people have personal needs and may want spiritual counseling. Spiritual counseling is often overlooked; a study from a UK hospital showed that the religious beliefs of people with dementia were documented less than those without dementia (Sampson et al. 2006). Spiritual care has been associated with an improved perception of quality of care from families at the end of life (Daaleman et al. 2008) and families' satisfaction with physicians' communication shortly after admission to a nursing home (van der Steen et al. 2014a).

It is very important for the nursing staff and medical team to explain the course of symptoms and possible treatment options to the family (including the presence of Cheyne-Stokes respiration, rattle, and time of death) and to make a clear description of medication with explanation what to give when and also if necessary extra medication which can be given. It is vital to include families as much as possible and to ask for the wishes of the family, when the team should contact the family and who. An end-of-life care plan can help to improve communication and care in the last days of life (Detering et al. 2010).

9.2.2 Pharmacological Treatment Options

Pain and shortness of breath are often treated with opioids; a high percentage of people use opioids on the last day before death, often requiring an increase on the last day (Hendriks et al. 2014, 2015; Klapwijk et al. 2014; Sandvik et al. 2016b). Agitation is treated with anxiolytics, but also palliative sedation may be initiated, with a Dutch study demonstrating palliative sedation was started in around 21% of cases (Hendriks et al. 2014, 2015).

Response to opioids should be closely monitored when prescribed for pain or shortness of breath to ensure effective response without excessive side effects. Special caution should be taken when prescribing for patients with renal failure as there is a risk of accumulation of renally excreted opioids.

Death rattle is sometimes treated with hyoscine (also known as scopolamine) subcutaneously; however, evidence is limited with a lack of consensus on the best approach (van der Maaden et al. 2015).

10 Conclusion

As this chapter demonstrates, palliative care for people with dementia shows similarities to palliative care for people with other conditions such as cancer in particular with relation to symptoms. However, there are also differences which make palliative care for people with dementia unique, including communication difficulties with the individual, recognition of dementia as a terminal illness, and large elements of uncertainty in several areas including patient wishes and prognosis. Advance care planning is important for people with dementia. Person-centered care should be adopted throughout the care journey, but in this chapter, we have also highlighted the importance of family caregivers. Families should be involved in care decisions and processes, but also we highlight their need for care themselves, as such palliative care for people with dementia is not a dyad relationship of health and care team and the person with dementia but a triad of the person with dementia, family, and the health and care team.

References

Agar MR, Lawlor PG, Quinn S, Draper B, Caplan GA, Rowett D, Sanderson C, Hardy J, Le B, Eckermann S, Mccaffrey N, Devilee L, Fazekas B, Hill M, Currow DC. Efficacy of oral risperidone, haloperidol, or placebo for symptoms of delirium among patients in palliative care: a randomized clinical trial. JAMA Intern Med. 2017; 177(1):34–42.

Alzheimer's Disease International. World Alzheimer report 2015: the global impact of dementia: an analysis of prevalence, incidence, cost and trends. In: Alzheimer's Disease International editors. London; 2015.

Boorsma M, Joling KJ, Frijters DH, Ribbe ME, Nijpels G, Van Hout HP. The prevalence, incidence and risk factors for delirium in Dutch nursing homes and residential care homes. Int J Geriatr Psychiatry. 2012;27: 709–15.

Borsje P, Wetzels RB, Lucassen PL, Pot AM, Koopmans RT. The course of neuropsychiatric symptoms in community-dwelling patients with dementia: a systematic review. Int Psychogeriatr. 2015;27:385–405.

Brodaty H, Donkin M. Family caregivers of people with dementia. Dialogues Clin Neurosci. 2009;11: 217–28.

Brown MA, Sampson EL, Jones L, Barron AM. Prognostic indicators of 6-month mortality in elderly people with advanced dementia: a systematic review. Palliat Med. 2013;27:389–400.

Casarett DJ, Farrington S, Craig T, Slattery J, Harrold J, Oldanie B, Roy J, Biehl R, Teno J. The art versus science of predicting prognosis: can a prognostic index predict short-term mortality better than experienced nurses do? J Palliat Med. 2012;15:703–8.

Cerejeira J, Lagarto L, Mukaetova-Ladinska EB. Behavioral and psychological symptoms of dementia. Front Neurol. 2012;3:73.

Chan D, Livingston G, Jones L, Sampson EL. Grief reactions in dementia carers: a systematic review. Int J Geriatr Psychiatry. 2013;28:1–17.

Daaleman TP, Williams CS, Hamilton VL, Zimmerman S. Spiritual care at the end of life in long-term care. Med Care. 2008;46:85–91.

Davies N, Maio L, Van Riet Paap J, Mariani E, Jaspers B, Sommerbakk R, Grammatico D, Manthorpe J, Ahmedzai S, Vernooij-Dassen M, Iliffe S. Quality palliative care for cancer and dementia in five European countries: some common challenges. Aging Ment Health. 2013;18:400–10.

Davies N, Maio L, Rait G, Iliffe S. Quality end-of-life care for dementia: what have family carers told us so far? A narrative synthesis. Palliat Med. 2014;28:919–30.

Davies N, Mathew R, Wilcock J, Manthorpe J, Sampson EL, Lamahewa K, Iliffe S. A co-design process developing heuristics for practitioners providing end of life care for people with dementia. BMC Palliat Care. 2016;15:68.

Davies N, Rait G, Maio L, Iliffe S. Family caregivers' conceptualisation of quality end-of-life care for people with dementia: a qualitative study. Palliat Med. 2017; 31(8): 726–733.

De Roo ML, Van der Steen JT, Galindo Garre F, Van den Noortgate N, Onwuteaka-Philipsen BD, Deliens L, Francke AL. When do people with dementia die peacefully? An analysis of data collected prospectively in long-term care settings. Palliat Med. 2014;28: 210–9.

Detering KM, Hancock AD, Reade MC, Silvester W. The impact of advance care planning on end of life care in elderly patients: randomised controlled trial. Br Med J. 2010;340:c1345 https://doi.org/10.1136/bmj.c1345.

Dixon J, Knapp M. The effectiveness of advance care planning in improving end of life outcomes for people with dementia and their carers: a systematic review and critical discussion. J Pain Symptom Manage. 2018;55(1):132–150.

Durepos P, Wickson-Griffiths A, Hazzan AA, Kaasalainen S, Vastis V, Battistella L, Papaioannou A. Assessing palliative care content in dementia care guidelines: a systematic review. J Pain Symptom Manag. 2017;53: 804–13.

Ellis-Smith C, Evans CJ, Bone AE, Henson LA, Dzingina M, Kane PM, Higginson IJ, Daveson BA. Measures to assess commonly experienced symptoms for people with dementia in long-term care settings: a systematic review. BMC Med. 2016;14:38.

Fabiszewski KJ, Volicer B, Volicer L. Effect of antibiotic treatment on outcome of fevers in institutionalized Alzheimer patients. J Am Med Assoc. 1990;263: 3168–72.

Fick DM, Agostini JV, Inouye SK. Delirium superimposed on dementia: a systematic review. J Am Geriatr Soc. 2002;50:1723–32.

Gill TM, Gahbauer EA, Han L, Allore HG. Trajectories of disability in the last year of life. N Engl J Med. 2010;362:1173–80.

Givens JL, Jones RN, Shaffer ML, Kiely DK, Mitchell SL. Survival and comfort after treatment of pneumonia in advanced dementia. Arch Intern Med. 2010;170: 1102–7.

Givens JL, Prigerson HG, Kiely DK, Shaffer ML, Mitchell SL. Grief among family members of nursing home residents with advanced dementia. Am J Geriatr Psychiatry. 2011;19:543–50.

Griffioen C, Willems EG, Husebo BS, Achterberg WP. Prevalence of the use of opioids for treatment of pain in persons with a cognitive impairment compared with cognitively intact persons: a systematic review. Curr Alzheimer Res. 2017;14:512–22.

Haasum Y, Fastbom J, Fratiglioni L, Kåreholt I, Johnell K. Pain treatment in elderly persons with and without dementia. Drugs Aging. 2011;28:283–93.

Harrison Dening K, King M, Jones L, Vickestaff V, Sampson EL. Advance care planning in dementia: do family carers know the treatment preferences of people with early dementia? PLoS One. 2016;11:e0159056.

Harrison Dening K, Greenish W, Jones L, Mandal U, Sampson EL. Barriers to providing end-of-life care for people with dementia: a whole-system qualitative study. BMJ Support Palliat Care. 2012;2:103–7.

Hendriks SA, Smalbrugge M, Hertogh CM, Van der Steen JT. Dying with dementia: symptoms, treatment, and quality of life in the last week of life. J Pain Symptom Manag. 2014;47:710–20.

Hendriks SA, Smalbrugge M, Galindo-Garre F, Hertogh CM, Van der Steen JT. From admission to death: prevalence and course of pain, agitation, and shortness of breath, and treatment of these symptoms in nursing home residents with dementia. J Am Med Dir Assoc. 2015;16:475–81.

Hendriks SA, Smalbrugge M, Van Gageldonk-Lafeber AB, Galindo-Garre F, Schipper M, Hertogh CM, Van der Steen JT. Pneumonia, intake problems, and survival among nursing home residents with variable stages of dementia in the Netherlands: results from a prospective observational study. Alzheimer Dis Assoc Disord. 2016;31(3):200–208.

Henry C., Seymour J.. Advance care planning: a guide for health and social care staff. In: National Council For Palliative Care, editors. London; 2007.

Hurley AC, Volicer BJ, Hanrahan PA, Houde S, Volicer L. Assessment of discomfort in advanced Alzheimer patients. Res Nurs Health. 1992;15:369–77.

Jones K, Birchley G, Huxtable R, Clare L, Walter T, Dixon J. End of life care: a scoping review of experiences of advance care planning for people with dementia. Dementia (London). 2016.

Klapwijk MS, Caljouw MA, Van Soest-Poortvliet MC, Van der Steen JT, Achterberg WP. Symptoms and treatment when death is expected in dementia patients in long-term care facilities. BMC Geriatr. 2014;14:99.

Lamahewa K, Mathew R, Iliffe S, Wilcock J, Manthorpe J, Sampson EL, Davies N. A qualitative study exploring the difficulties influencing decision-making at the end-of-life for people with dementia. Health Expect. 2018;21:118–127.

Lindgren CL. The caregiver career. J Nurs Scholarsh. 1993;25:214–9.

Lövheim H, Karlsson S, Gustafson Y. The use of central nervous system drugs and analgesics among very old people with and without dementia. Pharmacoepidemiol Drug Saf. 2008;17:912–8.

Mitchell SL, Lawson FM. Decision-making for long-term tube-feeding in cognitively impaired elderly people. Can Med Assoc J. 1999;160:1705–9.

Mitchell SL, Teno JM, Kiely DK, Shaffer ML, Jones RN, Prigerson HG, Volicer L, Givens JL, Hamel MB. The clinical course of advanced dementia. N Engl J Med. 2009;361:1529–38.

Mitchell SL, Mor V, Gozalo PL, Servadio JL, Teno JM. Tube feeding in us nursing home residents with advanced dementia, 2000–2014. JAMA. 2016;316:769–70.

Morandi A, Mccurley J, Vasilevskis EE, Fick DM, Bellelli G, Lee P, Jackson JC, Shenkin SD, Marcotrabucchi, Schnelle J, Inouye SK, Ely EW, Maclullich A. Tools to detect delirium superimposed on dementia: a systematic review. J Am Geriatr Soc. 2012;60:2005–13.

Morandi A, Han JH, Meagher D, Vasilevskis E, Cerejeira J, Hasemann W, Maclullich AMJ, Annoni G, Trabucchi M, Bellelli G. Detecting delirium superimposed on dementia: evaluation of the diagnostic performance of the Richmond agitation and sedation scale. J Am Med Dir Assoc. 2016;17:828–33.

Nakanishi M, Nakashima T, Shindo Y, Miyamoto Y, Gove D, Radbruch L, Van der Steen JT. An evaluation of palliative care contents in national dementia strategies in reference to the European Association for Palliative Care white paper. Int Psychogeriatr. 2015;27:1551–61.

Palecek EJ, Teno JM, Casarett DJ, Hanson LC, Rhodes RL, Mitchell SL. Comfort feeding only: a proposal to bring clarity to decision-making regarding difficulty with eating for persons with advanced dementia. J Am Geriatr Soc. 2010;58:580–4.

Pieper MJ, Van der Steen JT, Francke AL, Scherder EJ, Twisk JW, Achterberg WP. Effects on pain of a stepwise multidisciplinary intervention (STA OP!) that targets pain and behavior in advanced dementia: a cluster randomized controlled trial. Palliat Med. 2017:269216316689237.

Rait G., Walters K., Bottomley C., Petersen I., Iliffe S., Nazareth I.. Survival of people with clinical diagnosis of dementia in primary care: cohort study. BMJ. 2010; 341.

Rando TA. Clinical dimensions of anticipatory mourning: theory and practice in working with the dying, their loved ones, and their caregivers. Champaign: Research Press; 2000.

Reyniers T, Deliens L, Pasman HR, Morin L, Addington-Hall J, Frova L, Cardenas-Turanzas M, Onwuteaka-Philipsen B, Naylor W, Ruiz-Ramos M, Wilson DM, Loucka M, Csikos A, Rhee YJ, Teno J, Cohen J, Houttekier D. International variation in place of death of older people who died from dementia in 14 European and non-European countries. J Am Med Dir Assoc. 2015;16:165–71.

Robinson L, Dickinson C, Rousseau N, Beyer F, Clark A, Hughes J, Howel D, Exley C. A systematic review of the effectiveness of advance care planning interventions for people with cognitive impairment and dementia. Age Ageing. 2012;41:263–9.

Sampson EL, Gould V, Lee D, Blanchard MR. Differences in care received by patients with and without dementia who died during acute hospital admission: a retrospective case note study. Age Ageing. 2006;35:187–9.

Sampson E, Mandal U, Holman A, Greenish W, Dening KH, Jones L. Improving end of life care for people with dementia: a rapid participatory appraisal. BMJ Support Palliat Care. 2012;2:108–14.

Sanders S, Adams KB. Grief reactions and depression in caregivers of individuals with Alzheimer's disease: results from a pilot study in an urban setting. Health Soc Work. 2005;30:287–95.

Sanders S, Morano C, Corley CS. The expressions of loss and grief among male caregivers of individuals with Alzheimer's disease. J Gerontol Soc Work. 2003;39:3–18.

Sanders S, Butcher HK, Swails P, Power J. Portraits of caregivers of end-stage dementia patients receiving hospice care. Death Stud. 2009;33:521–56.

Sandvik R, Selbaek G, Kirkevold O, Aarsland D, Husebo BS. Analgesic prescribing patterns in Norwegian nursing homes from 2000 to 2011: trend analyses of four data samples. Age Ageing. 2016a;45:54–60.

Sandvik RK, Selbaek G, Bergh S, Aarsland D, Husebo BS. Signs of imminent dying and change in symptom intensity during pharmacological treatment in dying nursing home patients: a prospective trajectory study. J Am Med Dir Assoc. 2016b;17:821–7.

Seignourel PJ, Kunik ME, Snow L, Wilson N, Stanley M. Anxiety in dementia: a critical review. Clin Psychol Rev. 2008;28:1071–82.

Shega JW, Hougham GW, Stocking CB, Cox-Hayley D, Sachs GA. Patients dying with dementia: experience at the end of life and impact of hospice care. J Pain Symptom Manag. 2008;35:499–507.

Ticinesi A, Nouvenne A, Lauretani F, Prati B, Cerundolo N, Maggio M, Meschi T. Survival in older adults with dementia and eating problems: to PEG or not to PEG? Clin Nutr. 2016;35:1512–6.

Twigg J. Models of carers: how do social care agencies conceptualise their relationship with informal carers. J Soc Policy. 1989;18:53–66.

Van Dalen-Kok AH, Pieper MJ, De Waal MW, Lukas A, Husebo BS, Achterberg WP. Association between pain, neuropsychiatric symptoms, and physical function in dementia: a systematic review and meta-analysis. BMC Geriatr. 2015;15:49.

Van der Maaden T, Van der Steen JT, De Vet HC, Achterberg WP, Boersma F, Schols JM, Van Berkel

JF, Mehr DR, Arcand M, Hoepelman AI, Koopmans RT, Hertogh CM. Development of a practice guideline for optimal symptom relief for patients with pneumonia and dementia in nursing homes using a Delphi study. Int J Geriatr Psychiatry. 2015;30:487–96.

Van der Maaden T, Van der Steen JT, de Vet HC, Hertogh CM, Koopmans RT. Prospective observations of discomfort, pain, and Dyspnea in nursing home residents with dementia and pneumonia. J Am Med Dir Assoc. 2016;17:128–35.

Van der Steen JT. Dying with dementia: what we know after more than a decade of research. J Alzheimers Dis. 2010;22:37–55.

Van der Steen JT. Prolonged life and increased symptoms vs prolonged dying and increased comfort after antibiotic treatment in patients with dementia and pneumonia. Arch Intern Med. 2011;171:93–4.

Van der Steen JT, Mitchell SL, Frijters DH, Kruse RL, Ribbe MW. Prediction of 6-month mortality in nursing home residents with advanced dementia: validity of a risk score. J Am Med Dir Assoc. 2007;8:464–8.

Van der Steen JT, Lane P, Kowall NW, Knol DL, Volicer L. Antibiotics and mortality in patients with lower respiratory infection and advanced dementia. J Am Med Dir Assoc. 2012;13:156–61.

Van der Steen JT, Onwuteaka-Philipsen BD, Knol DL, Ribbe MW, Deliens L. Caregivers' understanding of dementia predicts patients' comfort at death: a prospective observational study. BMC Med. 2013;11:105.

Van der Steen JT, Gijsberts M-JH, Hertogh CM, Deliens L. Predictors of spiritual care provision for patients with dementia at the end of life as perceived by physicians: a prospective study. BMC Palliat Care. 2014a;13:61.

Van der Steen JT, Radbruch L, Hertogh CM, de Boer ME, Hughes JC, Larkin P, Francke AL, Junger S, Gove D, Firth P, Koopmans RT, Volicer L. White paper defining optimal palliative care in older people with dementia: a Delphi study and recommendations from the European Association for Palliative Care. Palliat Med. 2014b;28:197–209.

Van der Steen JT, Van Soest-Poortvliet MC, Hallie-Heierman M, Onwuteaka-Philipsen BD, Deliens L, de Boer ME, Van den Block L, Van Uden N, Hertogh CM, de Vet HC. Factors associated with initiation of advance care planning in dementia: a systematic review. J Alzheimers Dis. 2014c;40:743–57.

Van der Steen JT, Deliens L, Koopmans RT, Onwuteaka-Philipsen BD. Physicians' perceptions of suffering in people with dementia at the end of life. Palliat Support Care. 2017a;15(5):587-599.

Van der Steen JT, Van Soest-Poortvliet MC, Van der Wouden JC, Bruinsma MS, Scholten RJPM, Vink AC. Music-based therapeutic interventions for people with dementia. Cochrane Database Syst Rev. 2017b;5:CD003477.

Van der Steen JT, Giulio PD, Giunco F, Monti M, Gentile S, Vaillani D, Finetti S, Pettenati F, Charrier L, Toscani F. Pneumonia in nursing home patients with advanced dementia: decisions, intravenous rehydration therapy, and discomfort. Am J Hosp Palliat Med. 2018;35(3):423–430.

Van Soest-Poortvliet MC, Van der Steen JT, Gutschow G, Deliens L, Onwuteaka-Philipsen BD, de Vet HC, Hertogh CM. Advance care planning in nursing home patients with dementia: a qualitative interview study among family and professional caregivers. J Am Med Dir Assoc. 2015;16:979–89.

Vandervoort A, Van den Block L, Van der Steen JT, Volicer L, Vander Stichele R, Houttekier D, Deliens L. Nursing home residents dying with dementia in Flanders, Belgium: a nationwide postmortem study on clinical characteristics and quality of dying. J Am Med Dir Assoc. 2013;14:485–92.

Volicer L, Simard J. Palliative care and quality of life for people with dementia: medical and psychosocial interventions. Int Psychogeriatr. 2015;27:1623–34.

Winblad B, Amouyel P, Andrieu S, Ballard C, Brayne C, Brodaty H, Cedazo-Minguez A, Dubois B, Edvardsson D, Feldman H, Fratiglioni L, Frisoni GB, Gauthier S, Georges J, Graff C, Iqbal K, Jessen F, Johansson G, Jonsson L, Kivipelto M, Knapp M, Mangialasche F, Melis R, Nordberg A, Rikkert MO, Qiu C, Sakmar TP, Scheltens P, Schneider LS, Sperling R, Tjernberg LO, Waldemar G, Wimo A, Zetterberg H. Defeating Alzheimer's disease and other dementias: a priority for European science and society. Lancet Neurol. 2016;15:455–532.

Palliative Care and Stroke

60

Peter Eastman and Brian Le

Contents

Abstract

There have been significant advances in the prevention and management of stroke over the last few decades. Despite these important developments, stroke, both in the acute and chronic phases, remains a major cause of morbidity and mortality. The value of integrating palliative care principles and practices into stroke care management is being increasingly recognized across a range of domains including symptom management, assistance with complex decision-making, discharge planning, and end-of-life care. This chapter will explore the logistics, benefits, complexities, and challenges associated with the evolving relationship between stroke and palliative care services.

P. Eastman (✉)
Department of Palliative Care, Barwon Health, North Geelong, VIC, Australia

Department of Palliative and Supportive Care, Royal Melbourne Hospital/Melbourne Health, Parkville, VIC, Australia
e-mail: eastman@gmp.usyd.edu.au

B. Le
Department of Palliative and Supportive Care, Royal Melbourne Hospital/Melbourne Health, Parkville, VIC, Australia
e-mail: Brian.Le@mh.org.au

R. D. MacLeod, L. Van den Block (eds.), *Textbook of Palliative Care*,
https://doi.org/10.1007/978-3-319-77740-5_59

1 Introduction

There have been significant advances in the acute treatment and rehabilitation of stroke over the last few decades. Contributing factors include improved early detection/recognition, timely hospital presentation, the use of thrombolytic and endovascular therapies, early initiation of rehabilitation, and the introduction of organized stroke care. Ongoing improvements in stroke prevention, treatment, and rehabilitation are crucial as stroke prevalence is expected to increase with the aging population. The lifetime risk of having a stroke has been reported to be approximately one in five for females and one in six for males (Mozaffarian et al. 2015) although this figure was calculated from a predominantly Caucasian cohort within the United States and may therefore not be easily generalizable. Stroke incidence varies between countries and is influenced by a range of health, cultural, geopolitical, and socioeconomic factors. Globally the burden of stroke is increasing as measured by the absolute number of people affected, stroke survivors, and disability-adjusted life years lost (Feigin et al. 2014). Much of this burden is seen in low- to middle-income countries.

Strokes constitute a heterogeneous group of conditions which can be described by mechanism and/or location of injury. Approximately 80–85% of strokes are ischemic in nature, with the remainder being either intracerebral hemorrhage (ICH) or subarachnoid hemorrhage (SAH). ICH generally occurs following arterial wall rupture in vessels weakened by chronic hypertension while SAH typically follows aneurysmal rupture within the circle of Willis or trauma (Simmons and Parks 2008). Ischemic subtypes include thrombotic strokes due to occlusive arterial atherosclerotic disease, embolic strokes which are typically cardiac in origin, and lacunar infarcts which occur following the occlusion of the small arteries that supply deep brain structures. Broadly speaking the extent of injury or damage associated with a stroke will depend upon the blood vessels involved and the areas and extent of brain affected.

The most important factor in the initial management of acute stroke is time. The sooner a stroke is recognized and treatment commenced, the better the outcome is likely to be. Another key factor in optimizing chance of recovery is venue of care. There is clear evidence that patients who are managed in a designated stroke center or unit with a specialist multidisciplinary team do better than patients managed elsewhere. In a Cochrane review of 28 trials and 5855 participants which compared stroke care unit (SCU) care with alternative care, SCU was associated with significant reductions in the odds of death, dependency, and/or institutionalized care (Stroke Unit Trialists' Collaboration 2013). The benefits of management within a SCU have been demonstrated for all subtypes of ischemic strokes (Smith et al. 2010a) as well as for ICH (Langhorne et al. 2013).

After initial cardiorespiratory stabilization, immediate stroke management is individualized according to a range of factors including type and severity of stroke, presence of contraindications, medical comorbidities, and patient and family wishes. Following an ischemic stroke in appropriate patients who do not have contraindications, the initial goal is to provide intravenous (IV) thrombolytic therapy as quickly as possible. The provision of a single dose of IV recombinant tissue plasminogen activator (IV rt-PA) within 4.5 h of the commencement of symptoms has been associated with a substantially improved chance of independent function at 3 months post stroke (Maldonado et al. 2014). The use of endovascular therapies following ischemic stroke is an area of ongoing research and development. Therapies under this umbrella include endovascular thrombolysis, thrombectomy, and stent retriever technology. It has been suggested that these approaches may provide superior recanalization in situations such as proximal vessel occlusion when systemic thrombolysis may be less efficacious although until recently results from randomized trials were mixed. Two recently published trials however, both of which were stopped early due to efficacy, have shown significant improvements in functional outcome (Campbell et al. 2015; Goyal et al. 2015) as well as mortality (Goyal et al. 2015) for the combination of endovascular thrombectomy and IV rt-PA compared to IV rt-PA alone, in ischemic stroke with proximal cerebral arterial occlusion.

The management of ICH involves acute stabilization including management of blood glucose and temperature, careful blood pressure control, quality nursing care, prevention of complications, early rehabilitation, and prevention of recurrent hemorrhage (Hemphill et al. 2015). Time is again crucial as it is common for deterioration to occur in the period soon after an ICH. While the benefits of surgical removal of hemorrhage for most supratentorial ICH have not been proven, prompt surgical management is recommended for patients with a cerebellar ICH who are deteriorating neurologically or have brain stem compression (Simmons and Parks 2008; Hemphill et al. 2015). Emergent therapies under investigation in ICH include minimally invasive surgical techniques and the use of biological neuroprotective agents.

Despite advances in prevention, acute treatment, and rehabilitation, stroke remains a prominent cause of morbidity and mortality worldwide. It is a major cause of disability in the United States where up to a third of patients require admission to a long-term care facility following stroke (Mozaffarian et al. 2015). A range of psychological and physical sequelae have been reported by stroke survivors including anxiety and depression, pain syndromes, and communication difficulties. Not surprisingly high levels of distress and caregiver burden are also common among relatives and loved ones. The ideal model for managing the important physical and psychosocial needs of stroke survivors and their families is yet to be established, and it is not clear where palliative care services sit in this paradigm.

While mortality rates vary internationally and have decreased over the last 20 years (Feigin et al. 2014), stroke remains the second commonest cause of death worldwide (World Health Organization 2014). A range of important and diverse needs have been reported by dying patients and their families including symptom management, psychosocial support and assistance with prognostication, treatment decision-making, and future planning. The utilization of palliative care principles and practices would seem appropriate in meeting these needs, and there is increasing recognition, including from international guidelines, of the importance of integrating palliative care into stroke care (National Stroke Foundation 2010; Holloway et al. 2014; Casaubon et al. 2016; Intercollegiate Stroke Working Group 2016). However a range of challenges to effective integration have also been identified from both a stroke and palliative care perspective. The aim of this chapter is to explore the relationship between stroke services and palliative care in both the acute and longer-term setting. The current level of involvement and proposed models of integration will be discussed as well as some of the common palliative care needs and issues identified by patients, families, and health professionals. It is hoped this will provide a contemporaneous overview of the current situation and highlight some important areas for future thought, research, and investment.

2 Palliative Care and Acute Stroke

There is growing recognition that some patients and families following an acute stroke have needs that will be best met by integrating palliative care philosophies and practices into their stroke management.

2.1 Palliative Care Recognition Within International Stroke Guidelines

There is increasing recognition of the relevance of palliative care principles for some patients following a stroke within published international stroke guidelines. While the depth and breadth of information varies across guidelines, there is general agreement concerning the importance of high-quality end-of-life care within stroke services and some support for palliative care throughout the stroke care trajectory.

In a comprehensive scientific statement from the American Heart Association/American Stroke Association, Holloway and colleagues explored the dynamics, logistics, and complexities associated with palliative and end-of-life care in stroke (Holloway et al. 2014). The authors advocate for the availability of palliative care for all patients and their families following a severe or life-threatening stroke, throughout the disease course. In their proposed model, the management of most palliative care problems would be carried out by the stroke service multidisciplinary team with specialist palliative care services available for secondary consultation in situations of heightened complexity. Importantly, the authors provide evidence-based recommendations and guidance to aid implementation, including practical education regarding communication skills, goal setting, and symptom assessment and management.

The Canadian Stroke Best Practice Recommendations emphasize the importance of fostering palliative care expertise within stroke centers (Casaubon et al. 2016). The guidelines make a distinction between palliative care and end-of-life care noting that palliative care can occur in combination with life-prolonging therapies and is not reserved only for those who are imminently dying. A palliative approach is suggested in the setting of catastrophic stroke or multiple comorbidities in order to support both patient and family. Replicating the recommendations of Holloway and colleagues (2014), the guidelines make clear that the stroke service multidisciplinary team should have the appropriate palliative care skills to support dying stroke patients but also that there be access to specialist expertise. Specific indications for specialist palliative care referral include the management of unstable symptoms and assistance with decision-making and with managing complex family and psycho-social dynamics. Recommendations are also made in relation to Advance Care Planning (ACP), specifically that stroke survivors, their families, and caregivers should be supported to participate in it.

In Australia, the 2010 Clinical Guidelines for Stroke Management recommend that all patients dying following a stroke have access to care that is aligned with palliative care principles and practices (National Stroke Foundation 2010). This includes consideration of physical, psychosocial, spiritual, and cultural needs as well as guidance with prognostication and the diagnosis of dying in deteriorating patients or those following a severe stroke. The guidelines note that in many less complex situations, this care will be provided by stroke service staff, and these staff will require ongoing education and support in relation to end-of-life care. The importance of clear and timely communication between stroke services, patients, and families is stressed, and family meetings are suggested as an appropriate forum for these discussions.

The 2016 fifth edition of the UK National Clinical Guideline for Stroke include, among their key recommendations, the proposition that multidisciplinary stroke teams should consider high-quality end-of-life care as a core component of their work (Intercollegiate Stroke Working Group 2016). The need for enhanced education and support for stroke service staff in palliative care principles is emphasized, as is access to specialist palliative care and the opportunity for timely transfer to home if this is the desirable outcome. Among changes from the previous iteration, the 2016 guidelines caution against imposing burdensome restrictions upon patients dying from stroke with particular mention made about the pragmatic management of impaired swallowing and oral intake at end of life. The guidelines acknowledge the range of physical and psychological stressors that can occur following a large stroke and propose that the appropriate management of these problems can help ameliorate distress for patients and their families at end of life.

When considered together, a number of common themes are evident across the guidelines. These include:

- General support for palliative care principles as key components of stroke care.
- Recognition of the presence of multidimensional symptom issues for many patients and their families following a large stroke.
- The importance of clear and ongoing communication between stroke services, patients, and families particularly in relation to issues such as prognostication, goals of care, and management.
- Support for a service model in which the multidisciplinary stroke team provides the majority of palliative and end-of-life care with secondary support available from specialist palliative care services.

2.2 Integration of Stroke and Palliative Care

Although integrating palliative care and acute stroke services is considered important for patients, families, and health professionals alike, how this integration might actually take place is under-researched and not without its challenges. Establishing the palliative care needs of stroke patients and their families is a crucial first step in an integrated approach; however data addressing this question are limited and little is known about how these needs might change over time (Stevens et al. 2007).

Potential methods to assess palliative care needs might include triggers built into existing stroke care pathways – simple bedside prompts or more formal targeted needs assessment tools. Creutzfeldt and colleagues (2015) showed that the use of a simple four-question "palliative care needs checklist" during neurology ward rounds was an effective prompt for recognizing and meeting patient and family needs. Questions in the checklist addressed the presence of distressing symptoms, how the patient and family were coping, and whether the goals of care or treatment approach needed to be modified. Burton and colleagues (2010) used the Sheffield Profile for Assessment and Referral for Care (SPARC) tool to identify high levels of palliative care needs in a prospective study of 191 consecutive stroke admissions to two UK hospitals. The SPARC was developed to screen patients with a range of advanced diseases for specialist palliative care (SPC) referral and incorporates five domains covering physical, psychosocial, spiritual, and functional issues. The authors concluded that the use of the SPARC tool particularly in more disabled stroke patients provided a valuable trigger for staff to consider a range of palliative care issues.

In some ways acute stroke and palliative care might not be considered particularly compatible. The acute stroke environment is one of high-intensity neuro-restorative care with an emphasis on survival, while palliative care is commonly considered more meditative in approach with less concern placed upon survival and more on quality of life. Challenges in introducing palliative care into general stroke management are highlighted by qualitative studies in which stroke unit staff have questioned the juxtaposition of a simultaneous curative focused and palliative approach (Gardiner et al. 2013) and have viewed palliative care as being predominantly about end-of-life care and representative of failure of stroke management (Burton and Payne 2012). Beyond the acute stroke phase, categorizing a patient as "palliative" has been identified as a barrier to combining rehabilitation and palliative care (Burton and Payne 2012).

Traditional palliative care models developed predominantly for patients with malignant diseases may not be easily transferrable to stroke. With its typically sudden onset and decidedly unpredictable clinical course, stroke may behave differently to many cancers or other chronic non-malignant conditions in which palliative care is commonly involved. Such differences were highlighted by a study of 544 patients admitted to a tertiary SCU that found more than 50% of the 87 patients who died had been completely independent and well immediately prior to their stroke (Eastman et al. 2013). Caregivers of stroke survivors have also been noted to have different needs when compared to those of patients with cancer. They are typically older and frailer and as a result may lack important support and social networks (Stevens et al. 2007).

Despite a current lack of clarity concerning the characteristics and function of palliative care within acute stroke services (Burton and Payne 2012), there does appear to be general acceptance of a pragmatic service model in which the multidisciplinary stroke team provides the majority of palliative and end-of-life care with secondary support available from SPC (Holloway et al. 2014; Creutzfeldt et al. 2015; Casaubon et al. 2016). SPC services are also ideally placed to provide the necessary education, training, and support to enable the provision of high-quality nonspecialist palliative care. Importantly, for any model to be applicable to patients throughout the disease course as has been suggested (Holloway et al. 2014; Creutzfeldt et al. 2015), recognition will be required from stroke services that palliative care principles can be positive adjuncts to disease-modifying therapies rather than simply applying to end-of-life care. Additionally a model combining stroke and palliative care will need to consider important system issues such as avoiding overburdening already-stretched palliative care services and not deskilling stroke unit staff (Stevens et al. 2007).

Using qualitative data obtained from patients, families, and stroke service staff, Burton and Payne (2012) constructed a theoretical framework on how the integration of stroke services and palliative care might occur. They proposed that integration was underpinned by six key mechanisms, namely, *clinical legitimacy, capacity, family engagement, early integration, recognition of complexity,* and *recognition of dying.* These mechanisms could themselves be influenced by a range of clinical and organizational factors which vary according to the existing structures and processes within individual healthcare settings. Burton and Payne (2012) propose that analysis of the relationships and interactions influencing these six key mechanisms will facilitate service development and improve the care of patients and families following stroke.

Overall the development and optimization of integrative models will depend not only on the willingness of the stroke and palliative care sectors to embrace the process but also organizational and governmental support to ensure adequate funding and support. Underpinning the whole process is the requirement for ongoing collaborative quantitative and qualitative research focusing not just on outcomes but also factors such as needs assessment, appropriate patient stratification, timing and indication for SPC referral, cost/benefit analysis, and patient, family, and health professional experiences.

2.3 Specialist Palliative Care Utilization in Acute Stroke: A Review of the Current Literature

Data quantifying the level of SPC involvement in stroke are limited and predominantly focused on inpatient consultation services. While variability is seen between health organizations internationally, there is evidence to suggest that the overall uptake of palliative care services for patients following an acute stroke is increasing. In a large cross-sectional study investigating palliative care utilization in nontraumatic intracerebral hemorrhage (ICH), Murthy and colleagues (2016) analyzed admissions to over 1000 American hospitals using the National Inpatient Sample, the largest inpatient health database in the United States. Of the 311,217 included admissions, 32,159 (10.3%) received palliative care, with a substantial annual increase in palliative care involvement seen (4.3% in 2007 to 16.2% in 2011). In an analysis of administrative data of 4894 patients who died within 30 days of an ischemic stroke, 23% of all patients were enrolled in hospice for end-of-life care, a threefold increase from previously reported rates (duPreez et al. 2008).

A small amount of research has explored predictors for SPC involvement in patients following stroke as well as differences between referred and non-referred patients. The influence of both sociodemographic and clinical factors on referral patterns has been reported with data typically obtained from either large administrative dataset analyses or retrospective cohort studies.

In an analysis of palliative care involvement for patients following nontraumatic ICH (Murthy et al. 2016), significant predictors for palliative care involvement included ICH severity, associated comorbidities, female gender, advanced age, hospital location, and ethnicity. Several of these factors were also predictors for hospice utilization in 4894 patients who died within 30 days of an ischemic stroke (duPreez et al. 2008). Predictors which increased the likelihood of hospice utilization included older age, female gender, dementia, Caucasian descent, and hospital length of stay greater than 3 days. Mechanical ventilation, gastrostomy, and uncomplicated diabetes mellitus as a comorbidity correlated with decreased hospice enrolment.

Holloway and colleagues (2010) reviewed all patients referred to an inpatient palliative care consultation service within a large US teaching hospital over a 3-year period. Compared to patients with cancer or common nonmalignant diagnoses including chronic obstructive pulmonary disease (COPD), stroke patients tended to be more functionally impaired, less likely to have decision-making capacity, and were more likely to die in the hospital. For the 1551 stroke patients analyzed during the study period, 6.5% received palliative care consultation. Stroke patients seen by the palliative care service were older, stayed longer in the hospital, and were more likely to be discharged to hospice. However, the majority of stroke patients who died or were discharged to hospice were not seen by SPC.

In an Australian review of 544 admissions over a single year to a metropolitan, tertiary SCU, just over 11% of patients were referred to SPC (Eastman et al. 2013). The predominant reason for referral was end-of-life care, and a number of predictors for referral were identified. These included female gender, older age, increased disability pre stroke, ICH, and living alone or in a residential aged care facility prior to stroke. Sixteen per cent of all SCU admissions died during the review period with just over half seen by the palliative care team. This is approximately double the rate reported from both Swiss and Irish stroke services where only 26% and 24%, respectively, of decreased stroke patients received palliative care consultation (Mazzocato et al. 2010; Ntlholang et al. 2016). Stroke patients referred to the Australian SPC who died during the admission were older, more disabled, and had a significantly longer length of stay than those not referred. In contrast to the total SCU population, the proportion of patients with an ICH was higher in deceased stroke patients who did not receive palliative care consultation (50% vs. 37%). This in combination with the significantly shorter median survival of non-referred patients (2.5 days vs. 6 days) supports previous observations that stroke service staff are generally comfortable managing clearly terminal patients (Rogers and Addington-Hall 2005).

In a retrospective review of 54 consecutive deaths on an Irish teaching hospital stroke service over a 2-year period, several differences were found between patients referred and not referred to SPC (Ntlholang et al. 2016). Those patients whose cause of death was judged to be unrelated to their stroke were more likely to be seen by the SPC team. These patients also had a longer median time between stroke and death, again supporting the notion that stroke unit staff are more comfortable managing the palliative care needs of patients who die soon after a severe stroke, and less so in those who survive longer.

Taken together these data suggest that referrals to SPC, particularly to inpatient consultation services, following acute stroke are increasing. This may reflect increased recognition of the benefits associated with palliative care in areas such as symptom management, complex end-of-life decision-making, and communication. Referral to SPC is influenced by a range of clinical, sociodemographic, and health service factors, but not surprisingly stroke patients referred to palliative care tended to be older, frailer, and sicker. Importantly the majority of stroke patients, including those who were severely disabled or died, were not referred to SPC. While epidemiological data regarding referral rates and predictors are useful for service provision and planning, they do not answer important questions such as whether all patients with complex needs who would benefit from SPC input are currently being referred or whether non-referred "less complex" stroke patients are receiving timely and appropriate non-specialist palliative care (Stevens et al. 2007). This represents an area for ongoing research.

2.4 Shared Stroke and Palliative Care Issues in the Acute Setting

2.4.1 Prognostication

The prediction and communication of prognosis is an important but inherently difficult part of stroke care. Given the majority of patients will survive a stroke, prognostication is relevant to all stages of stroke care from initial acute presentation to post-acute recovery and finally to rehabilitation and/or discharge. Accurate prognostication provides a road map to guide treatment decision-making and allows patients and families to plan for the future. Inaccurate prognostication runs the risk of depriving some patients of the best chance of recovery while exposing others to burdensome treatments that may only prolong suffering. In essence prognostication attempts to provide some degree of certainty while being at the same time inherently uncertain. In a qualitative study that examined patient and family members' perspectives of acute stroke care, honest discussions around prognosis despite uncertainty were valued by relatives even when it was predicted that prognosis might be poor (Payne et al. 2010).

Studies investigating prognosis following stroke have tended to focus on mortality more than functional outcome or recovery. Numerous clinical, sociodemographic, and institutional predictors for mortality have been identified, with stroke severity and older age generally reported to have the strongest associations (Smith et al. 2010b). The National Institutes of Health Stroke Scale (NIHSS) provides a quantification of stroke severity and is a highly reliable predictor of mortality after stroke both on its own and in combination with other variables (Smith et al. 2010b; Frontera et al. 2015). It is a 15-item validated bedside assessment tool which incorporates testing of consciousness, language, sensation, and motor function.

Stroke type itself is also a strong predictor of mortality. This is illustrated by a Danish study of 39,484 hospitalized stroke patients in which intracerebral hemorrhage (ICH) was associated with a fourfold increased risk of dying compared to ischemic events in the immediate post-stroke period (Andersen et al. 2009). Interestingly the difference in mortality between the two stroke types progressively decreased over time until at 3 months, stroke type no longer correlated with mortality. Temporal differences in the factors associated with mortality have also been reported after ischemic stroke. In a Canadian study of 3631 patients following ischemic strokes, stroke severity was found to be a significant predictor of mortality at all time points, while clinician experience was only significant at seven and 30 days and age and medical comorbidities only significantly associated with 30-day and 1-year mortality (Saposnik et al. 2008).

Numerous multivariate prediction models for outcome and mortality following stroke are available although the quality and clinical utility of these models varies (Holloway et al. 2014). Examples include the Hunt-Hess scale for subarachnoid hemorrhage and the ICH score which incorporates Glasgow Coma Scale, ICH volume, intraventricular hemorrhage, age, and site of ICH origin. ICH scores of three or greater have been reported to have a sensitivity and specificity approaching 80% and 90%, respectively, for mortality following ICH (Simmons and Parks 2008).

The applicability of prognostic models to the real world is related in part to the commonality of the variables included and also by the sample from which the data are drawn. Prediction models, for example, generated using data from cohorts with high numbers of clinical trial participants or only patients managed in specialized stroke centers may not be easily applicable to a broader, community-based stroke population. Similarly models that include clinical information from imaging modalities that are not widely available may also lack generalizability.

One particular concern raised by a number of stroke researchers when considering mortality prediction models is the concept of "withdrawal bias." It is argued that because current models have incorporated patients who either never commenced or had life-sustaining therapies withdrawn, there is a potential bias toward mortality (or treatment withdrawal) as well as difficulty in establishing the true effect (positive or otherwise) of these therapies following severe stroke. This is likely to be particularly relevant for stroke types with poor prognosis such as ICH. Given this the importance for clinicians to understand the strengths and limitations of these models, when using them to establish and communicate prognosis to patients and families, has been highlighted (Holloway et al. 2014; Frontera et al. 2015). This may be particularly the case when considering instigating or transitioning to end-of-life care.

Prognostication based upon clinician experience and expertise is an alternative to a model-based approach. Unlike fixed mathematically generated models, clinicians have the advantage of being able to consider an individualized range of factors and adjust their estimations in real time. Clinician-based estimates however may vary considerably between individuals and be influenced by both optimistic and pessimistic judgements (Holloway et al. 2014; Frontera et al. 2015). The involvement of the multidisciplinary team and utilization of a second opinion (including from SPC) have been suggested as ways to overcome some of the issues with clinician-based estimates.

Despite the inherent difficulties associated with prognostication, the importance of providing patients and their families with a sense of the future cannot be underestimated. This is likely to be best achieved using a combination of clinician acumen and evidence-based estimation models individualized to each patient and their unique characteristics.

2.4.2 Limitations of Treatment

The majority of deaths after stroke follow either the limitation, cessation, or foregoing of potentially life-prolonging therapies (Kelly et al. 2012; Holloway et al. 2014; Creutzfeldt et al. 2015; Alonso et al. 2016). In the United States, up to 60% of all stroke deaths follow the removal of mechanical ventilation (Holloway et al. 2014) although this rate is likely to be different in other countries. Decision-making regarding limitations of treatment in acute stroke is complex as it needs to incorporate a range of patient, sociocultural, and clinical factors including autonomy, patient and family wishes, and prognostication. Additionally in the acute phase when uncertainty is high, management decisions need to be made quickly so as to maximize the chances of injury reversal and potential recovery. The acute stroke setting has been described as a "fast-paced, chaotic environment wrought with hope and disappointment, relief and anxiety" (Creutzfeldt et al. 2015), and therefore it is hardly surprising that decision-making in this setting is challenging. Complicating the situation further, many patients have impaired communication as a consequence of their stroke, meaning the responsibility for these complex and often life-and-death decisions will involve family and loved ones.

Treatment limitations can take numerous forms and may alter over time. In the acute setting, they may include decisions regarding thrombolytic and/or endovascular therapy or aggressive resuscitative approaches such as cardiorespiratory resuscitation or mechanical ventilation. In some patients, particularly the more elderly, frail, or those following a severe stroke, the decision to take a palliative approach with an emphasis on comfort might be taken at the outset. This might involve, among other things, the foregoing or withdrawal of antibiotic therapy, hydration, or supplementary feeding. In the majority of circumstances, these discussions and decisions will not involve SPC but be undertaken by members of the stroke team or emergency department. Relatives of stroke patients have reported experiencing discomfort when they felt excluded from the decision-making process, overly responsible for the decisions made (Cowey et al. 2015), or when participating in discussions if they knew do-not-resuscitate (DNR) orders had already been made by the medical team (Payne et al. 2010). This highlights the importance of mutual, shared decision-making between clinicians, patients, and families. The importance of good communication skills underpinned by an awareness of palliative care practice and philosophy has been advocated as a valuable component of both neurology practice and training (Holloway et al. 2014; Creutzfeldt et al. 2015).

The impact of treatment limitations on acute stroke outcomes has been fairly extensively studied with particular interest in the effect of early DNR orders (and other limitations) on stroke mortality. A number of papers have shown an association between DNR orders and increased mortality in both ICH and ischemic stroke independent of other established mortality predictors (Zahuranec et al. 2007; Holloway et al. 2014; Parry-Jones et al. 2016). In a study of 270 non-traumatic ICH, the presence of early treatment limitations (defined as DNR orders alone or in combination with early withdrawal and/or early deferral of other life-sustaining therapies) was associated with a twofold increase in mortality independent of a range of established predictors including age, Glasgow Coma Scale score, and ICH volume (Zahuranec et al. 2007). It has been suggested that the association between DNR orders and early mortality following stroke (and

ICH in particular) represents a "self-fulfilling prophecy" whereby the prediction of poor prognosis leads to limitations of care which ultimately produce a poor prognosis. Accordingly, and in the absence of clear advance care directives, caution is advised about making early treatment limitations decisions in the immediate post-stroke period.

Following the acute stroke phase, ongoing consideration of treatment goals is influenced by the evolving clinical picture, patient and family wishes, and expectations in relation to recovery. This can be a time of significant uncertainty for patients, families, and clinicians and one in which decision-making can be become more complex with emphasis on factors such as prognosis, potential withdrawal of life-prolonging therapies, and discharge planning (Rogers et al. 2005; Eastman et al. 2013). Decisions around the withdrawal of hydration and nutrition can be particularly challenging and were recorded as a source of conflict in nearly half of all interactions between family members and staff in a study of 104 patients who died in a Canadian SCU (Blacquiere et al. 2009). Assistance with this complex decision-making and communication is a common reason for SPC involvement following stroke and is valued by other health professionals. In one study, stroke staff noted that the benefits of access to SPC in these complex scenarios included "reassurance" and "support for decision-making" (Burton and Payne 2012).

For relatives of patients who have had a severe stroke, acting as a surrogate decision-maker can be a two-edged sword. On the one hand, feeling sufficiently involved in decision-making is a predictor of high satisfaction with end-of-life care for bereaved relatives of stroke patients (Young et al. 2009). On the other, when relatives have reflected upon their experiences as surrogates for patients who had suffered severe strokes, a number of conflicts and struggles were described (de Boer et al. 2015). These include the strain of making decisions under time pressure, feeling unprepared or underqualified to speak for their relative, and dealing with uncertainty and change. Despite differences in the experiences reported between interviewees, there was an overall tendency for surrogates to follow medical advice, highlighting again the importance of patient- and family-centered communication in this setting.

Longer-term positive and negative consequences have been reported for surrogates involved in making treatment decisions for others (not specific to stroke). In a systematic review (Wendler and Rid 2011) which included 2854 surrogates across 40 quantitative and qualitative studies, nine papers found that being involved in decision-making had beneficial effects for some surrogates. Importantly however up to a third of surrogates reported negative emotional consequences associated with making decisions for their loved one including stress, guilt, and doubt about whether they had done the right thing. These negative emotions were typically sustained for months and sometimes years which has important implications for bereavement services. Feeling confident they were following a treatment plan consistent with patient preferences seemed to mitigate some of the emotional burden on surrogates, perhaps highlighting the value of Advance Care Directives as a way of planning for future health care.

2.4.3 Symptom Burden Following Acute Stroke

The recognition and appropriate management of both physical and psychological symptoms has been highlighted as an unmet need for patients and their families following acute stroke (Addington-Hall et al. 1995; Stevens et al. 2007; Burton and Payne 2012). While published literature is limited, symptom burden has been reported in between 65% and 98% of dying stroke patients. A broad range of physical symptoms have been reported with varying frequency in patients following an acute stroke including fatigue, nausea, restlessness, and issues with urination and defecation. Pain has been variably described with reported prevalence rates of between 30% and 70% (Addington-Hall et al. 1995; Mazzocato et al. 2010; Ntlholang et al. 2016; Eriksson et al. 2016).

There is evidence that psychological distress is common in patients following an acute stroke, although differences in prevalence are noted in the limited available published literature. Psychological distress, including anxiety, dysthymia, and loneliness, was found to be present in almost half of 191 consecutive stroke admissions in one UK study (Burton et al. 2010) and in 25% of dying stroke patients referred to a Swiss palliative care consultation service (Mazzocato et al. 2010). By contrast, in a separate review of 54 consecutive deaths in an Irish specialist stroke service, psychological distress was reported in only one patient (Ntlholang et al. 2016). Investigating the palliative care needs of patients following an acute stroke, Burton and colleagues (2010) found that while spiritual or religious concerns were low, up to a 25% of patients were worried about death and dying. Additionally, many were concerned about ongoing dependence and disability and the impact this might have on their loved ones. About a quarter felt that their care needs would exceed the capabilities of their families creating the potential for additional distress and even disharmony in an already emotionally fraught time.

The importance of considering the psychological impact of stroke upon patients and families was highlighted in a study investigating bereaved family members' satisfaction with the care provided to patients palliated after ischemic stroke (Blacquiere et al. 2013). While overall satisfaction with palliative care was high, lower satisfaction rates were reported for treatment of anxiety and depression and for the level of emotional support provided to families. The impact of stroke upon loved ones and families is frequently profound, in large part due to the abrupt change in function and cognition often associated with stroke. In the longer term, a number of adverse outcomes have been identified in stroke caregivers including mental health issues, worsening physical health, and financial burden (van Heugten et al. 2006; Carod-Artal and Egido 2009). This potential for longer-term adverse sequelae adds further weight to the importance of considering the psychosocial needs of stroke patients and their families in the acute phase.

While variability in symptom burden following acute stroke has been reported, respiratory symptoms including dyspnea and secretions appear to be particularly prevalent. This is likely to be due, at least in part, to their demonstrability when compared to less visibly obvious symptoms such as pain and anxiety. In one prospective cohort study of 22 patients admitted to a SCU and felt likely to die within 3 months of admission, all of the 20 patients who subsequently died experienced respiratory symptoms during their last hours of life (Rogers and Addington-Hall 2005). Respiratory secretions or "death rattle" were recorded in just over 60% of 1626 dying stroke patients in a Swedish database review (Eriksson et al. 2016), and dyspnea was the commonest recorded symptom in 54 consecutive patients who died in an Irish hospital stroke service (Ntlholang et al. 2016) and in 81% of stroke patients referred to a Swiss palliative care consultation team (Mazzocato et al. 2010). The potential difficulty of managing dyspnea in dying patients was highlighted in this study as only 48% of patients were felt to be free from dyspnea during their last 48 h of life (compared to 81% who were assessed as being free from pain).

Using data from the Swedish Register of Palliative Care, Eriksson and colleagues (2016) compared the prevalence of six symptoms (pain, "death rattle," dyspnea, anxiety, confusion, and nausea) between 1626 patients who died following a stroke and 1626 patients dying from cancer. Interesting differences in symptom prevalence, awareness, and management were noted between the groups. While all symptoms were present in the stroke group (nausea 7.6%, confusion 7.9%, dyspnea 16.3%, anxiety 18.9%, pain 42.7%, and "death rattles" 60.7%) when compared with their matched counterparts with cancer, stroke patients were significantly more likely to experience "death rattles" but less likely to experience any of the other five symptoms. Importantly however, staff caring for stroke patients were significantly less likely to know whether a patient suffered from any of the target symptoms compared to staff caring for patients with malignant disease. It might be anticipated that this difference was related to higher rates of reduced consciousness in dying stroke patients; however this does not seem to have been the case as the ability to self-determine until the last days of life was equivalent between groups (73.3% of stroke patients, 74.3% in cancer). In keeping with the differences seen in symptom prevalence and staff awareness of symptoms, stroke patients were significantly more likely to have as-required medications charted for "death rattle" but less likely to have them for pain, nausea, or anxiety. Overall this study highlights the potential differences in palliative care needs between dying stroke and cancer patients and lends support to individualized approaches rather than assuming that one model of care will fit all. Crucially it also reinforces the importance of stroke service staff being appropriately educated and supported in the provision of general palliative care.

The considerable variability in symptom prevalence seen in the published literature is likely due to a range of factors including communication and consciousness impairment and inconsistent symptom assessment. Additionally accurate quantification of symptom burden for patients following an acute stroke is hampered at least in part by the fact that most studies addressing the question have been retrospective reviews of precollected data. Further prospective longitudinal research is required to expand the currently limited dataset addressing this question and to guide the development of appropriate interventions and approaches to meet the important needs of patients and their families.

2.4.4 End-of-Life Care and Dying Following Acute Stroke

The recognition or diagnosis of dying is complicated and largely arbitrary. Difficulties identifying the time point at which end-of-life care (EOLC) might be initiated are commonly reported by stroke care staff (Burton and Payne 2012; Gardiner et al. 2013; Cowey et al. 2015) leading to potential under- or overtreatment and delay in providing palliative and end-of-life care. A large contributor to this difficulty is the commonality between many of the features associated with dying and those seen in patients following a severe stroke who may subsequently recover. A range of factors have been used to identify dying stroke patients including stroke characteristics (including subtype and severity), clinical course (in particular the lack of meaningful recovery or ongoing deterioration), and physiological parameters (such as altered breathing patterns) (Cowey et al. 2015). In a study of patients who died in a stroke unit, disturbed consciousness, early dysphagia, and large supratentorial strokes were indications for initiation of EOLC (Alonso et al. 2016). In a separate mixed-methods study involving 23 Scottish stroke unit health professionals, over a quarter reported using intuition (at least in part) to recognize dying (Cowey et al. 2015).

The responsibility for decision-making regarding commencement of EOLC for hospitalized stroke patients has generally rested with the SCU medical team, although the importance of input and insight from other members of the multidisciplinary team cannot be underestimated. As we have seen due to the nature of stroke presentation and management, SPC services are infrequently and reactively involved in this process typically at times of increased complexity or significant uncertainty. Involvement of family members in decision-making around end-of-life care is important but not without its problems particularly if there is discordance between relatives and healthcare professionals (Rogers and Addington-Hall 2005). Feeding patients after a severe stroke has been highlighted as an area where motivations and opinions may differ between family members and staff. Rogers and Addington-Hall (2005) noted that while relatives and stroke unit staff shared the common motivation of wanting to avoid prolongation of suffering, stroke unit staff were also concerned about the patient starving or having their chance of recovery impinged due to lack of nutrition. Despite these difficulties family involvement allows a unique perspective on the patient and their place in the world and has been shown to be a predictor of high satisfaction with EOLC. As for all other areas of stroke care, the importance of clear, unambiguous, empathic, and effective communication cannot be overstated.

Two distinct patterns of dying following an acute stroke have been described, namely, a rapid, sudden death or prolonged dying. A prolonged dying phase can be particularly difficult for family members, and this is likely to be exacerbated if there was expectation of a quick death, they had not been informed of the possibility of prolonged dying, and in the setting of severe dysphagia (Cowey et al. 2015). Not surprisingly the transition from recovery-focused care to EOLC can be challenging for family members with feelings of isolation and abandonment reported (Payne et al. 2010). However when death is considered likely, the most important things identified by relatives and stroke unit staff alike are the avoidance of distress and the maintenance of comfort and dignity (Rogers and Addington-Hall 2005; Payne et al. 2010).

End-of-life care (EOLC) pathways have been used to guide and optimize multidisciplinary, holistic care for dying patients and their families including following stroke. In this setting EOLC pathways aim to cover not only physical symptoms but also psychological, spiritual, and cultural considerations, desired place of care, and after-death management. The Liverpool Care Pathway (LCP) is an example of an EOLC pathway which has been used worldwide in both malignant and nonmalignant conditions. Recently the LCP has attracted considerable media attention and controversy in part due to concerns about its perceived overapplication at times, the inappropriate denial of nutrition and hydration in some cases, and deficits in communication with patients and families about its use. A subsequent UK government-commissioned independent review, while acknowledging the principles underpinning the LCP, expressed among a range of concerns that it was too frequently used as a "tick-box" exercise and recommended that it be progressively phased out and replaced by individualized care plans (Neuberger et al. 2013).

There is limited evidence addressing the use of EOLC pathways following severe stroke with available data seeming to be generally supportive of their use. The Australian Clinical Guidelines for Stroke Management in a small section devoted to palliative care include a recommendation that pathways for stroke palliative care can be used to improve the care of people dying following a stroke but acknowledge that evidence to support this recommendation is weak (National Stroke Foundation 2010). Very little is known about the quantitative impact of EOLC pathways on care parameters following severe stroke although improvements in both documentation and clinical practice were observed in a small retrospective audit pre- and post the implementation of the LCP on a 12-bed stroke unit (Jack et al. 2004). Examples of the changes in clinical practice seen included increases in the discontinuation of inappropriate medications (from 40% to 100%), in the charting of subcutaneous medications (from 20% to 85%), and in the assessment of religious needs. While these results appear promising, they need to be interpreted cautiously given the retrospective study design and small sample size.

Two qualitative studies have addressed the perceptions of healthcare professionals regarding the use of the LCP in English and Scottish stroke units (Gardiner et al. 2013; Cowey et al. 2015). In general satisfaction has been reported with its use, with staff in one study suggesting that the LCP was a core element of high-quality palliative care (Gardiner et al. 2013). Surveyed family members were also generally satisfied with LCP-based care although tended to be more concerned with adequate control of problems rather than whether an EOLC pathway was used (Cowey et al. 2015). Importantly family members were able to influence EOLC including when the LCP was used. This meant that management plans, including components such as the ongoing provision of parenteral hydration, were adapted to incorporate their wishes. This negotiated mutual pragmatism is perhaps what Neuberger and colleagues (2013) were envisaging when they recommended the replacement of the LCP with individualized care plans. Interestingly while both of these studies undertook their qualitative data collection prior to the 2013 independent LCP review, the paper by Cowey and colleagues (2015) was published subsequent to it. In their conclusions, the authors acknowledged the withdrawal of the LCP in the UK but noted that it continued to be used worldwide. They reiterated that in their study, family members were more concerned with distressing stroke-related problems than the LCP. In a succinct summary encapsulating the complexity of EOLC following stroke, they concluded that "such problems are enduring in nature and remain as clinical challenges whether end-of-life care pathways are used or not."

3 Palliative Care in the Post-Stroke Phase

The last couple of decades have seen emerging recognition of the role palliative care can play beyond end of life. Earlier involvement in advanced malignant disease, for example, has been demonstrated to lead to improvements in symptom burden, quality of life, and psychological well-being. Increased awareness of the substantive symptom burden and distress associated with a range of noncancer conditions, including chronic respiratory, renal, and neurological disorders, has highlighted the benefits of multidisciplinary palliative care in symptom management, complex decision-making, and care facilitation. In stroke while there is a developing evidence base for palliative care in the acute phase, the picture is much less clear for the post-stroke period. This is worthy of further consideration because as previously discussed the majority of patients will ultimately survive an acute stroke.

For those people who survive their initial stroke, the focus of most clinical programs and the literature has understandably been on secondary prevention and stroke rehabilitation. Accordingly there is comparatively little published data evaluating the involvement or potential role of palliative care services in post-stroke care. While data examining palliative care in this setting are limited, there is evidence of a range of often under-recognized symptoms and morbidity in patients, families, and caregivers following stroke.

The symptoms and issues experienced by patients and their caregivers in the chronic post-stroke phase will be familiar to many palliative care clinicians. They can include pain, depression, functional disability, seizures, bladder and bowel dysfunction, and caregiver stress/fatigue. While these symptoms are likely to share similarities with those seen in patients with cancer, end-organ failure, and/or neurological degenerative disorders, they may also display features unique to stroke. For example, the immediate onset of profound change in physical and cognitive function that often accompanies acute stroke contrasts with the subacute development of illness and disability in other malignant and nonmalignant conditions. Additionally the management of symptom burden in an environment where patient survival might be measured in years rather than weeks or months is outside the traditional skill set of many palliative care clinicians.

In some ways the chronic post-stroke period might be considered analogous to cancer survivorship as both may share features of ongoing symptoms in the context of likely long-term survival. The role of palliative care in cancer survivorship, while variable worldwide, remains relatively undefined, debatably appropriate, and influenced by a broad range of clinical and structural factors including limitations in clinician experience, workforce issues, and funding models. It seems likely that involvement in the post-stroke phase will provide palliative care, at both a clinician and organizational level, with similar challenges regarding clinical appropriateness and service provision.

3.1 Pain Syndromes

The most common types of pain reported in stroke survivors are central post-stroke pain, hemiplegic shoulder pain, painful spasticity, musculoskeletal pain, and tension-type headache (Creutzfeldt et al. 2012). Accurate pain assessment following stroke can be challenging due to the consequent communication deficits that may include dysphasia and dysarthria and/or changes in consciousness that occur in some stroke survivors.

3.1.1 Central Post-Stroke Pain

Central post-stroke pain (CPSP) is a neuropathic pain syndrome that is both highly distressing and frequently refractory to treatment. Sometimes referred to as Dejerine-Roussy syndrome, it was first described in 1906 (Vartiainen et al. 2016). There is variability in the reported rates of CPSP development among stroke survivors as well as concerns that it may be under-recognized. In an Italian population-based study which included 1494 post-stroke patients, symptoms and sensory changes consistent with CPSP were present in 11% of stroke survivors (Raffaeli et al. 2013). Other authors have reported prevalence rates of between 3% and 8% when all stroke survivors are considered (Vartiainen et al. 2016) and up to 35% in those with specific thalamic lesions. While the pathogenesis of CPSP is not well established, postulated mechanisms for development include hyperexcitability of injured sensory networks, changes in central inhibitory mechanisms, or central nervous system neurotransmitter imbalances. The varying incidence and prevalence of CPSP is explained by the unclear etiology of this pain syndrome as well as the lack of universally accepted diagnostic criteria. The diagnosis of CPSP requires the exclusion of pain caused by joint contracture, peripheral nerve disorders, and spasticity.

The pain of CPSP may be spontaneous or evoked. Spontaneous pain can occur either continuously or intermittently, while evoked pain is typically precipitated by stimuli such as touch, movement, stress, or temperature change (Creutzfeldt et al. 2012; Vartiainen et al. 2016). Sensory abnormalities such as allodynia, dysesthesia, paresthesia, and hyperalgesia are common features (Creutzfeldt et al. 2012; Raffaeli et al. 2013). The pain is typically experienced within the area of sensory impairment and usually at the point of maximal deficit. Spinothalamic abnormalities such as temperature-sensory abnormality are frequently described. CPSP may develop at any time from immediately to years after a stroke; however onset most commonly occurs at 3–6 months (Raffaeli et al. 2013).

Management of CPSP is challenging as there is a paucity of evidence to guide practice. Optimal management is likely to be best achieved by utilizing a combination of pharmacological and non-pharmacological treatment approaches. A range of pharmacological agents have been trialed in the management of CPSP with a particular focus on antidepressants and anticonvulsants. The efficacy and tolerability of these agents has varied across trials. Amitriptyline at a final dose of 75 mg daily was associated with significant improvements in pain when compared to placebo in a small double-blind, placebo-controlled crossover study conducted in 15 nondepressed patients (Leigon and Boivie 1989). Importantly there was little in the way of adverse effect associated with amitriptyline. No statistically significant benefit was seen for carbamazepine (at doses of up to 800 mg/day) in the same study.

In terms of other agents, there is some evidence of benefit from both case series and a controlled trial for lamotrigine; however, there is limited evidence for gabapentin and none for opioids (Frese et al. 2006). The efficacy and safety of pregabalin in the management of CPSP was assessed in a double-blind, placebo-controlled randomized trial in 219 patients. The mean dose of pregabalin received was 356.8 mg, and after 13 weeks, pain had improved in both treatment arms (pregabalin baseline pain score 6.5, end-point pain score 4.9; placebo baseline pain score 6.3, end-point pain score 5.0); however there was no significant difference between the groups. Pregabalin was associated with improvements in sleep and anxiety in the study; however, more than 50% of patients in the pregabalin group reported some adverse effects (compared to 23% in the placebo group), with dizziness and somnolence being most common (Kim et al. 2011).

Non-pharmacological therapies including cognitive behavioral therapy and stimulation therapies including transcutaneous electrical nerve stimulation and acupuncture have been described in small case series; however, controlled trial evidence is lacking. Surgical pain therapies such as rhizotomy, sympathectomy, cordotomy, and deep brain stimulation have not been formally evaluated for the treatment of CPSP and should be considered only in the context of approved clinical trials.

3.1.2 Hemiplegic Shoulder Pain

Hemiplegic shoulder pain (HSP) is the most common post-stroke pain, occurring in 11–83% of patients (Creutzfeldt et al. 2012). The prevalence of HSP increases with worsening motor impairment. HSP occurs as a consequence of joint subluxation and sensory and motor deficits. Careful attention to joint positioning in hemiplegic patients and physical therapies are the mainstay of treatment, with some emerging data for intra-articular steroid injections and intramuscular injections of botulinum toxin-A. Analgesia with anti-inflammatory medications, paracetamol, and topical heat or ice and soft-tissue massage can also assist with initial pain management.

3.1.3 Spasticity and Musculoskeletal Pain

Pain due to contractures, pressure areas, and spasticity are best prevented through the use of physical and rehabilitative therapies, body positioning, and range of motion exercises. Baclofen and dantrolene are used for post-stroke spasticity; however, their side effects including sedation, confusion, and dizziness can limit their use. Botulinum toxin can be used, particularly in upper-limb spasticity, to improve functional outcome (Creutzfeldt et al. 2012).

3.2 Post-Stroke Depression

Depression is part of a constellation of neuropsychiatric disorders that are recognized to be associated with stroke. Estimates of the frequency of post-stroke depression (PSD) vary due to the heterogeneity of assessment and reporting approaches; however, a recent meta-analysis which included 61 studies and over 25,000 people found a frequency for PSD of 31% out to 5 years post stroke (Hackett and Pickles 2014). PSD onset can occur at any time following a stroke, with a prospective, longitudinal study of over 200 patients, observing rates of PSD to be relatively stable across a range of time points from 1 month to 18 months post stroke (De Ryck et al. 2014). Stroke severity and the resultant degree of physical and functional disability are the strongest predictors of post-stroke depression, with other recognized predictors including cognitive impairment, dysphasia and aphasia, apraxia, and premorbid history of depression or anxiety (De Ryck et al. 2014; Robinson and Jorge 2016). Evidence for the impact of social support and stroke lesion location upon PSD is conflicting; however, there are reports of association between left frontal and left basal ganglia lesions and PSD (Robinson and Jorge 2016).

Post-stroke depression is associated with increased mortality, poorer engagement in rehabilitation, decreased quality of life, and social isolation (Creutzfeldt et al. 2012; De Ryck et al. 2014; Robinson and Jorge 2016). An independent and direct association exists between depression severity and functional impairment although this relationship is likely to be reciprocal in many cases. The increased mortality associated with PSD has been reported to be due to greater cardiovascular mortality, with PSD associated disruptions in autonomic nervous system function postulated as a potential explanatory mechanism (Robinson and Jorge 2016).

A number of double-blind, placebo-controlled treatment trials for PSD have been undertaken using both tricyclic antidepressants and selective-serotonin uptake inhibitors (SSRI) since 1984 (Robinson and Jorge 2016). Although sample numbers were generally small across the trials, most reported improvements in depression scores when compared to placebo. A meta-analysis that included 17 trials (13 using pharmacological agents and 4 psychotherapy) and 1655 patients (Hackett et al. 2008) found that pharmacotherapy conferred a small but significant benefit in treating depression and reducing depressive symptoms; however, this was coupled with an increase in adverse effects. No evidence of benefit was demonstrated for psychotherapy; however, other studies have reported positive outcomes for brief psychosocial interventions (including psychoeducation and family support) when combined with antidepressants (Robinson and Jorge 2016). The impacts of antidepressant medications on physical and functional outcomes are less well described (Creutzfeldt et al. 2012); however, improvements in motor, cognitive, and functional capacity have been demonstrated (Robinson and Jorge 2016). There is emerging evidence that pharmacotherapy (in particular SSRIs) may have a preventative role in PSD as well as interesting data, suggesting antidepressants might improve stroke survival independent of either successful depression treatment or the presence of depression in the first place (Robinson and Jorge 2016).

3.3 Quality of Life

Of patients who survive 30 days following acute stroke, half will die within 5 years, and of the survivors, approximately 30% will remain disabled, with 14% requiring institutional care

(Hankey et al. 2002). Quality of life (QOL) while difficult to define and inherently subjective in nature is generally considered to be a multidimensional construct incorporating multiple broad domains including physical, social, and mental. Recognition of the potential impact of stroke upon QOL has seen the development of a number of stroke-specific health-related QOL scales in recent years. These scales include specific factors relevant to stroke patients including vision and language impairments, with examples being the Stroke Impact Scale and the Burden of Stroke Scale (Carod-Artal and Egido 2009).

A wide range of factors have been shown to impair QOL following stroke including dependency in activities of daily living (ADL), motor dysfunction, aphasia, presence of depression, CPSP, sexual dysfunction, and limited social supports (Carod-Artal et al. 2000; Choi-Kwon et al. 2006; Carod-Artal and Egido 2009). Reductions in QOL have been described by stroke survivors with differing levels of functional impairment from the profoundly disabled to those who regained independence in ADL function but did not get back to premorbid functional levels and in others who were not able to return to work. A Korean study that examined influences on QOL in 151 first-time stroke patients found that ADL dependency, CPSP, depression, and lower socioeconomic status were all important explanatory factors for lower QOL 3 years post stroke (Choi-Kwon et al. 2006). Although variation exists in the literature stroke type, lesion location, age, and gender have not consistently been associated with lower QOL (Choi-Kwon et al. 2006) although there is some evidence to suggest females have lower QOL following stroke than men (Carod-Artal et al. 2000; Carod-Artal and Egido 2009).

Importantly recognition of the negative influence of a broad range of factors upon QOL highlights the need for close attention to be paid to these things in the post-stroke period. In particular, vigilance when it comes to the assessment and treatment of depression and pain and rehabilitative efforts focused on maximizing functional outcomes and independence are crucial components in the preservation of QOL for patients following a stroke.

3.4 Caregiver Issues

While patients after stroke confront a myriad of issues, caregivers are also confronted with a new and often devastatingly different world. This is often exacerbated by the sudden onset of change which necessitates the rapid acquisition of new knowledge, skills, and acceptance of changed circumstances. This contrasts other more chronic illnesses where disease progression is typically gradual and predictable, allowing caregivers greater opportunity for adjustment and adaptation. Cognitive deficits including perceptual and language change along with motor deficits and functional dependency add additional complexity to the caregiver role. Additionally many caregivers are themselves elderly with their own health problems and often contracting social and support networks.

Worsening physical health, lower QOL, high levels of stress and mood disorder, social isolation, and financial burden have all been reported by stroke caregivers (van Heugten et al. 2006; Carod-Artal and Egido 2009). Anxiety and depression are common with rates of depression estimated to be upward of 25%. Given the recognized high levels of burden among stroke caregivers and the crucial role they play in supporting patients at home, increasing attention is being paid to assessing and managing stroke caregiver needs. Importantly despite the clear challenges that the caregiver role can bring, evidence suggests that many stroke caregivers still experience increased appreciation of life and role fulfillment.

A lack of attention to caregivers in established stroke guidelines prompted the development of evidence-based clinical practice guidelines specific to stroke caregivers in the Netherlands in the mid-2000s (van Heugten et al. 2006). These guidelines cover a range of topics including risk factors for caregiver burden, approaches to assessing burden, and possible caregiver interventions. Factors identified as predictive of increased caregiver burden include both patient characteristics (particularly limited functional capacity and significant cognitive impairment) and caregiver factors including preexisting psychological ill-health.

The impact of interventions upon stroke caregivers has been evaluated across a number of studies with varying degrees of benefit reported. Interventions identified to provide at least some improvement in caregiver wellbeing include the provision of information, social and practical supports, training in the caregiver role, attention to mental health issues, and counseling (Kalra et al. 2004; van Heugten et al. 2006). Clinicians have a key role to play in preparing caregivers for their role. In retrospective surveys of bereaved caregivers, satisfaction with care following a stroke is positively correlated with involvement of doctors and nurses who are knowledgeable about stroke, clinicians being open to discussing fears and concerns, and caregivers being involving in decision-making processes (Young et al. 2009).

While after-stroke care largely focuses on secondary prevention and rehabilitation, it is clear that symptoms and complex care needs including pain syndromes, depression, impaired quality of life, functional impairment, and caregiver issues are highly prevalent following stroke. These are all things familiar to multidisciplinary palliative care clinicians, who accordingly are conceivably well positioned to address them utilizing expertise and experience drawn from other chronic diseases, as well as collaboration with colleagues from stroke and rehabilitation teams.

4 Conclusions/Summary

Despite significant advances in prevention, recognition, and treatment, stroke remains a major cause of morbidity and mortality worldwide. The value of integrating palliative care principles and practices into stroke management is being increasingly recognized particularly in relation to issues such as symptom management, complex decision-making, and establishment of goals of care. Ongoing research is required addressing not only these important patient and family needs but also the theoretical basis, clinical requirements, and departmental structures required for successful integration. In the acute phase, the majority of palliative care is currently and likely to continue to be undertaken by members of the stroke team with secondary support available from specialist palliative care services on an as-needed basis. Additionally specialist palliative care is ideally placed to provide the necessary education and guidance to ensure the provision of high-quality care.

The role of palliative care in the more chronic post-stroke phase is less clear with little published data addressing the question. There is clear evidence of significant symptom burden, reduced quality of life, and caregiver distress for patients and their families in this period, and these are all things familiar to multidisciplinary palliative care teams. In many ways palliative care clinicians are well placed to take a lead role in the management of many of these problems although their chronicity is likely to impose clinical, organizational, and workforce challenges upon the profession.

The ongoing success of the integration of palliative care and stroke services will be contingent on a number of factors, not least of which being buy-in from both specialties. For palliative care this will perhaps require a conscious shift away from the cancer-related models and ideologies of the past and an acknowledgement that adaption, conciliation, and collaboration will be crucial in moving forward. This is relevant not just for stroke but also other nonmalignant diseases and the ever-changing cancer landscape. In essence this is the challenge for modern palliative care and the next generation of specialists.

References

Addington-Hall J, Lay M, Altmann D, McCarthy M. Symptom control, communication with health professionals, and hospital care of stroke patients in the last year of life as reported by surviving family, friends, and officials. Stroke. 1995;26(12):2242–8.

Alonso A, Ebert AD, Dörr D, Buchheidt D, Hennerici MG, Szabo K. End-of-life decisions in acute stroke patients: an observational cohort study. BMC Palliat Care. 2016; 15(1):1.

Andersen KK, Olsen TS, Dehlendorff C, Kammersgaard LP. Hemorrhagic and ischemic strokes compared stroke severity, mortality, and risk factors. Stroke. 2009;40(6): 2068–72.

Blacquiere DP, Gubitz GJ, Dupere D, McLeod D, Phillips S. Evaluating an organized palliative care approach in patients with severe stroke. Can J Neurol Sci. 2009; 36(06):731–4.

Blacquiere D, Bhimji K, Meggison H, Sinclair J, Sharma M. Satisfaction with palliative care after stroke. A prospective cohort study. Stroke. 2013;44:2617–9.

Burton CR, Payne S. Integrating palliative care within acute stroke services: developing a programme theory of patient and family needs, preferences and staff perspectives. BMC Palliat Care. 2012;11(1):1.

Burton CR, Payne S, Addington-Hall J, Jones A. The palliative care needs of acute stroke patients: a prospective study of hospital admissions. Age Ageing. 2010; 39(5):554–9.

Campbell BC, Mitchell PJ, Kleinig TJ, Dewey HM, Churilov L, Yassi N, et al. Endovascular therapy for ischemic stroke with perfusion-imaging selection. N Engl J Med. 2015;372(11):1009–18.

Carod-Artal FJ, Egido JA. Quality of life after stroke: the importance of a good recovery. Cerebrovasc Dis. 2009;27(Suppl 1):204–14.

Carod-Artal J, Egido JA, Gonzalez JL, de Seijas EV. Quality of life among stroke survivors evaluated 1 year after stroke. Stroke. 2000;12:2995–3000.

Casaubon LK, Boulanger J-M, Glasser E, Blacquiere D, Boucher S, Brown K, et al. Canadian stroke best practice recommendations: acute inpatient stroke care guidelines, update 2015. Int J Stroke. 2016;11(2):239–52.

Choi-Kwon S, Choi JM, Kwon SU, Kang DW, Kim JS. Factors that affect the quality of life at 3 years post-stroke. J Clin Neurol. 2006;2:34–41.

Cowey E, Smith LN, Stott DJ, McAlpine CH, Mead GE, Barber M, et al. Impact of a clinical pathway on end-of-life care following stroke: a mixed methods study. Palliat Med. 2015;29(3):249–59.

Creutzfeldt CJ, Holloway RG, Walker M. Symptomatic and palliative care for stroke survivors. J Gen Intern Med. 2012;27:853–60.

Creutzfeldt CJ, Holloway RG, Curtis JR, Palliative Care A. Core competency for stroke neurologists. Stroke. 2015;46(9):2714–9.

de Boer ME, Depla M, Wojtkowiak J, Visser MC, Widdershoven GA, Francke AL, et al. Life-and-death decision-making in the acute phase after a severe stroke: interviews with relatives. Palliat Med. 2015;29(5):451–7.

De Ryck A, Fransen E, Brouns R, Geurden M, Peij D, Marien P, et al. Post-stroke depression and its multifactorial nature: results from a prospective longitudinal study. J Neurol Sci. 2014;347:159–66.

duPreez AE, Smith MA, Liou JI, Frytak JR, Finch MD, Cleary JF, et al. Predictors of hospice utilization among acute stroke patients who died within thirty days. J Palliat Med. 2008;11(9):1249–57.

Eastman P, McCarthy G, Brand CA, Weir L, Gorelik A, Le B. Who, why and when: stroke care unit patients seen by a palliative care service within a large metropolitan teaching hospital. BMJ Support Palliat Care. 2013; 3(1):77–83.

Eriksson H, Milberg A, Hjelm K, Friedrichsen M. End of life care for patients dying of stroke: a comparative registry study of stroke and cancer. PLoS One. 2016;11(2):e0147694.

Feigin VL, Forouzanfar MH, Krishnamurthi R, Mensah GA, Connor M, Bennett DA, et al. Global and regional burden of stroke during 1990–2010: findings from the global burden of disease study 2010. Lancet. 2014;383(9913):245–55.

Frese A, Husstedt IW, Ringelstein EB, Evers S. Pharmacologic treatment of central post-stroke pain. Clin J Pain. 2006;22:252–60.

Frontera JA, Curtis JR, Nelson JE, Campbell M, Gabriel M, Mosenthal AC, et al. Integrating palliative care into the care of neurocritically ill patients: a report from the improving palliative care in the ICU project advisory board and the center to advance palliative care. Crit Care Med. 2015;43(9):1964–77.

Gardiner C, Harrison M, Ryan T, Jones A. Provision of palliative and end-of-life care in stroke units: a qualitative study. Palliat Med. 2013;27(9):855–60.

Goyal M, Demchuk AM, Menon BK, Eesa M, Rempel JL, Thornton J, et al. Randomized assessment of rapid endovascular treatment of ischemic stroke. NEJM. 2015;372(11):1019–30.

Hackett ML, Pickles K. Part I: frequency of depression after stroke: an updated systematic review and meta-analysis of observational studies. Int J Stroke. 2014; 9(8):1017–25.

Hackett ML, Anderson CS, House A, Xia J. Interventions for treating depression after stroke. Cochrane Database Syst Rev. 2008;(4):CD003437. https://doi.org/10.1002/14651858.CD003437.pub3.

Hankey GJ, Jamrozik K, Broadhurst RJ, Forbes S, Anderson CS. Long term disability after first-ever stroke and related prognostic factors in the Perth community stroke study 1989-1990. Stroke. 2002;33:1034–40.

Hemphill JC, Greenberg SM, Anderson CS, Becker K, Bendok BR, Cushman M, et al. Guidelines for the management of spontaneous intracerebral hemorrhage a guideline for healthcare professionals from the American Heart Association/American Stroke Association. Stroke. 2015;46(7):2032–60.

Holloway RG, Ladwig S, Robb J, Kelly A, Nielsen E, Quill TE. Palliative care consultations in hospitalized stroke patients. J Palliat Med. 2010;13(4):407–12.

Holloway RG, Arnold RM, Creutzfeldt CJ, Lewis EF, Lutz BJ, McCann RM, et al. Palliative and end-of-life care in stroke a statement for healthcare professionals from the American Heart Association/American Stroke Association. Stroke. 2014;45(6):1887–916.

Intercollegiate Stroke Working Group. National clinical guideline for stroke 5th edition [Online]. London: Royal College of Physicians; 2016. Available: www.strokeaudit.org/SupportFiles/Documents/Guidelines/2016-National-Clinical-Guideline-for-Stroke-5t-(1).aspx.

Jack C, Jones L, Jack BA, Gambles M, Murphy D, Ellershaw JE. Towards a good death: the impact of the care of the dying pathway in an acute stroke unit. Age Ageing. 2004;33(6):625–6.

Kalra L, Evans A, Perez I, Melbourn A, Pateal A, Knapp M, et al. Training carers of stroke patients: randomized controlled trial. BMJ. 2004;328:1099.

Kelly AG, Hoskins KD, Holloway RG. Early stroke mortality, patient preferences, and the withdrawal of care bias. Neurology. 2012;79(9):941–4.

Kim JS, Bashford G, Murphy TK, Martin A, Dror V, Cheung R. Safety and efficacy of pregabalin in patients with central post-stroke pain. Pain. 2011;152(5):1018–23.

Langhorne P, Fearon P, Ronning OM, Kaste M, Palomaki H, Vemmos K, et al. Stroke unit care benefits patients with intracerebral hemorrhage systematic review and meta-analysis. Stroke. 2013;44(11):3044–9.

Leigon G, Boivie J. Central post-stroke pain: a controlled trial of amitriptyline and carbamazepine. Pain. 1989;36:27–36.

Maldonado NJ, Kazmi SO, Suarez JI. Update in the management of acute ischemic stroke. Crit Care Clin. 2014;30(4):673–97.

Mazzocato C, Michel-Nemitz J, Anwar D, Michel P. The last days of dying stroke patients referred to a palliative care consult team in an acute hospital. Eur J Neurol. 2010;17(1):73–7.

Mozaffarian D, Benjamin SJ, Go AS, Arnett DK, Blaha MJ, Cushman M, et al. Heart disease and stroke Statistics-2015 update: a report from the American Heart Association. Circulation. 2015;131:e29–e322.

Murthy SB, Moradiya Y, Hanley DF, Ziai WC. Palliative care utilization in nontraumatic intracerebral hemorrhage in the United States. Crit Care Med. 2016;44: 575–82.

National Stroke Foundation. Clinical guidelines for stroke management. Melbourne; 2010.

Neuberger J, Guthrie C, Aaronovitch D. More care, less pathway: a review of the Liverpool care pathway. London: Department of Health; 2013.

Ntlholang O, Walsh S, Bradley D, Harbison J. Identifying palliative care issues in inpatients dying following stroke. Ir J Med Sci. 2016;185:741–4.

Parry-Jones AR, Paley L, Bray BD, Hoffman AM, James M, Cloud GC, et al. Care-limiting decisions in acute stroke and association with survival: analyses of UK national quality register data. Int J Stroke. 2016;11(3):321–31.

Payne S, Burton C, Addington-Hall J, Jones A. End-of-life issues in acute stroke care: a qualitative study of the experiences and preferences of patients and families. Palliat Med. 2010;24(2):146–53.

Raffaeli W, Minella CE, Magnani F, Sarti D. Population-based study of central post-stroke pain in Rimini District, Italy. J Pain Res. 2013;6:705–11.

Robinson RG, Jorge RE. Post-stroke depression: a review. Am J Psychiatry. 2016;173(3):221–31.

Rogers A, Addington-Hall J. Care of the dying stroke patients in the acute setting. J Res Nurs. 2005;10(2): 153–67.

Saposnik G, Hill MD, O'Donnell M, Fang J, Hachinski V, Kapral MK. Variables associated with 7-day, 30-day, and 1-year fatality after ischemic stroke. Stroke. 2008;39(8):2318–24.

Simmons BB, Parks SM. Intracerebral hemorrhage for the palliative care provider: what you need to know. J Palliat Med. 2008;11(10):1336–9.

Smith EE, Hassan KA, Fang J, Selchen D, Kapral MK, Saposnik G, Investigators of the Registry of the Canadian Stroke Network, Stroke Outcome Research Canada (SORCan) Working Group. Do all ischemic stroke subtypes benefit from organized inpatient stroke care? Neurology. 2010a;75(5):456–62.

Smith EE, Shobha N, Dai D, Olson DM, Reeves MJ, Saver JL, et al. Risk score for in-hospital ischemic stroke mortality derived and validated within the get with the guidelines–stroke program. Circulation. 2010b; 122(15):1496–504.

Stevens T, Payne SA, Burton C, Addington-Hall J, Jones A. Palliative care in stroke: a critical review of the literature. Palliat Med. 2007;21(4):323–31.

van Heugten C, Visser-Meily A, Post M, Lindeman E. Care for carers of stroke patients: evidence-based clinical practice guidelines. J Rehabil Med. 2006;38(3):153–8.

Vartiainen N, Perchet C, Magnin M, Creac'h C, Convers P, Nighoghossian N, et al. Thalamic pain: anatomical and physiological indices of prediction. Brain. 2016; 139(3):708–22.

Wendler D, Rid A. Systematic review: the effect on surrogates of making treatment decisions for others. Ann Intern Med. 2011;154(5):336–46.

World Health Organisation. The top 10 causes of death. 2014. http://www.who.int/mediacentre/factsheets/fs310/en/. Accessed 18 Nov 2016.

Young AJ, Rogers A, Dent L, Addington-Hall JM. Experiences of hospital care reported by bereaved relatives of patients after a stroke: a retrospective survey using the VOICES questionnaire. J Adv Nurs. 2009;65(10): 2161–74.

Zahuranec DB, Brown DL, Lisabeth LD, Gonzales NR, Longwell PJ, Smith MA, et al. Early care limitations independently predict mortality after intracerebral hemorrhage. Neurology. 2007;68(20):1651–7.

Palliative Care in Heart Failure

61

James M. Beattie and Jillian P. Riley

Contents

J. M. Beattie (✉)
Cicely Saunders Institute, King's College, London, UK
e-mail: jmbeattie@hotmail.com

J. P. Riley
National Heart and Lung Institute, Imperial College, London, UK
e-mail: jillian.riley@imperial.ac.uk

Abstract

Heart failure is a life limiting cardiovascular condition, frequently encountered in the increasingly aged population. People affected endure a symptomatic burden and mortality risk at least equivalent to those associated with common cancers. However, the clinical scenario is usually more complicated in that heart

R. D. MacLeod, L. Van den Block (eds.), *Textbook of Palliative Care*,
https://doi.org/10.1007/978-3-319-77740-5_60

failure tends to occur in multimorbid older individuals who exhibit an unpredictable disease trajectory. In most patients, cardiac function tends to decline inexorably, with a mortality of about 50% in the 5 years following diagnosis. An ever more complex evidence-based therapy, which likely materially benefits less than half of those with this clinical diagnosis, involves polypharmacy, implanted cardiac devices, and consideration for surgical intervention including cardiac transplantation. Acknowledging its prognostic ambiguity, the capricious nature of the heart failure state, and the relatively onerous treatment protocol may undermine care coordination, patient autonomy, and ultimately conflict with patients' and families' preferences for care along a progressively declining clinical course to the end of life. This chapter describes the challenges and opportunities in providing palliative care to this burgeoning clinical population.

1 Introduction

Heart failure is a common clinical and public health problem which occurs in epidemic proportions. Currently, about 38 million people suffer with heart failure worldwide, of whom approximately 6.5 million are affected in the United States, where there is an anticipated 46% increase in prevalence by 2030 (Roger 2013; Braunwald 2015; Benjamin et al. 2017). Heart failure accounts for a significant proportion of healthcare expenditure, and for 2012, the global economic burden of heart failure was estimated at nearly US$108 billion in direct and indirect costs (Cook et al. 2014). From the age of 45 years through to 95 years, the lifetime risk of heart failure is high, ranging from 20% to 45% depending on a spectrum of demographic, lifestyle, and cardiovascular risk factors (Huffman et al. 2013). Heart failure tends to occur in older individuals, being diagnosed in 1–2% of the general population, but rising to about 8% in people aged 80 years or more (Guha and McDonagh 2013). For males, the incidence of heart failure doubles for each decade between 65 and 85 years, while for females the incidence trebles over the same periods (Benjamin et al. 2017). Given the changing demography with a trend towards an aging population, the incidence of heart failure is now similar to that of breast, bowel, prostate, and lung cancers combined (Conrad et al. 2017). Despite our best efforts to address the needs of this increasingly dependent clinical cohort, heart failure remains a generally progressive condition and affected individuals are subject to a symptom burden, a poor quality of life, and a mortality risk at least equivalent to those resulting from the above cancers. Recognition of the comparable palliative care needs and the resulting literature base accruing over the past 20 years, it is evident that heart failure has been in the vanguard of the expansion of palliative care beyond its founding association with oncologic care. A suite of consensus documents and guidelines have been produced, but delivery of palliative care to the increasingly complex population diagnosed with this unpredictable clinical condition remains problematic (Goodlin et al. 2004: Jaarsma et al. 2009; McKelvie et al. 2011; Braun et al. 2016).

2 The Nature of Heart Failure

Forty years ago, Dr. Dean Mason, then chief of cardiovascular medicine at the University of California, Davis, penned a classic description of heart failure as "*the abnormal condition in which disturbed cardiac performance is primarily responsible for the inability of the heart to pump blood at a rate commensurate with systemic metabolic requirements at rest and during normal activity*" (Mason 1976). It is important to note that heart failure is not a disease per se but rather a group of acute and chronic syndromes arising from abnormalities of cardiac structure and function, representing the outcome of a diverse range of acquired or inherited cardiovascular diseases (Ponikowski et al. 2016). Given that these various etiologies result in a spectrum of disordered left ventricular physiology and remodeling, it is unsurprising that the clinical features of heart failure occur in the setting of both systolic and diastolic dysfunction.

The American College of Cardiology Foundation (ACCF), the American Heart Association (AHA), and the European Society of Cardiology (ESC) have characterized heart failure in terms of a constellation of classic symptoms and clinical signs, combined with objective assessment of ventricular function (Yancy et al. 2013; Ponikowski et al. 2016). The recent ESC guidelines have proposed a terminology describing left ventricular dysfunction with respect to the left ventricular ejection fraction (EF), that percentage volume of the blood pool within the relaxed ventricle ejected during each cardiac contraction. This is usually assessed by echocardiography or some other form of cardiac imaging. The most recent guidelines from the American Society of Echocardiography and European Association of Cardiovascular Imaging suggest that the EF should be considered abnormal if $\leq$52% for men and $\leq$54% for women (Lang et al. 2015). By the ESC criteria, symptomatic patients are said to exhibit heart failure with a reduced EF (HFrEF) when the left ventricular EF is less than 40%, commonly reflecting a background of coronary artery disease with segmental myocardial damage and eccentric remodeling.

Heart failure with a preserved EF (HFpEF) is said to apply when the EF is at least 50%. These patients predominantly exhibit diastolic dysfunction with impaired ventricular filling. In this situation, myocardial changes arise from a pro-inflammatory state linked to the commonly occurring comorbidities in obesity, diabetes mellitus, and hypertension (Paulus and Tschöpe 2013). Even in the absence of left ventricular hypertrophy, HFpEF patients may exhibit increased left ventricular mass resulting from an excess of collagen deposition in the extracellular matrix. Intrinsic cardiomyocyte stiffness might also stem from changes in the cytoskeletal protein titin, as well as slow myocyte relaxation due to impaired cross-bridge detachment and sarcoplasmic reticular Ca^{2+} reuptake (Borlaug and Paulus 2011). An intermediate group of patients has also been defined with a mid-range EF between 40% and 49% (HFmrEF) in which the heart failure state reflects a combination of systolic and diastolic dysfunction.

Table 1 The New York Heart Association classification

NYHA Functional Class	Patient symptoms
I	Objective evidence of ventricular dysfunction but no limitation of ordinary physical activity or induction of symptoms
II	Slight limitation of physical activity. Comfortable at rest. Ordinary physical activity results in fatigue, dyspnea, or palpitation
III	Significant limitation of physical activity. Comfortable at rest. Less than ordinary activity causes fatigue, dyspnea, or palpitation
IV	Unable to undertake any physical activity without discomfort. Symptoms of heart failure at rest

Table 2 The American College of Cardiology Foundation/American Heart Association stages of heart failure

ACCF/AHA Heart failure stage	Objective assessment
A	Risk factors but no objective evidence of established cardiovascular disease. No symptoms and no limitation of physical activity
B	Objective evidence of structural cardiac disease without signs or symptoms of heart failure
C	Objective evidence of structural heart disease with current or prior symptoms of heart failure
D	Refractory/advanced heart failure requiring consideration for specialized intervention

The long established New York Heart Association (NYHA) functional classification (Classes 1 to 4) and the ACCF/AHA heart failure staging system (Stages A to D) offer helpful complementary information in categorizing the impact and severity of heart failure at a given time (The Criteria Committee of the NYHA 1994; Hunt et al. 2001) (Tables 1 and 2). The former offers insight into the achievable level of exercise before symptom onset, and while this classification has been criticized as being relatively subjective and prone to inter-observer variation (Raphael et al. 2007), this metric of functional capacity remains useful and has the benefit of familiarity for many clinicians. The latter emphasizes the progressive nature of heart failure and aids in the selection of appropriate treatment options pertinent to the individual patient's heart failure stage and their changing needs.

Over the past 25 years or so, we have gained a significant understanding of the pathophysiology of heart failure, particularly in relation to HFrEF. Following an insult to cardiac function, a variety of compensatory cardiac and neurohumoral mechanisms come into play in an effort to maintain cardiac output and critical organ perfusion. These include an increase in vascular tone secondary to augmented sympathetic adrenergic activity, as well as activation of the renin-angiotensin aldosterone system (RAAS) and the release of cytokines such as interleukins and tumor necrosis factors. Responses to alterations in ventricular loading conditions are consistent with the Frank-Starling relationship. While initially protective, these various physiological responses ultimately become maladaptive and tend to promote progressive multisystem dysfunction and a spiral of decline. Elucidation of the background to this integrated cardiovascular adaptation has generated a series of landmark studies with a resultant raft of evidence-based pharmacological therapies.

Alongside these, protocols have been developed to further optimize treatment with the use of implanted electronic devices in the form of complex pacemakers as cardiac resynchronization therapy (CRT) to improve the efficiency of ventricular contraction and implantable cardioverter-defibrillator (ICDs) to reduce the risk of sudden death from malignant arrhythmias. Surgical strategies have also evolved for those with advanced HFrEF, including the use of mechanical circulatory support (MCS) in the placement of left ventricular assist devices (LVADs) as a bridge to recovery or cardiac transplantation, or long term as so-called destination therapy. The benefits of such a multifaceted approach to this life limiting condition are well established, and this is now enshrined in HFrEF treatment guidelines (National Heart Foundation of Australia 2011; Yancy et al. 2013; Ponikowski et al. 2016). In contrast, the complex mechanisms underlying the predominant diastolic dysfunction typical of those with HFpEF are only just coming to light and effective therapies to specifically modulate these are yet to emerge (Borlaug and Paulus 2011; Ponikowski et al. 2016).

In the clinical cohort exhibiting features of heart failure, 80–90% likely have HFrEF or HFpEF which are relatively evenly represented, the residual 10–20% being made up of those with HFmrEF (Lam and Solomon 2014). HFpEF is more common in the oldest old, and secular trends in age-related heart failure variants suggest that HFpEF may become the predominant clinical phenotype. It is also uncertain if the potential benefits of evidence-based HFrEF therapy are generalizable to those affected in the growing elderly population as this group was largely excluded from the pivotal clinical trials (Rich et al. 2016).

3 Health Burden of Heart Failure

Heart failure is the most common admission diagnosis in those aged 65 years or older in high income nations (Braunwald 2015). According to the National Heart Failure Audit in England and Wales, following hospital admission with acute heart failure, the projected 1-year mortality of those below and above 75 years of age has been estimated at 26% and 56%, respectively (Cleland et al. 2011). Analysis of data from the Olmsted County Registry on 4596 patients with chronic heart failure tracked by the Mayo Clinic suggested similar 1-year and 5-year mortality rates at 32% vs. 28% and 68% vs. 65% for HFrEF and HFpEF, respectively, using an EF of 50% as the cut point (Owan et al. 2006). Comparing modes of death, for both of these clinical subtypes, a cardiovascular cause predominates, manifest as refractory congestive heart failure or sudden cardiac death, but proportionately more of the HFpEF population die of non-cardiovascular comorbidities (Chan and Lam 2013).

4 Comorbidities

Given the typically elderly population affected by heart failure, many patients exhibit several comorbidities including frailty, cognitive impairment, anemia, diabetes, chronic obstructive pulmonary disease (COPD), renal dysfunction, and depression/anxiety (van Deursen et al. 2014). Some of these are discussed in more detail below. The Charlson Comorbidity Index may have limited prognostic utility in the chronic heart failure population, and evidence on how to manage comorbidities at the end of life is limited (Testa et al. 2009; Tevendale and Baxter 2011).

4.1 Frailty

In recent years, frailty has been increasingly recognized in those with heart failure and associated with greater symptom burden and poor outcomes such as increased rates of hospitalization and mortality (Chaudhry et al. 2013; Jha et al. 2015; Denfeld et al. 2018). This complex syndrome has been variously attributed to a specific age-related biological phenotype including sarcopenia, or alternatively, to the effects of composite physiologic deficits resulting in diminished reserve and increased vulnerability to stressors (Fried et al. 2001; Jermyn and Patel 2015). Significantly affected patients often struggle with mobility and the activities of daily living which can impact on self-care behaviors affecting nutrition and hydration, sometimes manifest as falls and delirium. While no frailty assessment instrument has been validated specifically for the heart failure population (McDonagh et al. 2018), evaluation tends to be focused on the five domains of the Fried Frailty Index: self-reported exhaustion, physical activity, walking speed, hand grip strength, and unintentional weight loss; parameters initially assessed in the Cardiovascular Health Study (Fried et al. 1991). Based on this model, a recent study of patients with advanced heart failure demonstrated that 65% of them were frail and 35% were prefrail (Madan et al. 2016).

4.2 Cognitive Impairment

Cognitive impairment is relatively common in those with heart failure, the reported prevalence varying between 25% and 75% by a range of assessments across diverse studies, and estimated to be about 40% overall in a recent meta-analysis (Ampadu and Morley 2015; Cannon et al. 2017). Both HFrEF and HFpEF patients may develop this (Alagiakrishnan et al. 2016). The spectrum of cognitive dysfunction is similar to that seen in non-heart failure patients and includes agitated delirium, as well as isolated memory or non-memory deficits through to dementia. The risk factors for cognitive impairment are similar for those with or without heart failure, and while we must be aware of the potential secondary effects of heart failure therapy on cerebral perfusion, to date no causal relationship to specific treatment has been identified. However, neprilysin is involved in clearing amyloid peptides from cerebral tissue. Theoretically, following the positive results of the PARADIGM HF trial, use of the recently licensed angiotensin receptor neprilysin inhibitor sacubitril/valsartan (Entresto®) might interfere with this (Cannon et al. 2017). Two clinical trials currently in progress may clarify this potential risk [ClinicalTrials.gov identifiers: NCT01920711, NCT02884206]. The presence of atrial fibrillation, whether permanent or paroxysmal, is strongly linked to cognitive decline, even when there is no evidence of a major stroke or imaging features characteristic of cerebral microembolic disease (Ampadu and Morley 2015). The effects of cognitive impairment may impact self-care decision making and are associated with a greater use of healthcare resources, higher rates of hospital readmission, and mortality (Riley and Arslanian-Engoren 2013; Alagiakrishnan et al. 2016).

4.3 Anemia and Iron Deficiency

Anemia, conventionally characterized as a hemoglobin of less than 13 g/dL and 12 g/dL for men and women, respectively, is relatively common in heart failure. However, even in the absence of clinically overt anemia, heart failure is associated with both absolute and functional iron deficiency (McDonagh and Macdougall 2015). Absolute iron deficiency occurs when iron stores are low, generally defined as a serum ferritin level below 100 ng/ml. This may occur as a consequence of nutritional deficiency, poor iron absorption through a congested gastrointestinal mucosa, or blood loss due to the effects of antiplatelet or anticoagulant therapy. In functional iron deficiency, typically defined as a serum ferritin greater than 200 ng/ml with a transferrin saturation (TSAT) below 20%, iron stores are replete, but iron utilization is insufficient to drive adequate erythropoiesis or normal cellular metabolism. This is often mediated by the response of hepcidin, a polypeptide and key regulator of iron metabolism. Hepcidin controls intestinal iron absorption, serum iron concentrations, and cellular iron distribution by inducing degradation of its receptor, the cellular iron exporter ferroportin (Ganz and Nemeth 2012). In the early phase of heart failure, the active inflammatory state results in high levels of hepcidin which may "trap" iron in macrophages and hepatocytes (McDonagh and Macdougall 2015). However, as heart failure progresses, hepcidin levels decline with impaired iron homeostasis and resultant anemia (Jankowska et al. 2013). Iron deficiency has been shown to occur in all heart failure variants (HFrEF, HFmrEF, and HFpEF) and is associated with poor quality of life and outcomes (Martens et al. 2017). Effective therapy is now available as intravenous ferric carboxymaltose as proposed in the ESC guidelines (Ponikowski et al. 2016). Although the mechanisms are different, iron deficiency may also arise in chronic kidney disease (CKD), a common comorbidity in those with heart failure.

4.4 Renal Dysfunction

Heart and kidney function are mutually interdependent. Cardiovascular physiology relies on the maintenance of salt and water balance by the kidney, and kidney function depends on adequate blood pressure and renal perfusion provided by the heart. Both organ systems share common risk factors and disturbances of pressure and volume homeostasis are typical of both acute and chronic heart failure (Boudoulas et al. 2017). The intimate relationship between cardiac and kidney function has seen evolution of the concept of the so-called *cardiorenal syndrome* which has been subclassified as occurring as five variants (Table 3). The pathophysiological mechanisms underlying this complex interplay remain incompletely understood but may be broadly summarized as relating to:

- Hemodynamic changes due to low cardiac output and deranged venous return
- Dysregulation of the neurohumoral axis with enhanced sympathetic drive and triggering of the RAAS system
- Other factors affecting heart and kidney function such as oxidative stress due to sepsis, inflammation, anemia, and cachexia

CKD, defined as a glomerular filtration rate (GFR) persistently less than 60 ml/min/1.73m^2, is demonstrable in 40–50% of heart failure patients (Schefold et al. 2016). This is an independent risk factor for cardiovascular disease including heart failure and for heart failure progression. For those with HFrEF, a declining GFR is a more powerful predictor of mortality than the EF. While a transient reduction in GFR is commonly observed after initiation of angiotensin converting enzyme inhibitor (ACEI) therapy or angiotensin receptor blockers (ARBs), this usually recovers. However, the presence of CKD often worries

Table 3 Variants of the cardiorenal syndrome. (Modified from Boudoulas et al. 2017)

Type	Cardiorenal syndromes
1	Acute heart failure or decompensation of chronic heart failure resulting in acute kidney injury or dysfunction
2	Chronic heart failure resulting in CKD
3	Acute decompensation of renal function inducing acute heart failure
4	CKD producing chronic heart failure
5	A variety of other conditions secondarily impacting heart and kidney function

clinicians and inhibits the optimal prescription of evidence-based heart failure therapy, including that for those on renal replacement therapy as hemodialysis. The adverse cardiovascular effects of long-term hemodialysis are well established, and while renal transplantation was previously considered contraindicated in those with significant HFrEF, this has now been shown to be beneficial. Indeed this intervention may promote recovery of ventricular function (Kute et al. 2014).

4.5 Depression and Anxiety

Depression appears to be relatively common being present in at least 1 in 5 of the clinical cohort with heart failure and may be proportionately greater in those with more advanced disease. This comorbidity is associated with increased healthcare utilization, and higher readmission rates and mortality (Moraska et al. 2013). In one study of 985 patients assessed by the Beck Depression Inventory Scale during their index heart failure admission and followed over a 12-year period, the mortality was 80% for those with depression against 73% for those without (Adams et al. 2012). Anxiety is said to be 60% more frequent in those with heart failure compared to the general population, and rates are considered at least comparable or possibly greater than those with cancer and pulmonary disease depending on the method of assessment. The effect of anxiety on outcomes is less certain than for depression (Sokoreli et al. 2016), but clearly these conditions frequently co-exist. Postulated mechanisms relevant to outcomes include both health behavioral and biological effects. Depression may result in poor adherence to heart failure medication, or anxiety-related sympathetic hyperactivity may reduce the threshold for significant arrhythmia, induce coronary vasospasm and ischemia, or promote a pro-thrombotic effect (Fan et al. 2014). Safe and effective treatments for depression in heart failure are available, either in the form of cognitive behavioral therapy or with the use of drugs such as selective serotonin reuptake inhibitors (Rustad et al. 2013).

5 The Heart Failure Disease Trajectory

Heart failure patients tend to deteriorate along a roller coaster disease trajectory of progressively declining physical capacity interspersed with distressing clinical crises (Fig. 1) (Goodlin et al. 2004). These inflection points may be markers of further cardiac events leading to incremental ventricular dysfunction, life-threatening episodes of acute decompensation, or arrhythmia. Although potentially lethal arrhythmias may occur at any stage along the course of the disease, these are more frequent in the earlier, milder phase of HfrEF, particularly when there is a background of coronary artery disease resulting in patchy scarring and electrophysiological instability. Notwithstanding the absence of an ICD, rates of sudden death have declined over the past 20 years or so consistent with a beneficial response to use of the evidence-based medication developed over that period (Fig. 2) (Udelson and Stevenson 2016; Shen et al. 2017). In advanced heart failure, the usual mode of death is through congestion and irreversible multiorgan failure, the terminal phase often preceded by a cluster of unplanned hospital admissions (Udelson and Stevenson 2016). Despite this, those close to the patient often perceive the death as unexpected. This may reflect a lack of appreciation of the nature and significance of this condition (Alonso et al. 2017), or inadequate communication between health care professionals, patients, and their families (Russ and Kaufman 2005; Allen et al. 2012). It is important to emphasize that while the schematic illness trajectory shown in Fig. 1 is a reasonable representation of clinical reality on a population basis, the pattern of decline and response to treatment is unique to each individual (Fig. 3) (Gott et al. 2007).

The fluctuating, inconsistent disease course and resultant uncertainty also constitute a barrier to discussion on end of life care as heart failure professionals find it difficult to discern specific transition points when this might be appropriate (Barclay et al. 2011). Having recovered from earlier high risk episodes, patients tend to overestimate life expectancy and assume they will

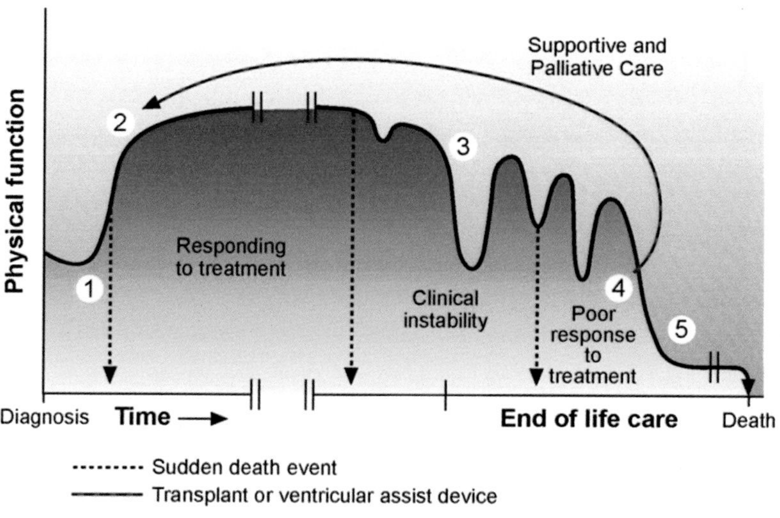

Fig. 1 A schematic of the heart failure disease trajectory (Modified from Goodlin et al. (2004) with permission)

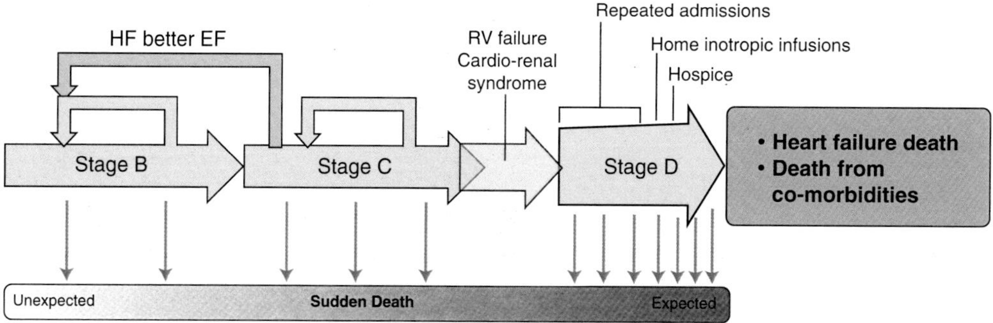

Fig. 2 The changing face of heart failure outcomes across the development of evidence-based heart failure therapy (From Udelson and Stevenson (2016) with permission)

survive against all the odds (Allen et al. 2008). While this intrinsic unpredictability needs to be acknowledged by the healthcare team, hope for the future should be maintained in fostering coping and adjustment strategies to deal with changing circumstances (Davidson et al. 2007). Themes important to those living with the uncertainty of chronic advanced illnesses, including

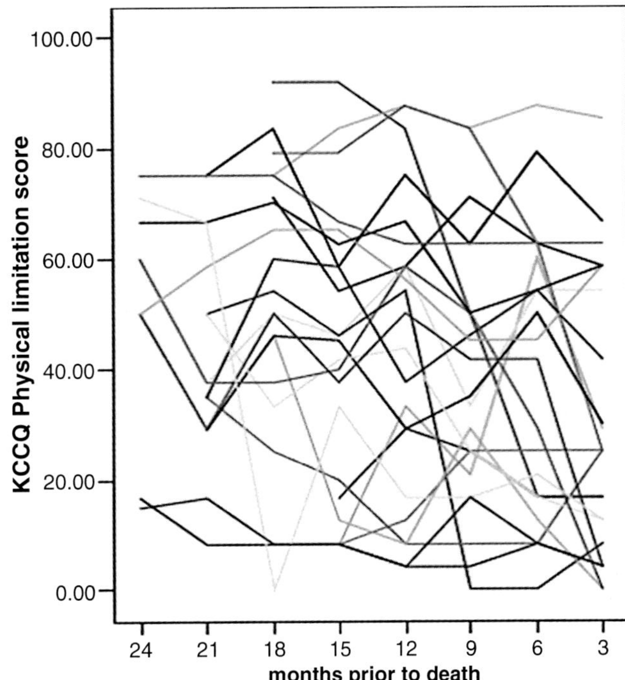

Fig. 3 The uniqueness of individual heart failure patients' disease trajectories (From Gott et al. (2007) with permission)

heart failure, have been evaluated (Etkind et al. 2017). These were shown to include their degree of engagement or control over the illness, temporal focus on the present and future, factors relating to communication, information needs and preferences, and a variety of priorities including quality of life, social factors, and concern about potential conflict between themselves and the health professionals responsible for their care.

6 Prognostication

Regardless of advances in cardiovascular therapy, heart failure in all its forms constitutes an increasingly encountered life limiting condition; about 50% of those diagnosed with heart failure die within 5 years of diagnosis (Gerber et al. 2015). Heart failure is documented on 1 in 8 death certificates in the United States (Benjamin et al. 2017). As outlined in a recent review, a variety of prognostic tools have been utilized in the assessment of survival in heart failure (Treece et al. 2017). Despite acknowledgment of subjectivity, functional assessment by the NYHA classification has been accepted as a strong prognostic indicator for both HFrEF and HFpEF (Raphael et al. 2007). In a study in England of 293 heart failure patients who self-assigned their NYHA class, subsequent mortality over 6–20 months was 19.6% for classes I/II, 34.3% for class III, and 39.2% for class IV (Holland et al. 2010).

The CardioVascular Medicine Heart Failure Index incorporates NYHA Class III/IV alongside 12 other variables related to cardiac conditions and comorbidities to stratify patients, treated across a variety of care settings, into low-, medium-, and high-risk for a 12-month mortality (Senni et al. 2006). The other variables include age, anemia, hypertension, COPD, complicated diabetes, moderate/severe CKD, metastatic cancer, absence of β-blocker, ACEI or ARB therapy, EF less $\leq$20%, and the presence of severe valvular heart disease or atrial fibrillation. A similar multivariate approach was adopted in the development of the Heart Failure Survival Score which uses 80 clinical attributes to characterize mortality risk, validated in a clinical cohort with advanced heart failure referred in consideration for heart transplantation (Aaronson et al. 1997).

The most widely used scoring system is the Seattle Heart Failure Model, developed by the

University of Washington, and validated in a cohort predominantly exhibiting HFrEF (Levy et al. 2006). This model, applicable to both ambulatory and hospitalized patients, is based on readily accessible clinical, laboratory, pharmacological, and device features and has been regularly updated to accommodate developments in heart failure therapy. More recently, a robust heart failure mortality risk assessment tool has been elaborated by the Meta-Analysis Global Group in Chronic Heart failure (MAGGIC) (Pocock et al. 2013). This is founded on 13 independent predictors derived from data collated from over 39,000 patients with HFrEF or HFpEF across 30 cohort studies comprising 6 clinical trials and 24 registries. The MAGGIC model is available via www.heartfailurerisk.org. While potentially useful on a population basis (Sartipy et al. 2014), this and the Seattle Heart Failure Model have not been specifically validated for the advanced heart failure population, and neither appear to be particularly reliable in predicting 12-month mortality for individual patients (Allen et al. 2017).

7 Palliative Care Needs Assessment

Acknowledging the underlying prognostic difficulties, and recognizing that those affected by heart failure are subject to a mortality risk and symptom burden at least equivalent to those with cancer (Xu et al. 2015), it is arguable that support should be offered at any point along the disease trajectory based on palliative care needs, rather than life-expectancy (Hogg and Jenkins 2012; Meyers and Goodlin 2016; Lewin et al. 2017). However, given the clinical complexity of the affected population and the ethos of the medical model in providing comprehensive guideline-directed heart failure therapy, of itself sometimes onerous (Jani et al. 2013), knowing when to trigger such palliative care involvement is difficult.

While potentially helpful in raising awareness, use of the "Surprise Question" – "*Would I be surprised if this patient died in the next 12 months*" – appears to offer little advantage when used alone in identifying heart failure patients who may benefit from palliative care (Small et al. 2010; White et al. 2017). Needs assessment involves comprehensive evaluation of symptom burden and functional status (Opasich et al. 2008). To some extent reflecting NYHA status, the Kansas City Cardiomyopathy Questionnaire (KCCQ) and the Minnesota Living with Heart Failure Questionnaire (MLHFQ) offer wide-ranging evaluation of heart failure-related physical and psychological symptoms, performance status, and health-related quality of life (Rector et al. 1987; Green et al. 2000). The KCCQ comprises a 21-item self-administered instrument which facilitates derivation of a summary score across domains of physical function, symptoms (frequency, severity, recent trends), social function, self-efficacy, knowledge, and quality of life. The higher summary score, the better the health status. The widely used MLHFQ is based on a psychometrically validated 21-item questionnaire covering the effects of heart failure on key elements of the physical, emotional, social, and psychological dimensions of quality of life. For each of the 21 variables, patients complete a 6-point Likert scale (0–5), indicating by how much heart failure impacts on living as they would wish. A lower score correlates with a better quality of life. The MLHFQ is available in many languages, validated against the original, and is curated by the Mapi Research Trust (www.mapi-trust.org).

A series of studies have demonstrated a moderate correlation between these heart failure instruments and palliative care assessment tools including the Karnofsky Performance Status Scale, the Palliative Performance Scale and the Edmonton Symptom Assessment Scale, but also suggest that combining these approaches might be useful in clarifying unmet palliative care needs (Opasich et al. 2008; Ezekowitz et al. 2011; Timmons et al. 2013; Johnson et al. 2014). Use of the Integrated Palliative care Outcomes Scale (IPOS) combined with specialist heart failure nurse education and training has been shown to be feasible and acceptable to patients exhibiting any of the heart failure phenotypes as HFrEF, HFmrEF, or HFpEF, as well as to their responsible health professionals (Kane et al. 2017). Similarly, an instrument specific to heart failure, the Needs

Assessment Tool: Progressive Disease – Heart Failure (NAT: PD – HF), developed in Australia, shows promise and is currently being piloted in Scotland (Waller et al. 2013; Campbell et al. 2015). In contrast, a recent review suggests that the RADboud indicators for PAlliative Care needs (RADPAC) and the NECesidades PALiativas (NECPAL), tools developed in the Netherlands and Spain, respectively, to assess the palliative care needs in those with chronic diseases, may have limited utility in those with heart failure (Thoonsen et al. 2012; Gómez-Batiste et al. 2013; Janssen et al. 2017). Palliative care needs assessment is particularly relevant to some increasingly used forms of heart failure therapy.

8 Implantable Cardioverter-Defibrillators

Since their first deployment in humans in 1980, implantable cardioverter-defibrillator (ICD) technology has been significantly refined and their use has increased exponentially in recent years (Hindricks et al. 2017; Benjamin et al. 2017). There is unequivocal evidence of their benefit in the primary or secondary prevention of sudden cardiac death in individuals deemed to be at risk from malignant ventricular arrhythmias (Russo et al. 2013; Epstein et al. 2013). These may be used as standalone ICDs or combined with cardiac resynchronization therapy (CRT-D) in appropriately selected patients with HFrEF (Yancy et al. 2013). In continuously monitoring cardiac rhythm, they offer a number of key responses:

- Automatic administration of defibrillation shocks to terminate ventricular fibrillation or fast ventricular tachycardia (VT)
- Antibradycardia pacing, often activated after a defibrillator shock as the heart transitions to normal rhythm
- Antitachycardia pacing to terminate slower VT
- Cardioversion of VT

Risks affecting quality of life sometimes accompany the benefits of these devices (Atwater and Daubert 2012). While ICD function offers no intrinsic symptomatic advantage, the discomfort associated with shock delivery, likened to being punched in the chest or kicked by a horse, or the anxiety engendered by shock anticipation, may be acceptable trade-offs in clinical scenarios when life extension is the primary goal. However, close to the end of life, when the patient is dying of progressive heart failure or an unrelated disease, futile ICD shocks constitute a painful and avoidable harm. The metabolic and biochemical derangement typical of this terminal phase may trigger arrhythmias and device activity, and such occurrences are well documented. An early study, based on experiences of bereaved families, reported that 20% of ICD patients received shocks as they were dying, and if device deactivation took place at all, this was only in a minority and very close to the point of death (Goldstein et al. 2004). In a more recent study, postmortem interrogation of explanted devices demonstrated that a third of decedents were subjected to a shock on their last day alive, often within an hour of death (Kinch Westerdahl et al. 2014). While more than half of these patients had a “Do not resuscitate” order in place, in about two-thirds of this group, the defibrillation mode of the device was still active at the time of death.

Clinical practice guidelines propose that discussion on the possibility of later device deactivation should be broached at the time of informed consent for the de novo ICD implant, and that this aspect of care should be revisited at intervals, particularly when considering device replacement due to generator battery depletion (Lewis et al. 2016). However, in real life clinical practice, these discussions are infrequent (Clark et al. 2011; Niewald et al. 2013; Hill et al. 2016). In contrast, by defaulting to a guideline-directed treatment protocol, cognitive bias has been demonstrated in that clinicians undertaking discussions before such procedures tend to over emphasize the benefits of initiating or maintaining ICD therapy (Hauptman et al. 2013; Matlock et al. 2017). A positive spin is also evident in educational materials relating to ICDs, some of which emanate from the device industry (Strachan et al. 2012). Given the framing effects evident in this information exchange, patients tend to regard the decision on ICD therapy as binary in life or death and do not seem to recall being offered alternatives to the primary implant or the option to decline device replacement (Agård et al. 2007; Carroll et al. 2013a). Data from the United States National ICD Registry have shown that 42% of new ICDs were implanted in those aged over 70 years and 12% in those more than 80 years, yet 51% of people receiving an ICD after the age of 65 years were either dead or in hospice 5 years after implantation (Wright et al. 2013; Kramer et al. 2016). Thus, for many, particularly the relatively elderly multimorbid heart failure patients, the benefits of ICD therapy are uncertain (Kaufman et al. 2011; Barra et al. 2015; Green et al. 2016; Rich et al. 2016). As highlighted at a recently convened Hartford Change Agents Symposium (Kramer et al. 2015), a more nuanced and values-based approach is required to ensure that treatment decisions are aligned with patient preferences for care and mode of death (Joyce et al. 2013). As such preferences are prone to change (Brunner-La Rocca et al. 2012), this discourse needs to be an iterative process rather than at a single point along the individual patient's disease trajectory.

Undertaking these difficult conversations can be uncomfortable for both patients and clinicians. Perhaps linked to the anchoring heuristic set at earlier discussions in consideration of ICD therapy, patients tend to overestimate the expected benefit derived from the device, and sometimes regard the notion of deactivation as akin to an act of suicide (Goldstein et al. 2008a; Stewart et al. 2010). When proposing this intervention, ideally prior to implantation as part of the informed consent process, it would be appropriate to highlight that the perceived benefits of ICD therapy are to some extent conditional, and should be subject to review in the face of disease progression, changes in attitude to device acceptability, or other circumstances. Impartial education should be provided to ICD eligible patients and their families (Dunbar et al. 2012). While some are in development, robust decision tools to facilitate this dialogue are not yet available (Clark et al. 2012; Carroll et al. 2013b). A group at the University of Colorado, Denver, are undertaking a pilot study of ICD patient decision aids [Clinical.Trials.org identifier: NCT02026102], and through the Colorado Program for Patient Centered Decisions, have developed a web-based informational/decision support tool for patients and their families considering an ICD as primary prevention (University of Colorado 2016). It is important to include family members in this process. They often provide significant informal care to heart failure patients and may have to assume the role of surrogate decision maker if the patient loses intellectual capacity. Cognitive decline has been demonstrated in ICD recipients as early as 12 months after implantation (Kim et al. 2013). Spouses have reported feeling unprepared to take on this responsibility and have sometimes been excluded from the formal follow up process (Fluur et al. 2014). While advance care planning, including the appointment of a proxy to make decisions if capacity is lost, might obviate some of the dilemmas which may arise later, few device-specific advance directives are enacted by the heart failure population (Dunlay et al. 2012; Merchant et al. 2017).

Health professionals are sometimes uncomfortable in initiating conversations about ICD deactivation. This can stem from difficulties in prognostication, their own attitudes to dying, or a fear that such conversations might impact patients' hopes for the future and undermine the clinician-patient relationship (Goldstein et al. 2008b). Alternatively, they may falsely perceive that effective communication has been achieved. A trial has just been completed exploring means of improving clinician–patient communication in respect of ICD therapy [ClinicalTrials.gov identifier NCT01459744] but has yet to report. Some clinicians may also have unfounded ethical concerns that ICD deactivation is equivalent to euthanasia (Kramer et al. 2010, 2011), but the ethical principles supporting appropriate device withdrawal have been fully established (Wright et al. 2013; Chamsi-Pasha et al. 2014). National and international guidelines for ICD deactivation have been developed, but it is important that clinicians ensure that their handling of device issues is compatible with local legislation relevant to the state or country where their clinical practice is based (Padeletti et al. 2010; Lampert et al. 2010;

Pitcher et al. 2016). While national guidance offers a benchmark, effective device management requires the formulation of institutional, local, and regional protocols, supported by regularly updated staff education and training, and with adequate provision and unrestricted access to the required trained personnel and equipment.

Palliative care involvement may facilitate clarification of goals of care or symptom management after device withdrawal (Pasalic et al. 2016), but hospice care may present significant difficulties to heart failure patients with these devices (Lum et al. 2015). Previous surveys of hospices in the United States and the United Kingdom have shown that while most admit patients with ICDs, there was poor documentation of this on admission, a paucity of deactivation protocols, deficiencies in staff training, and poor access to equipment to facilitate urgent device deactivation (Goldstein et al. 2010; Beattie et al. 2012). Compared to those in urban centers, hospices based in rural communities report particular difficulties (Fromme et al. 2011), Planned ICD deactivation can be achieved simply by device reprogramming, and in an emergency, the shocking function can be temporarily disarmed by placing a doughnut magnet on the chest wall over the device (Pitcher et al. 2016). It is also important to remember that, if not already completed, the device should be deactivated after death to avoid a shock risk to mortuary personnel or undertakers, and that the device should be removed prior to any planned cremation to prevent an explosion hazard.

9 Mechanical Circulatory Support and Transplantation

For patients with advanced HFrEF (Stage D), aggressive surgical options include ventricular reconstructive surgery – often a form of the Dor procedure, cardiac transplantation, or the placement of a left ventricular assist device (LVAD) (Fang et al. 2015). First implanted in 1984, a LVAD is a mechanical pump inserted via open heart surgery to supplement the poor contractile function of the failing ventricle. As with implanted electronic devices in ICDs or pacemakers, refinements in technology have led to the rather bulky early devices becoming more miniaturized, with improved biocompatibility, durability, and increased functional performance. Early LVADs provided pulsatile flow based on volume displacement, but currently used axial or centrifugal continuous flow rotary pumps have fewer moving parts and are designed to provide an augmented cardiac output of up to 10 L/min. At times, when there is also right ventricular dysfunction, biventricular support in the form of a total artificial heart is implanted (Wordingham et al. 2015). The evolution and outcomes from these mechanical circulatory support (MCS) devices are collated by the Interagency Registry for Mechanically Assisted Circulatory Support (INTERMACS) and are described in sequential reports (Kirklin et al. 2015).

The use of MCS devices in appropriately selected advanced heart failure patients offers a significant prognostic advantage compared to optimal medical therapy, with an 80% 1-year and a 70% 2-year survival compared to about 6 months without the implant (Kirklin et al. 2015). Initially, LVAD use was intended as a bridge to recovery, sometimes effective in acute heart failure states due to conditions such as viral myocarditis or postpartum cardiomyopathy (Kirkpatrick et al. 2015). At times temporary MCS is still indicated alongside pharmacologic inotropic support for patients with critical cardiogenic shock. Such devices can be placed percutaneously or surgically and are offered as a bridge to decision in terms of potentially receiving long-term device placement depending on the outcome with respect to recovery of ventricular function, or survival (Becnel et al. 2017). More commonly, surgically placed LVADs are used as a bridge to transplant (BTT) in those with chronic heart failure. While this policy continues, given the positive outcomes in improving symptoms and prognosis, together with the scarcity of donor organs, LVAD responsive patients may be assigned a lower priority on transplant waiting lists. Alternatively, some may choose not to go on to transplantation or become transplant ineligible as they age and develop comorbidities. Consequently, many patients now receive LVADs as a long-term MCS option in destination therapy (DT).

While there are noteworthy benefits of this intervention in improved quality of life and physical capacity, living with a LVAD as BTT or DT may also be burdensome for both patients and those close to them. Implantees must adhere to relatively complex medication regimes and are physically constrained in the need to maintain device functionality through an external driveline connecting the pump to the controller and battery pack. This limits day to day activities of both patients and families, impacting their broader social but also closer interpersonal relationships. There is also existential anxiety in an heightened awareness that life itself depends on the device. Despite the hemodynamic support derived from the implant, rehospitalization may be required due to recurrent heart failure or the occurrence of device-related infections, most often linked to the driveline (Goldstein et al. 2012). Devices are being developed that can be recharged transcutaneously which might supplant the need for this external power connection. There is also a substantial risk of gastrointestinal bleeding which appears to originate in mucosal arteriovenous malformations, developing as a form of angiodysplasia in response to the moderately low pulse pressure associated with continuous flow perfusion. An acquired form of von Willebrand syndrome may also be relevant here. These clinical situations can be challenging as all continuous flow devices require anticoagulation with warfarin, usually combined with aspirin because of device-mediated changes in platelet function. Despite this, there is also a relatively high incidence of pump thrombosis, with a cumulative risk of 14%, 24%, and 25%, at 1, 3, and 5 years, respectively (Stulak et al. 2016). This almost invariably requires pump replacement. Another feared complication is that of stroke, with an incidence of 11% at 1 year and 17% at 2 years (Kirklin et al. 2015). If clinically significant, this might require consideration for withdrawal of device therapy with a consequential rapidly fatal outcome. Most patients die within an hour of LVAD deactivation. In a recent review of DT-LVAD patients from the Mayo Clinic, the most common causes of death were multiorgan failure (26%), hemorrhagic stroke (24%), and progressive heart failure (21%) (Dunlay et al. 2016). Given the complexity of this clinical cohort, the vast majority of patients die in hospital, usually in the intensive care unit.

The development and progressively mainstream use of MCS for advanced heart failure offers significant opportunities to synergize the complementary expertise of cardiologists, cardiac surgeons, and palliative care professionals (Goldstein et al. 2011). Indeed, since 2014 in the United States, the Centers for Medicare and Medicaid Services have mandated that a palliative care professional is included in all DT-LVAD program teams (Centers for Medicare and Medicaid Services 2014). Palliative care involvement may facilitate preparedness planning and goal setting against the background of clinical issues which might play out for patients and families throughout the MCS journey from just considering LVAD support, through the implant procedure and any subsequent transplant, or living with a DT-LVAD to the end of life (Swetz et al. 2011; Luo et al. 2016; Nakagawa et al. 2017; Wordingham et al. 2017). The impact of including palliative care professionals was noteworthy in aiding decision making in patients and families dealing with complications of LVADS, including consideration for LVAD deactivation. They also strengthened the expertise of the MCS team in providing enhanced symptom relief and psychosocial support and facilitated hospice referral for suitably selected patients (Sagin et al. 2016). Further, there was a perception that integrating palliative care within the MCS team improved the experience of patients and families. Care structures vary between institutions, and bereaved caregivers of LVAD patients have also reported significant confusion and care fragmentation at the end of life which underscores the need to develop effective models of collaborative care, supported by robust outcome assessment to promote and spread best practice (McIlvennan et al. 2016).

Palliative care support is also relevant to those patients who follow the clinical continuum and go on to cardiac transplantation (Banner et al. 2011). This intervention is highly effective for the privileged few graft recipients. With a 1-year and 5-year survival of 84.5% and 72.5%, respectively

(Wilhelm 2015), current data from the International Society for Heart and Lung Transplantation registry suggest a median life expectancy of 10–15 years posttransplant. However, cardiopulmonary transplantation is still associated with significant morbidity, mortality, and unmet palliative care needs (McKenna and Clark 2015).

Pretransplantation, given the significant symptomatic burden and uncertainty while waiting for a suitable donor organ, patients and families have a poor quality of life and are in need of multimodal support. Data on the effects of intervention are limited (Muhandiramge et al. 2015; Bayoumi et al. 2017), but a small pilot study of palliative care consultations jointly undertaken by a palliative care physician and cardiologist in those referred for heart transplantation demonstrated benefits for both patients and families in better continuity of care, goal setting, and reduced opioid use (Schwarz et al. 2012).

Several issues affect outcomes in the peri- and post-transplantation phases. The 30-day mortality after heart or lung transplantation lies between 10% and 30% (McKenna and Clark 2015). Despite improvements in immunosuppression, there are still significant problems with rejection. This occurs in both acute and chronic forms through cell- or antibody-mediated responses and may be manifest as accelerated allograft vasculopathy which affects about 50% of graft recipients by 10 years post-transplant (Wilhelm 2015). Infection accounts for about 30% of deaths in the first year post-intervention, the risk reducing thereafter. Pharmacologic immunosuppression is associated with a higher incidence of malignancy and more aggressive tumor biology (Collett et al. 2010). Malignancies are evident in about 15% of heart transplant patients by 5 years out and account for around 22% of the annual mortality beyond this. Skin cancer is particularly common (Wilhelm 2015).

The evidence specifically relating to palliative care provision after heart transplantation is limited. Attitudinally, some transplant teams seem to regard palliative care as a last resort and only consider this when all other forms of therapy have been exhausted, limiting involvement to end of life care (McKenna and Clark 2015). This requires education in the broader reach of palliative care and the promotion of multidisciplinary working. There are undoubtedly significant parallels in the needs and intensity of care required of the populations these disciplines serve in their different ways. The evolving collaboration between palliative care and cardiac surgical professionals related to patients requiring MCS, and indeed in those undergoing transcatheter aortic valve implantation (TAVI), might provide a useful platform to meld and expand the remit of this shared expertise (Lauck et al. 2014; Steiner et al. 2017). It is also important to emphasize that palliative care provision should be central to the continuing care of those who are assessed and deemed to be transplant ineligible. Apart from patient choice, a variety of clinical and psycho-social features may be relevant to that decision and some are outlined in Table 4. Given the irreversible nature of heart failure disease progression, in the absence of potential rescue by transplantation, addressing symptom control and planning for end of life care are likely to become the dominant goals of treatment.

Table 4 Relative contraindications for cardiac transplantation. (Adapted from Banner et al. 2011)

Active infection Recent malignancy
Recent pulmonary embolism Significant pulmonary pathology Persistent severe pulmonary hypertension (>60 mmHg)
Severe obesity (>32 kg/m^2) Diabetes with significant extra-cardiac end-organ damage Symptomatic peripheral vascular disease Symptomatic cerebrovascular disease Irreversible significant renal impairment (GFR < 40 ml/min/m^2)
Cognitive impairment precluding consent Inadequate accommodation or social support History of non-adherence to therapy Substance abuse (active smoking, excessive alcohol, or illicit drug use)

10 Symptom Burden

Those living with heart failure experience a symptom burden similar to that associated with cancer and other progressive long-term conditions (Solano et al. 2006; Bekelman et al. 2009; O'Leary et al.

2009). In addition to the anticipated heart failure-related symptoms of breathlessness and congestion, over the past two decades a plethora of other debilitating features has also been described including gastrointestinal, spiritual, and psycho-social dysfunction, which may be under appreciated by cardiology focused healthcare providers (Murray et al. 2007; Bekelman et al. 2009).

Pain is particularly common in heart failure patients and is frequently poorly recognized and treated (Light-McGroary and Goodlin 2013). The symptomatic spectrum in heart failure has recently been summarized and this is shown in Table 5 (Riley and Beattie 2017). The prevalence of symptoms and the extent to which they are perceived as distressing appear to vary. For example, the background to breathlessness and fatigue in heart failure is complex, but the former is both highly prevalent and highly distressing, while the latter appears to be less associated with distress (Riley and Beattie 2017). Even towards the end of life when symptoms increase in prevalence and intensity, health-related quality of life may be relatively well preserved (Levenson et al. 2000). Comparing the postulated level of symptom impact across studies is hampered by inconsistencies in methods of assessment; however, the Memorial Symptom Assessment Scale – Heart Failure (MSAS-HF), and the MD Anderson Symptom Inventory-HF, modified from instruments initially developed for those with cancer, may be particularly useful (Zambroski et al. 2005; Lee and Moser 2013). A comprehensive review suggested that heart failure patients experienced a mean of 15 $\pm$ 8 symptoms (Zambroski et al. 2005), and these may be directly linked to the heart failure syndrome or to the patients' comorbidities, perhaps particularly relevant to those with HFpEF (Blinderman et al. 2008; Eckerblad et al. 2015).

Clinicians have tended to focus on individual symptoms as distinct clinical entities, but the malaise of heart failure is multidimensional and in recent years the concept of symptom clustering has come into play. Using registry data and symptom assessment from a quality of life tool, Jurgens et al. (2009) reported three distinct symptom clusters: an acute volume overload cluster (shortness of breath, fatigue, and sleeping difficulties), a chronic volume overload cluster (ankle swelling, need to rest, and breathlessness on exertion), and an emotional cluster (depression, memory loss, and worry). They reported these symptom clusters were more common in older persons but caused less functional limitation. Another survey of more than 700 patients from the United States, Europe, and Asia described clusters of physical symptoms that included dyspnea, difficulty walking, fatigue, and increased need to rest. Worrying, feeling depressed, cognitive problems, and difficulty sleeping formed another cluster of symptoms that the researchers termed an "emotional symptom cluster" (Moser et al. 2014). A recent review from Hong Kong offers some insight into features of symptom clustering that included the physical and emotional/cognitive domains exhibited by people with advanced heart failure and describes some patterns which may presage a poor outcome (Yu et al. 2017). It is important to note that attitudes and views on the meaning of symptoms vary with cultural norms and a transcultural comparison has demonstrated dissimilar symptom clustering and resultant degrees of distressful impact in matched heart failure populations (Park and Johantgen 2017). As our understanding of symptom clustering in heart failure continues to develop, it is important that health care professionals are aware of such disparities to allow them to better target the interrelated symptom groupings and anticipated effects relevant to their local populations.

11 Symptom Relief

Symptom relief can be approached in accordance with general palliative care principles (Johnson et al. 2012a; Stewart and McPherson 2017), but the management of congestion and breathlessness are worthy of special mention. Congestion, either pulmonary or peripheral, is a cardinal sign of acute and chronic heart failure, resulting in breathlessness, discomfort, and limited physical capacity. Intuitively, salt and water restriction have been facets of both the professional and self-care of those exhibiting heart failure-related congestion.

Table 5 Symptom spectrum and associated distress in heart failure (Modified from Riley and Beattie (2017), used with permission)

	Lokker et al. (2016) n = 230		Blinderman et al. (2008) n = 103		Zambroski et al. (2005) n = 53		Wilson and McMillan (2013) n = 40	
	Frequency (%)	High distress (%)	Frequency (%)	High distress (%)	Frequency (%)	High distress (%)	Frequency (%)	High distress (%)
Physical symptoms								Unreported
Shortness of breath	95.2	89	56.3	43.1	85.2	60.5	65	
Feeling drowsy/tired	93.0	83	52.4	24.1	67.9	37.1	72.5	
Pain	91.3	76	37.9	54.1	57.4	51.7	52.5	
"I don't look like myself"	90.4	81	25.2	23.1				
Weight loss	84.8	51	19.4	25	32.1	18.8	52.5	
Lack of energy	82.2	67	66	44.8	84.9	63.6	70	
Swelling arms/legs	81.3	70	32	33.3	47.2	30.4	47.5	
Difficulty sleeping	77.0	64	44.1	44.4	64.2	60.6	52.5	
Tingling hands/feet	73.5	66	48.5	22	46.2	47.8	55	
Changes in way food tastes	73.0	61	15.5	18.5	18.9	44.4	50	
Lack of appetite	72.2	53	31.1	25.8	30.2	40	37.5	
Difficulty concentrating	67.4	30	33	29.4	50	44	40	
Problems with sexual interest/activity	52.6	8	26	46.2	46.3	50	17.5	
Cough	49.1	33	40.8	16.7	57.4	14.8	45	
Nausea	42.2	23			41.5	19	20	
Dizziness	41.3	19	27.2	32.1	51.9	38.5	45	
Feeling bloated	36.1	19	28.2	17.2	51.9	40	25	
Dry mouth	35.7	15	62.1	14.1	74.1	33.3	72.5	
Problems urinating	32.2	16	26.2	29.6	24.1	27.3	17.5	
Itching	28.3	8	34.3	22.9	43.4	47.4	40	
Constipation	26.1	15	25.2	38.5	26.4	30.8	30	
Vomiting	25.7	13			24.1	33.3	10	
Sweats	25.2	15	21.4	18.2	53.7	42.9	27.5	
Diarrhea	12.2	18			22.2	10	17.5	
Psychological problems								
Worrying	94.3	30	43.7	33.3	61.5	53.3	50	
Feeling irritable	93.5	28	33	26.5	53.7	34.6	32.5	
Feeling sad	93	18	42.7	34.1	54.7	44	37.5	
Feeling nervous	92.2	50	35.9	38.9	53.7	38.5	30	

However, recent evidence suggests that this is of little benefit and a more liberal approach should be adopted to avoid exacerbating thirst, a significant symptom in heart failure patients (Aliti et al. 2013; Allida et al. 2015). The use of loop diuretics is the cornerstone of treatment, with the intention of restoring and maintaining euvolaemia (Ponikowski et al. 2016). Furosemide is the prototype of this drug group and may be administered by a variety of routes (Carone et al. 2016). Oral diuretics may be poorly absorbed via a congested gastrointestinal tract, when intravenous therapy may be more effective. In those with decompensated chronic heart failure, a useful start point might be to prescribe the same dose intravenously that the patient was taking orally. It remains unclear whether administration by intermittent bolus dosing or continuous intravenous infusion is the better strategy. Irrespective of the mode of delivery, the duration of therapy and the dose required will be determined by individual patient responses. Prolonged use of high dose loop diuretics is associated with worsening renal function and a high mortality (Palazzuoli et al. 2017). Close monitoring, ideally with daily weighing, is required to guide dose adjustment and maintain patient safety (Felker et al. 2011). The combination of a loop diuretic with a thiazide such as metolazone may be useful in resistant congestion, but should be used with caution due to a higher likelihood of adverse events. Delivery of drugs by the subcutaneous route has been widely adopted in palliative care practice. Given the relatively light evidence base, some concern has been raised about the effectiveness of furosemide when so administered (Beattie and Johnson 2012). However, data are starting to emerge that this approach may indeed be useful (Zacharias et al. 2011; Farless et al. 2013). Subcutaneous injection of generic furosemide is sometimes associated with a tissue reaction and discomfort at the infusion site. SC Pharmaceuticals® based in Burlington, MA, in the United States have developed a buffered preparation of furosemide, together with a customized infusion pump (sc2Wear®), which appears to show potential in early clinical trials [ClinicalTrials.gov identifier NCT02329834]. Permanent catheter drainage systems are sometimes required for the palliation of diuretic resistant ascites (Bevan et al. 2016).

Multiple mechanisms contribute to the sensation of breathlessness in heart failure (Johnson and Clark 2016). Exercise training, neuro-electrical stimulation of respiratory muscles, and mindfulness approaches have been shown to be of some benefit. Opioids appear to act, at least in part, through depression of cortical centers responsible for the perception of breathlessness. Evidence suggests that low dose opioids can be helpful, particularly in stable chronic heart failure, but there may be a time lag before drug efficacy is evident (Johnson et al. 2002; Oxberry et al. 2011, 2013). Because of the possible accumulation of active drug metabolites, caution is required in those with concomitant renal dysfunction (Stewart and McPherson 2017). In the absence of demonstrable hypoxemia, long-term oxygen therapy does not appear to offer symptomatic benefit in chronic heart failure (Davidson and Johnson 2011; Clark et al. 2015), but the use of a hand-held fan to blow air on the face may be effective, perhaps mediated by activation of afferent trigeminal receptors in the nasal mucosa and facial skin (Galbraith et al. 2010).

It is logical to assume that conventional evidence-based treatment for heart failure, at present predominantly relevant to HFrEF, "palliates" the effects of this syndrome to some extent in ameliorating heart failure-related symptoms, improving quality of life, and in reducing mortality. Therefore, there may be advantages in maintaining the prescription of ACEIs, ARBs, and ß-blockers where possible. Towards the end of life, when patients often develop relative hypotension or multiorgan failure including a cardiorenal syndrome, dose reduction or withdrawal of these agents may need to be considered. At that phase of the illness, when the emphasis shifts to symptom management rather than life extension, reconsideration of goals of treatment might deem acceptable the de-prescription of medication such as statins and antiplatelet therapy offered primarily for prognostic benefit. Decisions on cessation of anticoagulant therapy need to be carefully deliberated, cognizant of the specific indications for that treatment. For patients implanted with a mechanical prosthetic

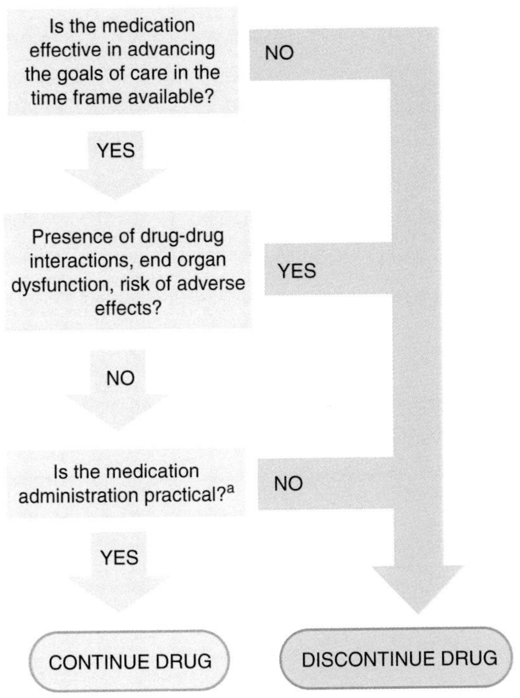

Is the medication effective in advancing the goals of care in the time frame available?

NO

YES

Presence of drug-drug interactions, end organ dysfunction, risk of adverse effects?

YES

NO

Is the medication administration practical?[a]

NO

YES

CONTINUE DRUG

DISCONTINUE DRUG

Fig. 4 An algorithm to determine appropriateness of maintaining drug therapy (From Spiess (2017) with permission)

heart valve or a LVAD, discontinuation of this therapy may be ill-advised. With such treatment dilemmas, involvement of the heart failure team may be helpful for palliative care staff. It might also be reassuring for patients to know that withdrawal of elements of their sometimes long established prescription medication was sanctioned by the team responsible for its initiation. Difficulties in routes of drug administration also arise at this terminal phase. In a recent review, Spiess (2017) has produced a useful algorithm (Fig. 4) to help guide decisions on therapy delivery through what may be the final clinical transition.

12 Palliative Care Service Provision

Providing effective heart failure palliative care relies on good communication, coordination, and timely access to specialist expertise to respond to the sometimes rapidly changing requirements of patients and families, including the opportunity for bereavement care (Low et al. 2011; Luckett et al. 2014; Siouta et al. 2016). This requires a flexible multidisciplinary approach to blend knowledgeable input from cardiology, palliative care, and other health professionals, as well as the provision of social care, to ensure optimal clinical management and support for patients and families. The composition of the multidisciplinary team and the relative contribution required of its members will be determined by the individual needs of the patient-carer dyad, but where possible, it is important that a single team member is designated as the interlocutor between the professionals and the family to ensure clear lines of communication (Ryder et al. 2011; Fendler et al. 2015). Even close to the end of life, when the emphasis of care might shift towards palliation to expertly address difficult symptoms, existential and psychosocial distress, it is important that the cardiology team remain closely involved. This will better secure the maintenance of optimal heart failure management, which might involve intermittent or chronic inotropic support (Hauptman et al. 2006). As alluded to above, this will facilitate shared decision making to determine the continuing role of established therapies, discernment of realistic ceilings of care, and definition of the preferred place of care and death. This also avoids the risk of patients and families feeling abandoned by clinicians familiar to them in this difficult final phase of the disease trajectory.

General palliative care in providing basic symptom control and supporting those with progressive disease in goal setting or advance care planning is a central tenet of general clinical care across all specialties. It has been estimated that about 5% of all heart failure patients require specialist palliative care involvement (Dunlay and Roger 2014). This would certainly be appropriate for those with refractory symptoms, complex care needs, or with features of advanced heart failure (Stage D). But it has been suggested that in other periods of the illness, generalist (primary) palliative care might be provided by those health professionals principally responsible for the patients' care. This could be their primary care physician, an internist, or a member of the heart failure team

(Gelfman et al. 2017a). This is consistent with a commentary proposing a practical model of palliative care delivery in a sometimes resource constrained specialty (Quill and Abernethy 2013), but is dependent on adequate undergraduate and postgraduate education, practical experience, and opportunities to maintain proficiency.

While palliative care teaching is increasingly featured in undergraduate medical school curricula, albeit varying widely in depth, this is yet to be offered by a third of European universities (Carrasco et al. 2015). A set of competencies for heart failure palliative care provision has been outlined for cardiology fellows in the United States, where benefits have also been demonstrated for communication skills training (Munoz-Mendoza 2015; Berlacher et al. 2017). Palliative care education is incorporated within the ESC heart failure subspecialty training program, but the reported experience of medical trainees suggests they still struggle to deliver this (McDonagh et al. 2014; Ismail et al. 2015). In contrast, sequential surveys of specialist heart failure nurses in the UK showed that after participation in palliative care training, they were better equipped to provide generalist palliative care, resulting in fewer referrals to specialist palliative care services (Johnson et al. 2012b). More research is required to define the potential role of generalist versus specialist palliative care in supporting people with heart failure.

Despite the widespread recognition of the need to include palliative care as part of a multidisciplinary approach within the clinical standards required of heart failure care, provision is inconsistent (Strachan et al. 2009; McDonagh et al. 2011; Kane et al. 2015). Service delivery is often provided on an ad hoc basis, largely supported by local champions, and subject to available resources. Unsurprisingly, care configuration is determined by the constitution of local health economies and a variety of arrangements may be applicable. This might be based on a consultancy service, in keeping with the approach in the ESC position statement (Jaarsma et al. 2009), co-management across different clinical settings including intensive care units, or in the use of dedicated palliative care units or independent hospices depending on the specific needs of patients and families. While there is increasing access to hospices by people with heart failure which may reduce acute medical service utilization and associated costs (Kheirbek et al. 2015; Taylor et al. 2017; Yim et al. 2017), numbers treated remain relatively low compared to those with cancer (Cheung et al. 2013; Cheang et al. 2015). The lack of staff experience with this condition might affect patient care. It is important to ensure that when patients are admitted to an independent palliative care unit or hospice, there is adequate transfer of clinical information, including agreed treatment policies, that any necessary heart failure therapy is readily available and that the means to deal expeditiously with any implanted cardiac devices are in place (Wingate et al. 2011; Fromme et al. 2011; Lum et al. 2016).

While some successful collaborative heart failure palliative care models have been developed (Davidson et al. 2004; Johnson et al. 2012c), there is a paucity of robust evidence from randomized clinical trials on which to base best practice (Xie et al. 2017; Gelfman et al. 2017b). However, results are accumulating confirming the benefits of a range of palliative care initiatives across inpatient, outpatient, and assisted living settings, including transitional programs between hospital and home (Pattenden et al. 2013; Evangelista et al. 2014; Brännström and Boman 2014; Sidebottom et al. 2015; Wong et al. 2016; Hopp et al. 2016; Diop et al. 2017; Gandesbery et al. 2017). While several trials are in progress and still to report, the recently published landmark PAL-HF study of 150 patients hospitalized with heart failure undertaken by Duke University and demonstrating improved quality of life by palliative care intervention provides a benchmark in taking this research forward (Rogers et al. 2017). We need to build on this growing evidence base as the foundation of quality assured comprehensive care delivered to affected patients and families.

13 Summary

Heart failure is an increasingly prevalent chronic progressive condition, occurring in epidemic proportions across the world. The widespread implementation of the current comprehensive heart failure treatment paradigm as espoused in clinical guidelines has improved the quality of life and longevity of some of those affected. While these benefits should be celebrated, such developments may contribute to the overall burden endured by those living in fragile health and declining with this cardiovascular disease, often set against the backdrop of comorbidities typical of the changing demography. Given the prognostic uncertainty, it can be difficult to recognize when established therapies have become futile, compounded by poor care co-ordination and communication, sometimes manifest in an unconscious collusion between health professionals, patients, and their families in avoiding difficult conversations. Over the last decade or so, while the palliative care needs of those living and dying with heart failure have been increasingly recognized, care provision remains difficult. At times, the professional ethos of heart failure and palliative care specialists seem to be at odds, when in reality we need to synergize our complementary skill sets to optimize patient care from diagnosis and throughout the disease trajectory. Treatment provision will be largely determined by local healthcare structures. As agents of change, providers should endeavor to develop bespoke models of collaborative interdisciplinary working, consolidated by mutual education, to facilitate effective and coherent delivery of the dual cardiology and palliative care approaches required of this life limiting condition, and best ensure that treatment goals remain consistent with the changing needs, preferences, and values of this vulnerable population.

References

Aaronson KD, Schwartz JS, Chen TM, Wong KL, Goin JE, Mancini DM. Development and prospective validation of a clinical index to predict survival in ambulatory patients referred for cardiac transplant evaluation. Circulation. 1997;95(12):2660–7.

Adams J, Kuchibhatla M, Christopher EJ, Alexander JD, Clary GL, Cuffe MS, et al. Association of depression and survival in patients with chronic heart failure over 12 years. Psychosomatics. 2012;53(4):339–46. https://doi.org/10.1016/j.psym.2011.12.002.

Agård A, Löfmark R, Edvardsson N, Ekman I. Views of patients with heart failure about their role in the decision to start implantable cardioverter defibrillator treatment: prescription rather than participation. J Med Ethics. 2007;33(9):514–8. https://doi.org/10.1136/jme.2006.017723.

Alagiakrishnan K, Mah D, Ahmed A, Ezekowitz J. Cognitive decline in heart failure. Heart Fail Rev. 2016;21(6):661–73. https://doi.org/10.1007/s10741-016-9568-1.

Aliti GB, Rabelo ER, Clausell N, Rohde LE, Biolo A, Beck-da-Silva L. Aggressive fluid and sodium restriction in acute decompensated heart failure: a randomized clinical trial. JAMA Intern Med. 2013;173(12):1058–64. https://doi.org/10.1001/jamainternmed.2013.552.

Allen LA, Yager JE, Funk MJ, Levy WC, Tulsky JA, Bowers MT, et al. Discordance between patient-predicted and model predicted life expectancy among ambulatory patients with heart failure. JAMA. 2008;299:2533–42. https://doi.org/10.1001/jama.299.21.2533.

Allen LA, Stevenson LW, Grady KL, Goldstein NE, Matlock DD, Arnold RM, American Heart Association; Council on Quality of Care and Outcomes Research, Council on Cardiovascular Nursing; Council on Clinical Cardiology, Council on Cardiovascular Radiology and Intervention, Council on Cardiovascular Surgery and Anesthesia, et al. Decision making in advanced heart failure: a scientific statement from the American Heart Association. Circulation. 2012;125(15):1928–52. https://doi.org/10.1161/CIR.0b013e31824f2173.

Allen LA, Matlock DD, Shetterly SM, Xu S, Levy WC, Portalupi LB, et al. Use of risk models to predict death in the next year among individual ambulatory patients with heart failure. JAMA Cardiol. 2017;2(4):435–41. https://doi.org/10.1001/jamacardio.2016.5036.

Allida SM, Inglis SC, Davidson PM, Lal S, Hayward CS, Newton PJ. Thirst in chronic heart failure: a review. Clin Nurs. 2015;24(7–8):916–26. https://doi.org/10.1111/jocn.12732.

Alonso W, Hupcey JE, Kitko L. Caregivers' perceptions of illness severity and end of life service utilization in advanced heart failure. Heart Lung. 2017;46:35–9. https://doi.org/10.1016/j.hrtlng.2016.09.001.

Ampadu J, Morley JE. Heart failure and cognitive dysfunction. Int J Cardiol. 2015;178:12–23. https://doi.org/10.1016/j.ijcard.2014.10.087.

Atwater BD, Daubert JP. Implantable cardioverter defibrillators: risks accompany the life-saving benefits. Heart. 2012;98(10):764–72. https://doi.org/10.1136/heartjnl-2012-301853.

Banner NR, Bonser RS, Clark AL, Clark S, Cowburn PJ, Gardner RS, et al. UK guidelines for referral and assessment of adults for heart transplantation. Heart. 2011;97(18):1520–7. https://doi.org/10.1136/heartjnl-2011-300048.

Barclay S, Momen N, Case-Upton S, Kuhn I, Smith E. End-of-life care conversations with heart failure patients: a systematic literature review and narrative synthesis. Br J Gen Pract. 2011;61(582):e49–62. https://doi.org/10.3399/bjgp11X549018.

Barra S, Providencia R, Paiva L, Heck P, Agarwal S. Implantable cardioverter-defibrillators in the elderly: rationale and specific age-related considerations. Europace. 2015;17:174–86. https://doi.org/10.1093/europace/euu296.

Bayoumi E, Sheikh F, Groninger H. Palliative care in cardiac transplantation: an evolving model. Heart Fail Rev. 2017;22(5):605–10. https://doi.org/10.1007/s10741-017-9613-8.

Beattie JM, Johnson MJ. Subcutaneous furosemide in advanced heart failure: has clinical practice run ahead of the evidence base? BMJ Support Palliat Care. 2012;2(1):5–6. https://doi.org/10.1136/bmjspcare-2011-000199.

Beattie JM, Butler J, MacCallum A, Fuller A, Johnson MJ. A national survey of the management of implantable cardioverter defibrillators in specialist palliative care settings. BMJ Support Palliat Care. 2012;2(Suppl 1):A101.

Becnel MF, Ventura HO, Krim SR. Changing our approach to stage D heart failure. Prog Cardiovasc Dis. 2017;60(2):205–14. https://doi.org/10.1016/j.pcad.2017.08.003.

Bekelman DB, Rumsfeld JS, Havranek EP, Yamashita TE, Hutt E, Gottlieb SH, et al. Symptom burden, depression, and spiritual well-being: a comparison of heart failure and advanced cancer patients. J Gen Intern Med. 2009;24:592–8. https://doi.org/10.1007/s11606-009-0931-y.

Benjamin EJ, Blaha MJ, Chiuve SE, Cushman M, Das SR, Deo R, American Heart Association Statistics Committee and Stroke Statistics Subcommittee, et al. Heart disease and stroke Statistics-2017 update: a report from the American Heart Association. Circulation. 2017;135(10):e146–603. https://doi.org/10.1161/CIR.0000000000000485.

Berlacher K, Arnold RM, Reitschuler-Cross E, Teuteberg J, Teuteberg W. The impact of communication skills training on cardiology fellows' and attending physicians' perceived comfort with difficult conversations. J Palliat Med. 2017;20:767–9. https://doi.org/10.1089/jpm.2016.0509.

Bevan J, Pen L-A, Mitchell ARJ. Permanent catheter drainage system for palliation of diuretic-resistant ascites. ESC Heart Fail. 2016;3:60–2. https://doi.org/10.1002/ehf2.12074.

Blinderman CD, Homel P, Billings A, Porenoy RK, Tennstedt SL. Symptom distress and quality of life in patients with advanced congestive heart failure. J Pain Symptom Manag. 2008;35:594–603. https://doi.org/10.1016/j.jpainsymman.2007.06.007.

Borlaug BA, Paulus WJ. Heart failure with preserved ejection fraction: pathophysiology, diagnosis and treatment. Eur Heart J. 2011;32:670–9. https://doi.org/10.1093/eurheartj/ehq426.

Boudoulas KD, Triposkiadis F, Parissis J, Butler J, Boudoulas H. The cardio-renal interrelationship. Prog Cardiovasc Dis. 2017;59(6):636–48. https://doi.org/10.1016/j.pcad.2016.12.003.

Brännström M, Boman K. Effects of person-centred and integrated chronic heart failure and palliative home care. PREFER: a randomized controlled study. Eur J Heart Fail. 2014;16:1142–51. https://doi.org/10.1002/ejhf.151.

Braun LT, Grady KL, Kutner JS, Adler E, Berlinger N, Boss R, American Heart Association Advocacy Coordinating Committee, et al. Palliative care and cardiovascular disease and stroke: a policy statement from the American Heart Association/American Stroke Association. Circulation. 2016;134(11):e198–225. https://doi.org/10.1161/CIR.0000000000000438.

Braunwald E. The war against heart failure: the lancet lecture. Lancet. 2015;385(9970):812–24. https://doi.org/10.1016/S0140-6736(14)61889-4.

Brunner-La Rocca HP, Rickenbacher P, Muzzarelli S, Schindler R, Maeder MT, Jeker U, TIME-CHF Investigators, et al. End-of-life preferences of elderly patients with chronic heart failure. Eur Heart J. 2012;33(6):752–9. https://doi.org/10.1093/eurheartj/ehr404.

Campbell RT, Jackson CE, Wright A, Gardner RS, Ford I, Davidson PM, et al. Palliative care needs in patients hospitalized with heart failure (PCHF) study: rationale and design. ESC Heart Fail. 2015;2:25–36. https://doi.org/10.1002/ehf2.12027.

Cannon JA, Moffitt P, Perez-Moreno AC, Walters MR, Broomfield NM, McMurray JJV, et al. Cognitive impairment and heart failure: systematic review and meta-analysis. J Card Fail. 2017;23(6):464–75. https://doi.org/10.1016/j.cardfail.2017.04.007.

Carone L, Oxberry SG, Twycross R, Charlesworth S, Mihalyo M, Wilcock A. Furosemide. J Pain Symptom Manag. 2016;52(1):144–50. https://doi.org/10.1016/j.jpainsymman.2016.05.004.

Carrasco JM, Lynch TJ, Garralda E, Woitha K, Elsner F, Filbet M, et al. Palliative care medical education in European universities: a descriptive study and numerical scoring system proposal for assessing educational development. J Pain Symptom Manag. 2015;50(4):516–23. https://doi.org/10.1016/j.jpainsymman.2015.04.019.

Carroll SL, Strachan PH, de Laat S, Schwartz L, Arthur HM. Patients' decision making to accept or decline an implantable cardioverter defibrillator for primary prevention of sudden cardiac death. Health Expect. 2013a;16(1):69–79. https://doi.org/10.1111/j.1369-7625.2011.00703.x.

Carroll SL, McGillion M, Stacey D, Healey JS, Browne G, Arthur HM, et al. Development and feasibility testing of decision support for patients who are candidates for a prophylactic implantable defibrillator: a study protocol for a pilot randomized controlled trial. Trials. 2013b;14:346. https://doi.org/10.1186/1745-6215-14-346.

Centers for Medicare & Medicaid Services, Dept of Health and Human Services. MLN matters: ventricular assist devices for bridge-to-transplant and destination therapy. https://www.cms.gov/Outreach-and-Education/Medicare-Learning-Network-MLN/MLNMattersArticles/Downloads/MM8803.pdf. Published 29 Aug 2014. Accessed 10 Oct 2017.

Chamsi-Pasha H, Chamsi-Pasha MA, Albar MA. Ethical challenges of deactivation of cardiac devices in advanced heart failure. Curr Heart Fail Rep. 2014;11(2):119–25. https://doi.org/10.1007/s11897-014-0194-8.

Chan MM, Lam CS. How do patients with heart failure with preserved ejection fraction die? Eur J Heart Fail. 2013;15:604–13. https://doi.org/10.1093/eurjhf/hft062.

Chaudhry SI, McAvay G, Chen S, Whitson H, Newman AB, Krumholz HM, et al. Risk factors for hospital admission among older persons with newly diagnosed heart failure: findings from the cardiovascular health study. J Am Coll Cardiol. 2013;61:635–42. https://doi.org/10.1016/j.jacc.2012.11.027.

Cheang MH, Rose G, Cheung CC, Thomas M. Current challenges in palliative care provision for heart failure in the UK: a survey on the perspectives of palliative care professionals. Open Heart. 2015;2(1):e000188. https://doi.org/10.1136/openhrt-2014-000188.

Cheung WY, Schaefer K, May CW, Glynn RJ, Curtis LH, Stevenson LW, et al. Enrolment and events of hospice patients with heart failure vs. cancer. J Pain Symptom Manag. 2013;45(3):552–60. https://doi.org/10.1016/j.jpainsymman.2012.03.006.

Clark AM, Jaarsma T, Strachan P, Davidson PM, Jerke M, Beattie JM, et al. Effective communication and ethical consent in decisions related to ICDs. Nat Rev Cardiol. 2011;8(12):694–705. https://doi.org/10.1038/nrcardio.2011.101.

Clark AM, Dryden D, Hartling L. Systematic review of decision tools and their suitability for patient-centered decision making regarding electronic cardiac devices. Rockville: Agency for Healthcare Research and Quality; 2012.

Clark AL, Johnson M, Fairhurst C, Torgerson D, Cockayne S, Rodgers S, et al. Does home oxygen therapy (HOT) in addition to standard care reduce disease severity and improve symptoms in people with chronic heart failure? A randomised trial of home oxygen therapy for patients with chronic heart failure. Health Technol Assess. 2015;19(75):1–120. https://doi.org/10.3310/hta19750.

Cleland JG, McDonagh T, Rigby AS, Yassin A, Whittaker T, Dargie HJ. The national heart failure audit for England and Wales 2008–2009. Heart. 2011;97(11):876–86. https://doi.org/10.1136/hrt.2010.209171.

Collett D, Mumford L, Banner NR, Neuberger J, Watson C. Comparison of the incidence of malignancy in recipients of different types of organ: a UK registry audit. Am J Transplant. 2010;10(8):1889–96. https://doi.org/10.1111/j.1600-6143.2010.03181.x.

Conrad N, Judge A, Tran J, Mohseni H, Hedgecott D, Crespillo AP, et al. Temporal trends and patterns in heart failure incidence: a population-based study of 4 million individuals. Lancet. 2017. https://doi.org/10.1016/S0140-6736(17)32520-5.

Cook C, Cole G, Asaria P, Jabbour R, Francis DP. The annual global economic burden of heart failure. Int J Cardiol. 2014;171(3):368–76. https://doi.org/10.1016/j.ijcard.2013.12.028.

Davidson PM, Johnson MJ. Update on the role of palliative oxygen. Curr Opin Support Palliat Care. 2011;5(2):87–91. https://doi.org/10.1097/SPC.0b013e3283463cd3.

Davidson PM, Paull G, Introna K, Cockburn J, Davis JM, Rees D, et al. Integrated, collaborative palliative care in heart failure: the St. George heart failure service experience 1999–2002. Cardiovasc Nurs. 2004;19:68–75.

Davidson PM, Dracup K, Phillips J, Padilla G, Daly J. Maintaining hope in transition. A theoretical framework to guide interventions for people with heart failure. J Cardiovasc Nurs. 2007;22(1):58–64.

Denfeld QE, Winters-Stone K, Mudd JO, Hiatt SO, Lee CS. Identifying a relationship between physical frailty and heart failure symptoms. J Cardiovasc Nurs. 2018;33(1):E1–7. https://doi.org/10.1097/JCN.0000000000000408.

Diop MS, Rudolph JL, Zimmerman KM, Richter MA, Skarf LM. Palliative care interventions for patients with heart failure: a systematic review and meta-analysis. J Palliat Med. 2017;20(1):84–92. https://doi.org/10.1089/jpm.2016.0330.

Dunbar SB, Dougherty CM, Sears SF, Carroll DL, Goldstein NE, Mark DB, American Heart Association Council on Cardiovascular Nursing, Council on Clinical Cardiology, and Council on Cardiovascular Disease in the Young, et al. Educational and psychological interventions to improve outcomes for recipients of implantable cardioverter defibrillators and their families: a scientific statement from the American Heart Association. Circulation. 2012;126(17):2146–72. https://doi.org/10.1161/CIR.0b013e31825d59fd.

Dunlay SM, Roger VL. Understanding the epidemic of heart failure: past, present, and future. Curr Heart Fail Rep. 2014;11(4):404–15. https://doi.org/10.1007/s11897-014-0220-x.

Dunlay SM, Swetz KM, Mueller PS, Roger VL. Advance directives in community patients with heart failure. Circ Cardiovasc Qual Outcomes. 2012;5(3):283–9. https://doi.org/10.1161/CIRCOUTCOMES.112.966036.

Dunlay SM, Strand JJ, Wordingham SE, Stulak JM, Luckhardt AJ, Swetz KM. Dying with a left ventricular assist device as destination therapy. Circ Heart Fail. 2016;9(10):e003096. https://doi.org/10.1161/CIRCHEARTFAILURE.116.003096.

Eckerblad J, Theander K, Ekdahl A, Unosson M, Wirehn AB, Milberg A, et al. Symptom burden in community-dwelling older people with multimorbidity: a cross-sectional study. BMC Geriatr. 2015;15:1. https://doi.org/10.1186/1471-2318-15-1.

Epstein AE, DiMarco JP, Ellenbogen KA, Estes NA 3rd, Freedman RA, Gettes LS, American College of

Cardiology Foundation, American Heart Association Task Force on Practice Guidelines, Heart Rhythm Society, et al. 2012 ACCF/AHA/HRS focused update incorporated into the ACCF/AHA/HRS 2008 guidelines for device-based therapy of cardiac rhythm abnormalities: a report of the American College of Cardiology Foundation/American Heart Association Task Force on Practice Guidelines and the Heart Rhythm Society. J Am Coll Cardiol. 2013;61(3):e6–75. https://doi.org/10.1016/j.jacc.2012.11.007.

Etkind SN, Bristowe K, Bailey K, Selman LE, Murtagh FEM. How does uncertainty shape patient experience in advanced illness? A secondary analysis of quantitative data. Palliat Med. 2017;31(2):171–80. https://doi.org/10.1177/0269216316647610.

Evangelista LS, Liao S, Motie M, De Michelis N, Lombardo D. On-going palliative care enhances perceived control and patient activation and reduces symptom distress in patients with symptomatic heart failure: a pilot study. Eur J Cardiovasc Nurs. 2014;13(2):116–23. https://doi.org/10.1177/1474515114520766.

Ezekowitz JA, Thai V, Hodnefield TS, Sanderson L, Cujec B. The correlation of standard heart failure assessment and palliative care questionnaires in a multidisciplinary heart failure clinic. J Pain Symptom Manag. 2011;42:379–87. https://doi.org/10.1016/j.jpainsymman.2010.11.013.

Fan H, Yu W, Zhang Q, Cao H, Li J, Wang J, Shao Y, Hu X. Depression after heart failure and risk of cardiovascular and all-cause mortality: a meta-analysis. Prev Med. 2014;63:36–42. https://doi.org/10.1016/j.ypmed.2014.03.007.

Fang JC, Ewald GA, Allen LA, Butler J, Westlake Canary CA, Heart Failure Society of America Guidelines Committee, et al. Advanced (stage D) heart failure: a statement from the Heart Failure Society of America Guidelines Committee. J Card Fail. 2015;21(6):519–34. https://doi.org/10.1016/j.cardfail.2015.04.013.

Farless LB, Steil N, Williams BR, Bailey FA. Intermittent subcutaneous furosemide: parenteral diuretic rescue for hospice patients with congestive heart failure resistant to oral diuretic. Am J Hosp Palliat Care. 2013;30:791–2. https://doi.org/10.1177/1049909112465795.

Felker GM, Lee KL, Bull DA, Redfield MM, Stevenson LW, Goldsmith SR, NHLBI Heart Failure Clinical Research Network, et al. Diuretic strategies in patients with acute decompensated heart failure. N Engl J Med. 2011;364:797–805. https://doi.org/10.1056/NEJMoa1005419.

Fendler TJ, Swetz KM, Allen LA. Team-based palliative and end-of-life care for heart failure. Heart Fail Clin. 2015;11(3):479–98. https://doi.org/10.1016/j.hfc.2015.03.010.

Fluur C, Bolse K, Strömberg A, Thylén I. Spouses' reflections on implantable cardioverter defibrillator treatment with focus on the future and the end-of-life: a qualitative content analysis. J Adv Nurs. 2014;70(8):1758–69. https://doi.org/10.1111/jan.12330.

Fried LP, Borhani NO, Enright P, Furberg CD, Gardin JM, Kronmal RA, et al. The cardiovascular health study: design and rationale. Ann Epidemiol. 1991;1:263–76.

Fried LP, Tangen CM, Walston J, Newman AB, Hirsch C, Gottdiener J, Cardiovascular Health Study Collaborative Research Group, et al. Frailty in older adults evidence for a phenotype. J Gerontol A Biol Sci Med Sci. 2001;56:M146–56.

Fromme EK, Stewart TL, Jeppesen M, Tolle SW. Adverse experiences with implantable defibrillators in Oregon hospices. Am J Hosp Palliat Care. 2011;28(5):304–9. https://doi.org/10.1177/1049909110390505.

Galbraith S, Fagan P, Perkins P, Lynch A, Booth S. Does the use of a handheld fan improve chronic dyspnea? A randomized, controlled, crossover trial. J Pain Symptom Manag. 2010;39:831–8. https://doi.org/10.1016/j.jpainsymman.2009.09.024.

Gandesbery B, Dobbie K, Gorodeski EZ. Outpatient palliative cardiology service embedded within a heart failure clinic: experiences with an emerging model of care. Am J Hosp Palliat Care. 2017. https://doi.org/10.1177/1049909117729478.

Ganz T, Nemeth E. Hepcidin and iron homeostasis. Biochim Biophys Acta. 2012;1823(9):1434–43. https://doi.org/10.1016/j.bbamcr.2012.01.014.

Gelfman LP, Kavalieratos D, Teuteberg WG, Lala A, Goldstein NE. Primary palliative care for heart failure: what is it? How do we implement it? Heart Fail Rev. 2017a;22(5):611–20. https://doi.org/10.1007/s10741-017-9604-9.

Gelfman LP, Bakitas M, Warner Stevenson L, Kirkpatrick JN, Goldstein NE, and on behalf of the Improving Palliative Care for Patients with Heart Failure and Their Families (IMPACT-HF) Working Group. The state of the science on integrating palliative care in heart failure. J Palliat Med. 2017b;20(6):592–603.

Gerber Y, Weston SA, Redfield MM, Chamberlain AM, Manemann SM, Jiang R, et al. A contemporary appraisal of the heart failure epidemic in Olmsted County, Minnesota, 2000 to 2010. JAMA Intern Med. 2015;175(6):996–1004. https://doi.org/10.1001/jamainternmed.2015.0924.

Goldstein NE, Lampert R, Bradley E, Lynn J, Krumholz HM. Management of implantable cardioverter defibrillators in end-of-life care. Ann Intern Med. 2004;141(11):835–8.

Goldstein NE, Mehta D, Siddiqui S, Teitelbaum E, Zeidman J, Singson M, et al. "That's like an act of suicide" patients' attitudes toward deactivation of implantable defibrillators. J Gen Intern Med. 2008a;23(Suppl 1):7–12. https://doi.org/10.1007/s11606-007-0239-8.

Goldstein NE, Mehta D, Teitelbaum E, Bradley EH, Morrison RS. "It's like crossing a bridge" complexities preventing physicians from discussing deactivation of implantable defibrillators at the end of life. J Gen Intern Med. 2008b;23(Suppl 1):2–6. https://doi.org/10.1007/s11606-007-0237-x.

Goldstein N, Carlson M, Livote E, Kutner JS. Brief communication: management of implantable cardioverter defibrillators in hospice: a nationwide survey. Ann Intern Med. 2010;152:296–9. https://doi.org/10.7326/0003-4819-152-5-201003020-00007.

Goldstein NE, May CW, Meier DE. Comprehensive care for mechanical circulatory support: a new frontier for synergy with palliative care. Circ Heart Fail. 2011;4:519–27. https://doi.org/10.1161/CIRCHEARTFAILURE.110.957241.

Goldstein DJ, Naftel D, Holman W, Bellumkonda L, Pamboukian SV, Pagani FD, et al. Continuous-flow devices and percutaneous site infections: clinical outcomes. J Heart Lung Transplant. 2012;31(11):1151–7. https://doi.org/10.1016/j.healun.2012.05.004.

Gómez-Batiste X, Martinez-Muñoz M, Blay C, Amblàs J, Vila L, Costa X, et al. Identifying chronic patients in need of palliative care in the general population: development of the NECPAL tool and preliminary prevalence rates in Catalonia. BMJ Support Palliat Care. 2013;3:300–8. https://doi.org/10.1136/bmjspcare-2012-000211.

Goodlin SJ, Hauptman PJ, Arnold R, Grady K, Hershberger RE, Kutner J, et al. Consensus statement: palliative and supportive care in advanced heart failure. J Card Fail. 2004;10(3):200–9.

Gott M, Barnes S, Parker C, Payne S, Seamark D, Gariballa S, et al. Dying trajectories in heart failure. Palliat Med. 2007;21:95–9. https://doi.org/10.1177/0269216307076348.

Green CP, Porter CB, Bresnahan DR, Spertus JA. Development and evaluation of the Kansas City cardiomyopathy questionnaire: a new health status measure for heart failure. J Am Coll Cardiol. 2000;35:1245–55.

Green AR, Leff B, Wang Y, Spatz ES, Masoudi FA, Peterson PN, et al. Geriatric conditions in patients undergoing defibrillator implantation for prevention of sudden cardiac death: prevalence and impact on mortality. Circ Cardiovasc Qual Outcomes. 2016;9(1):23–30. https://doi.org/10.1161/CIRCOUTCOMES.115.002053.

Guha K, McDonagh T. Heart failure epidemiology: European perspective. Curr Cardiol Rev. 2013;9(2):123–7.

Hauptman PJ, Mikolajczak P, George A, Mohr CJ, Hoover R, Swindle J, et al. Chronic inotropic therapy in end-stage heart failure. Am Heart J. 2006;152:1096.e1–8. https://doi.org/10.1016/j.ahj.2006.08.003.

Hauptman PJ, Chibnall JT, Guild C, Armbrecht ES. Patient perceptions, physician communication, and the implantable cardioverter-defibrillator. JAMA Intern Med. 2013;173(7):571–7. https://doi.org/10.1001/jamainternmed.2013.3171.

Hill L, McIlfatrick S, Taylor BJ, Dixon L, Cole BR, Moser DK, et al. Implantable cardioverter defibrillator (ICD) deactivation discussions: reality versus recommendations. Eur J Cardiovasc Nurs. 2016;15(1):20–9. https://doi.org/10.1177/1474515115584248.

Hindricks G, Camm J, Merkely B, Raatikainen P, Amar DO. The EHRA White Book, 10th ed. European Heart Rhythm Association. 2017. https://www.escardio.org/static_file/Escardio/Subspecialty/EHRA/Publications/Documents/2017/ehra-white-book-2017.pdf. Accessed 2 Nov 2017.

Hogg KJ, Jenkins SM. Prognostication or identification of palliative needs in advanced heart failure: where should the focus lie? Heart. 2012;98(7):523–4. https://doi.org/10.1136/heartjnl-2012-301753.

Holland R, Rechel B, Stepien K, Harvey I, Brooksby I. Patients' self-assessed functional status in heart failure by New York Heart Association class: a prognostic predictor of hospitalizations, quality of life and death. J Card Fail. 2010;16(2):150–6. https://doi.org/10.1016/j.cardfail.2009.08.010.

Hopp FP, Zalenski RJ, Waselewsky D, Burn J, Camp J, Welch RD, et al. Results of a hospital-based palliative care intervention for patients with an acute exacerbation of chronic heart failure. J Card Fail. 2016;22(12):1033–6. https://doi.org/10.1016/j.cardfail.2016.04.004.

Huffman MD, Berry JD, Ning H, Dyer AR, Garside DB, Cai X, et al. Lifetime risk for heart failure among white and black Americans cardiovascular lifetime risk pooling project. J Am Coll Cardiol. 2013;61:1510–7. https://doi.org/10.1016/j.jacc.2013.01.022.

Hunt SA, Baker DW, Chin MH, Cinquegrani MP, Feldman AM, Francis GS, American College of Cardiology/American Heart Association Task Force on Practice Guidelines (Committee to Revise the 1995 Guidelines for the Evaluation and Management of Heart Failure), International Society for Heart and Lung Transplantation, Heart Failure Society of America, et al. ACC/AHA guidelines for the evaluation and management of chronic heart failure in the adult: executive summary a report of the American College of Cardiology/American Heart Association task force on practice guidelines (Committee to revise the 1995 guidelines for the evaluation and management of heart failure): developed in collaboration with the International Society for Heart and Lung Transplantation; endorsed by the Heart Failure Society of America. Circulation. 2001;104(24):2996–3007. https://doi.org/10.1161/hc4901.102568.

Ismail Y, Nightingale AK, Shorthouse K. Trainee experience of delivering end-of-life care in heart failure: key findings of a national survey. Br J Cardiol. 2015;22:26. https://doi.org/10.5837/bjc.2015.008.

Jaarsma T, Beattie JM, Ryder M, Rutten FH, McDonagh T, Mohacsi P, Advanced Heart Failure Study Group of the HFA of the ESC, et al. Palliative care in heart failure: a position statement from the palliative care workshop of the heart failure Association of the European Society of cardiology. Eur J Heart Fail. 2009;11(5):433–43. https://doi.org/10.1093/eurjhf/hfp041.

Jani B, Blane D, Browne S, Montori V, May C, Shippee N, et al. Identifying treatment burden as an important concept for end of life care in those with advanced heart failure. Curr Opin Support Palliat Care. 2013;7(1):3–7. https://doi.org/10.1097/SPC.0b013e32835c071f.

Jankowska EA, Malyszko J, Ardehali H, Koc-Zorawska E, Banasiak W, von Haehling S, et al. Iron status in patients with chronic heart failure. Eur Heart J. 2013;34(11):827–34. https://doi.org/10.1093/eurheartj/ehs377.

Janssen DJA, Johnson MJ, Spruit MA. Palliative care needs assessment in chronic heart failure. Curr Opin Support Palliat Care. 2018;12(1):25–31. https://doi.org/10.1097/SPC.0000000000000317.

Jermyn R, Patel S. The biologic syndrome of frailty in heart failure. Clin Med Insights Cardiol. 2015; 8(Suppl 1):87–92. https://doi.org/10.4137/CMC.S15720.

Jha SR, Ha HS, Hickman LD, Hannu M, Davidson PM, Macdonald PS, et al. Frailty in advanced heart failure: a systematic review. Heart Fail Rev. 2015;20(5):553–60. https://doi.org/10.1007/s10741-015-9493-8.

Johnson MJ, Clark AL. The mechanisms of breathlessness in heart failure as the basis of therapy. Curr Opin Support Palliat Care. 2016;10(1):32–5. https://doi.org/10.1097/SPC.0000000000000181.

Johnson MJ, McDonagh T, Harkness A, MacKay S, Dargie H. Morphine for breathlessness in chronic heart failure. Eur J Heart Fail. 2002;4:753–6.

Johnson M, Hogg K, Beattie J. Heart failure: from advanced disease to bereavement. Oxford: Oxford University Press; 2012a.

Johnson MJ, MacCallum A, Butler J, Rogers A, Sam E, Fuller A, et al. Heart failure specialist nurses' use of palliative care services: a comparison of surveys across England in 2005 and 2010. Eur J Cardiovasc Nurs. 2012b;11(2):190–6. https://doi.org/10.1016/j.ejcnurse.2011.03.004.

Johnson MJ, Nunn A, Hawkes T, Stockdale S, Daley A. Planning for end of life care in people with heart failure: experience of two integrated cardiology-palliative care teams. Br J Cardiol. 2012c;19:71–5. https://doi.org/10.5837/bjc.2012.014.

Johnson MJ, Bland JM, Davidson PM, Newton PJ, Oxberry SG, Abernethy AP, et al. The relationship between two performance scales: New York Heart Association Classification and Karnofsky Performance Status Scale. J Pain Symptom Manag. 2014;47:652–8. https://doi.org/10.1016/j.jpainsymman.2013.05.006.

Joyce KE, Lord S, Matlock DD, McComb JM, Thomson R. Incorporating the patient perspective: a critical review of clinical practice guidelines for implantable cardioverter defibrillator therapy. J Interv Card Electrophysiol. 2013;36:185–97. https://doi.org/10.1007/s10840-012-9762-6.

Jurgens CY, Moser DK, Armola R, Carlson B, Sethares K, Riegel B, Heart Failure Quality of Life Trialist Collaborators. Symptom clusters of heart failure. Res Nurs Health. 2009;32:551–60. https://doi.org/10.1002/nur.20343.

Kane PM, Murtagh FE, Ryan K, Mahon NG, McAdam B, McQuillan R, et al. The gap between policy and practice: a systematic review of patient-centred care interventions in chronic heart failure. Heart Fail Rev. 2015;20:673–87. https://doi.org/10.1007/s10741-015-9508-5.

Kane PM, Daveson BA, Ryan K, Ellis-Smith CI, Mahon NG, McAdam B, BuildCARE, et al. Feasibility and acceptability of a patient-reported outcome intervention in chronic heart failure. BMJ Support Palliat Care. 2017:7(4):470–9. https://doi.org/10.1136/bmjspcare-2017-001355.

Kaufman SR, Meuller PS, Ottenberg AL, Koenig BA. Ironic technology: old age and the implantable defibrillator in US health care. Soc Sci Med. 2011;72(1):6–14. https://doi.org/10.1016/j.socscimed.2010.09.052.

Kheirbek RE, Fletcher RD, Bakitas MA, Fonarow GC, Parvtaneni S, Bearden D, et al. Discharge hospice referral and lower 30-day all-cause readmission in Medicare beneficiaries hospitalized for heart failure. Circ Heart Fail. 2015;8:733–40. https://doi.org/10.1161/CIRCHEARTFAILURE.115.002153.

Kim J, Pressler SJ, Groh WJ. Change in cognitive function over 12 months among patients with an implantable cardioverter-defibrillator. J Cardiovasc Nurs. 2013;28(6):e28–36. https://doi.org/10.1097/JCN.0b013e31829dfc6e.

Kinch Westerdahl A, Sjöblom J, Mattiasson AC, Rosenqvist M, Frykman V. Implantable defibrillator therapy before death. High risk of painful shocks near the end of life. Circulation. 2014;129:422–9. https://doi.org/10.1161/CIRCULATIONAHA.113.002648.

Kirklin JK, Naftel DC, Pagani FD, Kormos RL, Stevenson LW, et al. Seventh INTERMACS annual report: 15,000 patients and counting. J Heart Lung Transplant. 2015;34(12):1495–504. https://doi.org/10.1016/j.healun.2015.10.003.

Kirkpatrick JN, Wieselthaler G, Strueber M, St John Sutton MG, Rame JE. Ventricular assist devices for treatment of acute heart failure and chronic heart failure. Heart. 2015;101(14):1091–6. https://doi.org/10.1136/heartjnl-2014-306789.

Kramer DB, Kesselheim AS, Brock DW, Maisel WH. Ethical and legal views of physicians regarding deactivation of cardiac implantable electrical devices: a quantitative assessment. Heart Rhythm. 2010;7(11):1537–42. https://doi.org/10.1016/j.hrthm.2010.07.018.

Kramer DB, Ottenberg AL, Gerhardson S, Mueller LA, Kaufman SR, Koenig BA, et al. "Just because we can doesn't mean we should": views of nurses on deactivation of pacemakers and implantable cardioverter-defibrillators. J Interv Card Electrophysiol. 2011;32(3):243–52. https://doi.org/10.1007/s10840-011-9596-7.

Kramer DB, Matlock DD, Buxton AE, Goldstein NE, Goodwin C, Green AR, et al. Implantable cardioverter-defibrillator use in older adults: proceedings of a Hartford change AGEnts symposium. Circ Cardiovasc Qual Outcomes. 2015;8(4):437–46. https://doi.org/10.1161/CIRCOUTCOMES.114.001660.

Kramer DB, Reynolds MR, Normand SL, Parzynski CS, Spertus JA, Mor V, et al. Hospice use following implantable cardioverter-defibrillator implantation in older patients: results from the National Cardiovascular Data Registry. Circulation. 2016;133(21):2030–7. https://doi.org/10.1161/CIRCULATIONAHA.115.020677.

Kute VB, Vanikar AV, Patel HV, Gumber MR, Shah PR, Engineer DP, et al. Significant benefits after renal transplantation in patients with chronic heart failure and chronic kidney disease. Ren Fail. 2014;36(6):854–8. https://doi.org/10.3109/0886022X.2014.899474.

Lam CS, Solomon SD. The middle child in heart failure: heart failure with mid-range ejection fraction (40–50%). Eur J Heart Fail. 2014;16(10):1049–55. https://doi.org/10.1002/ejhf.159.

Lampert R, Hayes DL, Annas GJ, Farley MA, Goldstein NE, Hamilton RM, American College of Cardiology, American Geriatrics Society, American Academy of Hospice and Palliative Medicine, American Heart Association, European Heart Rhythm Association, Hospice and Palliative Nurses Association, et al. HRS expert consensus statement on the Management of Cardiovascular Implantable Electronic Devices (CIEDs) in patients nearing end of life or requesting withdrawal of therapy. Heart Rhythm. 2010;7(7):1008–26. https://doi.org/10.1016/j.hrthm.2010.04.033.

Lang RM, Badano LP, Mor-Avi V, Afilalo J, Armstrong A, Ernande L, et al. Recommendations for cardiac chamber quantification by echocardiography in adults: an update from the American Society of Echocardiography and the European Association of Cardiovascular Imaging. J Am Soc Echocardiogr. 2015;28(1):1–39.e14. https://doi.org/10.1016/j.echo.2014.10.003.

Lauck S, Garland E, Achtem L, Forman J, Baumbusch J, Boone R, et al. Integrating a palliative approach in a transcatheter heart valve program: bridging innovations in the management of severe aortic stenosis and best end-of-life practice. Eur J Cardiovasc Nurs. 2014;13:177–84. https://doi.org/10.1177/1474515114520770.

Lee KS, Moser DK. Heart failure symptom measures: critical review. Eur J Cardiovasc Nurs. 2013;12(5):418–28. https://doi.org/10.1177/1474515112473235.

Levenson JW, McCarthy EP, Lynn J, Davis RB, Phillips RS. The last six months of life for patients with congestive heart failure. J Am Geriatr Soc. 2000;48(5 Suppl):S101–9.

Levy WC, Mozaffarian D, Linker DT, Sutradhar SC, Anker SD, Cropp AB, et al. The Seattle heart failure model: prediction of survival in heart failure. Circulation. 2006;113(11):1424–33. https://doi.org/10.1161/CIRCULATIONAHA.105.584102.

Lewin WH, Cheung W, Horvath AN, Haberman S, Patel A, Sullivan D. Supportive cardiology: moving palliative care upstream for patients living with advanced heart failure. J Palliat Med. 2017;20(10):1112–9. https://doi.org/10.1089/jpm.2016.0317.

Lewis KB, Stacey D, Carroll SL, Boland L, Sikora L, Birnie D. Estimating the risks and benefits of implantable cardioverter defibrillator generator replacement: a systematic review. Pacing Clin Electrophysiol. 2016;39(7):709–22. https://doi.org/10.1111/pace.12850.

Light-McGroary K, Goodlin SJ. The challenges of understanding and managing pain in the heart failure patient. Curr Opin Support Palliat Care. 2013;7:14–20. https://doi.org/10.1097/SPC.0b013e32835c1f2f.

Lokker ME, Gwyther L, Riley JP, van Zuylen L, van fer Heide A, Harding R. The prevalence and associated distress of physical and psychological symptoms in patients with advanced heart failure attending a South African medical center. J Cardiovasc Nurs. 2016;31:313–22. https://doi.org/10.1097/JCN.0000000000000256.

Low J, Pattenden J, Candy B, Beattie JM, Jones L. Palliative care in advanced heart failure: an international review of the perspectives of recipients and health professionals on care provision. J Card Fail. 2011;17(3):231–52. https://doi.org/10.1016/j.cardfail.2010.10.003.

Luckett T, Phillips J, Agar M, Virdun C, Green A, Davidson PM. Elements of effective palliative care models: a rapid review. BMC Health Serv Res. 2014;14:136. https://doi.org/10.1186/1472-6963-14-136.

Lum HD, Jones J, Lahoff D, Allen LA, Bekelman DB, Kutner JS, et al. Unique challenges of hospice for patients with heart failure: a qualitative study of hospice clinicians. Am Heart J. 2015;170(3):524–30. https://doi.org/10.1016/j.ahj.2015.06.019.

Lum HD, Horney C, Koets D, Kutner JS, Matlock DD. Availability of heart failure medications in hospice care. Am J Hosp Palliat Care. 2016;33(10):924–8. https://doi.org/10.1177/1049909115603689.

Luo N, Rogers JG, Dodson GC, Patel CB, Galanos AN, Milano CA, et al. Usefulness of palliative care to complement the management of patients on left ventricular assist devices. Am J Cardiol. 2016;118:733–8. https://doi.org/10.1016/j.amjcard.2016.06.010.

Madan SA, Fida N, Barman P, Sims D, Shin J, Verghese J, et al. Frailty assessment in advanced heart failure. J Card Fail. 2016;22(10):840–4. https://doi.org/10.1016/j.cardfail.2016.02.003.

Martens P, Nijst P, Verbrugge FH, Smeets K, Dupont M, Mullens W. Impact of iron deficiency on exercise capacity and outcome in heart failure with reduced, mid-range and preserved ejection fraction. Acta Cardiol. 2017;21:1–9. https://doi.org/10.1080/00015385.2017.1351239.

Mason DT. Congestive heart failure: mechanisms, evaluation and treatment. New York: Yorke Medical Books; 1976.

Matlock DD, Jones J, Nowels CT, Jenkins A, Allen LA, Kutner JS. Evidence of cognitive bias in decision making around implantable-cardioverter defibrillators: a qualitative framework analysis. J Card Fail. 2017;23(11):794–9. https://doi.org/10.1016/j.cardfail.2017.03.008.

McDonagh T, Macdougall IC. Iron therapy for the treatment of iron deficiency in chronic heart failure: intravenous or oral? Eur J Heart Fail. 2015;17(3):248–62. https://doi.org/10.1002/ejhf.236.

McDonagh TA, Blue L, Clark AL, Dahlström U, Ekman I, Lainscak M, al w. European Society of Cardiology Heart Failure Association standards for delivering heart failure care. Eur J Heart Fail. 2011;13:235–41. https://doi.org/10.1093/eurjhf/hfq221.

McDonagh TA, Gardner RS, Lainscak M, Nielsen OW, Parissis J, Filippatos G, et al. Heart failure Association of the European Society of cardiology specialist heart failure curriculum. Eur J Heart Fail. 2014;16(2): 151–62. https://doi.org/10.1002/ejhf.41.

McDonagh J, Martin L, Ferguson C, Jha SR, Macdonald PS, Davidson PM, et al. Frailty assessment instruments in heart failure: a systematic review. Eur J Cardiovasc Nurs. 2018;17(1):23–35. https://doi.org/10.1177/1474515117708888.

McIlvennan CK, Jones J, Allen LA, Swetz KM, Nowels C, Matlock DD. Bereaved caregiver perspectives on the end-of-life experience of patients with a left ventricular assist device. JAMA Intern Med. 2016;176(4):534–9. https://doi.org/10.1001/jamainternmed.2015.8528.

McKelvie RS, Moe GW, Cheung A, Costigan J, Ducharme A, Estrella-Holder E, et al. The 2011 Canadian cardiovascular society heart failure management guidelines update: focus on sleep apnea, renal dysfunction, mechanical circulatory support, and palliative care. Can J Cardiol. 2011;27(3):319–38. https://doi.org/10.1016/j.cjca.2011.03.011.

McKenna M, Clark SC. Palliative care in cardiopulmonary transplantation. BMJ Support Palliat Care. 2015;5(4):427–34. https://doi.org/10.1136/bmjspcare-2014-000769.

Merchant FM, Binney Z, Patel A, Li J, Peddareddy LP, El-Chami MF, et al. Prevalence, predictors, and outcomes of advance directives in implantable cardioverter-defibrillator recipients. Heart Rhythm. 2017;14(6):830–6. https://doi.org/10.1016/j.hrthm.2017.02.022.

Meyers DE, Goodlin SJ. End-of-life decisions and palliative care in advanced heart failure. Can J Cardiol. 2016;32(9):1148–56. https://doi.org/10.1016/j.cjca.2016.04.015.

Moraska AR, Chamberlain AM, Shah ND, Vickers KS, Rummans TA, Dunlay SM, et al. Depression, healthcare utilization, and death in heart failure: a community study. Circ Heart Fail. 2013;6(3):387–94. https://doi.org/10.1161/CIRCHEARTFAILURE.112.000118.

Moser DK, Lee KS, Wu JR, Mudd-Martin G, Jaarsma T, Huang TY, et al. Identification of symptom clusters among patients with heart failure: an international observational study. Int J Nurs Stud. 2014;51:1366–72. https://doi.org/10.1016/j.ijnurstu.2014.02.004.

Muhandiramge D, Udeoji DU, Biswas OS, Bharadwaj P, Black LZ, Mulholland KA, et al. Palliative care issues in heart transplant candidates. Curr Opin Support Palliat Care. 2015;9(1):5–13. https://doi.org/10.1097/SPC.0000000000000112.

Munoz-Mendoza J. Competencies in palliative care for cardiology fellows. J Am Coll Cardiol. 2015;65:750–2. https://doi.org/10.1016/j.jacc.2014.12.030.

Murray SA, Kendall M, Grant E, Boyd K, Barclay S, Sheikh A. Patterns of social, psychological, and spiritual decline toward the end of life in lung cancer and heart failure. J Pain Symptom Manag. 2007;34(4):393–402. https://doi.org/10.1016/j.jpainsymman.2006.12.009.

Nakagawa S, Yuzefpolskaya M, Colombo PC, Naka Y, Blinderman CD. Palliative care interventions before left ventricular assist device implantation in both bridge to transplant and destination therapy. J Palliat Med. 2017;20(9):977–83. https://doi.org/10.1089/jpm.2016.0568.

National Heart Foundation of Australia and the Cardiac Society of Australia and New Zealand (Chronic Heart Failure Guidelines Expert Writing Panel). Guidelines for the prevention, detection and management of chronic heart failure in Australia. Updated October 2011. Document PRO-119.v2. https://www.heartfoundation.org.au/.../Chronic_Heart_Failure_Guidelines_2011.pdf. Accessed 12 Nov 2017.

Niewald A, Broxterman J, Rosell T, Rigler S. Documented consent process for implantable cardioverter-defibrillators and implications for end-of-life care in older adults. J Med Ethics. 2013;39:94–7. https://doi.org/10.1136/medethics-2012-100613.

O'Leary N, Murphy NF, O'Loughlin C, Tiernan E, McDonald K. A comparative study of the palliative care needs of heart failure and cancer patients. Eur J Heart Fail. 2009;11:406–12. https://doi.org/10.1093/eurjhf/hfp007.

Opasich C, Gualco A, De Feo S, Barbieri M, Cioffi G, Giardini A, et al. Physical and emotional symptom burden of patients with end-stage heart failure: what to measure, how and why. J Cardiovasc Med (Hagerstown). 2008;9(11):1104–8. https://doi.org/10.2459/JCM.0b013e32830c1b45.

Owan TE, Hodge DO, Herges RM, Jacobsen SJ, Roger VL, Redfield MM. Trends in prevalence and outcome of heart failure with preserved ejection fraction. N Engl J Med. 2006;355:251–9. https://doi.org/10.1056/NEJMoa052256.

Oxberry SG, Torgerson DT, Bland M, Clark AL, Cleland JG, Johnson MJ. Short-term opioids for breathlessness in stable chronic heart failure: a randomised controlled trial. Eur J Heart Fail. 2011;13:1006–12. https://doi.org/10.1093/eurjhf/hfr068.

Oxberry SG, Bland JM, Clark AL, Cleland JG, Johnson MJ. Repeat dose opioids may be effective for breathlessness in chronic heart failure if given for long enough. J Palliat Med. 2013;16:250–5. https://doi.org/10.1089/jpm.2012.0270.

Padeletti L, Arnar DO, Boncinelli L, Brachman J, Camm JA, Daubert JC, European Heart Rhythm Association, Heart Rhythm Society, et al. EHRA expert consensus statement on the management of cardiovascular implantable electronic devices in patients nearing end of life or requesting withdrawal of therapy. Europace. 2010;12(10):1480–9. https://doi.org/10.1093/europace/euq275.

Palazzuoli A, Ruocco G, Vescovo G, Valle R, Di Somma S, Nuti R. Rationale and study design of intravenous loop diuretic administration in acute heart failure: DIUR-AHF. ESC Heart Fail. 2017;4(4):479–86. https://doi.org/10.1002/ehf2.12226.

Park J, Johantgen ME. A cross-cultural comparison of symptom reporting and symptom clusters in heart failure. J Transcult Nurs. 2017;28(4):372–80. https://doi.org/10.1177/1043659616651673.

Pasalic D, Gazelka HM, Topazian RJ, Buchhalter LC, Ottenberg AL, Webster TL, et al. Palliative care consultation and associated end-of-life care after pacemaker or implantable cardioverter-defibrillator deactivation. Am J Hosp Palliat Care. 2016;33(10): 966–71. https://doi.org/10.1177/1049909115595017.

Pattenden JF, Mason AR, Lewin RJP. Collaborative palliative care for advanced heart failure: outcomes and costs from the "better together" pilot study. BMJ Support Palliat Care. 2013;3:69–76. https://doi.org/10.1136/bmjspcare-2012-000251.

Paulus WJ, Tschöpe C. A novel paradigm for heart failure with preserved ejection fraction comorbidities drive myocardial dysfunction and remodeling through coronary microvascular endothelial inflammation. J Am Coll Cardiol. 2013;62(4):263–71. https://doi.org/10.1016/j.jacc.2013.02.092.

Pitcher D, Soar J, Hogg K, Linker N, Chapman S, Beattie JM, CIED Working Group, et al. Cardiovascular implanted electronic devices in people towards the end of life, during cardiopulmonary resuscitation and after death: guidance from the Resuscitation Council (UK), British Cardiovascular Society and National Council for palliative care. Heart. 2016;102(Suppl 7):A1–A17. https://doi.org/10.1136/heartjnl-2016-309721.

Pocock SJ, Ariti CA, McMurray JJ, Maggioni A, Køber L, Squire IB, Meta-Analysis Global Group In Chronic Heart Failure, et al. Predicting survival in heart failure: a risk score based on 39 372 patients from 30 studies. Eur Heart J. 2013;34(19):1404–13. https://doi.org/10.1093/eurheartj/ehs337.

Ponikowski P, Voors AA, Anker SD, Bueno H, Cleland JG, Coats AJ, et al. 2016 ESC guidelines for the diagnosis and treatment of acute and chronic heart failure: the task force for the diagnosis and treatment of acute and chronic heart failure of the European Society of Cardiology (ESC). Developed with the special contribution of the heart failure association (HFA) of the ESC. Eur J Heart Fail. 2016;18(8):891–975. https://doi.org/10.1002/ejhf.592.

Quill TE, Abernethy AP. Generalist plus specialist palliative care – creating a more sustainable model. N Engl J Med. 2013;68(13):1173–5. https://doi.org/10.1056/NEJMp1215620.

Raphael C, Briscoe C, Davies J, Whinnett ZI, Manisty C, Sutton R, et al. Limitations of the New York heart association functional classification system and self-reported walking distances in chronic heart failure. Heart. 2007;93(4):476–82. https://doi.org/10.1136/hrt.2006.089656.

Rector TS, Kubo SH, Cohn JN. Patients self-assessment of their congestive heart failure: content, reliability and validity of a new measure, the Minnesota living with heart failure questionnaire. Heart Fail. 1987;3:198–209.

Rich MW, Chyun DA, Skolnick AH, Alexander KP, Forman DE, Kitzman DW, American Heart Association Older Populations Committee of the Council on Clinical Cardiology, Council on Cardiovascular and Stroke Nursing, Council on Cardiovascular Surgery and Anesthesia, and Stroke Council, American College of Cardiology, American Geriatrics Society, et al. Knowledge gaps in cardiovascular care of the older adult population: a scientific statement from the American Heart Association, American College of Cardiology, and American Geriatrics Society. Circulation. 2016;133(21): 2103–22. https://doi.org/10.1111/jgs.14576.

Riley PL, Arslanian-Engoren C. Cognitive dysfunction and self-care decision making in chronic heart failure: a review of the literature. Eur J Cardiovasc Nurs. 2013;12(6):505–11. https://doi.org/10.1177/1474515113487463.

Riley JP, Beattie JM. Palliative care in heart failure: facts and numbers. ESC Heart Fail. 2017;4(2):81–7. https://doi.org/10.1002/ehf2.12125.

Roger VL. Epidemiology of heart failure. Circ Res. 2013;113(6):646–59. https://doi.org/10.1161/CIRCRESAHA.113.300268.

Rogers JG, Patel CB, Mentz RJ, Granger BB, Steinhauser KE, Fiuzat M, et al. Palliative care in heart failure the PAL-HF randomized, controlled clinical trial. J Am Coll Cardiol. 2017;70(3):331–41. https://doi.org/10.1016/j.jacc.2017.05.030.

Russ AJ, Kaufman SR. Family perceptions of prognosis, silence, and the "suddenness" of death. Cult Med Psychiatry. 2005;29(1):103–23.

Russo AM, Stainback RF, Bailey SR, Epstein AE, Heidenreich PA, Jessup M, et al. ACC/HRS/AHA/ASE/HFSA/SCAI/SCCT/SCMR 2013 appropriate use criteria for implantable cardioverter-defibrillators and cardiac resynchronization therapy: a report of the American College of Cardiology Foundation appropriate use criteria task force, Heart Rhythm Society, American Heart Association, American Society of Echocardiography, Heart Failure Society of America, Society for Cardiovascular Angiography and Interventions, Society of Cardiovascular Computed Tomography, and Society for Cardiovascular Magnetic Resonance. Heart Rhythm. 2013;10(4):e11–58. https://doi.org/10.1016/j.hrthm.2013.01.008.

Rustad JK, Stern TA, Hebert KA, Musselman DL. Diagnosis and treatment of depression in patients with congestive heart failure: a review of the literature. Prim Care Companion CNS Disord. 2013;15(4). https://doi.org/10.4088/PCC.13r01511.

Ryder M, Beattie JM, O'Hanlon R, McDonald K. Multidisciplinary heart failure management and end of life care. Curr Opin Support Palliat Care. 2011; 5(4):317–21. https://doi.org/10.1097/SPC.0b013e32834d749e.

Sagin A, Kirkpatrick JN, Pisani BA, Fahlberg BB, Sundlof AL, O'Connor NR. Emerging collaboration between palliative care specialists and mechanical circulatory support teams: a qualitative study. J Pain Symptom Manag. 2016;52:491–7. https://doi.org/10.1016/j.jpainsymman.2016.03.017.

Sartipy U, Dahlström U, Edner M, Lund LH. Predicting survival in heart failure: validation of the MAGGIC heart failure risk score in 51,043 patients from the Swedish heart failure registry. Eur J Heart Fail. 2014;16(2):173–9. https://doi.org/10.1111/ejhf.32.

Schefold JC, Filippatos G, Hasenfuss G, Anker SD, von Haehling S. Heart failure and kidney dysfunction: epidemiology, mechanisms and management. Nat Rev Nephrol. 2016;12(10):610–23. https://doi.org/10.1038/nrneph.2016.113.

Schwarz ER, Baraghoush A, Morrissey RP, Shah AB, Shinde AM, Phan A, et al. Pilot study of palliative care consultation in patients with advanced heart failure referred for cardiac transplantation. J Palliat Med. 2012;15(1):12–15. https://doi.org/10.1089/jpm.2011.0256.

Senni M, Santilli G, Parrella P, De Maria R, Alari G, Berzuini C, et al. A novel prognostic index to determine the impact of cardiac conditions and co-morbidities on one-year outcome in patients with heart failure. Am J Cardiol. 2006;98(8):1076–82. https://doi.org/10.1016/j.amjcard.2006.05.031.

Shen L, Jhund PS, Petrie MC, Claggett BL, Barlera S, Cleland JGF, et al. Declining risk of sudden death in heart failure. N Engl J Med. 2017;377(1):41–51. https://doi.org/10.1056/NEJMoa1609758.

Sidebottom AC, Jorgenson A, Richards H, Kirven J, Sillah A. Inpatient palliative care for patients with acute heart failure: outcomes from a randomized trial. J Palliat Med. 2015;18:134–42. https://doi.org/10.1089/jpm.2014.0192.

Siouta N, van Beek K, Preston N, Hasselaar J, Hughes S, Payne S, et al. Towards integration of palliative care in patients with chronic heart failure and chronic obstructive pulmonary disease: a systematic literature review of European guidelines and pathways. BMC Palliat Care. 2016;15:18. https://doi.org/10.1186/s12904-016-0089-4.

Small N, Gardiner C, Barnes S, Gott M, Payne S, Seamark D, et al. Using a prediction of death in the next 12 months as a prompt for referral to palliative care acts to the detriment of patients with heart failure and chronic obstructive pulmonary disease. Palliat Med. 2010;24(7):740–1. https://doi.org/10.1177/0269216310375861.

Sokoreli I, de Vries JJ, Pauws SC, Steyerberg EW. Depression and anxiety as predictors of mortality among heart failure patients: systematic review and meta-analysis. Heart Fail Rev. 2016;21(1):49–63. https://doi.org/10.1007/s10741-015-9517-4.

Solano JP, Gomez B, Higginson IJ. A comparison of symptom prevalence in far advanced cancer, AIDS, heart disease, chronic obstructive pulmonary disease and renal disease. J Pain Symptom Manag. 2006;31:58–69. https://doi.org/10.1016/j.jpainsymman.2005.06.007.

Spiess JL. Hospice in heart failure: why, when, and what then? Heart Fail Rev. 2017;22(5):593–604. https://doi.org/10.1007/s10741-017-9595-6.

Steiner JM, Cooper S, Kirkpatrick JN. Palliative care in end-stage valvular heart disease. Heart. 2017;103(16):1233–7. https://doi.org/10.1136/heartjnl-2016-310538.

Stewart D, McPherson ML. Symptom management challenges in heart failure: pharmacotherapy considerations. Heart Fail Rev. 2017;22(5):525–34. https://doi.org/10.1007/s10741-017-9632-5.

Stewart GC, Weintraub JR, Patibhu PP, Semigran MJ, Camuso JM, Brooks K, et al. Patient expectations from implantable defibrillators to prevent death in heart failure. J Cardiac Fail. 2010;16:106–13. https://doi.org/10.1016/j.cardfail.2009.09.003.

Strachan PH, Ross H, Rocker GM, Dodek PM, Heyland DK, Canadian Researchers at the End of Life Network (CARENET). Mind the gap: opportunities for improving end-of-life care for patients with advanced heart failure. Can J Cardiol. 2009;25:635–40.

Strachan PH, de Laat S, Carroll SL, Schwartz L, Vaandering K, Toor GK, et al. Readability and content of patient education material related to implantable cardioverter defibrillators. J Cardiovasc Nurs. 2012;27(6):495–504. https://doi.org/10.1097/JCN.0b013e31822ad3dd.

Stulak JM, Davis ME, Haglund N, Dunlay S, Cowger J, Shah P, et al. Adverse events in contemporary continuous-flow left ventricular assist devices: a multi-institutional comparison shows significant differences. J Thorac Cardiovasc Surg. 2016;151(1):177–89. https://doi.org/10.1016/j.jtcvs.2015.09.100.

Swetz KM, Freeman MR, AbouEzzeddine OF, Carter KA, Boilson BA, Ottenberg AL, et al. Palliative medicine consultation for preparedness planning in patients receiving left ventricular assist devices as destination therapy. Mayo Clin Proc. 2011;86(6):493–500. https://doi.org/10.4065/mcp.2010.0747.

Taylor GJ, Lee DM, Baicu CF, Zile MR. Palliative care for advanced heart failure in a Department of Veterans Affairs regional hospice program: patient selection, a treatment protocol, and clinical course. J Palliat Med. 2017;20(10):1068–73. https://doi.org/10.1089/jpm.2017.0035.

Testa G, Cacciatore F, Galizia G, Della-Morte D, Mazzella F, Russo S, et al. Charlson comorbidity index does not predict long-term mortality in elderly subjects with chronic heart failure. Age Ageing. 2009;38(6):734–40. https://doi.org/10.1093/ageing/afp165.

Tevendale E, Baxter J. Heart failure comorbidities at the end of life. Curr Opin Support Palliat Care. 2011;5(4):322–6. https://doi.org/10.1097/SPC.0b013e32834d2ee4.

The Criteria Committee of the New York Heart Association. Nomenclature and criteria for diagnosis of diseases of the heart and great vessels. 9th ed. Boston: Little, Brown & Co; 1994. p. 253–6.

Thoonsen B, Engels Y, van Rijswijk E, Verhagen S, van Weel C, Groot M, et al. Early identification of palliative care patients in general practice: development of RADboud indicators for PAlliative care needs (RADPAC). Br J Gen Pract. 2012;62:625–3. https://doi.org/10.3399/bjgp12X654597.

Timmons MJ, MacIver J, Alba AC, Tibbles A, Greenwood S, Ross HJ. Using heart failure instruments to determine when to refer heart failure patients to palliative care. J Palliat Care. 2013;29:217–24.

Treece J, Chemchirian H, Hamilton N, Jbara M, Gangadharan V, Paul T, et al. A review of prognostic tools in heart failure. Am J Hosp Palliat Care. 2017. https://doi.org/10.1177/1049909117709468.

Udelson JE, Stevenson LW. The future of heart failure diagnosis, therapy, and management. Circulation. 2016;133(25):2671–86. https://doi.org/10.1161/CIRCULATIONAHA.116.023518.

University of Colorado. (2016) Patient Decision Aids – Implantable Cardioverter-Defibrillator (ICD). URL: http://www.patientdecisionaid.org Accessed 5 Nov 2017.

van Deursen VM, Urso R, Laroche C, Damman K, Dahlström U, Tavazzi L, et al. Co-morbidities in patients with heart failure: an analysis of the European heart failure pilot survey. Eur J Heart Fail. 2014;16(1):103–11. https://doi.org/10.1002/ejhf.30.

Waller A, Girgis A, Davidson PM, Newton PJ, Lecathelinais C, Macdonald PS, et al. Facilitating needs-based support and palliative care for people with chronic heart failure: preliminary evidence for the acceptability, inter-rater reliability, and validity of a needs assessment tool. J Pain Symptom Manag. 2013;45:912–25. https://doi.org/10.1016/j.jpainsymman.2012.05.009.

White N, Kupeli N, Vickerstaff V, Stone P. How accurate is the 'Surprise Question' at identifying patients at the end of life? A systematic review and meta-analysis. BMC Med. 2017;15(1):139. https://doi.org/10.1186/s12916-017-0907-4.

Wilhelm MJ. Long-term outcome following heart transplantation: current perspective. J Thorac Dis. 2015;7(3): 549–51. https://doi.org/10.3978/j.issn.2072-1439.2015.01.46.

Wilson A, McMillan S. Symptoms experienced by heart failure patients in hospice care. J Hosp Palliat Nurs. 2013;15:13–21. https://doi.org/10.1097/NJH.0b013e31827ba343.

Wingate S, Bain KT, Goodlin SJ. Availability of data when heart failure patients are admitted to hospice. Congest Heart Fail. 2011;7(6):303–8. https://doi.org/10.1111/j.1751-7133.2011.00229.x.

Wong FK, Ng AY, Lee PH, Lam PT, Ng JS, Ng NH, et al. Effects of a transitional palliative care model on patients with end-stage heart failure: a randomised controlled trial. Heart. 2016;102(14): 1100–8. https://doi.org/10.1136/heartjnl-2015-308638.

Wordingham SE, Kasten RM, Swetz KM. Total artificial heart #296. J Palliat Med. 2015;18(11): 985–6. https://doi.org/10.1089/jpm.2015.0243.

Wordingham SE, McIlvennan CK, Fendler TJ, Behnken AL, Dunlay SM, Kirkpatrick JN, et al. Palliative care clinicians caring for patients before and after continuous flow-left ventricular assist device. J Pain Symptom Manag. 2017;54(4):601–8. https://doi.org/10.1016/j.jpainsymman.2017.07.007.

Wright GA, Klein GJ, Gula LJ. Ethical and legal perspective of implantable cardioverter defibrillator deactivation or implantable cardioverter defibrillator generator replacement in the elderly. Curr Opin Cardiol. 2013;28:43–9. https://doi.org/10.1097/HCO.0b013e32835b0b3b.

Xie K, Gelfman L, Horton JR, Goldstein NE. State of research on palliative care in heart failure as evidenced by published literature, conference proceedings, and NIH funding. J Card Fail. 2017;23(2):197–200. https://doi.org/10.1016/j.cardfail.2016.10.013.

Xu J, Nolan MT, Heinze K, Yenokyan G, Hughes MT, Johnson J. Symptom frequency, severity, and quality of life among persons with three disease trajectories: cancer, ALS, and CHF. Appl Nurs Res. 2015;28(4): 311–5. https://doi.org/10.1016/j.apnr.2015.03.005.

Yancy CW, Jessup M, Bozkurt B, Butler J, Casey DE Jr, Drazner MH, et al. 2013 ACCF/AHA guideline for the management of heart failure a report of the American College of Cardiology Foundation/American Heart Association Task Force on practice guidelines. J Am Coll Cardiol. 2013;62(16):e147–239. https://doi.org/10.1016/j.jacc.2013.05.019.

Yim CK, Barrón Y, Moore S, Murtaugh C, Lala A, Aldridge M, et al. Hospice enrolment in patients with advanced heart failure decreases acute medical service utilization. Circ Heart Fail. 2017;10(3). https://doi.org/10.1161/CIRCHEARTFAILURE.116.003335.

Yu DS, Li PW, Chong SO. Symptom cluster among patients with advanced heart failure: a review of its manifestations and impacts on health outcomes. Curr Opin Support Palliat Care. 2017. https://doi.org/10.1097/SPC.0000000000000316.

Zacharias H, Raw J, Nunn A, Parsons S, Johnson M. Is there a role for subcutaneous furosemide in the community and hospice management of end-stage heart failure? Palliat Med. 2011;25:658–63. https://doi.org/10.1177/0269216311399490.

Zambroski C, Moser D, Bhat G, Ziegler C. Impact of symptom prevalence and symptom burden on quality of life in patients with heart failure. Eur J Cardiovasc Nurs. 2005;4:198–206. https://doi.org/10.1016/j.ejcnurse.2005.03.010.

Palliative Care of Respiratory Disease in Primary Care

62

Patrick White

Contents

Abstract

The palliative care of advanced progressive respiratory disease in the setting of a primary care team is concerned mainly with chronic obstructive pulmonary disease (COPD), idiopathic pulmonary fibrosis (IPF), and cystic fibrosis (CF). COPD is the commonest of these but it is perhaps the most difficult to identify in its final stages. IPF has a trajectory and prognosis more akin to malignant disease. Though relatively rare in general practice, IPF is the disease among these three that has the most easily definable terminal stage, and so primary care teams should be alert to the palliative care needs of these patients.

CF is a remarkable disease because life expectancy at birth with CF has changed from childhood or teenage years to 30 years now,

P. White (✉)
Primary Care Respiratory Medicine, School of Population Health and Environmental Science, King's College London, London, UK
e-mail: Patrick.white@kcl.ac.uk

R. D. MacLeod, L. Van den Block (eds.), *Textbook of Palliative Care*,
https://doi.org/10.1007/978-3-319-77740-5_61

and for those aged 30 years, life expectancy is now in mid-50s. Like COPD, prognosis in CF is difficult to define. Most people with advanced disease in both groups are living with the disease. Most of these people want to continue living in the face of considerable challenges. The task in both of these diseases is to develop an approach to the amelioration of symptoms and to the support of patients and carers, that is, in keeping with the personal objectives of the patients. Information about treatment, future exacerbations, and the risk of dying is all important. Symptom control is difficult, and for intractable breathlessness, oral morphine has a role in many patients.

End-stage progressive nonmalignant respiratory disease:

the challenge/the burden from a palliative care perspective/the symptoms/issues in specific diseases/the assessment and treatment of breathlessness in respiratory disease

1 The Challenge

The palliative care of respiratory disease presents the classic challenges of advanced progressive nonmalignant disease. The disease trajectory is often prolonged and uncertain. The transition between high dependency and dying may be imperceptible. In idiopathic pulmonary fibrosis (IPF), the end stage of the disease may resemble the terminal stage of a moderately progressive cancer. As symptoms become intractable, their management can be increasingly complex, and multidisciplinary input is likely to be needed.

In this chapter, the focus is on the advanced progressive nonmalignant diseases of the respiratory system. Lung cancer will not be treated as a separate issue here because the features of the terminal stages of lung cancer are largely indistinguishable from other malignant diseases in which metastasis to the lung is prominent.

The two most common progressive respiratory diseases that present to palliative care are chronic obstructive pulmonary disease (COPD) and idiopathic pulmonary fibrosis (IPF). They lead to contrasting experiences and different demands. COPD is likely to have progressed over 10 or 20 years. It usually does not progress to a clear terminal stage of the disease. Death may be relatively sudden from a severe acute exacerbation or pneumonia. IPF is likely to be more predictably progressive. The mean survival of IPF from diagnosis is 2.5–3.5 years. It usually has a more defined terminal stage and a more conventional opportunity for palliative care intervention than COPD.

Cystic fibrosis (CF), an inherited condition, has an altogether different onset and trajectory, from early life until premature death, which is usually in the 1950s nowadays. The need for palliative care of cystic fibrosis has only recently been addressed in the research literature. Despite its systemic effects, particularly in the gastrointestinal tract, the greatest threat in CF is progressive respiratory disease. Death may be from an acute infection. Many patients are selected for possible lung transplantation when respiratory function has been severely impaired. At that point the need for palliative and supportive care input is not likely to be in the domain of primary care.

The palliative care of advanced progressive respiratory disease shares the same basic aims of all palliative care. Timely planning and provision of clear information are the cornerstones of treatment. Neither should depend on being able to make an accurate prognosis. Symptom palliation should be determined by the severity of the symptom and the responsiveness of the underlying pathology to the treatment. Involvement of the patient, and their carers, in decisions about their care will help to ensure that care is appropriate. Providing an accurate prognosis may be challenging. That difficulty should not be used as an excuse for failing to prepare patients and their families for what lies ahead.

In advanced progressive nonmalignant respiratory disease, particularly in COPD and in CF, living with the disease is the dominant issue. The risk of death, rather than preparation for it, is the shadow that requires acknowledgment. In IPF, by contrast, the prognosis, all too clearly, is short.

The context of the stage of the disease in chronic nonmalignant respiratory disease is important to these discussions. For some clinicians, it may be more difficult to introduce this subject because of the greater uncertainty that exists over the disease prognosis. Acknowledgment that prognosis is not the key issue here may help. Putting the issue of prognosis to one side may allow clearer thinking to be done about the risks of the disease at this stage, including the risk of dying. Will it be useful for my patient if I raise the subject of the risks associated with their illness? Is my patient someone who would like to consider the risks that they face? Have they reached the stage that life has become precarious because of the risk that the next exacerbation will be fatal?

Symptom control is the second big challenge in advanced nonmalignant respiratory disease. Patients with advanced severe disease will survive at least 2 years on average. This is not the moment to exhibit all the drugs at the clinician's disposal in the attempt to ameliorate intractable breathlessness. There is a need for a careful structured approach to symptom palliation that adopts a realistic evaluation of the patient's position. This approach will be discussed more at length in the Sect. 3. At this point the clinician should review what has been provided so far.

In this chapter the prevalence, burden, and risk of death from respiratory disease is discussed from the perspective of primary care in the UK. The population of the UK is now more than 60 million people. Where figures for prevalence are given, readers should translate those to their own country or setting. Prevalence can vary significantly. The incidence of COPD, for example, is likely to fall progressively in the UK where rates of smoking have plummeted in the last 40 years to a low of 16%. Exposure to biomass fuels in the home is virtually unheard of in the UK. This contrasts to countries in which the promotion of cigarette smoking has continued unabated and biomass fuel is commonly used for cooking. In such circumstances death from COPD is likely to be much younger because the exposure to risk factors starts earlier in life.

This chapter is written for primary care, taken from the experience of primary care in the UK. It is not directed at a particular clinical group. The issues discussed should be as relevant to general practitioners or family physicians as they are to nurse specialists, practice nurses, community nurses, healthcare assistants, and other professional clinical groups caring for patients approaching the end of their lives in the community. In other countries the organization of healthcare may differ significantly from that in the UK. Readers should translate the ideas presented here to their own setting.

2 The Burden from a Palliative Care Perspective

2.1 Chronic Obstructive Pulmonary Disease (COPD)

COPD is common. About 2% (>1,000,000) of people have diagnosed COPD in the UK (British Lung Foundation 2018). Ten percent of these have very severe disease as defined by the spirometry criterion of forced expiratory volume in the first second (FEV_1) (White et al. 2013). The prevalence of COPD in the UK is based primarily on people who have symptomatic disease. The prevalence varies quite markedly from country to country depending on the cause of the disease and whether or not screening is carried out for COPD. In many of the people diagnosed with COPD through screening, the disease causes no symptoms and has no impact on quality of life at the time of screening.

In developed countries the main cause of COPD is tobacco smoking. Occupational exposures account for a small proportion of the prevalence. In countries with high rates of poverty or large rural communities, exposure to biomass fuels is a significant cause of the disease. Exposure to biomass fuels is usually through cooking with wood or animal waste. The cooking is done in the house with poor ventilation. The whole family is exposed to smoke and volatile materials from a young age.

About 30,000 people die from COPD in the UK every year, just under 1 death from COPD for every GP each year or 3–6 deaths for a primary care team per year. This depends on the number of patients registered with the team. This is not far below the rate of deaths from lung cancer. The mean age of death from COPD in the UK is 76 years. Comorbidities are likely to contribute to the risk of death. They may complicate the care of people with advanced COPD.

2.2 Idiopathic Pulmonary Fibrosis (IPF)

The symptoms of IPF are breathlessness, cough, and fatigue (Shaw et al. 2017). It affects more than 32,000 people in the UK or 1 in 2000 people. About 1 patient has IPF for every 30 patients with COPD. Worldwide the prevalence of IPF is 2.8–9.3 per 100,000 (Hutchinson et al. 2015). Each GP is likely to have a little less than one patient with IPF on his or her list in the UK at any one time. There are 5000 deaths from IPF in the UK each year (Navaratnam et al. 2011). On average a primary care team will have a patient who dies from IPF every 2–3 years. This is about a sixth of the deaths that might be expected from COPD.

In IPF, the diagnosis and severity are defined by the spirometric criterion of forced expiratory volume (FEV). The treatment of IPF has changed in the last 5 years with the publication of two trials of antifibrotic drugs. These two drugs, pirfenidone and nintedanib, have been shown to reduce the progression of the disease (NICE 2016; Nathan et al. 2017). It is not yet clear how well this treatment will control the impact of IPF. If successful it will significantly reduce the burden of IPF at the end of life.

2.3 Cystic Fibrosis

About 10,000 people in the UK have cystic fibrosis, the commonest inherited disease affecting Caucasians. It is a common reason for lung transplant. Dramatic changes have occurred in the life expectancy of CF (Keogh et al. 2018). At birth people with CF should now expect to live until their mid-40s. People with CF at 30 years should expect to live into their mid-50s. In 10 years life expectancy is projected to be in the mid-60s for people aged 30. Better understanding of the underlying mechanisms is likely to lead to significant improvements in the treatment of cystic fibrosis. For now, the most important intervention is early treatment of respiratory infections with the prevention of mucous plugging if possible. Respiratory failure is the commonest cause of death. It is difficult to define the burden of cystic fibrosis on palliative care services because deaths are sporadic, result from acute infections, or occur in people in lung transplant programs.

3 The Symptoms

In advanced respiratory disease, four symptoms dominate patients' experience: breathlessness, cough, weakness, and low mood.

Breathlessness is the central problem in loss of respiratory function, the chief impact of these diseases. In COPD breathlessness progresses gradually. Sometimes it deteriorates so slowly that it is the loss of functional capacity that makes the change apparent. Breathlessness is difficult to remedy. There is a variety of strategies that can ameliorate its impact in people with advanced disease, including exercise to improve muscular fitness, breath training to give greater control of the symptom, psychological strategies to reduce the anxiety that often accompanies the symptom, mechanical devices to distract from the symptom, and pharmacological interventions to reduce its perception. These are discussed in more detail later in the chapter.

Cough is usually a more prominent symptom in early disease. However, in IPF cough progresses with the disease, and 80% of patients with advanced IPF have cough (Shaw et al. 2017). In IPF the symptom is often intractable, and treatment is usually ineffective. In COPD cough is usually productive. It can become intractable in advanced disease especially when associated with difficulty in clearing secretions from the upper airway. There has been more interest in recent years in the use of mucolytics such as carbocysteine, but evidence for their effectiveness is moderate.

Weakness is the culmination of the downward spiral that results from progressive breathlessness. Breathlessness leads to reduced exercise that in turn leads to muscle deconditioning. With muscle deconditioning, there is less efficient use of oxygen so that more breathing is required to achieve the same functional result and the outcome is weakness. In advanced disease, exhaustion and demoralization can follow minor physical activity. In COPD, in IPF, or in CF, there is no evidence of inflammatory activity outside the respiratory system. The progressive weakness that occurs is not due to peripheral myopathy or neuropathy.

The most effective treatment of the progressive symptoms and disability of COPD and IPF, and possibly CF, is pulmonary rehabilitation, which converts the downward spiral of progressive weakness into a virtuous cycle (McCarthy et al. 2015). It improves breathlessness, exercise capacity, sense of mastery over the disease, and anxiety. Pulmonary rehabilitation is a treatment based on exercise, disease education, and social interaction. Participants usually attend between 8 and 12 classes spread over 6–10 weeks. The main effect of pulmonary rehabilitation is improved exercise capacity in the muscles, but there is now increased evidence, from brain scanning, that pulmonary rehabilitation is also associated with changes in the neural responses in the brain to breathlessness, which alter the perception of breathlessness (Herigstad et al. 2017). The challenge for clinicians in treating patients with advanced disease is to judge whether their patients can undertake pulmonary rehabilitation. Evidence for the effectiveness of pulmonary rehabilitation in moderate and severe disease is undisputed. There has been less study of its effect in patients with advanced disease, but such is its effectiveness in other groups; it should be considered in the most severely affected patients.

Low mood together with anxiety is a common accompaniment of chronic breathlessness and is frequently seen in COPD and IPF. The evidence for the effectiveness of the treatment of psychological symptoms in moderate or severe respiratory disease is limited. Chronic breathlessness often leads to social isolation and dependence on carers. The progressive deterioration seen in COPD, in IPF, and in cystic fibrosis is dispiriting. The chronic breathlessness also leads to insomnia and loss of established sleep patterns. In COPD, commonly caused by smoking, many patients will have suffered criticism from family, friends, and health professionals for failing to give up smoking. The implication of this criticism is that the disease has been self-inflicted, and some patients with advanced COPD feel undeserving of treatment or of the support of family and friends.

IPF by contrast with COPD is of unknown cause, has no specific treatment, and will be completely unfamiliar to most patients. IPF and CF patients may not share the sense of blame that is common in COPD. They are more likely to feel perplexed and hopeless. For all of these patients, the burden of the disease is immense, and patients' resilience is undermined further by low mood and anxiety.

4 Trajectory and Prognosis in Advanced Progressive Respiratory Disease

Prognosis is one of the more vexed areas in the management of advanced chronic respiratory disease. With IPF prognosis is worse than in many cancers. As respiratory function deteriorates, it is possible to predict roughly when a patient is likely to die (Shaw et al. 2017). The advantages that accompany this relative accuracy are the opportunities for informing patients and their families what is likely to lay ahead and for enabling patients and families to plan for the implications of the patient's death.

In cystic fibrosis prognosis is a much less precise possibility. While the disease is progressive, deterioration is determined by respiratory infection (Keogh et al. 2018). Damage is caused to the lung parenchyma by infection and mucous plugging. With each infection the process is accelerated. This is a well-documented trajectory. Death is unpredictable because it is likely to occur during an infection. The gaps between infections may be prolonged. However, the experience of people dying very prematurely from cystic fibrosis has led to little attention to the palliative care aspects of the disorder in the research literature. Recent research on palliative care of CF has suggested that the preoccupation with preventing further progression of the disease may have drawn attention from the need to prepare those for whom death was a likely possibility. Patients and families may be unprepared for deterioration and death.

The situation with COPD is strikingly different. For many years it was the hope of most people interested in improving the management of advanced chronic respiratory disease that with more careful assessment and more careful research, it would be possible to make the prediction of the risk of death more accurate. Alas we are now more confident than ever that there is little hope of predicting the risk of death within a year in COPD.

5 Issues in Specific Diseases

5.1 COPD

The clarity with which patients with advanced COPD have indicated breathlessness as their dominant symptom, while affirming their commitment to living presents a complex dilemma (White et al. 2011; Pinnock et al. 2011). Breathlessness is a very difficult symptom for which there are limited therapeutic options. Yet patients would prefer to take their chances with the next exacerbation, with the limited treatment available, than hope for their symptoms to be relieved by death. The severity of breathlessness in COPD has been compared with that in advanced cancer (Gore et al. 2000). How is it that COPD patients with breathlessness in advanced disease manage their everyday lives? Clearly it is not easy, but a number of factors distinguish patients with COPD from those with cancer and indeed patients with IPF. The breathlessness of COPD is slow in developing, often over more than 20 years. As it progresses it is likely that patients adjust to the symptom in their perception and in their expectations. If the status quo is breathlessness on exertion, then the symptom will have no surprise element, and impaired function will the norm. As breathlessness at rest increases then, there are the accompanying problems of exhaustion, low mood, and progressive immobility. But COPD patients are often remarkably phlegmatic and accept these changes as part of the disease.

Prognosis in COPD is a thorny issue. In a landmark study in the USA in 1996, of 1016 COPD patients admitted with Type II respiratory failure (hypercapnia ± hypoxia), 50% were still alive after 2 years (Connors et al. 1996). Six years later this study was effectively repeated on a smaller scale in Spain (Almagro et al. 2002). In the later study, the survival in a similar group of patients was 65%. In such severely affected patients, the most accurate prognosis possible was a risk of dying between 35% and 50% within 2 years.

Some 15 years ago, COPD patients were reported to have expressed an interest in knowing their prognosis when asked if they wanted their physician to discuss it with them (Curtis et al. 2004). There are concerns as to whether it is ethical to ask research participants this question when an accurate prognosis was beyond the capacity of specialists or generalists. A conclusion to this question has been effectively drawn by the latest work by Almagro and colleagues (2017). They have demonstrated that a prognosis of less than 1 year is impossible to make in advanced COPD with all the disease-specific and general demographic information available.

For patients with advanced COPD or CF, and their clinicians, introducing the subject of advance care planning may seem counter to the flow of communication. One of these exacerbations may be fatal. Has important communication of this risk been considered with dependents and key intimates in their lives? Do affairs need to be put in order? Are there treatment options that should be reviewed? This opportunity must be seized because it is unlikely that a definitive prognostic moment will present itself. The opportunity is the result of increasing risk in a long trajectory of risk.

The supportive care of advanced COPD and of CF should include discussion of the stage of the disease, the likely progression of symptoms, the potential complications, and the available treatments. Progression may be accelerated by exacerbations. The role of smoking cessation in advanced disease is uncertain. More than 40% of people with moderate, severe, or very severe disease, in whom smoking was the main cause of the disease, continue to smoke.

Since survival is important to people with advanced COPD, how can end-stage disease be identified? The terminal stage of COPD, the stage of imminent death, can be identified by a combination of conventional or generic signs of diminishing functional capacity. These include requirement of help with eating, drinking, washing, and toileting by becoming bedbound, by loss of appetite, and by severe weight loss or cachexia. In the presence of advanced COPD, with no other explanation, these signs are suggestive of imminent death. Such a case is presented in Box 1.

Box 1 A Story of Imminent Death in COPD

MD, a single man of 57 years, had COPD diagnosed at the age of 54. His COPD probably began in his mid-40s to judge from the onset of his cough and breathlessness. He was a scaffolder until 2 years ago, when his breathlessness stopped him from working. He had two hospital admissions due to his COPD in the previous 6 months. The most recent was associated with a marked deterioration. He had been ventilated during the admission and was in the hospital for nearly 3 months. No other cause was found. The doctors said there was nothing more that could be done, and he was at risk of readmission. On discharge from the hospital, he was breathless at rest and prone to confusion. He was on long-term oxygen therapy for chronic hypoxia. He was taking his inhaled drugs by nebulizer every 4 h.

He was looked after at home by his two sisters, one of whom had come to stay. Within 2 weeks of his discharge, he had deteriorated again. He was more short of breath and confused, and he was refusing food. With his sisters' help, he was using a commode. At this point his GP, who had known him for years, was shocked at his

Box 1 A Story of Imminent Death in COPD (continued)

cachectic state. He wanted to readmit him to the hospital. His sisters pleaded for him not to be readmitted because he had asked them to promise not to let him be sent back. They felt that he was dying.

The GP examined him. MD was confused. His heart rate was 104/min; his respiratory rate was 36/min. He was cyanosed. There was no fever and no evidence of pneumonia. After discussion with MD's sisters, it was agreed that MD would spend the night at home and that an urgent request for assessment by the palliative care team would be made. The GP told the sisters that MD may not survive for many days in this condition. They said they knew that already.

The following day a call came from MD's sisters. He had died during the night.

The uncertain trajectory of advanced COPD, the prolonged experience of severe symptoms, and the long-term adjustments that patients make demand a palliative care approach which is about support, symptom management, and psychological adjustment. End-of-life care is not the dominant concern in COPD for the main part. Patients with advanced COPD are more likely to see themselves living with their disease than dying from it. Until they enter that final period in which cachexia and rapid loss of function are the predominant features, it is more appropriate to provide palliative care that has an outlook that matches that of the patient. Interventions should be symptom-responsive. Talk about symptom management and supportive care should be the dominant component where appropriate, not preparation for the imminent end to life.

5.2 Idiopathic Pulmonary Fibrosis

IPF presents an altogether different challenge to that of COPD. It is a disease with a limited prognosis from the outset. The annual rate of decline of FEV_1 from diagnosis is usually between 10% and 20% of expected so that the progression of the symptoms is so rapid that there is much less time for adjustment than is seen in COPD. The loss of function is more obvious and more alarming to family and friends. The diagnosis is like that of a malignant disease, with moderate but relentless progression. As the disease progresses, so does functional impairment. The value of pulmonary rehabilitation at this stage should not be underestimated. It is common for the suggestion of the potential benefits of pulmonary rehabilitation to be lost on breathless patients. Recovering a small degree of functional improvement can make a surprising difference.

Early and effective information provision in IPF for the patient and for carers can allow for effective planning. Advance planning is needed to prepare for inevitable challenges at work, for financial commitments, for discussion with close family, and for the preparation of impending loss. Patients with IPF should be considered early for referral to multidisciplinary clinics for the management of breathlessness. The rapid deterioration in symptoms may mean that there is a greater role for psychological interventions for breathlessness and for the use of opioids.

The recent introduction of antifibrotic drugs, pirfenidone, and nintedanib, for IPF, has been shown to slow the progression of the disease in many patients (Nathan et al. 2017; NICE 2016). Should this intervention be shown to be effective in the later stages of the disease, there may be hope that its terminal stages can be postponed.

While the rate of deterioration in IPF is rapid by comparison to COPD, it is an uncommon disease, and little research has been done on the palliative care of the condition. Careful monitoring of change in FVC can be used, and from this the clinician can obtain a relatively accurate estimate of prognosis.

5.3 Cystic Fibrosis

Change in the last 50 years in the life expectancy of cystic fibrosis from birth has been remarkable. The progress of cystic fibrosis is usually intermittent, but 50 years ago the prognosis from birth was less than 15 years. Even before the disease becomes advanced, the life-threatening nature of acute infections may be unavoidable. Acute severe infections should provide a timely opportunity to consider how interventions can be optimized and the importance of early intervention with antibiotics in worsening breathlessness. They also show how such infections raise problems of antimicrobial resistance and the risk of dying. Advance care planning in CF requires good continuity of care especially as sufferers move through adolescence.

Little research has been published on the palliative care of CF. It seems likely that the patient, the carers, and the clinicians become preoccupied with early intervention and careful management of acute exacerbations of the disease. At some point there must be an opportunity to consider the increasing risk that the patient faces of an exacerbation being life-threatening. This may be addressed when patients are considered for lung transplant. There will have been appropriate and earlier occasions when the subject could have been raised. It would be remiss of services not to respond to the opportunity at the right time.

6 The Assessment and Treatment of Breathlessness

Breathlessness in advanced disease has a variable association with measures of respiratory function, particularly reductions in FEV_1 and FVC. The control of breathing and the experience of breathlessness are determined by a complex array of physiological and psychological influences and controls (Currow et al. 2016). These include the peripheral stimuli associated with movement in the muscles of respiration; the movement of air in the face, mouth, and pharynx; and drying of the mouth and pharynx with increased breathing. Internal factors include levels of oxygen, carbon dioxide and acid/base balance in the blood, and emotional factors, including expectations and learned responses. Such is the complexity of the interactions of these different elements that it is hardly surprising that people have very different experiences of breathlessness for the same levels of disease severity. To understand the role of treatments for breathlessness in advanced disease, it is worth considering the underlying issues of low oxygen (hypoxia) and raised carbon dioxide (hypercapnia) in advanced respiratory disease.

The effect of impaired breathing due to obstruction and parenchymal damage in COPD, and due to restriction of respiratory movement in IPF, is to reduce the delivery of oxygen (O_2) into the blood and to reduce the removal of carbon dioxide (CO_2). Patients with advanced COPD usually develop tolerance in the brain to increased CO_2 (hypercapnia). The main drive to breathing in established COPD is reduced oxygen in the blood, hypoxia. In such patients complete relief of hypoxia by giving O_2 diminishes the drive to breathe. If the drive to breathe is reduced, the CO_2 level in the blood may rise to dangerous levels. This can cause the patient to become drowsy or unconscious – CO_2 narcosis – and ultimately to be in danger of dying. Patients dependent on hypoxia for the drive to breathe may be at considerable risk in receiving unlimited O_2 for symptom relief.

On the other hand, patients with persistent hypoxia may require long-term oxygen therapy to prevent pulmonary hypertension. The identification of hypoxia, O_2, below a saturation of 92% on a pulse oximeter, should lead to specialist referral for consideration of long-term oxygen therapy.

For patients that become intermittently hypoxic on exercise, intermittent oxygen may be needed. In the unusual situation that a severely ill patient becomes hypoxic at rest, then low dose (2 L/min) oxygen can be administered to relieve breathlessness until the patient is assessed by a specialist. The relief obtained is likely to be small if any.

The perception of breathlessness in the brain is complex. It varies from person to person, some people appearing to tolerate breathlessness in more severe disease than others. Breathlessness perception and the tolerance of breathlessness can be markedly affected by anxiety. Understanding the mechanisms of breathlessness is tied to the therapies that are brought to bear on the symptom in advanced disease. These are pulmonary rehabilitation, breathing training and exercises, therapy for anxiety, handheld fan, neuromuscular electrical stimulation, and the suppression of the perception of breathlessness with drugs (Higginson et al. 2014; Farquhar et al. 2016; Maddocks et al. 2017). Pulmonary rehabilitation and a handheld fan can be prescribed in primary care. If the patient needs breathing training, therapy for anxiety, neuromuscular electrical stimulation, or the use of drugs, referral should be made to a multidisciplinary center.

Breathing training and exercises work by promoting more efficient posture for breathing and by reinforcing the sense of control of breathing when the patient is more breathless through specific physical strategies to manage the breathlessness. Some people experience a cycle of worsening breathlessness in which the breathlessness causes anxiety, which in turn leads to hyperventilation and a sensation of even worse breathlessness. This combination is difficult to identify. It may be evident from an exceptional response to breathing exercise which is accompanied by a marked reduction in anxiety. The handheld fan is of variable value. It probably works by blowing air across the lips and cheeks generating a sense of greater movement of air and of more effective breathing. Neuromuscular electrical stimulation is designed to improve breathlessness by improving peripheral muscle power (Maddocks et al. 2016). It is effective in reducing the effect of exercise on breathlessness. But how long the effect is sustained has not been assessed, and it is only available in specialist centers.

The suppression of breathlessness by opioids has been used for many years in people with advanced cancer, particularly in their last days. The development of tolerance and dependence is not an issue in such circumstances. In advanced respiratory disease, the circumstances are different. Evidence is slowly coming to light about appropriate dosing and the risks of prolonged use. The case in Box 2 highlights some of the issues.

Box 2 Opioids in Chronic Respiratory Breathlessness? A Case History

SB, a widower of 74 years, had COPD for 15 years. Having been a smoker since a teenager, he was still smoking three or four cigarettes a day. He lived alone and was a volunteer driver for the local hospital, taking patients to and from their appointments. He liked his voluntary work, but his breathlessness was increasingly troublesome. He had difficulty sleeping at night and had to sit up. He was on maximal treatment for his COPD. He was not hypoxic. His GP referred him to the local chest clinic to rule out lung cancer.

The chest physician investigated SB. No new problems were identified. There was no sign of cardiac disease. He was told to continue on his medications and discharged from the clinic. He had started pulmonary rehabilitation 6 months ago, but he did not think it was helping, so he stopped after two sessions.

After another 6 months, SB's breathlessness was worse. He now spent all of his time at home, breathless at rest. He was again referred to the chest physician who discharged him saying there was no further treatment that would help his COPD.

SB's GP did not know what to do next. She referred SB to the local palliative care breathlessness clinic. SB was seen there by a palliative care physician and palliative care nurse.

SB was referred to a psychologist to treat the anxiety associated with his breathing and to a physiotherapist for breathing exercises and breathing training. He was given a handheld fan. After 4 months there was little change. SB was then started on oral morphine 2.5 mg four times daily. His breathing improved for the first time in perhaps a year. His exercise capacity was no different, but he felt better and slept better. SB was admitted to the hospital with an exacerbation of COPD 9 months after starting morphine. He was taking 5 mg in

Box 2 Opioids in Chronic Respiratory Breathlessness? A Case History (continued)

the morning and the evening and 2.5 mg twice during the day. His breathlessness was still better. Sadly he developed pneumonia and died.

It is clear that this patient has advanced COPD. The multidisciplinary team had run out of options, and so morphine was started. He was taking relatively small amounts of morphine for a prolonged period of 9 months until an exacerbation led to his death. It is unclear if the morphine retained its effectiveness or whether the increase in dosing had an impact on his death in terms of his response to the exacerbation. The morphine had been very helpful in improving the symptom for a long period of time.

The usual dosage of morphine currently recommended for advanced respiratory disease is a starting dose of 10 mg daily as a sustained release preparation (Smallwood et al. 2015). This can also be administered as 2.5 mg of immediate acting morphine up to four times daily. The maximum dose should be 30 mg. There is no evidence of difference of effectiveness between different opioids, but most of the current evidence relates to morphine. Among the issues yet to be addressed with respect to morphine use in advanced respiratory disease are the long-term effects on survival, the development of tolerance, the sustained effect on symptoms, and the need for larger amounts during exacerbations. Within the dosage guidance described here, general practitioners may wish to start opioids for COPD patients with intractable. It may be wise to do so with the support of a palliative care team for those who are inexperienced. It should only be initiated for advanced respiratory disease in specialist centers until evidence for its use becomes clearer.

7 Supporting Carers in Respiratory Disease

Carers of people with advanced IPF have needs that are similar to those of carers with advanced cancer. The needs of carers of people with COPD and CF are different. It is only recently that the needs of this group have begun to be examined (Farquhar 2017). They relate to the slow progression of the disease, the lack of certainty about the prognosis, the frequency of exacerbations, and the isolation that comes with caring for a person with severe functional impairment who may be housebound. Spouses or partners do much of the caring. Just as many people with COPD have comorbidities, so do many of their carers.

8 Conclusion

The goal of treatment of advanced progressive respiratory disease must be in keeping with both the aspiration of patients and the practical realities of the stage of the disease. In COPD and in CF, defining prognosis is so difficult that priority should be given to informing patients and trying to meet their hopes and expectations. In IPF, prognosis may be so limited that clear information about the risk of impending death should be available to the patient and the relatives in line with their perceived need. In COPD and in CF, breathlessness may become slowly intractable over 20 or more years so that life eventually becomes barely tolerable. In IPF this is likely to be the case at a more rapid pace over 2–3 years. There are many remedies to be considered in the breathlessness of COPD and IPF. In all three diseases, morphine may have a role in reducing the perception of breathlessness. In IPF morphine may also have a role in cough which affects 80% of sufferers and is progressive. Morphine in low doses does not suppress breathing, does not appear to generate tolerance, and seems safe in the breathlessness of advanced respiratory disease.

References

Almagro PL, Calbo E, Ochoa de Echagüen A, Barreiro B, Quintana S, Heredia JL, Garau J. Mortality after hospitalization for COPD. Chest. 2002;121(5):1441–8.

Almagro P, Yun S, Sangil A, Rodríguez-Carballeira M, Marine M, Landete P, Soler-Cataluña JJ, Soriano JB, Miravitlles M. Palliative care and prognosis in COPD: a systematic review with a validation cohort. Int J Chron Obstruct Pulmon Dis. 2017;12:1721–9. https://doi.org/10.2147/COPD.S135657. eCollection 2017.

British Lung Foundation. Chronic obstructive lung disease statistics [online]. 2018. Available at https://statistics.blf.org.uk/copd. Accessed 2 Jan 2018.

Connors AF Jr, Dawson NV, Thomas C, Harrell FE Jr, Desbiens N, Fulkerson WJ, et al. Outcomes following acute exacerbation of severe chronic obstructive lung disease. The SUPPORT investigators (Study to Understand Prognoses and Preferences for Outcomes and Risks of Treatments). Am J Respir Crit Care Med. 1996;154(4 Pt 1):959–67.

Currow DC, Abernethy AP, Allcroft P, Banzett RB, Bausewein C, Booth S, et al. The need to research refractory breathlessness. Eur Respir J. 2016;47(1):342–3.

Curtis JR, Engelberg EL, Nielsen DH, Patrick DL. Patient-physician communication about en-of-life for patients with severe COPD. Eur Respir J. 2004;24:200–205. https://doi.org/10.1183/09031936.04.00010104.

Farquhar M. Assessing carer needs in chronic obstructive pulmonary disease. Chron Respir Dis. 2017. https://doi.org/10.1177/1479972317719086.

Farquhar MC, Prevost AT, McCrone P, Brafman-Price B, Bentley A, Higginson IJ, Todd CJ, Booth S. The clinical and cost effectiveness of a Breathlessness Intervention Service for patients with advanced non-malignant disease and their informal carers: mixed findings of a mixed method randomised controlled trial. Trials. 2016;17:185. https://doi.org/10.1186/s13063-016-1304-6.

Gore JM, Brophy CJ, Greenstone MA. How well do we care for patients with end stage chronic obstructive pulmonary disease (COPD)? A comparison of palliative care and quality of life in COPD and lung cancer. Thorax. 2000;55(12):1000–6.

Herigstad M, Faull OK, Hayen A, Evans E, Hardinge FM, Wiech K, et al. Treating breathlessness via the brain: changes in brain activity over a course of pulmonary rehabilitation. Eur Respir J. 2017;50(3):1701029. https://doi.org/10.1183/13993003.01029-2017

Higginson IJ, Bausewein C, Reilly CC, Gao W, Gysels M, Dzingina M, et al. An integrated palliative and respiratory care service for patients with advanced disease and refractory breathlessness: a randomised controlled trial. Lancet Respir Med. 2014;2(12):979–87.

Hutchinson J, Fogarty A, Hubbard R, et al. Global incidence and mortality of idiopathic pulmonary fibrosis: a systematic review. Eur Respir J. 2015;46:795–806.

Keogh RH, Szczesniak R, Taylor-Robinson D, Bilton D. Up-to-date and projected estimates of survival for people with cystic fibrosis using baseline characteristics: a longitudinal study using UK patient registry data. J Cyst Fibros. 2018. https://doi.org/10.1016/j.jcf.2017.11.019. pii: S1569-1993(17)30976-1. [Epub ahead of print].

Maddocks M, Nolan CM, Man WD, Polkey MI, Hart N, Gao W, et al. Neuromuscular electrical stimulation to improve exercise capacity in patients with severe

COPD: a randomised double-blind, placebo-controlled trial. Lancet Respir Med. 2016;4(1):27–36.

Maddocks M, Lovell N, Booth S, Man WD, Higginson IJ. Palliative care and management of troublesome symptoms for people with chronic obstructive pulmonary disease. Lancet. 2017;390(10098):988–1002.

McCarthy B, Casey D, Devane D, Murphy K, Murphy E, Lacasse Y. Pulmonary rehabilitation for chronic obstructive pulmonary disease. Cochrane Database Syst Rev. 2015;(2):CD003793. https://doi.org/10.1002/14651858.CD003793.pub3. Review.

Nathan SD, Albera C, Bradford WZ, et al. Effect of pirfenidone on mortality: pooled analyses and meta-analyses of clinical trials in idiopathic pulmonary fibrosis. Lancet Respir Med. 2017;5:33–41.

Navaratnam V, Fleming KM, West J, et al. The rising incidence of idiopathic pulmonary fibrosis in the UK. Thorax. 2011;66:462–7.

NICE (National Institute for Health and Care Excellence). Nintedanib for treating idiopathic pulmonary fibrosis (TA379). London: NICE; 2016.

Pinnock H, Kendall M, Murray SA, Worth A, Levack P, Porter M, et al. Living and dying with severe chronic obstructive pulmonary disease: multi-perspective longitudinal qualitative study. BMJ. 2011;342:d142. https://doi.org/10.1136/bmj.d142.:d142.

Shaw J, Marshall T, Morris H, Hayton C, Chaudhuri N. Idiopathic pulmonary fibrosis: a holistic approach to disease management in the antifibrotic age. J Thorac Dis. 2017;9(11):4700–7. https://doi.org/10.21037/jtd.2017.10.111.

Smallwood N, Le B, Currow D, Irving L, Philip J. Management of refractory breathlessness with morphine in patients with chronic obstructive pulmonary disease. Intern Med J. 2015;45(9):898–904. https://doi.org/10.1111/imj.12857.

White P, White S, Edmonds P, Gysels M, Moxham J, Seed P, Shipman C. Palliative care or end of life care in advanced COPD? A prospective community survey. Br J Gen Pract. 2011. https://doi.org/10.3399/bjgp11X578043.

White P, Thornton H, Pinnock H, Georgopoulou S, Booth H. Overtreatment of COPD with inhaled corticosteroids – implications for safety and costs: cross-observational study. PLoS One. 2013;8(10):e75221. https://doi.org/10.1371/journal.pone.0075221.

Palliative Care and Liver Diseases

63

Anne M. Larson

Contents

Abstract

Liver disease leads to over 4 million visits to medical practitioners and over 750,000 hospitalizations per year in the USA. Those with chronic liver disease frequently progress to cirrhosis, end-stage liver disease (ESLD), hepatocellular carcinoma, and death. Patients with ESLD experience numerous complications, including muscle cramps, confusion (hepatic encephalopathy), protein calorie malnutrition, muscle wasting, fluid overload (ascites, edema), bleeding (esophagogastric variceal hemorrhage), infection (spontaneous bacterial peritonitis), fatigue, anxiety, and depression. Despite significant improvements in palliation of these complications, patients with liver disease still suffer reduced quality of life and must confront the fact that their disease will often inexorably progress to death. Liver transplantation is a valid option in this setting, increasing the duration of survival and palliating many of the symptoms. However, many patients die waiting for an organ or are not candidates for transplantation due to comorbid illness or psychosocial issues. Others receive a transplant but succumb to complications of the transplant itself. Patients and families must struggle with simultaneously hoping for a cure while facing a life-threatening illness. Ideally, the combination of early palliative care with life-sustaining therapy can

A. M. Larson (✉)
Department of Internal Medicine, Division of Gastroenterology, University of Washington, NW Hepatology/UW Medicine, Seattle, WA, USA
e-mail: amlarson@uw.edu

R. D. MacLeod, L. Van den Block (eds.), *Textbook of Palliative Care*,
https://doi.org/10.1007/978-3-319-77740-5_62

maximize the patients' quality and quantity of life. If it becomes clear that life-sustaining therapy is no longer an option, these patients are then already in a system to help them with end-of-life care.

1 Introduction

1.1 The Scope of the Problem

Chronic liver disease affects 30–35 million persons in the USA, 29 million in the European region, and even more worldwide (Younossi et al. 2011). It leads to over 4 million US ambulatory physician visits annually, with >3.5 million visits for viral hepatitis alone. Chronic liver disease often progresses to cirrhosis and subsequent liver failure. There are 5.5 million cirrhotics in the USA, and the global prevalence of cirrhosis from autopsy series is as high as 712 million (9.5% of the population) (Scaglione et al. 2015; Lim and Kim 2008). Annually, over 750,000 US hospitalizations can be attributed to acute and chronic liver disease. US health-care costs in this population approach almost $4 billion annually, and the incidence of hospitalizations due to cirrhosis and its complications is rising significantly. Similar figures are seen worldwide. Within a month following discharge, up to 37% of cirrhotic patients are readmitted at a mean cost of nearly $30,000. The more frequent the readmission rate, the greater the risk of subsequent mortality. In 2014, 38,170 US deaths were attributed to chronic liver disease and cirrhosis – 26.4% per 2-year interval compared to 8.4% in matched controls (Scaglione et al. 2015; Kochanek et al. 2016). In 2010, over 1.0 million deaths (2% of all deaths) worldwide were attributable to hepatitis and cirrhosis (Mokdad and Lopez 2014; World Health Organization 2017). It is estimated that globally, another million deaths were due to liver cancer and acute hepatitis. This number is likely even greater, given the scarcity of mortality data in Sub-Saharan Africa and other countries (i.e., Pakistan, Bolivia, Laos, and North Korea) (Sankoh and Bypass 2012). Chronic liver disease and cirrhosis were the 12th leading cause of death in the USA, and the age-adjusted death rate has increased from 9.6/100,000 in 1999 to 10.4/100,000 in 2014 (Kochanek et al. 2016). In 2009, malignant liver neoplasms, cirrhosis, and alcoholic liver disease were the 3rd, 4th, and 5th leading causes of death due to gastrointestinal disease, respectively.

Both the incidence and the death rate of liver cancer have also gone up in the USA and worldwide (Fig. 1). From 2003 to 2012, the US incidence increased by 2.3% per year – an overall increase of 72% (Ryerson et al. 2016). Since 2003, there has been a 56% increase in deaths from liver cancer. In 2016, an estimated 39,230 persons were diagnosed with liver and bile duct cancer and 27,170 (69%) died from the disease (Howlader et al. 2016). Liver cancer was the 13th leading cause of cancer death in the USA and accounts for 750,000 to 788,000 deaths annually worldwide, the 2nd most common cause of cancer death. The relative 5-year survival rate for liver cancer is about 16–18% overall. For those whose cancer is discovered while still at a localized stage, the 5-year survival rate is still only 30.5%. The median age at death is 67 years and the rate is highest among persons aged 55–64 years (Fig. 2).

Chronic viral hepatitis is a major risk factor for hepatocellular carcinoma (HCC) and correlates with the increasing trends in HCC incidence. Approximately 50% of cases of liver cancer are related to chronic hepatitis C virus (HCV) infection and 15% to chronic hepatitis B virus (HBV) infection (Ryerson et al. 2016). There are millions of at-risk individuals with viral hepatitis. Up to 2.2 million persons in the USA and 350 million worldwide are living with chronic HBV infection, with a prevalence as high as 25% in some countries (Zampino et al. 2015). As many as 130 to 150 million worldwide are living the chronic HCV infection with 2.7–3.5 million persons in the USA. Additionally, cirrhosis and HCC secondary to nonalcoholic fatty liver disease are rapidly increasing. It is believed that at least a quarter of chronic HCV patients have yet to be diagnosed. Other important risk factors for development of hepatocellular carcinoma include chronic liver disease secondary to excessive alcohol consumption, nonalcoholic fatty liver disease (affecting

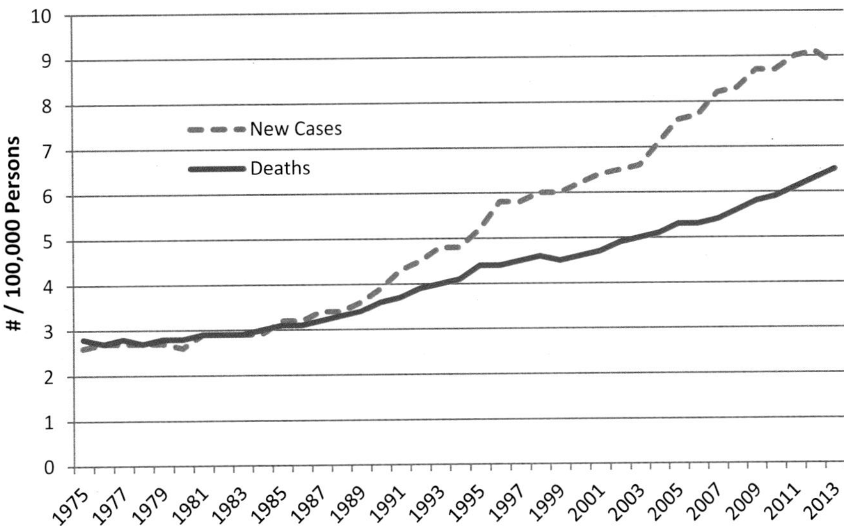

Fig. 1 New cases of hepatocellular carcinoma and age-adjusted death rate (From: SEER Cancer Statistics Factsheets: Liver and Intrahepatic Bile Duct Cancer. National Cancer Institute. Bethesda, MD, http://seer.cancer.gov/statfacts/html/livibd.html)

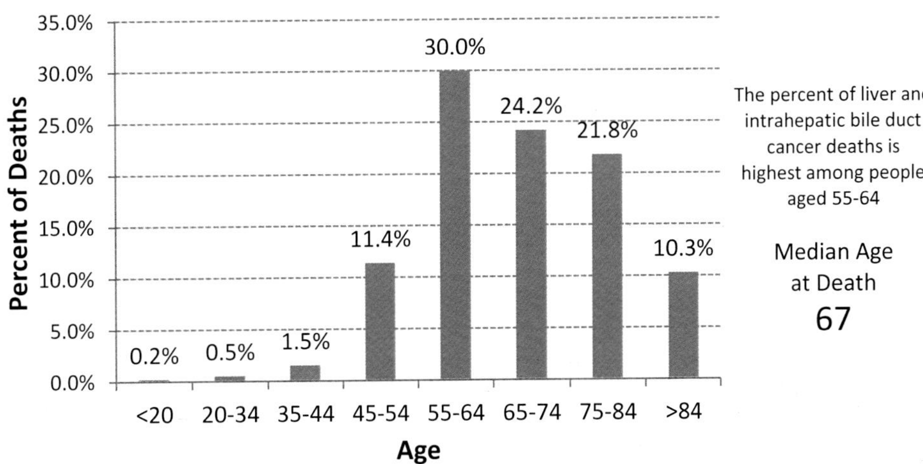

Fig. 2 Primary liver cancer death rate by age. From: SEER Cancer Statistics Factsheets: Liver and Intrahepatic Bile Duct Cancer. National Cancer Institute. Bethesda, MD, http://seer.cancer.gov/statfacts/html/livibd.html

20% of the worldwide population), and other metabolic and genetic disorders.

2 Palliative Care and Hospice Services

Palliative care (PC) is defined as an approach that improves the quality of life (QoL) of patients and families facing the problems associated with life-threatening illness. This is accomplished through the prevention and relief of suffering by means of early identification and impeccable assessment and treatment of pain and other problems – physical, psychosocial, and spiritual (World Health Organization 2017). Palliative care is a board-certified specialty in the USA, and between 2000 and 2010, there was nearly a 150% increase in palliative care teams (Wordingham and Swetz 2015). Across Europe and elsewhere, specialist palliative care (SPC) provides multidisciplinary specialist care – from a team with training and ongoing education in palliative care and working predominantly with this patient group. SPC physicians are specifically trained in the early recognition and management of both pain and non-pain symptoms, psychosocial and spiritual support, and advanced care planning. An experienced interdisciplinary PC team provides support not only to the patient and their family but to the primary team caring for the patient. Treatment is not excluded if it helps the patient and is in line with the goals of their care (Walling and Wenger 2014; Kelly and Rice 2015). Palliative care is designed to meet the preferences, goals, and values of the patient, and patient satisfaction is greater if these needs are met (Wordingham and Swetz 2015).

There is often confusion between palliative care and hospice or end-of-life care. In the USA, hospice has traditionally focused on comfort and quality of life, rather than disease-directed therapy (i.e., symptom management) (Wordingham and Swetz 2015), and hospice teams, although interdisciplinary, rely more on nursing assistants, volunteers, and bereavement specialists. Hospice is often considered a component of palliative care. In other countries, this may be seen as end-of-life care and usually is seen to be relevant in the last 6–12 months of life or more. For example, in the UK, end-of-life care is defined as "support for people who are in the last months or years of their life," and palliative care is considered a component of end-of-life care (National Health Service 2017). This confusion between palliative care and hospice/end-of-life care may lead to the avoidance of involvement of the palliative care team in patient with ESLD, particularly in the setting of potential liver transplantation. These specialists, however, can be of great assistance to patients and also help make the determination when the transition to hospice care would be beneficial for the ESLD patient (Brisebois and Tandon 2015).

Palliative care and hospice/end-of-life care are complementary entities, with palliative care supporting the quality of life and symptom burden of those with an ultimately terminal illness (Strand et al. 2014). Historically, there has been very little guidance for the use of palliative care in the setting of ESLD (Potosek et al. 2014). Palliative and hospice/end-of-life care have more traditionally been used in the setting of illnesses whose progressive disease course is clear, such as end-stage cancer. Patients with non-cancer illness such as ESLD are less likely to receive palliative care services than those with cancer (Wachterman et al. 2016; Walling et al. 2017). Palliative care is of significant value and ideally may be utilized at any stage of disease for any patient with a serious or life-threatening illness, including ESLD (Strand et al. 2014). Patients involved with palliative care experience improved quality of life, decreased depression and anxiety, and longer survival and feel that there is better alignment of their goals with their medical care (Kelly and Rice 2015; Strand et al. 2014). Early palliative care is also associated with reduced health-care costs (Harris and Murray 2013). Palliative care should therefore be considered compatible with the management of ESLD patients, including those listed for liver transplantation (Brisebois and Tandon 2015).

3 Discussing End-of-Life Issues in ESLD

Once the diagnosis of cirrhosis and end-stage liver disease is made or complications develop, patients are often frightened and wonder how they could have reached this point. They may be angry that they were unaware of the ultimate consequences of their illness. They often absorb only a small proportion of what is being told to them and have trouble piecing it all together. Patients must ultimately confront the fact that their disease will inexorably progress to death. Liver transplantation may be a valid treatment option in this setting, increasing the duration of survival and palliating many of the symptoms. These patients must be "sick enough to die" to be considered for transplant (Larson and Curtis 2006). Up to 10–15% listed for liver transplantation will die without receiving an organ, and there are many patients who are not candidates for liver transplantation.

There are medical and nonmedical contraindications to liver transplantation. The more common reasons include extrahepatic malignancy, comorbid medical disease (i.e., significant cardiopulmonary disease, active infection), multisystem organ failure, inadequate social support, inadequate finances, and ongoing alcohol or drug abuse. Furthermore, some patients will receive a liver transplant but succumb to complications of the transplant itself, including graft failure, infection, bile duct complications, or post-transplant cancers. The 1- and 3-year patient survival rates after liver transplant depend on many factors but in the USA they average about 90% and 80%, respectively.

Receiving news of a terminal or life-limiting diagnosis is stressful and evokes strong emotions such as fear, anxiety, anger, depression, despair, hopelessness, and helplessness. In addition to dealing with physical and life-threatening symptoms, patients experience psychological and emotional stress, financial concern, and worry about their family (Ryerson et al. 2016; Boyd et al. 2015). They must also deal with uncertainty regarding the development of acute, life-threatening complications (Hope and Morrison 2011; Boyd et al. 2015). Early discussion of end-of-life issues is thus essential in the management of all patients with ESLD, including those being evaluated for liver transplantation (Boyd et al. 2015). Palliative care specialists have expertise in communication, and their involvement in this setting provides benefit to both the patient and medical practitioner (Tulsky 2005; Brisebois and Tandon 2015), but all professionals seeing patients with ESLD should be able to provide honest and open communication, which improves understanding of patient's wishes and goal-oriented care (Lamba et al. 2012).

Patients and their families must fully understand the disease and its prognosis and be prepared for all potential outcomes to make realistic treatment decisions. These discussions need to occur early during the course of the disease, ideally prior to the development of significant complications such as hepatic encephalopathy, variceal hemorrhage, ascites, or hepatocellular carcinoma. Discussions become particularly challenging in the presence of hepatic encephalopathy which further impedes communication and the patient's ability to make decisions. Practitioners should anticipate this and engage the patient and their family early in advance care planning (Highet et al. 2014). Physicians face the additional challenge of supporting hope for a good outcome while providing patients with accurate prognostic information. These discussions are particularly difficult in the setting of ESLD because of its highly unpredictable trajectory. Patients often experience periods of relative health in between episodes of severe, life-threatening hepatic decompensation. Very often physicians and practitioners are overly optimistic regarding the prognosis, confusing patients further (Janssen et al. 2011; Abdul-Razzak et al. 2014; Parry et al. 2014).

There is also a substantial burden on the caregivers of patients in this setting, particularly if the patient has developed hepatic encephalopathy and can no longer adequately participate in decision-making (Bajaj et al. 2011; Rodrigue et al. 2011; Walling and Wenger 2014). Family members may be asked to be involved in helping to make decisions for the patient. Which family member is responsible for this assistance depends on country and local laws and whether there is a clear documentation as to who the patient prefers in this position. If clear documentation is not available, most governments determine who is legally responsible – i.e., in the USA it is the spouse followed by the children if no spouse is available, etc. The need for becoming the decision-maker is particularly stressful if the caregiver is unaware of the patient's wishes or family members have differing opinions on what should be done. Patients with liver disease associated with significant substance abuse may lack a strong social network. There are often inner-family disputes regarding the abuse. Family estrangement can be seen, particularly if there are feelings of abandonment, anxiety, blame, or anger toward the addicted patient. Thus, the lack of close family to provide support further complicates communication and long-term care planning (Walling and Wenger 2014).

Palliative care discussions can become particularly difficult if the ESLD patient is being considered for or has been listed for liver transplantation. Patients must face dealing with the risk of an early death while at the same time focusing on the hope of receiving a life-saving transplant – "hope for the best and prepare for the worst." The patient must be helped to understand that they may experience a catastrophic decline in their condition before transplant can be provided or may receive a transplant only to die of post-transplant complications. These competing outcomes lead to a "roller-coaster ride" of emotions which is difficult for all involved (Larson and Curtis 2006). Throughout the transplant evaluation process, patients and their families struggle with the uncertainty of whether they will ever receive a transplant (Boyd et al. 2015). Those for whom liver transplant is not available or has failed face having their hopes dashed and confronting their terminal illness head on.

The discussion regarding the use of do-not-attempt resuscitation (DNAR) orders in the setting of ESLD is even more controversial. Decompensated cirrhotics have lower rates of DNAR orders when compared to lung cancer patients or those with other chronic illnesses (Larson and Curtis 2006; Stotts et al. 2014; Brisebois and Tandon 2015; Wachterman et al. 2016). The possibility of receiving a liver transplant adds complexity to the discussion of DNAR, and many argue that liver transplant candidates should not carry this type of directive. There is often fear that the patient may be transitioned to hospice/end-of-life care prematurely while awaiting transplantation. Resuscitation may be reasonable for patients who are still healthy enough to survive resuscitation efforts without compromising future treatment options such as transplant. As ESLD progresses, however, and patients become more critically ill, the possibility of transplant futility must be addressed (Biggins 2012; Petrowsky et al. 2014). Resuscitation is rarely successful in the critically ill ESLD patient who experiences a catastrophic event (e.g., cardiopulmonary arrest) (Roth et al. 2000; Cholongitas et al. 2006; Stotts et al. 2014). Despite successful resuscitation, the event may further compromise transplant outcome or prevent transplant altogether. In this setting, DNAR orders may be appropriate.

4 Integrating Palliative Care with ESLD Management

At the time of this writing, there are no guidelines specific to the use of palliative care in the setting of end-stage liver disease (Brisebois and Tandon 2015). Aggressive medical care is generally aimed at improving both quantity and quality of life – both of which decline as the ESLD progresses. Most patients with chronic liver disease feel well for decades, often completely unaware of the progressive nature of their illness (Scaglione et al. 2015). As the disease relentlessly progresses, however, patients may develop nonspecific symptoms such as fatigue, even in the absence of cirrhosis or liver failure. Fatigue is in fact one of the most frequently identified symptoms of chronic liver disease and cirrhosis and can lead to a substantial decrease in quality of life.

Once chronic liver disease is diagnosed or complications abruptly develop, patients often experience psychological distress which further contributes to their poor quality of life (Nardelli et al. 2013). There may be little time to adjust to the diagnosis. If disease is perceived to be "self-inflicted," there are often issues of blame and anger. Depression and anxiety frequently follow (Nardelli et al. 2013; Perng et al. 2014). Self-reported quality of life is remarkably poor in cirrhotics. The cirrhotic liver eventually decompensates, leading to end-stage liver disease (ESLD), the final phase in disease trajectory. At this point, patients experience pronounced morbidity and develop a very high symptom burden. Symptoms and complications include pain, nausea, muscle cramps, dyspnea, cognitive dysfunction (hepatic encephalopathy), anorexia, malnutrition and cachexia, fluid overload (ascites, edema), profound fatigue, and pruritus (Larson and Curtis 2006; Potosek et al. 2014; Poonja et al. 2014; Cox-North 2015). Additionally, they may experience such life-threatening complications as variceal hemorrhage, spontaneous bacterial peritonitis, or hepatocellular carcinoma. Life-saving liver transplantation is available only to a small subset of these patients.

4.1 Barriers to Palliative Care Referral

There are many barriers to the consideration of palliative care in the setting of cirrhosis and ESLD. Although the field of PC is expanding, access remains limited for a considerable portion of patients, particularly in the outpatient setting (Rakoski and Volk 2015). In US hospitals with more than 50 beds, only two-thirds reported palliative care programs in 2012 (Rakoski and Volk 2015). In London, it was reported that there were 322 hospice beds (15 providers) for a population of 9,323,570 (Cox et al. 2016). Worldwide, it is estimated that only 14% of the 40 million people in need of palliative care receive it (Palliative Care 2017). In 2013, Lynch et al. found that 42% of 234 countries surveyed had no viable palliative care services and 32% reached only a small percentage of the population (Lynch et al. 2013). Palliative care is rare or nonexistent in Mexico, South America, Africa, and Russia.

Cirrhotic patients may not appear "sick" and, therefore, may not be considered to need help with symptoms or to be at risk of dying. The marked symptom burden in these patients is frequently not identified as an important issue by physicians, caregivers, family, or friends (Poonja et al. 2014). The trajectory of liver failure is unpredictable compared with that of other terminal illnesses, such as advanced cancer (Walling and Wenger 2014). This is particularly true earlier in the disease course or if symptoms (i.e., encephalopathy or ascites) have been medically well controlled. This waxing and waning of symptoms makes care planning and projection regarding end-of-life issues more complicated. This prognostic uncertainty, however, should not be a barrier to referral to either palliative care or hospice care (Wordingham and Swetz 2015).

Discussing palliative care and advance directives may appear to be at odds with pursuit of curative or life-prolonging therapies, such as liver transplant (Potosek et al. 2014; Brisebois and Tandon 2015). Patients often have a poor understanding of their disease severity and what palliative care entails (Rakoski and Volk 2015). The discussion can be complicated further if patients refuse to accept their prognosis and focus only on life-saving interventions. The practitioner, patient, or caregivers additionally may view palliative care as synonymous with hospice/end-of-life care and appropriate only during the final days of life – seeing PC as giving up, treatment withdrawal, or imminent death (Boyd et al. 2015; Rakoski and Volk 2015; Cagle et al. 2016; Beck et al. 2016). Additionally, practitioners may be uncomfortable with end-of-life discussions – leaving both the physician and the patient with confusion and uncertainty regarding long-term care goals (Rakoski and Volk 2015; Beck et al. 2016). Patients and caregivers must be helped to prepare for future decisions regarding their care (Boyd et al. 2015). This type of discussion requires excellent communication skills on the part of the practitioner (Brisebois and Tandon 2015).

End-of-life issues in ESLD are frequently not addressed at all or addressed far too late to be of benefit to the patient and their family (Larson and Curtis 2006; Walling et al. 2013; Rakoski and Volk 2015). Poonja et al. reported that only 11% of patients who were too sick for liver transplant were referred to palliative care, despite a high symptom burden (Poonja et al. 2014). They and others have also found that goals of care and do-not-resuscitate status were rarely discussed with these dying patients. Only 28% of those in the Poonja study were designated as DNAR. Hansen et al. followed six ESLD patients who were hospitalized in the ICU and were either on the liver transplant list or being considered for liver transplant. Interviews conducted with multiple staff and family members throughout the course of the hospitalization found that what mattered most to all participants was the goal of liver transplant (Hansen et al. 2012). There was no focus on patient comfort and goals of care until all treatment options had been exhausted, and none of the patients received a palliative care consultation. Kathpalia et al. found that only 17% of patients who died or were removed from the liver transplant list had a palliative care consultation (Kathpalia et al. 2016), and half of these consultations were within 72 h of death. A more alarming finding was that palliative care services were associated predominantly with younger or Caucasian patients. The lack of palliative and end-of-life care offered to those who are not candidates for liver transplant or have been removed from the liver transplant list often leads to feelings of abandonment by patients.

4.2 Benefit of Palliative Care Involvement in ESLD

The early integration of palliative care and medical care in the setting of ESLD provides great benefit to the patient and caregiver as well as the medical provider (Brisebois and Tandon 2015). The goals of palliative care often overlap the goals of medical care (Larson and Curtis 2006; Potosek et al. 2014; Brisebois and Tandon 2015). All practitioners involved in the patient's care can provide palliative services, including family physicians, nursing staff, transplant services staff and physicians, intensive care staff, and inpatient ward staff. Palliative care specialists provide added support for management of these complicated patients, particularly with regard to end-of-life discussions and psychologic and spiritual support (Brisebois and Tandon 2015). The palliative care specialist can also help the general clinician with the management of physical symptoms. The early integration of palliative care in the setting of chronic disease has been shown to improve QoL and results in longer patient survival. Patients have fewer emergency room visits, ICU admissions, and hospital deaths. Support for the concept of palliative care in the setting of ESLD is growing (Langberg and Taddei 2016). Palliative care services should therefore be considered in any patient who is at risk of dying within the next year from advanced liver disease.

As noted, the course of ESLD is much less predictable than many other chronic illnesses – patients experience episodic periods of exacerbation and recovery. This makes predicting the actual time course of progression to death difficult and contributes to the stress patients and caregivers feel. This also makes the timing of palliative care involvement unclear, most likely contributing to the lack of palliative care referrals in this population. However, survival significantly declines once hepatic decompensation develops (LaFond and Shah 2016). Following development of esophageal varices, the median patient survival is 7–10 years and each variceal hemorrhage carries a 10–20% risk of death (Kelly and Rice 2015). The 2-year survival following development of either hepatic encephalopathy or ascites is 50% (Potosek et al. 2014; LaFond and Shah 2016). Cirrhotics with hyponatremia (serum sodium <135 mmol/L) have a 23% 1-year survival. Patients who develop refractory ascites have a 1-year survival of 32% and those with type 2 hepatorenal syndrome have a 6-month median survival. Those with type 1 hepatorenal syndrome generally survive only a few weeks without transplantation. Thus, palliative care referral, based on needs and symptoms rather than prognosis, may be considered earlier in the disease progression when it becomes more obvious that not only are there increasing symptoms but the outlook is poor.

Early concurrent palliative care significantly benefits the patient with ESLD, and the health-care team providing this care must find ways to integrate palliative care with the possibility of life-prolonging therapy (Medici et al. 2008). It has been suggested that certain clinical findings could be used as triggers for palliative care consultation, including refractory ascites, hepatic encephalopathy, hepatorenal syndrome, bacterial peritonitis, and recurrent variceal bleeding. Additionally, symptoms such as pain, cramping, nausea, and emotional distress could also be used as a guide for referral. Patients with a high symptom burden (i.e., Edmonton Symptom Assessment Scale or SPICT™ clinical indicators) could also be referred. Prognostic scoring systems could also be utilized regarding referral timing. For patients with a model for end-stage liver disease (MELD) score > 20 as a trigger, a VA study showed an increase in PC referrals (62.5% vs 47.1%, $p = 0.38$) (Davila et al. 2012). Several have identified conditions for which a PC referral in an ESLD patient would be appropriate (Table 1) (Brisebois and Tandon 2015; Cox-North 2015; Rakoski and Volk 2015).

Table 1 Indications for palliative care in the setting of ESLD

Indication	Examples
At diagnosis	Patient and family education Planning strategies to improve functional capacity Education regarding advance care planning and goals of care Identify health-care proxies or surrogates
Physical symptoms	Uncontrolled pain Muscle cramping Hepatic encephalopathy Intractable ascites Nausea Anorexia and malnutrition Deterioration in performance status Dependence on others for care needs
Emotional or spiritual distress	Fear of dying Guilt about behaviors which may have caused the disease
Family/caregiver emotional or spiritual distress	Financial stress – time off from work to care for the patient; cost of medical care Exhaustion – continual care of a patient with hepatic encephalopathy Frustration – unpredictable hospitalizations; ups and downs of the liver disease itself
Interfamily conflict regarding goals of care	Family uncertain of patient's desires (severe encephalopathy, intubated, etc.) Family members disagree regarding patient management
Accelerating need for medical care or hospitalizations	Weekly paracenteses Modifying medications to reflect patient goals Frequent hospital readmissions
Curative care unavailable	Patient has been declined liver transplantation Patient has been removed from the liver transplant list
Patient requests palliative care	Patient does not wish to pursue life-sustaining treatment
Physician distress	Difficulty communicating a poor prognosis Lack of curative options Unable to manage symptoms appropriately

Adapted from: Highet et al. 2014, Cox-North 2015, Brisebois and Tandon 2015, Boyd et al. 2015, and Rakoski and Volk 2015

4.3 Palliative Care and Liver Transplant

Palliative care and consideration for liver transplantation are considered by many to be contradictory plans of management (Potosek et al. 2014). This often leads to PC involvement only after all medical options have been exhausted and the patient is near death. However, Baumann et al. showed that there was a clear benefit to combining palliative care with routine liver transplant care (Baumann et al. 2015). These patients had a 50% improvement in symptom scores and were more likely to have care plans in place in anticipation of further decline in health. Additionally, PC services are helpful to the patient for the management of feelings of uncertainty, fear, and the loss of control over their medical condition during the complicated liver transplant process. Goals of care and plans for future end-of-life care are more thoroughly addressed when PC services are involved. Therefore, patients should not be denied the benefit of palliative care while awaiting liver transplantation.

4.4 ESLD Symptoms Requiring Management

4.4.1 Quality of Life

Despite significant improvements in the medical management and the potential for life-saving liver transplant, ESLD patients still suffer a profoundly reduced QoL and have an increase in health-care utilization. They often have difficulty with activities of daily living, including bathing, dressing, managing money, cooking, shopping, and ambulating safely.

This poor QoL is comparable to that reported by patients suffering from advanced chronic obstructive pulmonary disease or heart failure. Additionally, patients are frequently anxious and depressed which contributes to worse QoL, contributing to more physical symptoms – a vicious cycle. As ESLD progresses, management of the complications of cirrhosis becomes a more time-consuming endeavor and is all too often left to the busy primary care clinician. Increased disease complexity is associated with increased hospitalizations (Strand et al. 2014). Aggressive management of the symptoms of ESLD improves patient QoL. Palliative care teams can assist with this management, as well as help address the patient goals and plans for managing ever-worsening disease (Brisebois and Tandon 2015). Quality of life can be improved and health-care utilization decreased for the ESLD patient with aggressive symptom control.

4.4.2 Ascites

Ascites is the most common complication of ESLD. The development of ascites is one of the most emotionally and physically distressing symptoms for the cirrhotic patient. At least 50% of patients will develop ascites over the 10-year period following the diagnosis of cirrhosis. Ascites leads to abdominal and back pain as well as emotional distress due to an altered body habitus and decrease in mobility. It is associated with about a 50% 2-year survival after onset. Therefore, it is associated not only with an increased short-term mortality but markedly a decreased QoL.

Management of ascites is labor intensive as it progresses, but crucial for patient well-being. Early in the course, it can often be managed with sodium restriction (<2000 mg/day) and oral diuretics. This controls and appreciably reduces the discomfort caused by the ascites in about 90% of patients. Approximately 17% of patients will develop refractory ascites within 5 years of initial ascites development (LaFond and Shah 2016). Refractory ascites fails to respond to sodium restriction and diuretics and leads to an even further decline in the patient's physical and psychosocial well-being. By this point, the placement of transjugular intrahepatic portosystemic shunts (TIPS) may be limited by the presence of encephalopathy and liver failure. The use of indwelling peritoneal catheters in this setting is limited by complications, including peritonitis in 10% within 72 h of placement. Those who develop peritonitis then have a 50% 5-month mortality (Kathpalia et al. 2016; LaFond and Shah 2016). If fluid restriction is ultimately required in the setting of cirrhotic or diuretic induced hyponatremia, the patient's QoL decreases further.

4.4.3 Hepatic Encephalopathy

Hepatic encephalopathy (HE) is one of the most debilitating complications of ESLD. HE presents with a wide spectrum of neurologic or psychiatric abnormalities which range from minimal (subclinical or covert) alterations to frank coma. Minimal HE, the earliest stage, is present in up to 80% of cirrhotics. It manifests with significant impairment in attention, psychomotor speed, visuospatial perception, response inhibition, and delayed information processing (Shaw and Bajaj 2017). These patients then begin to have problems with day-to-day functioning, but this is often completely unnoticed by those around them. The presence of HE, even at the subclinical level, fundamentally complicates the patient's QoL and their medical management. Patients may make mistakes at work, sometimes leading to loss of employment and insurance coverage. Studies have shown that even minimal HE impairs the patient's fitness to drive, particularly regarding car handling, adaptation, attention deficit, and cautiousness. Therefore, independence is lost – driving is not an option once HE develops. They may not take their medications appropriately, often forgetting them, further complicating their management.

The encephalopathic patient should always be accompanied to their physician visits by a trusted family member or friend – someone to help make decisions, write out plans, learn and understand the patient's medications, and remember details of the visit and discussions. Encephalopathy can generally be managed successfully with lactulose therapy and, if necessary, the addition of rifaximin. As the ESLD progresses, however, HE may become unmanageable and patients/caregivers may find the usual aspects of daily living very difficult. The patients may require ongoing institutional care, such as nursing homes, care homes, or skilled nursing facilities.

4.4.4 Pain Management

As many as 60–70% of patients with ESLD experience pain – at least a third of which rate this as moderately severe most of the time. In fact, patients with late ESLD report rates of moderate to severe pain like that reported by those with lung or colorectal cancer (Roth et al. 2000; Poonja et al. 2014). Pain adversely affects their QoL and often heightens other symptoms. Additionally, hospital utilization is significantly increased among ESLD patients with pain and among those who use opioids.

Pain is often undertreated in this setting for fear of complicating the liver disease. The failing liver makes pain management in the ESLD patient more complicated, and adverse events from analgesics can be seen (Soleimanpour et al. 2016). Most analgesics are metabolized through the liver, and therefore their metabolism may be altered. The alterations in hepatic blood flow, enzyme capacity, and plasma protein binding seen in cirrhosis all affect drug metabolism. As liver failure worsens, there is greater impairment in drug metabolism. The decrease in albumin synthesis by the failing liver may lead to an increased risk of adverse drug reactions by those drugs that require albumin for their metabolism (Soleimanpour et al. 2016).

Unfortunately, there are no evidence-based guidelines regarding the use of analgesics in these patients. The basic principles of pain assessment and management apply to these patients just as they do to those without ESLD; however, clinicians must often modify standard treatments (Chandok and Watt 2010). Palliative care physicians can be of assistance in this setting, having expertise in pain management as well as opioid and end-of-life medication use (Brisebois and Tandon 2015).

Acetaminophen/paracetamol is generally the preferred first-line analgesic. However, in those with cirrhosis, the half-life of the drug is double that seen in healthy controls. Its toxicity is dose dependent, and it is felt that it can be safely used in this population in daily doses of 2 g or less (Chandok and Watt 2010). However, there is no data regarding the safety of long-term use.

Selective and nonselective nonsteroidal anti-inflammatory drugs are metabolized by the hepatic cytochromes and are heavily protein bound – hepatotoxicity has been well described (Chandok and Watt 2010). These drugs should not be used in patients with cirrhosis. They inhibit platelet function and can cause gastrointestinal ulceration. The risk of gastrointestinal mucosal bleeding is even greater in patients with portal hypertension and varices, gastropathy, or gastric antral vascular ectasias. In addition, they can lead to acute renal failure, including hepatorenal syndrome, because they inhibit prostaglandin-regulated renal afferent arteriolar vasodilatation (Chandok and Watt 2010).

Opioids may be used cautiously, given that hepatic processing may be altered (Imani et al. 2014). Altered hepatic processing may result in decreased hepatic clearance (increased bioavailability) due to decreased first-pass metabolism (e.g., morphine, oxycodone, pentazocine, and tramadol). The half-life of morphine is doubled compared to healthy controls. Methadone clearance is also reduced in patients with severe liver insufficiency and drug half-life increases. Tramadol must be dose reduced in the setting of severe ESLD. Therefore, in the setting of severe ESLD, initial dosing of these drugs should be decreased by 30–50% and carefully titrated upward as needed for pain control (Soleimanpour et al. 2016). Patients should be cautioned about this and avoid taking extra pills or taking them more frequently than prescribed. As liver disease worsens, the interval between dosing may also need to be extended (Imani et al. 2014). For example, a drug normally dosed every 6 h may need to be dosed every 8 or 12 h.

Certain opioids (e.g., codeine) rely on hepatic transformation to active metabolites and therefore will be less effective. Codeine is metabolized to morphine in the liver and should not be used in the setting of ESLD due to decreased effectiveness. Meperidine is metabolized to normeperidine, the half-life of which is prolonged. Normeperidine carries severe central nervous system toxicity, and it should be avoided in cirrhotics, particularly those with renal insufficiency. Other opioids are unaffected by the underlying liver dysfunction (e.g., fentanyl, sufentanil). All opioids can complicate or precipitate hepatic encephalopathy, as can the opioid-related constipation (Bosilkovska et al. 2012). Therefore, dosing must be carefully considered and frequent patient monitoring is essential.

Table 2 Management of muscle cramps in the cirrhotic

Medications	Dose	Comments
Baclofen	300 mg daily	Improvement in cramps compared to placebo
Branched-chain amino acids (BCAA)	4 g granules three times daily	No side effects have been reported. Improved cramps. No control groups. Expensive
Gabapentin	600–900 mg daily	No data in ESLD
L-carnitine	900–1200 mg daily	Improvement in muscle cramps. No control groups
Magnesium	400 mg 1–2 times daily	Mild diarrhea. No data in ESLD
Taurine	3 g daily	No side effects have been reported. No control groups. Cramps improved
Vitamin B complex	1 tablet daily	Most helpful in nocturnal leg cramps. No data in ESLD
Vitamin E	200 mg three times daily	No side effects have been reported. Controlled trial suggests no benefit. Use with caution in cirrhosis
Quinine sulfate	200–300 mg at bedtime	No longer available over the counter due to adverse effects. FDA recommends against prescription forms for cramps
Zinc sulfate	220 mg twice daily	Improvement in cramps. Mild diarrhea. No control groups

Adapted from: Vidot et al. 2014, Cox-North 2015 (complete citations available upon request)

4.4.5 Muscle Cramps

Painful muscle cramps are reported in 67–90% of patients with cirrhosis. These cramps are unrelated to the use of diuretics, electrolyte imbalance, or minerals (i.e., zinc) and are correlated with the severity of liver disease. They contribute to a poor quality of sleep and QoL. They are unfortunately difficult to treat, although many therapies have been tried (Table 2).

A full review of the management of all complications of cirrhosis is beyond the scope of this chapter. However, these patients suffer from a wide spectrum of symptoms which need continual management. Careful attention to this management improves their quality and quantity of life.

5 Conclusion

Chronic liver disease carries significant morbidity and mortality. These patients suffer a markedly reduced quality and quantity of life. Their management is labor intensive for all involved and is constant throughout the course of their disease. The collaboration of palliative care with primary care and specialty physician management of potential life-sustaining therapy for the ESLD patient improves not only QoL but the length of survival as well. Involvement of the palliative care team should not be interpreted as "giving up" but as integral to management of these complicated patients. When life-sustaining therapy is no longer an option, these patients are already in a system to help them with further end-of-life care.

References

Abdul-Razzak A, You J, Sherifali D, Simon J, Brazil K. 'Conditional candour' and 'knowing me': an interpretive description study on patient preferences for physician behaviours during end-of-life communication. BMJ Open. 2014;4:e005653. https://doi.org/10.1136/bmjopen-2014-005653.

Bajaj JS, Wade JB, Gibson DP, Heuman DM, Thacker LR, Sterling RK, et al. The multi-dimensional burden of cirrhosis and hepatic encephalopathy on patients and caregivers. Am J Gastroenterol. 2011;106:1646–53. https://doi.org/10.1038/ajg.2011.157.

Baumann AJ, Wheeler DS, James M, Turner R, Siegel A, Navarro VJ. Benefit of early palliative care intervention in end-stage liver disease patients awaiting liver transplantation. J Pain Symptom Manag. 2015;50:882–6 e2. https://doi.org/10.1016/j.jpainsymman.2015.07.014.

Beck KR, Pantilat SZ, O'Riordan DL, Peters MG. Use of palliative care consultation for patients with end-stage liver disease: survey of liver transplant service providers. J Palliat Med. 2016;19:836–41. https://doi.org/10.1089/jpm.2016.0002. Epub 2016 Apr 19

Biggins SW. Futility and rationing in liver retransplantation: when and how can we say no? J Hepatol. 2012;56:1404–11. https://doi.org/10.1016/j.jhep.2011.11.027. Epub 2012 Feb 4

Bosilkovska M, Walder B, Besson M, Daali Y, Desmeules J. Analgesics in patients with hepatic impairment: pharmacology and clinical implications. Drugs. 2012;72(12):1645–69. https://doi.org/10.2165/11635500-000000000-00000.

Boyd K, Kimbell B, Murray S, Iredale J. A “good death” with irreversible liver disease: talking with patients and families about deteriorating health and dying. Clin Liver Dis. 2015;6:15–8. https://doi.org/10.1002/cld.479.

Brisebois AJ, Tandon P. Working with palliative care services. Clin Liver Dis. 2015;6:37–40. https://doi.org/10.1002/cld.493.

Cagle JG, Van Dussen DJ, Culler KL, Carrion I, Hong S, Guralnik J, et al. Knowledge about hospice: exploring misconceptions, attitudes, and preferences for care. Am J Hosp Palliat Care. 2016;33:27–33. https://doi.org/10.1177/1049909114546885.

Chandok N, Watt KD. Pain management in the cirrhotic patient: the clinical challenge. Mayo Clin Proc. 2010;85:451–8. https://doi.org/10.4065/mcp.2009.0534.

Cholongitas E, Senzolo M, Patch D, Kwong K, Nikolopoulou V, Leandro G, et al. Risk factors, sequential organ failure assessment and model for end-stage liver disease scores for predicting short term mortality in cirrhotic patients admitted to intensive care unit. Aliment Pharmacol Ther. 2006;23(7):883–93. https://doi.org/10.1111/j.1365-2036.2006.02842.x.

Cox S, Murtagh FEM, Tookman A, Gage A, Sykes N, McGinn M, et al. A review of specialist palliative care provision and access across London – mapping the capital. London J Prim Care (Abingdon). 2016;9:33–7. https://doi.org/10.1080/17571472.2016.1256045.

Cox-North P. Issues in the end-stage liver disease patient for which palliative care could be helpful. Clin Liver Dis. 2015;6:33–6. https://doi.org/10.1002/cld.492.

Davila JA, Duan Z, McGlynn KA, El-Serag HB. Utilization and outcomes of palliative therapy for hepatocellular carcinoma: a population-based study in the United States. J Clin Gastroenterol. 2012;46:71–7. https://doi.org/10.1097/MCG.0b013e318224d669.

Hansen L, Press N, Rosenkranz SJ, Baggs JG, Kendall J, Kerber A, et al. Life-sustaining treatment decisions in the ICU for patients with ESLD: a prospective investigation. Res Nurs Health. 2012;35:518–32. https://doi.org/10.1002/nur.21488. Epub 2012 May 11

Harris I, Murray SA. Can palliative care reduce futile treatment? A systematic review. BMJ Support Palliat Care. 2013;3(4):389–98. https://doi.org/10.1136/bmjspcare-2012-000343.

Highet G, Crawford D, Murray SA, Boyd K. Development and evaluation of the Supportive and Palliative Care Indicators Tool (SPICT): a mixed-methods study. BMJ Support Palliat Care. 2014;4:285–90. https://doi.org/10.1136/bmjspcare-2013-000488. Epub 2013 Jul 25

Hope AA, Morrison RS. Integrating palliative care with chronic liver disease care. J Palliat Care. 2011;27:20–7.

Howlader N, Noone AM, Krapcho M, Miller D, Bishop K, Altekruse SF, et al., editors. SEER Cancer Statistics Review, 1975–2013. Bethesda: National Cancer Institute; 2016. http://seer.cancer.gov/csr/1975_2013/, based on November 2015 SEER data submission, posted to the SEER web site

Imani F, Motavaf M, Safari S, Alavian SM. The therapeutic use of analgesics in patients with liver cirrhosis: a literature review and evidence-based recommendations. Hepat Mon. 2014;14:e23539. https://doi.org/10.5812/hepatmon.23539.eCollection 2014.

Janssen DJ, Curtis JR, DH A, Spruit MA, Downey L, Schols JM, et al. Patient-clinician communication about end-of-life care for Dutch and US patients with COPD. Eur Respir J. 2011;38:268–76. https://doi.org/10.1183/09031936.00157710.

Kathpalia P, Smith A, Lai JC. Underutilization of palliative care services in the liver transplant population. World J Transplant. 2016;6:594–8. https://doi.org/10.5500/wjt.v6.i3.594.

Kelly SG, Rice JP. Palliative care for patients with end-stage liver disease: the role of the liver team. Clin Liver Dis. 2015;6:22–3. https://doi.org/10.1002/cld.474.

Kochanek KD, Murphy SL, Xu J, Tejada-Vera B. Deaths: final data for 2014. Natl Vital Stat Rep. 2016;65:1–122.

LaFond JP, Shah NL. Bursting with symptoms: a review of palliation of ascites in cirrhosis. Clin Liver Dis. 2016;8:10–2. https://doi.org/10.1002/cld.559.

Lamba S, Murphy P, McVicker S, Harris Smith J, Mosenthal AC. Changing end-of-life care practice for liver transplant service patients: structured palliative care intervention in the surgical intensive care unit. J Pain Symptom Manag. 2012;44:508–19. https://doi.org/10.1016/j.jpainsymman.2011.10.018. Epub 2012 Jul 4

Langberg KM, Taddei TH. Balancing quality with quantity: the role of palliative care in managing decompensated cirrhosis. Hepatology. 2016;64:1014–6. https://doi.org/10.1002/hep.28717. Epub 2016 Aug 5

Larson AM, Curtis JR. Integrating palliative care for liver transplant candidates: “too well for transplant, too sick for life”. JAMA. 2006;295(18):2168–76. https://doi.org/10.1001/jama.295.18.2168.

Lim YS, Kim WR. The global impact of hepatic fibrosis and end-stage liver disease. Clin Liver Dis. 2008;12:733–46. https://doi.org/10.1016/j.cld.2008.07.007.

Lynch T, Connor S, Clark D. Mapping levels of palliative care development: a global update. J Pain Symptom Manag. 2013;45:1094–106. https://doi.org/10.1016/j.jpainsymman.2012.05.011.

Medici V, Rossaro L, Wegelin JA, Kamboj A, Nakai J, Fisher K, et al. The utility of the model for end-stage liver disease score: a reliable guide for liver transplant candidacy and, for select patients, simultaneous hospice referral. Liver Transpl. 2008;14:1100–6. https://doi.org/10.1002/lt.21398.

Mokdad AA, Lopez AD, Shahraz S, et al. Liver cirrhosis mortality in 187 countries between 1980 and 2010: a systematic analysis. BMC Med. 2014;12:145. https://doi.org/10.1186/s12916-014-0145-y.

Nardelli S, Pentassuglio I, Pasquale C, Ridola L, Moscucci F, Merli M, et al. Depression, anxiety and alexithymia symptoms are major determinants of health related quality of life (HRQoL) in cirrhotic patients. Metab Brain Dis. 2013;28:239–43. https://doi.org/10.1007/s11011-012-9364-0.

National Health Service. 2017. http://www.nhs.uk/Planners/end-of-life-care/Pages/what-it-involves-and-when-it-starts.aspx. Last accessed June 2017.

World Health Organization. Palliative Care. 2017. At http://www.who.int/ncds/management/palliative-care/en/. Last accessed 21 Jan 2018.

Parry R, Land V, Seymour J. How to communicate with patients about future illness progression and end of life: a systematic review. BMJ Support Palliat Care. 2014;4:331–41. https://doi.org/10.1136/bmjspcare-2014-000649.

Perng CL, Shen CC, LY H, Yeh CM, Chen MH, Tsai CF, et al. Risk of depressive disorder following non-alcoholic cirrhosis: a nationwide population-based study. PLoS One. 2014;9:e88721. https://doi.org/10.1371/journal.pone.0088721.

Petrowsky H, Rana A, Kaldas FM, Sharma A, Hong JC, Agopian VG, et al. Liver transplantation in highest acuity recipients: identifying factors to avoid futility. Ann Surg. 2014;259:1186–94. https://doi.org/10.1097/SLA.0000000000000265.

Poonja Z, Brisebois A, van Zanten SV, Tandon P, Meeberg G, Karvellas CJ. Patients with cirrhosis and denied liver transplants rarely receive adequate palliative care or appropriate management. Clin Gastroenterol Hepatol. 2014;12(4):692–8. https://doi.org/10.1016/j.cgh.2013.08.027. Epub 2013 Aug 24

Potosek J, Curry M, Buss M, Chittenden E. Integration of palliative care in end-stage liver disease and liver transplantation. J Palliat Med. 2014;17(11):1271–7. https://doi.org/10.1089/jpm.2013.0167.

Rakoski MO, Volk ML. Palliative care for patients with end-stage liver disease: an overview. Clin Liver Dis. 2015;6:19–21. https://doi.org/10.1002/cld.478.

Rodrigue JR, Dimitri N, Reed A, Antonellis T, Hanto DW, Curry M. Quality of life and psychosocial functioning of spouse/partner caregivers before and after liver transplantation. Clin Transpl. 2011;25:239–47. https://doi.org/10.1111/j.1399-0012.2010.01224.x.

Roth K, Lynn J, Zhong Z, Borum M, Dawson NV. Dying with end stage liver disease with cirrhosis: insights from SUPPORT. Study to understand prognoses and preferences for outcomes and risks of treatment. J Am Geriatr Soc. 2000;48(5 Suppl):S122–30.

Ryerson AB, Eheman CR, Altekruse SF, Ward JW, Jemal A, Sherman RL, et al. Annual report to the nation on the status of cancer, 1975–2012, featuring the increasing incidence of liver cancer. Cancer. 2016;122:1312–37. https://doi.org/10.1002/cncr.29936.

Sankoh O, Bypass P. The INDEPTH network: filling vital gaps in global epidemiology. Int J Epidemiol. 2012;41:579. https://doi.org/10.1092/ije/dys081.

Scaglione S, Kliethermes S, Cao G, Shoham D, Durazo R, Luke A, et al. The epidemiology of cirrhosis in the United States: a population-based study. J Clin Gastroenterol. 2015;49:690–6. https://doi.org/10.1097/MCG.0000000000000208.

Shaw J, Bajaj JS, Covert Hepatic Encephalopathy. J Clin Gastroent 2017; 51(2):118–126. https://doi.org/10.1097/MCG.0000000000000764.

Soleimanpour H, Safari S, Shahsavari Nia K, Sanaie S, Alavian SM. Opioid drugs in patients with liver disease: a systematic review. Hepat Mon. 2016;16:e32636. https://doi.org/10.5812/hepatmon.32636.

Stotts MJ, Hung KW, Benson A, Biggins SW. Rate and predictors of successful cardiopulmonary resuscitation in end-stage liver disease. Dig Dis Sci. 2014;59:1983–6. https://doi.org/10.1007/s10620-014-3084-8.

Strand JJ, Mansel JK, Swetz KM. Department of medicine SoPMMC. The growth of palliative care. Minn Med. 2014;97:39–43.

Tulsky JA. Beyond advance directives: importance of communication skills at the end of life. JAMA. 2005;294:359–65. https://doi.org/10.1001/jama.294.3.359.

Vidot H, Carey S, Allman-Farinelli M, Shackel N. Systematic review: the treatment of muscle cramps in patients with cirrhosis. Aliment Pharmacol Ther. 2014;40:221–32. https://doi.org/10.1111/apt.12827.

Wachterman MW, Pilver C, Smith D, Ersek M, Lipsitz SR, Keating NL. Quality of end-of-life care provided to patients with different serious illnesses. JAMA Intern Med. 2016;176:1095–102. https://doi.org/10.1001/jamainternmed.2016.1200.

Walling AM, Wenger NS. Palliative care and end-stage liver disease. Clin Gastroenterol Hepatol. 2014;12:699–700. https://doi.org/10.1016/j.cgh.2013.11.010.

Walling AM, Asch SM, Lorenz KA, Wenger NS. Impact of consideration of transplantation on end-of-life care for patients during a terminal hospitalization. Transplantation. 2013;95:641–6. https://doi.org/10.1097/TP.0b013e318277f238.

Walling AM, Ahluwalia SC, Wenger NS, Booth M, Roth CP, Lorenz K, et al. Palliative care quality indicators for patients with end-stage liver disease due to cirrhosis.

Dig Dis Sci. 2017;62:84–92. https://doi.org/10.1007/s10620-016-4339-3.
World Health Organization. 10 Facts on the state of Global Health. 2017. http://www.who.int/features/factfiles/global_burden/en/. Last accessed January 2018.
Wordingham SE, Swetz KM. Overview of palliative care and hospice services. Clin Liver Dis. 2015;6:30–2. https://doi.org/10.1002/cld.486.
World Health Organization. WHO definition of palliative care. 2017. http://www.who.int/cancer/palliative/definition/en/. Accessed 21 Jan 2018.
Younossi ZM, Stepanova M, Afendy M, Fang Y, Younossi Y, Mir H, et al. Changes in the prevalence of the most common causes of chronic liver diseases in the United States from 1988 to 2008. Clin Gastroenterol Hepatol. 2011;9:524–30 e1.; quiz e60. https://doi.org/10.1016/j.cgh.2011.03.020.
Zampino R, Boemio A, Sagnelli C, Alessio L, Adinolif LE, Sagnelli E, et al. Hepatitis B virus burden in developing countries. World J Gastroenterol. 2015; 21(42):11941–53. https://doi.org/10.3748/wjg.v21.i42.11941.

Palliative Care in Kidney Disease

64

Fliss E. M. Murtagh

Contents

F. E. M. Murtagh (✉)
Wolfson Palliative Care Research Centre, Hull York Medical School, University of Hull, Hull, UK
e-mail: fliss.murtagh@hyms.ac.uk

Abstract

This chapter first provides evidence about identifying which patients with kidney disease might need palliative or supportive care. Although care should be based on needs and not on prognosis, it

R. D. MacLeod, L. Van den Block (eds.), *Textbook of Palliative Care*,
https://doi.org/10.1007/978-3-319-77740-5_63

is nevertheless important to consider palliative needs in the context of the number of weeks, months, or years which remain. What needs to be addressed only weeks from death is often very different – and more urgent – than what needs to be addressed if there are years ahead. For this reason, there is a comprehensive overview of evidence on survival, so that the context of care can be understood.

Then a more detailed examination of how to identify and manage common symptoms is included, although details of management may vary from country to country, according to local guidelines and availability of individual medicines. Pain, constipation, breathlessness, nausea, vomiting, itch, restless legs, and fatigue are all considered. The last days of life may sometimes prove challenging in terms of symptom management, yet it is important to provide best possible care at this time, so this stage of illness is considered in further detail.

Finally, team working, communication, and planning ahead – all crucial for effective and coordinated care – are then explored, to help facilitate best palliative and supportive care for this population.

1 Introduction

As the world's population ages, the number of older adults is projected to increase dramatically; this will result in a marked increase in the incidence and prevalence of end-stage kidney failure (Stevens et al. 2010). While some reaching end-stage kidney failure will go on to have renal replacement therapy in the form of dialysis, others may choose (or be advised) not to have dialysis because it may have little to offer in terms of added survival or improved quality of life. Those receiving dialysis, often with multiple co-morbid conditions, who are doing less well and those managed without dialysis – called "comprehensive conservative care" (Davison et al. 2015) – often have complex palliative and supportive care needs (Kane et al. 2013; Wasylynuk and Davison 2015).

This chapter aims to present some of the existing and recent evidence, to inform best care and management of this population. Providing the best possible supportive and palliative care for people with advanced kidney failure and their families has the potential to markedly improve patient and family wellbeing over the last months and weeks of life, yet it has not always had sufficient attention alongside the more technological interventions available in nephrology.

2 Identifying Which Patients with Kidney Disease Need Palliative and Supportive Care

Kidney patients whose palliative and supportive care needs should be considered are those with end-stage kidney disease who:

1. Have been on dialysis but are increasingly less well (with either increasing or unstable symptoms, declining functional ability, or deteriorating overall wellbeing)
2. Are on dialysis but with a poor prognosis, often because of co-morbid conditions (especially cardiac disease, but sometimes with a new diagnosis of cancer or other life-limiting condition)
3. Are on dialysis, but finding it hard to tolerate dialysis and they and/or their kidney team are considering withdrawal from dialysis
4. Are reaching end-stage kidney disease but have declined renal replacement therapy (dialysis or transplant) through their own preference
5. Are advised against renal replacement therapy because the burden of frequent dialysis is likely to outweigh survival and quality of life benefits

These last two categories are considered to be "comprehensive conservative care" (Davison et al. 2015).

3 Survival and Prognosis

For a professional delivering palliative care to a person with end-stage kidney disease, it is important to understand, and be able to communicate, the evidence on survival, as this provides the context for decisions about dialysis, as well as the context for preparation for ongoing care and advance care planning. It is also helpful for professionals to be familiar with the evidence about trajectory of illness and likely prognosis, and to communicate this sensitively to patients and their families, in accordance with information preferences.

One of the key questions in kidney care is whether those who are 75 years and older should have dialysis or not. While there is clear evidence that – in general – those over 75 years receiving dialysis live longer than those managed without dialysis (Foote et al. 2016), the increased survival associated with dialysis reduces substantially, or possibly disappears altogether, with increasing co-morbidity and worsening functional status. The evidence is evolving fast in this emergent field of research and is changing continually.

The recent systematic review of survival outcomes in dialysis versus conservative (non-dialytic) care for older people revealed 89 studies reporting evidence on survival, relating to 294,921 older people with end-stage kidney disease. Initial survival for older patients was similar, regardless of management type: one-year survival was 73% (95% confidence intervals 66–80%) for dialysis (type of dialysis unspecified); 78% (95% confidence intervals 75–82%) for hemo-dialysis; 78% (95% confidence intervals 74–82%) for peritoneal dialysis; and 71% (95% confidence intervals 63–78%) for those managed conservatively, without dialysis. In contrast, 2-year survival showed a marked difference; at 62% (95% confidence intervals 55–69%) for dialysis (type unspecified); 64% (95% confidence intervals 60–69%) for hemo-dialysis; 63% (95% confidence intervals 58–68%) for peritoneal dialysis; and 44% (95% confidence intervals 36–53%) for those managed without dialysis (Foote et al. 2016). However, there was very little evidence in respect of those receiving conservative care (only 724 patients or 0.2% of the total number of participants included in the review). The few studies which do include conservatively managed participants suggest that any survival advantage gained from dialysis is lost or very much reduced in those with multiple co-morbidities (especially heart disease) and/or frailty (Foote et al. 2016).

Nevertheless, it can be concluded that, regardless of whether they are receiving dialysis or not, about 1 in 4 older patients will not live more than 1 year from starting dialysis, or from an equivalent time-point if not receiving dialysis, and this falls to about 1 in 3 who will not live more than 2 years, two in three for those managed conservatively. There is a wide range however, with considerable heterogeneity among the end-stage kidney disease population, and the underlying reason for kidney failure, plus co-morbidities play a big part in understanding prognosis. It is important that more research is conducted, and better understanding of the heterogeneity of this population is gained.

4 Recognition of Palliative and Supportive Care Needs

Detailed evidence about palliative needs and interventions among people with advanced kidney disease is somewhat limited, but we do know that symptom burden in end-stage kidney failure is high (Murtagh et al. 2007a; Davison 2003a), psychological and social impacts are considerable (Murtagh et al. 2010), and there are complex transitions to be negotiated (Hutchinson 2005), especially as the illness advances towards end of life.

Communication, especially about dialysis decision-making and to support advance care planning, is very important (Davison and Torgunrud 2007) and may set the scene to facilitate or inhibit patient and family understanding of deterioration, preparation for progression of illness, and future access to palliative and supportive care services (Tonkin-Crine et al. 2015). As kidney disease advances and life expectancy reduces, the priorities and preferences of kidney patients may change, especially to take account of increasing caring burden on families. But contrary to the expectations of professionals, many patients place notably greater priority on better quality of life, improved symptom control, and accessing family support, than they do on extending life at any cost (Steinhauser et al. 2000; Morton et al. 2012). Therefore, professionals should talk early to individual patients, and families, where appropriate, about their information preferences and care priorities, and carefully – in close communication with the patient – work to adjust the goals of care over time to match these changing preferences and priorities in the context of progressive illness.

As for any patient, palliative and supportive care assessment in kidney disease requires a holistic and patient-centered approach (Richardson 2007). This includes detailed assessment of:

- Physical symptoms
- Emotional and psychological symptoms
- Social support and networks
- Family well-being, especially in the context of informal care provision
- Preferences and priorities for communication, decision-making, and goals of care
- Planning ahead as the illness advances, in accordance with preferences

Once each of these areas has been identified and fully assessed, interventions to address the concerns and priorities raised should then be implemented.

Excellent symptom management is particularly important for those with kidney failure. These patients are among the most symptomatic of any chronic disease group (Murtagh et al. 2007a; Solano et al. 2006; Murtagh and Weisbord 2010) and are often even more symptomatic than cancer patients (Saini et al. 2006). Renal replacement therapy may improve symptoms, but it does not completely abolish them and may sometimes exacerbate overall symptom burden.

There are several factors which prevent good symptom management for those with advanced kidney disease. Symptoms may not be routinely assessed by kidney professionals and are often under-recognized (Weisbord et al. 2007; Davison 2003a). Also, patients do not always raise their symptoms for discussion spontaneously as they may be unsure whether to attribute them to kidney disease or not, and symptoms may be more often related to co-morbidities (Murtagh et al. 2016b; Davison and Jassal 2016). In addition, professionals – especially non-renal professionals – do not have the knowledge or experience in prescribing medication in end-stage kidney disease, when renal clearance is much reduced and adverse effects more likely (Douglas 2014).

5 Identifying Symptoms

Regular, proactive assessment of symptoms is therefore important. If possible, an appropriate, clinically relevant, and valid measure of symptoms and other palliative care concerns should be used for all patients at regular intervals or at least with any change in health status. There are four measures in regular use which have been adapted and validated specifically for use in those with renal disease. These are:

(i) The Palliative (or Patient) Outcome Scale symptom module (POS-S Renal), developed in the UK (see www.pos-pal.org). This assesses the full range of physical and psychological symptoms in kidney disease and has been validated in end-stage kidney disease (Murphy et al. 2009).

(ii) The renal version of the Integrated Palliative (or Patient) Outcome Scale (see www.pos-pal.org), also developed in the UK. This measure captures not only physical and psychological symptoms but also family anxiety, practical matters, information needs, and existential distress: it is a brief measure which covers the global domains most relevant in advanced disease. It has been validated in advanced disease (Schildmann et al. 2016; Murtagh et al. 2016a) and is undergoing further validation in advanced kidney disease.

(iii) The Modified Edmonton Symptom Assessment Scale (ESAS). This is a measure of physical and psychological symptoms, derived from the well-validated original ESAS measure, and which has been adapted and validated in Canada for dialysis patients (Davison et al. 2006b; Davison et al. 2006a).

(iv) The Dialysis Symptom Index (DSI), again a measure of physical and psychological symptoms, but which was developed and tested in the USA (Weisbord et al. 2004).

6 Symptom Management

Once symptoms are identified, they need to be actively managed. In this chapter, the focus is on pharmacological management, but non-pharmacological management may be equally or more important, especially for symptoms such as itch, anxiety, depression, and sleep disturbance, which have major psychological and social impact.

The aim of symptom management is to improve symptoms to a level acceptable to the patient while minimizing any adverse effects of medication. The pharmacokinetic impact of renal disease is considerable, because drug metabolism is altered, renal clearance reduced or absent, and the risk of toxicity from accumulation of renally excreted drug and/or metabolites is very high. If estimated glomerular filtration rate is $\leq$30 mL/min/1.73m^2, then prescribing needs to take into account the impact of reduced renal clearance, as well as other pharmacokinetic alterations.

In addition, for those still on dialysis, the effects of dialysis on the drug need to be factored in too. Removal of a medication from systemic circulation during dialysis depends on the molecular size of the drug, the degree of water solubility of the drug, the extent of protein binding of the drug, and a range of dialysis-related factors (such as frequency, duration, type of dialysis, type of dialyzer membrane). Handbooks such as *Dialysis of Drugs* (updated annually and now available as an app) should be used for reference.

7 Pain

Pain is common among those on dialysis (Davison 2003a), those managed without dialysis (Murtagh et al. 2007b), and those who withdraw from dialysis (Germain et al. 2007). As for any other palliative care patient, pain needs to be carefully assessed to identify the underlying cause(s), and remove or ameliorate each as much as possible in a logical and stepwise fashion. Multiple pains are common, and frequently from non-renal causes such as musculoskeletal, cardiac, or other co-morbidities (Davison 2003b).

The commonest question in managing pain among kidney patients is "which opioid to use?" It is important to fully assess the opioid-responsiveness of each pain, as general pains will be less opioid responsive than among other palliative care populations, such as those with cancer.

The World Health Organization analgesic ladder (Azevedo Sao Leao et al. 2006) suggests a step-wise use of analgesics and the Step 2 opioids, codeine, and dihydrocodeine should generally not be used if estimated glomerular filtration rate is $\leq$15 mL/min/1.73m^2 (and only with extreme caution if estimated glomerular filtration rate is between 30 mL to 15 mL/min/1.73m^2). This is because of the evidence on rapid accumulation and toxicity (Davies et al. 1996), with prolonged sedation, respiratory depression, and narcosis (Murtagh et al. 2007e).

Tramadol is a better option but is still problematic. If estimated glomerular filtration rate is $\leq$15 mL/min/1.73m^2, the dose of tramadol should be kept to a maximum of 50 mg 12 hourly (Broadbent et al. 2003). Even at this lower level, adverse effects are common, especially among older people.

All of the Step 3 opioids can cause significant toxicity, but some are less problematic. Most undergo metabolism in the liver to either active or inactive metabolites. These compounds, as well as some of the unchanged opioid, are usually excreted by the kidneys. If a significant proportion of the unchanged opioid is excreted by the kidneys and the metabolites are active, then the opioid is highly likely to cause toxicity when the estimated glomerular filtration rate is less than 30 mL/min.

Alfentanil and fentanyl are cautiously recommended and may be the preferred opioids to use towards end-of-life when an injectable strong opioid is needed, although some clinicians use low-dose oxycodone, with reduced doses and increased dose interval (King et al. 2011). Methadone has also been recommended because of its fecal route of excretion (King et al. 2011), although it should not be used unless the clinician is knowledgeable and skilled in use of methadone more generally as titration and use are complex. Several clinical and practical considerations (other than safety) need to be taken into consideration: for instance, the short half-life of alfentanil makes it less practical for break-through pain, although it is more appropriate for continuous infusion.

Further information is available from several reviews (Murtagh et al. 2007c; Dean 2004; Broadbent et al. 2003; Mercadante and Arcuri 2004; Murtagh et al. 2007e; King et al. 2011), but all Step 3 opioids should be used cautiously, with dose reduction and increase in dosing interval, and morphine and diamorphine should be avoided in severe renal impairment because of their accumulation and adverse effects. Whichever opioid is prescribed, early review and regular monitoring is critical. Accumulation and adverse effects will occur quickly, within a matter of hours. For this reason, long-acting preparations should also be avoided.

Transdermal fentanyl patches may be useful for the ambulant patient earlier in the disease trajectory. However, professionals unfamiliar with prescribing these should recognize that even lowest strength patches represent quite a high-opioid dose and careful titration of immediate-acting oral opioids is usually needed before commencing fentanyl patches.

Transdermal buprenorphine is increasingly widely used clinically, without reports of adverse effects, although the evidence to support this remains limited. There is some evidence of biliary excretion of buprenorphine (Boger 2006) which may reduce any accumulation, but the metabolites may also be relatively inactive (Pergolizzi et al. 2008).

For oral immediate-acting preparations, oxycodone, hydromorphone, and buprenorphine all have very limited evidence to indicate whether they are safe or not, although buprenorphine is increasingly used clinically, and both hydromorphone and oxycodone are likely to be a better choice than morphine or diamorphine.

Musculoskeletal pain: Musculoskeletal pain is perhaps the most common cause of pain in patients with end-stage kidney disease (Davison 2007), and opioids are less suited to manage it, partly because of limited responsiveness and partly because of the adverse effects. Nonsteroidal anti-inflammatory drugs are likely to be beneficial for musculoskeletal or bone pain, but carry high risk of adverse effects in severe renal impairment, including risk of loss of any residual renal function. This consideration may be critical and prevent use of nonsteroidal anti-inflammatory drugs completely, but each case should be reviewed by an experienced clinician in order to make the best judgment. Sometimes, a short course of nonsteroidal anti-inflammatory drugs are prescribed as a considered risk in the absence of any residual renal function, or towards the end-of-life.

Neuropathic pain: Neuropathic (nerve) pain is unlikely to respond to opioids alone. Certain Step 3 opioids may be more useful than others in neuropathic pain. For instance, methadone may be appropriate but should only be prescribed by someone experienced in its use, usually pain or palliative care specialists. Anticonvulsants and antidepressants in low dose are commonly used as adjuvant medication to improve pain control. Antidepressants can be used in end-stage kidney disease, but it is better to avoid longer-acting preparations, reduce the dose, and/or increase the dosing interval. Anticonvulsants are more problematic, particularly gabapentin and pregabalin which accumulate markedly in renal impairment to cause adverse effects. While they can be used cautiously in those on dialysis, their use in those managed without dialysis is limited.

8 Constipation

Constipation is common among patients with end-stage kidney disease. The causes are most often from a combination of several factors, including fluid restriction to help manage kidney function; impaired mobility; a range of different medications (such as iron supplements, opioids, aluminium, or calcium phosphate binders); limited dietary intake; reduced muscle tone through edema and/or through muscle wasting; and dietary restriction of high potassium fruits and vegetables, leading to reduced fiber intake.

As for other symptoms, a detailed assessment is needed to identify causes and contributing factors, bearing in mind the likely causes listed above. Each of the reversible causes needs to be addressed where appropriate or possible, and this will depend of the stage of illness and what causes can realistically be addressed or modified.

To address constipation, other than mild constipation, usually needs both rectal measures and oral laxatives, in combination. Moderate, severe, or established constipation is rarely addressed by oral laxatives alone, and rectal measures will not prevent recurrence without oral laxatives. Useful interventions include: improving mobility, even standing regularly for a very ill and immobile patient is helpful; increasing dietary intake with sufficient fiber and fluid, within the constraints of reduced fluid intake for kidney management – clinical judgment is needed on how important this is, according to level and rate of change of renal impairment, symptoms, co-morbidity, and prognosis; oral laxatives; and rectal measures.

Laxatives, such as softeners or osmotic laxatives, and stimulant laxatives can be used, and often a combination of softener or osmotic laxative with a stimulant is required. Laxatives which contain magnesium, citrate, or phosphate should be avoided in end-stage kidney disease. Polyethelene glycol is not ideal for renal patients because it requires high-concurrent fluid intake and also contains potassium, but it may be useful short term for constipation which does not respond to other measures.

9 Dyspnea

Dyspnea or breathlessness in the patient with end-stage kidney disease may be due to anemia, pulmonary edema (related to fluid overload or to coexisting cardiovascular disease), or co-morbidity (cardiac or respiratory disease). Identifying and treating the underlying cause is the most important, appropriate, and effective management approach. Diuretic use and fluid restriction may or may not be appropriate, depending on the clinical circumstances.

If the breathless patient is anemic, it is often hard to decide how much correction of anemia may improve the symptom, since the correlation between breathlessness and fatigue, and degree of anemia is unclear (see Sect. 13, for more on anemia management).

If all possible and appropriate treatment for underlying causes has been put in place, there may still be a degree of chronic breathlessness remaining. In this situation, an approach to symptom control of breathlessness based on the Breathing, Thinking, Functioning model of breathlessness (Spathis et al. 2017) is helpful (see Fig. 1).

All three areas in Fig. 1 are important. Physical measure to help breathing, such as sitting upright rather than lying, thus increasing vital capacity, using a fan or stream of cool air to provide effective symptom relief, and physiotherapy techniques to manage breathing are helpful. However, without also considering the anxiety, cognitive processing, and emotional experience of breathing, it is unlikely that physical measures alone will be enough. It is also critical that attention is paid to functioning and mobility and occupational therapy can help to maximize mobility and provide appropriate aids, and deconditioning may need addressing to maintain and improve mobility, and so improve breathlessness. Appropriate information, education, and support of patient and family are also a key component, including using this tripartite model to communicate and explain the important elements of management.

As end-stage kidney disease advances and breathlessness may be more severe, disease management options become limited, general and nonpharmacological measures will have less to offer, and pharmacological management of breathlessness become more appropriate. This applies only when treatment of the underlying causes of breathlessness have been exhausted. Severe breathlessness towards end of life is very distressing and should be treated actively. It is important to plan with the patient who has had one or more episode of acute breathlessness (or steadily increasing breathlessness over time) how they would like to be treated if they become more symptomatic in the future. Not all patients will, for instance, choose to be admitted for maximal treatment with intravenous diuretics in the last days or weeks of life.

Pharmacological treatments directed specifically at breathlessness include opioids. Low-dose opioids (up to the equivalent of 30 mg morphine daily) may

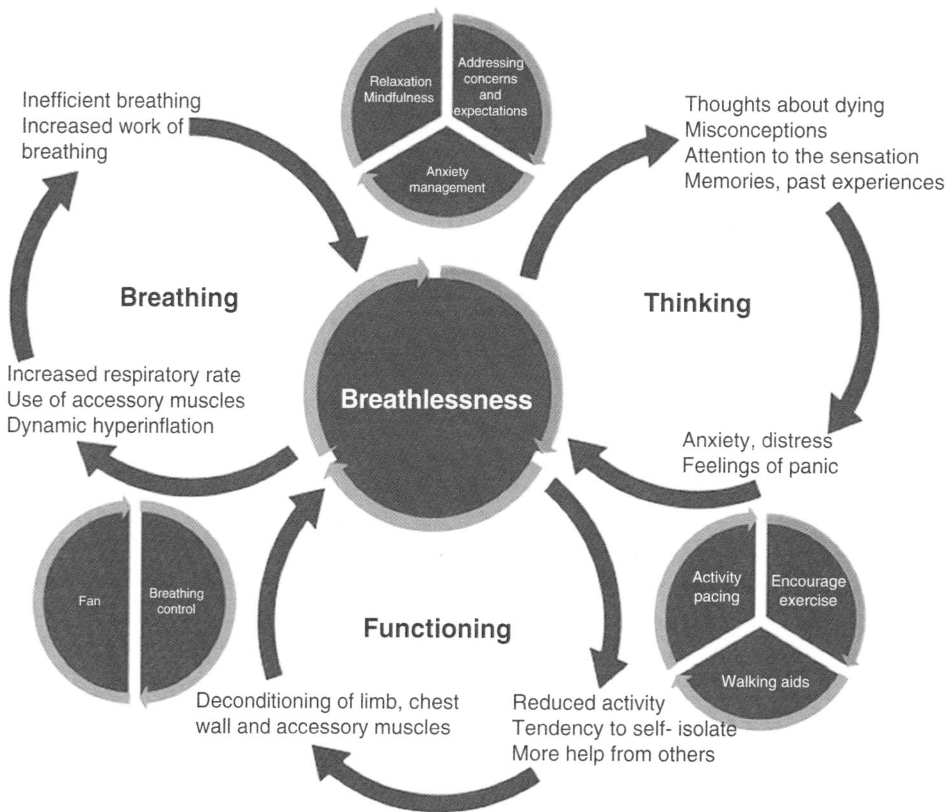

Fig. 1 The Breathing, Thinking, Functioning model to support management of breathlessness. References: see Spathis et al. (2017) and Chin and Booth (2016) for further details (Available under Creative Commons Licence at http://creativecommons.org/licenses/by/4.0/)

be helpful in relieving breathlessness near the end of life in end-stage cardiac and respiratory disease (Jennings et al. 2001) and clinical experience suggests that this also true for patients with kidney disease, although, as discussed in the Sect. 7, morphine should be avoided in end-stage kidney disease. A recent Cochrane review looking at the effectiveness of opioids to relieve breathlessness in advanced disease (Barnes et al. 2016) found evidence to suggest opioids improve the symptom of breathlessness, although the evidence was graded "low." As might be expected, the adverse effects reported included drowsiness, nausea and vomiting, and constipation. A second systematic review found no evidence of significant or clinically relevant ***respiratory*** adverse effects of opioids for chronic breathlessness (Verberkt et al. 2017), although this was not specific to end-stage renal disease.

10 Nausea and Vomiting

Nausea and vomiting are distressing symptoms. Often, the cause may be multifactorial, making these symptoms harder to manage. As with all symptoms, assessment requires a detailed history to understand the history and pattern of nausea and vomiting, considering both symptoms separately. The relationship between nausea and vomiting should also be established, as well as whether there is associated constipation, and a complete medication history. Profound nausea and/or repeated vomiting will prevent absorption of medications taken orally, and alternative routes will therefore need to be considered, at least until nausea and vomiting is controlled.

Management which is specifically directed to the underlying cause(s) is most likely to succeed. If medication or toxins are causing nausea, then nausea is usually persistent and unremitting, and sometimes without accompanying vomiting. Uremia and a variety of drugs, such as opioids, anticonvulsants, antibiotics, and antidepressants, can all cause persistent nausea. Gastroparesis or delayed gastric emptying, which may be caused by drugs such as opioids, as well as occurring secondary to uremic or diabetic autonomic neuropathy, for instance, usually presents with a history of postprandial nausea or vomiting of undigested food which relieves nausea. Bloating, epigastric fullness, flatulence, hiccough, or heartburn may also occur. Nausea related to gastritis is often associated with epigastric pain or discomfort, heartburn, or dyspepsia. Constipation exacerbates nausea and vomiting.

If gastroparesis or delayed gastric emptying is suspected, then domperidone, which increases increase gastric motility, may be preferred. If uremia is a suspected cause, then haloperidol or possibly a 5HT3 (a serotonin receptor subtype) antagonist may be the best choice. However, 5HT3 antagonists, such as ondansetron and granisetron, cause moderate or sometimes severe constipation – this must be a consideration when weighing up if they are the best choice. Drug-induced nausea can be relieved by stopping the causative drug but when this is not feasible, haloperidol is often effective. Gastritis, of which there is much higher risk in uremia, may sometimes contribute to nausea and should be actively treated with a proton pump inhibitor, to help control the related nausea. Towards the end of life, low-dose haloperidol or low-dose levomepromazine, a "broad-spectrum" antiemetic which works on several of the relevant receptors, can be effective to control nausea and vomiting. However, levomepromazine can be very sedative; it is used second or third line, and higher doses should be avoided if possible.

For all antiemetics used in end-stage kidney disease, lower than standard starting doses should be used, and then cautiously titrated to response. End-stage kidney disease patients are at greater risk than those with normal renal function of an enhanced central depressant effect, because of reduced protein binding in uremia and increased cerebral sensitivity to medication, especially where the drug crosses the blood–brain barrier (Wilcock et al. 2017). There is also higher chance of prolongation of the QT interval (risking ventricular arrhythmia) with domperidone, haloperidol, levomepromazine, and ondansetron (Wilcock et al. 2017).

11 Pruritus or Itch

Uremic itch has complex pathophysiology, and this pathophysiology is poorly understood and elucidated. Given this complexity, it is no surprise that it can occasionally be a very challenging symptom to manage. There is a very wide range of drug treatments proposed, often with limited evidence of effectiveness.

The first step is to optimize renal management. High phosphate levels may contribute to pruritus, therefore reducing phosphate levels may be important, with the consideration of dietary advice and the use of phosphate-binders. Hyperparathyroidism may also contribute and should also be considered and actively managed. Xerosis or dry skin, especially in older people, may both cause and contribute to pruritus and so should be treated actively with liberal emollients if dry skin is present. Older people living alone may find it hard to apply emollients easily and spray applications are often helpful in this instance. Preventive measures, such as nail care (keeping nails short), keeping cool (light clothing, and tepid baths or showers) are useful concurrent measures.

It is difficult to recommend specific pharmacological measures given the lack of clear evidence to support any one management over another. UVB light has good supporting evidence but may not be readily available. For those on dialysis, gabapentin may be the best choice, with some supporting evidence (Cheikh Hassan et al. 2015), including randomized controlled trial evidence (Gunal et al. 2004). However, gabapentin accumulates rapidly in those managed conservatively, without dialysis, and quickly causes adverse effects such as drowsiness or sedation; some authorities recommend avoiding gabapentin completely in the conservatively managed population, while others propose very small doses (such as 50 mg or 100 mg alternate days), used with caution and careful monitoring. There is even more limited evidence on the clinical effectiveness of mirtazapine (Davis et al. 2003), and the dose should be reduced in renal impairment. Antihistamines are widely used, but there is little supporting evidence, and – if there is any benefit at all – it may be through the effect of a sedating antihistamine, such as chlorpheniramine, at night in helping a patient to sleep better, since itch often disturbs sleep.

12 Restless Legs

Restless legs syndrome is characterized by the urge to move the legs, uncomfortable sensations in the legs, and worsening of symptoms at rest, especially during the night. The formal International Restless Legs Syndrome Study Group (IRLSSG) criteria (Walters et al. 2003) for diagnosis are:

- Urge to move the legs, usually with unpleasant sensations in the legs
- Worse during periods of rest or inactivity like resting or sitting
- Partial or total relief by physical activity
- Worse symptoms in the evening or night rather than the day

The exact cause for restless legs is not understood as yet; it is widely accepted, however, that the dopaminergic system in the central nervous system is disrupted. There is limited evidence in uremic restless legs that iron deficiency, low parathyroid hormone, hyperphosphatemia, and psychological factors may play a role. Treatment should involve correction of these factors and reduction of potential exacerbating agents, such as caffeine, alcohol, nicotine, and medications (tricyclic antidepressants, calcium antagonists, sedative antihistamines, metoclopramide, selective serotonin uptake inhibitors, and lithium and dopamine antagonists).

There is very limited evidence about treatment of restless legs in people with end-stage kidney disease and much of the evidence is extrapolated from idiopathic restless legs. Gabapentin or pregabalin can be used with those receiving dialysis and are often effective. Dopamine agonists, pergolide or pramipexole, are also effective, although nausea is common, especially with pergolide, as are other adverse effects such as dreams or nightmares. There is also uncertainty about the use of dopamine agonists longer term, because of an association with restrictive cardiac disease and pulmonary fibrosis. Co-careldopa can be used for restless legs and is effective at low dose. However, augmentation, with the return of the symptom, often at a worse level, is very problematic, and 80% will eventually experience augmentation with co-careldopa. Augmentation does occur with dopamine agonists, although much less so than with co-careldopa. In treating restless legs, the choice of drug management should be tailored to the individual and will depend on the presence of other symptoms, age and tolerance of side effects, and whether the patient is receiving dialysis or not.

13 Fatigue

Fatigue or tiredness is highly prevalent in end-stage kidney disease (Karakan et al. 2011) – see Table 1 – and has major impact on quality of life (Bonner et al. 2010). It impairs function and mobility, and can be one of the most devastating adverse influences on quality of life (Lowney et al. 2015). Interventions to alleviate fatigue center around management of anemia and

Table 1 Mean prevalence of symptoms in end-stage kidney disease - weighted by size of study (%) (Murtagh et al. 2007d)

	Percentage
Fatigue	71%
Pruritus	55%
Constipation	53%
Anorexia	49%
Pain	47%
Poor sleep	44%
Anxiety	38%
Dyspnea	37%
Nausea	33%
Restless legs	30%
Depression	27%

supportive interventions such as rehabilitation and practical aids. However, much of the evidence on these interventions is extrapolated from other populations. Rehabilitation-based interventions currently have the best supporting evidence.

Anaemia is a common complication in end-stage kidney disease and is associated with fatigue. It is not clear whether or how much erythropoiesis-stimulating agents – acting to replace endogenous erythropoietin – may or may not be helpful in alleviating fatigue in the palliative end-stage kidney population or not. A small retrospective study in renal palliative care patients suggests fatigue and hospitalizations are reduced (Cheng et al. 2017), but more substantive and robust evidence is needed.

14 Symptom Management at the End of Life

It was believed that a uremic death was relatively symptom-free, but the evidence does not support this. Where studies have specifically reported symptoms in the last day of life, a significant minority experience severe or distressing symptoms (Cohen and Germain 2004; Cohen et al. 1995). Pain, breathlessness, nausea, retained respiratory tract secretions, and terminal agitation are all reported.

These symptoms can be relatively well controlled in the majority of patients. Agitation usually responds to low dose of anxiolytics, such as midazolam. Retained respiratory tract secretions can be improved, although not always resolved, by glycopyrronium or hyoscine butylbromide, and treatment is optimal if commenced early. Pain or breathlessness can be effectively managed with opioid medications, and often only low doses are required, although morphine and diamorphine should be avoided in severe renal impairment because of the accumulation of metabolites and subsequent adverse effects (see Sect. 7, in this chapter). If the patient has been on regular strong opioids orally and can no longer take oral medication, then convert the total daily dose of strong opioid to the equivalent for subcutaneous fentanyl or alfentanil over 24 h and start a subcutaneous infusion.

15 Team Working

Multi-disciplinary team working is inherent to the palliative care approach. For patients with end-stage kidney disease, it is important to ensure excellent liaison, not only within the palliative care team but between the nephrology team, the specialist palliative care team, care of the elderly teams, other disease-based teams, and the primary care or community-based teams. Coordination of care across providers is always important, but it becomes critically so when caring for these, usually, older people with multiple conditions.

Primary care or community-based teams may see patients with end-stage kidney disease rarely; in the UK, deaths with end-stage kidney disease represent only 1–2% of all deaths (Murtagh and Higginson 2007). Each general practitioner will care for a patient with end-stage kidney disease only once every few years; and until recently, the care and deaths of these patients has largely been in acute hospitals (Lovell et al. 2017). This may be changing however, as conservative management programs expand (Lovell et al. 2017) and home deaths increase (Okamoto et al. 2015); nevertheless, primary care teams may need specialist supportive to deliver excellent end of life care.

There are a variety of models of care of those with end-stage kidney disease, as evidenced in a recent UK-wide study (Roderick et al. 2015). However, there is little evidence to suggest which model is most effective or cost-effective. Shared care models, with collaborations between primary, palliative, and nephrology providers to optimize recognition, assessment, and management of supportive and palliative care needs, would, at present, seem to be the most highly rated by patients, families, and professionals (Murtagh et al. 2016c).

16 Advance Care Planning

Planning ahead in end-stage kidney disease is important, especially given the high levels of cognitive impairment as the disease progresses. There is good evidence of benefit from advance care planning in a range of advanced illnesses

(Weathers et al. 2016; Houben et al. 2014) but wide variation in patients' perspectives on advance care planning (Ke et al. 2017). Most are keen to discuss and plan ahead, but small proportions prefer not to discuss.

This indicates that advance care planning needs to be done in such a way as to be highly individualized. Open questions, such as "What do you understand about your illness (or health) at present?"; "Do you have any concerns about how it might change in the future?"; or "Do you have any worries about the next weeks [or months or years, as appropriate]?," are invaluable ways to open up discussions at a pace or in a way which can be led by the patient. It is always hard to make opportunities for these discussions, but the conversation can readily be dropped if it is too soon or not currently desired, whereas considerable harm can be caused by not addressing important issues in time.

The overall evidence for advance care planning in hamodialysis patients remains inconclusive (Lim et al. 2016), but this is because the research has not yet been done. Several studies are currently underway, so the evidence may emerge soon which clarifies the effectiveness (or not). The economic benefits are particularly unclear (Dixon et al. 2015), but despite this uncertainly, if advance care planning is done well, with sensitivity to individual preferences and priorities.

17 Conclusion and Summary

Although those with end-stage kidney disease represent only about 2% of all deaths, there are major challenges to delivering effective palliative care to this population. This is accompanied by an increasing awareness among clinicians and health services of the complexity of their supportive and palliative care needs. This chapter outlines the current evidence on identification, assessment, and management of these supportive and palliative care needs, as well as the gaps in that evidence, in order to inform the best ways to overcome the challenges and deliver high-quality palliative care for those with end-stage kidney disease.

References

Azevedo Sao Leao FK, Kimura M, Jacobsen TM. The who analgesic ladder for Cancer pain control, twenty years of use: how much pain relief does one get from using it? Support Care Cancer. 2006;14(11):1086–93.

Barnes H, Mcdonald J, Smallwood N, Manser R. Opioids for the palliation of refractory breathlessness in adults with advanced disease and terminal illness. Cochrane Database Syst Rev. 2016;3:Cd011008.

Boger RH. Renal impairment: a challenge for opioid treatment? The role of buprenorphine. Palliat Med. 2006;20:S17–23.

Bonner A, Wellard S, Caltabiano M. The impact of fatigue on daily activity in people with chronic kidney disease. J Clin Nurs. 2010;19:3006–15.

Broadbent A, Khor K, Heaney A. Palliation and chronic renal failure: Opoid and other palliative medications – dosage guidelines. Prog Palliat Care. 2003;11:183–90.

Cheikh Hassan HI, Brennan F, Collett G, Josland EA, Brown MA. Efficacy and safety of gabapentin for uremic pruritus and restless legs syndrome in conservatively managed patients with chronic kidney disease. J Pain Symptom Manag. 2015;49:782–9.

Cheng HWB, Chan KY, Lau HT, Man CW, Cheng SC, Lam C. Use of erythropoietin-stimulating agents (Esa) in patients with end-stage renal failure decided to forego Dialysis: palliative perspective. Am J Hosp Palliat Med. 2017;34:380–4.

Chin C, Booth S. Managing breathlessness: a palliative care approach. Postgrad Med J. 2016;92:393–400.

Cohen LM, Germain MJ. Measuring quality of dying in end-stage renal disease. Semin Dial. 2004;17:376–9.

Cohen LM, Mccue JD, Germain M, Kjellstrand CM. Dialysis discontinuation. A 'good' death? Arch Intern Med. 1995;155:42–7.

Davies G, Kingswood C, Street M. Pharmacokinetics of opioids in renal dysfunction. Clin Pharmacokinet. 1996;31:410–22.

Davis MP, Frandsen JL, Walsh D, Andresen S, Taylor S. Mirtazapine For Pruritus. J Pain Symptom Manag. 2003;25:288–91.

Davison SN. Pain in hemodialysis patients: prevalence, cause, severity, and management. Am J Kidney Dis. 2003a;42:1239–47.

Davison SN. Pain in hemodialysis patients: prevalence, cause, severity, and management. Am J Kidney Dis. 2003b;42(6):1239–47.

Davison SN. The prevalence and management of pain in end-stage renal disease. J Palliat Med. 2007;10:1277–86.

Davison SN, Jassal SV. Supportive care: integration of patient-centered kidney care to manage symptoms and geriatric syndromes. Clin J Am Soc Nephrol. 2016;11:1882–91.

Davison SN, Torgunrud C. The creation of an advance care planning process for patients with Esrd. Am J Kidney Dis. 2007;49:27–36.

Davison SN, Jhangri GS, Johnson JA. Cross-sectional validity of a modified Edmonton symptom assessment system in Dialysis patients: a simple assessment of symptom burden. Kidney Int. 2006a;69:1621–5.

Davison SN, Jhangri GS, Johnson JA. Longitudinal validation of a modified Edmonton symptom assessment system (Esas) in Haemodialysis patients. Nephrol Dial Transplant. 2006b;21:3189–95.

Davison SN, Levin A, Moss AH, Jha V, Brown EA, Brennan F, Murtagh FE, Naicker S, Germain MJ, O'donoghue DJ, Morton RL, Obrador GT, Kidney Disease: Improving Global Outcomes. Executive summary of the Kdigo controversies conference on supportive care in chronic kidney disease: developing a roadmap to improving quality care. Kidney Int. 2015;88:447–59.

Dean M. Opioids in renal failure and Dialysis patients. J Pain Symptom Manag. 2004;28:497–504.

Dixon J, Matosevic T, Knapp M. The economic evidence for advance care planning: systematic review of evidence. Palliat Med. 2015;29(10):869–84.

Douglas CA. Palliative care for patients with advanced chronic kidney disease. J Roy Coll Phys Edinburgh. 2014;44:224–31.

Foote C, Kotwal S, Gallagher M, Cass A, Brown M, Jardine M. Survival outcomes of supportive care versus Dialysis therapies for elderly patients with end-stage kidney disease: a systematic review and meta-analysis. Nephrology. 2016;21:241–53.

Germain MJ, Cohen LM, Davison SN. Withholding and withdrawal from Dialysis: what we know about how our patients die. Semin Dial. 2007;20:195–9.

Gunal AI, Ozalp G, Yoldas TK, Gunal SY, Kirciman E, Celiker H. Gabapentin therapy for pruritus in Haemodialysis patients: a randomized, placebo-controlled, double-blind trial. Nephrol Dial Transplant. 2004;19:3137–9.

Houben CHM, Spruit MA, Groenen MTJ, Wouters EFM, Janssen DJA. Efficacy of advance care planning: a systematic review and meta-analysis. J Am Med Dir Assoc. 2014;15:477–89.

Hutchinson TA. Transitions in the lives of patients with end stage renal disease: a cause of suffering and an opportunity for healing. Palliat Med. 2005;19:270–7.

Jennings AL, Davies AN, Higgins JP, Broadley K. Opioids for the palliation of breathlessness in terminal illness. Cochrane Database Syst Rev. 2001;4:Cd002066.

Kane PM, Vinen K, Murtagh FE. Palliative care for advanced renal disease: a summary of the evidence and future direction. Palliat Med. 2013;27:817–21.

Karakan S, Sezer S, Ozdemir FN. Factors related to fatigue and subgroups of fatigue in patients with end-stage renal disease. Clin Nephrol. 2011;76:358–64.

Ke LS, Huang X, Hu WY, O'connor M, Lee S. Experiences and perspectives of older people regarding advance care planning: a meta-synthesis of qualitative studies. Palliat Med. 2017;31:394–405.

King S, Forbes K, Hanks GW, Ferro CJ, Chambers EJ. A systematic review of the use of opioid medication for those with moderate to severe Cancer pain and renal impairment: a European palliative care research collaborative opioid guidelines project. Palliat Med. 2011;25:525–52.

Lim CED, Ng RWC, Cheng NCL, Cigolini M, Kwok C, Brennan F. Advance care planning for Haemodialysis patients. Cochrane Database Syst Rev. 2016;2016(7): CD010737.

Lovell N, Jones C, Baynes D, Dinning S, Vinen K, Murtagh FE. Understanding patterns and factors associated with place of death in patients with end-stage kidney disease: a retrospective cohort study. Palliat Med. 2017;31:283–8.

Lowney AC, Myles HT, Bristowe K, Lowney EL, Shepherd K, Murphy M, O'brien T, Casserly L, Mcquillan R, Plant WD, Conlon PJ, Vinen C, Eustace JA, Murtagh FE. Understanding what influences the health-related quality of life of hemodialysis patients: a collaborative study in England and Ireland. J Pain Symptom Manag. 2015;50:778–85.

Mercadante S, Arcuri E. Opioids and renal function. J Pain. 2004;5:2–19.

Morton RL, Snelling P, Webster AC, Rose J, Masterson R, Johnson DW, Howard K. Factors influencing patient choice of Dialysis versus conservative care to treat end-stage kidney disease. CMAJ. 2012;184:E277–83.

Murphy EL, Murtagh FE, Carey I, Sheerin NS. Understanding symptoms in patients with advanced chronic kidney disease managed without Dialysis: use of a short patient-completed assessment tool. Nephron Clin Pract. 2009;111:C74–80.

Murtagh FE, Higginson IJ. Death from renal failure eighty years on: how far have we come? J Palliat Med. 2007;10:1236–8.

Murtagh FEM, Weisbord S. Symptoms in renal disease: their epidemiology, assessment and management. In: Chambers EJ, Germain M, Brown E, editors. Supportive care for the renal patient. 2nd ed. Oxford: Oxford University Press; 2010.

Murtagh FE, Addington-Hall J, Higginson IJ. The prevalence of symptoms in end-stage renal disease: a systematic review. Adv Chronic Kidney Dis. 2007a;14:82–99.

Murtagh FE, Addington-Hall JM, Edmonds PM, Donohoe P, Carey I, Jenkins K, Higginson IJ. Symptoms in advanced renal disease: a cross-sectional survey of symptom prevalence in stage 5 chronic kidney disease managed without Dialysis. J Palliat Med. 2007b;10:1266–76.

Murtagh FE, Chai MO, Donohoe P, Edmonds PM, Higginson IJ. The use of opioid analgesia in end-stage renal disease patients managed without Dialysis: recommendations for practice. J Pain Palliat Care Pharmacother. 2007c;21:5–16.

Murtagh FEM, Addington-Hall J, Higginson IJ. The prevalence of symptoms in end-stage renal disease: a systematic review. Adv Chronic Kidney Dis. 2007d; 14:82–99.

Murtagh FEM, Chai MO, Donohoe P, Edmonds PM, Higginson IJ. The use of opioid analgesia in end-stage renal disease patients managed without Dialysis: recommendations for practice. J Pain Palliat Care Pharmacother. 2007e;21(2):5–16.

Murtagh FE, Addington-Hall J, Edmonds P, Donohoe P, Carey I, Jenkins K, Higginson IJ. Symptoms in the month before death for stage 5 chronic kidney disease patients managed without Dialysis. J Pain Symptom Manag. 2010;40:342–52.

Murtagh F, Ramsenthaler C, Firth A, Groeneveld EI, Lovell N, Simon S, Denzel J, Bernhardt F, Schildmann E, Bausewein C, Higginson IJ. A brief, patient- and proxy-reported outcome measure for the adult palliative care population: validity and reliability of the integrated palliative outcome scale (Ipos) (in Eapc 2016: abstracts). Palliat Med. 2016a;30(6):NP11.

Murtagh FE, Burns A, Moranne O, Morton RL, Naicker S. Supportive care: comprehensive conservative care in end-stage kidney disease. Clin J Am Soc Nephrol. 2016b;11:1909–14.

Murtagh FEM, Burns A, Moranne O, Morton RL, Naicker S. Supportive care: comprehensive conservative care in end-stage kidney disease. Clin J Am Soc Nephrol. 2016c;11:1909–14.

Okamoto I, Tonkin-Crine S, Rayner H, Murtagh FE, Farrington K, Caskey F, Tomson C, Loud F, Greenwood R, O'donoghue DJ, Roderick P. Conservative care for Esrd in the United Kingdom: a National Survey. Clin J Am Soc Nephrol. 2015;10:120–6.

Pergolizzi J, Böger RH, Budd K, Dahan A, Erdine S, Hans G, Kress HG, Langford R, Likar R, Raffa RB, Sacerdote P. Opioids and the management of chronic severe pain in the elderly: consensus statement of an international expert panel with focus on the six clinically most often used World Health Organization step III opioids (buprenorphine, fentanyl, Hydromorphone, methadone, morphine, oxycodone). Pain Pract. 2008;8:287–313.

Richardson A. Holistic common assessment of supportive and palliative care needs for people with Cancer: report to the National Cancer Action Team. London: Kings College London; 2007.

Roderick P, Rayner H, Tonkin-Crine S, Okamoto I, Eyles C, Leydon G, Santer M, Klein J, Yao GL, Murtagh F, Farrington K, Caskey F, Tomson C, Loud F, Murphy E, Elias R, Greenwood R, O'donoghue D. A National Study of Practice Patterns in Uk Renal Units in the use of Dialysis and Conservative Kidney Management to Treat People Aged 75 years and over with chronic kidney failure. Southampton: National Institute For Health Research; 2015.

Saini T, Murtagh FE, Dupont PJ, Mckinnon PM, Hatfield P, Saunders Y. Comparative pilot study of symptoms and quality of life in Cancer patients and patients with end stage renal disease. Palliat Med. 2006;20:631–6.

Schildmann EK, Groeneveld EI, Denzel J, Brown A, Bernhardt F, Bailey K, Guo P, Ramsenthaler C, Lovell N, Higginson IJ, Bausewein C, Murtagh FE. Discovering the hidden benefits of cognitive interviewing in two languages: the first phase of a validation study of the integrated palliative care outcome scale. Palliat Med. 2016;30:599–610.

Solano JP, Gomes B, Higginson IJ. A comparison of symptom prevalence in far advanced Cancer, aids, heart disease, chronic obstructive pulmonary disease and renal disease. J Pain Symptom Manag. 2006;31(1):58–69.

Spathis A, Booth S, Moffat C, Hurst R, Ryan R, Chin C, Burkin J. The breathing, thinking, functioning clinical model: a proposal to facilitate evidence-based breathlessness management in chronic respiratory disease. NPJ Prim Care Respir Med. 2017;27:27.

Steinhauser KE, Christakis NA, Clipp EC, Mcneilly M, Mcintyre L, Tulsky JA. Factors considered important at the end of life by patients, family, physicians, and other care providers. JAMA. 2000;284:2476–82.

Stevens LA, Viswanathan G, Weiner DE. Chronic kidney disease and end-stage renal disease in the elderly population: current prevalence, future projections, and clinical significance. Adv Chronic Kidney Dis. 2010;17:293–301.

Tonkin-Crine S, Okamoto I, Leydon GM, Murtagh FE, Farrington K, Caskey F, Rayner H, Roderick P. Understanding by older patients of Dialysis and conservative management for chronic kidney failure. Am J Kidney Dis. 2015;65:443–50.

Verberkt CA, Van Den Beuken-Van Everdingen MHJ, Schols J, Datla S, Dirksen CD, Johnson MJ, Van Kuijk SMJ, Wouters EFM, Janssen DJA. Respiratory adverse effects of opioids for breathlessness: a systematic review and meta-analysis. Eur Respir J. 2017;50(5). https://doi.org/10.1183/13993003.01153-2017.

Walters AS, Lebrocq C, Dhar A, Hening W, Rosen R, Allen RP, Trenkwalder C. Validation of the international restless legs syndrome study group rating scale for restless legs syndrome. Sleep Med. 2003;4:121–32.

Wasylynuk BA, Davison SN. Palliative care in patients with advanced chronic kidney disease. CANNT J. 2015;25:28–32.

Weathers E, O'caoimh R, Cornally N, Fitzgerald C, Kearns T, Coffey A, Daly E, O'sullivan R, Mcglade C, Molloy DW. Advance care planning: a systematic review of randomised controlled trials conducted with older adults. Maturitas. 2016;91:101–9.

Weisbord SD, Fried LF, Arnold RM, Rotondi AJ, Fine MJ, Levenson DJ, Switzer GE. Development of a symptom assessment instrument for chronic hemodialysis patients: the Dialysis symptom index. J Pain Symptom Manag. 2004;27:226–40.

Weisbord SD, Fried L, Mor MK, Resnick AL, Unruh ML, Palevsky PM, Levenson DJ, Cooksey SH, Fine MJ, Kimmel PL, Arnold RM. Renal provider recognition of symptoms in patients on maintenance hemodialysis. Clin J Am Soc Nephrol. 2007;2:960–7.

Wilcock A, Charlesworth S, Twycross R, Waddington A, Worthington O, Murtagh FEM, Beavis J, King S, Mihalyo M, Kotlinska-Lemieszek A. Prescribing non-opioid drugs in end-stage kidney disease. J Pain Symptom Manag. 2017;54(5):776–87.

Palliative Care and Endocrine Diseases 65

Pallavi D. Rao and K. M. Prasanna Kumar

Contents

Abstract

Palliative care in endocrine diseases is similar to palliative care in any other disease. The aim will be to reduce the symptoms, avoid short-term complications and improve or maintain the quality of life by minimal interference and with least inconvenience to the patient. Palliative care in diabetes mellitus aims at avoiding hypoglycemia and symptomatic hyperglycemia, and not necessarily achieving euglycemia or postponing/preventing chronic complications of diabetes. Palliative care in thyroid disorders aims to help the patient remain asymptomatic in both hypothyroidism and hyperthyroidism and not normalizing the TSH. Palliative care in all other endocrine diseases like Cushing's disease, pheochromocytoma, pituitary tumor, insulinoma, and hyperparathyroidism is also mostly minimal medical intervention to alleviate symptoms and improve quality of life. Replacing endocrine deficiency as in Addisons disease, hypothyroidism, hypocalcemia due to hypoparathyroidism is important and similarly managed to any other endocrine deficiency.

P. D. Rao (✉) · K. M. Prasanna Kumar
Centre for Diabetes and Endocrine Care, Bengaluru, India
e-mail: pdrao27@gmail.com; dr.kmpk@gmail.com

R. D. MacLeod, L. Van den Block (eds.), *Textbook of Palliative Care*,
https://doi.org/10.1007/978-3-319-77740-5_112

1 Introduction

Palliative care aims to provide comfort care, supportive care, and symptoms management, and its goal is not to cure the disease but to prevent or treat, as early as possible, and to alleviate the symptoms of the disease and side effects of its treatment.

In this chapter, we aim to discuss treatment of diabetes and other endocrine disorders in life limiting disorders and towards the end-of-life.

2 Diabetes Mellitus

Diabetes mellitus is a chronic relentless disorder, needing major lifestyle changes and maintaining them as the years go by. Patients are encouraged to manage their disease, with close monitoring of the blood glucose, with the aim of reducing morbidity, further complications, and mortality.

However, the most important goal of management of diabetes in palliative care is to avoid hypoglycemia and symptomatic hyperglycemia. Tight control of diabetes is not necessary in palliative care as the life span is limited in these patients. When it comes to managing diabetes in life limiting illnesses, the targets obviously need to change, as with the medications. The majority of patients in palliative care do not need to achieve a target Hb A1C below 7%.

Strict avoidance of added sugars is often impractical, when food choices are already limited. Patients may request "sugary" nutrients, which should be provided. Calorie-dense foods (including chocolate) are encouraged despite their adverse impact on glucose concentration. Adjusting medication is preferable to limiting the diet but therapy will have to match small frequent meals· (End of life diabetes care 2013).

A set of key principles underlie high quality diabetes care at the end-of-life and these have been summarized as:

- Provision of a painless and symptom-free death
- Tailored glucose-lowering therapy and minimize diabetes-related adverse treatment effects
- Avoid metabolic de-compensation and diabetes-related emergencies: frequent and unnecessary hypoglycemia, diabetic ketoacidosis, hyperosmolar hyperglycemic state, persistent symptomatic hyperglycemia
- Avoidance of foot complications in frail, bed-bound patients with diabetes
- Avoidance of symptomatic clinical dehydration
- Provision of an appropriate level of intervention according to stage of illness, symptom profile, and respect for dignity
- Supporting and maintaining the empowerment of the individual patient (in their diabetes self-management) and carers to the last possible stage. (End of life diabetes care 2013)

The goal of diabetes management in palliative care is not achieving euglycemia. Blood glucose above 5.6 mmole/l (100 mg/dl) is acceptable to prevent hypoglycemia. Blood glucose below 14 mmole/l (250 mgm/dl) is acceptable to prevent symptoms of hyperglycemia in palliative care of diabetes. In many ways, it is important to keep the blood glucose level at a level of 10–15 mmole/l so that if there are problems such as vomiting or reduced oral intake, hypoglycemia is less likely.

The palliative care of diabetes should be a team work involving care providers, endocrinologist or diabetologist, diabetes nurse educator, dietitian, primary care team, palliative care specialist, and the family of the patient.

2.1 Patients on Oral Antidiabetic Treatment

Patients who are on oral antidiabetic agents can continue medication, provided there is no hypoglycemia. However, if appetite is poor or the patients unable to eat adequately long-acting sulfonylureas need to be avoided (End of life diabetes care 2013). Repaglinide or Nataglinide can be useful for patients managing small regular meals with the dose carefully adjusted according to intake (End of life diabetes care 2013).

With liver impairment and cirrhosis, compensatory mechanisms are altered due to reduced or lack of neo-glucogenesis and glycogenolysis, and hence sugar targets will need to be relaxed to reduce the risk of severe hypoglycemia.

Similarly, with renal impairment, many of the oral hypoglycemics cannot be continued and insulin doses may need to be reduced or a change in insulin regime may be warranted.

Low-dose insulin may be the only option for patients whose glucose levels are high despite a significantly reduced oral intake.

2.2 Patients on Insulin Regimes

In persons with Type 1 diabetes (T1DM), however, insulin will definitely need to be continued to avoid ketoacidosis, as a basal insulin.

Persons with T2 DM on insulin may not need basal bolus regimens or even pre-mixed insulin, as these are likely to cause hypoglycemia. Symptom control may be achieved with once-a-day basal insulin.

2.3 End-of-Life Care

Towards the last few weeks and days of life, the focus in diabetes mellitus treatment should shift from tight control to symptom control only. Hyperglycemic symptoms that need to be addressed and treated are excessive thirst and excessive urination.

Many factors associated with end-of-life care may precipitate hyperglycemia (steroids, concurrent infection, tumor-specific effects, and the stress response) and/or hypoglycemia (loss of appetite, weight loss, and renal or hepatic failure).

Dexamethasone or prednisolone is often used for symptom control in palliative care. Regardless of the indication, the impact of steroids on glucose control can contribute to hyperglycemic symptoms. Regular monitoring of blood sugars may be helpful, particularly if there are symptoms of hyperglycemia. Once daily steroid therapy taken in the morning tends to cause a late afternoon or early evening rise in glucose levels which can be managed by a morning sulfonylurea (such as gliclazide) or morning isophane insulin (including NPH, Detemir, Glargine, Degludac); If steroids are to be given twice daily, twice daily gliclazide or isophane insulin can be effective but early morning hypoglycemia may occur and the dose must be adjusted with this risk in mind (End of life diabetes care 2013).

3 Other Endocrine Disorders

There are no guidelines available for the management of endocrine disorders towards the end-of-life. As with diabetes mellitus, management should aim to ensure that side-effects are kept to the minimum and management is to maintain comfort and quality of life.

3.1 Thyroid Disorders

3.1.1 Hypothyroidism

The etiology of hypothyroidism in oncology patients may be pre-existing auto-immune hypothyroidism, as a result of chemotherapy agents or radiation to thyroid. In these cases, replacement thyroxine will be necessary.

In pre-existing hypothyroidism, Levothyroxine should be continued with an aim to maintain the TSH within normal ranges as before or below10 mIU/L is good enough. Changes in Levothyroxine doses, dosing schedules (weekly or bi-weekly rather than daily) and route of administration (oral/nasogastric tube) may need to be considered. Changes in the route depend on the ability of the patient to swallow tablets, absorption of levothyroxine in conditions affecting the gastrointestinal tract, and possible interaction with the chemotherapy agents (Jonklaas et al. 2014).

Management of hypothyroidism secondary to chemotherapy agents or radiation therapy is similar to that of autoimmune hypothyroidism.

Towards the end-of-life however, like in many other disorders, symptom control should take priority. There is no evidence to suggest increase in mortality or death being caused as a result of stopping thyroxine towards end-of-life.

3.1.2 Hyperthyroidism

Long-term anti-thyroid drugs (ATD), like carbimazole ormethimazol 10–15 mgm once a day-treatment of toxic multinodular goitre (TMNG) or toxic adenoma (TA), may be indicated in some elderly or otherwise ill patients with limited life expectancy, in patients who are not good candidates for surgery or ablative therapy, and in patients who prefer this option (Jonklaas et al. 2014; Ross et al. 2016).

The required dose of ATD to restore the euthyroid state in TMNG or TA patients is usually low (5–15 mg/d). Because long-term, low-dose ATD treatment in nodular hyperthyroidism can be difficult to regulate, frequent (every 3 months) monitoring is recommended initially, especially in the elderly until stability has been documented, after which testing frequency can be decreased (Takats et al. 1999).

3.2 Parathyroid Disorders

3.2.1 Hyperparathyroidism

Hyperparathyroidism could be primary, where it is due to a parathyroid adenoma, or secondary, where it develops secondary to vitamin D deficiency or chronic kidney disease. Treating vitamin D deficiency and chronic kidney disease is the treatment of choice for secondary hyperparathyroidism. Surgery is the treatment of choice in primary hyperparathyroidism. In patients who are not fit for surgery or those who choose medical management over surgery, cinacalcet, a calcimimetic, may be used.

Cinacalcet, a calcimimetic, reduces both serum calcium and parathyroid hormone (PTH) levels and raises serum phosphorus. Cinacalcet inhibits parathyroid cell function and reduces PTH secretion by altering the function of parathyroid calcium-sensing receptors, normalizes serum calcium in PHPT, both mild and more severe, for sustained periods (Griebeler et al. 2016).

Cinacalcet can be considered for patients with hypercalcemia secondary to parathyroid carcinoma, secondary hyperparathyroidism, and primary hyperparathyroidism.

3.2.2 Hypoparathyroidism

Hypoparathyroidism is a condition of parathyroid hormone (PTH) deficiency. Primary hypoparathyroidism is a state of inadequate PTH activity. In the absence of adequate PTH activity, the ionized calcium concentration in the extracellular fluid falls below the reference range. Primary hypoparathyroidism results from iatrogenic causes or from a few rare disorders.

Secondary hypoparathyroidism is a physiological state in which PTH levels are low in response to a primary process that causes hypercalcemia.

Treatment of patients with hypoparathyroidism involves correcting the hypocalcemia by administering calcium and vitamin D. Recombinant human PTH is indicated as an adjunct to calcium and vitamin D to control hypocalcemia in patients with hypoparathyroidism.

Vitamin D supplementations needs to be in a daily dose of 400–800IU to patients treated with activated vitamin D analogues. In a patient with hypercalciuria, it is important to consider a reduction in calcium intake, a sodium-restricted diet, and/or treatment with a thiazide diuretic (Bollerslev et al. 2015). Calcium excretion is increased by loop diuretics and diminished by thiazide-type diuretics and amiloride (Rose 1991).

3.3 Adrenal Disorders

3.3.1 Hypoadrenalism

Hypoadrenalism will need to be treated even towards the end-of-life to avoid adrenal crisis, as the patient does not produce corticosteroids and is dependent on the administered replacement therapy. Depending on the severity of the terminal illness, the dose will need to be adjusted to accommodate for the stress response as a result of the illness per se. Parenteral administration of hydrocortisone may be necessary if the patient is unable to take oral medication. 200 mgm i.v. bolus followed by 100 mgm i.v. 6–8th hourly.

3.3.2 Cushing's Syndrome (Steroid Excess)

Cushing's syndrome occurs when there is an excess of steroids. This may be due to administration of corticosteroids. If the etiology is unclear, the investigation and the cause may be against the principles of palliative care, and the aim is to ensure symptom control. Controlling hyperglycemia, hypertension, and hyperlipidemia with medications as needed should be the goal.

Ketoconazole, an imidazole derivative, inhibits steroid synthesis through inhibition of cytochrome P450 enzymes 17,20-lyase, 11-B hydroxylase, 17-hydroxylase, and side chain cleavage. These effects are dose dependent and completely and rapidly reversible upon drug discontinuation (Liu et al. 2007; Sonino et al. 1991).

Metyrapone blocks the production of cortisol through the inhibition of 11B-hydroxylase, resulting in a dramatic rise in 11-deoxycortisol, a precursor steroid with mineralocorticoid activity formed immediately proximal to cortisol in the steroid biosynthesis pathway (Rizk et al. 2012; Jeffcoate et al. 1977).

Dopamine agonists are widely available and used clinically for the treatment of prolactinomas and occasionally for acromegaly. However, use in Cushing's syndrome has shown variable results possibly with better short-term than long-term results (Sonino and Boscaro 1999; Boscaro et al. 1983).

Etomidate inhibits cholesterol side chain cleavage and 11-B hydroxylase. It has been successfully used as a short-term treatment in critically ill patients with Cushing's syndrome unable to take oral medications (Krakoff et al. 2001).

Mitotane reduces cortisol synthesis through the inhibition of 11B-hydroxylase, 18-hydroxylase, 3-α hydroxylase, hydroxysteroid dehydrogenase, and several cholesterol side chain cleavage enzymes. It is also an adrenolytic agent at doses greater than 4 g per day and is used most often for the treatment of adrenocortical carcinoma (Crane and Harris 1970).

Mineralo-corticoid excess in patients where there is no indication for surgery or who, choose not to undergo surgery, can be treated with eplerenone or spironolactone (Lim et al. 2001). When blood pressure is not controlled with spironolactone or eplerenone, or side-effects limit tolerability, the addition of other antihypertensive therapies may be required.

Mineralocorticoid deficiency in life-limiting illness is best managed again with replacement with fludrocortisone to control symptoms of postural hypotension. Mineralocorticoid excess in the same way could be to control with ACE-inhibitors and aldactone.

3.4 Pituitary Disorders

3.4.1 Hypopituitarism

Treatment of hypopituitarism is by the replacement of the hormones that are not being produced. Patients with pan hypopituitarism will need to be treated with hydrocortisone until the very end, similar to the treatment with insulin in patients with insulin-dependent diabetes mellitus, and steroids for hypoadrenalism and Addisons disease.

Thyroid hormone replacement though is not as crucial as cortisone, but thyroxine should be given in adequate doses to keep serum T4 levels in the normal range.

Hypogonadism need not be treated in life-limiting disorders. Testosterone and estrogen therapy need not be started or may be stopped.

3.5 Pituitary Tumors

3.5.1 Prolactinoma

A prolactinoma leads to excess prolactin secretion with symptoms of galactorrhea/amenorrhea in women and erectile dysfunction in men. Macroadenomas can also present with visual field defects if large enough to compress the optic chiasm.

Treatment with dopamine agonists needs to be continued in macroadenomas, especially sight threatening macroadenomas. Cabergoline or bromocryptine could be stopped in post-menopausal women. In patients who do not respond to either and who are in-operable, temozolomide, a chemotherapeutic alkylating agent, could be tried.

Hormonal deficiencies as a result of compression on the normal pituitary will need to be dealt with individually as explained above.

3.5.2 Acromegaly

In acromegaly, there is excessive growth hormone (GH) secretion, leading to growth of bone soft tissue. This results in enlarged hands and feet; protruding lower jaw and brow; an enlarged nose; thickened lips and wider spacing between your teeth; coarsened, enlarged facial features; coarse, oily, thickened skin; small outgrowths of skin tissue (skin tags); fatigue and muscle weakness; deepened, husky voice due to enlarged vocal cords and sinuses; severe snoring due to obstruction of the upper airway from soft tissue growth; impaired vision; headaches; enlarged tongue; pain and limited joint mobility; menstrual cycle irregularities in women; erectile dysfunction in men; enlarged liver, heart, kidneys, spleen, and other organs; increased chest size (barrel chest).

This condition is often diagnosed late and morbidity and mortality rates are high, particularly as a result of the associated cardiovascular, cerebrovascular, respiratory complications, metabolic, bone, and endocrine complications and malignancies. Hypopituitarism may also develop as a result of the tumor mass.

Medical management would be the treatment of choice in a subgroup of patients. These are patients who are not willing for surgery, are not fit enough for surgery, patients in whom the tumor is deemed in-operable, patients with postoperative relapse.

Medical management is with somatostatin analogues (Octreotide, Lanreotide, Pasireotide) and dopamine analogues (Bromocryptine, Cabergoline) and GH receptor antagonist (Pegvisomant).

4 Summary

In summary, palliative care of endocrine disorders and diabetes focuses on symptom control, as is more appropriate in life-limiting conditions and towards the end-of-life. The monitoring of diabetes and the endocrine condition per se should be kept to the minimum and aims to guide treatment towards symptom control only, reducing adverse effects and maintaining quality of life.

References

Bollerslev J, Rejnmark L, Marcocci C, Shoback DM, Sitges-Serra A, van Biesen W, et al. European Society of Endocrinology Clinical Guideline: treatment of chronic hypoparathyroidism in adults. Eur J Endocrinol. 2015;173(2):G1–G20.

Boscaro M, Benato M, Mantero F. Effect of bromocriptine in pituitary-dependent Cushing's syndrome. Clin. Endocrinol. (Oxf.). 1983;19(4):485–91.

Crane MG, Harris JJ. Effect of spironolactone in hypertensive patients. Am J Med Sci. 1970;260:311–30.

End of life Diabetes care. Clinical care recommendations 2nd ed. 2013.

Griebeler ML, Kearns AE, Ryu E, Thapa P, Hathcock MA, Melton LJ 3rd, et al. Thiazide-associated hypercalcemia: incidence and association with primary hyperparathyroidism over two decades. J Clin Endocrinol Metab. 2016;101(3):1166–73.

Jeffcoate WJ, Rees LH, Tomlin S, Jones AE, Edwards CR, Besser GM. Metyrapone in long-term management of Cushing's disease. Br Med J. 1977;2(6081):215–7.

Jonklaas J, Bianco AC, Bauer AJ, Burman KD, Cappola AR, Celi FS, Cooper S, Kim W, Peeters P, Rosenthal MS, Sawka AM. Guidelines for the Treatment of Hypothyroidism: Prepared by the American Thyroid Association Task Force on Thyroid Hormone Replacement. Thyroid. 2014;24(12):1670–751.

Krakoff J, Koch CA, Calis KA, Alexander RH, Nieman LK. Use of a parenteral propylene glycol-containing etomidate preparation for the long-term management of ectopic Cushing's syndrome. J Clin Endocrinol Metab. 2001;86(9):4104–8.

Lim PO, Young WF, MacDonald TM. A review of the medical treatment of primary aldosteronism. J Hypertens. 2001;19:353–61.

Liu JK, Fleseriu M, Delashaw JB Jr, Ciric IS, Couldwell WT. Treatment options for Cushing disease after unsuccessful transsphenoidal surgery. Neurosurg Focus. 2007;23(3):E8.

Rizk A, Honegger J, Milian M, Psaras T. Treatment options in Cushing's disease. Clin Med Insights Oncol. 2012;6:75–84.

Rose BD. Diuretics. Kidney Int. 1991;39:336–52.

Sonino N, Boscaro M, Paoletta A, Mantero F, Ziliotto D. Ketoconazole treatment in Cushing's syndrome: experience in 34 patients. Clin Endocrinol. 1991;35(4):347–52.

Sonino N, Boscaro M. Medical therapy for Cushing's disease. Endocrinol Metab Clin N Am. 1999;28(1): 211–22.

Ross DS, Burch B, Cooper David S, Greenlee MC, Laurberg P, Maia AL, Rivkees SA, Samuels M, Sosa JA, Stan MN, Walter MA. 2016 American Thyroid Association Guidelines for Diagnosis and Management of Hyperthyroidism and Other Causes of Thyrotoxicosis. Thyroid. 2016;26(10):1343–421.

Takats KI, Szabolcs I, Foldes J, Foldes I, Ferencz A, Rimanoczy E, Goth M, Dohan O, Kovacs L, Szilagyi G. The efficacy of long term thyrostatic treatment in elderly patients with toxic nodular goitre compared to radioiodine therapy with different doses. Exp Clin Endocrinol Diabetes. 1999;107:70–4.

Palliative Care in Chronic Illness and Multimorbidity

66

Tim Luckett, Meera Agar, and Jane J. Phillips

Contents

T. Luckett
Improving Palliative, Aged and Chronic Care through Clinical Research and Translation, Faculty of Health, University of Technology Sydney, Sydney, NSW, Australia
e-mail: Tim.Luckett@uts.edu.au; tim.luckett@uts.edu.au

M. Agar (✉)
Faculty of Health, University of Technology Sydney, Ultimo, NSW, Australia

South Western Sydney Clinical School, School of Medicine, University of New South Wales (UNSW), Sydney, NSW, Australia

Ingham Institute for Applied Medical Research, Liverpool, NSW, Australia

Palliative Care Service, South Western Sydney Local Health District, Sydney, NSW, Australia
e-mail: Meera.Agar@uts.edu.au

J. J. Phillips
Faculty of Health, Improving Palliative, Aged and Chronic Care Through Clinical Research and Translation, University of Technology Sydney, Ultimo, NSW, Australia

School of Nursing, University of Notre Dame Australia-Sydney, Darlinghurst, NSW, Australia
e-mail: Jane.Phillips@uts.edu.au

R. D. MacLeod, L. Van den Block (eds.), *Textbook of Palliative Care*,
https://doi.org/10.1007/978-3-319-77740-5_64

Abstract

Extended chronic phases of life-limiting illness and increasing multimorbidity present growing challenges that require a new approach to healthcare. A population-based approach is needed to harmonize policies, systems and services relating to chronic and palliative care. Partnerships are needed between different healthcare disciplines and specialties, and between health services and communities. Technology is likely to play an increasingly important role in transfer of information (including advance care plans) and enabling coordination of care. During periods of stability, patients and families should be actively involved in keeping well and helped to "hope for the best while preparing for the worst" to support sustained coping. A rapid response is needed to clinical events that helps people return to stability and takes preventive action against future events wherever possible. Transitions between chronic and terminal phases of illness and different settings (community, residential and hospital) need focal support to prevent people "falling through the gaps." The optimal timing of referral to specialist palliative care services is the subject of ongoing debate and research. Consumer advocacy may play an important role in raising awareness and advocating for appropriate resourcing and changes to policy and legislation.

1 Introduction

Aging of the population and medical advances are leading to ongoing changes to the community who have palliative care needs. Illnesses that once were a major cause of sudden death have become progressive and chronic in nature, resulting in many people living with extended and unpredictable cycles of wellness and disability. With increased longevity, people are also accumulating more than one chronic illness, together with associated symptoms and treatment side effects and progressive disability. This changing epidemiology demands innovative models of care. This chapter will use the World Health Organization (WHO) Framework for Innovative Care for Chronic Conditions to consider the implications of these changes for a needs-based approach to care from the perspectives of the patient/family, health organization, wider community, and policy.

2 World Health Organization (WHO) Framework for Innovative Care for Chronic Conditions

The WHO Framework for Innovative Care for Chronic Conditions (ICCC) is the most widely accepted framework for chronic care (World Health Organization (WHO) 2002). This framework identifies that people with chronic illness and their families require support not only from formal healthcare services but also their communities and the wider policy environment (see Fig. 1). Healthcare enablers are focused on promoting continuity and coordination, organizing and equipping healthcare teams and communities, using information systems to support coordination and communication, and supporting patients and families to self-manage health within the context of everyday life. This framework provides a useful lens for considering the supports required

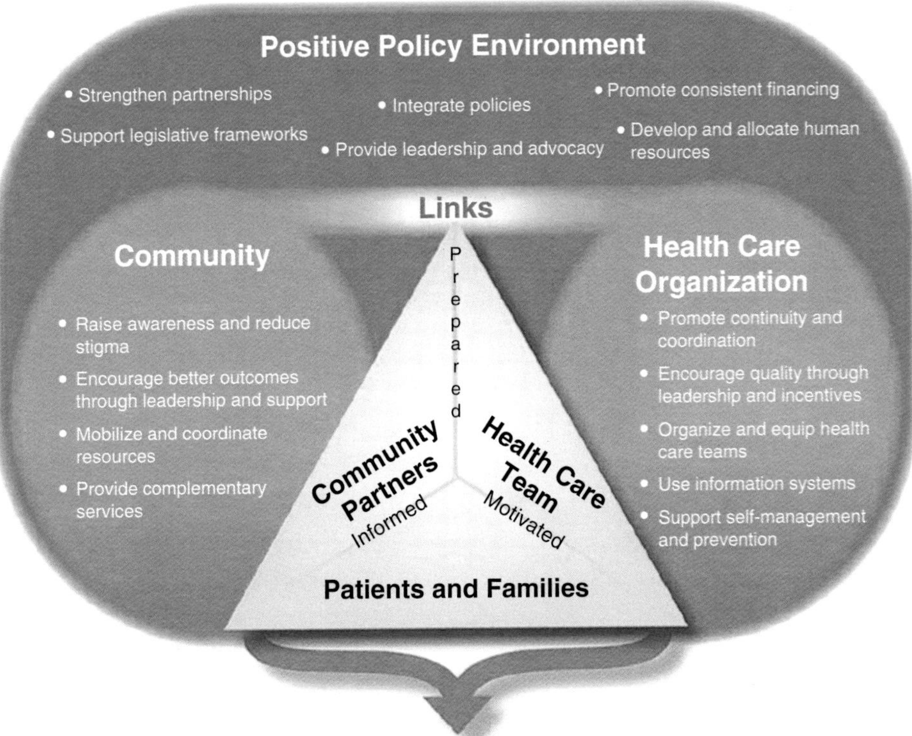

Fig. 1 World Health Organization's Framework for Innovative Care for Chronic Conditions (World Health Organization (WHO) 2002)

by patients and families during the chronic phase of a life-limiting illness.

3 Defining Chronic Illness and Multimorbidity

3.1 Chronic Life-Limiting Illness

Treatment advances are enabling people with life-limiting illness to live for many years longer than previous generations (Canadian Hospice Palliative Care Association 2013). Life-limiting illnesses that are now frequently described as chronic include respiratory, heart, cerebrovascular, and kidney disease, HIV/AIDS, dementia and other neurodegenerative disorders (e.g., Parkinson's disease), and many types of cancer. Worldwide, the most common chronic life-limiting illness is chronic obstructive pulmonary disease (COPD), affecting 26.6 million people in 2004 (World Health Organization 2004). An analysis from the UK found cancer to be the most costly for healthcare services but dementia to have the greatest social care costs (Luengo-Fernandez et al. 2012).

For some of these diseases, such as dementia, medical advances have led to incremental rather than exponential benefits. But for cancer in particular, developments over the past decade in targeted therapies have been profound. This has led to more recent and explicit consideration of what is meant by "chronic" for cancer than for other life-limiting illnesses. While references to cancer as a chronic illness go back more than half a century, definitions have changed over time to reflect developments both in treatment and healthcare (Harley et al. 2015; McCorkle et al. 2011; Phillips and Currow 2010). The most recent definition by Harley et al. (2015) refers to a "chronic phase" that is finite, unpredictable, and associated with a burden of symptoms, treatment side effects, and medical appointments (see Box 1).

Box 1 Working definition of the chronic phase of cancer provided by Harley et al. (2015), p. 344)

- A diagnosis of active, advanced, or metastatic cancer that cannot be cured.
- Active anticancer treatments are available that can lead to symptom control, slow disease progression, or prolong life.
- The patient is not considered to be at the end stage of cancer.
- The chronic cancer phase ends when the cancer no longer responds to treatment and there are no treatment options available that are expected to slow disease progression or prolong life. Patients will leave the chronic phase when they are expected to have only months to live.

The expansion of genomics, proteomics and metabolomics will continue to impact on improved cancer diagnosis, prognostication and treatment decisions (Roychowdhury and Chinnaiyan 2016). In the future, advances are likely to result in better matching between therapeutic agents and the molecular characteristics of the individual patient. Currently, however, the new generation of advanced cancer treatments are available for only some tumor types and have variable efficacy between individuals. For many, treatment response leads to recovery commensurate with prior functional status. However, for others, adverse effects such as febrile neutropenia can sometimes confer a similar trajectory to that traditionally associated with heart and lung failure (see Fig. 2).

Advances in treatments for heart and lung failure have also extended life and increased the variability in trajectories, decreasing the likelihood of acute events but often at the expense of significant disability. The field of mechanical circulatory support for heart disease has seen particular growth, with important developments in pacemakers, implantable cardioverter defibrillators (ICDs), and ventricular assist devices (VADs). Most recently, VADs have transitioned from being "bridge to transplantation" devices to destination therapy for critically ill patients with heart failure, allowing individuals to live at home (Abraham and Smith 2013). While organ transplant success rates have improved and eligibility criteria have expanded, those with multimorbidity are less likely to benefit, and an inadequate supply of organs means that many people die on the waiting list. Emergent developments in dialysis include wearable artificial kidneys that may lead to much less interruption of everyday functioning during dialysis.

The healthcare needs conferred by benefits and burdens associated with expanding chronic phases of life-limiting illnesses will be discussed in the next section, which is concerned with the "healthcare organization" component of the WHO's ICCC Framework.

3.2 Multimorbidity

In the absence of a clear definition, the term "multimorbidity" is typically operationalized as the coexistence of two or more long-term health conditions (National Institute for Health and Care Excellence 2016). The related term "comorbidity" assumes that a particular condition is the main focus and refers to each "additional co-existing ailment" (Feinstein 1970, p. 455). Distinctions between constructs such as "health condition" or "ailment" and developmental disorders (e.g., learning disability), symptoms (e.g., chronic pain), functional status (e.g., cognitive impairment), geriatric syndromes (e.g., frailty, falls), sensory impairment, and alcohol/substance misuse vary between conceptualizations; sometimes, it may also be difficult to distinguish these based on aetiology. Multimorbidity in the context of chronic life-limiting illness may either refer to more than one life-limiting disease (e.g., lung cancer and COPD) or else to diseases that have potential to become life-limiting (e.g., chronic renal disease) or non-life-limiting diseases (e.g., skin conditions) presenting comorbidly with a life-limiting illness. Chronic illnesses that are not normally life-limiting but may increase symptom burden and the complexity of care needs include diabetes, musculoskeletal disease, and mental health disorders.

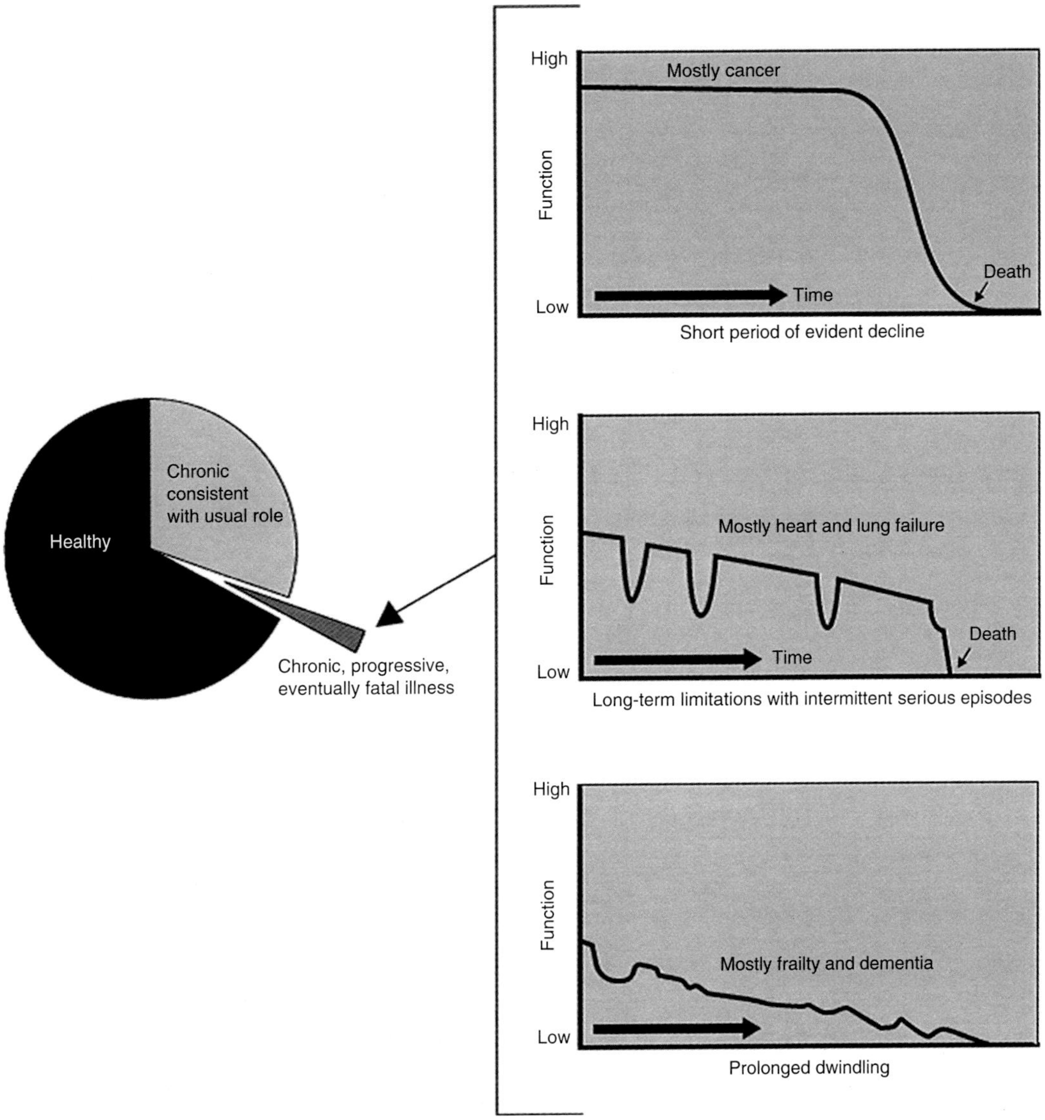

Fig. 2 Chronic illness in the elderly typically follows three trajectories (Lynn and Adamson 2003). Note that adverse effects associated with new treatments for some advanced cancer types mean the trajectory can sometimes resemble "long-term limitations with intermittent serious episodes"

Estimates of the prevalence of multimorbidity in clinical populations have varied from 20% to 98% depending on the population and definition of morbidity, but are generally more than 50% – higher than the prevalence of any single chronic disease (Marengoni et al. 2011). Multimorbidity has consistently been associated with higher age, female sex, and lower socioeconomic status. Multimorbidity is also increasing in prevalence, with the US National Health Interview Survey data collected over two time periods demonstrating a 37% increase in multimorbidity in adults aged 65 years of age and older between 1999–2000 and 2009–2010 based on self-reports of two or more of nine listed conditions (hypertension, heart disease, diabetes, cancer, stroke, chronic bronchitis, emphysema, current asthma, and kidney disease) (Freid et al. 2012). Increases over time were especially notable in hypertension, diabetes, and cancer. Multimorbidities involving life-limiting illness identified as common in either this study or others have included hypertension combined with heart disease or cancer, and angina with asthma and COPD.

Measurement of multi- or comorbidity has tended to focus on relative burden (de Groot et al. 2003). Many such measures weight comorbidities according to their association with mortality. However, the burden for any given condition is highly variable, especially where the additional impact of each new morbidity is synergistic with others, resulting in greater overall burden than expected based on simple accumulation (Verbrugge et al. 1989). Understanding the mechanisms by which these synergies occur is a priority for future research because of its potential for informing which interventions may offer the most cost-effective opportunities for improvement in outcomes.

4 Elements of the WHO's Framework for Innovative Care for Chronic Conditions as Applied to Chronic Life-Limiting Illness and Multimorbidity

4.1 Healthcare Organization

4.1.1 Self-Management

The problems experienced by patients and families in each of the domains of palliative care – physical, psychological, social, and spiritual (World Health Organization 2002) – will vary according to a large range of factors, including the life-limiting illness in question, comorbidities, living situation, occupational roles, financial status and social support (Murray et al. 2005). However, for most people most of the time, support will be delivered within a self-management paradigm. Self-management is best promoted within a partnership or collaborative model, in which patients are considered experts on the experience of illness and its relationship to their daily life, while health professionals assume a coaching role aimed at building confidence in one's ability to manage ("self-efficacy") as well as necessary skills themselves (McCorkle et al. 2011). As well as practical aptitude in disease and symptom management, self-management skills include more generic abilities in: problem-solving; decision-making; finding and using information, services, and other resources; and building further partnerships with health professionals as needed (Lorig and Holman 2003). In addition to benefits to quality of life from improved symptom and disease management, development of self-efficacy has itself been associated with a range of positive psychosocial outcomes, perhaps because of an increased sense of control (Marks et al. 2005).

Self-Management in the Context of Multiple Comorbidities

Limited evidence is available for self-management interventions designed specifically for people with multiple comorbidities. However, a layered approach may be required where a foundation of generic skills is developed alongside skills in managing each disease and its interactions with others (see Fig. 3). An initial focus on each separate disease should be aimed at helping patients better understand the processes and consequences of each before considering the reasons and ways that management needs to be modified to accommodate interactions between symptoms and side effects from other illnesses. Developing an understanding of this kind is needed to identify safety considerations and clarify which aspects of the self-management plan are most important. Rather than expecting patients to "comply with doctor's orders," the partnership model of care supports patients in developing their own management goals and making informed choices among management options according to their priorities and preferences. Regardless of whether doctors are collaborative or paternalistic, patients will often seek participation and control by modulating the medication dose to find an appropriate balance between symptoms and side effects (Luckett et al. 2013) or by using complementary and alternative medicines in addition to, or in place of, those prescribed (Bishop et al. 2007). Encouraging open, honest communication about these decisions will not only improve management safety and quality but also foster patients'

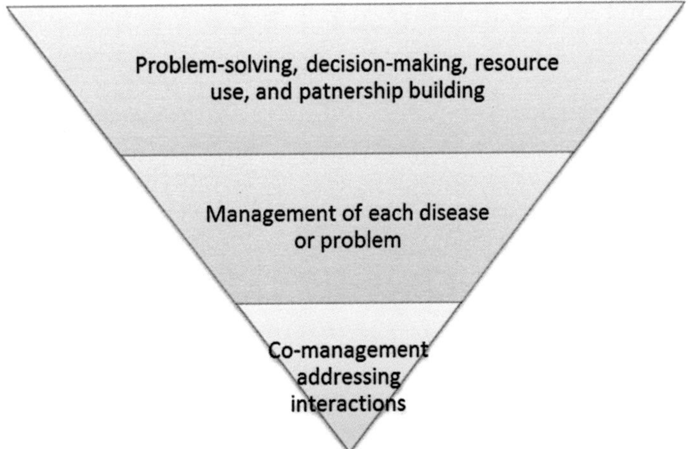

Fig. 3 Suggested foci for self-management support in people with multimorbidity, starting with generic skills identified by Lorig and Holman (2003)

feelings of participation, control, and shared responsibility in "co-producing" their own healthcare and health (Batalden et al. 2016). A partnership approach is especially essential in the context of multimorbidity because the feasibility of treatment for any given condition often becomes questionable due to competing priorities and burden from managing others (Petrillo and Ritchie 2016). Guideline recommendations also note that treatments approved for individual health conditions should be used with caution because the evidence on which approval is based has often been collected in samples specifically excluding those with multimorbidities (National Institute for Health and Care Excellence 2016).

Self-Management in the Context of Palliative Care

Self-management pertains not only to the medical aspects of illness and symptoms but also to managing changes in everyday functioning and the psychosocial consequences of chronic illness (Corbin and Strauss 1988). Unpredictability of prognosis and daily fluctuations in symptoms have led people living with chronic life-limiting illness to liken the experience to being on a "roller coaster" (Brannstrom et al. 2006). Even in the terminal phase, patients and families may continue to hope for a cure (Clayton et al. 2008); in the chronic phase, there are likely to be several transitions in hope as new treatments succeed or fail and symptoms worsen or abate. The "long-haul" nature of the chronic phase also means that maintaining a degree of normalcy is likely to be a priority for many people (Ohman et al. 2003). Where there are periods of stability, daily concerns may shift away from health altogether either because life events take precedence or people actively seek respite from the "medicalization" of their lives (Mendes 2015). However, even during periods where people are well enough to carry on everyday roles such as working and parenting, there may be insidious impacts from illness. For example, healthcare costs can sometimes mean that patients have to extend their working hours at a time when they might otherwise be reducing them to enjoy other aspects of life while they remain well (Zafar et al. 2013). This challenge is likely to become increasingly common even in countries with universal healthcare because of the delay in approval for new treatments and their high associated costs. The psychological impact on dependent children may also be especially complex during the chronic phase because of periodic reversals in the role of parents as the giver versus recipient of care and associated expectations placed on children (Kennedy and Lloyd-Williams 2009). While evidence is lacking, it may also be that "false hope" during periods of wellness and consequent disruption of anticipatory grief can have a negative impact on bereavement outcomes after a parent dies.

4.1.2 Advance Care Planning

Psychosocial impacts of the above kinds require a balanced approach to support that empowers patients and families to self-manage their response to the challenges of chronic illness by helping them "hope for the best while preparing for the worst" (Feuz 2012). Evidence suggests that patients and families tend to welcome honest and accurate information communicated with empathy and understanding. Formally structuring this through a process of advance care planning (ACP) will enable information to be contextualized within an individualized discussion regarding patient and family values and preferences for the future. Clinicians are often reluctant to discuss ACP with people before the terminal phase for fear of undermining hope and demotivating self-management (Luckett et al. 2014b). However, when appropriately facilitated, ACP is viewed by patients as empowering rather than damaging to hope (Davison and Simpson 2006). Delaying ACP may also mean that patients lack time to thoroughly consider and discuss their wishes and risk a loss of decision-making capacity, especially for people with organ failure or respiratory disease who may face a sudden clinical crisis or increasing cognitive impairment (Shen et al. 2016).

Key considerations for ACP during the chronic phase concern the unpredictability of the disease course and likelihood that preferences for life-sustaining treatment may change dramatically in response to clinical events. These considerations warrant a "slow start" and iterative approach to ACP that:

- Helps patients consider the relative possibilities of a range of future scenarios that may each become more or less likely over time
- Enables "death awareness" to develop gradually, allowing time for adjustment (Sanders et al. 2008)
- Ensures that ensuing directives are both well considered and current

Approaches should be aimed at anticipating, identifying, and providing focal support during transitions from the chronic to terminal phases of life-limiting illness, which may otherwise lack the same attention as diagnosis. A good example of this kind of transition concerns the decision to withdraw medicines aimed at treating underlying disease. Advance discussion regarding the net benefits of continuing or discontinuing such medications as goals of care change may help frame this decision as a positive choice rather than "giving up" and decrease the likelihood that patients continue medications inappropriately (Reeve et al. 2017).

Patients with organ failure commencing life-sustaining treatment require special consideration for ACP. The dynamic ratio of benefit to adverse effects for treatments like dialysis needs careful discussion, especially in the context of increasing age and multimorbidity (Dasgupta and Rayner 2009). Patients awaiting transplant and their families will also require specific information and support to deal with uncertainties regarding organ availability and transplant outcomes (Larson and Curtis 2006). Finally, ACP for people with heart failure may need to include consideration of resuscitation status and device therapy at the end of life. Recent studies found that the majority (85%) of ICD recipients believed that "switching off" the device equated to immediate death (Stromberg et al. 2014), and few realized that almost a third (31%) of dying patients with ICDs receive shock therapy in the last 24 hours of life (Kinch Westerdahl et al. 2014). Shock therapy at the end of life is likely to cause discomfort to patients and distress to family, highlighting the importance of developing a deactivation plan.

While self-management and patient empowerment through choice are key principles in the care of people with chronic life-limiting illness, it is important to recognize that:

- Some patients will want more of an active role than others
- There is a risk of overburdening patients and families
- Caution is needed to avoid any sense of blame being attached to perceived failures in self-management or "bad" choices (Thorne et al. 2016)

4.1.3 Services and Coordination

Care Coordination

Care coordination is the most significant challenge in delivering healthcare to people with chronic life-limiting illness and multimorbidity. Unlike people at the end of life, those in the chronic phase are likely to require treatment from one or more specialties focused on their underlying condition – for example, oncology, cardiology, or respiratory medicine. At the same time, care for people with multimorbidity requires a shift from single disease practices to a patient-centered framework that recognizes the broad range of services that are likely to be needed, the burden faced by the patient and family both from the illness itself and its management, and the duration of time people will be living with the illness (National Institute for Health and Care Excellence 2016; Petrillo and Ritchie 2016). The complexity of care needs and difficulty in successfully integrating care associated with multimorbidity is evidenced by the higher rates of unplanned and emergency care seen in this population (Lehnert et al. 2011; Marengoni et al. 2011).

Case management is the service element with perhaps the most evidence for coordinating care and improving outcomes: in chronic illness (Ouwens et al. 2005); during the chronic phase of life-limiting illness (Aiken et al. 2006); for people with multimorbidity (Smith et al. 2012); and at the end of life (Luckett et al. 2014a). Case management has been found cost-effective for older people living in the community over 1 year due to avoided hospitalizations and GP visits (Black 2007). However, cost-effectiveness for people with chronic life-limiting illness has yet to be evaluated and is likely to be a "moving target" as the chronic phase becomes further extended through medical advancements in the future. Given the likelihood of exacerbations and decline in people with life-limiting illness, case management needs to pay special attention to timely prevention, response to acute events, and support for transitions to and from hospital as needed, in addition to helping patients maintain health and functioning during periods of stability.

A special challenge is faced by healthcare services trying to provide integrated care to people with chronic life-limiting illness and multimorbidity living in nursing homes. Models tested by research have typically involved in-reach from a specialized healthcare team either to deliver direct care or to train and support clinical champions within the nursing home (Goodman et al. 2016). To effect more sustainable change, models of care are needed that value and motivate nursing home personnel, support joint priority setting, and foster ongoing relational working. Successful models will likely need to make use of systems and processes for encouraging regular communication and shared decision-making, such as case conferencing (Phillips et al. 2013). Systems also need to be in place for formally monitoring changes in residents' needs and communicating information between nursing homes and acute care during transitions.

Managing the Transition from Chronic to Palliative Care

Changes in the trajectories of life-limiting illnesses mean that the optimal timing of transition from a chronic to palliative approach to care may be becoming increasingly difficult to identify and will vary between individuals (Burge et al. 2012). For many people, the optimal transition may be gradual and draw on elements of both approaches concurrently for much of the trajectory (see Fig. 4).

Involvement of Specialist Palliative Care Services

While palliative care has traditionally focused on the last 6 to 12 months of life, its ethos has much to offer those with complex care needs at any stage of the disease trajectory (Agar et al. 2015). Palliative care has an established philosophy that aims to help people focus on "living with" rather than "dying from" advanced illness. It focuses on the whole person rather than disease and is needs-based rather than discipline-based in its approach to delivering care. Indeed, if we assume that palliative care should be assigned according to needs rather than prognosis, it may be that a palliative approach is relevant from diagnosis onward for patients with life-limiting illness of any kind (Beernaert et al. 2016).

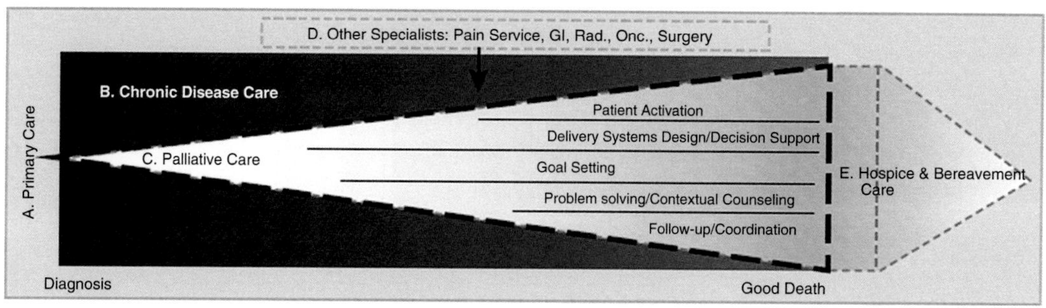

Fig. 4 Model of concurrent chronic disease palliative care for people with cancer (Canadian Hospice Palliative Care Association 2013, p. 5)

At the same time, it is important to distinguish between palliative care as an approach to care versus specialist palliative care services (SPC). Worldwide, resourcing of SPC is insufficient to enable its provision to everyone with life-limiting illness from the time of diagnosis; nor is this necessarily desirable (Glare and Virik 2001). In Australia, the New South Wales Department of Health (2007) has identified three populations of people with life-limiting illness with differing levels of need regarding input from SPC, namely, (A) those whose needs can be met almost entirely within primary care, (B) those who are predominantly managed within primary care but who experience exacerbations that require support or intervention from SPC, and (C) those with complex needs who require direct and intensive intervention from SPC. It seems likely that people in the chronic phase of life-limiting illness will generally be included in the first or second of these categories and will also be spending most of their time in the community rather than in the hospital. For these people, the responsibility for care coordination will likely sit with primary care. Indeed, it could be said that primary care health professionals are themselves the "specialists" in managing chronic illness.

The question of appropriate timing for SPC referral is the subject of much ongoing debate. Interest in "early" referral was sparked by the 2010 publication of a landmark trial which found this contributed not only to quality of life but also survival for people with advanced lung cancer (Temel et al. 2010). However, the mechanism by which early referral might have contributed to this outcome remains unclear (Irwin et al. 2013), and little research is available on referral even earlier in the disease trajectory or for other disease groups. Published guidance has tended to make use of the question "would you be surprised if this patient died in the next 6 or 12 months?" taking into account disease progression and general indicators such as functional decline, weight loss, and unplanned admissions (Boyd and Murray 2010). However, the UK Gold Standards Framework has acknowledged increasing difficulties with predicting prognosis and now advocates "instinctive, anticipatory and insurance-type thinking" which lowers the threshold at which end-of-life care planning and referral to SPC should be undertaken (National Gold Standards framework 2011). Based on this reasoning, there may be many patients with chronic illness and multimorbidity not traditionally considered life-limiting who might meet criteria for – and benefit from – referral to SPC, including people with diabetes and nonhealing foot disease (Calam et al. 2012).

A special role for SPC in the care of people with multimorbidity is supported by research suggesting that cost savings may increase with the number of comorbidities (May et al. 2016). However, further discussion is needed both within SPC and across specialties to better define the parameters of optimal SPC service provision and, if necessary, inform advocacy for funding to increase capacity. Promotion of earlier referral to SPC would also need to change perceptions among people with chronic illness and health professionals that palliative care is reserved for people who are imminently dying (Mason et al. 2016). US research suggests that both patients and health professionals may favor the term supportive rather than palliative care even during the terminal phase (Maciasz et al. 2013). While a change in terminology of this kind is controversial in the context of end-of-life care, the fact that supportive care is currently used in oncology to refer to management of problems associated with active treatment suggests it may be a good fit for the chronic phase of life-limiting illness.

4.1.4 Information Systems

The WHO's ICCC Framework identifies information systems as being critical in organizing care for people with chronic illness. In the context of life-limiting illness, these need to include systems for sharing up-to-date information about ACP at the point of care. Transitions between care settings (e.g., aged care and hospital) are especially notorious for hampering communication about ACP as well as current care plans, test results, and medication management (Coleman 2003). Little evidence is available to support particular information system approaches, although several countries have implemented national patient healthcare information systems that enable patients to upload and share ACP information along with other medical records if they so wish. Uptake of these systems to date has been limited, and little research has been conducted on the impact on processes and outcomes of care. A recent systematic review of personal health records found evidence of benefit for chronic conditions such as HIV, asthma, and diabetes but none for cancer or multiple sclerosis (Price et al. 2015). Benefit seemed to be related to personal health records' potential for monitoring and informing self-management.

4.2 Community Perspective

The WHO ICCC Framework recognizes the need to build community capacity to support people with chronic illness in addition to formal health services. Recently, a global movement called Compassionate Communities has emerged with the aim of developing community "death literacy" and capacity to support people who are dying and their families. The movement is based on a premise that, compared with previous generations, modern communities tend to have less awareness about death and dying and weaker local networks to provide support in times of need. Research has consistently found the public to have a limited understanding of advanced illness and palliative care (Cox et al. 2013).

Initiatives aimed at improving death literacy include those promoted by the Compassionate Cities program which include "death cafe" and "death over dinner" events where people talk about their experiences of bereavement or caring for someone who is dying or death and dying more generally, visual and performing art projects, initiatives within workplaces and schools to raise awareness, and memorial events. Initiatives of this kind may be run by local government, healthcare organizations, or citizen groups. One of the largest and longest running public health and advocacy campaigns of this kind has been the Project on Death in America (PDIA) run by the nonprofit foundation, the Open Society Institute (Aulino and Foley 2001), which from 1994 to 2001 funded 94 projects to a sum of US$34 million.

Initiatives developing community capacity to support people who are dying and their families have been primarily aimed at enabling people to die at home through establishment and support of social networks that meet practical needs (e.g., preparing food, shopping), sharing knowledge about services, and, in some areas, healthcare professionals to provide training to help carers deliver care (Sallnow et al. 2016).The optimal interface between formal healthcare and community initiatives of this kind is the subject of ongoing debate. A central tenet of the Compassionate Communities movement is that care for people with life-limiting illness is "everybody's business." For some, a goal of demedicalizing death and dying is a natural corollary. Healthcare services may be viewed as "essential but not central" to care for people who are dying, with some arguing that their role is primarily to equip communities with the skills to care for themselves, providing as little direct intervention as possible (Abel 2017). This view differs from the partnership model to self-management introduced above in that service provision is seen as community-centered rather than patient- or even family-centered.

It is unclear whether public awareness has kept pace with changes in disease trajectories, but it seems likely that this will be similar to death literacy in needing focal education and support to increase community capacity. Nongovernment organizations (NGOs) (e.g., Macmillan Cancer Support [UK], Lung Foundation Australia) may play an important role in raising awareness and advocating for resources to meet the needs of this population. Many NGOs already provide support well-suited to the needs of people during the chronic phase of life-limiting illness, including telephone helplines, wellness programs, and peer support networks. These interventions have potential to respond more quickly than healthcare systems to changing illness trajectories. They also present immediate opportunities for community engagement and leadership.

4.3 Policy Perspective

Community initiatives form just one part of a public health approach long since advocated for both palliative and chronic care (Institute of Medicine 2012; Sepulveda et al. 2002). A population-level approach that integrates policies in these two domains is needed to ensure coherence, efficiency, and progress toward addressing disparities in access to services and outcomes (Murray et al. 2009). A population-based approach will also distil the special requirements of the burgeoning population of people with chronic life-limiting illness and how these differ from palliative and chronic care populations more generally. Surveillance measures are also needed to measure progress, including a composite of patient-reported measures (e.g., life satisfaction and well-being), healthcare system (e.g., access), and population-level measures (e.g., clinical, access, and funding policies) (Institute of Medicine 2012). Cost-effectiveness analyses are needed that compare different public health models and take into account societal costs and benefits at a population level (Dzingina and Higginson 2015).

The ICCC Framework emphasizes the need to support chronic care through policies aimed at appropriate financing and partnership building. Many of the world's health systems remain geared toward a single-disease model rather than integrated care (Bayliss et al. 2007). Funding models are needed that acknowledge multidisciplinary contributions and clinician time spent on preventive healthcare, psychosocial support, and self-management. In practice, this may mean moving remuneration away from a fee-for-service basis to the patient or population level (Oliver-Baxter et al. 2013). This approach is being adopted by a new Australian initiative called "Health Care Homes," which aims to integrate care for people with chronic and complex care needs across community and acute settings. Bundled payments, made to general practices and Aboriginal Medical Services, can be managed between services as needed and are responsive to changes in patients' needs over time, making this model especially suited to people with chronic life-limiting disease whose needs are likely to fluctuate.

Legislative frameworks presenting a barrier to outcomes for people with chronic life-limiting illness include those relating to approval and funding of new treatments. The need for these frameworks to be more responsive to emerging evidence has become an increasing focus in the popular press. Consumer advocacy is likely to be key in driving changes to policy and legislation to better align these with the needs of people with chronic life-limiting illness, as it has been in recognizing other patient populations, such as cancer survivors.

5 Conclusion and Summary

This review of the changing nature of life-limiting illness and associated healthcare needs with reference to the WHO's Framework for Innovative Care for Chronic Conditions shows the need for advocating a population-based approach aimed at harmonizing policies, systems, and services relating to chronic and palliative care. Elements of the

ICCC model requiring special support include healthcare coordination and community awareness and capacity building. More evidence and debate is needed to inform the question of optimal timing for referral to specialist palliative care services. NGOs and consumer advocacy will be expected to play an important role in advocating for appropriate resourcing and changes to policy and legislation.

References

Abel J. How to build compassionate communities at the end of life. Compassionate communities symposium; 20–21 Feb; Sydney 2017.

Abraham WT, Smith SA. Devices in the management of advanced, chronic heart failure. Nat Rev Cardiol. 2013;10(2):98–110.

Agar M, Luckett T, Phillips J. Role of palliative care in survivorship. Cancer Forum. 2015;39(2):90–4.

Aiken LS, Butner J, Lockhart CA, Volk-Craft BE, Hamilton G, Williams FG. Outcome evaluation of a randomized trial of the PhoenixCare intervention: program of case management and coordinated care for the seriously chronically ill. J Palliat Med. 2006;9(1):111–26.

Aulino F, Foley K. The project on death in America. J R Soc Med. 2001;94(9):492–5.

Batalden M, Batalden P, Margolis P, Seid M, Armstrong G, Opipari-Arrigan L, Hartung H. Coproduction of healthcare service. BMJ Qual Saf. 2016;25(7):509–17.

Bayliss EA, Bosworth HB, Noel PH, Wolff JL, Damush TM, McIver L. Supporting self-management for patients with complex medical needs: recommendations of a working group. Chronic Illn. 2007;3 (2):167–75.

Beernaert K, Deliens L, De Vleminck A, Devroey D, Pardon K, Block LV, Cohen J. Is there a need for early palliative care in patients with life-limiting illnesses? Interview study with patients about experienced care needs from diagnosis onward. Am J Hosp Palliat Care. 2016;33(5):489–97.

Bishop FL, Yardley L, Lewith GT. A systematic review of beliefs involved in the use of complementary and alternative medicine. J Health Psychol. 2007;12(6):851–67.

Black DA. Case management for elderly people in the community. BMJ. 2007;334(7583):3–4.

Boyd K, Murray SA. Recognising and managing key transitions in end of life care. BMJ. 2010;341:c4863.

Brannstrom M, Ekman I, Norberg A, Boman K, Strandberg G. Living with severe chronic heart failure in palliative advanced home care. Eur J Cardiovasc Nurs. 2006;5 (4):295–302.

Burge F, Lawson B, Mitchell G. How to move to a palliative approach to care for people with multimorbidity. BMJ. 2012;345:e6324.

Calam MJ, Gwynn A, Perkins P. The role of specialist palliative care in managing patients with multimorbidity. BMJ Support Palliat Care. 2012;2(1):48–50.

Canadian Hospice Palliative Care Association. Integrating a palliative approach into the management of chronic, life-threatening diseases: who, how and when? Ottawa: CHPCA; 2013.

Clayton JM, Hancock K, Parker S, Butow PN, Walder S, Carrick S, Currow D, Ghersi D, Glare P, Hagerty R, Olver IN, Tattersall MHN. Sustaining hope when communicating with terminally ill patients and their families: a systematic review. Psychooncology. 2008;17 (7):641–59.

Coleman EA. Falling through the cracks: challenges and opportunities for improving transitional care for persons with continuous complex care needs. J Am Geriatr Soc. 2003;51(4):549–55.

Corbin J, Strauss A. Unending work and care: managing chronic illness at home. San Francisco: Jossey-Bass; 1988.

Cox K, Bird L, Arthur A, Kennedy S, Pollock K, Kumar A, Stanton W, Seymour J. Public attitudes to death and dying in the UK: a review of published literature. BMJ Support Palliat Care. 2013;3(1):37–45.

Dasgupta I, Rayner HC. In good conscience – safely withholding dialysis in the elderly. Semin Dial. 2009;22 (5):476–9.

Davison SN, Simpson C. Hope and advance care planning in patients with end stage renal disease: qualitative interview study. BMJ. 2006;333(7574):886.

de Groot V, Beckerman H, Lankhorst GJ, Bouter LM. How to measure comorbidity. A critical review of available methods. J Clin Epidemiol. 2003;56(3):221–9.

Dzingina MD, Higginson IJ. Public health and palliative care in 2015. Clin Geriatr Med. 2015;31(2):253–63.

Feinstein AR. The pre-therapeutic classification of co-morbidity in chronic disease. J Chronic Dis. 1970;23 (7):455–68.

Feuz C. Hoping for the best while preparing for the worst: a literature review of the role of hope in palliative cancer patients. J Med Imag Radiat Sci. 2012; 43:168–74.

Freid VM, Bernstein AB, Bush MA. Multiple chronic conditions among adults aged 45 and over: trends over the past 10 years. NCHS Data Brief. 2012;100:1–8.

Glare PA, Virik K. Can we do better in end-of-life care? The mixed management model and palliative care. Med J Aust. 2001;175(10):530–3.

Goodman C, Dening T, Gordon AL, Davies SL, Meyer J, Martin FC, Gladman JR, Bowman C, Victor C, Handley M, Gage H, Iliffe S, Zubair M. Effective health care for older people living and dying in care homes: a realist review. BMC Health Serv Res. 2016; 16(1):269.

Harley C, Pini S, Bartlett YK, Velikova G. Defining chronic cancer: patient experiences and self-management needs. BMJ Support Palliat Care. 2015;5(4):343–50.

Institute of Medicine. Living well with chronic illness: a call for public health action. Washington, DC: The National Academies Press; 2012.

Irwin KE, Greer JA, Khatib J, Temel JS, Pirl WF. Early palliative care and metastatic non-small cell lung cancer: potential mechanisms of prolonged survival. Chron Respir Dis. 2013;10(1):35–47.

Kennedy VL, Lloyd-Williams M. How children cope when a parent has advanced cancer. Psychooncology. 2009;18(8):886–92.

Kinch Westerdahl A, Sjöblom J, Mattiasson A-C, Rosenqvist M, Frykman V. Implantable cardioverter-defibrillator therapy before death: high risk for painful shocks at end of life. Circulation. 2014;129(4):422–9.

Larson AM, Curtis JR. Integrating palliative care for liver transplant candidates: "too well for transplant, too sick for life". JAMA. 2006;295(18):2168–76.

Lehnert T, Heider D, Leicht H, Heinrich S, Corrieri S, Luppa M, Riedel-Heller S, Konig HH. Review: health care utilization and costs of elderly persons with multiple chronic conditions. Med Care Res Rev. 2011;68 (4):387–420.

Lorig KR, Holman H. Self-management education: history, definition, outcomes, and mechanisms. Ann Behav Med. 2003;26(1):1–7.

Luckett T, Davidson PM, Green A, Boyle F, Stubbs J, Lovell M. Assessment and management of adult cancer pain: a systematic review and synthesis of recent qualitative studies aimed at developing insights for managing barriers and optimizing facilitators within a comprehensive framework of patient care. J Pain Symptom Manag. 2013;46(2):229–53.

Luckett T, Phillips J, Virdun C, Agar M, Green A, Davidson PM. Elements of effective palliative care models: a rapid review. BMC Health Serv Res. 2014a;14(136). https://doi.org/10.1186/472-6963-14-136.

Luckett T, Sellars M, Tieman J, Pollock CA, Silvester W, Butow PN, Detering KM, Brennan F, Clayton JM. Advance care planning for adults with CKD: a systematic integrative review. Am J Kidney Dis. 2014b;63 (5):761–70.

Luengo-Fernandez R, Leal J, Gray AM. UK research expenditure on dementia, heart disease, stroke and cancer: are levels of spending related to disease burden? Eur J Neurol. 2012;19(1):149–54.

Lynn J, Adamson DM. Living well at the end of life. Adapting health care to serious chronic illness in old age. Washington, DC: Rand Health; 2003.

Maciasz RM, Arnold RM, Chu E, Park SY, White DB, Vater LB, Schenker Y. Does it matter what you call it? A randomized trial of language used to describe palliative care services. Support Care Cancer. 2013;21 (12):3411–9.

Marengoni A, Angleman S, Melis R, Mangialasche F, Karp A, Garmen A, Meinow B, Fratiglioni L. Aging with multimorbidity: a systematic review of the literature. Ageing Res Rev. 2011;10(4):430–9.

Marks R, Allegrante JP, Lorig K. A review and synthesis of research evidence for self-efficacy-enhancing interventions for reducing chronic disability: implications for health education practice (part II). Health Promot Pract. 2005;6(2):148–56.

Mason B, Nanton V, Epiphaniou E, Murray SA, Donaldson A, Shipman C, Daveson BA, Harding R, Higginson IJ, Munday D, Barclay S, Dale J, Kendall M, Worth A, Boyd K. 'My body's falling apart.' Understanding the experiences of patients with advanced multimorbidity to improve care: serial interviews with patients and carers. BMJ Support Palliat Care. 2016;6(1):60–5.

May P, Garrido MM, Cassel JB, Kelley AS, Meier DE, Normand C, Stefanis L, Smith TJ, Morrison RS. Palliative care teams' cost-saving effect is larger for cancer patients with higher numbers of comorbidities. Health Aff (Millwood). 2016;35(1):44–53.

McCorkle R, Ercolano E, Lazenby M, Schulman-Green D, Schilling LS, Lorig K, Wagner EH. Self-management: enabling and empowering patients living with cancer as a chronic illness. CA Cancer J Clin. 2011;61(1):50–62.

Mendes A. Demedicalising the cardiac patient. Br J Cardiac Nurs. 2015;10:577.

Murray MA, Fiset V, Young S, Kryworuchko J. Where the dying live: a systematic review of determinants of place of end-of-life cancer care. Oncol Nurs Forum. 2009;36 (1):69–77.

Murray SA, Kendall M, Boyd K, Sheikh A. Illness trajectories and palliative care. BMJ. 2005;330(7498): 1007–11.

National Gold Standards framework. Prognostic Indicator Guidance 4th Edition. 2011 [cited Feb 22 2017]; Available from: http://www.goldstandardsframework.org.uk/cd-content/uploads/files/GeneralFiles/Prognostic Indica tor Guidance October 2011.pdf

National Institute for Health and Care Excellence. Multimorbidity: clinical assessment and management. London: NICE; 2016. https://www.nice.org.uk/guidance/ng56

Ohman M, Soderberg S, Lundman B. Hovering between suffering and enduring: the meaning of living with serious chronic illness. Qual Health Res. 2003;13 (4):528–42.

Oliver-Baxter J, Bywood P, Brown L. Integrated care: what policies support and influence integration in health care across New Zealand, England, Canada and the United States? PHCRIS policy issue review. Adelaide: Primary Health Care Research & Information Service; 2013.

Ouwens M, Wollersheim H, Hermens R, Hulscher M, Grol R. Integrated care programmes for chronically ill patients: a review of systematic reviews. Int J Qual Health Care. 2005;17(2):141–6.

Petrillo LA, Ritchie CS. The challenges of symptom management for patients with multimorbidity in research and practice: a thematic review. Prog Palliat Care. 2016;24:262–7.

Phillips JL, Currow DC. Cancer as a chronic disease. Collegian. 2010;17:47–50.

Phillips JL, West PA, Davidson PM, Agar M. Does case conferencing for people with advanced dementia living in nursing homes improve care outcomes: evidence from an integrative review. Int J Nurs Stud. 2013;50(8): 1122–35.

Price M, Bellwood P, Kitson N, Davies I, Weber J, Lau F. Conditions potentially sensitive to a personal health record (PHR) intervention, a systematic review. BMC Med Inform Decis Mak. 2015;15:32.

Reeve E, Thompson W, Farrell B. Deprescribing: a narrative review of the evidence and practical recommendations for recognizing opportunities and taking action. Eur J Intern Med. 2017;38:3–11.

Roychowdhury S, Chinnaiyan AM. Translating cancer genomes and transcriptomes for precision oncology. CA Cancer J Clin. 2016;66(1):75–88.

Sallnow L, Richardson H, Murray SA, Kellehear A. The impact of a new public health approach to end-of-life care: a systematic review. Palliat Med. 2016;30(3): 200–11.

Sanders C, Rogers A, Gately C, Kennedy A. Planning for end of life care within lay-led chronic illness self-management training: the significance of 'death awareness' and biographical context in participant accounts. Soc Sci Med. 2008;66(4):982–93.

Sepulveda CM, Yoshida A, Ulrich T. Palliative care: the World Health Organisation's global perspective. J Pain Symptom Manag. 2002;24:91–6.

Shen Z, Ruan Q, Yu Z, Sun Z. Chronic kidney disease-related physical frailty and cognitive impairment: a systemic review. Geriatr Gerontol Int. 2016;17:529.

Smith SM, Soubhi H, Fortin M, Hudon C, O'Dowd T. Managing patients with multimorbidity: systematic review of interventions in primary care and community settings. BMJ. 2012;345:e5205.

Stromberg A, Fluur C, Miller J, Chung ML, Moser DK, Thylen I. ICD recipients' understanding of ethical issues, ICD function, and practical consequences of withdrawing the ICD in the end-of-life. Pacing Clin Electrophysiol. 2014;37(7):834–42.

Temel JS, Greer JA, Muzikansky A, Gallagher ER, Admane S, Jackson VA, Dahlin CM, Blinderman CD, Jacobsen J, Pirl WF, Billings JA, Lynch TJ. Early palliative care for patients with metastatic non-small-cell lung cancer. N Engl J Med. 2010;363(8):733–42.

Thorne S, Roberts D, Sawatzky R. Unravelling the tensions between chronic disease management and end-of-life planning. Res Theory Nurs Pract. 2016;30(2):91–103.

Verbrugge LM, Lepkowski JM, Imanaka Y. Comorbidity and its impact on disability. Milbank Q. 1989;67(3–4): 450–84.

World Health Organization. WHO definition of palliative care. 2002 [cited Feb 22 2017]; Available from: http://www.who.int/cancer/palliative/definition/en/

World Health Organization. The global burden of disease: 2004 update. Geneva: WHO; 2004.

World Health Organization (WHO). Innovative care for chronic conditions: building blocks for action. Geneva: WHO; 2002.

Zafar SY, Peppercorn JM, Schrag D, Taylor DH, Goetzinger AM, Zhong X, Abernethy AP. The financial toxicity of cancer treatment: a pilot study assessing out-of-pocket expenses and the insured cancer patient's experience. Oncologist. 2013;18(4):381–90.

Part VI

Palliative Care in Specific Populations

Palliative Care, Frailty, and Older People

67

Caroline Nicholson, Catherine Evans, and Sarah Combes

Contents

C. Nicholson (✉)
King's College London, Florence Nightingale Faculty of Nursing, Midwifery and Palliative Care, London, UK

St Christopher's Hospice, London, UK

Supportive and End of Life Care (Nursing), St. Christopher's Hospice/King's College, London, UK
e-mail: caroline.nicholson@kcl.ac.uk

C. Evans
King's College London, Cicely Saunders Institute of Palliative Care, Policy and Rehabilitation, London, UK

Sussex Community NHS Foundation Trust, Brighton General Hospital, Brighton, UK

S. Combes
King's College London, Florence Nightingale Faculty of Nursing, Midwifery and Palliative Care, London, UK

St Christopher's Hospice, London, UK

R. D. MacLeod, L. Van den Block (eds.), *Textbook of Palliative Care*,
https://doi.org/10.1007/978-3-319-77740-5_66

Abstract

This chapter provides an overview of the symptoms of frailty, the tools used to recognize and assess older people living with frailty such as the frailty phenotype and frailty index, and some of their common palliative care needs. Further, it details some of the perceived challenges of frailty to current palliative care practice, namely, recognizing dying, multiple morbidities and symptom burden, and the focus or goals of care. Palliative care for older people with frailty requires a broader disability rather than a single disease focus. Coordination and interdependencies with other care providers become as important as the discrete patient/professional clinical encounter. The centrality of the older person with frailty and their "family" living and dying over time means the social environment becomes paramount local resources; support and the interplay between services and community are vital. While evidence on the best ways to provide palliative care to this population is still developing, the chapter offers some examples of current services and suggests key elements derived from the literature and practice. The authors suggest there is a moral and clinical imperative for palliative care services to engage with older people with frailty and their caregivers, both lay and professional. This imperative brings opportunities and challenges, including revaluing living and dying rather than an overemphasis on care in the last days of life and remodeling palliative care services to focus more on need than diagnosis and the reorientation of palliative care, so that it can be integrated with older people's services.

1 Introduction

1.1 Frailty and Palliative Care

Frailty is a complex medical syndrome, combining the effects of natural aging with the outcomes of multiple long-term conditions and loss of fitness and reserve. Frailty has been termed "the most problematic expression of population ageing" (Clegg et al. 2013) and, as such, is an increasingly important consideration for palliative care. Globally, the number of people living and dying in old age is growing; by 2050 21.5% of the world's population will be aged over 60. People living into late old age are the fastest growing sector of the population (particularly in more economically developed regions),with the number of people aged over 80 growing at twice the rate of people over 60 years (McNicoll 2002). Most people who need palliative care are older adults. Increasingly, the need will be for palliative care associated with older people dying with multiple, long-term conditions and frailty (World Health Organization 2015).

Yet older people with frailty are sometimes called the "disadvantaged dying." They constitute a section of society with poorer end-of-life care experiences and less access to palliative care than other groups (Gott and Ingleton 2011). Reasons for this include siloed services related to singular diseases, perceptions that palliative care referrals relate to medical condition rather than need arising from the interplay of multiple conditions, and under-recognition of palliative care needs in older people, including from older people themselves (Hall et al. 2011). Precisely because people have lived with their symptoms for so long, older people and those around them might overlook needs, normalizing them as part of growing old (Teunissen et al. 2006). Palliative care with the emphasis on quality of life and person-centered approaches is a vital intervention for older people with frailty; indeed Morrison et al. (2003) PX111 (Morrison et al. 2003) note "*frailty is the quintessential model for palliative care in older adults as optimal medical treatment for the frail patient typically includes preventive, life-prolonging, rehabilitative, and palliative measures in varying proportion and intensity based on the individual patient's needs.*"

Older people living and dying with frailty for palliative care raise both challenges and opportunities. This chapter provides an overview of the symptom complex of frailty, the tools required to recognize and assess older people living with frailty, and the potential need for palliative care. Further, it details some of the perceived challenges of frailty to current palliative care practice, namely, recognizing dying, multiple morbidities and symptom burden, and the focus or goals of care. We argue there is a moral and clinical imperative for palliative care services to engage with older people with frailty and their caregivers, both lay and professional. Such an imperative will help to bring the realization of the WHO 2014 palliative care resolution (WHO 2014) – to be an essential healthcare service for people with chronic and life-limiting illness. Palliative care needs to move its focus from a discrete service with an overemphasis on care in the last few days of life to a service integrated with the treatment of long-term conditions and with older peoples' services.

1.2 What Is Frailty?

In practice, the term frailty is used as both a general descriptor and to signify a discrete medical syndrome. Individuals whose health status indicates they may be susceptible to decline may be described as "becoming frail." Those people who meet specific diagnostic criteria are identified as having the medical syndrome of frailty. This chapter focuses on the latter. Hence, while cognitive decline is a component of frailty (considered later in the chapter), the distinctive palliative care needs of people with severe cognitive impairment or dementia are discussed elsewhere within this publication.

Frailty is a distinctive health state related to the aging process in which multiple body systems gradually lose their inbuilt reserves, leaving a person vulnerable to dramatic, sudden changes in health triggered by seemingly small events such as a change in medication or an infection (Clegg et al. 2013). Figure 1 illustrates the reduced recovery potential of older people with frailty following a seemingly minor illness. The red line demonstrates the longer recovery time with incomplete return to levels of functional ability for a person with frailty compared to an older person without frailty.

While not all older people become frail, frailty becomes more prevalent with age. Choi et al.'s (2015) study using national population-based surveys in the UK, Europe, United States, Taiwan, and Korea found frailty prevalence was between 4.9% and 27.3% in the total population. Figures

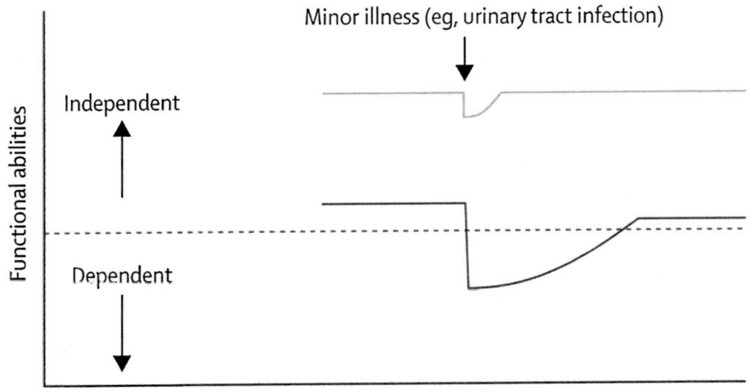

Fig. 1 Vulnerability of frail elderly people to a sudden change in health status after a minor illness (Clegg et al. 2013)

Minor illness (eg, urinary tract infection)
Functional abilities
Independent
Dependent

from the UK suggest frailty affects around 10% of those over 65 increasing to around 65% of those 90 and above (Clegg et al. 2013). Frailty is a dynamic state and is known to change over time, mostly worsening rather than improving (the red line in Fig. 1 does not come back to the previous level). Frailty in old age is often characterized by a progressive decline in physical, mental (Rockwood et al. 2005), and social functions (van Campen 2011), increased vulnerability to sudden deterioration (Covinsky et al. 2003), and reduced recovery potential (Turner and Clegg 2014). Typical signs and symptoms of frailty include sarcopenia, anorexia, exhaustion, and low mood. Evidence of the pathophysiology of frailty is growing, and chronic systemic inflammation leading to neurological and immunological dysfunction is a major contributor, as is cardiovascular degeneration and genetic predisposition (Fulop et al. 2010). Frailty biomarkers are being studied. Velissaris et al.'s (2017) systematic review explores the relationship between older people with frailty and systemic inflammation. C-reactive protein is an easily measurable biomarker, but not consistently associated with frailty. However, robust evidence demonstrates the association between morbidity and mortality with frailty, which increases as an older person becomes progressively more frail. Compared to fit older people, those with frailty are at greater risk of disability, nursing home admission, hospitalization, and death (Fried et al. 2001). Those with even mild frailty have almost twice the mortality risk of a fit older person; for those severely frail, the risk is almost five times higher (Clegg et al. 2016).

1.3 Identifying Frailty

It is important to identify frailty because it is predictive of adverse outcomes. While there is currently no robust evidence of the reversibility of frailty, research does demonstrate that the side effects of frailty, e.g., weakness and fatigue, can be lessened with intervention, particularly in the early stages. Frailty identification means we can deliver the most appropriate therapeutic interventions, including palliative care to those with severe frailty. The evidence on recognition, effects, and treatment for the symptom complex of frailty has grown exponentially over the last 10 years; however, it is still a concept in evolution. The two most common ways of operationally defining frailty are (1) the frailty phenotype (Fried et al. 2001) and (2) the frailty index (Rockwood et al. 2005) (see Table 1). It is useful to see the phenotype and frailty index as complementary rather than opposing approaches to identifying frailty (Cesari et al. 2013). The frailty phenotype assesses five dimensions that are hypothesized to reflect systems whose impaired regulation underlies the syndrome. These five dimensions are unintentional weight

Table 1 Comparing the frailty phenotype and frailty accumulation of deficit index approaches to identify frailty

Identifying frailty – table comparing the frailty phenotype and frailty accumulation of deficit index approaches	
Frailty phenotype	Frailty index
Frailty as a pre-disability syndrome Signs, symptoms relating to sarcopenia	Frailty as an accumulation of deficits using a combination of factors including symptoms, diseases, activities of daily living, and results of holistic clinical assessments
Categorical variable – five dimensions with set criteria: pre-frail meets one or two criteria, frailty requires satisfaction of three or more	Continuous variable which describes a risk profile moving from pre- to severely frail depending upon the accumulation of deficits
Five predefined dimensions with criteria: involuntary weight loss, exhaustion, slow gait speed, poor handgrip strength, and sedentary behavior	Predefined set of deficits identified over physical, psychological (including memory and cognitive problems), and social domains
Identification possible outside of a full clinical assessment	Identification part of a comprehensive clinical assessment or through an Electronic Frailty Index (EFI) (Clegg et al., 2016) calculated through routinely collected patient data in primary care

loss, exhaustion, muscle weakness, slowness while walking, and low levels of activity. Those who meet at least one or two of the criteria for these dimensions are defined as pre-frail, and those meeting three or more of the criteria are defined as frail. The frailty index is based on the concept that frailty is a consequence of interacting physical, psychological, and social factors. As deficits accumulate, people become increasingly vulnerable to adverse outcomes, moving from mild to moderate and then to severely frail. The number of deficits that are needed to indicate the presence and grade of frailty has changed with further research from the original 70 items of the earliest version of the frailty index (Rockwood et al. 2005). The Electronic Frailty Index eFI (Clegg et al. 2016) identifies 36 deficits across physical, psychological, and social domains to calculate a frailty risk value (an eFI) from data collected routinely from community-dwelling older people. The eFI is calculated by the number of deficits the patient has, divided by the number of deficits considered. Such indices can be used to identify the possible presence and grade of frailty, confirmed by a clinical assessment thus tailoring clinical services.

Clinically, there are many ways to recognize frailty. The NICE Multi-morbidity Guidelines (https://www.nice.org.uk/guidance/ng56) argue for two main approaches: (1) assessment through simple instruments based on the two main ways of identifying frailty discussed above, e.g., timed get up and go test (taking more than 10 s to get up from a chair walk 3 m and sit down again) is based on the frailty phenotype approach, or (2) through routinely collected data such as the Electronic Frailty Index which draws on the accumulation of deficits frailty index (Clegg et al. 2016). The choice of instrument is informed by purpose of identification, clinical setting, and availability. Simple tools are often a useful clinical starting point. The Clinical Frailty Scale, see Fig. 2 (The Clinical Frailty Scale), is a pictorial scale based on activities of daily living (ADLs) which

Clinical Frailty Scale*

1 **Very Fit** – People who are robust, active, energetic and motivated. These people commonly exercise regularly. They are among the fittest for their age.

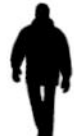

2 **Well** – People who have **no active disease symptoms** but are less fit than category 1. Often, they exercise or are very **active occasionally**, e.g. seasonally.

3 **Managing Well** – People whose **medical problems are well controlled**, but are **not regularly active** beyond routine walking.

4 **Vulnerable** – While **not dependent** on others for daily help, often **symptoms limit activities.** A common complaint is being "slowed up", and/or being tired during the day.

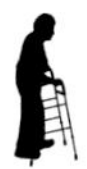

5 **Mildly Frail** – These people often have **more evident slowing,** and need help in **high order IADLs** (finances, transportation, heavy housework, medications). Typically, mild frailty progressively impairs shopping and walking outside alone, meal preparation and housework.

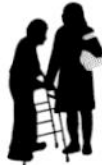

6 **Moderately Frail** – People need help with **all outside activities** and with **keeping house**. Inside, they often have problems with stairs and need **help with bathing** and might need minimal assistance (cuing, standby) with dressing.

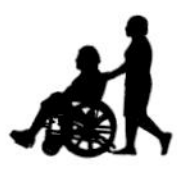

7 **Severely Frail** – **Completely dependent for personal care**, from whatever cause (physical or cognitive). Even so, they seem stable and not at high risk of dying (within ~ 6 months).

8 **Very Severely Frail** – Completely dependent, approaching the end of life. Typically, they could not recover even from a minor illness.

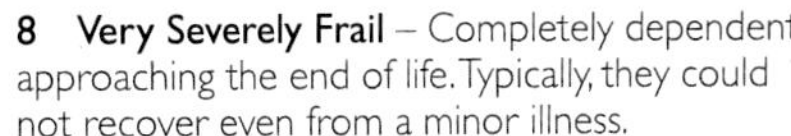

9. Terminally Ill - Approaching the end of life. This category applies to people with **a life expectancy <6 months**, who are **not otherwise evidently frail.**

Scoring frailty in people with dementia

The degree of frailty corresponds to the degree of dementia. Common **symptoms in mild dementia** include forgetting the details of a recent event, though still remembering the event itself, repeating the same question/story and social withdrawal.

In **moderate dementia**, recent memory is very impaired, even though they seemingly can remember their past life events well. They can do personal care with prompting.

In **severe dementia**, they cannot do personal care without help.

* 1. Canadian Study on Health & Aging, Revised 2008.
2. K. Rockwood et al. A global clinical measure of fitness and frailty in elderly people. CMAJ 2005;173:489-495.

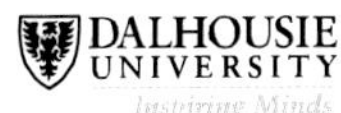

Fig. 2 The Clinical Frailty Scale. (http://camapcanada.ca/Frailtyscale.pdf)

categorizes frailty on a scale of 0–9 into mild, moderate, and severe frailty (see Fig. 2). It is a pragmatically useful tool to identify people in with frailty and appropriate therapeutic interventions, including palliative care.

2 Frailty and Multi-morbidity

While frailty might be the sole long-term condition with which an older person presents, it is often the case that it is the interplay between a combination of long-term conditions, called multi-morbidities, which are life threatening. The UK NICE guidelines (https://www.nice.org.uk/guidance/ng56) define multiple morbidity as a combination of two or more physical and mental health conditions such as diabetes or dementia, ongoing conditions such as learning disability, symptom complexes such as frailty, sensory impairment, and substance misuse. Fortin et al.'s (2012) systematic review of prevalence of multimorbidity in European and North American countries suggests there is marked variation between the prevalence of multiple morbidities due to methodological and definitional differences. However, the prevalence of multi-morbidities was associated with increased age in both general population and community-only studies. Barnett et al.'s (2012) much cited cross-sectional study across 314 community practices in Scotland suggests by age 65, 75% of the population are multimorbid, and for those 85 and over, 55% will be living with at least three long-term conditions, the number of conditions rising with age. As well as frailty, common morbidities identified by NICE from physical and mental health conditions include dementias, respiratory disease, urinary incontinence, and depression. Evidence is growing about the interplay between the frailty syndrome and cognitive decline, e.g., frailty is a risk factor for dementia (Searle and Rockwood 2015), there is a shared mechanism of pathophysiology (Sampson 2012), and cognitive decline is one of the deficits included in the frailty index accumulation of deficit approach to frailty. Pragmatically, clinicians will see many older people with frailty who have a component of cognitive decline. However, severe cognitive impairment, such as Alzheimer's disease, is a distinct condition.

The complexity of symptom burden and need over time for older adults with frailty cannot be fully captured by a biological disease model alone. This underlines the need for holistic assessment, incorporating medical, spiritual, social, and psychological care needs. Palliative care is such an approach, working with the whole person and addressing need rather than solely focusing on pathology.

3 Frailty: Moving Beyond a Biomedical Approach

Moving frailty beyond a biomedical deficit, conceptualization requires an acknowledgment of the resilience and resources of older people with frailty within the communities in which they are living and dying (Nicholson et al. 2012). An alternative conceptualization of frailty is also one where an older person is in a state of imbalance, experiencing simultaneously accumulated biopsychosocial losses while working to sustain and create new ways of connecting to their surroundings. Achieving balance between loss and continuity is crucial for the well-being of older people with frailty and is supported, or undermined, by the quality of their interactions with health and social care and the wider contexts of their lives (Nicholson et al. 2013). This approach moves beyond the dichotomies of independent/dependent or coping/requiring care to a person-centered approach, recognizing capabilities as well as potential needs, even when severely frail. It seeks to recapture McCue's (1995) insight of life naturally moving toward closure in old age. In this formulation, severe frailty is engaged with holistically and not, without careful thought, resisted biologically. However, while the case for palliative care involvement with frailty is clear, what is not so evident is robust data to describe or quantify specific palliative care needs. The following section of this chapter details some of the main issues identified to date in meeting the palliative care needs of older people with frailty.

4 Palliative Care for Older People with Frailty

4.1 Identification of Palliative Care Needs

Recognizing where a person might be in their dying trajectory is an increasingly important marker of potential care need and referral to palliative care. It also aids communication across teams and supports person-centered decision-making at end of life. Lunney et al. (2003) (ref) explores functional decline in four disease-based trajectories: sudden death, malignancy, organ failure, and frailty. The functional trajectory of frailty describes a progressive decline or prolonged dwindling over several months or years, punctuated by episodes of acute illness. This unpredictable trajectory makes it difficult to diagnose when people are nearing the end of life, and their increasing vulnerability to sudden health changes means dying might be characterized as unexpected. This is confirmed by Gill et al.'s (2010) retrospective study of disability trajectories of community-dwelling older people in the last year of life. They note considerable heterogeneity in the sample of frail older people; 25% of older people with frailty had progressive, severe disability in the last year of life, compared with 70% of people with advanced dementia. The authors conclude that the findings indicate the need for services to assist at end of life is at least as great in frailty as for those with a defined terminal condition. However recognizing this need is difficult. Pailoux et al. (2013) note that the sum of several illnesses or syndromes encompassing frailty is often looked at as separate diseases (rather than an accumulation of deficits), and thus, "practitioners have difficulty integrating the inevitably fatal nature of the situation" (p. 3). Nicholson et al. (2018) illustrate this in their work comparing patient needs and concerns of older people within an innovative new palliative care service with those of the conventional specialist palliative population (typically those with malignancy). Surprisingly similar needs were identified at first contact however Older people entered palliative care with a much lower performance status and remained in a longer period of stable deterioration than those with malignancies. Consequently, the dying phase can be very short or indeed unrecognized by clinicians. Murray et al. (2017) explore trajectories of decline with a more holistic perspective. The authors posit three main functional end-of-life trajectories: rapid, often associated with malignancy; intermittent, often associated with organ failure or multiple morbidities; and gradual, often associated with frailty or cognitive decline. For each pattern, the authors describe the likely pattern of physical, psychological, social, and spiritual decline and set out the implications for palliative care. They argue such an approach may help clinicians to identify, plan, and involve palliative care earlier.

What is clear is that in order to receive palliative care, older people with frailty need to be identified as having palliative care needs. There are a number of prognostication tools to help identify people in need of palliative care. However, evidence of reliability and validity for older people with frailty is sparse. Maas et al.'s (2013) systematic review of European and North American studies identified tools commonly used for identification of community palliative care. These include the RADPAC, Radboud Indicators for Palliative Care Need (Thoonsen et al. 2011) (which contains disease-specific assessment criteria for cancer, COPD, and heart failure); the SPICT Tool (the Supportive and Palliative Indicators Tool, a combination of general indicators, and disease-specific assessment criteria) (Highet et al. 2014), and the Gold Standards Framework Prognostic Guidance (Gold Standard Framework (GSF)) (based on three triggers that suggest that patients are nearing the end of life: the surprise question and general and specific clinical indicators for decline in organ failure, dementia, and frailty trajectories). The surprise question, "*Would I be surprised if this patient died in the next 12 months?*" has been shown to be of poor to moderate performance in specificity and sensitivity in identifying people in the last year of life (Downar et al. 2017). This is particularly the case in older people with frailty where lack of underlying pathology, and unpredictable illness trajectories, means some doctors are less likely to use the surprise question with this patient population (Elliott and Nicholson 2017).

The SPICT Tool (Highet et al. 2014) has been validated in hospitalized geriatric patients (De Bock et al. 2017), demonstrating a significant association with 1 year mortality. The Dementia/Frailty specific section of SPICT uses functional decline, activities of daily living, and frequent falling as clinical indicators of deterioration. As such, it links well to frailty syndrome. Multiple hospitalizations (Kelley et al. 2017) and recurrent infections (Leibovici 2013) have been evidenced a marker of poor prognosis in older people with frailty. While such clusters of triggers may be helpful in identifying need for older people with frailty, they are service dependent. Studies (Campbell et al. 2004; Ávila-Funes et al. 2008) suggest it is often a complex interplay of variables that coalesce to contribute to poor prognosis. These variables might include, for example, the effect of hospital admission, multiple morbidity, as well as frailty, age, gender, cognitive function, and sociodemographic factors on baseline before admission to hospital.

4.2 Specific Palliative Care Needs of Older People with Frailty

The principles of symptom assessment remain constant, focusing on relief of discomfort and enhancing quality of life. The gold standard in geriatric care for the assessment and management of frailty in older adults is a process of care known as the comprehensive geriatric assessment (CGA) (Ellis et al. 2011). CGA has been defined as a "multidimensional and usually interdisciplinary diagnostic process designed to determine a frail older person's medical conditions, mental health, functional capacity and social circumstances" (Ellis et al. 2011). CGA has much in common with palliative care holistic assessment. The application of both geriatric and end-of-life expertise is often beneficial because of the complexity of coexisting social, psychological, and medical needs in older people with frailty.

4.3 Defining Symptoms

4.3.1 Sarcopenia, Falling, and Fatigue

Sarcopenia is the loss of skeletal muscle mass and function with old age. Frailty shares common biomedical determinants with rapid muscle aging, i.e., inflammation, malnutrition, changes in neuromuscular function, and structure, and both are closely linked with falling and exhaustion. Muscle fatigue is a common symptom associated with older people with frailty at the end of life. It can be measured through low grip strength, walking speed, or balance. The management of sarcopenia includes leucine-enriched protein and vitamin D supplements (Morley 2016). Evidence over decades suggest that exercise involving strength and balance, even those who are very frail, is the key intervention component (Cadore et al. 2013). In older people with frailty, functionality, rather than diagnosis of disease, is one of the best indicators of health status. De Labra et al. (2015) systematic review of RCTs of exercise interventions in older people with frailty noted improvement in mobility balance, strength, body composition, and falls. However, the optimal exercise program is not yet clear. A Pan-European intervention program, the VIVIfrail project, has devised a range of resources including a practical exercise guide, including those with severe frailty and at risk of falling (http://www.vivifrail.com/resources). A Cochrane systematic review of the effect of functional rehabilitation programs in older people living in long-term care showed improvements in physical function (Gold Standard Framework (GSF)) such as strength, flexibility, and balance, as well as the potential to improve mood (Crocker et al. 2013). Pulmonary rehabilitation in particular may be helpful for older people living with frailty, as it targets key frailty symptoms such as fatigue, weakness, and dyspnea and encourages physical activity (Maddocks et al. 2016).

4.3.2 Polypharmacy

An important aspect of assessment of older people with frailty is medicine optimization: there is a strong association between polypharmacy (four or more medications) and falling in old age (Ziere et al. 2006). Palliative care clinicians need to be aware both of the medications they may prescribe and the need to optimize medications to decrease the risk of inadvertently increasing the burden of symptoms for older people with frailty including falling. Sedative hypnotics, antidepressants, cardiovascular drugs, and cardiovascular medication are of particular concern. Validated tools, e.g., the START/STOP tool (O'mahony et al. 2015), can be of use. Additionally, an important and an often underutilized expert is the pharmacist, both in the hospital and community.

4.3.3 Weight Loss

Given the interconnection between weight loss, sarcopenia, and frailty, anorexia is a powerful, independent predictor of poor quality of life, morbidity, and mortality in older persons (Morley 2003). One of the most important goals in the management of older, frail people is to optimize their nutritional status. Nutritional interventions may include smaller, more frequent meals, high caloric foods, altering consistency and referrals to speech and/or occupational therapists, and dietitians. Evidence supporting the use of nutritional supplements for older people with weight loss is mixed, in part because the underlying frailty pathology, rather than an inadequate intake, may cause the loss of weight. However, the importance of accessible nutritious food, assistance, and teeth and oral hygiene is interventions that can be overlooked. Morley (2003) notes the importance of enhancing the environment for older people and the importance of breakfast as a meal – circadian shifts in old age mean people eat more in the morning.

4.3.4 Depression

Depression is a major cause of weight loss in older people and there is a strong association between frailty and depression (Brown et al. 2014). Older adults with depressive symptoms have poorer functioning compared to those with chronic medical conditions such as lung disease, hypertension, or diabetes. Depression also increases the perception of poor health, the utilization of medical services, and healthcare costs. It is important to treat depression, as it is associated with increased mortality and risk of physical illness. Older people who attempt suicides are more likely to die than younger people, while in those who survive, prognosis is worse for older adults (Rodda et al. 2011). While not all older people with frailty who attempt suicide are depressed, treating depression is often overlooked in assessments. The British Geriatric Society (BGS) suggests medication should not be offered as a first-line treatment. Psychosocial interventions such as increasing social contact and physical exercise are first line. See http://www.bgs.org.uk/depression/cga-toolkit-category/how-cga/cga-assessment/cga-assessment-mental/cga-management-of-depression for further details. It is beyond this chapter to discuss physician-assisted suicide across differing cultures and contexts. However, it is important sensitively to addresses the fears of some older people with frailty.

5 Quality of Life and Goals of Care

Older people with frailty are frequently evidenced as having a significantly lower quality of life, compared with non-frail counterparts (Kojima et al. 2016). However, quality of life and health status are often narrowly measured, which has led to an increasing call for better measures including social, community, and psychological domains (Malley et al. 2012). Puts et al. (2007) used qualitative methods to explore the meaning of quality of life for older frail and non-frail people. Five common themes emerged, physical health, psychological well-being, social contacts, activities, and home/communities. Quality of life was derived through comparison to others, and adapted, dependent on the degree of frailty. When health was poor, there was a shift from health to social contacts as the most important factor, although poor health was not completely accepted and social goals, e.g., helping other people, checking on neighbors and friends, feelings of safety, and living conditions, became important. This adaptive shift has much in common with Knight and Emmanuel's (2007) reintegration of loss theory in palliative care. Building from literature on loss and adjustment, they describe a conceptual framework of key adjustment processes that allow for a shift in self-concept that supports quality of life while becoming more dependent, as one approaches death.

This approach is congruent with the focus of rehabilitative palliative care (Leslie et al. 2014), an essential approach to enable goals and preferences of older people to influence quality of care. Rehabilitation aims to improve quality of life by enabling people to be as active and productive as possible with minimum dependence on others, regardless of life expectancy. In the context of palliative rehabilitation, Jennings (2013) highlights the alternative term "habilitation" to dispel any unrealistic expectations of returning to premorbid levels of function which the "re" of rehabilitation may imply. However, rehabilitation is broader than symptom management alone, focusing on enabling people with long-term conditions or a terminal diagnosis to live well, and as independently as possible, until they die. Those with long-term conditions, such as frailty, are empowered to set goals to achieve their personal priorities with the support of those important to them and with adaptations to surroundings as necessary. The centrality of such approaches for older people with frailty cannot be underestimated, the importance of independence, dignity, and continuity of personhood providing a vital counterpoint to being frail (Lloyd et al. 2014).

6 Advance Care Planning

Promoting the empowerment of older people and their surrogate decision-makers in healthcare decisions through advance care planning can also aid quality of life. Advance care planning (ACP) is an ongoing conversation between professionals and someone nearing the end of life, often with family involvement (Thomas 2011). This dialogue provides an opportunity to discuss and document what matters most about future care, including preferred care, place of care and death, unwanted treatments, and proxy decision-makers. When successful, ACP decreases inappropriate emergency admissions and invasive procedures and improves quality of life by ensuring care represents the dying person's wishes (Sudore et al. 2017). However, while ACP is reasonably embedded for diseases such as cancer and within palliative services, it is seldom used with older people with frailty, due to its complex systems and personal and family challenges (Brinkman-Stoppelenburg et al. 2014). As previously discussed, prognostication is challenging in frailty, with its repeated episodes of deterioration and subsequent recovery. It is therefore unclear when best to start ACP discussions. Further, evidence suggests older peoples' engagement with ACP is mixed, as they have a different set of preoccupations and concerns to those traditionally associated with planning future care. Older people with frailty often make decisions within their social network, a shared ecology of decision-making, which is processual and develops and changes over time (Musa et al. 2015). Decisions about preferred place of treatment and care may focus more on not wanting to be a burden to others, as well as on where the older person with frailty feels most safe and secure. This may include a preference for dying in hospital (Barclay and Arthur 2008). Further, when older people with frailty are managing well, they, and their significant others, do not always wish to discuss future planning, and there are often misunderstandings around what ACP might mean (Sharp et al. 2013).

Consequently, while ACP is particularly relevant for this population, often their priorities have not been discussed prior to a significant deterioration. This leads to crisis decision-making, for which the person may not have capacity, and often means older people with frailty are under- or overtreated and experience unnecessary hospital admissions or inappropriate, invasive procedures. Critics of ACP often relate to the process; too often ACP is defined as a stand-alone activity, with its focus frequently being only on future care decisions. However, ACP, when carried out well, should be an ongoing process, not a one-off event, a realistic and supportive conversation between professionals, the older person, and their significant others. It should focus on the persons' goals for their care, both now and in the future, and, in that way, promotes the fundamental aim of palliative care, "*to live until you die.*" Engaging in ACP does not guarantee that the dying person's wishes are realistic or possible and acknowledges that priorities may change. However, only by enabling people to make informed decisions, to articulate and record these, can we hope to deliver person-centered end-of-life care (Sudore et al. 2017). Working with older people and their significant others in partnership enables professionals to provide person-centered end-of-life care. Further, enhancing the idea of ACP as a process rather than a single event enables the focus to be on living well now, as well as planning for future terminal care needs.

7 Revaluing Living with Dying in Frailty

Frailty's dwindling trajectory fits poorly with the popular idea of a "good death in old age," in which awareness of dying, choice, communication, and control are central (Seymour et al. 2005). The idea of dying in old age with frailty as an "event" is therefore perhaps less useful than thinking of dying as a process (Martin et al. 2018). With this framing, the idea of "living as well as possible until you die" seems relevant. It is helpful to think of the concept of supportive care. This model maximizes quality of life in life-limiting illness by giving equal importance to the palliative, end-of-life approach and appropriate medical treatments, to meet patients' overall needs from diagnosis to bereavement (NICE 2004). Sometimes an open awareness of dying requires time for patients and the people, including professionals, caring for them. Supportive care can provide a bridging language and practice between curative and end-of-life discourses (Nicholson et al. 2017). Reframing language around uncertainty allows for a different praxis. Parallel planning, an approach from pediatric palliative care (Wolff and Browne 2011), acknowledges there may be numerous possibilities; some become more obvious over time, while other outcomes become less likely. Crucially, these discussions are with the family, and acknowledging honestly that this is an uncertain journey builds partnership between the clinical team, child, and family. While older people with frailty are in no way children, the degree of dependency on others for fundamentals of care and centrality of family and friends in coordinating care resonates.

A revaluation of living and dying with frailty requires a reconfiguration of partnerships and expert knowledge in palliative care. Evidence reveals that friends and family of older people with frailty are often unrecognized, unsupported, and overlooked as they care for people at the end of life (Lloyd et al. 2016). They are often coordinating a number of services, carrying out physical and emotional care over many weeks or months, and living with the uncertainty of a person dying in a protracted and often erratic way (Grande GaK 2011). While carers are often "the conductor of the orchestra" (Lowson et al. 2013), evidence (Thomas 2011; Sudore et al. 2017) highlights that their knowledge and resources are overlooked by health services. Living and dying partnerships align to health-promoting approaches to end-of-life care (Sallnow et al. 2016) in which citizens are actively engaged in their own care, drawing on partnerships between services and communities, and building on their existing strengths and skills, rather than replacing them with professional care. The focus of outcomes of care then shifts to enhancing capacity, resilience, and empowerment at an individual, social network, and wider community level, alongside more traditional palliative care outcomes.

8 Service Models to Meet the Palliative Care Needs of Older People with Frailty

Older people with frailty challenge our assumptions about who palliative care is for and where it should be delivered. Specialist of palliative care could be censured for delivering a discrete service, largely unconnected to, rather than integrated into, wider systems of health and social care. Jerant et al. (2004) criticize this model of palliative care for an emphasis on symptomatic and disease-focused treatment, resulting in a reactive and crisis-driven approach. Older people with frailty require a focus on both living and dying well within prolonged and uncertain disease trajectories. This reorientation of palliative care models, integrating across geriatric and palliative care, supports the wider World Health Assembly (WHA) (Organization WH 2015) position for palliative care to be considered internationally as an essential health service for all people living with chronic and life-limiting conditions. Increasingly there are shared goals in geriatric and end-of-life care, to improve quality of life and to enable people to die "well" based on benefit rather than prognosis. However, what is underdeveloped is evidence on the "best" systems and models of service delivery, which and how to tailor care to meet the complex health needs associated with frailty. Sawatsky et al. (2016) argue that extending a palliative care approach to others with life-limiting and chronic conditions, such as older people with frailty, requires clear delineation of the underlying concepts of a palliative care approach. Their systematic review identified three core concepts: (1) upstream orientation toward the needs of people who have life-limiting conditions and their families, (2) adaptation of palliative care knowledge and expertise, and (3) operationalization of a palliative approach through integration into systems and models of care that do not specialize in palliative care.

The recent WHO Evans et al. (2018) scoping review of systematic reviews on service models to maximize quality of life for older people at end of life builds on Sawatzky's approach. The scoping review identified end-of-life service models as being on a continuum. At one end of the spectrum is integrated geriatric care, conceptualized as person-centered care, mainly given at an earlier trajectory of functional decline, focusing on quality of life with emphasis on strengthening and maintaining function. At the other end of the spectrum is integrated palliative care, conceptualized as person-centered care commonly accessed at a later trajectory of functional decline and dying, focusing on quality of life with emphasis on reducing symptom distress and concerns. This service continuum and the interface between integrated geriatric and palliative care balance functionality, quality of life, and quality of dying for older people with frailty and multiple morbidity. Key components across the service models reviewed were (1) multiple service providers, (2) person-centered care targeting quality of life, and (3) education of service users and providers (conceptualized in Fig. 3). However, the heterogeneity of the data within the review did not allow for detailed analysis of key components or processes to support sustainability/transferability of service models. Common outcome measures identified were quality of life, function, and impact of symptoms. However, there was insufficient data consistently to analyze outcomes and patient benefit in relation to particular service models. Health economic data was reported in less than half the reviews and results were inconclusive. Data for the review was derived mainly from high-income countries. The report argues that service delivery models must build on specific population needs, characteristics, and resources, e.g., using volunteers to deliver an end-of-life service in low- and

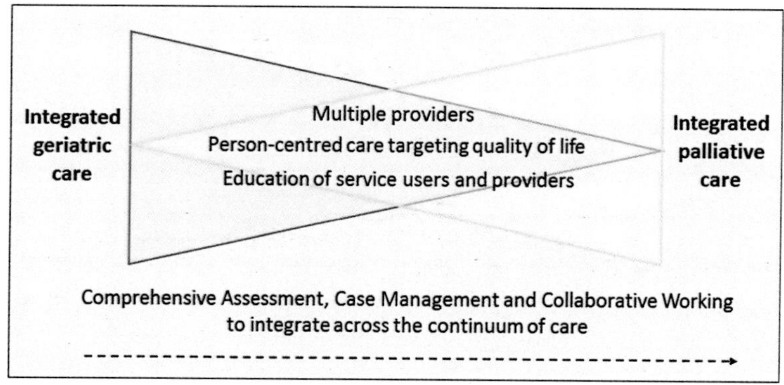

Fig. 3 Overarching integrated service delivery models and processes to maximize quality of life for older people in the last years of life (Evans et al. 2018, Adapted from Hawley 2014)

middle-income populations and consideration of the amount of primary/community palliative care available.

We consider here three examples of models of end-of-life care for older people with frailty and progressive conditions. These models seek to improve quality of life and quality of dying across the continuum of integrated palliative care and integrated geriatric care. These are as follows: first, short-term integrated palliative and supportive care, SIPScare (Bone et al. 2016); second, ongoing shared care coordination within primary care with community doctors (Bromley Care Coordination (BCC)) service via St Christopher's Hospice (Nicholson et al. 2018); and, third, skilling up the acute older adult workforce via the Assessment; Management; Best practice; Engagement and Recovery (AMBER) care bundle (Carey et al. 2014).

SIPScare (Sawatzky et al. 2016) aims to provide specialist palliative care using an approach of a consult service to assess and improve management and treatment of physical, emotional social, and other concerns and act as a catalyst to access health and social care services. Service provision is based on potential for benefit at points of actual or anticipated deterioration, with a presentation of two or more symptoms or concerns for the patient and/or their carer(s). The service is delivered "short-term" with the palliative care team providing one to three visits to assess and review concerns with expectation that the patient is discharged within 3 months. The service is integrated with the existing community services, notably GP and community nursing and other specialist nursing services (e.g., respiratory nurse). Patients/carers and practitioners re-refer at future points when care needs indicate likely benefit from palliative care services. This may be at points of anticipated or actual decline (e.g., an unplanned hospital admission), unstable symptoms, and/or concerns and care in the dying phase. The central tenets are to provide palliative care early in an individual's illness/condition based on potential for benefit and integrated professional working with the palliative care team working with the existing main provider of care. The addition of supportive care increases the emphasis on enabling individuals to live life well. Findings from the phase II trials indicate the acceptability of SIPScare for patients, families, and staff and potential for patient benefit in improving the key symptoms identified as the respective main outcome and evidence of cost saving.

Bromley Care Coordination (Nicholson et al. 2018) was commissioned by a community care-commissioning group in December 2013 to enable patients with progressive and advanced illness or frailty, thought to be in the last year of life, to receive timely and coordinated end-of-life care. The majority of patients are older and would not have met the referral criteria for "specialist palliative care" services. The service aims to address the inequalities of access to services for dying patients to prevent unnecessary hospital admissions, to help people die with dignity in their place of choice, and to provide support for their families and carers. BCC is a nursing-led service, with the community doctor taking medical responsibility for the patient. The team consists of clinical nurse specialists, community staff nurses, and administrators. Other hospice services are available as necessary to meet patient needs. Those using the service can access advice and help around the clock, 365 days a year. The service averages 280 people on the caseload at any 1 time, of which 85% have a non-cancer diagnosis and 63% are over 85 years of age. To date, outcomes include reduction of deaths in hospital (76% of patients have died at home, compared with the average in the borough of 23%) and reduction in inappropriate hospital admissions. It also increased patient and family satisfaction and anticipatory care planning. Resource implications to the proposed model include an increase in key working some patients, rather than the original plan to assess and refer onto other services. This is in part due to the lack of services for some patient groups, e.g., people with dementia and long-term neurological disorders who have high levels of dependency and uncertainty around deterioration. In part, the nonexistent or fragile social networks of people living on their own make the ongoing connection or "watchful waiting" aspect of hospice care of extra importance.

The AMBER care bundle was developed and piloted in the UK for patients in hospital whose clinical situation was uncertain in terms of recovery or continued decline, increasing risk to end of life. The model of care was in response to inconsistencies in the quality of care for patients presenting with decline and clinical uncertainty as to recovery and risk to end of life. Typically, these were older patients with frailty and multi-morbidities presenting with signs and symptoms not defined by a chronic illness. The AMBER care bundle follows an algorithmic approach to encourage clinical teams to develop and document a clear medical plan, considering anticipated outcomes and resuscitation and escalation status and revisiting the plan daily. The AMBER care bundle encourages staff, patients, and families to continue with treatment in the hope of a recovery while talking openly about preferences and priorities for end-of-life care and increasing nearness to end of life. It aims to increase and improve communication, support shared decision-making, reduce patient and family anxiety and distress, and increase attainment of preferences for end-of-life care and reduced unplanned hospital admission. Evaluation of a single site demonstrated increased communication between clinical staff and patients on prognosis and reduced length of hospital stay. However, the quality of the communication was not assessed, and relatives of patients supported by AMBER reported more unresolved concerns about providing care at home. A cluster feasibility trial is underway.

Key features of palliative care provision for older people with frailty exemplified in these models are summarized as follows:

1. Partnership with the older person and their family to enable hopeful and realistic conversations about living and dying with frailty. There is a delicate balance between perseverance/continuity and adaption to loss/dying in old age.
2. The importance of goals of care which maintain function and center on the quality of everyday life of the older person in their community as well as future planning for the last few days of life.
3. Early introduction and revisiting of advance care planning during an unpredictable and possible prolonged dying trajectory.
4. Integration and interdependencies with other care providers is an essential component as assessment and care focus on living and dying with frailty.
5. Early identification and involvement of palliative care which requires close collaboration and discussion.
6. A dynamic model which involves palliative, older person and their family, voluntary, health, and social care providers. With shifting service provision aligned to a person's needs and goals of care.
7. Proactive care – Health service care tends to manage points of decompensation on the frailty trajectory as "event-based care" by treating and managing the cause of the decline, e.g., an infection (see Fig. 1). Equal attentiveness is required to the older person's gradual deterioration with each event increasing their risk to unplanned hospital attendance, and requirement for long-term care and end of life. Regular planned assessment and use of identification tools, e.g., Electronic Frailty Index (Clegg et al. 2016)

This chapter has argued that person-centered palliative care demands a meaningful engagement with the older person with frailty within the social networks in which they are both living and dying. An understanding and valuing of capacity and strategies of continuity, alongside older people's potential and actual vulnerability, is crucial as older people with frailty reach the end of their life. However, living and dying with frailty does not always fit well within current palliative care policy and practice. This chapter argues for a flexible practice that works with uncertainty, transitions, and need, rather than a defined prognosis. The invitation to palliative care with the rise and need of older people living and dying with frailty can be framed within the potential to flourish within dying. Illes (2016) suggests that dying is the most grown up thing we will ever do, moving the focus away from productivity, external validation of worth, and the future to a more conscious habitation of the present. Such flourishing requires an integration of palliative and older people's care crucially working with older people and the communities in which most older people will live and die.

References

Ávila-Funes JA, Helmer C, Amieva H, Barberger-Gateau P, Goff ML, Ritchie K, et al. Frailty among community-dwelling elderly people in France: the three-city study. J Gerontol: Ser A. 2008;63(10):1089–96.

Barclay S, Arthur A. Place of death—how much does it matter? Br J Gen Pract. 2008;58:229.

Barnett K, Mercer SW, Norbury M, Watt G, Wyke S, Guthrie B. Epidemiology of multimorbidity and implications for health care, research, and medical education: a cross-sectional study. Lancet. 2012;380:37.

Bone AE, Morgan M, Maddocks M, Sleeman KE, Wright J, Taherzadeh S, et al. Developing a model of short-term integrated palliative and supportive care for frail older people in community settings: perspectives of older people, carers and other key stakeholders. Age Ageing. 2016;45(6):863–73.

Brinkman-Stoppelenburg A, Rietjens JA, van der Heide A. The effects of advance care planning on end-of-life care: a systematic review. Palliat Med. 2014;28(8): 1000–25.

Brown PJ, Roose SP, Fieo R, Liu X, Rantanen T, Sneed JR, et al. Frailty and depression in older adults: a high-risk clinical population. Am J Geriatr Psychiatry. 2014;22(11):1083–95.

Cadore EL, Rodríguez-Mañas L, Sinclair A, Izquierdo M. Effects of different exercise interventions on risk of falls, gait ability, and balance in physically frail older adults: a systematic review. Rejuvenat Res. 2013;16(2): 105–14.

Campbell SE, Seymour DG, Primrose WR. A systematic literature review of factors affecting outcome in older medical patients admitted to hospital. Age Ageing. 2004;33(2):110–5.

van Campen C. Frail older persons in the Netherlands. Summary. The Hague: Netherlands Institute for Social Research, SCP; 2011.

Carey I, Shouls S, Bristowe K, Morris M, Briant L, Robinson C, et al. Improving care for patients whose recovery is uncertain. The AMBER care bundle: design and implementation. BMJ Support Palliat Care. 2014;5:12. https://doi.org/10.1136/bmjspcare-2013-000634

Cesari M, Gambassi G, Abellan van Kan G, Vellas B. The frailty phenotype and the frailty index: different instruments for different purposes. Age Ageing. 2013;43(1): 10–2.

Choi J, Ahn A, Kim S, Won CW. Global prevalence of physical frailty by Fried's criteria in community-dwelling elderly with national population-based surveys. J Am Med Dir Assoc. 2015;16(7):548–50.

Clegg A, Young J, Iliffe S, Rikkert MO, Rockwood K. Frailty in elderly people. Lancet. 2013;381(9868): 752–62.

Clegg A, Bates C, Young J, Ryan R, Nichols L, Ann Teale E, et al. Development and validation of an electronic frailty index using routine primary care electronic health record data. Age Ageing. 2016;45(3):353–60.

Covinsky KE, Palmer RM, Fortinsky RH, Counsell SR, Stewart AL, Kresevic D, et al. Loss of independence in activities of daily living in older adults hospitalized with medical illnesses: increased vulnerability with age. J Am Geriatr Soc. 2003;51(4):451–8.

Crocker T, Young J, Forster A, Brown L, Ozer S, Greenwood DC. The effect of physical rehabilitation on activities of daily living in older residents of long-term care facilities: systematic review with meta-analysis. Age Ageing. 2013;42(6):682–8.

De Bock R, Van Den Noortgate N, Piers R. Validation of the supportive and palliative care indicators tool in a geriatric population. J Palliat Med. 2017.

de Labra C, Guimaraes-Pinheiro C, Maseda A, Lorenzo T, Millán-Calenti JC. Effects of physical exercise interventions in frail older adults: a systematic review of randomized controlled trials. BMC geriatrics. 2015;15 (1):154.

Downar J, Goldman R, Pinto R, Englesakis M, Adhikari NK. The "surprise question" for predicting death in seriously ill patients: a systematic review and meta-analysis. Can Med Assoc J. 2017;189(13):E484–E93.

Elliott M, Nicholson C. A qualitative study exploring use of the surprise question in the care of older people: perceptions of general practitioners and challenges for practice. BMJ Support Palliat Care. 2017;7(1):32–8.

Ellis G, Whitehead MA, Robinson D, O'Neill D, Langhorne P. Comprehensive geriatric assessment for older adults admitted to hospital: meta-analysis of randomised controlled trials. BMJ. 2011;343:d6553.

Evans CJ, Ison L, Ellis-Smith C, Nicholson C, Costa A, Oluyase AO, Namisango E, Bone AE, Brighton LJ, Yi D, Combes S, Bajwah S, Gao W, Harding R, Ong P, Higginson IJ, Maddocks M. Rapid scoping review of service delivery models to maximise quality of life for older people at the end of life prepared for the World Health Organisation (WHO). King's College London; 2018. Available from: http://www.who.int/kobe_centre/mediacentre/news/EOLC_report/en/.

Fortin M, Stewart M, Poitras M-E, Almirall J, Maddocks H. A systematic review of prevalence studies on multimorbidity: toward a more uniform methodology. Ann Fam Med. 2012;10(2):142–51.

Fried LP, Tangen CM, Walston J, Newman AB, Hirsch C, Gottdiener J, et al. Frailty in older adults: evidence for a phenotype. J Gerontol Ser A Biol Med Sci. 2001;56(3): M146–M57.

Fulop T, Larbi A, Witkowski JM, McElhaney J, Loeb M, Mitnitski A, et al. Aging, frailty and age-related diseases. Biogerontology. 2010;11(5):547–63.

Gill TM, Gahbauer EA, Han L, Allore HG. Trajectories of disability in the last year of life. N Engl J Med. 2010;362(13):1173–80.

Gott M, Ingleton C. Living with ageing and dying: palliative and end of life care for older people. Oxford: Oxford University Press; 2011.

Grande GaK J. Needs, access, and support for older carers. Living with ageing & dying: palliative and end of life care in older people. In: Gott M, Ingleton C, editors. Living with ageing and dying: palliative and end of life care for older people. Oxford: Oxford University Press; 2011. p. 158–69.

Hall S, Petkova H, Tsouros AD, Costantini M, Higginson IJ. Palliative care for older people: better practices. Copenhagen: World Health Organization; 2011.

Hawley PH. The bow tie model of 21st century palliative care. J Pain Symptom Manag. 2014;47(1):e2–5.

Highet G, Crawford D, Murray SA, Boyd K. Development and evaluation of the Supportive and Palliative Care Indicators Tool (SPICT): a mixed-methods study. BMJ Support Palliat Care. 2014;4(3):285–90.

Iles V. Dying is the most grown-up thing we ever do: but do health care professionals prevent us from taking it seriously? Health Care Anal. 2016;24(2):105–18.

Jennings R. Who is the palliative care physiotherapist? In: Taylor J, Simander R, Nielan P, editors. Potential and possibility: rehabilitation at the end of life. Munich: Elveseir; 2013.

Jerant AF, Azari RS, Nesbitt TS, Meyers FJ. The TLC model of palliative care in the elderly: preliminary application in the assisted living setting. Ann Fam Med. 2004;2(1):54–60.

Kelley AS, Covinsky KE, Gorges RJ, McKendrick K, Bollens-Lund E, Morrison RS, et al. Identifying older adults with serious illness: a critical step toward improving the value of health care. Health Serv Res. 2017;52(1):113–31.

Knight SJ, Emanuel L. Processes of adjustment to end-of-life losses: a reintegration model. J Palliat Med. 2007;10(5):1190–8.

Kojima G, Iliffe S, Jivraj S, Walters K. Association between frailty and quality of life among community-dwelling older people: a systematic review and meta-analysis. J Epidemiol Community Health. 2016;70(7):716–21.

Leibovici L. Long-term consequences of severe infections. Clin Microbiol Infect. 2013;19(6):510–2.

Leslie P, Sandsund C, Roe J. Researching the rehabilitation needs of patients with life-limiting disease: challenges and opportunities. Prog Palliat Care. 2014;22(6): 313–8.

Lloyd L, Calnan M, Cameron A, Seymour J, Smith R. Identity in the fourth age: perseverance, adaptation and maintaining dignity. Ageing Soc. 2014;34(1):1–19.

Lloyd AKM, Cardiff E, Cavers D, Kimball B, Murray SA. Why do older people get less palliative care than younger people? Eur J Palliat Care. 2016;23(3):132–7.

Lowson E, Hanratty B, Holmes L, Addington-Hall J, Grande G, Payne S, et al. From 'conductor' to 'second fiddle': older adult care recipients' perspectives on transitions in family caring at hospital admission. Int J Nurs Stud. 2013;50(9):1197–205.

Lunney JR, Lynn J, Foley DJ, Lipson S, Guralnik JM. Patterns of functional decline at the end of life. J Am Med Assoc. 2003;289:2387.

Maas EAT, Murray SA, Engels Y, Campbell C. What tools are available to identify patients with palliative care needs in primary care: a systematic literature review and survey of European practice. BMJ Support Palliat Care. 2013;3(4):444–51.

Maddocks M, Kon SS, Canavan JL, Jones SE, Nolan CM, Labey A, et al. Physical frailty and pulmonary rehabilitation in COPD: a prospective cohort study. Thorax. 2016;71:988–95. https://doi.org/10.1136/thoraxjnl-2016-208460.

Malley JN, Towers A-M, Netten AP, Brazier JE, Forder JE, Flynn T. An assessment of the construct validity of the ASCOT measure of social care-related quality of life with older people. Health Qual Life Outcomes. 2012;10(1):21.

Martin J, Nicholson, Caroline and George, Rob. The approach of dying and death, and the mourning process of the survivors. Oxford textbook of geriatric medicine third edition. Jean-Pierre Michel BLB, Finbarr C. Martin, and Jeremy D. Walston, Oxford: Oxford University Press; 2018.

McCue JD. The naturalness of dying. JAMA. 1995;273 (13):1039–43.

McNicoll G. World population ageing 1950–2050. Popul Dev Rev. 2002;28(4):814–6.

Morley JE. Anorexia and weight loss in older persons. J Gerontol Ser A Biol Med Sci. 2003;58(2):M131–M7.

Morley JE. Frailty and sarcopenia: the new geriatric giants. Rev Investig Clin. 2016;68(2):59–67.

Morrison RS, Meier DE, Capello C, editors. Geriatric Palliative Care. Oxford University Press 2003.

Murray SA, Kendall M, Mitchell G, Moine S, Amblàs-Novellas J, Boyd K. Palliative care from diagnosis to death. BMJ: Br Med J (Online). 2017;356:j878.

Musa I, Seymour J, Narayanasamy MJ, Wada T, Conroy S. A survey of older peoples' attitudes towards advance care planning. Age Ageing. 2015;44(3):371–6.

National Institute for Clinical Improvement. Improving supportive and palliative care for adults with cancer NICE guidelines. London, 2004.

Nicholson C, Meyer J, Flatley M, Holman C, Lowton K. Living on the margin: understanding the experience of living and dying with frailty in old age. Soc Sci Med. 2012;75(8):1426–32.

Nicholson C, Meyer J, Flatley M, Holman C. The experience of living at home with frailty in old age: a psychosocial qualitative study. Int J Nurs Stud. 2013;50(9):1172–9.

Nicholson C, Morrow EM, Hicks A, Fitzpatrick J. Supportive care for older people with frailty in hospital: an integrative review. Int J Nurs Stud. 2017;66:60–71.

Nicholson C, Davies, J, Smith, B, Pace, V, Harris, L, George, R, Noble, J, Hansford, P, Murtagh, F. What are the main palliative care symptoms and concerns of older people with multimorbidity? A service evaluation using routinely collected Phase of Illness, Australian Karnofsky Performance Status and Integrated Palliative Care Outcome Scale data. Ann Palliat Med. 2018 (In Press).

O'mahony D, O'sullivan D, Byrne S, O'connor MN, Ryan C, Gallagher P. STOPP/START criteria for potentially inappropriate prescribing in older people: version 2. Age Ageing. 2015;44(2):213–8.

World Health Organization. World report on ageing and health. Geneva: World Health Organization; 2015.

Pialoux T, Goyard J, Hermet R. When frailty should mean palliative care. J Nurs Educ Pract. 2013;3(7):75.

Puts M, Shekary N, Widdershoven G, Heldens J, Lips P, Deeg D. What does quality of life mean to older frail and non-frail community-dwelling adults in the Netherlands? Qual Life Res. 2007;16(2):263–77.

Rockwood K, Song X, MacKnight C, Bergman H, Hogan DB, McDowell I, et al. A global clinical measure of fitness and frailty in elderly people. Can Med Assoc J. 2005;173(5):489–95.

Rodda J, Walker Z, Carter J. Depression in older adults. BMJ-Br Med J. 2011;343(8):d5219.

Sallnow L, Richardson H, Murray SA, Kellehear A. The impact of a new public health approach to end-of-life care: a systematic review. Palliat Med. 2016;30(3): 200–11.

Sampson EL. Frailty and dementia: common but complex comorbidities. Aging Ment Health. 2012;16(3): 269–272.

Sawatzky R, Porterfield P, Lee J, Dixon D, Lounsbury K, Pesut B, et al. Conceptual foundations of a palliative approach: a knowledge synthesis. BMC Palliat Care. 2016;15(1):5.

Searle SD, Rockwood K. Frailty and the risk of cognitive impairment. Alzheimers Res Ther. 2015;7(1):54.

Seymour J, Witherspoon R, Gott M, Ross H, Payne S. Dying in older age: end-of-life care. Bristol: Policy Press; 2005.

Sharp T, Moran E, Kuhn I, Barclay S. Do the elderly have a voice? Advance care planning discussions with frail and older individuals: a systematic literature review and narrative synthesis. Br J Gen Pract. 2013;63(615): e657–e68.

Sudore RL, Lum HD, You JJ, Hanson LC, Meier DE, Pantilat SZ, et al. Defining advance care planning for adults: a consensus definition from a multidisciplinary Delphi panel. J Pain Symptom Manag. 2017;53(5): 821–32. e1

Teunissen SC, de Haes HC, Voest EE, de Graeff A. Does age matter in palliative care? Crit Rev Oncol Hematol. 2006;60(2):152–8.

The Clinical Frailty Scale. http://camapcanada.ca/Frailtyscale.pdf.

Thomas K. The Gold Standards Framework (GSF) in community palliative care. Eur J Palliat Care. 2003;10: 113–115.

Thomas K. Overview and introduction to advance care planning. In: Advance care planning in end of life care. Oxford, UK: Oxford University Press; 2011. p. 3–15.

Thoonsen B, Groot M, Engels Y, Prins J, Verhagen S, Galesloot C, et al. Early identification of and proactive palliative care for patients in general practice, incentive and methods of a randomized controlled trial. BMC Fam Pract. 2011;12(1):123.

Turner G, Clegg A. Best practice guidelines for the management of frailty: a British Geriatrics Society, Age UK and Royal College of General Practitioners report. Age Ageing. 2014;43(6):744–7.

Velissaris D, Pantzaris N, Koniari I, Koutsogiannis N, Karamouzos V, Kotroni I, et al. C-reactive protein and frailty in the elderly: a literature review. J Clin Med Res. 2017;9(6):461.

WHO. WHA67.19. W. Strengthening of palliative care as a component of comprehensive care throughout the life course. Geneva: World Health Organization; 2014.

Wolff T, Browne J. Organizing end of life care: parallel planning. Paediatr Child Health. 2011;21(8):378–84.

Ziere G, Dieleman J, Hofman A, Pols HA, Van Der Cammen T, Stricker B. Polypharmacy and falls in the middle age and elderly population. Br J Clin Pharmacol. 2006;61(2):218–23.

Palliative Care of Pediatric Populations

68

Ross Drake and Emily Chang

Contents

R. Drake (✉) · E. Chang
Starship specialist paediatric palliative care service,
Auckland City Hospital, Auckland, New Zealand
e-mail: RossD@adhb.govt.nz; EChang@adhb.govt.nz

R. D. MacLeod, L. Van den Block (eds.), *Textbook of Palliative Care*,
https://doi.org/10.1007/978-3-319-77740-5_67

Abstract

Pediatric palliative care clinicians care for children with life-limiting illnesses – ranging from the unborn child through to young adulthood. It is a unique specialty that shares some concepts with adult palliative care but also important differences. The range of diagnoses, illness trajectories, and prognoses are very different to the diseases of adults. In addition, children are developing with changes in cognition, psychological and emotional maturity, spiritual and cultural influences, and behavior. The evolving roles of the child and family through illness, end-of-life care, death, and bereavement also influence palliative care provision.

Multidisciplinary pediatric teams provide family-centered care, in the setting of the child and family's choice. Core responsibilities include symptom management, psychological and emotional care, advocacy, and spiritual and cultural care. Advance care planning and decision-making are fluid processes that require attention to the child's level of understanding, capacity to make decision, his/her role in the family, parental views, and the child's condition.

Due to a low prevalence compared with adult patients, geographical distance, and resourcing limitations, not all children with palliative care needs will have access to a specialist pediatric palliative care team. Care can be provided by general pediatric and adult palliative care teams working together and complimenting each other's skill sets where there is an absence of a specialist pediatric palliative care team.

Research in this area is in a phase of development. Ethical considerations of conducting research in children and with families who are considered vulnerable make study design and recruiting challenging. However, there is a great need for evidence to enable high-quality palliative care provision in this population.

1 Introduction

Providing palliative care to children and young people with life-limiting illnesses has similarities with adult palliative care, but also significant differences (Hynson et al. 2003; Dingfield et al. 2015), enough to make it a related but separate discipline. Shared principles of care include attention to quality of life, symptom management, and psychosocial and spiritual care. However, delivery of care is greatly affected by the diagnosis, illness trajectory, developmental needs of the child, and his/her place within the family and wider community.

Children requiring palliative care have a wide range of diagnoses, each with a different and sometimes very uncertain prognosis (Serwint and Nellis 2005; Brook and Hain 2008). The illness trajectory and palliative care needs of a child with acute lymphoblastic leukemia or neuroblastoma, for example, are very different to those with neurological disability arising from rare genetic or metabolic disorders.

In addition, the child is continuously developing, undergoing remarkable physical, social, and cognitive changes throughout childhood. He/she starts life as an unborn baby and progresses through infancy, childhood, and eventually to being a self-aware, autonomous young adult. His/her perception and understanding of life, illness, and death are, through this time, formative and malleable. At the same time, his/her role and relationships within the family and wider community is shaped by the culture of the family and society and evolves over time. In contrast, a significant proportion of children accessing palliative care services have varying degrees of neurological disability and cognitive impairment. This affects the degree of dependence on caregivers, their role within the family and community, and his/her awareness and understanding of illness and death.

Diagnosis of a life-limiting condition has far-reaching physical, psychosocial, emotional and spiritual, and cultural ramifications on the child, parents, siblings, grandparents, and other members of the extended family and community. Children and young people are dependent to varying degrees on their caregivers to provide the essentials of life, love, security, and increasingly, complex medical and nursing interventions.

This chapter outlines the principles and practicalities of pediatric palliative care provision and the epidemiology, special considerations, and challenges of research in this population.

2 Principles of Pediatric Palliative Care Provision

The World Health Organization (WHO) defines pediatric palliative care as:

"the total active care of the child's body, mind and spirit, and also involves giving support to the family.

- It begins when the illness is diagnosed and continues regardless of whether or not a child receives treatment directed at the disease.
- Health providers must evaluate and alleviate a child's physical, psychological and social distress.
- It makes use of available community resources; it can be successfully implemented even if resources are limited.
- It can be provided in tertiary care facilities, in community health centres and even in children's homes" (Sepúlveda et al. 2002).

Another frequently quoted definition from the Association for Children with Life-Threatening or Terminal Conditions and Their Families (ACT, now known as Together for Short Lives) and the Royal College of Paediatrics and Child Health (RCPCH) is given below:

"Palliative care for children and young people with life-limiting conditions is an active and total approach to care, embracing physical, emotional, social and spiritual elements. It focuses on quality of life for the child and support for the family and includes the management of distressing symptoms, provision of respite and care through death and bereavement" (Association for Children with Life-threatening or Terminal Conditions and their Families and Baum 1997).

Both these definitions acknowledge the importance of multidimensional care and the need to support both the child and family.

3 Referring to Palliative Care

In general, pediatric palliative care services will take referrals for children from before they are born through to late adolescence and increasingly young adulthood. Both the WHO and the American Academy of Pediatrics support the introduction of components of palliative care at diagnosis of a life-limiting illness (American Academy of Pediatrics Committee on Bioethics 2000; Feudtner 2007).

In 1997, the Association for Children's Palliative Care (ACT) and the Royal College of Paediatrics and Child Health (RCPCH) published a system identifying life-limiting illness in childhood. Four distinct categories (groups) were identified (Association for Children with Life-threatening or Terminal Conditions and their Families and Baum 1997). These categories were found to apply well to the pediatric palliative care population (Wood et al. 2010).

Group 1

Life-threatening conditions for which curative treatment may be feasible but can fail. Palliative care may be necessary during periods of prognostic uncertainty and when treatment fails. Children in long-term remission or following successful curative treatment are not included.

Examples include cancer and severe organ failure: heart, liver, or kidneys. Case 1 illustrates this concept.

Case 1

J, a previously healthy 11-year-old Maori (New Zealand indigenous peoples) boy presented with a 2-week history of abdominal pain and jaundice. An ultrasound and endoscopic retrograde cholangiopancreatography (ERCP) showed dilated bile ducts and polyps in the stomach and duodenum. A mediastinal mass and pleural and pericardial effusions were found on computed tomography (CT) imaging. A full blood count showed circulating blast cells and he was diagnosed with high-risk acute myeloblastic leukemia.

He was started on chemotherapy with curative intent and disease remission was achieved. He proceeded to a matched

(*continued*)

unrelated bone marrow transplant but relapsed 46 days after transplant. A referral to the palliative care team was made.

J's disease progressed rapidly. He developed breathlessness from leukemic infiltration of his lungs and bone pain in his legs. Both of these problems responded well to opioid medications. The palliative care team met with his parents and extended family who expressed a desire to take him home for end-of-life care. An advance care plan was created with his parents. He was discharged home with palliative care and pediatric community nursing support for end-of-life care. His pain and breathlessness escalated rapidly requiring frequent morphine and midazolam boluses and continuous subcutaneous infusions. He died 1 day after discharge surrounded by his family.

Group 2
Conditions where there may be long periods of intensive treatment aimed at prolonging life and allowing participation in normal childhood activities, but premature death is still possible.

Muscular dystrophy and other neuropathies causing respiratory failure fall into this category. Attention to nutrition and noninvasive ventilation have led to longer life expectancy but premature death is still likely.

Case 2
H, a 10-month-old New Zealand European girl was referred to the pediatric neurology service for delayed gross motor development. She was not able to hold her head up in the prone position consistently (a milestone normally attained at 3 months old) or roll over (usually 4 months old). Her social and language development were normal. She was profoundly weak and hypotonic on examination.

Genetic testing showed she had a homozygous deletion of the SMN1 gene, giving a diagnosis of spinal muscular atrophy (SMA) Type 1. This is an autonomic recessively inherited disease resulting in death of the anterior horn cells in the spinal cord. Life expectancy is limited by respiratory failure from muscle weakness. Impaired cough, hypoventilation, and chest and lung underdevelopment contribute to recurrent life-threatening respiratory tract infections. Prognosis is poor with a natural age of death younger than 2 years. Noninvasive ventilation and enteral nutrition can prolong life but premature death is still likely (Wang et al. 2007).

H was referred to respiratory, neurodevelopmental therapy and disability services as well as the pediatric palliative care team.

H's respiratory function and oral intake began to decline after diagnosis. At 12 months of age, she developed respiratory failure and started nocturnal noninvasive ventilation. Soon afterwards, she required a nasogastric tube to support her growth and nutrition. At 22 months old, she suffered her first life-threatening respiratory tract infection with admission to the intensive care unit, intubation, and mechanical ventilation. She developed several more serious lower respiratory tract infections over the next 2 months requiring long hospital admissions, without full recovery in between.

Just before her 2nd birthday, H suffered a series of life-threatening respiratory tract infections. She did not improve with maximal therapy on the ward. With the support of the palliative care team and the respiratory team, her parents made an advance care plan that avoided further intensive care admissions, intubation, mechanical ventilation or cardiopulmonary resuscitation. Her noninvasive ventilation was stopped and replaced with low flow oxygen. A continuous

(*continued*)

subcutaneous morphine infusion was started with provision for frequent morphine boluses for breathlessness.

Surprisingly, her symptoms improved dramatically on this regimen, from being obtunded to being able to play and interact. She steadily improved and was discharged home.

She is now 4 years old, relatively stable and well with excellent quality of life. Her advance care plan was changed at the age of 32 months to include full resuscitation and intensive care admission.

Group 3
Progressive conditions without curative treatment options, where treatment is exclusively palliative and may commonly extend over many years.

Some metabolic disorders such as Batten's disease fall into this group. Batten's disease is an autosomal recessive disorder affecting the lysosome. Progressive neurological disability results from a buildup of lipofuscins, causing developmental regression, seizures, and death. Palliative care can involve treating pain, muscle spasms, seizures, nutrition, and other disability-related problems. Care of these children and their families often involves several pediatric multidisciplinary teams, including neurology, rehabilitation, and general pediatric community teams, with whom palliative care work closely in a coordinated fashion. Prognosis and illness trajectory can be uncertain with plateaus and acute or more gradual episodes of decline.

Incurable cancers such as some childhood brain tumors also fall into this category. Tumor-directed therapy including debulking surgery, chemotherapy, and radiotherapy can control pain and other symptoms and prolong life expectancy.

Case 3
B was diagnosed at 6 months of age with a peroxisomal biogenesis disorder. She had been hypotonic since birth with difficulty feeding. Previously showing signs of having intact vision and hearing, both of these abilities had declined over the preceding 2 months. Her gross motor and language development had both regressed over the same time course. Her liver function tests were abnormal, putting her at risk for coagulopathy.

There is no known treatment for her condition. Her prognosis is uncertain but she could develop progressive degeneration of the white matter with increasing disability and shortened life expectancy. A referral to the palliative care was made to support her family with grief and loss issues, advocacy obtaining respite and suitable housing and advance care planning.

Over the next 4 years, B developed a series of neurological, respiratory, and gastrointestinal complications. She developed recurrent life-threatening respiratory tract infections and compromised liver function. Her vision and development regressed. Distressingly she developed severe muscle spasms, intractable irritability, gastrointestinal pseudo-obstruction, and gastric bleeding of unknown cause.

B's family had moved to another town and her care was transferred to the local pediatric team. However her parents brought her back to the metabolic team at the children's tertiary hospital where she had been cared for previously.

During her prolonged admission, she was cared for by the pediatric metabolic team, pediatric palliative care team, pediatric neurology team and pediatric gastroenterology teams, and child liaison psychiatry and ward nursing teams. She had a team of allied health practitioners including a physiotherapist, occupational therapist, and dietician to help support her development, seating aids, and nutrition. They did not have suitable housing or adequate respite

(*continued*)

care in their hometown, and the palliative care social worker advocated for access to these during her admission.

When she was ready for discharge, several videoconferences were held with the local general pediatric and palliative care teams to ensure a smooth coordinated handover of care. A detailed symptom management plan was drawn up by the palliative care and metabolic teams. A contact and communication system was set up so her parents knew who to call and where to get help.

Group 4
Conditions with severe neurological disability which may cause weakness and susceptibility to health complications and may deteriorate unpredictably, but are not usually considered progressive.

Children with severe cerebral palsy or have multiple disabilities from head or spinal cord injury fall into this group. Although the neurological lesion itself is nonprogressive, the child may suffer from frequent, worsening respiratory tract infections or seizure disorders which can cause premature death.

Case 4
E was born by emergency cesarean section at term after placental abruption. She required extensive resuscitation at birth and mechanical ventilation for 6 days. Magnetic resonance imaging (MRI) showed severe cerebral edema, consistent with severe hypoxic ischemic encephalopathy. She developed seizures and her EEG was profoundly abnormal. In discussion with her parents, mechanical ventilation was withdrawn with the expectation that she would not survive. However, surprisingly, she established spontaneous respirations and some oral feeding skills and was discharged home with palliative care and general pediatric support.

Shortly before discharge, E developed moderate irritability. This escalated sharply after she went home. Her high-pitched screaming cry lasted 20 h a day, causing much distress and fatigue for her parents and extended family members. She lost the ability to bottle-feed and became fully nasogastrically fed. Several full pediatric assessments failed to reveal any cause. Treatments for infantile colic and gastroesophageal reflux disease were not effective.

A diagnosis of cerebral irritability following hypoxic ischemic encephalopathy was made. Gabapentin was titrated up with initial improvement but irritability increased again.

Her parents were sleep deprived, exhausted, and distressed. Respite was slow to become available and was far from adequate. The palliative care social worker obtained some short-term night nursing and advocated for the parents with the local needs assessment agency for an increase in respite hours.

Several more possible causes of pain and irritability emerged over several months, prolonged oral candidiasis, projectile vomiting, seizure activity, dystonic posturing, and muscle spasms. Each of these were investigated and treated with varying levels of effectiveness on her irritability.

Agents trialed include gabapentin and morphine for cerebral irritability and central pain; diazepam, clonazepam, baclofen, and midazolam for dystonia and spasms; ranitidine, omeprazole, and gaviscon antacid liquid for reflux oesophagitis; a change of enteral feed to elemental formula for milk protein intolerance; carbamazepine, sodium valproate, and topiramate for seizures; and fluconazole for oral candidiasis.

(*continued*)

Her parents and grandparents became exhausted and experienced feelings of helplessness, despair, and anger. The healthcare professionals also felt frustrated and helpless.

After 3 months, her irritability slowly settled but continued to fluctuate for the first year of her life causing much distress.

4 Epidemiology

4.1 Prevalence

There is evidence that the prevalence of children needing palliative care is increasing. In England, the prevalence was estimated at 10 per 10,000 children in 1997 (Association for Children with Life-threatening or Terminal Conditions and their Families and Baum 1997). This figure had risen to 25 per 10,000 in the year 2000, then increased again by 33% to 32 per 10,000 by 2010 (Fraser et al. 2012). The groups with the highest prevalence were those less than 1 year old. However, the 16–19-year-old age group showed the greatest increase, rising by 45% over the 10-year period between 2000 and 2010. This suggests that increasing survival times, possibly from medical interventions, accounts for at least some of the increase in overall prevalence.

Exploring the young adult group in more detail, a study from the University of York, England, demonstrated a linear relationship between prevalence and deprivation. Those who were most deprived had the highest rates of life-limiting illness. Variation between ethnic groups was also found, with those of black or South East Asian descent having significantly higher rates of life-limiting illness (Fraser et al. 2014).

4.2 Diagnosis

The majority of referrals consist of children with non-cancer diagnoses, a departure from the traditional adult palliative care population. In a prospective observational cohort study (Feudtner et al. 2011) of children served by 6 hospital-based services in the United States and Canada, 515 new (35.7%) or established (64.3%) patients were identified over a 3-month period. Of these, the predominant primary clinical conditions were genetic/congenital (40.8%), neuromuscular (39.2%), cancer (19.8%), respiratory (12.8%), and gastrointestinal (10.7%). Similar patterns have been recorded in England (Fraser et al. 2012). Most patients were reliant on some form of medical technology, with gastrostomy tubes (48.5%) being the most common, and 47.2% of the children had cognitive impairment.

Similarly, children with non-cancer diagnoses accounted for over 70% of deaths in a New Zealand study (Chang et al. 2013). Children with non-cancer diagnoses often have a less predictable illness trajectory and prognosis, resulting in greater uncertainty and often require palliative care for a number of years (Brook and Hain 2008). More detailed discussion of the challenges of working with this group is covered in following sections of this chapter.

5 Illness Trajectories

How children progress from health, through illness, and finally death can be roughly divided into 4 patterns – sudden death, steady decline, fluctuating decline, and fragile with repeated risk of decline and death (Feudtner 2007). These do not completely correlate with the four diagnostic categories outlined by the ACT/RCPCH. There are some common elements of disease trajectory which cross all categories as well as some distinct to certain categories (Wood et al. 2010).

5.1 Sudden Death

A previously healthy child experiences a sudden event, such as an accident or previously asymptomatic undiagnosed medical illness such as hypertrophic cardiomyopathy. Other than bereavement care, there is no opportunity to benefit from palliative care.

5.2 Steady Decline

A previously healthy child is diagnosed with a life-limiting illness such as a cancer with poor prognosis. There may be some decline in quality of life and health status before diagnosis and some improvement with treatments such as chemotherapy, radiotherapy, and surgery. However, once there are no further treatments that can modify disease progression, the child's condition declines until the child dies.

Case 1, J with acute myelocytic leukemia from Group 1 (above) followed this type of course.

5.3 Fluctuating Decline

Children from Groups 2 and 3 (above) often have a turbulent course with periods of acute illness and decline followed by recovery. After each episode of illness, however, the recovery is incomplete and the child may not return to his/her previous health status or quality of life. This is common in children with non-cancer conditions, but increasingly, with development of novel cancer therapies, children who die from cancer can also follow such a course. Diagnosis is followed by chemotherapy, radiotherapy, and sometimes surgery resulting in periods of recovery followed by relapse. Second-line treatments can be introduced to prolong life or enhance quality of life for a limited time before the child's condition declines and eventually they die.

5.4 Fragile

Children from Group 4 often experience a compromised level of quality of life and health status from the start due to disability and can plateau for long periods of time. Events such as aspiration pneumonia, intractable seizures, cerebral irritability, and spasticity can lead to acute decline in quality of life. If these are treated, the child can recover to some extent and plateau but is always vulnerable to further complications.

6 Settings

Palliative and end-of-life care can be provided wherever the child is. The three main settings are the child's home, in hospital, or in a children's hospice. Rates of death in these settings vary internationally. This may be influenced by availability of services and facilities, e.g., children's hospice, community outreach teams, etc. Cultural beliefs about the place of death may also influence where children are cared for at the end of life.

In a large multicenter trial looking at place of death of children referred to pediatric palliative care services in Canada, Australia, and the United Kingdom, the numbers of children dying at home, in hospital, and in a children's hospice were equally divided between the three settings (Siden et al. 2008). Rates of death in hospital have been shown to vary by age, diagnosis, and ethnic group (Feudtner et al. 2002; Cochrane et al. 2007; Chang et al. 2013). Infants (children under 1 year old) have higher odds of dying in hospital as do children with non-cancer diagnoses. Referral to a pediatric palliative care team has been shown to decrease the odds of dying in hospital (Chang et al. 2013).

7 The Palliative Care Team

The World Health Organization, as mentioned before, refers to palliative care of children as the "total active care of the child's body, mind and spirit" and "health providers must evaluate and alleviate a child's physical, psychological and social distress" (Sepúlveda et al. 2002). Caring for the child also means caring for the family, consisting of parents, siblings of varying ages, grandparents, and other significant members. Providing effective, quality palliative care to the child therefore means providing family-centered care. This approach equips families to care for their children through diagnosis and palliative and end-of-life care and provides support into bereavement. Not included in the WHO definition, but of increasing importance with globalization and immigration, is providing care that meets the cultural needs of each family.

Such an all-encompassing job description means that no single practitioner or discipline is able to acquire all the skills needed. An interdisciplinary team working closely in a coordinated fashion is most likely to provide quality palliative care. This team can then be truly responsive to the requirements of the individual child and their family by effectively communicating with the family unit about anxieties, fears, and misconceptions and, in so doing, openly discuss treatment strategies.

Team members in pediatric palliative care services around the world vary according to training and resources. In general, however, most teams will have, as a minimum, pediatric nurses and pediatricians with some expertise in children's palliative care. Psychologists, social workers, psychotherapists, psychiatrists, play specialists, physiotherapists, and occupational therapists are among the other members of the interdisciplinary team (Knapp et al. 2012).

In conjunction with the palliative care team, children and their families are cared for by other pediatric teams, disability support services, and cultural and spiritual support services. General and/or subspecialty multidisciplinary teams may have cared for them since diagnosis and can remain involved through palliative and end-of-life care.

Often, one member of the palliative care team acts as a key or link worker. This strategy gives the family a point of contact to assist with coordination and planning of care, particularly as this group of children often have a large number of care providers and agencies involved across a range of care settings (Hynson et al. 2003). Case 3, the child with a peroxisomal biogenesis disorder illustrates the large number of teams and healthcare professionals that are typically involved with pediatric palliative care patients and now care needs to be carefully coordinated.

8 Special Considerations in Children

8.1 Developmental Issues

The most obvious difference between children and adults is the considerable physical, cognitive, and emotional change that occurs as a child moves from infancy through childhood then into adolescence. This is by no means a linear process and neither is it determined by the age of the child. Rather "milestones" are achieved within a likely age range and developmental gains are followed by periods of plateau whether that is physical, cognitive, or emotional. This is seen in full clarity during the adolescent years, internationally recognized as ranging from 10 to 25 years, when adult physical attributes are gained relatively quickly compared to the staggered and slower cognitive and emotional changes with connection of the executive functioning of the frontal lobes to the deeper emotional centers of the limbic system.

This then requires the pediatric healthcare clinician to be able to determine the child's developmental level at the time of assessment. This is not a skill gained by having your own children but gained by years of interaction with acutely and chronically ill children of all ages where age-appropriate development is the norm and through this experiential foundation being able to determine when a child is outside the expected. The additional nuance brought to the table by working with seriously ill children is when development out of keeping for the child's age is acceptable. For example, the 7-year-old child with intestinal failure from birth who appears physically frail but through years of interaction with the medical system has advanced cognitive and emotional skills, or the 15-year-old physically well-developed adolescent with cancer shows regression in behavior consistent with a 10-year-old at a time of an acute deterioration requiring hospitalization for further evaluation.

This means assessing children across the age range requires a large array of approaches to allow a therapeutic relationship to be established with not only the child but their family as well. This raises the fundamental need to see the child not only as an individual but a unit involving their parents (and not uncommonly in today's Western society separated but equally concerned parent's), their siblings, and, in many cultural settings, the wider family unit of grandparents, aunts, uncles, etc. who may also be the main point of communication or decision-making rather than the parents (Craig et al. 2007; Bradford et al. 2014).

8.2 Symptom Management

As in adult palliative care, management of physical symptoms is a core part of providing quality care. However, the range of symptoms faced by children is very much determined by the mix of conditions cared for by pediatric palliative care specialist services. Children often present with multiple symptoms. The most common symptoms identified were cognitive impairment, speech impairment, fatigue and sleep problems, low enteral intake, and seizures (Feudtner et al. 2011).

Pain was less common with approximately 20% presenting with somatic pain, 10% visceral pain, and another 10% with neuropathic pain. The assessment and management of pain in children is a good example of the specialized skills and knowledge required in this field (Feudtner et al. 2011).

8.2.1 Pain

Even though a relatively small proportion of children present with pain, it is consistently the most concerning for children and their families during palliative and end-of-life care. Good pain management plays a central role in maintaining a satisfactory quality of life. It also exemplifies many of the issues involved in working with children during palliation and provides a good window onto managing any symptom a child may experience.

The clinician requires a sound knowledge of pathophysiology, child development and behavior, pain responses and family dynamics, children's spirituality, and cultural influences to elicit and interpret a history given by the child and caregivers. Case 4, the newborn with hypoxic brain injury during birth, illustrates some of the complexity involved in assessing pain and irritability in an infant.

Pain is subjective; it is "what the child says it is," but it is not uncommon for children to underreport pain. The reasons for this can be simple or more complex. A simple explanation being the child underreports pain to avoid a possible or perceived painful experience as they fear this will lead to an injection. An example of a more complex issue is seen when the child plays their part in "mutual pretense" (Bluebond-Langner et al. 2005); a situation where the child and parent(s) guard against the disclosure to each other that the child will eventually die to avoid distressing the other party with this extending to the child underreporting pain.

The assessment of pain needs to be thorough and, if suspected but not revealed, specifically asked about. This can be particularly challenging when the child is not fully able to express themselves. However, the lack of verbal ability does not preclude assessment as several validated, observational pain assessment tools are available. The FLACC Behavioral Pain Assessment Tool is suitable for infants and toddlers (Voepel-Lewis et al. 1997), the Premature Infant Pain Profile for preterm neonates (Stevens et al. 1996; Voepel-Lewis et al. 1997), and the Non-Communicating Children's Checklist, the Paediatric Pain Profile, and the revised FLACC for children with disability (Breau et al. 2002; Hunt et al. 2004; Malviya et al. 2006). These tools can be applied in any setting by the child's caregiver or health professional and, for most, only take a few minutes. The child is observed for signs and behaviors that indicate pain and a score is generated which indicates the likely level of pain the child is experiencing. Pain behaviors in children with cognitive impairment can differ from those of other children and not easily recognized. For example, a sign of moderate pain could be "tense or guarded movements; mild agitation (e.g. head moved back and forth, aggression); shallow splinting respirations and intermittent sighs." Another example could be an "increase in spasticity, constant tremors or jerking of the legs" (Voepel-Lewis et al. 1997). The use of a validated pain tool is a prerequisite to effective pain assessment and management and the onus is on clinicians to be aware of, and use these tools, appropriately.

In addition, if pain is seen purely as a physical phenomenon, then the ramifications and impact on the child's emotional, psychosocial, and existential or spiritual domains will be missed. Furthermore, this Cartesian view, where the mind is separate from the body, also overlooks the likelihood that a disease in any one of these domains can influence pain. This reinforces the need for a holistic approach to symptom assessment and for these to be pitched at a level of understanding harmonious with the individual child. This requires therapeutic actions to employ a combination of pharmacological and nonpharmacological approaches and any endeavors failing to take this into account are less likely to be successful (McGrath 1996).

The value of any chosen therapy should be carefully considered by weighing up potential benefits against burdens. This requires the clinician to have knowledge about the disease process, pathophysiology of pain (or symptom being addressed), and the pharmacolical and nonpharmacological methods used to treat it. As always, basing this on published evidence is the ideal. The problem is children are "therapeutic orphans" where investigation of treatment options to base management decisions is generally lacking. This does not mean medications should be denied because of absent published studies or the availability of poor data. What it does mean is use can be informed by inference from adult data and moderated by clinical experience of tolerability and effectiveness in children.

8.3 Prescribing in Children

The key distinction of growth and development as linked processes between working with children and adults is illustrated by prescribing medication. Historically, dosing has been based on body weight or the use of body surface area for drugs with a low therapeutic index. The problem with these methods is body weight can underestimate while surface area overestimate dosing in children. However, there are many formularies that offer suitable instructions based on the supposition that the volume of distribution per kilogram is the same in children as for adults. These "per kilogram of weight" dosing recommendations, while approximations, work reasonably well (Hain 1999; Hunt et al. 1999). However, there is a third, more complicated model, **allometric power model**, which has been found useful in normalizing a large number of physiological and pharmacokinetic variables. Essentially, this model uses an exponent of weight to derive a potentially more appropriate dose of a drug for children (Anderson and Meakin 2002).

8.4 Communication and Decision-Making

One specific difference to adult care is how the healthcare professional communicates with the child and family. Primary communication is not always going to be with the child, regardless of age, it is going to be with their caregivers. This requires the child health worker to be able to change their style of communication to not only talk at a level consistent with child's cognitive ability, which is not necessarily the same as their chronological age, but to connect with and inform parents, grandparents, and siblings alike. This may raise concern about the child's autonomy (right to self-determination) which means one must act with intention, with understanding, and without controlling influences. Children requiring palliative care may not be able to fulfill these requirements because of the effects of the illness, or they may not wish to have the additional burden of decision-maker on their shoulders, even if able to do so, making them reliant on their caregivers as surrogate decision-makers.

No one would dispute that the infant is fully dependent on its caregivers, particularly their mother, for food, warmth, shelter, and safety. This requires the health worker in children's palliative care to work with, at least, the mother to ascertain the needs of the baby and, in many ways, the parent(s) becomes a vital interpreter of the baby's welfare, for example, interpreting mannerisms that are out-of-keeping for their baby and indicative of troublesome symptoms or changes in behavior that are more reflective of emotional or psychological distress. In some cases, such changes may not be related to the disease process at all; rather they are consistent with a known developmental phenomenon such as colic vs. pain from a disease entity or movements at night being a normal part of the sleep cycle vs. movements associated with age-related reflux vs. seizures or dystonia associated with the child's disease state.

Switch to the other end of the developmental trajectory and you could be confronted by the reticent, if not patently disrespectful, adolescent who in the face of distressing symptoms ignores effective medications out of a need to have, at least, some form of control and independence in a situation that is trying to rob them of this desired goal attainment. Yet, the adolescent in this situation is not fully equipped to be truly autonomous as they are not free of influences such as undertreated symptoms that can affect their ability to make decisions. However, within the context of children's palliative care, experience indicates that even older adolescents do not necessarily wish to be the sole architect of their fate, preferring to defer to their parents for decisions about their care. This can lead to a harmful misinterpretation by the healthcare worker that the parents are controlling the young person's decision-making against their will unless time is taken to determine the actual circumstances.

In the medical context, respect for autonomy involves allowing a person to make informed choices, a nebulous concept, about their care. The Royal College of Paediatrics and Child Health among others (Royal College of Paediatrics and Child Health London 2004; Jacobs et al. 2015; Xafis et al. 2015; Day et al. 2016) advocate strongly for participation of children in decision-making to the extent their ability allows, and they identify four levels of decision-making in pediatric care:

1. The child being informed
2. The child being consulted
3. The child's views being taken into account
4. The child being respected as the main person in decision-making (Royal College of Paediatrics and Child Health London 2004)

This translates to even young children having the right to be informed about decisions affecting their future with this communicated in a way that is appropriate to their level of understanding. It is also important that no matter what the child's ability or inability to communicate or participate is, it does not mean their suffering should be excluded from benefit vs. burden considerations. Facilitation of information also requires the child and their family to be free of conditions such as fear, pain, and depression which may compromise their capacity to make truly autonomous decisions. The obligation on the pediatric palliative care worker is to ascertain if they are free of such encumbrances.

The other important concept in palliative care for children as compared to adult care with respect to decision-making capacity is competence. Assessing a child's competence requires the ability to ascertain the child's cognitive ability. At its simplest, this can be determined by their ability to provide a clinical history, understand their condition and treatment options, and have an appreciation of the consequences of choosing one treatment approach over another. These factors then need to be considered in the context of their level of education, verbal skills, and previous demonstrations of their capacity to make decisions. All in the presence or absence of disturbed thinking that could be part of a psychiatric disorder or psychological diagnosis.

To this point, an attempt has been made to downplay age as a determining factor, but this is the very thing turned to if a legal perspective is sought. At least in the United Kingdom and in its legal system, the following concept has some influence.

There is an assumption that children <14 years of age are not competent to make decisions while young adults, 18 years and over, are considered adult with full decision-making capacity. Between these bookends of age, a gray zone exists where children between 16 and 18 years are known as mature minors and legally considered able to consent to treatment but not able to consent to withdrawal of life-sustaining treatment against their parents' wishes, while children aged between 14 and 16 years require careful assessment as to what level of decision-making they fulfill. However, this viewpoint is not universally accepted. Cultural views on childhood and coming of age vary around the world. For example, an Islamic perspective of adulthood is tied to the ability to reproduce. Thus, menarche in girls and first ejaculation in boys signals the onset of adulthood, a view not commonly accepted in Western societies (Gatrad and Sheikh 2001).

In practice though, the majority of children and their parents agree about the most appropriate way to make decisions. A young adult may wish to make some or all decisions during palliation and end-of-life care but may also wish for his/her parents to do this on their behalf.

8.4.1 Advance Care Planning and Illness Trajectories

Illness trajectories seen in pediatrics lead to further challenges in decision-making. For many children, their clinical course and rate of decline is uncertain and unpredictable. He/she may suffer several life-threatening episodes where end-of-life care is started, only to survive and recover. Advance care plans need to factor in this unpredictability and encompass the hope for recovery and longer survival as well as symptom management, emotional, psychosocial, spiritual, and cultural support for the end of life. One scenario in which the advance care plan needs to encompass a range of possibilities is when a fetus is diagnosed with a life-limiting condition.

Case 2, the child with spinal muscular atrophy, shows how advance care plans need to be changed according to the child's condition and the hopes of the child and family.

9 Collaboration Between Adult and Pediatric Services

Although pediatric palliative care is distinct from adult palliative care, the number of specialist clinicians in pediatric palliative care, medical and nonmedical, is limited. Children often live geographically distant from specialist pediatric palliative care services as teams are mostly based in larger towns and cities. Currently and in the near future, the pediatric palliative care workforce is unlikely to reach a number sufficient to care for, in any country, every child eligible for palliative care support (Knapp et al. 2012).

This requires a pragmatic approach to providing an alternative model of care. It is not entirely surprising that a reasonably consistent attitude has developed where specialist services promote supporting health professionals in the pediatric healthcare and adult palliative care sectors.

Ideally, these two groups will collaborate to ensure their particular skills and knowledge are used to complement each other. The pediatrician and pediatric multidisciplinary team have in-depth knowledge of the child's disease, prognosis, likely complications, and management strategies. This knowledge is essential for good symptom management and decision-making. He/she may have established a significant relationship with the family from many years of involvement. This enhances communication and provision of psychological and emotional support. The adult palliative care physician and team have experience in symptom management and end-of-life care and regularly provide psychological, emotional, and spiritual support to family members through grief and bereavement. A combination of these two skill sets can result in good quality palliative, end-of-life care, and bereavement care.

For the reasons outlined in this chapter, it cannot be recommended that the adult palliative care workers operate in isolation to pediatric teams. Lack of expertise in normal child development, pediatric pathophysiology, and assessment of symptoms in children can mean misdiagnosis and incorrect treatment with consequent suffering. Practicing without experience and understanding of cognitive and emotional development and family dynamics can lead to miscommunication, anger, and a compromised therapeutic relationship with long-lasting effects in bereavement.

If you work in isolation by choice, no matter your profession, training, or experience, then consider Alexander Pope's quote in "An Essay on

Criticism." "Of all the causes which conspire to blind man's erring judgment and misguide the mind, what the weak head with strongest bias rules, is pride, the never-failing vice of fools."

10 Research

As a relatively new specialty, pediatric palliative care research is still developing. Currently, much of the literature comprises of case series and descriptive studies with small numbers of participants (Ullrich et al. 2013). Clinical guidelines rely strongly on expert opinion and experience and studies on the adult population which have been extrapolated to children, which for various reasons are of limited use. The evidence base is weak and this is well recognized. Why then is research so underdeveloped?

The patient population itself presents a hurdle to high-quality research. Children with palliative care needs have a diverse range of diagnoses, illness trajectories, and potential symptoms, making it difficult to compare one group of children with another (Ullrich et al. 2013). Rarity of diagnoses with small numbers of potential participants can mean that studies are underpowered to look for desired outcomes. The emotionally charged nature of this field and ethical considerations pose an additional challenge.

One barrier to research is difficulty recruiting children and families (Ullrich et al. 2013). Fear of causing distress and adversely affecting a family's journey through grief and bereavement is a valid concern. Selection of potential participants is often done via palliative care team members who have cared for the patient and family. This can lead to "gatekeeping" where eligible children and families are not approached to participate out of concern for the distress this is perceived to cause. For example, in a recent study looking at parents' experiences of advance care planning, only 5% of eligible families currently receiving palliative care were invited to participate. The rate was a little higher with recently bereaved families with 29% invited to participate (Crocker et al. 2014).

Looking at clinician's field notes of how they chose families to approach, several factors were identified. The perceived well-being of the family, how they may react to being approached, and their previous engagement with healthcare professionals were important. How likely they were to contribute to the study, e.g., communication abilities and relevant experience, is also featured.

Recruitment was affected by the relationship between family and clinician. Clinicians felt they could invite families with whom they had a good established relationship. Concern that the relationship could be adversely affected by recruitment led to non-recruitment. As a result, families who had had more contact with clinicians and in particular out of hours contact were more likely to be invited. (Crocker et al. 2014) This leads to potential bias, with those considered well adjusted, articulate, and able to engage clinicians more likely to be selected. Therefore, the needs of families who have been less able to access palliative care services are not well identified, and little is written about how to engage this population.

How well founded are the concerns of clinicians and researchers? A survey of parents looking at the effect of participation from the Dana Farber Cancer Institute suggests that this is not as great an issue as feared. One hundred and ninety-four parents (70% response rate) who had taken part in a study about discussion of their child's prognosis were asked about the positive and negative effects of participating (Olcese and Mack 2012).

Only 1% found research participation very distressing. Sixty-two percent indicated that they were not at all distressed and 69% felt it was useful to them personally to have participated. Overall, 18% of parents gave higher ratings for distress than utility. Parents were more likely to have found it distressing if the research was done less than 100 days since the child's diagnosis and less likely if they felt a sense of peace about the child's illness. This suggests that a lower than anticipated number of parents would find participation distressing. The majority also found participation useful even if it caused distress. Paying attention to factors such as the timing of the research could help lower distress.

So what is the future for pediatric palliative care research? A Delphi study involving clinicians and researchers identified family experiences, pain and symptom management, bereavement, and suffering at the end of life as priority topics (Steele et al. 2008). More recently, an editorial from the *Journal of Palliative Medicine* further clarifies these priorities. Research should focus either on child-specific issues or areas in palliative care for children that would contribute to palliative care provision for children as well as adults. In addition, the needs of the very young (perinatal palliative care) and the young adult need to be highlighted. Lastly, adequate funding, research training, and expertise are essential for these priorities to result in quality pediatric palliative care research (Ullrich et al. 2013).

11 Summary

Children with life-limiting illnesses have unique palliative care needs that are distinct from adults. Pediatric palliative care services care for children with life-limiting illnesses, from the unborn baby through to the young adult. A wide range of conditions, some rare with unpredictable and changing illness trajectories, require expert knowledge in childhood conditions and a flexible approach to symptom management, goals of care, and advance care planning. The child's developmental needs and his/her place in the family and society change through the lifespan and must be considered at all times when assessing and communicating with the child and family. The child or young person's ability and willingness to participate in their own care and in advance care planning can vary widely depending on age, intellectual ability, cultural influences, family dynamics, and past experiences. Care of the child and the whole family through illness, end of life, and bereavement is essential when delivering quality pediatric palliative care.

References

American Academy of Pediatrics Committee on Bioethics. Palliative care for children. Pediatrics. 2000;106(2):351–7.

Anderson BJ, Meakin GH. Scaling for size: some implications for paediatric anaesthesia dosing. Pediatr Anesth. 2002;12(3):205–19.

A guide to the development of children's palliative care services. Report of a joint working party of the Royal College of Paediatrics and Child Health and the Association for Chidlren with Life-threatening or Terminal Conditions and their Families. London: RCPCH; 1997

Bluebond-Langner M, DeCicco A, Belasco J. Involving children with life-shortening illnesses in decisions about participation in clinical research: a proposal for shuttle diplomacy and negotiation. In: Kodish E, editor. Ethics and research with children. New York: Oxford University Press; 2005. p. 323–44.

Bradford N, Herbert A, Mott C, Armfield N, Young J, Smith A. Components and principles of a pediatric palliative care consultation: results of a Delphi study. J Palliat Med. 2014;17(11):1206–13.

Breau LM, McGrath PJ, Camfield CS, Finley GA. Psychometric properties of the non-communicating children's pain checklist-revised. Pain. 2002;99(1):349–57.

Brook L, Hain R. Predicting death in children. Arch Dis Child. 2008;93(12):1067–70.

Chang E, MacLeod R, Drake R. Characteristics influencing location of death for children with life-limiting illness. Arch Dis Child. 2013;98(6):419–24.

Cochrane H, Liynage S, Nantanmbi R. Palliative care statistics for children and young adults: health and care partnerships analysis. London: Department of Health; 2007.

Craig F, Abu-Saad Huijer H, Benini F, Kuttner L, Wood C, Feraris P, Zernikow B, Steering Committee of the EAPC task force on palliative care for children and adolescents. IMPaCCT: standards for paediatric palliative care in Europe. Eur J Palliat Care. 2007;14:109–14.

Crocker JC, Beecham E, Kelly P, Dinsdale AP, Hemsley J, Jones L, Bluebond-Langner M. Inviting parents to take part in paediatric palliative care research: a mixed-methods examination of selection bias. Palliat Med. 2014;29:231. https://doi.org/10.1177/0269216314560803.

Day E, Jones L, Langner R, Bluebond-Langner M. Current understanding of decision-making in adolescents with cancer: a narrative systematic review. Palliat Med. 2016;30(10):920–34.

Dingfield L, Bender L, Harris P, Newport K, Hoover-Regan M, Feudtner C, Clifford S, Casarett D. Comparison of pediatric and adult hospice patients using electronic medical record data from nine hospices in the United States, 2008–2012. J Palliat Med. 2015;18(2): 120–6.

Feudtner C. Collaborative communication in pediatric palliative care: a foundation for problem-solving and decision-making. Pediatr Clin N Am. 2007;54(5):583–607.

Feudtner C, Silveira MJ, Christakis DA. Where do children with complex chronic conditions die? Patterns in Washington state, 1980–1998. Pediatrics. 2002;109 (4):656–60.

Feudtner C, Kang TI, Hexem KR, Friedrichsdorf SJ, Osenga K, Siden H, Friebert SE, Hays RM, Dussel V, Wolfe J. Pediatric palliative care patients: a prospective multicenter cohort study. Pediatrics. 2011;127(6):1094–101.

Fraser LK, Miller M, Hain R, Norman P, Aldridge J, McKinney PA, Parslow RC. Rising national prevalence of life-limiting conditions in children in England. Pediatrics. 2012;129(4):e923–9.

Fraser L, Miller M, Aldridge J, McKinney PA, Parslow RC. Prevalence of life-limiting and life-threatening conditions in young adults in England 2000–2010. Palliat Med. 2014;28:513–20.

Gatrad A, Sheikh A. Medical ethics and Islam: principles and practice. Arch Dis Child. 2001;84(1):72–5.

Hain RD. Morphine and morphine-6-glucuronide in the plasma and cerebrospinal fluid of children. Br J Clin Pharmacol. 1999;48(1):37–42.

Hunt A, Joel S, Dick G, Goldman A. Population pharmacokinetics of oral morphine and its glucuronides in children receiving morphine as immediate-release liquid or sustained-release tablets for cancer pain. J Pediatr. 1999;135(1):47–55.

Hunt A, Goldman A, Seers K, Crichton N, Mastroyannopoulou K, Moffat V, Oulton K, Brady M. Clinical validation of the paediatric pain profile. Dev Med Child Neurol. 2004;46(01):9–18.

Hynson JL, Gillis J, Collins JJ, Irving H, Trethewie SJ. The dying child: how is care different? Med J Aust. 2003;179(6):S20.

Jacobs S, Perez J, Cheng YI, Sill A, Wang J, Lyon ME. Adolescent end of life preferences and congruence with their parents' preferences: results of a survey of adolescents with cancer. Pediatr Blood Cancer. 2015;62(4):710–4.

Knapp C, Madden V, Fowler-Kerry S. Pediatric palliative care: global perspectives. Dordrecht: Springer; 2012.

Malviya S, VOEPEL-LEWIS T, Burke C, Merkel S, Tait AR. The revised FLACC observational pain tool: improved reliability and validity for pain assessment in children with cognitive impairment. Pediatr Anesth. 2006;16(3):258–65.

McGrath PA. Development of the World Health Organization guidelines on cancer pain relief and palliative care in children. J Pain Symptom Manag. 1996;12(2):87–92.

Olcese ME, Mack JW. Research participation experiences of parents of children with cancer who were asked about their child's prognosis. J Palliat Med. 2012;15(3):269–73.

Royal College of Paediatrics and Child Health. Withholding and Withdrawing life saving treatment in children: A framework for practice. 2nd edn. London: RCPCH; 2004

Sepúlveda C, Marlin A, Yoshida T, Ullrich A. Palliative care: the World Health Organization's global perspective. J Pain Symptom Manag. 2002;24(2):91–6.

Serwint JR, Nellis ME. Deaths of pediatric patients: relevance to their medical home, an urban primary care clinic. Pediatrics. 2005;115(1):57–63.

Siden H, Miller M, Straatman L, Omesi L, Tucker T, Collins J. A report on location of death in paediatric palliative care between home, hospice and hospital. Palliat Med. 2008;22(7):831–4.

Steele R, Bosma H, Johnston MF, Cadell S, Davies B, Siden H, Straatman L. Research priorities in pediatric palliative care: a Delphi study. J Palliat Care. 2008;24(4):229.

Stevens B, Johnston C, Petryshen P, Taddio A. Premature infant pain profile: development and initial validation. Clin J Pain. 1996;12(1):13–22.

Ullrich C, Morrison SAE, Sean R. Pediatric palliative care research comes of age: what we stand to learn from children with life-threatening illness. J Palliat Med. 2013;16(4):334–6.

Voepel-Lewis T, Shayevitz JR, Malviya S. The FLACC: a behavioral scale for scoring postoperative pain in young children. Pediatr Nurs. 1997;23:293–7.

Wang CH, Finkel RS, Bertini ES, Schroth M, Simonds A, Wong B, Aloysius A, Morrison L, Main M, Crawford TO. Consensus statement for standard of care in spinal muscular atrophy. J Child Neurol. 2007;22(8):1027–49.

Wood F, Simpson S, Barnes E, Hain R. Disease trajectories and ACT/RCPCH categories in paediatric palliative care. Palliat Med. 2010;24(8):796–806.

Xafis V, Gillam L, Hynson J, Sullivan J, Cossich M, Wilkinson D. Caring decisions: the development of a written resource for parents facing end-of-life decisions. J Palliat Med. 2015;18(11):945–55.

Palliative Care and Intellectual Disability

69

Irene Tuffrey-Wijne

Contents

I. Tuffrey-Wijne (✉)
Faculty of Health, Social Care and Education, Kingston University and St George's, University of London, London, UK
e-mail: I.Tuffrey-Wijne@sgul.kingston.ac.uk

R. D. MacLeod, L. Van den Block (eds.), *Textbook of Palliative Care*,
https://doi.org/10.1007/978-3-319-77740-5_69

Abstract

People with intellectual disabilities make up an estimated 1–3% of the population. This is an aging population, with an associated increasing need for palliative care provision.

However, many do not have equitable access to palliative care services, for a variety of reasons. They often have issues, challenges, and circumstances that make it particularly difficult to meet their palliative care needs. This includes communication difficulties which affect all the aspects of palliative care provision; difficulties around insight and the ability to participate in decision making; unconventional ways of expressing signs and symptoms of ill health and distress; multiple comorbidities; complex family and social circumstances; and higher levels of behavioral or psychiatric problems.

This chapter describes the unique challenges in meeting the needs of people with intellectual disabilities at the end of life. It is based on the White Paper on Intellectual Disabilities, published by the European Association of Palliative Care in 2015. It addresses the following key areas: equity of access; communication; recognizing the need for palliative care; assessment of total needs; symptom management; end of life decision-making; involving those who matter; collaboration; support for families and carers; preparing for death; bereavement support; education and training; developing and managing services. This provides a comprehensive overview of the current state of the art.

1 Introduction

There has been a growing recognition in recent years of the importance of focusing attention on the palliative care needs of people with intellectual disabilities. The life expectancy of people with intellectual disabilities has increased significantly over the past 50 years (Patja et al. 2000). The increase in life expectancy for people with Down syndrome has been particularly marked, from 12 in 1949 to nearly 60 in 2004 (Bittles and Glasson 2004). This dramatic shift has been attributed to reduced childhood mortality and to better knowledge, healthcare, advocacy, and services (Yang et al. 2002; Haveman et al. 2009).

As people with intellectual disabilities are living longer, they are more likely to die of illnesses usually associated with old age, and they more likely to need a period of palliative care (Tuffrey-Wijne 2003). The aim of this chapter is to describe the unique challenges in meeting the needs of people with intellectual disabilities who require palliative care, as well as important considerations in addressing those challenges. It is based on the White Paper published by the European Association for Palliative Care (EAPC) in 2015, which sets out aspirational norms in 13 areas of practice. These norms were reached through using the Delphi method to reach consensus, involving 92 professionals in 15 countries who had expertise in the fields of palliative care, intellectual disabilities, or both. The full methods and detailed norms can be found in the White Paper itself (Tuffrey-Wijne and McLaughlin 2015) and an accompanying open access paper (Tuffrey-Wijne et al. 2015). Here, the focus is on describing the relevant issues under the following headings, in line with the 13 norms:

1. Equity of access
2. Communication
3. Recognizing the need for palliative care
4. Assessment of total needs
5. Symptom management
6. End-of-life decision making
7. Involving those who matter: families, friends, and carers
8. Collaboration
9. Support for families and carers
10. Preparing for death
11. Bereavement support
12. Education and training
13. Developing and managing services

First, the context of these issues will be set out through describing the prevalence of intellectual disabilities and the profile of illness and dying among this population.

2 Background

2.1 Definition

Intellectual disability is characterized by significantly impaired intellectual and adaptive functioning. Someone has intellectual disabilities if the following three aspects are present simultaneously: (1) a significantly reduced ability to understand new or complex information and to learn and apply new skills (impaired intelligence); (2) a significantly reduced ability to cope independently, expressed in conceptual, social, and practical adaptive skills (impaired adaptive functioning); and (3) onset before the age of 18, with a lasting effect on development (American Association on Intellectual and Developmental Disabilities 2013a).

This definition covers a large and heterogeneous group of people with a wide range of skills and limitations. On one end of the spectrum, it includes people with mild intellectual disabilities who may be able to function in society with little or no support and may have good communication skills. Sometimes, it is only when the equilibrium of life is disturbed (e.g., when their health fails) that their independent coping is challenged. On the other end of the spectrum, people with profound intellectual disabilities have significant and multiple impairments, usually including physical impairments; they will need 24 h support.

The term "intellectual disability" is currently most widely accepted across the world, replacing earlier terms including "mental retardation" (Schalock et al. 2010). In the UK, the term "learning disabilities" is used synonymously with "intellectual disabilities," but this can be confusing internationally. In the USA, for example, "learning disabilities" refers simply to weaknesses in certain academic skills, such as reading or writing. "Developmental disabilities" is an umbrella term that includes intellectual disabilities but also includes other disabilities that are apparent during childhood, such as cerebral palsy or epilepsy; they are severe chronic disabilities that can be physical, cognitive, or both (American Association on Intellectual and Developmental Disabilities 2013b).

An estimated 20–30% of adults with intellectual disabilities also have an autistic spectrum disorder (ASD). ASD is a lifelong condition that affects how a person communicates with, and relates to, other people. It is characterized by difficulties with social communication, social interaction, and social imagination (Emerson and Baines 2010). Not all people with ASD have intellectual disabilities. For example, people with Asperger's syndrome (a form of autism) have average or above-average intelligence, and therefore do not have intellectual disabilities.

2.2 Prevalence

Intellectual disability affects an estimated 1–3% of the population (Mash and Wolfe 2004). The exact prevalence is unknown, as there is little standardization of definitions or methods of data collection and there is a general lack of statistical information.

People with mild intellectual disabilities make up around 85% of the total population of people with intellectual disabilities (Department of Health 2001). There is a higher incidence of mild to moderate intellectual disabilities in deprived areas. It is difficult to establish causal effects with certainty. Exposure to socioeconomic adversity prenatally and in the early years of development is likely to increase the incidence of intellectual disability. It is also possible that the heritability of intellectual ability, and the link between low intellectual ability and social position, contributes to a higher incidence of intellectual disabilities in the areas of social and economic deprivation (Emerson 2012).

Many people with intellectual disabilities, especially those with mild and moderate intellectual disabilities, are not known to specialist services and may never have been diagnosed as having intellectual disabilities (Learning Disabilities Observatory 2016). This is therefore a largely hidden population. The fact that people's disabilities may not be recorded, supported, or even recognized creates particular challenges for services trying to meet their needs at the end of life. Some risk being labelled as "difficult" or "uncooperative," whereas their behavior or coping strategies may simply be due to undiagnosed intellectual disabilities.

2.3 Death and People with Intellectual Disabilities

2.3.1 Life Expectancy

Although life expectancy for people with intellectual disabilities has increased dramatically over the past century, it is still significantly below that of the general population. A recent government inquiry in England investigated the deaths of 247 people with intellectual disabilities between 2010 and 2012 (the CIPOLD study: Heslop et al. 2013). This important study, which was comprehensive and methodologically sound, has informed several parts of the EAPC White Paper and this chapter. A key finding was that the median age of death for people with intellectual disabilities (65 years for men; 63 years for women) was, on average, 16 years younger than the general population. Similar statistics have been found in the USA, where there have been mortality reviews for people with intellectual disabilities since 2004. The average age of death in 2014 was 59 (Connecticut State Department of Developmental Services 2015).

This shorter life expectancy may be partly due to factors related to the intellectual disability itself. For example, some conditions that cause intellectual disabilities can also cause significant physical health issues, which may be life-shortening. Some are related to the premature birth of babies that would not have survived in the past, but are now living into childhood or beyond. A significant proportion of the population of people with intellectual disabilities have a specific syndrome, which can be genetic (Down syndrome is the most common chromosomal disorder) or caused by toxins, injuries, infections, and genetic/metabolic disorders which can affect the central nervous system or other organ systems during the developmental period. These effects can become evident during the person's life (Evenhuis et al. 2001). For example, there are high rates of cardiovascular disease and diabetes among adults with Prader-Willi syndrome, arising from morbid obesity (Greenswag 1987).

However, there is sound evidence that the shorter life expectancy of people with intellectual disabilities is not just related to factors inherent in the presence of intellectual disabilities itself. This population experiences substantial health inequalities, leading to poorer outcomes (Emerson and Hatton 2013). There are inequalities in healthcare provision, including poorer access to palliative care services. People with intellectual disabilities, therefore, are at risk of premature death that could be amenable to better healthcare provision (Heslop et al. 2013).

2.3.2 Causes of Death

Leading causes of death among people with intellectual disabilities are respiratory disease, heart disease, and cancer. International data on cancer deaths among people with intellectual disabilities are lacking. In the CIPOLD study, cancer accounted for 20% of deaths among people with intellectual disabilities. The cancer profile is slightly different from the general population, with a higher than average incidence of gastrointestinal cancers (Hogg and Tuffrey-Wijne 2008). People with Down syndrome have a significantly increased risk of leukemia and a lower risk of many solid tumors (Satgé and Vekemans 2011).

The incidence of dementia is higher among people with intellectual disabilities (Strydom et al. 2010). In particular, the incidence of Alzheimer's disease is high among people with Down syndrome, with incidence rising sharply between the ages of 40 and 60. Around 40% of people with Down syndrome aged 60 and over suffer from the condition (although exact prevalence estimates vary). It is thought that there is an association between the presence of the third chromosome 21 and the production of the beta-amyloid protein which is involved in Alzheimer's disease.

3 Palliative Care for People with Intellectual Disabilities

Palliative care sets out to preserve the best possible quality of life until death. This involves management of pain and other symptoms, and of social, psychological, and spiritual problems. It requires an approach that encompasses the patient, the family, and the community in its scope (European Association for Palliative Care 1998).

The palliative care needs of people with intellectual disabilities are, on the face of it, no different from those of the general population. However, they often present with unique issues, challenges, and circumstances that make it much more difficult to meet those needs. This includes, for example: communication difficulties which affect all aspects of palliative care provision; difficulties around insight and the ability to participate in decision-making; unconventional ways of expressing signs and symptoms of ill health and distress; multiple comorbidities; complex family and social circumstances; and higher levels of behavioral or psychiatric problems.

In order to promote best practice, it is worth considering the 13 areas of practice and service delivery that are set out below.

The scope of the White Paper on which this chapter is based includes patients who are *adults* (children require a particular and additional focus); across *the entire spectrum of intellectual disabilities* (ranging from mild to profound); and *in a wide range of settings*, including the family home, independent living arrangements, residential care settings, nursing homes, hospitals, and specialist palliative care settings.

3.1 Equity of Access

3.1.1 Barriers

The barriers people with intellectual disabilities face in accessing health services, including palliative care services, arise from a number of different sources (Emerson and Hatton 2013). Some of these are related to late diagnosis of life-limiting illness such as cancer. People with intellectual disabilities themselves may not recognize the signs and symptoms of ill health, or they may be less able to communicate these signs effectively to others. They may also not appreciate the importance of taking up health screening.

It has often been asserted that late diagnosis is due, in large part, to family members or paid caregivers not realizing that something was wrong (Tuffrey-Wijne et al. 2007b). However, the CIPOLD study found that the majority of people with intellectual disabilities who died had been identified as being unwell prior to the diagnosis and treatment of their final illness, either by themselves, a family member or a paid carer; in most cases, medical attention had been sought in a timely way. However, there were significant problems with making a correct diagnosis. Frequently, the investigations that were needed to diagnose the problem were not done or posed difficulties. Physicians were more likely to take a "wait and see" approach. In a quarter of those identified as being unwell and who responded appropriately, the concerns of the person with intellectual disabilities, their family, or paid care staff were reportedly not taken seriously enough by medical professionals. Families of people with intellectual disabilities were significantly more likely than those of people without intellectual disabilities to not feel listened to; this finding echoed previous reports (Michael 2008).

Barriers can be created by attitudes and a lack of knowledge of clinicians and carers. Those working in generic health or social care settings may lack training and knowledge of intellectual disabilities. There is a risk of professionals attributing the signs and symptoms of ill health (which may take uncharacteristic forms of expression) to the intellectual disability itself rather than to the underlying illness – a phenomenon known as "diagnostic overshadowing" (Reiss and Syzszko 1983).

Another barrier may simply be that those working in palliative care services do not know the population of people with intellectual disabilities in their catchment areas and are therefore unlikely to reach out to them. Among those working with people with intellectual disabilities, there may be a misconception about hospice and palliative care services as being concerned only with the final stages of dying, rather than with helping people to live and cope with the life they have left. It may not be known to families and support staff that palliative care can be provided within people's own homes.

3.1.2 Reasonable Adjustments

Equitable access to health care is an internationally recognized human right (United Nations 2006). In Great Britain, the requirement to make "reasonable adjustments" to healthcare services, in order to make them accessible to people with disabilities, is enshrined in law (Disability Discrimination Act 2005). The underlying principle of equality is not usually disputed, but it can be difficult for palliative care services to know what changes they have to make in order to provide equal access to all patients. The need to remove physical barriers (such as providing lifts and ramps) may be easily understood, but it is important also to include changes to the ways in which services are delivered, so they work well for people with intellectual disabilities. In order to do so, services will have to recognize the specific additional needs of people with intellectual disabilities. Examples of reasonable adjustments for people with intellectual disabilities, which can be made by generic healthcare services or specialist palliative care services, include:

- Giving people information that is tailored to their communication needs (e.g., providing easy-read materials and pictures, or opportunities to see clinical areas or equipment beforehand)
- Allowing more time
- Involving family and other care givers
- Providing staff training about the needs of people with intellectual disabilities
- Accessing expertise about intellectual disability when needed (e.g., by engaging with intellectual disability nurses)

It is important to acknowledge that different countries have different ways in which health services are delivered to people with intellectual disabilities, which may affect the kinds of adjustments that may be needed. In the UK, Public Health England (2016) has an online database of reasonable adjustments provided by healthcare services, including tools and resources (Public Health England 2016).

3.2 Communication

Most people with intellectual disabilities, even at the mild or moderate end of the spectrum, will have some difficulty with communication. This can include any or a combination of the following (Iacono and Johnson 2004):

- Speech that is difficult to understand
- Problems in understanding what is said
- Problems in expressing themselves because of limited (or even absent) vocabulary and sentence formulation skills

These problems need to be recognized and taken into consideration. It is not surprising that difficulties with communication are often highlighted as one of the main reasons why palliative care provision for people with intellectual disabilities is so difficult (Tuffrey-Wijne and McEnhill 2008). It affects assessment of pain and other symptoms; the provision of emotional, social, and spiritual support; truth disclosure; and issues around consent and decision making.

Many people with intellectual disabilities benefit from communication aids to augment their spoken language, such as *objects of reference* (e.g., being shown a cup to signify drinks), *signs* (there are some specific sign languages used by people with intellectual disabilities, such as Makaton and Signalong), or *symbol-based systems* (including photograph and line drawings). Picture books, such as *Am I Going To Die?* from the *Books Beyond Words* series (books designed to help adults with intellectual disabilities understand and talk about difficult issues, see www.booksbeyondwords.org) can be useful.

However, some people with intellectual disabilities, especially those at the severe and profound end of the spectrum, do not easily understand either words or pictures. They have high individual communication needs, and it is imperative to involve family and other care givers in interpreting their behavior. As Thurman et al. (2005) describe:

> They may be unable to ask for things that are not actually present and are dependent on others to present them with the real tangible items... [they] can only react to situations as they arise. Such reactive communicative behaviour is often interpreted as challenging (for example, "He spits his food out on purpose").

It is important, therefore, to see any unconventional or "challenging" behavior as a possible message that the person is trying to communicate

– and to become a "detective," trying to interpret this unconventional communication correctly, together with those who know the person well.

3.2.1 Truth Disclosure

Many people with intellectual disabilities are being protected from knowing that their illness is expected to lead to their death. In one study, staff and families gave the following reasons for non-disclosure: "He will get upset"; "I will get upset"; "He can't understand"; "He has no concept of time"; and "Others don't want him told." Reasons for disclosure were related to the person's rights ("He has a right to know"), their coping ("Understanding will help him cope"), and involvement ("He needs to be able to plan and make decisions") (Tuffrey-Wijne et al. 2013). Similarly, people with intellectual disabilities are often not prepared for the death of someone close to them. Staff who work with people with intellectual disabilities usually talk to them about death *after* the death of someone close to them has occurred, but not beforehand (Ryan et al. 2011). This is especially poignant for people with intellectual disabilities who are themselves dying; they are not offered opportunities to engage with the topic of death unless they themselves initiate the conversation (Wiese et al. 2013).

It is important to make no assumptions about how much someone has understood. It is important to take people's life experiences into account, which will affect how someone makes sense of new information. This is illustrated by the following example:

> Dale, living with and caring for his remaining terminally ill parent told me in response to the question 'What is cancer?' that he had learned about it at school and that it was 'a disease the grows in your body, in your lungs and other places'. When I asked him whether it a serious illness he said 'Yes, very serious' but when I asked him whether he had then expected that his father would die of the disease, he said 'No I never expected that, no one told me'. Now faced with his mother's illness I asked him what he had thought when he had been told that she had cancer, he said 'I just froze, I thought, I am going to be on my own'. (McEnhill 2008).

There is little evidence within the literature that truth disclosure can be harmful for people with intellectual disabilities who are at the end of life, but research in this area is very limited. One study has suggested that for some people, full knowledge of what will happen in the future could be overwhelming, particularly if they are unable to put the information into the perspective of a time frame. The concepts of illness, treatments, and deaths might be too abstract to understand, which could cause severe distress for some people. Some people have high levels of anxiety, which makes it difficult to cope with distressing information. Any decision *not* to disclose the truth needs to be taken in the person's best interest, after careful consideration by everyone involved (especially those who know the person well), and reviewed regularly (Tuffrey-Wijne et al. 2013).

In recent years, a new model has been developed for breaking bad news to people with intellectual disabilities (Tuffrey-Wijne et al. 2012; www.breakingbadnews.org). This is based on evidence that the widely taught step-by-step approach to breaking bad news (Kaye 1996; Baile et al. 2000) doesn't work well for people with intellectual disabilities. For example, "finding out how much the patient already knows" can be difficult. "Warning shots" preceding disclosure of bad news can be confusing or even alarming for people with intellectual disabilities. Traditional models for breaking bad news do not take into consideration that people with intellectual disabilities usually begin to make sense of their situation (and the bad news) in their own environment, rather than in a doctor's office. Families and other care givers are often involved in disclosure of bad news, and they may find this particularly challenging. The new model takes account of the person's understanding and capacity, the people involved in the situation, and everyone's support needs. It is based on the premise that news needs to be broken down in very small chunks and added gradually, in order to build someone's understanding. This is different from "warning shots," even if it looks similar. Warning shots tend to be given in order to make the person aware that the news is bad. Telling someone "Dad is not going to get better" as a way of getting someone to ask or understand "Dad is going to die" is a warning shot – it's much better, in that case, simply to say "Dad is going to die." However, "Dad is not going to get better" could also be used in order to help someone understand what is happening with Dad's illness. It may be too early to tell someone "Dad is going to die" (especially if they have a poor sense of time), but when that time comes, this earlier bit of information will help the person to make sense of the situation.

3.3 Recognizing the Need for Palliative Care

Poor access to palliative care services may be due to a lack of recognition by those that support people with intellectual disabilities that palliative care is needed – or even, that palliative care services exist.

Predicting a need for palliative care can be particularly difficult when someone has intellectual disabilities (Vrijmoeth et al. 2016). This is complicated by the fact that prognostication can be challenging, as many people with intellectual disabilities have a range of comorbidities, such as epilepsy. Those with congenital conditions may have had complex health problems throughout their lives, so it can be hard to know when life-long and ongoing management of these problems turns into a need for palliative and end-of-life care.

It may be much more important, therefore, to take an approach that does not rely too heavily on prognostic indicators. Commonly used indicators for identifying those in need of palliative care can still be very useful in predicting mortality, including the "Surprise Question" ("Would you be surprised if this person were to die in the next 6–12 months?" (Moss et al. 2010). General and specific indicators can all lead to the answer being "No, I wouldn't be surprised": general physical decline, decreasing activity, progressive weight loss, repeated hospital admissions; cancer, organ failure, dementia). But more important is the anticipation and meeting of likely needs, "hoping for the best but preparing for the worst." There should be a proactive, even instinctive prediction of the rate and course of decline, and a regular review of the situation (Thomas et al. 2011).

3.4 Assessment of Total Needs

The unconventional way in which many people with intellectual disabilities express their emotional, social, spiritual, and physical needs means that their needs can be easily overlooked. In addition, their emotional capacities – including the capacity to cope with illness, death, and loss – are often underestimated.

In assessing someone's needs, it is essential to have an understanding of that person's experience of life. Here are some examples of relevant past life experience:

- Many people with intellectual disabilities have a life-long experience of being dependent on others. For some, this can lead to resilience and an ability to accept the need for increased care. Others, particularly those on the autistic spectrum, may find a change of circumstances and routines much more difficult to cope with.
- Many people with intellectual disabilities have not had extensive opportunities to make even the most basic of choices. Discussing different care or treatment options may not make much sense to people who have never been involved in deciding what to have for dinner.

There is evidence that spirituality plays a significant role in the lives of people with intellectual disabilities (Swinton 2001) and, therefore, they may need to be facilitated in expressing their spiritual needs at the end of life, like anyone else.

It is always worth remembering that challenging behavior in someone with intellectual disabilities may be a way of communicating pain. It is also worth paying attention to comorbidities that may be painful, especially if these are long-standing (e.g., contractures, sensory or motor impairments and postural problems). People who have experienced persistent and chronic pain throughout their lives may have been conditioned not to express their pain, or may express pain in unconventional ways.

There are some specific tools available. The Disability Assessment and Distress Tool (DisDAT) (Regnard et al. 2007) is particularly useful for people with intellectual disabilities, including those with severe and profound disabilities. The DisDAT is intended to help identify distress cues people who have severely limited communication. It is designed to describe a person's usual content cues, thus enabling distress cues to be identified more clearly. For example, a hospice nurse may not realize that someone who sits calmly and quietly in her chair is actually severely distressed; but her carers will know that this person usually rocks backward and forward, and therefore carers will realize her stillness is a cause for concern. Documenting this will help all professionals. Identification of the distress is only the beginning of the assessment; unless the person is able to tell you clearly what is causing the distress, this still needs to be determined and can often be no more than an "educated guess" (See also Sect. 3.5).

3.4.1 Tips for Effective Assessment

The following may be useful in assessing the needs of someone with intellectual disabilities (see also Tuffrey-Wijne and McEnhill 2008).

- Get to know the person. The earlier palliative care professionals can be involved, the better, as this provides opportunities to build a relationship of trust, which will be crucial in future needs assessment.
- Involve families and others who know the person well. They can be effective "interpreters" of the person's verbal and nonverbal communication, and should be part of your team.
- Take plenty of time, and accept that this is an ongoing process, to be refined over the coming days, weeks, or even months.
- Always speak to the person with intellectual disabilities first (even if they don't use verbal communication), and only then refer to the person's carer. Even if most of the assessment will need to be through the carer (e.g., if the person's communication is only understood by the carer, or if the person is too anxious to speak to those they don't know well), refer to the person frequently. This will build trust and confidence, not only for the person with intellectual disabilities but also for their carer.
- Use simple and straightforward questions. Never use more than one concept per sentence. Don't ask: "How are you, do you have pain today?", but rather, "How are you?" (wait for response), "Do you have pain today?" (wait for response).
- Allow the person plenty of time to respond. Do not fill necessary silence with another question.
- Many people with intellectual disabilities are eager to please and will tell you what they think you want to hear.
  - It is not unusual for people with intellectual disabilities to answer "yes" regardless of the question. Closed questions ("Do you have pain today?") may be important in assessments, but should be used with care. It is worth asking the opposite question as well, to see if you get a similar response ("Has the pain gone away?")
  - When presented with different options, some people with intellectual disabilities tend to repeat the final option ("Is the pain there all the time or only sometimes?" "Sometimes," so try repeating the question with the options the other way round, to see if you get the same response.
- Abstract concepts are much more difficult to understand than concrete ones. Concepts of time can be particularly difficult. Therefore, try to be as specific and concrete as you can. Instead of "How long have you had the pain," you could ask, "Did you have the pain when you went to church?"
- Do not assume that the person understands the connection between the symptoms and the illness.

3.5 Symptom Management

Pain and symptom management can be particularly complex in people with intellectual disabilities, many of whom have a range of chronic medical conditions and comorbidities; multi-pharmacy is not uncommon (Symons et al. 2008).

Pain is often not recognized, validated, or treated in people with intellectual disabilities. The CIPOLD study (Heslop et al. 2013) found that they receive less opioid analgesia in their final illness than the general population. The belief still exists that people with intellectual disabilities feel less pain than the general population. Pain assessment is complicated by the fact that self-reporting of pain can be difficult, and conventional pain assessment tools may not work well for this population.

It is important to try and determine the most likely cause of someone's distress. This is an imprecise art, but it is unacceptable to leave pain and other symptoms untreated because of uncertainty. Professionals need to use their clinical expertise and judgement to make an "educated guess" about the most likely cause. For example, is the symptom or the distress cue caused by the disease itself? The treatment of the disease? Debility or comorbidities? The impact of the symptom or illness on the person's life?

Treatment should be instigated accordingly and the result should be monitored, to see if the distress signs diminish over time. If they don't, then the situation needs to be reconsidered and another possible cause may be treated or managed. Consider both pharmacological and nonpharmacological treatments, including complementary therapies, emotional and spiritual support, the use of life stories and reminiscence therapy, relaxation exercises, etc.

The DisDAT assessment tool (See Sect. 3.4) includes a useful clinical decision checklist to help decide the cause of the distress. This is not an exhaustive list, and there is a strong emphasis on physical causes of distress; but it is important to exclude underlying physical causes, especially in this group where there is a risk of "diagnostic overshadowing."

IS THE NEW SIGN OR BEHAVIOR. . .

- **Repeated rapidly?**
  Consider pleuritic pain (in time with breathing); colic (comes and goes every few minutes); repetitive movement due to boredom or fear.
- **Associated with breathing?**
  Consider: infection, COPD, pleural effusion, tumor.
- **Worsened or precipitated by movement?**
  Consider: movement-related pains.
- **Related to eating?**
  Consider: food refusal through illness, fear or depression; food refusal because of swallowing problems; upper GI problems (oral hygiene, peptic ulcer, dyspepsia) or abdominal problems.
- **Related to a specific situation?**
  Consider: frightening or painful situations.
- **Associated with vomiting?**
  Consider: causes of nausea and vomiting.
- **Associated with elimination (urine or fecal)?**
  Consider: urinary problems (infection, retention); GI problems (diarrhea, constipation).
- **Present in a normally comfortable position or situation?**
  Consider: anxiety, depression, pains at rest (e.g., colic, neuralgia), infection, nausea.

Taken from **DisDAT** © 2006 Northumberland Tyne & Wear NHS Trust and St. Oswald's Hospice.

3.6 End of Life Decision-Making

People with intellectual disabilities have a right to be facilitated in making choices about care and treatment, where possible. People with intellectual disabilities are particularly vulnerable and can be excluded from conversations that they may be able to have which could help plan the palliative and end-of-life care that they wish to receive. There is evidence that medical decision making is sometimes based on misguided assumptions about the quality of life of people with intellectual disabilities, their ability to comply and cope with treatments, or their ability to consent to treatment and be involved in the decision making process. This can lead to people with intellectual disabilities not receiving potentially lifesaving treatment (Mencap 2007; Michael 2008; Wagemans et al. 2010). There should be no assumptions about their capacity to make decisions due to the label "intellectual disability" (Johnson 2010).

Professionals should be aware of the fact that capacity may be an issue and needs to be assessed. They should also be aware of, and adhere to, national and local laws and regulations around capacity, consent, and advance decision making.

3.6.1 Assessing Capacity

With the right support, many people with intellectual disabilities are able to make at least some decisions. A person's capacity needs to be assessed for each situation. Capacity is "decision specific," and some decisions are easier than others. A decision to start on opioid analgesia for pain may be easier than a decision to start (or continue with) chemotherapy for an invisible cancer. In the UK, a person is deemed to lack capacity if he or she is unable to do at least one of the following:

(a) Understand the information relevant to the decision
(b) Retain the information (for long enough to be able to make the decision)
(c) Balance the information (in other words, use the information to weigh up the options)
(d) Communicate the decision

It is important that people are given relevant information in a format that they can understand. Professionals must consider, therefore, what information is needed to enable informed decision making. It may be necessary to restrict information to the most essential. It is also important to remember that people have a right to make a decision that others may perceive as "unwise." In order to assess whether the person has been able to use the information to weigh up the options, it can be useful to ask them how they have come to their decision. This could show that someone does indeed have capacity to make the decision, but it could also demonstrate that someone who makes a seemingly clear decision has not, in fact, understood the full implications of the decision. It is not unusual for someone to be clear that he doesn't want surgery, and for this choice to be respected; but it may be that he has not understood that surgery could be life-saving and not having the surgery will eventually lead to his death – and therefore, he either has not been adequately informed, or he did not have the capacity to make this decision due to an inability to weigh up the information.

If someone lacks capacity, then someone else needs to make the decision for them. Who the surrogate decision maker is will depend on national laws, but an important general principle is that decisions are made *in the person's best interest*. All relevant circumstances, as wells as the person's wishes, feelings and values, must be taken into consideration. Even if it is decided that complying with their wishes is not in their best interest, people's wishes clearly matter. The important question to ask is: "If this person had capacity, and could understand all the relevant issues, what do we think he or she would choose?"

3.7 Involving those Who Matter: Families, Friends, and Carers

Involving families, friends, and carers is particularly important for people with intellectual disabilities. Families and carers are often effective advocates and can play an important role in reassuring the person, providing communication support, contributing expert knowledge, and participating in decision-making. Studies that have included the voices of people with intellectual disabilities themselves, ascertaining their views on support at the end of life, have shown how important it is for them to have familiar people around (Tuffrey-Wijne et al. 2007a; McLaughlin et al. 2015). Furthermore, it has been shown that a lack of effective carer involvement leads to poorer outcomes for people with intellectual disabilities (Heslop et al. 2013; Tuffrey-Wijne et al. 2016b).

The important relationships of people with intellectual disabilities ("significant others") should therefore be identified, with the help of the people themselves if at all possible. This could include family, partners, friends, informal (unpaid) carers, paid support staff, and professionals. The profile of this social network is likely to be different from that of the general population. Those in the general population often rely on the support of partners and children when they develop a serious illness, but for people with intellectual disabilities, family bonds tend to consist mostly of siblings and elderly parents (Tuffrey-Wijne 2010). It is often much more difficult for people with intellectual disabilities to create new bonds, including new family bonds, as they get older. It is also worth noting that many people with intellectual disabilities consider their professional support staff as their friends.

Some people with intellectual disabilities have lived with their parents all their lives and have developed interdependent relationships. Others may have been separated from their families at an early age and spent a lifetime in institutional care. Sometimes, relatives who have had little contact during the person's lifetime would like to be more involved at the end of life, which can at times cause tensions with those who have supported the person on a daily basis. It is important to consider the wishes and perspectives of the people with intellectual disabilities themselves. Family bonds may be crucially important to them, even if there has been a lack of contact (Hubert and Hollins 2006).

The risk that people with intellectual disabilities lose contact with the people that are important to them is heightened during a (final) illness, when they may not be able to organize visits or phone calls independently. Those who need to move into a new care setting are particularly vulnerable to losing contact with friends and familiar care staff.

3.8 Collaboration

Collaboration between services is key to successful provision of palliative care for people with intellectual disabilities. The importance of collaboration has been consistently highlighted in the literature as essential in ensuring that people with intellectual disabilities are well supported at the end of life (Read 2006; Cross et al. 2012; Friedman et al. 2012). Collaborative working should also include family carers and people with intellectual disabilities themselves; in fact, people with intellectual disabilities should be at the center of partnerships at all times.

Collaboration between palliative care services and intellectual disability services is particularly important. Developing a relationship with other services, built on mutual trust and respect for each other's knowledge base and skills, can enable a more robust assessment of the needs of people with intellectual disabilities. This can ensure better outcomes for this population, such as continuity of care and dying peacefully in their place of care with people familiar to them (McLaughlin et al. 2014). Building collaborative links may involve a concerted effort, in particular if professionals are not aware of each other's existence or range of services and expertise. It is important, therefore, that palliative care services and intellectual disability services actively reach out to each other. Often, a particularly complex situation with a person with intellectual disabilities in need of palliative care leads to services getting to know each other and work together. However, it is much better not to wait for a crisis, but to get to know other services within a catchment area in advance. The effectiveness of a proactive approach to collaborative working has been highlighted by the Palliative Care for People with Learning Disabilities Network (PCPLD Network 2016), which encourages an exchange of best practice. One example of a good practice initiative is a group of nurses and social workers from the community intellectual disability teams, who meet monthly with local palliative care specialists, to discuss service users who are known to be at the end of life or suspected to die within a year. The group follows nationally established frameworks and pathways and has developed these to suit the needs of people with intellectual disabilities. Each service user within their catchment area is now offered and of life planning, with a clearly recognizable folder for their health action planning and communication tool (PCPLD Network 2013).

3.9 Support for Families and Carers

3.9.1 Families

Families and carers are usually deeply affected when someone with intellectual disabilities reaches the end of life. This person has often been at the center of their family's or carer's life, sometimes for decades. Their death is a significant and difficult loss. For families of those who have needed active support throughout their lives, the death also signifies a loss of their role and identity as a care giver (Todd 2007; Young et al. 2014). All family carers need considerable and sensitive support, a recognition of their expertise in relation to the cared-for person, and a regular assessment of their needs (Payne and Morbey 2013). For carers of people with intellectual disabilities, whose situation is so much more complex, this is especially important.

The grief of families and carers is sometimes "disenfranchised" (where the relationship is not recognized, the loss is not recognized or the mourner is not recognized) (Doka 2002). Carers (and especially parents) of people with intellectual disabilities can experience their deaths as a painful physical loss of part of themselves. However, families may be given the message that the death of their relative is "for the best" or even a blessing (Young et al. 2014).

3.9.2 Paid Support Staff

The extent to which professional care givers are affected by the death of a person with intellectual disabilities is often under-estimated. Staff can form strong attachments with the people they support, and sometimes see themselves as surrogate family members, building relationships that last many years (Tuffrey-Wijne 2010). The death of a client of resident with intellectual disabilities can have a complex physical and emotional dimension for staff that is seldom recognized (Todd 2013). Many such staff have little experience of death and dying, and are likely to find the situation difficult on both a professional and a personal level. It is important that the grief of all those who loved and supported the person with intellectual disabilities is recognized and validated, including not only family carers but also paid support staff. Staff working with people with intellectual disabilities who are dying will benefit from training on self-care.

3.9.3 People with Intellectual Disabilities

The caring role of people with intellectual disabilities can go unrecognized. Sometimes, the carers of people with intellectual disabilities who need palliative care have intellectual disabilities themselves: they may be partners, friends, housemates, or adult children, for example. They will need a significant amount of support to cope with changing needs and impending losses.

It is also worth noting that people with intellectual disabilities who live at home with elderly parents often become carers within highly interdependent relationships, but they are often invisible to services because of a lack of recognition of mutual caring (Department of Health 2009). In a study of people with intellectual disabilities who were affected by a relative with cancer (usually a parent or partner), most had taken on a caring role (Tuffrey-Wijne et al. 2012). Palliative care services should be alert, therefore, to the possibility that adults with intellectual disabilities who live with a patient (including patients without intellectual disabilities) may need support as carers.

3.10 Preparing for Death

If people with intellectual disabilities are protected from knowledge about death, including their own impending death (See Sect. 3.2), it will be very difficult for them to prepare themselves for the future or be involved in care planning, if they so wish. Giving people opportunities to participate in decision making around their care and treatment, or discuss funeral wishes and make a will, it is necessary to have a culture of openness and inclusion. Conversations about death should happen throughout the life cycle, in order to build a foundation to help prepare people for their own final illness.

Discussions about the person's preferences could take place as early as is appropriate, even before the need for palliative care arises. Once the need for palliative care has been identified, a care plan should be put into place, taking into consideration any anticipated future needs for treatment and care.

3.10.1 Advance Care Planning

Within the field of palliative care, there is growing emphasis on Advance Care Planning (ACP). This has been described as a process where a patient's current condition and prognosis is reviewed, and likely dilemmas and options discussed with the patient and their family. It is a structured way of eliciting their wishes and thoughts for the future (goldstandardframework.org.uk). Important elements of ACP include:

- *Deciding what you want* – what care elements are important now and in the future? What is the preferred place of care?
- *Deciding what you don't want* – this can include legally binding statements, such as Do Not Attempt Cardiopulmonary Resuscitation orders
- *Who will speak for you* – e.g., appointing a proxy spokesperson or legal representative (the terminology and powers of others to decide for you will vary in different countries)

With the person's permission, all those involved in their care should be made aware of the patient's wishes and advance decisions.

There are several easy-read advance care planning documents available online. Within some of these documents, there tends to be a focus on funeral planning rather than care planning. These resources have not yet been properly evaluated. In order to use advance care planning documents, professionals and carers must have an understanding of the process of advance care planning, including an appreciation of the fact that it is indeed a *process* – it is not a one-off event, but involves discussions over time and should be revisited regularly. How advance care planning with people with intellectual disabilities is best instigated and supported needs further investigation.

3.11 Bereavement Support

The importance of supporting families, carers, and staff through a person's final illness and after their death has already been highlighted (See Sect. 3.9). This section deals specifically with the need for people with intellectual disabilities to receive bereavement support. People with intellectual disabilities often experience more losses than the general population. Most children within the general population will not have experienced the death of a friend; but it is not unusual for children who attend special schools to experience the deaths of their peers, not just once but repeatedly.

The impact of losing a significant person is always enormous, but can be particularly devastating for people with intellectual disabilities who may have been dependent on the deceased person in many ways. If the death of a relative precipitates a move into a care setting, there are multiple losses associated with the bereavement, including the loss of home and all that was familiar.

There is growing recognition of the bereavement support needs of people with intellectual disabilities. This is a relatively recent development; until the 1990s, it was assumed that people with intellectual disabilities did not experience grief (Oswin 1991). Even today, people with intellectual disabilities do not always get recognition for their loss and are not always given opportunities to talk about it or express their feelings (Tuffrey-Wijne et al. 2012). The grief responses of people with intellectual disabilities can be delayed, prolonged, or expressed in atypical ways, so it may not be recognized as a grief reaction (Hollins and Esterhuyzen 1997).

3.11.1 Risk of Complicated Grief

Not all people with intellectual disabilities need specific or specialist bereavement support, but the possibility of difficult grief processes must be borne in mind. A number of risk factors make people with intellectual disabilities more vulnerable than the general population to complicated grief reactions, including (McHale and Carey 2002; Blackman 2008; Blackman 2003):

- Social isolation
- High dependency on a small group (or even a single) significant other(s), with limited opportunities for developing new roles and relationships
- Exclusion from death rituals (such as attending funerals or visiting the grave)
- Difficulties with attachment in early life
- Low self-esteem
- Limited power or control over one's situation
- Associated, often hidden and multiple losses that accompany the death of a parent or close relative (e.g., loss of home)

In assessing the need for bereavement support, is can be useful to focus on how the loss has affected the following three areas of someone's life (Blackman 2008):

- The person's ability to communicate with others (e.g., a parent who dies may have been the only person who could interpret their adult son or daughter's communication)
- The impact on the person's familial network
- The person ability to recognize and express their emotions

3.11.2 Providing Bereavement Support

The following hints and tips can be helpful in providing support for people with intellectual disabilities who have been bereaved or for whom bereavement is anticipated (Blackman 2003; Read 2005; Read 2007).

- Prepare the person for the loss if at all possible. People with intellectual disabilities are often protected from knowing that someone close of them is going to die (perhaps because those around them want to spare them distress), but if they are unprepared, the death will be experienced as an unexpected, sudden death. Sudden death is usually more difficult to cope with and increases the risk of complicated grief (Murray Parkes 1998).
- Ensure that the person participates in death rituals, such as funerals. It can also be very helpful to hold additional rituals, such as memorial events, planting a tree in someone's memory, etc. People with intellectual disabilities are often excluded from active involvement in rituals, including the planning of funerals and memorial events. They are also less likely to have opportunities to share their grief with others, for example, through seeing others cry about the loss or through receiving cards of condolence.
- Provide information about bereavement in a format that the person can understand. This may need to be repeated often. Be open and honest. Often, the truth is easier to cope with than uncertainties.
- Tangible ways of remembering are often helpful. Consider the use of life story books, memory books, or memory boxes. These can also help the person talk about the loss with others; for example, taking photographs at a funeral and showing these to others afterward can help to process what has happened.
- Bereavement counsellors may also need to use a variety of approaches to help someone with an intellectual disability experiencing grief, such as art work, creating family trees, use of pictures, photographs, videos, poetry, and reminiscence work.

Supporting people with profound intellectual disabilities in grief can be particularly complex. They will need to be provided with supportive relationships and sensory experiences in order to increase their sense of safety, enhance a sense of security, and facilitate expression of their grief. The resource created by PAMIS is particularly useful for this group (Young et al. 2014).

For some people with complicated grief responses, specialist bereavement support is indicated. In one randomized controlled trial, bereavement counsellors who worked with the general population received training on intellectual disabilities and then worked with bereaved people in one-to-one sessions; staff working within intellectual disability services received training on providing bereavement support, and worked with bereaved people within their own settings. The study found that the generic bereavement counsellors were able to improve outcomes for people with intellectual disabilities, while many of the staff within intellectual disability services dropped out of the program (Dowling et al. 2006). It seems that engaging with issues of death, dying, and loss is very difficult for staff working with people with intellectual disabilities on a daily basis; a finding that has been confirmed in later studies (Ryan et al. 2011; Tuffrey-Wijne and Rose 2017).

There are very few specialist bereavement services available for people with intellectual disabilities, but it is worth looking for generic bereavement services willing to take on clients with intellectual disabilities. They may need to know how to use different approaches, such as art work, creating family trees, using pictures, photographs, videos, poetry, and reminiscence work.

3.12 Education and Training

3.12.1 Training for Staff Providing Generic Palliative Care Services

Staff working in palliative care services have consistently reported that they lack of confidence, knowledge, and skills in supporting people with intellectual disabilities. They find assessment and communication issues particularly difficult (Tuffrey-Wijne et al. 2008; McLaughlin et al. 2014). Palliative care professionals may see relatively few people with intellectual disabilities, so their knowledge and skills are not being developed. The following areas are not exhaustive, but are important training priorities:

- What are intellectual disabilities and how does it affect people's lives?
- How are people with intellectual disabilities supported within the local area? Where do they live, who provides them with daily support, what specialist intellectual disability services are available? How skilled or experienced are these services or carers in providing end-of-life support, and what help do they need?
- Communication needs; interpreting communication; alternative communication methods; breaking bad news
- Assessment of symptoms and other problems

3.12.2 Training for Staff in Intellectual Disability Services

Staff working in intellectual disability services may not have any experience of death and dying, and may be frightened by it (Todd 2005; Tuffrey-Wijne 2010). Many will be unfamiliar with the needs of people at the end of life. It is easy to assume that people with intellectual disabilities who live within staffed homes or institutions are well supported, but such assumptions may be erroneous. In the UK, for example, support staff for people with intellectual disabilities tend to have very little training; most have limited knowledge of looking after people with failing health. In addition, they may experience anticipatory grief reactions themselves (See Sect. 3.9), making the delivery of support at the end-of-life challenging on many levels – practical as well as emotional. Training and support may be best delivered by outside experts (such as community palliative care nurses or district nurses) on an as-needed basis, showing staff who to support specific individuals. Generally, the following areas are important in training staff in intellectual disability services:

- Thinking about death and dying in general; your own attitudes, issues, reactions, fears, etc. In order for staff to be able to provide good support for others, it is usually helpful for them to think about and articulate these issues.
- What support services are available locally for people who need palliative care? Who is in the multidisciplinary team? (This could include: primary care services including general practitioners and district nurses; specialist services, including hospices and community palliative care services)
- The process of dying: what to expect, how you can help, when to ask for support
- How to communicate about death and dying with people with intellectual disabilities
- Loss and bereavement, and how people with intellectual disabilities can be supported

Cross-fertilization of knowledge and skills between palliative care staff and intellectual disability staff is particularly effective and useful. This could be through formal mutual training sessions and through informal exchange of expertise around a particular individual with intellectual disabilities. It can also be also highly effective to include carers and people with intellectual disabilities themselves, as experts-by-experience. Hearing their stories and perspectives can have a powerful impact on staff.

Training for People with Intellectual Disabilities

People with intellectual disabilities themselves often lack essential and basic knowledge around illness, death, and dying, and will benefit from education in this area. It is possible, and important, to create opportunities for them to learn about death and dying throughout their lives. Families and carers may need help and support in encouraging such discussions. Open discussions at home are particularly important; for example, the death of a celebrity or a soap opera character may prompt conversations about illness, dying, and funerals. There could also be planned sessions at day centers or special educational facilities.

3.13 Developing and Managing Services

In order to ensure that people with intellectual disabilities are adequately supported at the end of life, in the place that is most appropriate to their needs (and that is, ideally, their preferred place of care), it is essential to know where and how they die. Services need to be able to anticipate the likely need. Many people with intellectual disabilities may wish to choose to remain in their existing home environment. If this is a residential care setting, provision will have to be made to make that possible. This is likely to need advance planning, as it will require adequate resources in terms of staff and physical environment. Such services need to anticipate, therefore, the likelihood that their clients reach the end of life with an associated need for increased support. This will reduce the need for hospital admissions or a last minute search for a nursing home able to cater for the person's changed needs.

Palliative care services will need to consider whether they are sufficiently prepared to have patients with intellectual disabilities on their caseload. This is likely to require extra resources. They may need extra staff time, additional resources to help them communicate and additional time to manage their often complex needs. There may be a wide range of carers and professionals involved. Policy makers should commit adequate resources to this.

The following are particularly important in ensuring high-quality care for people with intellectual disabilities at end of life:

- Develop and encourage continuity of care across settings
- Ensure that good basic palliative care skills and knowledge are held within staff teams working in intellectual disability services
- Facilitate collaborative partnerships among palliative care programs, community hospices, and a wide range of other healthcare delivery settings.

4 Conclusion and Summary

Ensuring that people with intellectual disabilities are well supported at the end of life is highly challenging and needs focused attention. One key challenge is the "invisibility" of this population within health and social care services. The vast majority of people with intellectual disabilities are on the mild end of the spectrum, and this group may be particularly difficult to identify. Their needs are largely hidden, but their problems may be significant, and require skilled support. Even if the problems are identified and known, many staff, services, and systems are unprepared for meeting the needs of this population. Across Europe, good practice often depends on the dedication of individual practitioners, rather than effective services and systems (Tuffrey-Wijne and McLaughlin 2015).

4.1 Recommendations

The EAPC White Paper has set out key areas for practice, which have been discussed in this chapter. It also makes the following recommendations.

- **Palliative care services should actively reach out** to *find* the population of people with intellectual disabilities within their catchment areas.
- **Ongoing exchange** of experiences, expertise, and best practice should be encouraged on a range of levels:
  - Locally, between palliative care and intellectual disability services
  - Nationally, between individuals and organizations involved in supporting people with intellectual disabilities at the end of life
  - Internationally within Europe

- **International exchange of expertise,** for example through:
  - An ongoing, regularly updated online multilanguage resource, signposting relevant literature, resources, contacts, etc.
  - A dedicated person or team who can act as a "point of contact" for palliative care provision to people with intellectual disabilities in Europe. Their role could include: collating relevant information and resources (see above online resource); facilitating contact between different services in different countries; organizing exchange visits; signposting training opportunities.

4.2 Future Research

The following areas have been identified as priorities for future research by an international group of academics and practitioners (Tuffrey-Wijne et al. 2016a):

- Investigating issues around end-of-life decision making
- Mapping the scale and scope of the issue (in order to be able to plan adequate care provision)
- Investigating the quality of palliative care for people with intellectual disabilities, including the challenges in achieving best practice
- Developing outcome measures and instruments for palliative care of people with intellectual disabilities.

4.3 Benefits for Everyone

Is it worthwhile spending time and resources on supporting people with intellectual disabilities at the end of life, even for services who may see relatively few such patients? Practitioners, service managers, policy makers, and funders may well raise this question. Clearly, there is an argument for ensuring that the most vulnerable people in society are provided with the same quality of palliative care as the rest of the population. But the benefits of focusing on the needs of people with intellectual disabilities, and ensuring that staff and services are ready to meet those needs, go well beyond this. The skills needed to care for people with intellectual disabilities are transferrable and will benefit all patients. Services that can care for people with very severe communication problems, complex social situations, multiple comorbidities, unconventional ways of expressing symptoms, and perhaps high levels of anxiety, can probably care for all patients, whatever their complexities. Such services need flexibility. Their service delivery needs to be highly adaptable to individual need.

The quality of a palliative care services could be measured by the way in which they are able to support people with intellectual disabilities. It is worth the effort to "get it right."

References

American Association on Intellectual and Developmental Disabilities. Definition of intellectual disability. 2013a. Available at http://aaidd.org/intellectual-disability/definition#.WD2pNk0SGUk. Accessed 29 Nov 2016.

American Association on Intellectual and Developmental Disabilities. Frequently asked questions on intellectual disability. 2013b. Available at https://aaidd.org/intellectual-disability/definition/faqs-on-intellectual-disability#. Accessed 20 Dec 2016.

Baile W, et al. SPIKES – a six-step protocol for delivering bad news: application to the patient with cancer. Oncologist. 2000;5(4):302–11.

Bittles A, Glasson E. Clinical, social, and ethical implications of changing life expectancy in down syndrome. Dev Med Child Neurol. 2004;46:282–6.

Blackman N. Loss and learning disability. London: Worth Publishing; 2003.

Blackman N. The development of an assessment tool for the bereavement needs of people with learning disabilities. Br J Learn Disabil. 2008;36:165–70.

Connecticut State Department of Developmental Services. Mortality annual report 2014. Hartford: CT.GOV State of Connecticut; 2015.

Cross H, et al. Practical approaches toward improving end-of-life care for people with intellectual disabilities: effectiveness and sustainability. J Palliat Med. 2012;15(3):322–6.

Department of Health. Valuing people: a new strategy for learning disability for the 21st century. A white paper, London: Department of Health; 2001.

Department of Health. Valuing people now: a new three-year strategy for people with learning disabilities. 2009. Available at https://www.gov.uk/government/uploads/system/

uploads/attachment_data/file/250877/5086.pdf. Accessed 29 Nov 2016.

Disability Discrimination Act. Chapter 13, Disability discrimination act 2005. London: The Stationery Office. 2005. Available at http://www.legislation.gov.uk/ukpga/2005/13/introduction. Accessed 29 Nov 2016.

Doka K. Disenfranchised grief: new directions, challenges and strategies for practice. Champaign: Research Press; 2002.

Dowling S, et al. Bereaved adults with intellectual disabilities: a combined randomized controlled trial and qualitative study of two community-based interventions. J Intellect Disabil Res. 2006;50(Pt 4):277–87.

Emerson E. Deprivation, ethnicity and the prevalence of intellectual and developmental disabilities. J Epidemiol Community Health. 2012;66:218–24.

Emerson E, Baines S. The estimated prevalence of autism among adults with learning disabilities in England. Cambridge: Public Health England; 2010.

Emerson E, Hatton C. Health inequalities and people with intellectual disabilities. Cambridge: Cambridge University Press; 2013.

European Association for Palliative Care. EAPC definition of palliative care. 1998. Available at http://www.eapcnet.eu/Corporate/AbouttheEAPC/Definitionandaims.aspx. Accessed 29 Nov 2016.

Evenhuis H, et al. Healthy ageing – adults with intellectual disabilities: physical health issues. J Appl Res Intellect Disabil. 2001;14(3):175–94.

Friedman SL, Helm DT, Woodman AC. Unique and universal barriers: hospice care for aging adults with intellectual disability. Am J Intellect Dev Disabil. 2012;117(6):509–32.

Greenswag L. Adults with Prader-Willi syndrome: a survey of 232 cases. Dev Med Child Neurol. 1987;29: 145–52.

Haveman M, et al. Report on the state of science on health risks and ageing in people with intellectual disabilities. Dortmund: University of Dortmund: IASSID Special Interest Research Group on Ageing and Intellectual Disabilities/Faculty Rehabilitation Sciences; 2009.

Heslop P, et al. Confidential inquiry into premature deaths of people with learning disabilities (CIPOLD). Bristol; 2013. Available at http://www.bris.ac.uk/cipold/reports/index.html. Accessed 29 Nov 2016.

Hogg J, Tuffrey-Wijne I. Cancer and intellectual disability: a review of some key contextual issues. J Appl Res Intellect Disabil. 2008;21(6):509–18.

Hollins S, Esterhuyzen A. Bereavement and grief in adults with learning disabilities. Br J Psychiatry. 1997;170: 497–501.

Hubert J, Hollins S. Men with severe learning disabilities and challenging behaviour in long-stay hospital care. Br J Psychiatry. 2006;188:70–4.

Iacono T, Johnson H. Patients with disabilities and complex communication needs. The GP consultation. Aust Fam Physician. 2004;33(8):585–9.

Johnson B. Practical guide to health care decision making. In: Friedman S, Helm D, editors. End-of-life care for children and adults with intellectual and developmental disabilities. Washington, DC: American Association on Intellectual and Developmental Disabilities; 2010. p. 133–46.

Kaye P. Breaking bad news: a 10 step approach. Northampton: EPL Publications; 1996.

Learning Disabilities Observatory. People with learning disabilities in England 2015: Main report. London: Public Health England; 2016. Available at https://www.improvinghealthandlives.org.uk/securefiles/161129_1604//PWLDIE%202015%20final.pdf. Accessed 29 Nov 2016.

Mash E, Wolfe D. Abnormal child psychology. Belmont: Thomson Wadsworth; 2004.

McEnhill LS. Breaking bad news of cancer to people with learning disabilities. Br J Learn Disabil. 2008;36(3):157–64.

McHale R, Carey S. An investigation of the effects of bereavement on mental health and challenging behaviour in adults with learning disability. Br J Learn Disabil. 2002;30:113–7.

McLaughlin D, et al. Developing a best practice model for partnership practice between specialist palliative care and intellectual disability services: a mixed methods study. Palliat Med. 2014;28(10): 1213–31.

McLaughlin D, et al. Service user perspectives on palliative care education for health and social care professionals supporting people with learning disabilities. BMJ Support Palliat Care. 2015;5:531–7.

Mencap. Death by indifference. London Mencap; 2007. Available at https://www.mencap.org.uk/sites/default/files/2016-06/DBIreport.pdf. Accessed 29 Nov 2016.

Michael J. Healthcare for all: report of the independent inquiry into access to healthcare for people with learning disabilities. London; 2008. Available at http://webarchive.nationalarchives.gov.uk/20130107105354/http:/www.dh.gov.uk/prod_consum_dh/groups/dh_digitalassets/@dh/@en/documents/digitalasset/dh_106126.pdf. Accessed 29 Nov 2016.

Moss A, et al. Prognostic significance of the "surprise" question in cancer patients. J Palliat Med. 2010;13(7): 837–40.

Murray Parkes C. Bereavement in adult life. Br Med J. 1998;316(7134):856–9.

Oswin M. Am I allowed to cry? A study of bereavement amongst people who have learning difficulties. London: WBC Print; 1991.

Patja K, et al. Life expectancy of people with intellectual disability: a 35-year follow-up study. J Intellect Disabil Res. 2000;44(5):591–9.

Payne S, Morbey H. Supporting family carers report on the evidence of how to work with and support family carers. Lancaster, England; 2013.

PCPLD Network. Linda McEnhill Award 2012 winner. 2013. Available at http://www.pcpld.org/linda-mcenhill-award/2012-winner/. Accessed 20 Dec 2016.

PCPLD Network. Palliative care for people with learning disabilities network. 2016. Available at http://www.pcpld.org/. Accessed 20 Dec 2016.

Read S. Loss, bereavement and learning disabilities: providing a continuum of support. Learn Disabil Pract. 2005;8(1):31–7.

Read S. Communication in the dying context. In: Read S, editor. Palliative care for people with learning disabilities. London: Quay Books; 2006. p. 93–106.

Read S. Bereavement counselling for people with learning disabilities: a manual to develop practice. London: Quay Books; 2007.

Regnard C, et al. Understanding distress in people with severe communication difficulties: developing and assessing the disability distress assessment tool (DisDAT). J Intellect Disabil Res. 2007;51(4):277–92.

Reiss S, Syzszko J. Diagnostic overshadowing and professional experience with mentally retarded persons. Am J Ment Defic. 1983;87:396–402.

Ryan K, et al. Communication contexts about illness, death and dying for people with intellectual disabilities and life-limiting illness. Palliat Support Care. 2011;9(2): 201–8.

Satgé D, Vekemans M. Down syndrome patients are less likely to develop some (but not all) malignant solid tumours. Clin Genet. 2011;79(3):289–90.

Schalock R, et al. Intellectual disability: definition, classification, and systems of supports. 11th ed. Washington, DC: American Association on Intellectual and Developmental Disabilities; 2010.

Strydom A, et al. Dementia in older adults with intellectual disabilities – epidemiology, presentation, and diagnosis. J Policy Pract Intellect Disabil. 2010;7(2):96–110.

Swinton J. Spirituality and the lives of people with learning disabilities. London: Foundation for People with Learning Disabilities/Mental Health Foundation; 2001.

Symons F, Shinde S, Gilles E. Perspectives on pain and intellectual disability. J Intellect Disabil Res. 2008;52(4):275–86.

Thomas K et al. The gold standards framework prognostic indicator guidance. 4th ed. 2011. Available at http://www.goldstandardsframework.org.uk/cd-content/uploads/files/General Files/Prognostic Indicator Guidance October 2011.pdf. Accessed 29 Nov 2016.

Thurman S, Jones J, Tarleton B. Without words – meaningful information for people with high individual communication needs. Br J Learn Disabil. 2005;33(2): 83–9.

Todd S. Surprised endings: the dying of people with learning disabilities in residential services. Int J Palliat Nurs. 2005;11(2):80–2.

Todd S. Silenced grief: living with the death of a child with intellectual disabilities. J Intellect Disabil Res. 2007;51(Pt 8):637–48.

Todd S. "Being there": the experiences of staff in dealing with matters of dying and death in services for people with intellectual disabilities. J Appl Res Intellect Disabil. 2013;26(3):215–30.

Tuffrey-Wijne I. The palliative care needs of people with intellectual disabilities: a literature review. Palliat Med. 2003;17(1):55–62.

Tuffrey-Wijne I. Living with learning disabilities, dying with cancer: thirteen personal stories. London: Jessica Kingsley Publishers; 2010.

Tuffrey-Wijne I, McEnhill L. Communication difficulties and intellectual disability in end-of-life care. Int J Palliat Nurs. 2008;14(4):192–7.

Tuffrey-Wijne I, McLaughlin D. Consensus norms for palliative care of people with intellectual disabilities in Europe: EAPC White Paper. London/Milan: European Association for Palliative Care (EAPC); 2015. Available at http://www.eapcnet.eu/LinkClick.aspx?fileticket=Iym7SMB78cw%3d. Accessed 29 Nov 2016.

Tuffrey-Wijne I, Bernal J, et al. Using nominal group technique to investigate the views of people with intellectual disabilities on end-of-life care provision. J Adv Nurs. 2007a;58(1):80–9.

Tuffrey-Wijne I, Hogg J, Curfs L. End-of-life and palliative care for people with intellectual disabilities who have cancer or other life-limiting illness: a review of the literature and available resources. J Appl Res Intellect Disabil. 2007b;20(4):331–44.

Tuffrey-Wijne I, Curfs L, Hollins S. Providing palliative care to people with intellectual disabilities and cancer. Int J Disabil Hum Dev. 2008;7(4):365–70.

Tuffrey-Wijne I, et al. People with intellectual disabilities who are affected by a relative or friend with cancer: a qualitative study exploring experiences and support needs. Eur J Oncol Nurs. 2012;16(5):512–9.

Tuffrey-Wijne I, et al. Developing guidelines for disclosure or non-disclosure of bad news around life-limiting illness and death to people with intellectual disabilities. J Appl Res Intellect Disabil. 2013;26(3): 231–42.

Tuffrey-Wijne I, et al. Defining consensus norms for palliative care of people with intellectual disabilities in Europe, using Delphi methods: a white paper from the European Association of Palliative Care (EAPC). Palliat Med. 2015;30(5):446–55.

Tuffrey-Wijne I, Wicki M, et al. Developing research priorities for palliative care of people with intellectual disabilities in Europe: a consultation process using nominal group technique. BMC Palliat Care. 2016a;15(36)

Tuffrey-Wijne I, Abraham E, et al. Role confusion as a barrier to effective carer involvement for people with intellectual disabilities in acute hospitals: findings from a mixed-method study. J Adv Nurs. 2016b;72(11): 2907–22.

Tuffrey-Wijne I, Rose T. Investigating the factors that affect the communication of death-related bad news to people with intellectual disabilities by staff in residential and supported living services: an interview study. J Intellect Disabil Res. 2017;61(1):727–736.

United Nations. Convention on the rights of persons with disabilities. 2006. Available at http://www.un.org/disabilities/convention/conventionfull.shtml. Accessed 29 Nov 2016.

Vrijmoeth C, et al. Physicians' identification of the need for palliative care in people with intellectual disabilities. Res Dev Disabil. 2016;59:55–64.

Wagemans A, et al. End-of-life decisions: an important theme in the care for people with intellectual disabilities. J Intellect Disabil Res. 2010;54(6):516–24.

Wiese M, et al. "If and when?": the beliefs and experiences of community living staff in supporting older people with intellectual disability to know about dying. J Intellect Disabil Res. 2013;57(10):980–92.

Yang Q, Rasmussen S, Friedmann J. Mortality associated with Down's syndrome in the USA from 1983 to 1997: a population-based study. Lancet. 2002;359(9311):1019–25.

Young H, Garrard B, Lambe L. Bereavement and loss: supporting bereaved people with profound and multiple learning disabilities and their parents. Dundee: PAMIS; 2014. Available at http://www.pamis.org.uk/_page.php?id=70. Accessed 29 Nov 2016.

Pou Aroha: An Indigenous Perspective of Māori Palliative Care, Aotearoa New Zealand

70

Tess Moeke-Maxwell, Kathleen Mason, Frances Toohey, and Jaimee Dudley

Contents

T. Moeke-Maxwell (✉)
School of Nursing, Faculty of Medical and Health Sciences, University of Auckland, Auckland, New Zealand
e-mail: t.moeke-maxwell@auckland.ac.nz

K. Mason
School of Nursing, University of Auckland, Auckland, New Zealand
e-mail: k.mason@auckland.ac.nz

F. Toohey
Faculty of Medical and Health Sciences, University of Auckland, Auckland, New Zealand
e-mail: ftoo846@aucklanduni.ac.nz

J. Dudley
University of Auckland, Auckland, New Zealand
e-mail: jdud012@aucklanduni.ac.nz

R. D. MacLeod, L. Van den Block (eds.), *Textbook of Palliative Care*,
https://doi.org/10.1007/978-3-319-77740-5_121

Abstract
An indigenous perspective of palliative care is not commonly known. The aim of this chapter is to describe key caregiving strengths of New Zealand Māori whānau (family) to illustrate how they draw on their cultural customs at end of life. Cultural customs are informed by knowledge passed down from tūpuna (ancestors) and the relationship with the whenua (land). End of life cultural care customs ensure the highest quality of care is provided to the ill and dying person and their bereaved whānau. Whānau are critical "pou aroha" (care stalwarts); they carry out the bulk of end of life care. Whānau ensure the best physical, emotional/mental, and spiritual care is received before the person dies, no matter what healthcare setting they are in. A holistic healthcare approach is required at this time as this supports whānau cultural aspirations to prepare the person's spirit to pass through the ārai (veil) as they transition from the physical realm to the metaphysical realm at time of death. The chapter highlights the need for care that is genuinely holistic and relational as this is most likely to meet the needs of indigenous peoples. The facilitators and barriers associated with providing care are discussed within the context of a set of complex end of life circumstances. Barriers include health inequities, racism, poor access to palliative care and statutory (government) support, inadequate information, and poor communication. Whānau carers often experience high levels of stress and have too few informal family carers to share the care responsibility and the high financial costs associated with end of life care (Gott et al., Palliat Med 29:518–528, 2015a). However, the values of aroha (compassion, empathy, concern), whanaungatanga (relationships and connections), manaakitanga (caring for the mana (status, prestige, authority)) of the dying, kotahitanga (collective decision-making processes), and wairuatanga (spirituality) are introduced as guiding forces that protect and strengthen whānau carers.

1 Introduction

Increasing the health and palliative care sectors' understanding of indigenous peoples' end of life care needs and preferences is essential for designing palliative care services that are aligned with the aspirations of indigenous peoples. The aim of this chapter is to provide a description of indigenous end of life care by exploring Māori whānau (family, including extended family) experiences of caregiving. We introduce some strengths that support whānau to do this critical work, and we identify some of the challenges families encounter. Research evidence is drawn on to highlight the needs of Māori whānau (referred to as "whānau" henceforth). We highlight that whānau carers are *pou aroha* (care stalwarts) for family members who have a life-limiting illness.

Changes in the population of New Zealand will have significant future health policy, funding, and planning implications (Associate Minister of Health 2016) as well as implications for whānau in relation to the future palliative care needs of Māori. For example, the total number of deaths each year is projected to increase in New Zealand by 47.5% between 2016 and 2038. While the proportion of Māori deaths relative to the total deaths in New Zealand is expected to remain reasonably constant (10.9% by 2038) (McLeod 2016), the Māori population is projected to grow at a higher rate than non-Māori (Statistics New Zealand 2015) and is expected to exceed one million by 2038 (Statistics New Zealand 2017). An important feature of this period for both future health and palliative care services and whānau is not only the expected increase in the number of Māori deaths but also the significant shift in the age structure of Māori deaths where it is expected that there will be a large increase in the number of Māori deaths in all age bands above 75 years (McLeod 2016). The anticipated rise in the number of Māori deaths and the increasing age of Māori deaths over the next 20–30 years means that it is crucial for health and palliative care services to increase their cultural responsiveness to better support Māori whānau to care for their own at end of life.

Research evidence identifies that Māori whānau, like other families, carry out the majority of end of life care, not health and palliative care services (Gott et al. 2015a, 2018; Moeke-Maxwell et al. 2014). To die symptom- and pain-free is a strategic goal of the New Zealand Palliative Care Strategy (Ministry of Health 2001). However, in New Zealand, the biomedical approach often remains dominant, and the psychosocial (relational, cultural, psychological, and spiritual) aspects of care, if offered, appear to be included as an addendum or optional to the medical model of care provided. By and large, the indigenous desire for complimentary comfort treatments such as rongoā Māori (Māori herbal medicines and other complimentary therapies such as mirimiri/massage) is often unsupported within the mainstream health system. Rongoā Māori remains unregulated, and therefore these types of indigenous palliative care approaches are unavailable, resulting in the continued use of Western medical interventions and medications.

2 The New Zealand Palliative Care Context

Under the strategic provision of New Zealand's palliative care funding initiatives, the New Zealand Palliative Care Strategy (Ministry of Health 2001) requires that "[all] people who are dying and their family/whānau who could benefit from palliative care have timely access to quality palliative care services that are culturally appropriate and are provided in a co-ordinated way" (p. 7). Palliative care in this context includes care that is carried out by primary and secondary health services as well as specialist palliative care services (hospices). It comprises all health providers and health professionals including pharmacists, ambulance services, volunteer workforces (Palliative Care Subcommittee 2007), emergency departments (Laurenson et al. 2013), and statutory support from the social service sector (such as Work and Income, New Zealand) and Māori health providers. Collectively, these services provide support within the community (at home care), hospitals, hospices, and aged residential care facilities. Despite the implementation of cultural frameworks that govern the generalist palliative care sector (e.g., administered within public hospitals and services), the demands of busy medical services can mean that holistic cultural care may be lacking.

3 Palliative Care and Māori

Palliative care is a new concept for Māori. Within a relatively short period of New Zealand colonial history, indigenous New Zealanders have undergone significant cultural changes that have impacted their traditional caregiving and customs. Many challenges continue to confront Māori, such as institutionalized and personally mediated racism (Jones 2000) within the health system. According to Jones (2000), institutionalized racism is defined as "...differential access to the goods, services, and opportunities of society by race...[that] is normative, sometimes legalized, and often manifests as inherited disadvantage...[and] is often evident as inaction in the face of need..." (p. 1212). Jones (2000) defines personally mediated racism as "...prejudice and discrimination, where prejudice means differential assumptions about the abilities, motives, and intentions of others according to their race, and discrimination means differential actions towards others according to their race..." (pp. 1212–1213). Pascoe and Smart Richman (2009), in a meta-analysis of discrimination and health, link repeated exposure to experiences of perceived discrimination, such as racism, to an increased risk of mental and physical ill health. Māori are also confronted by other complications of colonization that have resulted in disproportionately poorer health outcomes than their non-Māori counterparts. According to Reid (2011), "...the state of Māori health is exemplified by systemic inequities..." (p. 40) evidenced by higher morbidity and mortality rates across most measures; lower utilization of health services relative to need; unequal distribution of socioeconomic, environmental, and political determinants of health; as well as issues pertaining to the delivery of quality health services that are accessible, affordable, effective, and nondiscriminatory (Reid and Robson 2007).

The individual end of life circumstances and preferences of whānau are diverse (Moeke-Maxwell et al. 2014; Reid 2005). For Māori it is essential that care administered at end of life is inclusive of their whānau and is culturally informed, relevant, and well-supported by health professionals. As indigenous people, Māori are at risk of not receiving the full range of benefits from palliative care due to late diagnosis resulting in less opportunity to access and benefit from treatment (Ministry of Health 2001). As descendants of ancestors whose language was subjugated to the dominance of the English language, and whose lands were confiscated or stolen during the colonial epoch, Māori have experienced significant changes to their economic livelihoods and communal lifestyles directly influencing upon their health determinants. Māori are also further marginalized by a wider health system that, despite becoming more holistic in its palliative care approach, still privileges a biomedical model of healthcare. The delivery of palliative care is marginalized as a result of the focus of the wider system. The current health systems' strategic goals are obliged to ensure Māori needs are met within the provisions set by the Treaty of Waitangi (1840) whereby the Crown has an obligation to care for Māori taonga (treasured objects) of which health is a vital taonga. But in reality, despite the improvements made to the health system in recent years, very little is known about what Māori need to support them to provide the type of end of life care congruous with their customary values, beliefs, processes, and cultural practices.

New Zealand hospices provide specialist palliative care services in New Zealand (Palliative Care Subcommittee 2007). Specialist palliative care services may also offer psychosocial services such as bereavement support for the ill person and their whānau. While specialist palliative care services have made efforts to practice compassionate holistic care, the degree that individual hospices effectively respond to the cultural aspirations or needs of Māori who are dying, and their whānau carers, may be variable. Often this will depend on access to and relationships with local Māori healthcare workers or kaumātua (elders) to guide the service.

Hospice professionals work in expert interdisciplinary teams. Hospice staff receive specific training and are accredited in palliative care and/or medicine. The use of the Whare Tapa Whā health model (Durie 1994) guides hospice practice. The increased presence of Māori staff within hospices and the introduction of specific cultural training to ensure staff are upskilled to be inclusive of Māori peoples has gone a long way to ensure a more inclusive approach to tangata whenua (people of the land) (Hospice New Zealand 2012). Importantly, the introductory spiritual care training program developed by Hospice New Zealand (2012) has started to increase an awareness and understanding of the cultural differences between Māori and non-Māori among staff (Mcleod et al. 2015). It has also made a start toward strengthening the capacity of health professionals to discuss spirituality with colleagues. Further, it has begun to increase confidence in recognizing spiritual distress and working more empathically with patients and their whānau (Mcleod et al. 2015). However there is still much to learn about Māori identity, culture, cultural diversity, and needs at end of life.

While specialist palliative care has made effort to practice compassionate holistic care, this does not necessarily reflect the unique cultural aspirations or needs of Māori at end of life or their whānau carers. Holistic care offered within primary and secondary healthcare may include initiatives to create welcoming cultural environments; observing hosting obligations and appropriate ways of greeting and working respectfully with Māori and offering environments that are spatially set up to accommodate whānau are often greatly appreciated.

Today, Māori, like everyone else, are reliant on medical services to ensure they live for as long as possible and remain symptom- and pain-free until death. Whānau generally assume end of life care either from the time of diagnosis or when the whānau member who has a life-limiting illness can no longer manage their own care. When informal carers become involved, the decision is usually determined by the wishes of the ill person. In this context, whānau includes close biological relatives, non-biological family, extended kin, and close friends. The combination of both indigenous and Western palliative care approaches is anticipated to bring the best outcomes for Māori whānau.

4 Historic Māori End of Life Care Traditions

Traditional customs associated with caring for the ill and dying are described to provide a foundation to understand the values Māori place on end of life caregiving. The aim of this section is to provide a general account enabling an understanding of Māori cultural values that inform their end of life requirements. Much of the references drawn upon reflect historical ethnographic accounts recorded by non-Māori academics. The authors provide the information to give an overview of the literature while recognizing that tribal differences prevailed. Optimal palliative care approaches and models of care are described as these influence the best outcomes for Māori before, during, and following death. Recommendations to improve end of life care for Māori are also identified.

Contemporary models of Māori end of life care generally highlight that Māori want to die at home surrounded by family who love and care for them (Ministry of Health 2001; Ngata 2005). An indigenous Māori model of care places the ill or dying person firmly at the heart of their whānau and their hapū (community) (Brown 1851; Dieffenbach 1843; Hiroa 1950). Historically, care was often carried out by older women or tohunga (spiritual experts) although there were tribal differences between iwi (tribes). Sickness was attributed to the transgression of tapu (breach of spiritual lore) (Brown 1851; Dieffenbach 1843; Polack 1840). Because treating illness and death was considered a spiritual phenomenon, male and female specialists were on hand to administer spiritual care (karakia; prayers, incantations, chants) to remove tapu and restore health. The practice of immersing the sick in wai tapu (purified water) at dawn was one method used to cleanse and heal the sick; the sick were often placed in temporary shelters to ensure the tapu would not contaminate the broader whānau (Phillipps 1954). Rongoā (natural medicine) was also used to provide comfort at end of life (Hiroa 1950; Jones 2012; Tregear 1890).

Traditional end of life care was also based on hierarchical status and was generally informed by whakapapa (Brown 1851; Dieffenbach 1843; Polack 1840). Best (1934) asserts that when death was inevitable, the dying did not fear death and on their deathbed were made to feel calm and clear-minded; this enabled them to express their last wishes, or in the case of an infectious illness, they may have been taken to a cave to avoid the spread of sickness (Hiroa 1950). A temporary shelter was usually erected some distance to the main living site outside the village. Māori preferred to die in the open air so they could greet the world one last time "mihi ki te ao marama" (Best 1934). Sometimes the person would die peacefully, unattended. Another important death wish was to return the dying to their ancestral land, and often they were carried long distances to achieve this.

Historically, major illnesses Māori encountered were attributed to the action of malignant spirits, usually the result of breaking the laws of tapu (sacred/restricted); the treatment of illness came under the jurisdiction of tohunga (spiritual experts). Lange (2011) explains that when caring for the sick and dying, the emphasis of the tohunga's actions was to rid of the malignant spirit or to remove the transgression responsible for it, rather than on patient care. Of central concern was the well-being of the entire settlement and people.

By the early 1900s, the traditional lifestyles of Māori tribal peoples had changed significantly in response to the prevalence of sickness and the efforts of Māori leaders to encourage people to seek medicine to treat illnesses such as tuberculosis (Ngata 1939). Tohunga and rongoā specialists were perhaps less visible following the Tohunga Suppression Act in 1907; however, they continued to provide spiritual healthcare to support their communities. This Act helped to place the medicalization of dying in the hands of Western medical discourse (Walker 1990). During the early 1900s, based on the observations of Beaglehole and Beaglehole (1945), the practice of "death watching" was undertaken by women of the pa (ancestral communal homes). By the 1940s and 1950s, influenced by Christianity and conforming to a Western work ethic, Māori men worked outside the home; death care primarily became the domain of women who had specific cultural knowledge and skills in this end of life area.

As stated above, the provision of care for Māori who were dying in the 1900s has been described by non-Māori scholars as "death watching" (Beaglehole and Beaglehole 1945). For Māori this involves the practice of helping to prepare the spirit for death and is congruous with other indigenous peoples' end of life care aims (Duggleby et al. 2015). This activity may include sitting with the ill, observing them, and tending to their physical, emotional, and spiritual needs. This custom tended to have greater significance depending on the rank of the dying person. The status of the ill person coincided with the number of visitors they would receive in their final days of life. Farewell speeches poroporoaki or ohaki were commonplace and considered an important part of the dying ritual (Reed 1963). The importance of Oo Matenga (death journey food) aimed to fortify the person for the death journey (Oppenheim 1973).

The increasing need for land by new European settlers led to conflicts between British government forces and tribes. Despite the signing of the peace treaty between the British Crown and Māori chieftain/chieftainess (Treaty of Waitangi 1840), the ensuing swell of British immigrants and the legal and illegal procurement of Māori lands resulted in a bloody land war (Walker 1990). At the turn of the twentieth century, Māori iwi and hapū were at risk of becoming extinct from colonial diseases such as the flu epidemic and tuberculosis (Walker 1990). This led Māori health professionals to politically advocate for Māori to adopt more Western lifestyles to ensure the survival of the Māori. Initiatives such as the Tohunga Suppression Act (1907) were believed to help Māori to survive decimation due to illness; tohunga (spiritual experts and healers) provided healing based on traditional philosophies and practices. However a small group of prominent Māori at that time believed that Māori Western medical interventions were needed to cure these new diseases (Durie 1994). This helped to further displace traditional customs and collective tribal lifestyles that were already being eroded through the discursive forces of neocolonialism. Despite these restrictions, tohunga and lay healers continued to work for their communities (Durie 1994).

5 An Indigenous Model of Illness and Death

Indigenous peoples share in common core beliefs about illness, dying, and death that are contrasted to a Western model (Hampton et al. 2010). A critical and overarching theme is the relationship indigenous people have with the land and the importance of the land to the ill and dying person. A second belief concerns the philosophy that life and death is part of the continuum of life and is an accepted and normal part of the life cycle (Dembinsky 2014). A meta-synthesis review of indigenous palliative care literature by Duggleby et al. (2015) discovered that the key commonality among indigenous peoples was the belief in the spirit and the transition of the spirit to the afterlife. For indigenous peoples then, the purpose of palliative care is to provide physical, emotional, and spiritual comfort to support the ill and dying person and their family; when combined, the

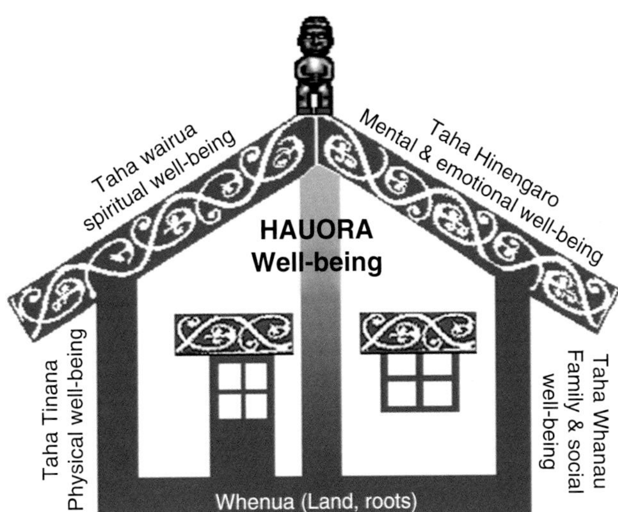

Fig. 1 Whare Tapa Whā (Durie 1994)

activation of these health domains helps to prepare the dying person's spirit to transition through the ārai (the veil between the physical and metaphysical realms) at time of death.

Māori are not dissimilar to other indigenous peoples when it comes to end of life care. Māori whānau prefer to care for their own. Caring for a loved one who is dying is a profound expression of aroha (love, empathy, compassion, concern), where the emotional, physical, familial, and, most importantly, spiritual needs of the ill or dying person are foremost (Moeke-Maxwell et al. 2013). In terms of any care provided by health and palliative care professionals, Māori prefer a holistic approach where the whole person is placed at the center of care. In this context, the desire for holistic care fits well in principle, with a palliative care approach.

Philosophically a palliative model of care is relationally driven and is focused on an inclusive holistic approach informing a "good death" (Clark 2002). This holistic model of a good death is based on a Western concept of palliative care but may not sit congruously with indigenous peoples' culturally diverse end of life care preferences. For example, New Zealand Māori favor a holistic model of care that takes into account their cultural values, spiritual beliefs, and customs (Ngata 2005). However, in reality the current palliative care approach is influenced by the cultural values of the dominant white cultural majority. Four healthcare domains are critically important to a holistic Māori healthcare model; these are the tinana (physical), hinengaro (mental and emotional), whānau (social and relational), and wairua (spiritual) domains; these are best represented in the Māori health model, Te Whare Tapa Whā (Four-Sided House) (Durie 1994), featured in the illustration below (Fig. 1):

5.1 Care Māori whānau Provide at End of Life

At times Māori whānau can be very resourceful; however, the capacity of individual whānau can vary in their ability to access information about palliative care support (Kidd et al. 2014; Moeke-Maxwell et al. 2014). When someone in the whānau has knowledge of the health system or has the ability to source information, there is a greater opportunity for whānau to navigate the health sector and statutory support services to seek the support and resources they require to help them carry out their caregiving activities. In the following example Moeke-Maxwell et al. (2014) provide an example of this.

Tia spoke about the end of life care she and her siblings carried out to care for their mother at home. Tia's brother's provided financial support while she and her sisters set up a care management plan; Tia stated:

Ariana [sister] was in charge of making sure that her medication was [taken care of]. . .She was in charge of taking Mum to the doctor to her appointments and what have you. Moana's [midwife] role was everything; it was making sure that the house was well looked after for our mother's comfort . . . I was sort of like a floater, I would sort of float, but if it was anything to do with her medication. . . anything to do with that it was primarily Ariana. (Tia) (p. 144)

Whānau provide the bulk of caregiving (Gott et al. 2015b, 2018). They provide a broad range of caregiving tasks including the provision of personal and spiritual cares as well as attending appointments with health providers and hosting visitors (Angelo and Wilson 2014). Whānau are diverse and have various capacities and resources to provide care to a dying loved one (Reid 2005). Large whānau can span several generations and include 200 relatives or more, particularly if they are involved with their iwi (tribes). Whānau may be well connected to te ao Māori (the Māori world) and cultural resources (land, marae, language, and traditional customs); they may be well organized and able to share the care duties across the broader whānau and navigate health services effectively (Moeke-Maxwell et al. 2014). However, sometimes whānau are a lot smaller, and at times there may be only a sole caregiver with limited or no whānau support (Johnston Taylor et al. 2014; Moeke-Maxwell et al. 2014). Or, on occasion, an individual Māori person with palliative care needs may wish to be independent, and therefore they do not require their whānau to provide their end of life care (Moeke-Maxwell and Nikora 2015).

Whānau draw on their cultural knowledge, values, and practices to inform end of life caregiving practices. This point is reflected on by Gott et al. (2015b):

Māori participants' caregiving commitment was often informed by cultural values steeped in āroha (compassion) and manaakitanga (preservation of mana and dignity), which were prioritised over care costs. Many participants' invoked notions of reciprocity in their discussions:

The way I see it is a parent raises a child, their whole role is to look after the child until they become an adult and then I see it, once you're an adult we should repay that back. You know, because your parent's health and everything starts to fail as they get older. So my obligation is to them. (STA, Māori daughter) (p. 521)

Johnston Taylor et al. (2014) identified a range of traditional Māori end of life cultural care customs carried out by whānau that benefited the ill and dying person and their whānau:

- The use of te reo Māori (Māori language)
- The incorporation of rongoā (traditional healing) including mirimiri (massage)
- The observance of tapu (protocols and practices that govern things restricted, profane)
- The observance of noa (protocols and practices that return a state of tapu back to its ordinary state, safe)
- The inclusion of karakia (incantations, prayers, chants)
- Inclusion of waiata (songs, singing)
- The presence of Māori kaumātua (older Māori) who oversee and provide cultural guidance and support
- The use of kai (food)
- Taking care of personal taonga (treasured objects)
- Observance of hygiene principles; for example, cleanliness with linen
- Correct disposal of body tissue

Moeke-Maxwell et al. (2014) identified that the use of traditional customs sustained and strengthened families who were tasked with providing care, often over weeks or months. By drawing on their vital cultural language, knowledge, values, and customs, whānau were fortified to manage with the demands placed on them, such as coping with poverty, too few carers, and limited knowledge of the health and palliative care systems as well as being confronted with structural and systemic inequities.

5.2 Dying and Caring for the Body Following Death

Death and post-death care (funeral customs) are part of an indigenous caregiving continuum. Caring for the dying and caring for the body following death are important cultural markers that reflect differences between cultural groups (Dembinsky 2014). In common with other indigenous peoples, Māori like to attend to and companion the ill and dying day and night; many gather at the bedside to say their farewells and to encourage the person to leave their body (Duggleby et al. 2015; McGrath and Holewa 2006; Ngata 2005). Whānau are responsible for providing aroha, manaakitanga (practical support based on reciprocity), and relational and spiritual care, before, during, and following death. Despite the pressures imposed by colonial domination on iwi (tribes), hapū (sub-tribes), and whānau, Māori have retained their tangihanga (customary funeral rituals). According to Nikora and Te Awekotuku (2013), tangihanga (ritualized mourning) practices have evolved, with contemporary practices adapting to both new environments and technologies while resonating with customary ways. Traditional caregiving practices of whānau have also changed in response to the assimilating forces that have shaped contemporary Māori lifestyles.

The important cultural criterion is that the care environment, no matter what setting, is flexible enough to become a culturally responsive home deathscape (Moeke-Maxwell and Nikora 2015). A home death may not be a preferred place of death if urgent medical care is required or if the home is not big enough to host visitors before or after death or if whānau are under resourced to provide this critical care (Gott et al. 2014; Moeke-Maxwell and Nikora 2015). Sometimes dying in a hospice, hospital, or residential care facility is preferable to the ill person and their whānau due to personal reasons (living at distance to family) or for complex medical issues (Moeke-Maxwell and Nikora 2015).

The Western health system can impede the death rituals of indigenous people and care needs to be taken to enable cultural processes to be carried out (Hampton et al. 2010). Māori whānau appreciate having the use of whānau rooms at hospitals and hospices where the whānau can stay to support their loved person to die. Whānau are crucial in helping to prepare the wairua to transition to the spiritual realm. However, many whānau are still reluctant to use hospitals or hospices because they view these places as spaces to die in as opposed to places to help people live longer or to have a better quality of life (Dembinsky 2014; Johnston Taylor et al. 2014).

The spiritual health domain is extremely important to indigenous peoples at end of life. Health providers can benefit from engaging in cultural competency training to strengthen their knowledge of traditional end of life customs (McGrath and Holewa 2006). Increasing awareness of traditional healing is also essential to forge a bicultural health framework to meet the multicultural needs of all New Zealanders. Underpinning traditional end of life care is a strong emphasis on wairuatanga (indigenous spiritual belief system) (Ngata 2005). Hampton et al. (2010) research emphasized that improving indigenous care will require health professionals to work together with traditional healers, patients, and family carers.

6 Barriers Māori Encounter at End of Life Care

Palliative care must take into consideration the culture and cultural needs of the person with a life-limiting illness and their whānau who care for them by preventing and relieving suffering (World Health Organisation 2002); this is more likely to be achieved when the culture and cultural needs of Māori are recognized and supported. Culture is recognized as an important determinant of health because it can positively or negatively influence health (National Advisory Committee on Health and Disability 1998). Culture influences attitudes, views, beliefs, and behaviors including those associated to health. Despite the fluidity of culture and cultural identity, Dein (2006) argues that the concept of "culture" is helpful in understanding the needs of different groups of people:

> . . . It [culture] is an important variable in the perception, experience and expression of suffering. There are very real differences between cultural groups. . . People actively draw on elements of their culture to manage life stresses. Culture influences, rather than determines, the way people live.

> It provides ideas about the appropriate behaviour in a given situation, their response to illness and to medical ideas about treatment. (p. 20)

As colonized people, Māori share a number of things in common with other indigenous people at end of life (McGrath and Holewa 2006; Moeke-Maxwell et al. 2014; O'Brien 2012).

- Poverty.
- High financial burden of care.
- Lack of adequate whānau support people due to smaller whānau; whānau living away from home.
- Carer burden and stress.
- Poor communication from health and palliative care service providers (assistance to discuss and explore preferences for place of care and death).
- Lack of support from health and palliative care services.
- Lack of community services (particularly relevant for rural and remote places).
- Whānau cultural preferences differ to palliative care provided by Western healthcare providers.
- Lack of support for caregivers (financial, respite, information).
- Lack of bereavement support (counseling).

Māori whānau may prefer to provide care for their relations who are terminally ill or have high needs at home or in a hospital or hospice setting. But there are many barriers in support provided by the state and in the services provided within hospitals or hospices. Improvements to palliative care services are urgently required, and these need to be flexible in terms of how and where the services are provided. We have to ensure that whānau are supported in carrying out their care obligations. Treating whānau on a "whānau-by-whānau" basis and ensuring services are flexible enough to respond to the diverse circumstances and needs of whānau are essential to providing good end of life care. Reid (2005) states:

> Māori whānau often want to provide care for their relations who are terminally ill or have high needs—either at home, or in a hospital or hospice. But there are many barriers still in the way of this, in the kind of state support provided, and in the services in hospitals or hospices. We have to improve the palliative care services themselves, and the flexibility of how and where the services are provided. And we have to ensure that whānau are supported in their care for family members. That's not only providing real choice—it's also meeting needs and rights. (p. 45)

It is generally accepted by the palliative care sector that Māori want to die at "home" (Ministry of Health 2001; Ngata 2005). A home death is generally considered an important cultural preference for Māori. However, not all Māori want to die at home indicating there is diversity of end of life preferences (Moeke-Maxwell et al. 2014). In the following quote, a bereaved woman reflects on her perception that her husband's preference was to avoid dying at home:

> I didn't have the facilities here [at home] either, and I know that's what [he], I know he would have been thinking that . . . "I don't want to die at home." . . . Not that he said it, not that he said it. But I know, knowing [him], he wouldn't have wanted to die at home. (Moeke-Maxwell et al. 2014, p. 147)

Health providers may have a different concept of home than Māori. Māori have multiple homes; these can include a kainga (house whānau dwell in), ancestral landscapes, and tribal homes (marae) as well as the homes of other whānau (Gott et al. 2014; Moeke-Maxwell and Nikora 2015). Returning home to die or visiting an ancestral home or special place such as a graveyard before death helps to settle the wairua for the journey home to the spiritual realm (Moeke-Maxwell et al. 2014). Similarly Yamatji people felt that to die "in country" was essential for completing the cycle of life and death. Here the Yamatji would be reunited with ancestors which brought deep peace (Dembinsky 2014).

6.1 Access to Services and End of Life Support

Living rurally can present a challenge for whānau as palliative care support is limited, particularly in remote areas. Difficulties have been identified with accessing hospitals, specialists, and specialist palliative care services (Penney et al. 2009). However, living in an urban environment can also prove challenging, particularly for whānau who have moved away from their ancestral homes. They may find it difficult if there are not enough whānau available to support their care requirements. Sometimes friends and neighbors may fill the gap, or a local health service or hospice may be accessed (Moeke-Maxwell and Nikora 2015).

6.2 Personal Factors Affecting Palliative Care Among Older Māori

There are unique challenges for Māori kaumātua (older Māori), particularly for those of advanced age (over 80). Moeke-Maxwell et al. (2014) highlighted the diverse needs of Māori kaumātua. For example, many older Māori continue to be connected to their tribal roots, and they remain active within their whānau, communities, ancestral homes, and tribal groups (Dyall et al. 2011). Similarly, Moeke-Maxwell et al. (2014) identified that some Māori were socially well connected with their communities, and they relied on their whānau to support them at end of life; however, a small number of kaumātua resisted whānau support and were determined to care for themselves. Self-determination, particularly for older Māori, challenged their cultural connections and relationships with whānau (Oetzel et al. 2015b), highlighting differences between Māori as well as different end of life priorities between people of advanced age. Furthermore, whānau associate kaumātua with leadership qualities and cultural knowledge, and as such they are imbued with mana (authority, prestige, and spiritual status). Kaumātua may even find it difficult to receive caregiving support from whānau when they require end of life care as the relational balance of power is jeopardized (Oetzel et al. 2015b). Another reason older Māori may resist their whānau being involved in caregiving is to protect them against the burden of caregiving particularly when there are other concerns (financial, housing, other care obligations, work). For example, Gott et al. (2017) found in a New Zealand longitudinal study, Te Puawaitanga o Ngā Tapuwae Kia Ora Tonu – Life and Living in Advanced Age – that older Māori wished "... to not be a burden to family..." (p. 3). This may reflect the ill person trying to protect their whānau from enduring additional stress. This point is highlighted in a qualitative study of Māori end of life experiences and needs (Moeke-Maxwell and Nikora 2018). The findings revealed that kaumātua recognized their whānau were already burdened with responsibilities (work, caring for others, unwell themselves) and financial hardship. Kaumātua believed that the family's stressful circumstances would be further exacerbated by caring for their end of life needs. Therefore, despite whānau desperately wanting to help the older person, three kaumātua resisted their informal support until death was near (Moeke-Maxwell and Nikora 2018).

6.3 Financial Costs of End of Life Care

The financial costs associated with caring for someone at end of life are intensified at a time when whānau are already under pressure. A pilot bicultural study by Gott et al. (2015a) on the financial costs of care at end of life revealed that the 11 whānau who took part experienced financial hardships associated with meeting the demands of end of life caregiving. Direct costs to whānau, such as medical expenses, pharmaceutical costs, transport, hospital' parking fees, complementary therapies, and linen, were exacerbated by specific cultural care imperatives. These are costs related to cultural obligations associated with care practices such as hosting visitors, travel, and special foods. The costs associated with tangihanga are also high:

> For Māori, the cultural obligation and preference to return to ancestral homes before death and/or post-death (tangihanga) incurred additional transport costs and other expenses associated with meeting these cultural end-of-life needs. In several cases, customary funeral traditions were interrupted due to a lack of resources. Some participants also reported that caring had negatively affected their own health and well-being. (Gott et al. 2015a, p. 521)

Manaakitanga is a social and cultural responsibility (Moeke-Maxwell et al. 2013) that whānau, as hosts, express by taking care of visitors. The study (Gott et al. 2015a) found that feeding manuhiri (visitors) of a dying whānau member at a private home or in a hospital setting can become a very costly expense associated with end of life care. Further, the study highlighted that cultural obligations such as manaakitanga take place before, during, and following death. Other financial costs of care in Gott et al.'s (2015a) study included travel expenses associated with a dying loved one to visit their ancestral lands, homes, or a sacred place before death (e.g., ancestral gravesites) and purchasing kai rangatira (special foods consumed by someone prior to death). Kai rangatira may include delicacies that a kaumātua enjoyed in their youth such as seafood (e.g., crayfish, oysters, kina) and can come at considerable cost to whānau if they are unable to gather these foods themselves. As a result, some caregivers experienced significant debt associated to the financial costs of caregiving at end of life (Gott et al. 2015a). To provide end of life care requires at least one person to support the ill person on their journey. This can have a huge financial and personal impact on the carers, especially when they have to give up work to provide care:

> For example, a Māori participant terminated paid employment to provide full-time care for her older mother, knowing that it would incur financial hardship to nurse her at home: So I gave up my [job]; I resigned from my job which, yeah, which I knew would put me in a position where I wouldn't be able to cope financially. (CTH, Māori daughter) (Gott et al. 2015a, p. 523)

Moeke-Maxwell et al. (2014) similarly identified in a study of Māori end of life experiences that seeking support is not always easy for Māori. For example, accessing respite in a hospice setting may be challenging for whānau, particularly as whānau often have great attachments to their own homes. Financial hardships can make the decision to use hospice services almost essential, especially when the pressure to meet cultural obligations (e.g., such as hosting visitors) is an important, yet often expensive, cultural custom:

> It was brave [to go to hospice]. Boy I cried. It made me think as if I didn't want him [husband], I didn't love him, but I told him . . . I said, "Gee I'm tired." He said, "Tired of what?" I said, "I'm tired, there's too much going on. Your family's coming 'round, I've got to feed them, plus feed our kids and then—we've got nothing to feed them on." (Moeke-Maxwell et al. 2014, p. 146)

Furthermore, costs associated with cultural end of life care can be prohibitive. For example, the preference to use complementary therapies can be expensive for whānau. For example, a participant in Gott et al. (2015a) stated, "That was really costly, alternative medication, it was a Chinese herbalist, I think it cost us about $340 or $350 per week for 4 weeks" (MR, Māori daughter caring for father) (p. 522).

6.4 Māori Health Literacy

Māori carers have a greater opportunity to access palliative care and statutory services support (such as Work and Income, New Zealand) when they have the knowledge or skill to access information (Moeke-Maxwell et al. 2014). Confidence is increased when whānau carers know what is available and how to access it (Kidd et al. 2014). Through necessity whānau often have to rely on their own resources and informal community networks to access palliative care and statutory support information (Kidd et al. 2014). Whānau struggle to access information often due to a lack of the competency of health and palliative care providers to confidently lead and carry out a process of informational exchange between whānau and health professionals.

Hospices can provide invaluable support as they can often be a one-stop-shop of information and referrals. Increased understanding of services can lead to better opportunities to discuss with health professionals critical issues concerning diagnosis, prognosis, treatment, and end of life decision-making and to convey what the needs of the ill person are. Conversations that are helpful require a two-way dialogical process. To be effective, health professionals need to understand the Māori patient and their whānau's needs as much as the patient and their whānau need to understand the health and palliative care systems. For example, positive experiences among Māori whānau are often associated with accessing and receiving hospice support. A kaupapa Māori qualitative study by Johnston Taylor et al. (2014) examined Māori perspectives of hospice care in a large urban city in New Zealand. In line with the benefits enjoyed by Māori New Zealanders, the study highlighted that hospice benefited Māori carers by providing respite care, caregiving equipment, resources, and information and by offering a compassionate service including bereavement and spiritual care. Other benefits hospice provides to Māori have been identified by Slater et al. (2015) and include good communication that is inclusive and supportive of whānau, responsive in-patient units that can cater for whānau, after-hour services and continuity of care, and support with post-death arrangements.

7 Improvements Needed in Palliative Care Services

There are some specific areas in the current palliative care services provided to Māori that need addressing to redress health inequities at end of life. Reducing the gaps is critical given that Māori are often resource-poor and are likely not to be well-informed about the provisions provided by the health and palliative care sectors and statutory support services (Johnston Taylor et al. 2014; Penney et al. 2009).

A Māori preference for a holistic and relational model of healthcare that takes into consideration the mind, body, and spirit has largely been obscured within the mainstream healthcare system. Historically, the healthcare system's medical paradigm has privileged the medical domain almost to the exclusion of the psychosocial and cultural domain. The current health system arguably has some way to go to ensure its services are holistic and that healthcare professionals are equipped to meet the cultural end of life needs of Māori. The indigenous values that are critically important to Māori at end of life are often obscured beneath a preoccupation with the aWestern societal medicalization of dying (Duggleby et al. 2015; Ngata 2005).

A key principle of good palliative care is that people have access to information (Johnston Taylor et al. 2014; Kidd et al. 2014; Ministry of Health 2001; Penney et al. 2009). However, cultural differences between health providers and those receiving services create an additional barrier for Māori accessing and using palliative care services (Frey et al. 2013). In a study by Frey et al. (2013), the researchers discovered that New Zealanders were often unaware of specialist palliative care and that Māori participants had misconceptions about palliative care. This can lead to misunderstanding, further obstructing access to quality care (Frey et al. 2013). Study participants also found it difficult to access information, and prior experiences or knowledge of discrimination encountered within the sector also acted as a barrier.

7.1 Quicker Referrals to Palliative Care Services

Quicker referrals to palliative care services will result in whānau being able to access support and resources much earlier. Research evidence in one rural study highlighted concern over late presentations, late referrals, and late diagnoses delaying the palliative care pathway (Penney et al. 2009). Similarly, a study undertaken by Koti (2013) found that despite numerous visits to a primary healthcare provider over several years for the same health issue, a general practitioner failed to refer the patient to a specialist within a reasonable time-frame. A core component of good palliative care is the delivery of support within a timely manner (Ministry of Health 2001).

7.2 Communication and Information

Of vital importance is the information whānau need to prepare them make informed decisions about the end of life trajectory (Kidd et al. 2014; Penney et al. 2009) and what whānau need to support them to provide care. Closely associated with this is the level of communication needed to convey information to whānau. To date, communication from health providers has at times been of a variable and even disrespectful quality (Koti 2013). Commonly reported issues reflect the use of jargon, lack of information being shared, and the form in which the information is given (Penney et al. 2009). Whānau respond to effective communication employing multiple methods (verbal, pictorial, written) across the care continuum, at the time of diagnosis, during treatment, prior to death, and following death (Moeke-Maxwell et al. 2014; Oetzel et al. 2015a; Penney et al. 2009).

7.3 Racism and Palliative Care

From an indigenous Māori perspective, palliative care should aim to support families to whakamana (uplift the status, authority, and prestige) of an ill or dying family member. Racism acts as a barrier to Māori accessing and receiving end of life care (Harris et al. 2006; Moeke-Maxwell et al. 2014; Penney et al. 2009). Frey et al. (2013) identified that Māori can also be influenced by experiences of discrimination within the health system shared by other Māori.

Racism is broad-based and can include inequitable access to services or discriminatory treatment based on ethnicity that can lead to stereotypes, negative assumptions, and treatment toward Māori. For example, a young kaumātua in the study conducted by Moeke-Maxwell et al. (2014) experienced personal discrimination from hospital staff who stereotyped the unwell man as a drug user. The withholding of his pain medication caused him to suffer unnecessary physical, emotional, and spiritual pain.

8 Conclusion

Māori are culturally and ethnically diverse. Given this heterogeneity, there are often diverse care preferences within and between whānau at end of life (Moeke-Maxwell et al. 2014; Reid 2005). Despite colonialism and the disruptions Māori have faced, many whānau have held on tightly to their mātauranga Māori (knowledge), tikanga (customs), and kawa (protocols) as these fortify and guide Māori caregiving practices (Mead 2003). These customs must actively be retained within the health and palliative care sectors (Durie 1998). The prioritization of the care of the ill and dying remains a critical and core cultural custom of Māori whānau, and it is one that is driven by indigenous cultural and spiritual values, including the cultural imperative to prepare the spirit to transition (Duggleby et al. 2015). A critical role of whānau is to ensure the ill and dying person has their physical, medical, mental and emotional, relational, social, and spiritual needs met.

The New Zealand government has an obligation under the Treaty of Waitangi (1840) to ensure health equity for Māori. This is urgently needed to reduce disparities and the high need for palliative care among Māori. Attention must be focused on ensuring Māori are supported to seek help early to reduce the high numbers of late admissions and the shortened opportunity to access palliative care support. Whānau also desperately need support from health and palliative care services and statutory services (government) to resource them to carry out their caregiving activities (Gott et al. 2015a). These services have a responsibility to fully align their palliative care approach within a framework that is congruous with Māori culture and customs to ensure the best end of life health outcomes for Māori. However, there are critical issues that need improving to reduce the burden on Māori whānau. Whānau often encounter obstacles on the end of life journey (Gott et al. 2015a; Moeke-Maxwell and Nikora 2015; Johnston Taylor et al. 2014; Moeke-Maxwell et al. 2014; Koti 2013; Penny et al. 2009; Harris et al. 2006) including difficulty accessing and receiving the benefits of palliative care (e.g., rural New Zealanders), and there are reduced opportunities via late admissions to palliative care. Furthermore, as a result of neocolonial forces, many whānau have social and economic hardships making the task of caregiving difficult due to the high financial costs associated with end of life care (Gott et al. 2015a; Moeke-Maxwell 2014). Giving up paid work to provide caregiving adds extra financial pressure on whānau carers.

Specifically focused Māori palliative care cultural competency training will help to ensure that health professionals have an understanding of New Zealand history, Māori language, local tribal knowledge and traditional end of life care customs (rongoā Māori – Māori medicines), spiritual practices, and customary rituals. Training in these areas will support health and palliative care services and statutory services to make cultural improvements and to continue to develop services that are aligned with Māori cultural aspirations. Additionally, health provider cultural literacy and communication must also be improved to ensure that communication is simple and straightforward to assist whānau to navigate the health system and access services and statutory support as required (Kidd et al. 2014). Furthermore, once help is accessed, there must be clear, direct, and respectful communication from health professionals toward whānau (Kelly et al. 2009).

The four Te Whare Tapa Whā (Durie 1994) healthcare domains work in synergy with each other and are not separate health fields. The Te Whare Tapa Whā holistic health model "whare" (meeting house) is symbolically viewed by tangata whenua (people of the land) as a place of well-being, safety, and protection. The whare symbolizes the body of a woman; it is protective as it is filled with the spiritual energy forces of the spiritual realms, atua (gods), deities, and ancestors. As such, the Te Whare Tapa Whā health model predates a holistic Western palliative care approach. There is not *one* specific healthcare domain that requires strengthening to support Māori whānau carers to meet the increasing caregiving demands anticipated over the next 30 years. *Every* healthcare domain needs to be strengthened and united to ensure the cultural customs of Māori whānau are supported. This is required to uphold the mana of the dying Māori individual and their whānau carers at end of life. These initiatives will go some way to ensuring there is the desired balance between the physical, emotional, relational, social, and spiritual healthcare domains. A strong community public health approach could help support whānau carers to undertake this critical and sacred end of life work by increasing the opportunity for local psychosocial support (counseling, bereavement, financial assistance, care navigation).

Living with a life-limiting illness and the process of dying are critically important times in the human life span for Māori; it is the sacred time when the wairua is prepared for its journey across the ārai during its transition to the spiritual realm. Whānau, health and palliative care providers, and statutory support services all play an interconnected and critical role on this journey. Their combined efforts will ensure whānau are able to fulfill their cultural obligations as *pou aroha*. The popular Māori adage is relevant here, "if we get this right for Māori, we will get it right for everyone."

References

Angelo J, Wilson L. Exploring occupational roles of hospice family caregivers from Māori, Chinese and Tongan ethnic backgrounds living in New Zealand. Occup Ther Int. 2014;21(2):81–90.

Associate Minister of Health. Healthy aging strategy. Wellington: Ministry of Health; 2016.

Beaglehole E, Beaglehole P. Contemporary Maori death customs. J Polyn Soc. 1945;54(2):91–116.

Best E. The Maori as he was: a brief account of Maori life as it was in pre-European days. Wellington: Dominion Museum; 1934.

Brown W. New Zealand and its Aborigines. London: J. & D.A. Darling; 1851.

Clark D. Between hope and acceptance: the medicalisation of dying. BMJ. 2002;324(7342):905–7.

Dein S. Culture and cancer care: anthropological insights in oncology. Maidenhead: Open University Press; 2006.

Dembinsky M. Exploring Yamatji perceptions and use of palliative care: an ethnographic study. Int J Palliat Nurs. 2014;20(8):387–93.

Dieffenbach E. Travels in New Zealand: with contributions to the geography, botany, and natural history of that country, vol. 2. London: John Murray; 1843.

Duggleby W, et al. Indigenous people's experiences at the end of life. Palliat Support Care. 2015;13:1721–33.

Durie M. Whaiora: Māori health development. Auckland: Oxford University Press; 1994.

Durie M. Whaiora: Māori health development. 2nd ed. Auckland: Oxford University Press; 1998, viii, 244.

Dyall L, et al. Pinnacle of life – Māori living to advanced age. N Z Med J. 2011;124(1331):1–12.

Frey R, et al. 'Where do I go from here'? A cultural perspective on challenges to the use of hospice services'. Health Soc Care Community. 2013; 21(5):519–29.

Gott M, Williams L, Moeke-Maxwell T. The paradoxes of 'home' within a palliative care context. In: Roche M, et al., editors. Engaging geographies: landscapes, lifecourses and mobilities. Cambridge: Cambridge University Press; 2014. p. 137–51.

Gott M, et al. 'No matter what the cost': a qualitative study of the financial costs faced by family and whānau caregivers within a palliative care context. Palliat Med. 2015a;29(6):518–28.

Gott M, et al. Te Pakeketanga: living and dying in advanced age – a study protocol. BMC Palliat Care. 2015b;14(74):21.

Gott M, et al. End of life care preferences among people of advanced age: LiLACS NZ. BMC Palliat Care. 2017;16(1):19.

Gott M, et al. What is the role of community at the end of life for people dying in advanced age? A qualitative study with bereaved family carers. Palliat Med. 2018;32(1):268–75.

Hampton M, et al. Completing the circle: elders speak about end-of-life care with aboriginal families in Canada. J Palliat Care. 2010;26(1):6–14.

Harris R, et al. Racism and health: the relationship between experience of racial discrimination and health in New Zealand. Soc Sci Med. 2006;63:1428–11.

Hiroa TR. The coming of the Maori. Wellington: Thomas Avery & Sons; 1950.

Johnston Taylor E, et al. Māori perspectives on hospice care. Divers Equity Health Care. 2014;11:61–71.

Jones C. Levels of racism: A theoretic framework and a gardener's tale. Am J Public Health. 2000;90(8): 1212–5.

Jones R. Rongoā – medicinal use of plants – the impact of colonisation. In: Te Ara – the encyclopedia of New Zealand. New Zealand: New Zealand Government; 2012.

Kelly L, et al. Palliative care of First Nations people: a qualitative study of bereaved family members.[Erratum appears in Can Fam Physician. 2009 Jun;55(6):590 Note: Gilles, Chris [corrected to Giles, Chris]]. Can Fam Physician. 2009;55(4):394–5.

Kidd J, et al. Kia mau te kahu whakamaru: health literacy in palliative care. Wellington: Ministry of Health; 2014.

Koti DM. Te Tatau o te Pō: perceptions and experiences of palliative care and hospice – a Māori perspective. Massey University: Manawatū Campus, New Zealand; 2013.

Lange R. Story: Te hauora Māori i mua – history of Māori health – re-European health. In: Te Ara – the Encyclopedia of New Zealand. New Zealand: New Zealand Government; 2011.

Laurenson R, et al. Palliative care patients use of emergency departments. N Z Med J. 2013;126(1372):80–8.

McGrath P, Holewa H. The living model: a resource manual for indigenous palliative care service delivery. Toowong: Researchman; 2006.

McLeod H. The need for palliative care in New Zealand. Technical report prepared for the Ministry of Health. Wellington: Ministry of Health; 2016.

Mcleod R, et al. Foundations of spiritual care professional development programme: evaluation report. Wellington: Hospice New Zealand; 2015.

Mead SM. Tikanga Māori: living by Māori values. Wellington: Huia; 2003 x, 398.

Ministry of Health. The New Zealand palliative care strategy. Wellington: Ministry of Health; 2001.

Moeke-Maxwell T, Nikora LW. Homedeathscapes: Māori end-of-life decision-making processes. In: Kepa M, McPherson M, Manu'atu L, editors. Home: here to stay. Wellington: Huia; 2015.

Moeke-Maxwell T, Nikora LW, Te Awekotuku N. Manaakitanga: ethical research with Māori who are dying. In: Agee M, et al., editors. Pacific identities and well-being – cross-cultural perspectives. London: Routledge; 2013. p. 188–203.

Moeke-Maxwell T, Nikora LW, Te Awekotuku N. End-of-life care and Māori Whānau resilience. Mai J. 2014;3(2):140–52.

National Advisory Committee on Health and Disability. The social, cultural and economic determinants of health in New Zealand: action to improve health. Wellington: National Advisory Committee on Health and Disability; 1998.

Ngata AT. Report of Young Maori conference. Auckland: Auckland University College; 1939.

Ngata P. Death, dying and grief. In: Schwass M, editor. Last words: approaches to death in New Zealand's cultures and faiths. Wellington: Bridgett Williams Books with the Funeral Directors Association of New Zealand; 2005. p. 29–41.

Nikora LW, Te Awekotuku N. Tangihanga: the ultimate form of Māori cultural expression – an overview of a research program. In: Agee M, et al., editors. Pacific identities and well-being. Cross-cultural perspectives. New York: Routledge; 2013. p. 169–73.

O'Brien V. Person-centred palliative care: a First Nations perspective. Hamilton, Ontario: McMaster University; 2012.

Oetzel J, et al. Differences in ideal communication behaviours during end-of-life care for Māori carers/ patients and palliative care workers. Palliat Med. 2015a;29(8):764–6.

Oetzel J, et al. Managing communication tensions and challenges during the end-of-life journey: perspectives of Māori kaumātua and their whānau. Health Commun. 2015b;30(4):350–60.

Oppenheim RS. Maori death customs. Wellington: A.H. & A.W. Reed Ltd.; 1973.

Palliative Care Subcommittee. New Zealand palliative care: a working definition. Wellington: NZ Cancer Treatment Working Party; 2007.

Pascoe EA, Smart Richman L. Perceived discrimination and health: a meta-analytic review. Psychol Bull. 2009; 135(4):531–54.

Penney L, Fieldhouse W, Kerr S. Te Hononga a Te Hekenga o Te Rā: connections at the going down of the sun: improving Māori access to palliative care/ tapuhi hunga roku in Te Tai Tokerau. Kerikeri: Kiwikiwi Research and Evaluation; 2009.

Phillipps WJ. European influences on tapu and the tangi. J Polyn Soc. 1954;63(3):147–63.

Polack JS. Manners and customs of the New Zealanders: with notes corroborative of their habits, usages, etc., and remarks to intending emigrants, with numerous cuts drawn on wood, vol. 2. London: J. Madden & Company; 1840.

Reed AW. An illustrated encyclopedia of Māori life. Wellington: A.H. & A.W. Reed Ltd.; 1963.

Reid P. Contemporary perspectives. In: Schwass M, editor. Last words: approaches to death in New Zealand's cultures and faiths. Wellington: Bridgett Williams Books with the Funeral Directors Association of New Zealand; 2005. p. 41–9.

Reid P. Good governance: the case of health equity. In: Tawhai V, Gray-Sharp K, editors. "Always speaking": the Treaty of Waitangi and public policy. Wellington: Huia; 2011.

Reid P, Robson B. Understanding health inequalities. In: Robson B, Harris J, editors. Hauora Māori standards of health IV. Wellington: Te Rōpu Rangahau Hauora a Eru Pomare; 2007.

Slater T, et al. Exploring Māori cancer patients', their families', community and hospice views of hospice care. Int J Palliat Nurs. 2015;21(9):439–45.

Statistics New Zealand. How is our Māori population changing? 2015. http://archive.stats.govt.nz/browse_for_stats/people_and_communities/maori/maori-population-article-2015.aspx. Accessed

Statistics New Zealand. Ethnic population projections to grow across New Zealand. 2017. https://www.stats.govt.nz/news/ethnic-populations-projected-to-grow-across-new-zealand. Accessed

Tregear E. The Maoris of New Zealand. J Anthropol Inst G B Irel. 1890;19:96–123.

Walker R. Ka whawhai tonu matou: struggle without end. Auckland: Penguin Books; 1990.

World Health Organisation. National cancer control programmes: policies and managerial guidelines. 2nd ed. Geneva: World Health Organisation; 2002.

Hospice New Zealand. Hospice New Zealand standards for palliative care. Wellington: Hospice New Zealand; 2012.

Moeke-Maxwell T, Nikora LW. Wairua manuake: Māori end of life preferences. Forthcoming 2018.

Moeke-Maxwell T, Nikora LW. Wairua manuake: flight of the wairua: Māori end of life preparations. Forthcoming 2018.

End-of-Life Healthcare Experiences of Indigenous People and Ethnic Minorities: The Example of Canada

71

Carrie Bourassa, Eric Oleson, and Janet McElhaney

Contents

Abstract

This chapter will explore understandings of culture, ethnicity, indigeneity, intergenerational trauma, and othering and how they relate to health outcomes, experiences with illness and death, accessing healthcare and palliative care, and patient/practitioner interactions predominantly in Canada. Discussions will define indigenous and ethnic minorities and examine the commonalities in health disparities experienced by both groups. Although commonalities will be discussed, they will be paired with the continual need to avoid "pan-Indigenous" or

C. Bourassa (✉)
Indigenous and Northern Health, Health Sciences North Research Institute, Sudbury, ON, Canada

Institute of Indigenous Peoples' Health, Canadian Institute of Health Research, Sudbury, ON, Canada
e-mail: cbourassa@hsnri.ca

E. Oleson
First Nations University of Canada, Regina, SK, Canada

J. McElhaney
Health Sciences North Research Institute, Sudbury, ON, Canada

R. D. MacLeod, L. Van den Block (eds.), *Textbook of Palliative Care*,
https://doi.org/10.1007/978-3-319-77740-5_65

"pan-cultural" understandings that oversimplify the reality of diverse populations. Culture, spirituality, the desire to provide palliative care within the home and community, and subsequent barriers to doing so will be introduced. Though rumblings of culturally safe models of care continue to grow throughout the country, they are often overpowered by stories of mistreatment, discrimination, and colonial behaviors in the healthcare system. In an effort to overcome these barriers and provide the best possible end-of-life care to individuals, a brief overview of cultural safety and culturally safe models of palliative care will be introduced. Finally, recommendations and best practices are presented along with a case study highlighting the importance of patient/practitioner communication when offering culturally safe palliative care.

1 Introduction

The introduction of cultural safety and cultural awareness models into healthcare practice over the past few decades has brought about a much-needed conversation on the roles of culture and othering that inform patient/practitioner interactions in palliative care and healthcare in general. Culture plays an important role in palliative care, as one's understanding of, and approach to, end of life is largely determined by their cultural upbringing. By incorporating the principles of cultural safety into healthcare provision, the patient and their family may guide the process, enabling healthcare practitioners to provide care that aligns with the beliefs of the individual patient. The progress toward implementing these models, including recommendations made by guiding bodies for healthcare practitioners, has seen the widespread enactment of, and support for, training programs for practitioners to ensure relevant and appropriate care for diverse groups of patients, including Indigenous populations and other ethnic or cultural minorities. Existing cultural safety training in Canada approaches training with a focus on the historical experiences of Indigenous peoples in Canada, specifically discussing the colonial efforts to "kill the Indian to save the child" mentality of residential schools, criminalization of Indigenous spiritual practices, and attempted eradication of languages and cultural practices. While this is an excellent way to educate non-Indigenous Canadians on our colonial history, its focus on Indigenous experiences does not address the experiences of immigrants or non-Indigenous ethnic minorities. As is often the case in intercultural relationship building, there is a tendency to skew toward painting marginalized groups with broad brushstrokes, assuming that a homogenous solution may be applied to all members. Indigenous people in Canada hold a vast array of beliefs, traditions, practices, and experiences, yet most of the training programs and recommendations for implementing culturally safe practices assume a shared history and experiences. Add to this the attempt to prescribe the same cultural safety model to other minority and immigrant groups, and it begs the question: is cultural safety doing more harm than good, as it tries to improve patient outcomes and experiences? How is this model enacted with palliative care patients and their families? Are the changes actually accommodating cultural needs, or is lip service being paid to the unique experiences and needs of individuals?

This chapter will explore understandings of culture, ethnicity, indigeneity, intergenerational trauma, and othering and how they relate to health outcomes, experiences with illness and death, accessing healthcare and palliative care, and patient/practitioner interactions. Discussions will pull information from specific Indigenous communities and will also highlight high-level commonalities that are relevant when examining current and potential models of end-of-life care for Indigenous communities. Although commonalities will be discussed, they will be paired with the continual need to avoid "pan-Indigenous" or "pan-cultural" understandings that oversimplify the reality of diverse populations. Indigenous groups and individuals have a vast array of cultures, traditions, beliefs, practices, and experiences. Like all palliative care provision, each individual, family, and community will have unique understanding of death and what they desire for end-of-life care.

2 Defining Indigenous

Indigenous populations live across the globe and are defined by their long-standing connections to the land. Throughout the course of history, Indigenous populations have adapted and migrated, but a vast majority have been displaced or significantly impacted by Euro-western colonization of their lands. This chapter will focus largely on Canada but will also include reference to the British colonized areas of the United States, New Zealand, and Australia, as a result of commonalities in colonial histories, as well as some similarities in their healthcare systems and the way care is provided. This is not to say that there is not vast importance in palliative care models of other Indigenous countries across the globe, but in an area where research is often limited, this serves as a starting point and a foundation to begin identifying specific effective recommendations for communities and geographic locations.

Indigenous peoples are a dynamic and diverse group with their own unique cultural traditions and practices, languages, histories, and ways of knowing. For many Indigenous people in Canada, their sense of identity is connected to definitions created through Canada's colonial history and the creation of legislation such as the *Canadian Constitution Acts of 1867* and *1982*, *the Indian Act*, and subsequent amendments to these documents (Palmater 2011). The Canadian Constitution recognizes three groups of Indigenous people in Canada: Indians (commonly referred to as First Nations), Métis, and Inuit. Currently, many Indigenous people and communities throughout Canada have been granted "Indian status" under *the Indian Act*, while others have not. This is significant as status determines whether or not individuals, even those within the same family and community, can access land rights, band membership, and treaty benefits. Furthermore, creating divisive categories of who is considered Indigenous and who is not demonstrates the Canadian government's continued control over Indigenous peoples, their rights, and their identities (Palmater 2011).

Data from the National Household Survey (NHS) of 2011 reports that 4.3% of the total Canadian population self-identified as Indigenous. Of these citizens, 60.8% are identified as First Nations (this could include status or non-status First Nations), 32.3% identified as Métis, while another 4.2% identified as Inuit (Statistics Canada 2013). The total number of Indigenous peoples in Canada has increased from 3.8% of the population enumerated in the 2006 Census, 3.3% in the 2001 Census, and 2.8% in the 1996 Census (Statistics Canada 2013). Furthermore, Canada's Indigenous population increased by 20% between 2006 and 2011, compared with just over 5% for the non-Indigenous population. The largest numbers of Indigenous people live in Ontario and the western provinces (Manitoba, Saskatchewan, Alberta, and British Columbia) (Statistics Canada 2013).

Indigenous identity has been utilized for centuries to assist colonial efforts, which first aimed to take imperial control of land, and later strove to limit treaty and legally prescribed Indigenous rights. Limiting the power of Indigenous peoples was essential to colonization, and defining and controlling who they were was a strategy consistently employed by colonizers. Although the umbrella term of "Indigenous" refers to connections to a portion of land for a long period of time, centuries of assimilation policies and intentional suppression of Indigenous identities have generated circumstances where indigeneity has become riddled within complex legal and political discourse. And, ultimately, the political and social impacts on identity move into the everyday lives of Indigenous populations and are tied directly to health and wellness. Identity is central to holistic well-being for individuals and communities. Indigenous populations and other minorities face realities where they are "othered" and are socially categorized outside the mainstream.

Despite the complex legal and political discourse surrounding indigeneity, many Indigenous people feel they are able to define their own identity and determine what it means to be Indigenous in Canada. According to Palmater (2011), there is no need to maintain the archetypal "Indian," and Indigenous peoples are free to grow and expand their identities while still having a connection to shared history, ancestors, and traditional territories. As such, palliative care models for Indigenous populations require flexible definitions of indigeneity and should work from an inclusive model that allows for self-identification. Indigenous populations were, and continue to be, disempowered through the denial of their ability to self-identity. They also faced blatant oppression as a result of their identities, as well as subliminal oppression through the exclusion of identities in mainstream discourse. To counter this oppression, models that empower self-identification are of the utmost importance, and the development of any care model should ensure that the power associated with identity is placed with the patient, their family, and their community.

Indigeneity, as discussed, refers to people who have a connection with land. It is distinct from ethnicity and culture but yet remains intertwined with both of these concepts. Ethnicity and culture are two different notions, and it is important to create this distinction when discussing culturally responsive healthcare models. Ethnicity is categorized as the distinctive shared origins or social backgrounds and traditions of a group of people that are maintained between generations. It should not be confused with race, migration, or nationality. Ethnicity is fluid and creates a sense of identity that may include a common language and religion (Busolo and Woodgate 2015). Culture, on the other hand, refers to beliefs, values, and customs expressed in daily living including diet, clothing, or rituals. It also influences language and social or political systems. In this way, culture may be fluid because of developments in people's lives (Busolo and Woodgate 2015).

Identity and culture evolve and are re-negotiated and recreated over time. Aggressive colonial practices have created identities for Indigenous people, which has resulted in Indigenous identities and cultures being framed as homogenous, static, and valued through another society's agenda. This has led to a lack of agency and created health inequities that still exist today (King et al. 2009). For example, trauma histories are highly prevalent among Canadian Indigenous populations and occur from collective and individual experiences with discrimination and social exclusion, poverty, emotional abuse, physical violence, sexual assault, torture, and war (Guilfoyle et al. 2008). For Indigenous Canadians, these traumatic experiences are not merely historical and relegated to the experiences of past generations. Rather, these traumatic experiences are intergenerational, meaning the psychological, spiritual, emotional, and physical pain and suffering continues today and is experienced by each new generation of Indigenous youth (Browne 2006; Guilfoyle et al. 2008). As a result of this deep historical trauma, health disparities cannot merely be mitigated by matching socioeconomic status or altering individual lifestyle factors. Intergenerational trauma is a collective experience that has created and continues to create structural inequalities and violence in the healthcare context.

3 Indigenous and Ethnic Minority Disparities in Healthcare

In addition to the increasing population of Indigenous peoples around the globe, globalization is driving immigration, with millions of people uprooting from their birthplaces to seek greener pastures and brighter futures. In 2011, Canada had a foreign-born population of nearly seven million people, representing 20.6% of the total population. In the past 5 years, the majority of newcomers have come from Asia and the Middle East (Statistics Canada 2013). Furthermore, 19.1% of Canadians identified themselves as a member of a visible minority group, and only 30.9% were born in Canada, while 65.1% were born outside the country and came to live in Canada as immigrants. Visible minorities also experience health disparities that may be the result of the direct effects of discrimination or unequal treatment by healthcare providers, or indirectly, through the effects of race-related socioeconomic inequalities (Khan et al. 2015). However, there is a lack of data and research on the role of race or visible minority status on health in Canada compared to Indigenous peoples and the impacts of applying universal cultural safety models to visible minorities, despite similar healthcare disparities or experiences (Khan et al. 2015). The continuous impact of colonization leaves Indigenous and non-Indigenous people in a deep-rooted systemic issue around healthcare. Healthcare professionals are encouraged to be mindful not to "homogenize" an individual's end-of-life care plan based on cultural heritage alone, as many individual differences need to be taken into consideration (Bellamy and Gott 2013).

Both Indigenous and immigrant Canadians experience health inequalities compared to their non-Indigenous, Canadian-born counterparts (Anderson et al. 2015; Kirmayer and Brass 2016). Through the destructive process of "othering," racial, cultural, and ethnic stereotypes are enacted in healthcare creating a social distance that marginalizes and disempowers Indigenous people and immigrants. Othering marks certain individuals and devalues their identity as it is continually created and recreated in the eyes of those who are unmarked or valued in society, producing positions of domination and subordination (Barter-Godfrey and Taket 2009; Johnson et al. 2009). In the healthcare context, othering has led to large health disparities for Indigenous peoples and newcomers. Several Canadian studies have found that both Indigenous and foreign-born Canadians face barriers to accessing healthcare services (Guilfoyle et al. 2008).

The impacts of these disparities between Indigenous people and ethnic minorities share a common connection. Much like how Indigenous people in Canada can trace a decline in their health to European contact, new immigrants also face a decline in health upon entering the country. Research suggests that those new to Canada actually enter the country with high levels of health but experience a deterioration in their health status after settling in the country (De Maio and Kemp 2008). The reasons for this change in health from the so-called healthy immigrant are often the results of discrimination and inequitable experiences in healthcare but are also due to difficulties transitioning to a new country (De Maio and Kemp 2008). Therefore, the healthcare rhetoric of "treating everyone the same" runs counter to the experiences of marginalized groups, claiming they are "being treated differently" by healthcare providers because of their identity (Tang and Browne 2008).

Despite the commonalities, there are some differences to consider when examining health disparities among Indigenous and immigrant Canadians. Studies highlight one area where there is a critical divergence in the healthcare status and experiences between the two populations. The health inequities between foreign-born Canadians and those born here converge after controlling for sociodemographic and socioeconomic status and lifestyle factors (Kobayashi et al. 2008). When these factors are controlled for Indigenous people, disparities still remain (Browne et al. 2012). This can partially be attributed to the intersection of race with other social categories including class, substance use, and history that creates inequitable access to health and healthcare for Indigenous people (Tang and Browne 2008). Specifically, it is the historical intergenerational trauma that continues to entrench these health disparities into contemporary contexts (Browne et al. 2012; Guilfoyle et al. 2008).

4 Culture, Spirituality, and Dignity in Dying

The experiences of each person, family, community, and culture throughout, and at the end of one's life, are unique. Everyone will experience death differently, and people will require different supports at the end of life. There are similar characteristics and experiences among Indigenous groups; there is also significant variation between regions and communities. When discussing or providing palliative care for Indigenous people and ethnic minorities, it is essential to avoid the assumption that everyone will have the same understandings and experiences. Care models should avoid generalist approaches that assess diverse individuals and groups strictly based on their cultural identity. Space must be generated that allows for cultural and communal similarities and subsequent connections but, at the same time, allows for diversity and individual care needs. Creating this balance is necessary to providing anti-oppressive healthcare.

This chapter will further address this concept, and its practical applications, through discussions of cultural safety. To further examine the intricacies of implementing cultural safety, the following sections will highlight some high-level concepts of how culture and indigeneity influence dying and the end of life and, subsequently, palliative care.

Culture influences the way we see and experience the world; therefore, one's culture influences understandings of death and dying. The experiences of all people, including Indigenous peoples, at the end of life are connected to their cultural understandings of life, death, and health. The meaning of health, life, and death is influenced by familial, social, and cultural experiences, and therefore it is not only individual but also social and cultural. One cannot detach meanings of death, dying, grief, and care from family, community, and culture.

For many Indigenous populations, health is holistic and involves a cyclical journey that incorporates death as a meaningful and important part of this journey (Clarke and Holtslander 2010). Despite cultural differences between many groups, preparing the personal spirit for end-of-life journeys is a shared worldview that is important for connection, healing, and protection during this time (Duggleby et al. 2015). Elders and traditional teachers from communities in Saskatchewan, Canada, emphasized that death was a necessary part of completing the circle. It was an essential part of the life cycle and was not necessarily seen as an end – it was seen as essential to living (Hampton et al. 2010). This sentiment was echoed, and highlighted, by community-based researchers in Northern Alaska as well (DeCourtney et al. 2010b). These traditional views impact not only the emotional and mental state of the individual near the end of their life but also those of family members and community members.

The value of balance, and the understanding that life and death are all part of the same process, is foundational to how someone approaches death. In some instances, traditional elders speak of a "good death." The very fact that the concept of moving on to the "spirit world" and having a "good death" demonstrates how understandings of end-of-life processes are rooted in culture and how one sees the world. In some instances, dying well is connected to living well (Baydala et al. 2006). If death is part of completing the circle of life, then living in balance, and living a good life, is the foundation of a good death. In some cultural discourses, including biomedical ones, life and death are seen as opposites, and the belief that a good life means a good death would be counterintuitive. Different worldviews and different cultural teachings, including those from Indigenous communities, emphasize the spectrum that exists for how people experience death. When asked for their traditional views on death and dying, the elders from Saskatchewan, referenced earlier, were quick to point out that they could only relay what they knew, their own experiences, and the teachings they had been handed down from their ancestors. This reiterates that cultures and communities may share common teachings and traditions but that one cannot generalize assumptions of beliefs or experiences onto entire groups.

Spirituality may also play a significant role for many Indigenous populations at the end of life. For some, death is the process of traveling to the spirit world (Duggleby et al. 2015). Some Mi'kmaq communities explain death as a journey to the spirit world that is taken alongside your ancestors and kin who have already passed (Johnston et al. 2012). In line with this belief is a story from Alaska that outlines a young Indigenous girl's experience caring for her grandmother on the day she died. She remembers helping her grandmother get dressed for tea. The visitors that came for tea were her grandmother's previously deceased husband and son. Once the tea was drunk, she assisted her grandmother to her bed where she then died (DeCourtney et al. 2010a). This story is just one anecdotal example, but it highlights how spirituality and ancestral traditions will greatly impact experiences around end-of-life care.

5 Care in the Community and Dying at Home

Family and community often play an important role at the time of death, and culture also impacts the role they play at the end of life. An important consideration is that the definition of family is influenced by culture. For many Indigenous communities, the extended family and community played a large role in palliative care (McGrath 2010). For some Indigenous communities, the gathering of the community in a person's final days is very important (Hampton et al. 2010). As palliative care facilities are not always located within their communities, the thought of physically moving a patient would be conflicting with their desires to die at home or die in an environment that allows for the gathering of community members. Preparing the spirit for the journey ahead is very important for many Indigenous people. Duggleby et al. (2015) discusses the positive impact that hospital staff could have if they truly understood where (Indigenous) patients came from. Family and community members may also provide a key role in providing care for someone at the end of life. A study conducted in Ontario outlined aboriginal women as the primary caregivers of aboriginal elderly in geographically isolated areas. The value of passing on tradition and caring for the elderly started when women were young. Caring was perceived as a traditional role for women as they are strong and fundamental to holding their communities together (Crosato et al. 2007). These beliefs surrounding care were mirrored in both Alaska and Australia. In Alaska, traditional beliefs outlined that taking care of the elderly was both an obligation and a source of pride and joy (DeCourtney et al. 2010b). Research in the Northern Territory of Australia found strong value associated with caring for your own family members, and within some communities, it is strongly believed that families should look after the elderly. In this region, kinship rules outline who the most appropriate person would be to look after someone at the end of their life (McGrath 2008). The role of family members and community members in care provision influences experiences of care both in the community and in healthcare settings.

Many people wish to spend the time at the end of their life in their homes and in their communities, but most patients in palliative care in Canada die in hospital (Canadian Hospice Palliative Care Association 2007). This trend is consistent across most populations; however, there are some additional considerations that are particularly relevant for both ethnic minorities, as well as Indigenous populations. It has been recommended that enabling family members to provide "hands-on" care to their older relatives in an institutional setting creates a collaborative environment for the patient (Bellamy and Gott 2013). There are obvious comforts to familiar surroundings, as well as familiar people at the end of life. However other influences could be included: preferences for speaking and hearing traditional language, passing on traditional knowledge to community members, strong connections to the land they lived once, and accessing culturally relevant care, including traditional medicine.

6 Barriers to Providing End-of-Life Care at Home

There are several barriers that emerge when patients and families choose to provide palliative care at home. Some of these factors are similar to all individuals and families regardless of culture or ethnicity. These include the unpredictable time length of care, isolation and caregiver fatigue, financial strain, and the potential comorbidity with other illnesses that may require interventions and care. However, the largest barrier to dying at home for all Canadians is the inadequacy of home care and other forms of support for families caring for a dying person. Individuals and families that wish to have a home death need to be aware that the demands may be greater than their abilities and resources and they might be unable to satisfy a loved one's wish to die at home (Arnup 2013).

The physical environment of some institutional care settings can be a barrier to culturally appropriate palliative and end-of-life care. In one particular study, this was seen as an unwelcoming environment for some cultural groups, having historically served the needs of those from primarily white, Christian middle-class backgrounds (Bellamy and Gott 2013). For Indigenous Canadians, the choice to die at home becomes even more challenging and can be attributed to the complex historical, social, and political dynamics that have hindered Indigenous people's agency and control. For many Indigenous Canadians and other ethnic minorities, this means relocating to hospitals and care facilities far from home and away from their families (Bellamy and Gott 2013). Furthermore, family members may lack the financial resources needed to relocate with their loved one (Castleden et al. 2009). A lack of quality housing necessary to provide home care services and sustain the dying at home process is also a barrier for many Indigenous Canadians. Intergenerational trauma, systemic racism, and low socioeconomic status may mean that many families do not meet the necessary criteria for keeping a loved one in the home (Arnup 2013).

7 Cultural Safety in Healthcare

Cultural safety was developed during the 1980s in New Zealand as a concept in nursing, specifically as a result of observed inequities in healthcare services being offered to Māori, the Indigenous peoples of New Zealand. At that time the nursing profession, and most of the healthcare field, was focused on "transcultural" care or, as was the case in Canada, the notion of offering services in a multicultural context. Transcultural healthcare or offering healthcare in multicultural context considers all cultures as having an equal claim on government services and societal attention and downplays differences and historical context (Brascoupe and Waters 2009; Kirmayer 2012). This model of healthcare invalidates the unique experiences of Indigenous people because it assumes that health inequalities can, and should, be overcome by merely acknowledging cultural differences. It does not, however, acknowledge the power dynamics present. Healthcare staff should be cognizant of widespread variations of culture to be able to facilitate end-of-life care; it is a major challenge to care delivery when a heterogeneous approach is taken (Bellamy and Gott 2013). In Canada, cultural safety has been included in many health discourses, proving its applicability to a multicultural policy context. However, while cultural safety has been applied across ethnic and culturally diverse populations, the main focus in Canada has been on cultural safety in relation to Indigenous peoples (Brascoupe and Waters 2009).

In contrast, cultural safety requires the explicit and detailed recognition of the cultural identity of healthcare practitioners and patients. Cultural safety acknowledges the power imbalance present in healthcare and demands the transfer of this power to Indigenous people so that they might determine the quality and type of care services available. It recognizes that the current circumstances of Indigenous people are the result of contact and colonial history and that aggressive assimilation policies, the legacy of residential schools, and cultural genocide have resulted in power structures that continue to limit Indigenous peoples' agency in their own healthcare. Canadian healthcare practitioners have implemented it in conjunction with community-based healthcare and offering traditional healing methodologies in communities to increase positive health outcomes and mitigate risk (Brascoupe and Waters 2009; Kirmayer 2012).

A respectful, responsible, reciprocal, and relevant safe healthcare model must focus on a strategic and practical plan to change how healthcare is delivered to Indigenous people. The focus on the word safety is purposeful, and unlike previously utilized models of healthcare such as transcultural, cross-cultural, cultural sensitivity, or cultural competency, it involves the notion of safety as a critical part of delivering culturally based care and the harm that may occur in its absence (Brascoupe and Waters 2009; Kirmayer 2012). For example, cultural competency and cultural sensitivity ensure that service providers acknowledge cultural differences but still retain all of the power. Cultural safety realigns the power structure so that trust and positive relationships play a central role in the quality of care administered. It aims for equality and shared responsibility and allows patients to determine their needs rather than enforce the previously acknowledged western medical professional-client relationships with unilateral, practitioner-based decision-making (Brascoupe and Waters 2009; Kirmayer 2012).

In order to create culturally safe healthcare models, healthcare professionals must identify their own values, beliefs, and assumptions and then engage in a reflective practice that encourages honesty, active listening, and the sharing of power and knowledge. Education in healthcare must focus on training about Indigenous peoples and the social determinants of health in order to implement best practices for ensuring culturally safe healthcare practice. These best practices include understanding colonization and post-colonial forces and their impacts; principles of reciprocity, respect, inclusivity, community, and self-determination; culturally safe communication and language; and acknowledging Indigenous knowledge and practices in terms of health/healing/wellness (Brascoupe and Waters 2009; McGrath 2010).

8 Creating a Culturally Safe Palliative Care Model

Ethnocultural meaning of illness, suffering, and dying define the relationship foundations that patients and healthcare providers draw upon during interactions. Recent research demonstrates that ethnocultural factors influence the provision and receipt of palliative care more than age, education, gender, or socioeconomic status. Therefore, when they are overlooked or not acknowledged, inferior or unsafe care occurs (Busolo and Woodgate 2015). Given the importance of culture on an individual's well-being, healthcare professionals have recognized the need for a culturally safe palliative care model when working with Indigenous patients and their families. Though still in its infancy, a fluid, living model has emerged that can be adapted to meet the unique needs of the individual as well as the community (McGrath 2010). It rejects the notion of pan-Indigeneity, acknowledging that not all people will require the same end-of-life care and support in the same ways simply because they are Indigenous and that individuals are complex with varying healthcare needs (Kelly and Minty 2007).

This model is based on the principles of equity, autonomy, trust, nonjudgment, continuity of care, an emphasis on living rather than dying, and cultural respect. A more Indigenous holistic model differs from western medical palliative care models in that it places the individual and their family or kinship network at the center of the model rather than just the individual patient (McGrath 2010). In this way, it recognizes the importance of family and community in the healthcare and lives of individuals. Specifically, culturally safe palliative care models center on notions of choice, empowerment, and community participation. There is a deep respect for family and community relationships and effective communication. Palliative care models that are culturally safe must ensure respect for Indigenous languages, build community practices, attempt to offer on-site services, educate healthcare providers, understand and support cultural issues, develop culturally appropriate facilities, offer transportation services, deal with relocation issues, provide respite, and respect the importance of Indigenous grief practices (Kelly and Minty 2007; McGrath 2010).

One example of creating a culturally safe model that pertains to palliative care is the *Aboriginal Home Care Project*. The Regina Qu'Appelle Health Region (RQHR) operating in Saskatchewan identified a gap in home care service delivery and First Nations and Métis people living in the region. People were not accessing home care supports prompting RQHR to partner with the Eagle Moon Health Office, a local, Indigenous-based health services agency, initiating an *Aboriginal Home Care Project*. Following a community-based, culturally safe model of practice, the partnership assembled a working group with representation from First Nations, Métis, government, and home care to meet with community members and identify key issues. The barriers identified by this working group included a lack of case management and restrictive policies preventing home care access for Indigenous patients. This discovery allowed RQHR to adapt home care services to make them more culturally safe by offering additional services not utilized or valued in western practices (i.e., elder consultations, traditional healing, ceremony, etc.) and changing how practitioners work and communication with patients.

Specifically, RQHR Home Care created new staff positions and incorporated cultural practices into management, as all Indigenous patients using home care services now have more comprehensive case management and are linked to an Indigenous liaison worker (Health Council of Canada 2012).

9 Regulatory Bodies and Recommendations: Creating Best Practices in Culturally Safe Palliative Care

Kelly et al. (2009) sought the advice of palliative care patients and their families, and they found the recommendations ranged from intensive training of all staff that would interact with patients and their families to larger rooms for extended family and friends to visit with patients and to simply providing tea and cookies to visitors. Above all other recommendations, however, was communicating directly and clearly. Incorporating the former recommendations and excluding the latter would be an example of a homogenous approach to cultural safety: prescribing the same treatment to all perceived members of an ethnic group minimizes the importance of their individual experiences, traditions, and beliefs. There have been important elements of the intentions behind cultural safety that have been lost in the translation to enacting it in a broad system. Focusing training and policy on clear and direct communication (if this itself is culturally appropriate) puts the power in the hands of patients and their support networks to feel safe in communicating their wishes and needs.

Case Study: Communication as a Central Goal of Care

A 75-year-old woman from a rural First Nation community was transferred to a tertiary care center for heart valve replacement. She had experienced significant functional decline due to shortness of breath on exertion and associated weakness since she was unable to remain active because of her shortness of breath. By the time of admission to the rural hospital, she was bedbound, but her heart condition was stabilized enough for transfer to a tertiary care center so she could be assessed for a possible heart valve replacement. Her condition continued to deteriorate during the course of the work-up, and the heart valve replacement surgery was considered to be too high risk. In the intensive care setting, she required intravenous medications to support her blood pressure, but she became delirious and her level of consciousness continued to deteriorate. At this time, her treatment orders included full cardiopulmonary resuscitation in the event that her heart or breathing stopped. This included chest compressions, electric shocks to restart the heart, and ventilator support through a breathing tube. She would be unlikely to survive this intervention, and the chances of her surviving to return to her community were extremely poor. The patient was unable to participate in any discussions regarding goals of care, and there were no advance directives to limit the level of treatment being provided.

As the geriatrician consulted, I initiated discussions with her family (her husband who had traveled with her and her adult children who lived locally) to establish goals of care and the approach to care that would best support their goals. Her husband and adult children understood that she had been flown to the tertiary care hospital to have her heart problem "fixed"; in essence, the possibility of a miracle had been offered, and now the medical team realized that a palliative approach to end-of-life care was needed. In this situation, the patient's husband becomes the substitute decision-maker, but he spoke The (native) Language and had a limited understanding of the English language. Although the children spoke some of The Language and could interpret for their father, they felt that incorporating some of the "old" words of The Language would be important for the discussion of goals of care and levels of treatment. Thus, an interpreter was arranged. Through this discussion, the patient's husband and children came to understand that cardiopulmonary resuscitation would most likely be futile and would prevent her from dying in peace. They also understood that some of her current medications kept her blood pressure within a range that would keep her alive for a while, but they make no difference to her mental status or to her inevitable death. The level of treatment changed to no cardiopulmonary resuscitation but to continue full medical treatment including the medications to stabilize her blood pressure. While they recognized that their mother was nearing the end of her end-of-life care, they wanted to have time for the rest of the family to gather at her bedside and hoped that by continuing the blood pressure medication, there would be time for this to happen. This gathering was not a simple matter of having family quickly drive to the hospital – it involved applications for and approval of travel grants and other arrangements that would allow for the rest of the family to be with her. The family was also referred to the Medicine Lodge for any ceremony that they wanted, including preparations for a cedar bath for their mother. As each of the member of the family arrived, clinical staff were available to review the patient's condition and answer any questions.

Once the family had gathered without restrictions on the number of visitors that could be in the room, the intravenous treatments were discontinued and the patient crossed to the spirit world a few hours later. The family remained with her through this journey and was supported in the room with her for many hours after her passing. Arrangements were then made to have her body transported back to her home community for the wake that followed.

Reflecting on the lessons learned from discussions with Indigenous people regarding palliative care in their communities, I can understand that the healthcare system often serves Indigenous people poorly – particularly at the end of life. This can be related to many factors, such as a lack of cross-cultural awareness, poor cross-cultural communication, and a lack of flexibility within the healthcare system. Issues of racism, discrimination, and bias manifest as culturally unsafe practices and result in delays in Indigenous people seeking healthcare and in the failure of the health system to recognize and effectively and respectfully integrate the essential role of traditional healing and need for spirituality during their journey to the spirit world (Duggleby et al. 2015).

In this case, it was important to communicate with the patient's husband (through an interpreter) in a way that all of the family members and the providers could understand – especially her substitute decision-maker – her husband, who in this case understood very little English. Goals of care decisions are as important to the family as they are to the patient and help them with the processes of grieving and healing from the loss of a loved one. Having clarified that the goal of care was to support a good death, the next task was to determine how the patient could be medically supported until the rest of her children arrived and her whole family could gather at her bedside. It was important to ask about cultural and religious traditions that were not only important for the patient but also her family. Cultural traditions to provide care and comfort to all through the transition and honoring the need of her family to be with her in the moments and hours after her passing were supported.

Respectful, compassionate, and culturally appropriate care may be more time-consuming. Healthcare systems may be reluctant to take the extra time required or to be flexible on rules that more typically govern practices, such as limiting the number of visitors or moving the body quickly after death. Yet, our commitment to "Patients First" and to compassionate care that appropriately meets the needs of individual patients demands that we take the time and commit to our own learning with respect to the provision of culturally sensitive care.

10 Conclusion

While many attempts have been made to remedy the existing issues of discrimination, racism, bias, and the ignorance of the complexities of intercultural healthcare provision, the absence of a guiding policy or overarching framework tells us much about the current healthcare system in Canada. Though rumblings of culturally safe models of care, especially near the end of life, continue to grow throughout the country, they are often overpowered by stories of mistreatment, discrimination, and colonial behaviors in the healthcare system, whether in emergent care or through long-term hospice supports. Attempting to solve these issues through cultural competency, transcultural awareness, and other pan-Indigenous and pan-immigrant models falls flat in the face of the diversity of which Canada tries so hard to be inclusive. The disparity between ethnic groups and Indigenous peoples, and non-Indigenous Canadians, is the symptom of a deeper malady, one which stems from a common approach to healthcare that punishes those who do not conform to the majority. Palliative care endeavors to provide truly person-centered care but may still fall short in many instances. The message, then, is loud and clear: there is still more work to be done globally for our Indigenous communities and ethnic minorities that represent each distinct group in a culturally safe way.

Appendix

For further information regarding conversation on palliative care with Indigenous people, please see the *Completing the Circle* video series at https://www.youtube.com/user/EndofLifeCareProject.

References

Anderson LM, Adeney KL, Shinn C, Safranek S, Buckner-Brown J, Krause LK. Community coalition-driven interventions to reduce health disparities among racial and ethnic minority populations. Cochrane Database Syst Rev. 2015;6. Retrieved from http://onlinelibrary.wiley.com/store/10.1002/14651858.CD009905.pub2/asset/CD009905.pdf?v=1&t=j3gbpho4&s=291adc390c578895da6e001e23e3655211305159

Arnup K. Death, dying and Canadian families: contemporary family trends. Ottawa: The Vanier Institute of the Family; 2013.

Barter-Godfrey S, Taket A. Othering, marginalisation and pathways to exclusion in health. In: Taket A, Crisp BR, Nevill A, Lamaro G, Graham M, Barter-Godfrey S, editors. Theorising social exclusion. Abingdon: Routledge; 2009. p. 166–72.

Baydala A, Hampton M, Kinunwa L, Kinunwa G, Kinunwa L. Death, dying, grieving and end of life care: understanding personal meanings of aboriginal friends. Humanist Psychol. 2006;34:159–76.

Bellamy G, Gott M. What are the priorities for developing culturally appropriate palliative and end-of-life care for older people? The views of healthcare staff working in New Zealand. Health Soc Care Commun. 2013; 21:26–34.

Brascoupe S, Waters C. Cultural safety: exploring the applicability of the concept of cultural safety to aboriginal health and community wellness. J Aborig Health. 2009;5(2):6–41.

Browne AJ. Critical cultural perspectives and health care involving aboriginal peoples. Contemporary Nurse. 2006;22(2):155–67.

Browne AJ, Varcoe CM, Wong ST, Smye VL, Lavoie J, Littlejohn D, et al. Closing the health equity gap: evidence-based strategies for primary health care organizations. Int J Equity Health. 2012;11:15–1.

Busolo D, Woodgate R. Palliative care experiences of adult cancer patients from ethnocultural groups: a qualitative systematic review protocol. JBI Database System Rev. Implement Rep. 2015;13:99–111.

Canadian Hospice Palliative Care Association. Hospice palliative care in Canada: a brief to the Special Senate Committee on Aging. 2007. Retrieved from http://www.chpca.net/media/7487/Brief_to_Spec_Sen_Comm_on_Aging-HPC_in_Canada.pdf

Castleden H, Crooks VA, Morgan VS, Schuurman N, Hanlon N, Inter Tribal Health Authority. Dialogues on aboriginal-focused hospice palliative care in rural and remote British Columbia, Canada. Halifax: Dalhousie University; 2009.

Clarke V, Holtslander LF. Finding a balanced approach: incorporating medicine wheel teachings in the care of aboriginal people at end of life. J Palliat Care. 2010;26(1):34–6

Crosato K, Ward-Griffin C, Leipert B. Aboriginal women caregivers of the elderly in geographically isolated communities. Rural Remote Health. 2007; 7:796.

De Maio FG, Kemp E. The deterioration of health status among immigrants to Canada. Glob Public Health. 2008;5:462–78.

DeCourtney C, Branch PK, Morgan K. Eleanor McMullen's story. J Palliat Care. 2010a;26:67.

DeCourtney C, Branch P, Morgan K. Gathering information to develop palliative care programs for Alaska's aboriginal peoples. J Palliat Care. 2010b;26:22–31.

Duggleby W, Kuchera S, MacLeod R, Holyoke P, Scott T, Holtslander L, Chambers T. Indigenous people's experiences at the end of life. Palliat Support Care. 2015;13(6):1721–33.

Guilfoyle J, Kelly L, St Pierre-Hansen N. Prejudice in medicine: our role in creating health care disparities. Can Fam Physician. 2008;54:1511–3.

Hampton M, Baydala A, Bourassa C, McKay-McNabb K, Placsko C, Goodwill K, Boekelder R. Completing the circle: elders speak about end-of-life care with aboriginal families in Canada. J Palliat Care. 2010;26:6–14.

Health Council of Canada. Empathy, dignity, and respect: Creating cultural safety for Aboriginal people in urban health care. 2012. Retrieved from http://www.healthcouncilcanada.ca/tree/Aboriginal_Report_EN_web_final.pdf

Johnson JL, Bottorff JL, Browne AJ, Grewal S, Hilton BA, Clarke H. Othering and being othered in the context of health care services. J Health Commun. 2009;16:255–71.

Johnston G, Vukic A, Parker S. Cultural understanding in the provision of supportive and palliative care: perspective in relation to an indigenous population. Support Palliat Care. 2012. https://doi.org/10.1136/bmjspcare-2011-000122.

Kelly L, Minty A. End-of-life issues for aboriginal patients: a literature review. Can Fam Physician. 2007; 53:1459–65.

Kelly L, Linkewich B, Cromarty H, St. Pierre-Hansen N, Antone I, Gilles C. Palliative care of first nations people: a qualitative study of bereaved family members. Can Fam Physician. 2009;55:394–5.

Khan M, Kobayashi K, Kee S, Vang Z. (In)visible minorities in Canadian health data and research. Population Change and Lifecourse Strategic Knowledge Cluster Discussion Paper Series. 2015; 3 (1)

King M, Smith A, Gracey M. Indigenous health part 2: the underlying causes of the health gap. Lancet. 2009; 374:76–85.

Kirmayer LJ. Rethinking cultural competence. Transcult Psychiatry. 2012;49:149–64.

Kirmayer LJ, Brass G. Addressing global health disparities among indigenous peoples. Lancet. 2016;388:105–6.

Kobayashi KM, Prus S, Lin Z. Ethnic differences in self-rated and functional health: does immigrant status matter? Ethn Health. 2008;13:129–47.

McGrath P. Family caregiving for aboriginal peoples during end-of-life: findings from the northern territory. J Rural Trop Public Health. 2008;7:1–10.

McGrath P. The living model: an Australian model for aboriginal palliative care. J Palliat Care. 2010;26:59–64.

Palmater PD. Beyond blood: rethinking indigenous identity. Saskatoon: Purich Publishing; 2011.

Statistics Canada. Aboriginal peoples in Canada: first nations people, Métis and Inuit National Household Survey, 2011. 2013. Retrieved from http://www12.statcan.gc.ca/nhs-enm/2011/as-sa/99-011-x/99-011-x2011001-eng.pdf

Tang SY, Browne AJ. 'Race' Matters: racialization and egalitarian discourses involving aboriginal people in the Canadian health care context. Ethn Health. 2008; 13:109–27.

Part VII

Palliative Care Emergencies

Hypercalcemia of Malignancy

72

Kathryn A. Tham and Davinia S. E. Seah

Contents

K. A. Tham
Royal Melbourne Hospital Palliative Care, Parkville, VIC, Australia
e-mail: katie.a.tham@gmail.com

D. S. E. Seah (✉)
Sacred Heart Health Service, St Vincent's Hospital, NSW, Australia

School of Medicine, University of Notre Dame Australia, Darlinghurst, NSW, Australia

St Vincent's Clinical School, University of New South Wales, NSW, Australia
e-mail: davinia.seah@svha.org.au

R. D. MacLeod, L. Van den Block (eds.), *Textbook of Palliative Care*,
https://doi.org/10.1007/978-3-319-77740-5_70

Abstract

This chapter discusses hypercalcemia of malignancy which is the commonest biochemical complication of cancer and recognized as a medical emergency. Hypercalcemia presents with a wide range of clinical symptoms which in some cases can be severe and life-threatening. It is essential for clinicians to consider hypercalcemia as a differential diagnosis in patients with nonspecific symptoms, as hypercalcemia is potentially reversible. The following sections will review normal calcium homeostasis and discuss the mechanisms of how cancer disrupts this tightly regulated system. It is recognized that hypercalcemia is normally associated with advanced disease and, unless antineoplastic treatments are available, is a poor prognostic sign. It is therefore important to consider the individual clinical situation before deciding on an appropriate management plan. Hypercalcemia results in hypovolemia, and the initial management should consist of rehydration. Following this, specific calcium-lowering treatment should be considered. Following rehydration, bisphosphonates have been the treatment of choice for the last 20 years and are effective in the initial treatment for the majority of cases. Unfortunately, it is common for hypercalcemia to relapse, and the best approach to treatment of recurrent and refractory hypercalcemia is not clear. Denosumab is an emerging option, and the initial evidence appears favorable. Further research regarding the use of denosumab for hypercalcemia of malignancy is warranted.

1 Introduction

Malignant hypercalcemia is a common metabolic complication of cancer seen in oncology and palliative care. It is important for clinicians to remain vigilant as its presentation can often be insidious and mimic general disease progression. It may cause significant symptoms that can often be reversed, resulting in major improvements in quality of life. The occurrence of malignant hypercalcemia is a poor prognostic marker with or without treatment. Despite a number of anti-hypercalcemic agents available, bisphosphonates are currently considered the mainstay of treatment.

2 Epidemiology

Hypercalcemia is a common presentation seen both in primary care and in the emergency department. Ninety percent of cases are due to either primary hyperparathyroidism or malignancy (Lafferty 1991). Hypercalcemia due to malignancy typically evolves rapidly and often leads to significant symptoms and therefore acute clinical presentation. Patients admitted to the hospital with hypercalcemia have an almost 50% chance of having a malignancy, compared with those that present to primary care where hyperparathyroidism is the most likely cause (Lindner et al. 2013).

Malignant hypercalcemia is reported to develop in up to 40% of all cancer patients, although incidence varies quite widely depending on the literature (Burt and Brennan 1980; Vassilopoulou-Sellin et al. 1993; Alsirafy et al. 2009). This may be in part due to the variation in defining hypercalcemia. It is also dependent upon which patient group is included, as it is more common in advanced disease and in certain malignancies. The most common solid malignancies associated with malignant hypercalcemia are breast, renal, lung, and squamous cell cancers where the incidence may be close to 50% (Alsirafy et al. 2009). Multiple myeloma, leukemia, and non-Hodgkin's lymphoma are the most common hematological malignancies associated with malignant hypercalcemia (Burt and Brennan 1980; Vassilopoulou-Sellin et al. 1993).

The presence of malignant hypercalcemia is recognized as a marker of advanced disease and is a poor prognostic sign (Stewart 2005; Rosner and Dalkin 2012). Up to 50% of patients with treated hypercalcemia will have died within 1 month and 75% within 3 months (Ralston et al. 1990; Stewart 2005). Treating hypercalcemia alone has a limited impact on the overall prognosis as it does not modify the underlying advanced malignancy. Antineoplastic treatments together with anti-hypercalcemia management offer the best chance of a longer survival time (Ralston et al. 1990; Kristensen et al. 1998).

3 Pathophysiology

3.1 Normal Homeostasis of Calcium

Calcium is an essential element that is important in maintaining normal cellular function and signalling and maintaining physiological processes, e.g., neuromuscular signalling, hormonal secretion, and blood coagulation (Kasper et al. 2015). As a result, calcium homeostasis to maintain the extracellular calcium ions (ca^{2+}) is tightly regulated. Broadly, calcium levels are controlled by four organs: small intestine, bones, kidneys, and the parathyroid glands. About 10–20% of dietary calcium is absorbed by the small intestine, and the rest is excreted in feces.

Over 90% of the calcium in the body is stored as hydroxyapatite in the skeleton, acting as a reservoir. The remaining 10% is present in the plasma via two forms: the physiologically active calcium ions (ca^{2+}) and calcium bound to carriers, particularly albumin.

Several hormonal systems are involved in controlling the level of calcium ions in the plasma. The main systems affect the bone remodeling process to increase or decrease the release of calcium from skeletal stores, as well as affect the kidneys to increase or decrease renal calcium excretion. Fig. 1 shows the basic mechanism.

The most significant system is a negative feedback mechanism regulated by two main hormones, parathyroid hormone (PTH) and the active vitamin D metabolite 1,25-dihydroxyvitamin D [Calcitriol] (Kasper et al. 2015).

Calcium sensors on the parathyroid glands activate the release of parathyroid hormone (PTH) when the levels of extracellular calcium ion are low. PTH acts on the kidneys and bones to increase the extracellular calcium levels. PTH affects the kidneys in two ways to increase calcium levels: the reduction of calcium excretion and the production of Calcitriol. The renal production of Calcitriol assists the PTH in mobilizing calcium release from bones and also stimulates the small intestine to increase calcium absorption.

The release of PTH triggers calcium release from the bones by altering bone remodeling, a process that is complex and involves bone-forming cells (osteoblasts) and bone-resorbing cells (osteoclasts). It is the balance between osteoblasts and osteoclasts that controls the rate of bone turnover and calcium release. An important element of this process involves the receptor activator of nuclear factor kappa-B (RANK). This receptor is carried on the osteoclast precursor cells and when stimulated by a ligand (RANKL), which is expressed on the osteoblast, results in the formation of mature osteoclasts leading to increased bone resorption and calcium release (Kasper et al. 2015).

The final important hormone of note is calcitonin, which is produced by thyroid C cells in response to increased calcium levels. The effect of calcitonin reduces bone turnover and calcium reabsorption in the kidneys, which in turn reduce serum calcium.

Understanding this complex relationship between calcium levels, PTH, active vitamin D, and bone cells have allowed effective treatments to be developed that modify this system.

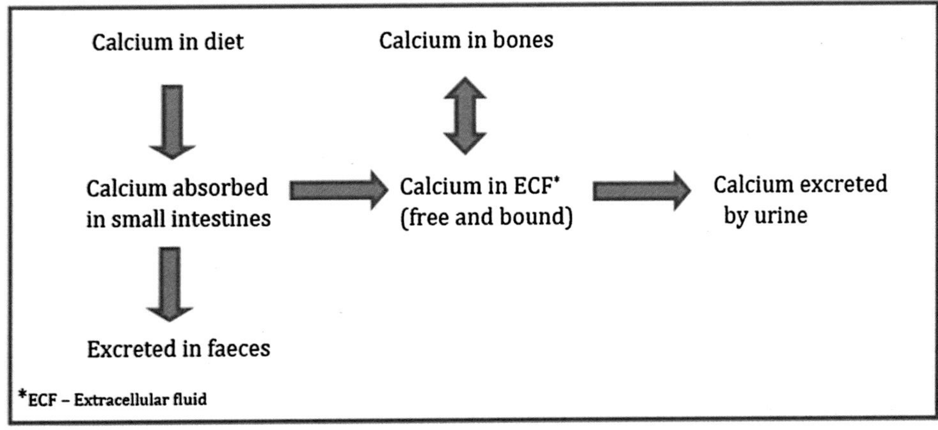

Fig. 1 Physiological schema of calcium

3.2 Mechanism of Malignant Hypercalcemia

The role of bone remodeling and PTH in calcium homeostasis is important in the understanding of the pathophysiology of hypercalcemia in malignancy. Normal calcium homeostasis is disrupted in advanced cancer through two main mechanisms described below.

3.2.1 Humoral Hypercalcemia of Malignancy

The humoral mechanism is responsible for approximately 80% of hypercalcemia related to malignancy, via an increased release of parathyroid hormone-related protein (PTHrP) from the tumor. PTHrP is structurally similar to PTH and initiates calcium release from the bones through increased osteoclastic activity, as well as reduced excretion from the kidneys, causing increased extracellular calcium levels. Unlike PTH, it does not influence the production of Calcitriol and hence has minimal influence on small bowel absorption of calcium (Horwitz et al. 2005). PTHrP acts on osteoblasts, which in turn increase the production of RANKL, and activates osteoclasts and bone resorption. The humoral mechanism does not depend upon the presence or absence of bone metastases and is most commonly seen in breast cancer, squamous cell cancers (e.g., head and neck, esophagus, cervix, or lung), and endometrial and renal cell cancers (Stewart 2005).

3.2.2 Local Osteolytic Hypercalcemia

Patients who have high volume metastatic, osteolytic bone involvement may develop hypercalcemia, via the production of local cytokines from increased osteoclastic activity (Francini et al. 1993). Osteoblastic metastatic disease, such as those typically seen in prostate cancer, is not associated with increased risk of hypercalcemia of malignancy. PTHrP is also a likely mediator of this mechanism, acting on the microenvironment within the bone; hence systemic PTHrP levels may not be raised (Rosner and Dalkin 2012). Metastatic breast and lung cancers, as well as myeloma, commonly involve an osteolytic mechanism which is causing hypercalcemia.

Other rare causes of malignant hypercalcemia include those mediated by increased active vitamin D production, seen most commonly in lymphoma (Seymour and Gagel 1993). In addition, parathyroid carcinoma can cause ectopic PTH production leading to hypercalcemia (VanHouten et al. 2006). A combination of mechanisms may occur simultaneously. In one study of 443 patients with cancer and hypercalcemia, 53% of patients had osteolytic hypercalcemia, 35% had humoral hypercalcemia, and 12% had both osteolytic and humoral factors (Soyfoo et al. 2013).

4 Clinical Presentation

Clinical presentation and development of symptoms in hypercalcemia are related to the rate of increase in serum calcium, rather than simply the absolute value. Hypercalcemia may be asymptomatic in severe levels if it has evolved slowly (Stewart 2005). This is particularly true in younger patients that have no pre-existing comorbidities. Hypercalcemia may therefore be only diagnosed due to an incidental finding on a blood test. It can however also present with very severe symptoms requiring urgent treatment.

The well-known mnemonic often associated with hypercalcemia of "painful **bones**, renal **stones**, abdominal **groans**, and psychic **moans**" is typically associated with the presentation of primary hyperparathyroidism. Hypercalcemia due to primary hyperparathyroidism often develops over a longer period, allowing for a patient to remain relatively well, but resulting in the development of complications such as renal stones and peptic ulceration.

In hypercalcemia of malignancy, the rapid rise in calcium level results in a patient becoming more constitutionally unwell. A combination of neurological and gastrointestinal symptoms is most common, especially confusion, somnolence, nausea, and constipation. Patients are often significantly dehydrated due to many factors: reduced oral intake, vomiting, and polyuria. In the most

Table 1 Symptoms and signs of hypercalcemia

	Mild	Severe
Neurological	Fatigue Mental dullness Muscle weakness Headache	Confusion Delirium Reduced conscious state Seizures
Gastrointestinal	Anorexia Constipation	Nausea Vomiting Abdominal pain
Renal	Thirst Polyuria (often not present)	
Cardiac	Shortened QT interval on ECG	Arrhythmias Bradycardia Hypertension Bundle branch/AV blocks Cardiac arrest (in most severe)

severe cases, cardiac complications and seizures may occur. Table 1 details the mild and severe symptoms and signs of hypercalcemia.

5 Diagnosis and Investigation

As the symptoms can be varied and nonspecific, often the most important element of diagnosis is in ensuring that it is part of the differential diagnosis. A patient's corrected calcium levels should be checked if there is a clinical suspicion that it may be raised. Serum calcium is present in two forms: calcium that is bound to protein, predominantly albumin, and ionized calcium. The physiologically active form is the ionized calcium, and this is maintained despite fluctuations in albumin levels. Laboratories routinely test total serum calcium levels. In healthy individuals, 45% of total calcium is in the active ionized form and 55% bound to carriers. Reference ranges for normal total calcium levels are made assuming an albumin level of 40 g/L (4 g/dL). In patients where albumin levels are low, this ratio is disrupted, and therefore a total serum calcium level will not reflect the active ionized calcium level. Some laboratories can directly measure ionized calcium; however in most

Table 2 Severity of hypercalcemia based on serum ionised levels

Mild	<3 mmol/L or <12 mg/dL
Moderate	3.0–3.5 mmol/L or 12–14 mg/dL
Severe	>3.5 mmol/L or >14 mg/dL

cases, it is calculated from the total serum calcium level using the following formula to give a corrected calcium level:

$$\begin{aligned}&\text{Corrected calcium } [\text{mmol/L}]\\&\quad = \text{Measured total calcium } [\text{mmol/L}]\\&\qquad + 0.02(40 - \text{albumin } [\text{g/L}])\end{aligned}$$

As patients with advanced malignancy commonly have low albumin levels, it is important to ensure that the *corrected calcium level* is known before a diagnosis of malignant hypercalcemia is made or excluded.

There can be variation in the diagnostic level of hypercalcemia, depending on local guidelines, but it is often classified as mild, moderate, or severe based on the serum ionized calcium level below (Stewart 2005). See Table 2.

In patients who have advanced cancer, it may not be necessary or appropriate to investigate the mechanism of hypercalcemia once it has been diagnosed, particularly as the treatment in most situations is the same regardless of cause. There are occasional situations where there is uncertainty or there is a suspicion of simultaneous mechanisms occurring. Primary hyperparathyroidism is a relatively common diagnosis across the general population with around 20 cases per 100,000 (Ayuk et al. n.d.). Therefore, primary hyperparathyroidism may occur concurrently with hypercalcemia of malignancy, and there is evidence that it may be more common in certain tumor types than the general population (Fierabracci et al. 2001). Primary hyperparathyroidism can be successfully treated with surgical resection of the parathyroid glands. Therefore, in a patient who has a low disease burden and a favorable prognosis, it may be of benefit to confirm the underlying cause of the hypercalcemia. Fig. 2 represents an approach to the diagnosis. In summary, serum PTH level will be raised in primary

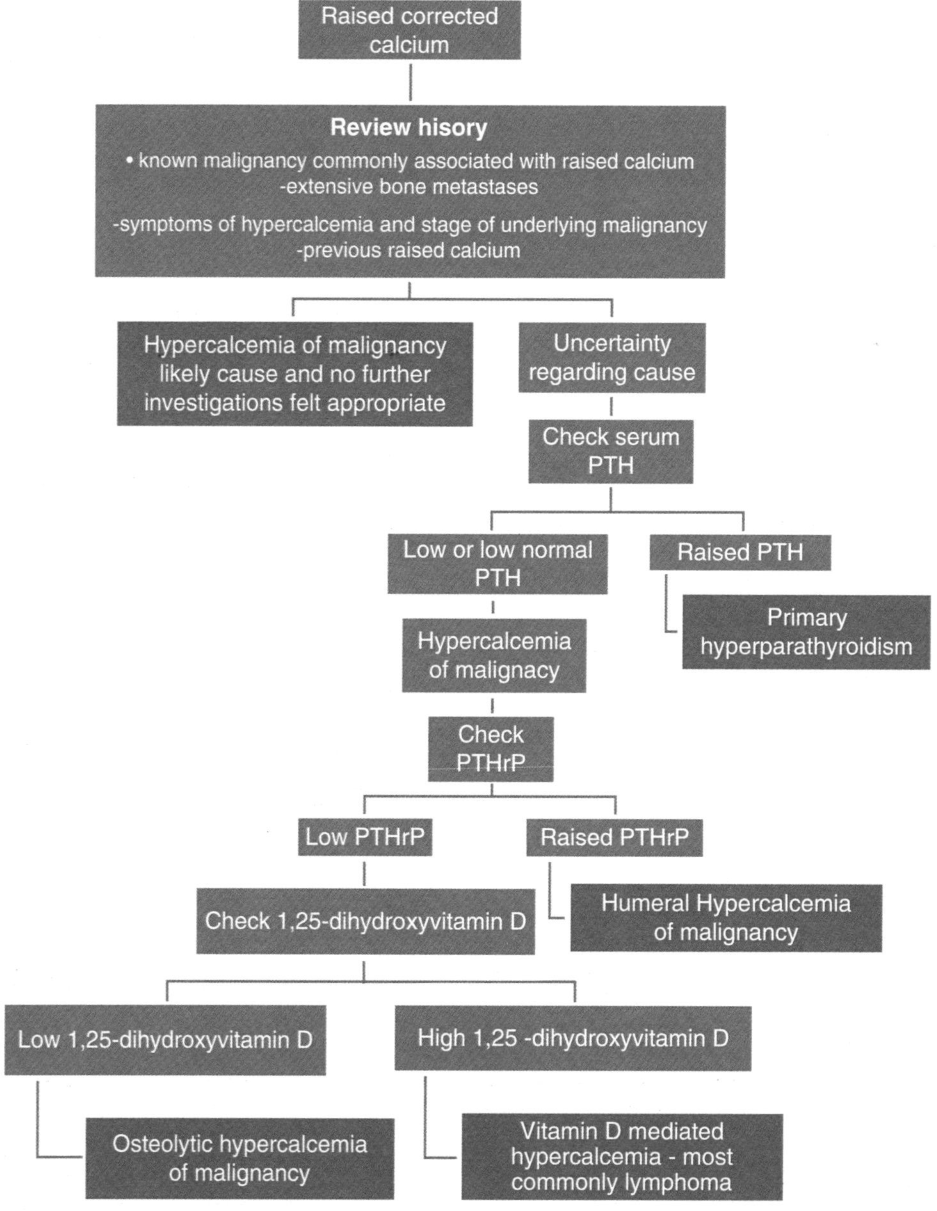

Fig. 2 Diagnostic approach to investigating hypercalcaemia

hyperparathyroidism and suppressed in hypercalcemia of malignancy. It is also possible to check PTHrP levels which can help confirm the underlying mechanism involved in those who have hypercalcemia of malignancy.

While PTH or PTHrP is not routinely requested for a patient with advanced cancer, one study suggests that the level of PTHrP may inform prognostication and predict likely response to the common treatment of bisphosphonates (Wimalawansa 1994b). In this study it was suggested that higher PTHrP levels would result in a poorer response to bisphosphonates treatment possibly due to the nonskeletal effects of PTHrP, such as the renal response, which bisphosphonates will not modify.

6 Treatment

6.1 General Approach

Multiple factors should be considered before deciding on a treatment plan. These include goals of care, severity of hypercalcemia, symptomatology, previous episodes of hypercalcemia (including response to treatment), and finally patient wishes.

Firstly, it is important to establish whether treatment is appropriate. If a patient is moribund due to their advanced malignancy, then treatment is likely to be futile. The difficulty can be distinguishing between disease progression and reversible symptoms secondary to hypercalcemia. Treatment may also not be appropriate in patients who have recently been treated for hypercalcemia and have either rapidly relapsed or been refractory to treatment. In these uncertain situations, a frank discussion about the limitations about efficacious treatments with a patient and their family is required.

When the treatment of the hypercalcemia is considered appropriate, the severity of the hypercalcemia and the symptom burden should be considered next. In asymptomatic patients with mildly raised hypercalcemia, conservative measures can be taken. These measures may include ensuring sufficient parenteral hydration, as well as stopping any contributory medications, e.g., calcium, vitamin D supplements, and thiazide diuretics.

In symptomatic patients with calcium levels greater than 3.0 mmol/L (12 mg/dL), further management is indicated. This initially involves parenteral rehydration, followed by specific anti-hypercalcemic treatments. The most commonly used agents are the bisphosphates and more recently denosumab. Calcitonin is frequently given, although it has limited benefits due to its short-acting effects. There are a number of other medications that are mentioned in the literature, including loop diuretics, gallium nitrate, and octreotide (Stewart 2005; Mirrakhimov 2015; Rosner and Dalkin 2012).

If a more active management approach is warranted, then antineoplastic treatments should also be considered to maintain normocalcemia after hypercalcemia is treated. Antineoplastic treatments such as chemotherapy provide optimal long-term treatment of hypercalcemia and offer the best prognosis (Ralston et al. 1990; Kristensen et al. 1998).

Regardless of the decisions pertaining to the goals of care, the occurrence of hypercalcemia of malignancy is a marker of poor prognosis and a harbinger of death within a few months in the majority of patients. Clear and sensitive information regarding the patient's advanced illness should be communicated to the patient and their family. It is important to explain to them that the correcting of the calcium levels is a temporizing measure, with the management and control of their underlying malignancy offering the best chance in prolonging survival. Patients and their family are also often fearful of the symptoms caused by hypercalcemia. Irrespective of the decision to treat the hypercalcemia, reassurance should be provided to the patient and the family that the treating team will endeavor to ensure the patient's comfort by managing the patient's symptoms utilizing other medications.

6.2 Intravenous Hydration and Role of Loop Diuretics

Hypercalcemia causes significant hypovolemia through a combination of mechanisms. Firstly, raised calcium results in an acquired nephrogenic diabetes insipidus cause polyuria. Secondly, gastrointestinal symptoms may result in nausea, reduced fluid intake, and vomiting. Finally, the hypovolemia itself results in a reduced glomerular filtration rate and therefore reduces the kidney's ability to excrete calcium. In all cases of symptomatic hypercalcemia, intravenous fluid hydration should be given to correct the volume deficit and to treat the hypercalcemia. The volume and rate of fluid replacement administered should be considered according to the clinical picture, severity of hypercalcemia, renal dysfunction, and cardiac insufficiency. In severe hypercalcemia, the fluid deficit can be profound, and aggressive fluid replacement is required. Current evidence recommends the use of intravenous normal saline at a rate of 200–300 mls/h (Mirrakhimov 2015). The total volume required may be as much as 4–6 l; however caution must be given to avoid fluid overload, particularly in the elderly. Historically, loop diuretics have been used to treat hypercalcemia to promote renal calcium loss. With the availability of more effective treatments, loop diuretics are now only indicated in situations of fluid overload following rehydration (Stewart 2005; Mirrakhimov 2015).

All current evidence recommends the intravenous route for rehydration. In the palliative care population, intravenous access can often be challenging, and the administration of fluids via the subcutaneous route is commonly utilized. The evidence regarding the benefits of administration of subcutaneous fluids is limited, and there is no research available at present assessing the use of subcutaneous fluids in the treatment of hypercalcemia. As most calcium-lowering treatments are given intravenously, using the same route for rehydration would be a sensible option, particularly as aggressive fluid replacement is often required. In situations where intravenous access is challenging, 2 l of normal saline can be administered subcutaneously in 24 h (Barton et al. 2004).

6.3 Specific Calcium-Lowering Treatments

6.3.1 Bisphosphonates

Bisphosphonates have been the mainstay in the treatment of malignant hypercalcemia for over 20 years (Saunders et al. 2004). As pyrophosphate analogs, bisphosphonates inhibit intracellular osteoclast activity, as well as bind to hydroxyapatite and stabilize the bone matrix (Rogers et al. 2000). Following administration, about 50% of the drug is selectively retained in the skeleton, and the remainder is eliminated in the urine without being metabolized. Skeletal uptake and retention are dependent on bisphosphonate potency for bone matrix, as well as patient factors including renal function, rate of bone turnover, and binding site availability. This adhesion to the bone matrix results in a prolonged half-life and mechanism of action. It is this enduring effect that has made bisphosphonates so important in the management of hypercalcemia of malignancy.

There are two groups of bisphosphonates: first-generation, non-nitrogen-containing bisphosphonates which include etidronate and clodronate; and the second-generation, nitrogen-containing bisphosphonates which include pamidronate, ibandronate, and, most recently, zoledronate. The second-generation bisphosphonates are considered more potent. There are both oral and parenteral bisphosphonates available. In the treatment of hypercalcemia, they are always given parenterally to ensure absorption and to avoid gastrointestinal side effects often seen with oral preparations. While most parenteral bisphosphonates can only be given intravenously, clodronate can be given intravenously or subcutaneously (Roemer-Bécuwe et al. 2003). The subcutaneous route may be useful in cases where intravenous access is difficult or when the patient is seen in the community setting.

Although extremely well-tolerated, bisphosphonates do have potential adverse effects. The most significant adverse effect is the risk of renal injury with possible nephrotic syndrome. To prevent renal toxicity, intravenous rehydration prior to the administration of bisphosphonates is always recommended. Where renal impairment also exists, a dose reduction may be considered to reduce the risk of further renal damage. A rare, but significant, adverse effect of bisphosphonates is osteonecrosis of the jaw. This is typically associated with prolonged and repeated use of bisphosphates (greater than 4 months). In the acute management of hypercalcemia of malignancy, the risk of osteonecrosis of the jaw is low (Saad et al. 2012). It may be worthwhile assessing the dentition of the patient prior to administration; however there is no evidence to support this approach when bisphosphonates are being used in the treatment of hypercalcemia. Other reported adverse effects include drug-related induced fevers, hypophosphatemia, and hypocalcaemia (Major et al. 2001). The drug-related induced fever is part of an acute phase reaction that causes transient flu-like symptoms. The true incidence of hypocalcaemia associated with bisphosphonate use in the treatment of hypercalcemia is unknown due to underreporting of cases. However, in clinical trials comparing zoledronate versus denosumab in the prevention of skeletal-related events in cancer patients, hypocalcaemia occurred in about 3.4–5.8% of patients treated with zoledronate (Body et al. 2015; Dranitsaris and Hatzimichael 2012). Although the frequency of bisphosphonate administration in the prevention of skeletal-related events is different compared to the treatment of hypercalcemia, clinicians should be vigilant of the possible complications of bisphosphonate-related symptomatic hypocalcaemia if using a bisphosphonate.

When selecting a bisphosphonate, the systematic review by Saunders et al. provides some limited guidance. The review showed that all bisphosphonates are effective when compared with placebo, with normal calcium being achieved in at least 70% of cases, regardless of which drug was used (Saunders et al. 2004). Table 3 details typical dose and administration regimes.

Pamidronate and zoledronate are the most commonly used bisphosphonates in the treatment of hypercalcemia. Although both drugs are effective in achieving normocalcemia, zoledronate tends to be favored for its ease in administration (15 min for zoledronate versus 2 h for pamidronate), potency, and efficacy (Major et al. 2001). In a pooled analysis of two randomized controlled trials involving 275 patients with hypercalcemia of malignancy, 87–88% of patients achieved normocalcemia after a single dose of zoledronate (4 mg or 8 mg) compared to 70% of patients who were treated with pamidronate. The mean duration of normocalcemia in patients who had received zoledronate was 32–43 days, compared to 18 days in patients who had received pamidronate (Major et al. 2001).

Although pamidronate and zoledronate have been shown to have a similar side effect profile, the 8 mg dose of zoledronate has shown an increased risk of causing renal injury compared to the 4 mg zoledronate dose and pamidronate (Major et al. 2001; Saunders et al. 2004). It is generally not recommended for patients with severe renal impairment (creatinine clearance <30 mL/min) to receive bisphosphonates. However, in some clinical situations where patients have limited effective options, the use of bisphosphonates may be indicated. Limited data suggests that ibandronate may be the safest option

Table 3 Bisphosphonates dosing and regimes

Bisphosphonate	Initial dose	Route/diluent/rate	Renal adjustment	
			CC[a]	Dose
Second generation				
Pamidronate	60–90 mg	IV, 375–500 ml 0.9% saline or 5% dextrose, over 90 min	30–90	No dose adjustment infusion rate of 4 h
			<30	Not recommended
Zoledronate	4 mg (consider 8 mg in refractory hypercalcemia)	IV, 100 ml 0.9% saline or 5% dextrose, over 15 min	>60	4 mg
			50–60	3.5 mg
			40–49	3.3 mg
			30–39	3 mg
			<30	Not recommended
Ibandronate	4 mg	IV, 500 ml 0.9% saline or 5% dextrose, over 2 h	No dose adjustment needed (Limited data suggest that this may be well tolerated in patients with renal impairment)	
First generation				
Clodronate	1500 mg	IV or SC, 50–250 ml 0.9% saline or 5% dextrose, over 2–3 h	Minimal data available	
Etidronate	7.5 mg/kg/day	IV, 250 ml of saline infused, over 2 h for 3 consecutive days	Minimal data available	

[a]*CC* Creatinine clearance mL/min

(Jackson 2005). Dose reduction, slowing the rate of the infusion, and the addition of increased hydration therapy can also be considered; however there is minimal literature to support this (Conte and Guarneri 2004; Kyle et al. 2007). Denosumab may potentially be an option in this scenario, and this will be discussed later.

Manufacturers suggest that the dose of pamidronate administered should depend on the severity of hypercalcemia. However, a systematic review from 2004 suggests that higher doses of bisphosphonates correlate with increased efficacy and therefore recommend use of the highest dose irrespective of the calcium level (Saunders et al. 2004). Given this review, pamidronate 90 mg or zoledronate 4 mg are appropriate first-line options in the treatment of malignant hypercalcemia.

Ibandronate and etidronate are less commonly used bisphosphonates. Ibandronate is a second-generation bisphosphonate and has been shown to be as effective as pamidronate. It appears to have a lower risk of renal injury; however there is limited data (Jackson 2005). Etidronate is a first-generation bisphosphonate and one of the first bisphosphonates to show efficacy in the treatment of hypercalcemia of malignancy. As it is administered via a 2-h intravenous infusion on 3 consecutive days, it has been superseded by newer more potent drugs that can be administered over a shorter time frame.

Regardless of which bisphosphonate is used, the reduction in calcium levels takes approximately 2–4 days to occur with the maximum effect between 4 and 7 days (Major et al. 2001). It is recommended that the serum-corrected calcium is rechecked 5–7 days following treatment with a bisphosphonate (Fleisch 1998). In most cases, intravenous rehydration given prior to bisphosphonate reduces the calcium level sufficiently while waiting for the bisphosphonates to act. In patients who have severe symptoms, needing immediate calcium reduction, calcitonin may be used. (See section below for further details.)

Up to 30% of cases of hypercalcemia are refractory to treatments with a bisphosphonate (Major et al. 2001; Saunders et al. 2004). There is limited evidence about which drug should be used in these cases. In the pooled analysis of the two randomized controlled trials by Major et al., patients who were refractory to zoledronate (4 or 8 mg) or pamidronate were retreated with 8 mg of zoledronate. Up to 55% of patients with refractory hypercalcemia responded to retreatment with zoledronate (Major et al. 2001). It is important to note that with time, hypercalcemia will usually become more difficult to treat and eventually may become resistant to bisphosphonate treatment. It is uncertain exactly why this occurs, but it is thought most likely related to the advancing underlying disease. In situations of refractory hypercalcemia, there is emerging evidence that the use of denosumab may be effective and is discussed further below. In patients with refractory hypercalcemia, zoledronate 8 mg may be trialled following initial treatment (Major et al. 2001).

Despite relapse being common in those who achieve normal calcium levels, there are no clear guidelines regarding how often serum calcium levels should be checked. However, given that the median time for relapse is between 2 and 4 weeks (Major et al. 2001; Wimalawansa 1994a), calcium levels could be checked 2–4 weeks posttreatment. A more conservative option would be to retest only if symptoms reoccur.

Finally, there is limited evidence to support the regular administration of bisphosphonates rather than waiting for relapse. One small study with 34 patients, investigating optimal frequency of pamidronate in the treatment of hypercalcemia, showed that a regular infusion every 2 weeks decreased the incidence of symptomatic hypercalcemia and prolonged survival compared to the regular infusion every 3 weeks (Wimalawansa 1994a). Until further evidence becomes available, the decisions regarding follow-up and the best drug to use in retreatment should be determined on an individual basis.

6.3.2 Denosumab

Denosumab is the latest treatment option in the management of hypercalcemia of malignancy. It is a human monoclonal antibody that specifically binds human RANKL. Denosumab inhibits osteoclast activity resulting in reduced bone resorption. Originally developed as an alternative option in the prevention and treatment of osteoporosis, it was subsequently used in the management and prevention of skeletal complications in cancer.

Currently, there are no randomized controlled trials comparing denosumab and bisphosphonates as first-line therapy for the management of hypercalcemia of malignancy. There is one single-arm study carried out by Hu et al. involving 33 patients who had bisphosphonate refractory hypercalcemia. The patients in this study had to have a corrected serum calcium level of >3.1 mmol/L (12.5 mg/dL) despite intravenous bisphosphonate treatment within 7–30 days. In this study, 64% of patients had serum calcium levels below 3.0 mmol/L (11.5 mg/dL) by day 10 after receiving denosumab. An improvement in symptoms was observed in over 50% of patients. The treatment effects were durable with an estimated median duration for compete response being 34 days (Hu et al. 2014). In this study the dose used was 120 mg given subcutaneously, every 4 weeks, with additional loading doses of 120 mg on days 8 and 15 of the first month. A repeat dose of denosumab was given successfully to patients who had relapsed. About 80% of the patients responded to the repeat dose. Therefore, a repeat dose of denosumab treatment on day 8 and 15 after initial treatment could be considered if calcium levels have not previously responded.

A retrospective case series of seven patients treated with single doses of denosumab for the management of hypercalcemia was described. In this small study, six of the seven patients had received bisphosphonates prior to treatment with denosumab. The mean corrected calcium levels were 3.06 mmol/L (12.24 mg/dL) on the day of the denosumab administration, and the last mean corrected calcium while in the hospital was 2.48 mmol/L (9.92 mg/dL) (Dietzek et al. 2015).

With the exception of the study by Hu et al. and Dietzek et al., the vast majority of the research performed utilizing denosumab is in the context of the management or prevention of skeletal-related events, and these results have been extrapolated to the management of hypercalcemia. Although the administration and dose of the drug are similar in both clinical scenarios, and the patient population appears similar, one must exercise caution in presuming that the use of denosumab in both clinical situations are identical. Patients with hypercalcemia typically have advanced disease, a different calcium metabolism profile and a poor prognosis, and may be different from patients who only have metastases to bones.

However, because of the scarcity of studies with the primary purpose of determining the role of denosumab in the management of hypercalcemia, understanding the effects of denosumab in the management and prevention of skeletal-related events will inform clinicians about the issues to be aware of when using denosumab for management of hypercalcemia.

In studies comparing denosumab and zoledronate in the prevention of skeletal complications in advanced cancer, the denosumab arm had fewer episodes of hypercalcemia compared to the zoledronate arm. Furthermore, the time to hypercalcemia was also delayed with the use of denosumab compared to zoledronate (Martin et al. 2012; Stopeck et al. 2010; Diel et al. 2015; Henry et al. 2011).

In regard to its safety and adverse effects, denosumab was well-tolerated in the management of osteoporosis and the skeletal complications of cancer. The most serious risk is that of osteonecrosis of the jaw; however this is rare, and rates appear similar to that of bisphosphonates (Stopeck et al. 2010; Fizazi et al. 2011; Henry et al. 2011; Martin et al. 2012; Dranitsaris and Hatzimichael 2012). The most clinically relevant risk is hypocalcaemia, extrapolated from studies where denosumab has been used in management of malignant bone disease and not in hypercalcemia. Up to 12.8% of patients treated with denosumab for skeletal complications develop significant hypocalcaemia, compared with 1–5% of those treated with zoledronate (Henry et al. 2011; Fizazi et al. 2011; Body et al. 2015; Dranitsaris and Hatzimichael 2012). In one study in patients with skeletal-related events, the median time to first occurrence of hypocalcaemia was 3.8 months with denosumab and 6.5 months with zoledronate (Body et al. 2015). It is worth noting that the highest incidence of hypocalcaemia was in the treatment of metastatic prostate cancer. As discussed, prostate cancer is associated with osteoblastic bone metastases, which in themselves may contribute to development of hypocalcaemia (Henry et al. 2011; Fizazi et al. 2011). In the context of the management of hypercalcemia, it is unclear what the clinical impact of denosumab-induced hypocalcaemia has. In a case series where denosumab was used for the management of hypercalcemia, one of seven patients developed symptomatic hypocalcaemia (Dietzek et al. 2015).

In a study by Body et al. (2015), the pooled results of three randomized controlled trial comparing the efficacy and safety of denosumab versus zoledronate in the prevention of skeletal-related events in metastatic bone disease showed that patients who took calcium and/or vitamin D supplements had a lower incidence of hypocalcaemia. This may suggest that adequate supplementation of both vitamin D and calcium reduced the risk of hypocalcaemia in patients treated with either denosumab or zoledronate. Patients with skeletal-related events have a different calcium profile compared with patients with hypercalcemia. There is no evidence for the routine monitoring of vitamin D levels and its replacement in the patients with hypercalcemia treated with denosumab. Indeed, the replacement of vitamin D has the potential to exacerbate hypercalcemia by mobilizing calcium release from bones and also stimulating the small intestine to increase calcium absorption.

In addition, the study found that patients who were at risk of developing hypocalcaemia include patients with prostate cancer or small cell lung cancer, reduced creatinine clearance (30 to <60 mL/min), and higher baseline values of urinary *N*-telopeptide of type 1 collagen and bone-specific alkaline phosphatase (Body et al. 2015). Given these findings, it would be prudent to monitor the calcium levels in patients who have these risk factors who are treated with denosumab regardless of reason.

Despite the limited information about the use of denosumab, there are some definite advantages identified. Denosumab is less likely to cause the acute phase reactions that are commonly seen with bisphosphonates (Henry et al. 2011; Fizazi et al. 2011; Stopeck et al. 2010; Dranitsaris and Hatzimichael 2012). It is also safer in renal impairment and not associated with renal injury (Henry et al. 2011; Stopeck et al. 2010; Martin et al. 2012; Dranitsaris and Hatzimichael 2012). In addition, it is administered via the subcutaneous route which may facilitate the use of denosumab in the community. Despite denosumab being more expensive compared to zoledronate, the ability to administer it at home subcutaneously may save on hospitalization costs.

6.3.3 Calcitonin

Calcitonin is a hormone produced by the parafollicular C cells of the thyroid gland. It inhibits the resorption of the bone by reducing both the number and activity of osteoclasts. Calcitonin also acts on the kidneys to reduce calcium reabsorption and inhibits intestinal calcium absorption. Administration of calcitonin occurs subcutaneously or intramuscularly every 12 h, with an initial dose of 4 international units/kg that can be increased up to 8 international units/kg every 6 h. As calcitonin works rapidly within 4–6 h (Vaughn and Vaitkevicius 1974), it may be used in combination with another anti-hypercalcemic agent such as bisphosphonates or glucocorticoids (Binstock and Mundy 1980; Sekine and Takami 1998).

Tachyphylaxis, the rapid reduction in the efficacy of a drug with repeated doses, seems to occur, therefore limiting long-term use after approximately 48–72 h (Vaughn and Vaitkevicius 1974). The reasons for tachyphylaxis are unclear and controversial but thought to be due to the formation of antibodies against heterologous calcitonins like salmon calcitonin (Grauer et al. 1995). The co-administration of glucocorticosteroids may prevent tachyphylaxis (Binstock and Mundy 1980). The main side effects of calcitonin include flushing, nausea, and vomiting.

6.3.4 Corticosteroids

Corticosteroids are most likely to benefit patients who have hypercalcemia as a result of increased Calcitriol production, as seen in some patients with lymphoma or chronic granulomatous disease. Steroids inhibit 1-alpha-hydroxylase conversion of 25-hydroxyvitamin D into Calcitriol, where reduced Calcitriol levels cause a decrease in intestinal absorption of calcium. In patients with hypercalcemia due to granulomatous diseases, prednisolone 20–40 orally daily would be a reasonable starting dose. The calcium levels should decrease within 3–5 days (Sharma 1996).

6.3.5 Gallium Nitrate

Gallium nitrate was initially developed because of its anticancer effect but was observed to cause a transient hypocalcaemia. Gallium nitrate works by inhibiting the release of calcium from the bone, but the mechanisms by which gallium nitrate exerts its effects are unclear (Warrell et al. 1984). It appears to have multiple effects such as the inhibition of osteoclast-mediated bone resorption, stimulation of bone formation, and alteration of the mineral composition and properties of bone.

The usual dose of gallium nitrate is a 5-day continuous intravenous infusion of 200 mg/m^2 per day. It is the long duration of treatment that limits its clinical use. There have been three randomized controlled trials comparing gallium nitrate and pamidronate, etidronate, and calcitonin. Gallium nitrate was effective in achieving normocalcemia and appeared to have a longer duration of normocalcemia compared to the bisphosphonates (Cvitkovic et al. 2006; Warrell et al. 1991). In a phase two randomized, double-blind trial of gallium nitrate versus pamidronate, 69% of the patients treated with gallium nitrate achieved normocalcemia compared with 56% of patients who were treated with pamidronate. The duration of normocalcemia was 14 days in patients who responded to gallium nitrate compared to 10 days in patients who responded to pamidronate (Cvitkovic et al. 2006). Gallium nitrate is generally well-tolerated, with the main side effects being asymptomatic hypophosphatemia (Warrell et al. 1991).

6.3.6 Mithramycin

Mithramycin is an antineoplastic antibiotic used as a chemotherapy agent. It is works by reducing both bone resorption and renal tubular calcium reabsorption (Ralston et al. 1985). It is usually administered as a single intravenous injection of 25 mcg/kg in 500 ml dextrose and can be repeated after 2 days. The serum calcium levels fall within 24–48 h of administration with a maximal effect at 2–4 days and a duration of action of 9–10 days (Godfrey 1971). The side effects of mithramycin include nausea, vomiting, fatigue, thrombocytopenia, and worsening liver function (Ralston et al. 1985). As the bisphosphonates are more efficacious and safer, mithramycin is rarely used in practice today.

6.3.7 Ocreotide

The evidence supporting the use of octreotide for the management of hypercalcemia is weak. Most of the evidence in the literature is based on single case reports (Mantzoros et al. 1997; Shiba et al. 1996).

6.3.8 Dialysis

Dialysis is effective in reducing serum calcium levels by hemodialysis with little or no calcium in the dialysate fluid. It is usually only used if no other options are available and has to be considered in the context of the clinical goals of treatment. Dialysis is likely to be considered when a patient has renal impairment or cardiac failure and where aggressive fluid hydration may be challenging.

7 Conclusion and Summary

Hypercalcemia of malignancy is a common condition and must be considered in a patient who presents with nonspecific symptoms and functional deterioration. The symptoms of hypercalcemia may be reversible with a number of treatments. Initial treatment should include intravenous hydration, followed by bisphosphonates. If urgent reduction of calcium levels is required and the patient is distressed by the symptoms, commencing calcitonin could be considered. Bisphosphonates such as zoledronate 4 mg or pamidronate 90 mg are currently the main medications of choice in the management of hypercalcemia of malignancy. The evidence for the use of denosumab is limited but can be considered if the hypercalcemia is refractory to bisphosphonates or if the patient has renal impairment.

Hypercalcemia signifies a poor prognosis and antineoplastic treatments to manage the underlying cancer which has the best chance of improving survival where appropriate.

References

Alsirafy SA, Sroor MY, Al-Shahri MZ. Hypercalcemia in advanced head and neck squamous cell carcinoma: prevalence and potential impact on palliative care. J Support Oncol. 2009;7(5):154–7.

Ayuk J, Gittoes N, Acknowledgements. Primary hyperparathyroidism. http://bestpractice.bmj.com/best-practice/monograph/133/basics/epidemiology.html. (n.d.). Accessed 28 Feb 2017.

Barton A, Fuller R, Dudley N. Using subcutaneous fluids to rehydrate older people: current practices and future challenges. QJM Int J Med. 2004;97(11):765–8. https://doi.org/10.1093/qjmed/hch119.

Binstock ML, Mundy GR. Effect of calcitonin and glucocorticoids in combination on the hypercalcemia of malignancy. Ann Intern Med. 1980;93(2):269–72.

Body J-J, Bone HG, de Boer RH, Stopeck A, Van Poznak C, Damião R, Fizazi K, et al. Hypocalcaemia in patients with metastatic bone disease treated with denosumab. Eur J Cancer (Oxford, England: 1990). 2015;51(13):1812–21. https://doi.org/10.1016/j.ejca.2015.05.016.

Burt ME, Brennan MF. Incidence of hypercalcemia and malignant neoplasm. Arch Surg (Chicago, Ill.: 1960). 1980;115(6):704–7.

Conte PF, Guarneri V. Safety of intravenous and oral bisphosphonates and compliance with dosing regimens. Oncologist. 2004;9(Suppl 4):28–37. https://doi.org/10.1634/theoncologist.9-90004-28.

Cvitkovic F, Armand J-P, Tubiana-Hulin M, Rossi J-F, Warrell RP. Randomized, double-blind, phase II trial of gallium nitrate compared with pamidronate for acute control of cancer-related hypercalcemia. Cancer J (Sudbury, Mass). 2006;12(1):47–53.

Diel IJ, Body J-J, Stopeck AT, Vadhan-Raj S, Spencer A, Steger G, von Moos R, Goldwasser F, Feng A, Braun A. The role of denosumab in the prevention of hypercalcaemia of malignancy in cancer patients with metastatic bone disease. Eur J Cancer. 2015;51(11):1467–75.

Dietzek A, Connelly K, Cotugno M, Bartel S, McDonnell AM. Denosumab in hypercalcemia of malignancy: a case series. J Oncol Pharm Pract. 2015;21(2):143–7. https://doi.org/10.1177/1078155213518361.

Dranitsaris G, Hatzimichael E. Interpreting results from oncology clinical trials: a comparison of denosumab to zoledronic acid for the prevention of skeletal-related events in cancer patients. Support Care Cancer. 2012;20(7):1353–60. https://doi.org/10.1007/s00520-012-1461-4.

Fierabracci P, Pinchera A, Miccoli P, Conte PF, Vignali E, Zaccagnini M, Marcocci C, Giani C. Increased prevalence of primary hyperparathyroidism in treated breast cancer. J Endocrinol Investig. 2001;24(5):315–20. https://doi.org/10.1007/BF03343867.

Fizazi K, Carducci M, Smith M, Damião R, Brown J, Karsh L, Milecki P, et al. Denosumab versus zoledronic acid for treatment of bone metastases in men with castration-resistant prostate cancer: a randomised, double-blind study. Lancet. 2011;377(9768):813–22. https://doi.org/10.1016/S0140-6736(10)62344-6.

Fleisch H. Bisphosphonates: mechanisms of action. Endocr Rev. 1998;19(1):80–100. https://doi.org/10.1210/edrv.19.1.0325.

Francini G, Petrioli R, Maioli E, Gonnelli S, Marsili S, Aquino A, Bruni S. Hypercalcemia in breast cancer. Clin Exp Metastasis. 1993;11(5):359–67. https://doi.org/10.1007/BF00132979.

Godfrey TE. Mithramycin for hypercalcemia of malignant disease. Calif Med. 1971;115(4):1–4.

Grauer A, Ziegler R, Raue F. Clinical significance of antibodies against calcitonin. Exp Clin Endocrinol Diabetes. 1995;103(6):345–51. https://doi.org/10.1055/s-0029-1211376.

Henry DH, Costa L, Goldwasser F, Hirsh V, Hungria V, Prausova J, Scagliotti GV, et al. Randomized, double-blind study of denosumab versus zoledronic acid in the treatment of bone metastases in patients with advanced cancer (excluding breast and prostate cancer) or multiple myeloma. J Clin Oncol. 2011;29(9):1125–32. https://doi.org/10.1200/JCO.2010.31.3304.

Horwitz MJ, Tedesco MB, Sereika SM, Syed MA, Garcia-Ocaña A, Bisello A, Hollis BW, et al. Continuous PTH and PTHrP infusion causes suppression of bone formation and discordant effects on 1,25(OH)2 Vitamin D. J Bone Miner Res. 2005;20(10):1792–803. https://doi.org/10.1359/JBMR.050602.

Hu MI, Glezerman IG, Leboulleux S, Insogna K, Gucalp R, Misiorowski W, Yu B, et al. Denosumab for treatment of hypercalcemia of malignancy. J Clin Endocrinol Metabol. 2014;99(9):3144–52. https://doi.org/10.1210/jc.2014-1001.

Jackson GH. Renal safety of ibandronate. Oncologist. 2005;10(Suppl 1):14–8. https://doi.org/10.1634/theoncologist.10-90001-14.

Kasper D, Fauci A, Hauser S, Longo D, Jameson J. Harrison's principles of internal medicine. New York: McGraw-Hill Education; 2015.

Kristensen B, Ejlertsen B, Mouridsen HT, Loft H. Survival in breast cancer patients after the first episode of hypercalcaemia. J Intern Med. 1998;244(3):189–98. https://doi.org/10.1046/j.1365-2796.1998.00355.x.

Kyle RA, Yee GC, Somerfield MR, Flynn PJ, Halabi S, Jagannath S, Orlowski RZ, et al. American Society of Clinical Oncology 2007 clinical practice guideline update on the role of bisphosphonates in multiple myeloma. J Clin Oncol. 2007;25(17):2464–72. https://doi.org/10.1200/JCO.2007.12.1269.

Lafferty FW. Differential diagnosis of hypercalcemia. J Bone Miner Res. 1991;6(Suppl 2):S51–9; discussion S61. https://doi.org/10.1002/jbmr.5650061413.

Lindner G, Felber R, Schwarz C, Marti G, Leichtle AB, Fiedler G-M, Zimmermann H, Arampatzis S, Exadaktylos AK. Hypercalcemia in the ED: prevalence, etiology, and outcome. Am J Emerg Med. 2013;31(4): 657–60. https://doi.org/10.1016/j.ajem.2012.11.010.

Major P, Lortholary A, Hon J, Abdi E, Mills G, Menssen HD, Yunus F, et al. Zoledronic acid is superior to pamidronate in the treatment of hypercalcemia of malignancy: a pooled analysis of two randomized, controlled clinical trials. J Clin Oncol. 2001;19(2):558–67.

Mantzoros CS, Suva LJ, Moses AC, Spark R. Intractable hypercalcaemia due to parathyroid hormone-related peptide secretion by a carcinoid tumour. Clin Endocrinol. 1997;46(3):373–5.

Martin M, Bell R, Bourgeois H, Brufsky A, Diel I, Eniu A, Fallowfield L, et al. Bone-related complications and quality of life in advanced breast cancer: results from a randomized phase III trial of denosumab versus zoledronic acid. Clin Cancer Res. 2012;18(17):4841–9. https://doi.org/10.1158/1078-0432.CCR-11-3310.

Mirrakhimov AE. Hypercalcemia of malignancy: an update on pathogenesis and management. N Am J Med Sci. 2015;7(11):483–93. https://doi.org/10.4103/1947-2714.170600.

Ralston SH, Gardner MD, Dryburgh FJ, Jenkins AS, Cowan RA, Boyle IT. Comparison of aminohydroxypropylidene diphosphonate, mithramycin, and corticosteroids/calcitonin in treatment of cancer-associated hypercalcaemia. Lancet (London, England). 1985;2(8461):907–10.

Ralston SH, Gallacher SJ, Patel U, Campbell J, Boyle IT. Cancer-associated hypercalcemia: morbidity and mortality. Clinical experience in 126 treated patients. Ann Intern Med. 1990;112(7):499–504.

Roemer-Bécuwe C, Vigano A, Romano F, Neumann C, Hanson J, Quan HK, Walker P. Safety of subcutaneous clodronate and efficacy in hypercalcemia of malignancy: a novel route of administration. J Pain Symptom Manag. 2003;26(3):843–8. https://doi.org/10.1016/S0885-3924(03)00252-5.

Rogers MJ, Gordon S, Benford HL, Coxon FP, Luckman SP, Monkkonen J, Frith JC. Cellular and molecular mechanisms of action of bisphosphonates. Cancer. 2000;88(Suppl 12):2961–78.

Rosner MH, Dalkin AC. Onco-nephrology: the pathophysiology and treatment of malignancy-associated hypercalcemia. Clin J Am Soc Nephrol. 2012;7:1722. https://doi.org/10.2215/CJN.02470312.

Saad F, Brown JE, Van Poznak C, Ibrahim T, Stemmer SM, Stopeck AT, Diel IJ, et al. Incidence, risk factors, and outcomes of osteonecrosis of the jaw: integrated analysis from three blinded active-controlled phase III trials in cancer patients with bone metastases. Ann Oncol. 2012;23(5):1341–7. https://doi.org/10.1093/annonc/mdr435.

Saunders Y, Ross JR, Broadley KE, Edmonds PM, Patel S, Steering Group. Systematic review of bisphosphonates for hypercalcaemia of malignancy. Palliat Med. 2004;18(5):418–31.

Sekine M, Takami H. Combination of calcitonin and pamidronate for emergency treatment of malignant hypercalcemia. Oncol Rep. 1998;5(1):197–9.

Seymour JF, Gagel RF. Calcitriol: the major humoral mediator of hypercalcemia in Hodgkin's disease and non-Hodgkin's lymphomas. Blood. 1993;82(5):1383–94.

Sharma OP. Vitamin D, calcium, and sarcoidosis. Chest. 1996;109(2):535–9.

Shiba E, Inoue T, Akazawa K, Takai S. Somatostatin analogue treatment for malignant hypercalcemia associated with advanced breast cancer. Gan to Kagaku Ryoho Cancer Chemother. 1996;23(3):343–7.

Soyfoo MS, Brenner K, Paesmans M, Body JJ. Non-malignant causes of hypercalcemia in cancer patients: a frequent and neglected occurrence. Support Care Cancer. 2013;21(5):1415–9. https://doi.org/10.1007/s00520-012-1683-5.

Stewart AF. Clinical practice. Hypercalcemia associated with cancer. N Engl J Med. 2005;352(4):373–9. https://doi.org/10.1056/NEJMcp042806.

Stopeck AT, Lipton A, Body J-J, Steger GG, Tonkin K, de Boer RH, Lichinitser M, et al. Denosumab compared with zoledronic acid for the treatment of bone metastases in patients with advanced breast cancer: a randomized, double-blind study. J Clin Oncol. 2010;28(35):5132–9. https://doi.org/10.1200/JCO.2010.29.7101.

VanHouten JN, Yu N, Rimm D, Dotto J, Arnold A, Wysolmerski JJ, Udelsman R. Hypercalcemia of malignancy due to ectopic transactivation of the parathyroid hormone gene. J Clin Endocrinol Metab. 2006;91(2): 580–3. https://doi.org/10.1210/jc.2005-2095.

Vassilopoulou-Sellin R, Newman BM, Taylor SH, Guinee VF. Incidence of hypercalcemia in patients with malignancy referred to a comprehensive cancer center. Cancer. 1993;71(4):1309–12.

Vaughn CB, Vaitkevicius VK. The effects of calcitonin in hypercalcemia in patients with malignancy. Cancer. 1974;34(4):1268–71.

Warrell RP, Bockman RS, Coonley CJ, Isaacs M, Staszewski H. Gallium nitrate inhibits calcium resorption from bone and is effective treatment for cancer-related hypercalcemia. J Clin Invest. 1984;73(5): 1487–90. https://doi.org/10.1172/JCI111353.

Warrell RP, Murphy WK, Schulman P, O'Dwyer PJ, Heller G. A randomized double-blind study of gallium nitrate compared with etidronate for acute control of cancer-related hypercalcemia. J Clin Oncol. 1991;9(8): 1467–75. https://doi.org/10.1200/JCO.1991.9.8.1467.

Wimalawansa SJ. Optimal frequency of administration of pamidronate in patients with hypercalcaemia of malignancy. Clin Endocrinol. 1994a;41(5):591–5.

Wimalawansa SJ. Significance of plasma PTH-Rp in patients with hypercalcemia of malignancy treated with bisphosphonate. Cancer. 1994b;73(8):2223–30. https://doi.org/10.1002/1097-0142(19940415)73:8<2223::AID-CNCR2820730831>3.0.CO;2-C.

Thromboembolism and Bleeding

73

Simon Noble

Contents

S. Noble (✉)
Marie Curie Palliative Care Research Centre, Division of Population Medicine, Cardiff University, Cardiff, UK
e-mail: simon.noble@wales.nhs.uk

R. D. MacLeod, L. Van den Block (eds.), *Textbook of Palliative Care*,
https://doi.org/10.1007/978-3-319-77740-5_71

Abstract

While thromboembolism and bleeding appear, at first glance, to be hematological processes at opposite ends of the clinical spectrum, they share many commonalities of relevance to palliative care teams. Both are increased in the malignant state, particularly with metastatic disease, and consequently confer a significant symptom burden, resulting in high level of distress for patients and carers. Furthermore, they are often the cause, or contributory cause, of death and frequently complicate care at the end of life.

The evidence base for the management of cancer-associated thrombosis (CAT) has increased significantly over the past 15 years, yet few studies have included or considered patients with advanced cancer or those nearing the end of life. With respect to the management of bleeding at the end of life, particularly terminal hemorrhage, management is informed by little more than case reports and expert opinion.

This chapter will comprise of two sections. First, it will provide an overview of the management of bleeding in the palliative setting with particular focus on terminal hemorrhage. The second section will focus on the treatment and prevention of venous thromboembolism in the advanced cancer setting, including the management of patients with recurrent thrombosis, thrombocytopenia, and bleeding. It will also review the new oral anticoagulants and consider their place in CAT management.

1 Introduction

Among the many physiological processes affected by the presence of malignancy, a derangement in the hemostatic system is characteristic and predisposes patients to both thrombosis and hemorrhage. Not only do these complications of hemostasis impact on the cancer journey; they also may even herald an as yet undiagnosed malignancy. Bleeding is a common presentation of many new cancers including bowel, bladder, renal, and lung, with tests for fecal occult blood or urinalysis for hematuria being commonplace in detecting early malignancy. Likewise, the presence of venous thromboembolism (VTE) without any obvious precipitating risk factors may indicate the presence of cancer. Data suggests 4–10% of patients will be diagnosed with cancer within a year of developing a VTE (Carrier et al. 2015).

For the palliative care team, bleeding and thrombosis will complicate the journey of many patients with advanced cancer, be it during palliative chemotherapy or at the end of life. The management will be determined by several factors including the severity of the event, the clinical environment, the presence of reversible factors, the overall prognosis of the patient, and the agreed ceilings of care. For some patients, complications of hemostasis may be anticipated. In such situations, wherever possible, teams should discuss the likelihood of bleeding or VTE with patients in order to ensure the treatment plan is congruent with their wishes.

2 Thrombosis and Hemorrhage Two Sides of the Same Coin

While this chapter will cover the management of thrombosis and bleeding separately, it is important to recognize that these two conditions are inextricably linked in both healthy people and those with cancer. Furthermore, these processes do not always occur in isolation; many cancer patients will have a level of disseminated intravascular

Table 1 Cancer associated mechanisms of increased risk of thrombosis and bleeding (TNF-α = tumor necrosis factor alpha, IL-1 = interleukin-1)

Risk factors	Increased risk of thrombosis	Increased risk of bleeding
Alteration of hemostatic system	Local release of procoagulants by tumor Tissue factor Local release of inflammatory cytokines TNF-α, IL-1 Increase platelet activity Disseminated intravascular coagulation	Reduction of vitamin K dependent clotting factors Thrombocytopenia due to marrow failure Disseminated intravascular coagulation
Anticancer treatments	Chemotherapy and targeted anticancer treatments Surgery Radiotherapy Central venous access	Chemotherapy Surgery
Local tumor effects	Reduction in venous return Pelvic tumors Lymphadenopathy	Local bleeding from vascular tumor Erosion of tumor into local blood vessel
Concurrent medications	Estrogen containing contraceptive pill Hormone therapies	Antiplatelet agents Non-steroidal anti-inflammatory drugs
Concurrent illness	Any inflammatory condition including Infection Congestive heart failure	Liver disease Hypersplenism

coagulation (DIC), a coagulopathy which causes widespread thromboembolic phenomena and, as platelets and clotting factors are consumed, bleeding at multiple sites. In addition, several mechanisms by which cancer cells are known to disseminate and metastasize are integral within the hemostatic system, particularly through clotting-dependent and clotting-independent activities of tissue factor, thrombin, and fibrin.

Abnormal coagulation tests will be common in cancer patients, regardless of the presence of thrombosis and/or bleeding. The results of laboratory tests demonstrate that a process of fibrin formation and fibrinolysis parallels the development of malignancy, increasingly in those with metastases, thereby worsening as the cancer progresses. Subtle hemostatic alterations may be identified, including high levels of plasma by-products of clotting reactions (i.e., prothrombin fragment 1 + 2 [F1 + 2], fibrinopeptide A [FPA], thrombin–antithrombin complex [TAT], and D-dimer) or an acquired protein C resistance, as well as high levels of circulating microparticles (MP) shed by cancer cells and platelets (Rickles and Falanga 2009). In addition to cancer-associated alterations to the hemostatic system, there are many other factors that may increase the risk of thrombosis and bleeding, and these are summarized in Table 1.

3 Section 1: Management of Hemorrhage

3.1 Risk Factors

Bleeding or hemorrhage occurs in 6–14% of advanced cancer patients and is the immediate cause of death in approximately 6% of these (Pereira and Phan 2004). Its presentation will depend on the site and severity of the bleed, although overt bleeds are a cause of significant distress for patients, carers, and even their healthcare professionals. The incidence varies according to the type of cancer, its stage, its anatomical site, hemostatic derangement, concurrent drug use, and the current (or previous) use of cancer-modifying treatments. Such factors will also influence whether the bleeding is clinically apparent or internal. Knowledge of the factors that influence the likelihood of bleeding will allow the team to identify those at greatest risk of bleeding and make anticipatory plans accordingly.

3.2 Alterations in Hemostatic System

3.2.1 Disseminated Intravascular Coagulation

As mentioned previously, many cancer patients will have DIC although it is important to recognize that this term covers a broad spectrum of clinical and hematological parameters ranging from asymptomatic to catastrophic hemorrhage. In the otherwise healthy person, hemostasis is a dynamic process involving the formation of a stable fibrin clot through coagulation followed by breakdown and reabsorption through fibrinolysis. In DIC, these processes are dysregulated, resulting in widespread thromboembolism in the small blood vessels. The ongoing coagulation consumes clotting factors and platelets, thereby leading to abnormal clotting and bleeding. In clinical practice, bleeding is a later manifestation of DIC, which is usually identified first in the laboratory. Several diagnostic criteria have been suggested which are usually based around scoring points, depending upon the presence of certain hematological blood parameters including the platelet count, presence of fibrin degradation products, prothrombin time, and fibrinogen level (Gando 2012). These are summarized in Table 2.

Table 2 Scoring tool for diagnosis of disseminated intravascular coagulation (DIC). (Score of 5 or more is suggestive of diagnosis of DIC)

Factor	Potential points
Presence of underlying disorder known to be associated with DIC	Yes = 2 No = 0
Platelet count	$>100 \times 10^9$/L = 0 $<100 \times 10^9$/L = 1 $<50 \times 10^9$/L = 2
Fibrin degradation products e.g., D-dimer	No ↑= 0 Moderate ↑= 2 Strong ↑= 3
Prolonged prothrombin time	< 3 s = 0 > 3 s = 1 > 6 s = 2
Fibrinogen level	> 1.0g/L = 0 < 1.0g/L = 1

3.2.2 Thrombocytopenia

Thrombocytopenia and platelet dysfunction is commonly seen in hematological malignancies such as leukemia and lymphoma. While less common in solid tumors, it may also occur if metastases are present in the spleen or the marrow of hematopoietically active bones.

3.2.3 Vitamin K-Dependent Clotting Factors

The liver is responsible for the synthesis of the vitamin K-dependent clotting factors II, VII, IX, and X. Liver dysfunction or biliary obstruction secondary to metastatic disease can lead to deficiencies in these clotting factors, with an increased bleeding tendency.

3.3 Anticancer Treatments

The myelosuppressive effects of certain chemotherapy agents will result in a nadir, 8–14 days after chemotherapy is given, leading to a temporary thrombocytopenia. The degree of thrombocytopenia will depend upon the agent used, doses administered, and if used in combination. While the list is not exhaustive, thrombocytopenia is typically seen with the use of gemcitabine, carboplatin, dacarbazine, docetaxel, and platinum-based compounds. Myelosuppression is also seen in patients who have received radiotherapy to the larger marrow-producing bones such as the pelvis.

3.4 Local Tumor Effects

Bleeding from highly vascular tumors may be the initial presenting symptom for several cancers including lung, bowel, nasopharyngeal, bladder, and cervical. Other patients will not show visible signs of blood loss but will bleed internally. Many patients will continue to show signs of hemorrhage throughout their illness. The risk of bleeding increases with disease progression, be it through the increase in the size of the primary or the development of metastases.

Table 3 Drugs that interfere with platelet function

Adenosine diphosphate (ADP) receptor inhibitor	Inhibition of prostaglandin pathways	Inhibition of platelet phosphodiesterase
Clopidogrel Prasugrel Ticagrelor Ticopidine	Aspirin Non-steroidal anti-inflammatory drugs	Dipyridamole Aminophylline Theophylline Vincristine Vinblastine Colchicine Caffeine

Some tumors may be anatomically or radiologically located in close proximity to a major blood vessel, where direct infiltration can lead to a sudden catastrophic bleed. This is a particular risk in locally recurring head and neck cancers, particularly following localized radiotherapy. Warning signs of visible pulsations in malignant wounds, herald bleeds, or a sudden increase in pain should prompt a swift assessment of the patient.

Table 4 Anticoagulants used in medical practice

Coumarins (vitamin K antagonists)
Warfarin
Heparin and derivative substances
Unfractionated heparin
Low molecular weight heparin
Bemiparin
Dalteparin
Enoxaparin
Nandroparin
Tinzaparin
Ultra low molecular weight heparin
Semuloparin
Synthetic pentasaccharide inhibitors of factor Xa
Fondaparinux
Idraparinux
Direct factor Xa inhibitors
Apixaban
Edoxaban
Rivaroxaban
Direct thrombin inhibitors
Dabigatran

3.5 Concurrent Medications

There are many drugs that interfere with platelet function, and these are summarized in Table 3. The use of anticoagulants will also increase bleeding risk and is summarized in Table 4.

3.6 Concurrent Illness

Local infection within tumor cavities can also increase the risk of bleeding. If infection is suspected, antibiotic therapy should be considered in order to reduce this risk and also help alleviate other symptoms of infection such as pain.

4 General Principles for Bleeding Management

4.1 Ceilings of Care

The scope of patient conditions falling under the care of palliative care teams has extended far beyond those requiring end of life care. Even within the hospice setting, it is not unusual to admit patients for whom escalation of care would be appropriate, in the event of a deterioration in their condition. Facilities for interventions such as surgery, radiotherapy, or interventional radiology may not be readily available in small or stand-alone centers. Likewise, escalation of care or transfer to another site may not be appropriate for patients at the end of life if there is no certainty of significant survival benefit or improvement in quality of life. For patients with a history of bleeding, or who have been identified at risk, a decision regarding what should be done in the event of a further bleed should be made as early as possible, so that clinical teams can act appropriately in the patient's best interests. Where appropriate, steps should be taken to minimize the likelihood of bleeding, including consideration of preemptive interventions to prevent crises arising.

4.2 Principles of Management

The management of a bleeding episode should be individualized and based on the following factors:

- The underlying cause(s)
- The likelihood of reversing or controlling the underlying cause
- The burden/benefit ratio of the interventions
- The patient's wishes within the context of disease burden, life expectancy, and goals of care

For patients in whom, aggressive management of bleeding is warranted, an acute bleeding episode may require general resuscitative measures, such as volume and fluid replacement, and specific measures to stop the bleeding. For those whose care is solely palliative/symptom control, management may include measures to stop the bleeding but not involve full resuscitative measures. In the case of irreversible catastrophic bleeds and anticipated terminal hemorrhage, comfort measures only may be most appropriate, and these will be covered separately within the chapter.

As a general principle, management should focus on identifying the underlying cause(s) and, where possible, controlling the bleeding. This should include:

- Resuscitation as appropriate
- Examination/investigations to:
  - Identify site of bleeding
  - Severity of bleed
- Stopping the bleeding:
  - Local measures/hemostatic agents
  - Correct reversible abnormalities:
    Correct coagulopathies
    Stop medicines which may worsen bleeding
  - Systemic interventions:
    Blood products
    Antifibrinolytics
    Vasoconstrictors
  - Interventions as appropriate:
    Interventional radiology
    Radiotherapy
    Endoscopy

A review of concurrent medications and other illnesses may identify the etiology or contributing factors, such as the concurrent use of nonsteroidal anti-inflammatory drugs, antiplatelets, and anticoagulants. Many inpatients will be on primary thromboprophylaxis. However, the risks of prophylactic anticoagulation may outweigh the potential benefits in patients with very advanced disease; one study suggested 10% of palliative care patients experience clinically relevant bleeding with primary thromboprophylaxis (Tardy et al. 2017).

Investigations should be considered, dependent upon how aggressive the management is intended. For most patients, full blood counts and clotting profiles may reveal systemic problems, while in some cases endoscopy or angiography may be appropriate in order to identify bleeding sites.

4.3 Local Measures/Hemostatic Agents

Where a bleeding point can be visualized, application of a dressing, with or without pressure, may be sufficient to achieve hemostasis. However, if simple dressings do not control bleeding, many different hemostatic agents have been reported to assist hemostasis or promote vasoconstriction. The myriad of predominantly topical agents that have been used to manage bleeding are outlined in Table 5. The evidence base is predominantly limited to case reports or series, and the type of agent used will vary according to the bleeding area, severity of the bleeding, and tumor type. For example, hemostasis can be facilitated by coating dressings with acetone in vaginal packing but cocaine in nasal packing. Wherever possible, the frequency of dressing changes should be reduced and non-adherent dressings used. In severe epistaxis, catheters with inflatable balloons may be used to control the bleeding. However, balloon tamponade should be considered a temporary measure since prolonged pressure may cause local ischemia. Many agents are derived from known coagulation factors, while some will form a scaffold upon which platelets or fibrin may allow a clot to form. Other agents, such as silver nitrate, are used topically to cauterize bleeding vessels, while topical epinephrine may be used on dressings as a vasoconstriction agent for localized capillary-based bleeding such as cutaneous melanoma.

Table 5 Hemostatic agents

Agent	Composition/derivation	Application	Uses
Thromboplastin	Powder Bovine derived	Topical	Wound healing
Oxidized cellulose	Cellulose derivative	Topical	Promotes local clotting Wound dressing
Collagen	Structural protein Bovine derived mesh dressing	Topical	Wound dressing
Epinephrine	Naturally occurring hormone Solution	Topical	Cutaneous
Silver nitrate	Inorganic silver salt	Topical	Nasal
Formalin	2% or 4% solution	Topical	Rectal Bladder
Prostaglandins E2 and F2	Naturally occurring hormone	Intravenous	Hemorrhagic cystitis
Alum	1% solution Aluminum derived	Continuous irrigation	Bladder
Sucralfate	Tablet Powder Solution/ gel	Oral Topical	Upper GI bleeds Cutaneous oozing
Gelatin Gelatin	Sponge like dressing or powder	Topical	Nasal Rectal Vaginal

4.4 Systemic Interventions: Blood Products

4.4.1 Packed Red Cells

Packed red cells are the most commonly administered blood product in the hospice setting, usually for fatigue and dyspnea. However, blood transfusions are potentially hazardous as well as beneficial, so should only be undertaken when the perceived clinical benefits to the patient outweigh the likely risks. The evidence base supporting the use of blood transfusions for the improvement of symptomatic anemia is limited to "before and after studies," with variable methods of evaluation. Transfusion is associated with a 31–70% subjective improvement in fatigue and dyspnea, although its effects tend to wane after 14 days (Preston et al. 2012). Furthermore, there is a risk of harm from blood transfusion in frail patients nearing the end of life, due to fluid overload or higher plasma viscosity.

4.5 Platelets

Thrombocytopenia is commonly encountered in advanced cancer and associated with an increased risk of bleeding. The frequency and severity of bleeding episodes increase as the platelet count drops below 20×10^9/L with severe bleeding associated with counts below 10×10^9/L. Platelet transfusion in the setting of advanced cancer should be on a case-by-case basis with the aim of controlling symptoms. Since platelets have a half-life of 4 days, their utility in severely thrombocytopenic end-stage cancer patients is limited. Criteria for platelet transfusions in end-stage hematological cancers have been proposed and include continuous bleeding of the mouth or gums, epistaxis, extensive and painful hematomas, severe headaches, or disturbed vision of recent onset, as well as continuous bleeding through the gastrointestinal, gynecological, or urinary systems (Schiffer et al. 2001). As a "rule of thumb," prophylactic platelet transfusion is only reserved for counts below 10×10^9/L or 20×10^9/L in the presence of sepsis. However, assuming normal splenic pooling, a single unit of platelets will increase the platelet count by 6–10 $\times 10^9$/L in an average adult, and four to six units are usually required to control bleeding.

From a practical perspective, the decision to commence platelet support should also involve consideration criteria for stopping platelet transfusions. These decisions pose ethical challenges, since ongoing transfusions may become futile. However, the patient or their family may perceive cessation of transfusions as withdrawal of life-sustaining therapy.

4.6 Fresh Frozen Plasma

Fresh frozen plasma, the liquid component of whole blood, can be used to correct deficiencies of coagulation factors such as factor V and VIII and other proteins. Its clinical uses are limited, and guidelines only recommend their use in the management of bleeding in patients on warfarin, with DIC, and as a plasma exchange medium for thrombotic thrombocytopenic purpura (O'Shaughnessy et al. 2004). In patients with advanced cancer, its use is limited to patients with a prognosis of several weeks or more.

4.7 Systemic Interventions: Drugs

4.7.1 Vitamin K

Vitamin K deficiency occurs in over 20% of advanced cancer patients, with 6.5% having evidence of clotting dysfunction (Harrington et al. 2008). This may include prolonged prothrombin time (PT) or international normalized ratio (INR) and partial thromboplastin time (PTT) with normal thrombin time, fibrinogen, and serum fibrin-fibrinogen degradation products. While there is little to be gained in the use of prophylactic vitamin K based solely on abnormal clotting studies, replacement therapy may help further bleeding in patients with previous bleeding episodes. The recommended dose varies between 2.5 and 10 mg depending on the severity of clotting dysfunction and should ideally be given orally or by the subcutaneous route. Intravenous vitamin K is associated with anaphylactoid reactions in 2% of patients and should be used with caution and administered slowly, at a rate no faster than 1 mg per min.

4.8 Antifibrinolytics

Plasmin is a serum protease that degrades fibrin in a process called fibrinolysis. It is formed when the liver-derived zymogen plasminogen is converted by tissue plasminogen activator (TPA) to plasmin. Tranexamic acid is a synthetic antifibrinolytic agent that blocks the plasminogen binding sites, thereby inhibiting the conversion of plasminogen into plasmin by TPA. This results in a decreased lysis of fibrin and a consequent reduction in clot breakdown and resorption (Hunt 2015). Tranexamic acid has been reported to reduce bleeding from several metastatic cancers including lung, esophageal, gynecological, colorectal, and prostate. The evidence base in this population is limited to case reports and case series, but tranexamic acid has recently been evaluated in two large RCTs (CRASH-2 and WOMAN) comprising 20,000 participants in each study (Roberts et al. 2013). These studies were undertaken in different populations (trauma and postpartum hemorrhage), and both saw significant reductions in bleeding and mortality. Importantly, they also demonstrated no increase in thrombotic events (venous or arterial). These data strongly suggest that concerns about tranexamic acid having a procoagulant effect are unfounded.

Tranexamic acid is usually given orally 1 g three times a day or intravenously as 10 mg/kg three to four times a day, infused over about 1 h. There are also case reports of it being administered topically, rectally, or by intrapleural instillation.

4.9 Interventional Radiology

Developments in interventional radiology have led to transcutaneous arterial embolization (TAE) becoming a readily available option in the palliative treatment to control hemorrhage, pain, reduce tumor bulk, and lower hormone production in hormone-secreting tumors (Broadley et al. 1995). Its role in the control of bleeding has been reported in cancers of the head and neck

(Dequanter et al. 2013), pelvis (Nabi et al. 2003), lung (Kawaguchi et al. 2001), liver, and upper gastrointestinal tract (Eriksson et al. 2008). The procedure is usually performed under local anesthetic via a femoral or axillary approach. The blood vessel supplying the affected site is first identified by arteriography and then occluded by particles (e.g., polyvinyl alcohol), mechanical devices (e.g., coils), or liquids (e.g., glue, alcohol). Embolization is not suitable for all cases; it is restricted to areas where blood vessels are accessible by catheter and where embolization will not result in ischemia of key organs. Furthermore, embolization is not without its risks; there are complications associated with the puncture site bruising/hematoma, bleeding, or vessel occlusion. To minimize bleeding complications, coagulopathies should be reversed wherever possible. Any embolization procedure may be associated with the post-embolization syndrome, which comprises varying degrees of pain at the site of embolization, nausea/vomiting, and flu-like symptoms. These are related to tissue ischemia/necrosis and may last for several days following embolization. Readily available analgesia or a patient-controlled analgesia (PCA) pump should be considered. Careful liaison with a suitably experienced interventional radiologist is essential and best considered sooner rather than later.

4.10 Radiotherapy

The use of external beam and internal radiotherapy in management of bleeding in cancer patients can be highly effective. External beam radiotherapy (EBRT) may control hemoptysis caused by lung cancer in up to 80% of patients (A Medical Research Council (MRC) 1992; Langendijk et al. 2000). The optimal dose and fractionation is best guided according to patient performance status and prognosis. Studies suggest that higher dose/fractionation palliative EBRT regimens (e.g., 30 Gy/10 fractions equivalent or greater) are associated with modest improvements in survival and total symptom score, particularly in patients with good performance status. However, these improvements are associated with an increase in esophageal toxicity. Shorter EBRT dose/fractionation schedules (e.g., 20 Gy in five fractions, 17 Gy in 2-weekly fractions, 10 Gy in one fraction), which provide good symptomatic relief with fewer side effects, can be used for patients requesting a shorter treatment course and/or in those with a poor performance status (Rodrigues et al. 2011). The literature reports the successful use of radiotherapy for the control of bleeding from cancers of the bladder (Abt et al. 2013), vagina (Eleje et al. 2015), and rectum (Cameron et al. 2014).

4.11 Endoscopy

Endoscopy has been successfully used for the control of bleeding from upper gastrointestinal, lung, and bladder cancers. This approach allows the additional benefit of direct visualization of the bleeding site, enabling the endoscopist to undertake diagnostic biopsies and direct therapeutic interventions. Historically bleeding sites have been injected with ethanol, gelatin, and epinephrine. Bleeding from upper gastrointestinal tumors is most commonly cauterized by argon laser coagulation (Martins et al. 2016). For hematuria, the urologist may use cystoscopy when bladder irrigation has failed in order to inspect the bladder lining and cauterize any bleeding points identified. In cases of hemoptysis, bronchoscopy may be used to perform ice-cold saline lavages, balloon tamponade, laser phototherapy, or apply topical thrombin or fibrinogen to the bleeding site (Sakr and Dutau 2010).

4.12 Terminal Hemorrhage

Terminal hemorrhage is defined as a major hemorrhage, usually from an artery, which results in death. Death typically occurs within a period of time that may be as short as minutes, because of the rapid internal or external loss of circulating blood volume. The incidence of terminal hemorrhage from published data varies from 3% in lung cancers, 6% in hematological malignancy, to 12% in head and neck cancers (Pereira and Phan 2004). Qualitative data reports terminal hemorrhage to be a distressing experience for both patients and staff although its management has historically been intuitive. A survey of UK palliative care teams suggested the management of patients considered to be at risk of terminal hemorrhage that would include the provision of what is known as "emergency" or "crisis" medication. Based on the understanding that a catastrophic bleed in a patient known to be at risk of exsanguination will be the terminal event, dominated by distressing symptoms, a consensus management is to administer high doses of sedatives with the intention of rendering the patient unconscious and unaware. However, a recent qualitative study of healthcare professionals' experiences of managing terminal hemorrhage directly challenges this approach on several levels (Harris et al. 2011). Firstly, the majority of patients experiencing terminal hemorrhage had not been identified as at risk, while those identified at risk of did not progress to bleeding. Secondly the average time from the initial bleed to loss of consciousness/death averaged at 60 s. In this context, if patients were administered emergency medication at the moment they bled, they would inevitably be unconscious before the sedative effects were realized. Finally, in circumstances where the emergency medicine was not kept close to the patient (i.e., in a controlled drugs cupboard), healthcare professionals may leave the patient to access the drugs, thereby leaving the patient dying alone.

In view of this data, while the principles of managing terminal hemorrhage remain the same, there is a greater emphasis on remaining with the patient and using supportive measures over the administration of crisis medication. Principles of managing terminal hemorrhage are identifying patients at risk of terminal hemorrhage, general supportive measures, and appropriate sedative medication (often termed as "emergency" or "crisis" medication). These principles are summarized in Table 6, and while they focus on carotid artery hemorrhage, also known as carotid blowout, they can be applied to all forms of terminal hemorrhage.

Table 6 Management of terminal hemorrhage

Identifying patients at risk of terminal hemorrhage
For head and neck cancers, the main risk factors are surgery (e.g., radical neck dissection)
Radiotherapy (the most implicated risk factor), postoperative healing problems
Visible arterial pulsation
Presence of a pharyngocutaneous fistula
Fungating tumors with artery invasion
Other systemic factors
Age above 50 years
10–15% loss of body weight
Diabetes mellitus
Immunodeficiency
Generalized atherosclerosis
Malnourishment
General supportive measures
Ensure a nurse stays with the patient (if in hospital/ hospice)
Provide psychological support to patients and their significant others
Call for nursing and medical assistance (if in hospital/ hospice)
Apply pressure to external bleeding if possible
Use dark towels to camouflage blood loss
Use suction if possible
Place the patient in the lateral position
Administer oxygen
Use of sedative medication
Where possible, the drug should be given intravenously in order to get into the systemic circulation as quickly as possible. In the absence of venous access, the drug should be given intramuscularly rather than subcutaneous
Midazolam: 5–10 mg IV, IM, SC
Ketamine: 150–250 mg IV
Diamorphine: 10 mg IV, IM, SC

5 Section 2: Management of Venous Thromboembolism

Venous thromboembolism (VTE), comprising of deep vein thrombosis (DVT) and pulmonary embolism (PE), occurs in 1 in 1000 people per annum, affecting 6.5 million people worldwide (Cohen et al. 2007; Torbicki et al. 2008). Its incidence is higher in cancer patients, occurring in up to 20% of patients during their lifetime. Cancer-associated thrombosis (CAT) is the commonest cause of chemotherapy-related death and the second commonest cause of cancer mortality overall (Khorana et al. 2007a). It also confers a significant symptom burden, both physical and psychological, which clinicians often find challenging to diagnose and manage (Johnson et al. 2012; Sheard et al. 2013; Johnson and Sherry 1997).

The symptoms attributable to VTE depend upon the location of the thrombosis and the volume of thrombus burden. An occlusive DVT may cause a spectrum of severity of symptoms including pain, swelling, and erythema. Untreated, a DVT risks propagating and ultimately breaking off and travelling to the pulmonary arteries causing a PE (Kakkar et al. 1969). Up to 80% of patients with pulmonary emboli report no symptoms suggestive of DVT. Therefore, the absence of DVT symptoms should not lower the index of suspicion of PE in a breathless patient (Meignan et al. 2000). As with DVT, the symptomatology of PE will vary from few, if any, attributable symptoms to severe dyspnea associated with chest pain, cardiovascular collapse, and death.

While the increased mortality due to VTE is considered to be of less relevance in the hospice setting, the symptom burden of fatal PE cannot be underestimated (Noble et al. 2008). Rather than being a sudden asymptomatic experience, the majority of fatal pulmonary emboli are associated with progressive "breathlessness dominated by tachycardia and fever" taking an average of 2 h to die (Havig 1977). In this cohort, only 10% of patients were diagnosed with a PE, the remainder being managed as heart failure, atrial fibrillation, and pneumonia. Breathlessness is often attributed to other pathologies without considering VTE as a diagnosis. These conditions may not only occur concurrently with VTE but also independently increase the VTE risk (Table 7).

Table 7 Attributable pathologies which mimic symptoms of pulmonary embolism

Attributable pathology	Can occur concurrently with PE	Increases risk of PE
Anemia	Yes	Yes: through release of erythropoietin or use of granulocyte colony stimulators
Pneumonia	Yes	Yes: pro-inflammatory condition
Left ventricular failure	Yes	Yes: venous stasis, increased viscosity with diuretic use and pro-inflammatory condition
Pulmonary metastases/ lymphangitis	Yes	Yes: cancer is prothrombotic
Malignant pleural effusion	Yes	Yes: cancer is prothrombotic

5.1 Epidemiology

It is highly likely that palliative care teams will see an increase in the number of patients with VTE, owing to the changing cancer population. Within the western world, people are living longer and a greater proportion of adults are being classed as obese. Both are independent risk factors for VTE, which along with people living longer with chronic illnesses establishes a highly thrombotic baseline risk. Specific to cancer patients, CAT rates have risen in parallel with increased chemotherapy use and are expected to grow further as people live longer with metastatic disease and receive ongoing cancer treatments until later in life (Khorana et al. 2007b).

The sequelae of VTE are not limited to the physical. Research has identified that patients who have been treated for VTE often go on to develop symptoms of post-traumatic stress disorder, and such complications are not limited to high thrombotic burden events (Noble et al. 2014; Bennett et al. 2016). Specific to CAT, research has suggested the symptomatic and psychological burden is such that some consider the experience more distressing than the cancer itself (Noble et al. 2014; Seaman et al. 2014). As such, a holistic approach to CAT is essential, particularly as these patients will also have needs within the context of their cancer journey (Noble et al. 2015b).

5.2 Treatment of VTE

The treatment and secondary prophylaxis of VTE in nonmalignant disease remains relatively straightforward; warfarin has been the mainstay of anticoagulants for decades but is likely to be superseded in most patients by the new direct-acting oral anticoagulants (DOACs) (Wells et al. 2014). However, there are some risks in the frail patient population where the bleeding risk is believed to be higher; DOAC elimination is reduced in renal impairment and should be avoided in those with creatinine clearance <30 ml/min.

Clinical guidelines for the treatment of CAT recommend between 3 and 6 months anticoagulation with weight-adjusted LMWH (Table 8). This is based on meta-analysis of randomized control trials, which have shown LMWH to reduce the rate of recurrent VTE when compared with warfarin, with no increase in bleeding rate. Additional benefits of LMWH are the lack of need for routine monitoring, absorption of the drug even in patients with vomiting, and few drug-drug interactions. Despite requiring a daily injection, qualitative data suggests that LMWH is acceptable within the context of the cancer journey (Seaman et al. 2014). Furthermore, warfarin's appeal as a tablet is undermined by its increased need for INR monitoring, which has been reported to lessen quality of life (Noble 2005). A recent study using conjoint methodology evaluated the preference of patients being treated for CAT (Noble et al. 2015a). Patients considered the most important attribute of their anticoagulant to be that it did not interfere with their ongoing cancer treatment. The second and third most important attributes were efficacy and safety, respectively, followed by the fourth most important attribute being a preference for a tablet over an injection. The authors concluded that patients saw themselves as cancer patients first and foremost, and their main concern was whether the VTE would affect or worsen their ability to receive the best cancer treatment possible. This is reflected in a single institution experience; patients will demonstrate considerable resilience to the side effects of their cancer treatments, in order to receive the best long-term outcome. Thus, they will also be willing to undergo similar inconvenience in the treatment of their CAT to ensure they receive the best treatment possible. Optimal compliance to LMWH is strongly improved by giving patients a full explanation of the importance of CAT treatment and the rationale for using LMWH (Noble et al. 2016).

5.3 Management of CAT when the Evidence Is Lacking

The heterogeneity of CAT goes beyond the different thrombogenicities and risk factors for VTE, conferred by each tumor type and chemotherapy regime. All of the LMWH studies in CAT had exclusion criteria: patients with poor performance status, life expectancy of less than 3 months, thrombocytopenia, increased bleeding risk, renal impairment, and weight less than 40 kg (Lee et al. 2003, 2015; Hull et al. 2006; Meyer et al. 2002). However, these patients are commonly seen by specialist palliative care teams, and up to 9% of patients receiving LMWH experience recurrent VTE, thereby requiring modification of their anticoagulation. Recurrent VTE is seen most commonly in those with advanced disease, in particular lung, ovarian, brain, and pancreatic cancer (Chee et al. 2014; Louzada et al. 2012). Up to 21% of CAT patients are managed outside of the standard treatment of weight-adjusted LMWH. These include patients with recurrent VTE despite anticoagulation, patient with thrombocytopenia, and those with bleeding complications. The management of such cases is covered in a guidance document recently published by the International Society on Thrombosis and Haemostasis Scientific Sub-Committee (ISTH SSC) for Malignancy and Haemostasis (Carrier et al. 2014). However, it is important to recognize that not all patients will be adequately managed with standard weight-adjusted LMWH, and such situations are summarized in Table 8.

The ISTH SSC makes only brief mention of using a twice day dosing of LMWH due to little supporting data. However, it is worth acknowledging a subgroup analysis of 149 cancer patients

Table 8 Management of challenging cases of CAT: ISTH SSC recommendations, Johnson et al. (2012)

Recurrent VTE despite anticoagulation
1. If on warfarin, switch to therapeutic LMWH
2. If already on LMWH, increase dose by 25% or increase back up to therapeutic weight adjusted dose if they are receiving nontherapeutic dosing.
3. If no symptomatic improvement, use peak anti-Xa level to estimate next dose escalation.
Management of CAT in thrombocytopenia
1. For platelet count $>50 \times 10^9\ L^{-1}$ give full therapeutic dose LMWH
2. For acute CAT and platelet count $<50 \times 10^9\ L^{-1}$
a. Full anticoagulation with platelet transfusion to maintain platelet count $>50 \times 10^9\ L^{-1}$
b. If platelet transfusion is not possible, consider retrievable IVC filter
3. For subacute or chronic CAT and thrombocytopenia (platelet count $<50 \times 10^9\ L^{-1}$)
a. Reduce therapeutic dose by 50% or use prophylactic dose for platelet count 25–50 $\times 10^9\ L^{-1}$
b. Omit LMWH if platelet count $<25 \times 10^9\ L^{-1}$
Bleeding while anticoagulated
1. Assess each bleeding episode to identify bleeding source, severity, impact, and reversibility
2. Provide supportive measures to stop bleeding including transfusion where indicated
3. For a major or life-threatening bleeding episode: withhold anticoagulation
a. Consider IVC filter insertion in patients with acute or subacute CAT with a major or life-threatening bleeding episode.
b. Do not consider IVC filter insertion in patients with chronic CAT.
c. Once bleeding resolves: remove retrievable filter (if inserted) and resume/initiate anticoagulation

in a study of 900 VTE patients randomized to receive enoxaparin 1.5 mg/kg SC once daily or enoxaparin 1 mg/kg SC twice daily. The study showed a higher yet statistically nonsignificant rate of recurrent VTE in cancer patients dosed with enoxaparin 1.5 mg/kg SC once daily (6/49 patients, 12.2%) as compared to patients given enoxaparin 1 mg/kg SC twice daily (3/47 patients, 6.4%). Interestingly, the subgroup analysis also found that none of the 49 patients (0%) in the once daily arm died during the study, while 4/47 (8.5%) deaths were reported in the twice-daily arm.

5.4 Prevention of VTE

The prevention of VTE in hospitalized patients has gained increasing attention within clinical research and health policy. VTE prevention is a priority for quality improvement projects within many international health settings and has been covered in a myriad of clinical guidelines.

There has been considerable debate as to whether the data informing VTE prevention (Noble et al. 2008; Noble 2005; Noble and Finlay 2006; Pace et al. 2006; Noble and Johnson 2010; Ambrus et al. 1975) in a largely general medicine population can be applied to specialist palliative care units (SPCU), be it in hospital or hospice settings. In the past, patients admitted to hospices had a fairly short life expectancy and did not expect to be discharged. In this context, the majority of these patients would not benefit from primary thromboprophylaxis since any attributable symptoms could be managed with end of life, symptom control medicines. In more recent years, the population of patients being admitted to what have become SPCUs has changed. Now, patients are often admitted for a period of symptom control, earlier in their disease trajectory. It is not unusual for such patients to have a good performance status and have months or even years to live.

There are limited data pertaining to the prevalence and incidence of VTE in hospice inpatients. One study using light-reflection-rheography to detect obstruction to lower limb venous flow of 258 inpatients suggested findings consistent with the presence of DVT in 135 (52%; 95% confidence interval 46–58) (Johnson et al. 1999). This study acknowledged several limitations, while a highly sensitive test, light-reflection-rheography, is unable to identify the site or cause of obstruction to venous flow. However, the study identified changes consistent with bilateral DVT, and thus potentially more extensive thrombosis, in 17% and 9% had VTE confirmed on imaging.

Practice in hospices has changed over the past 10 years, possibly due to increased awareness of the risks of VTE with advanced cancer (Noble and Finlay 2006; NICE 2018). Even so, the uptake of thromboprophylaxis remains relatively low in hospices despite qualitative data, which suggests that resistance to thromboprophylaxis does not lie with the patients (Noble et al. 2006). Reasons explaining this are complex but predominantly reflect a view that we do not have hard data pertaining to the true prevalence/incidence of VTE in the hospice/SPCU population or studies conducted in representative populations, reporting patient-relevant outcome measures (Noble et al. 2008).

Whatever the reasons for current practice, there appears to be a measurable prevalence of new symptoms attributable to VTE in patients admitted to SPCUs who would qualify for primary thromboprophylaxis if admitted through the medical on-call process. An audit of 1164 case notes from 5 UK hospices suggested that a temporary elevation of VTE risk factors was associated with a prevalence of VTE attributable symptoms in 21% of patients (Johnson et al. 2014). From a practical perspective, over 50% of SPCU admissions were identified as having contraindications to thromboprophylaxis. It is clear, therefore, that the impact of VTE in palliative care patients requires clarification with respect to prevalence, incidence, symptom burden, and impact on quality of life, before thromboprophylaxis guidance can be provided for clinicians caring for cancer patients in this setting (Noble and Johnson 2010). An outline of priorities for research that identifies these important issues has been suggested as follows:

- Identify the true prevalence and natural history of VTE in the palliative care setting.
- Develop appropriate outcome measures.
- Identify the clinical and symptom burden of VTE.
- Establish a consensus on what clinical/symptomatic outcome difference would be required to change thromboprophylaxis practice.
- Establish the clinical and cost-effectiveness of thromboprophylaxis.

At the time of writing, the Hospice Inpatient Deep vein thrombosis Detection Study (HIDDEN) is being conducted in order to establish the prevalence of VTE and evaluate the incidence of VTE during an inpatient stay. This study, in which hospice inpatients undergo a Doppler ultrasound on admission, and at weekly intervals, will provide data on the prevalence and incidence of VTE. These data, married with an appreciation of the symptom burden conferred by VTE, will help establish the need to evaluate the role of thromboprophylaxis. Until then, consensus recommends that hospice patients be considered on an individual basis. For patients admitted for terminal care, prevention of VTE is not a priority since symptoms attributable to VTE could be managed with end of life drugs. However, for the population of patients admitted for symptom control or rehabilitation, the prevention of VTE may be appropriate, especially in those with a longer life expectancy than days. For such patients, the strongest data still lies with LMWH.

5.5 New Anticoagulants and the Palliative Care Patient

The introduction of the oral factor IIa inhibitor (dabigatran) and the factor Xa inhibitors, i.e., rivaroxaban, apixaban, and edoxaban, offers an alternative to patients who would otherwise be treated with warfarin (Schulman et al. 2009; Prins et al. 2014; EINSTEIN Investigators et al. 2010; Agnelli et al. 2013; Hokusai et al. 2013). Collectively termed direct-acting oral anticoagulants (DOACs), they have demonstrated non-inferiority with warfarin for the treatment of conventional VTE, and some show a superior safety profile with respect to major bleeding. They require no monitoring or dose adjustments and have fewer drug-drug interactions than warfarin. As such, they have potential as an attractive alternative to current practice particularly in patients with nonmalignant disease. However, this assertion comes with certain caveats; to date it is not possible to accurately monitor their anticoagulation effect and no readily available reversal agent, should the patient bleed. Furthermore,

Table 9 Proportion of patients in clinical studies with metastatic disease

Study	LMWH (%)	Warfarin (%)	DOAC (%)
CLOT Lee et al. (2003)	66	69	–
LITE Hull et al. (2006)	47	36	–
CATCH Lee et al. (2015)	55	54	–
ONCENOX Meyer et al. (2002)	54	52	–
EINSTEIN DVT/PE Prins et al. (2014)	–	26	19
HOKUSAI VTE Hokusai et al. (2013)	–	22	24

all these drugs rely on the renal system for clearance and are contraindicated, or to be used with caution, in renal failure (creatinine clearance <30 ml/min). Finally, real-world data has suggested caution should be exercised with the use of DOACs particularly in the frail and elderly (Harper et al. 2012). While a case-by-case evaluation of their use in patients with advanced incurable illness is wholly justifiable, a working understanding of factors that increase bleeding risk is essential. Since increased bleeding with DOACs is associated with frailty, increased age, renal impairment, and polypharmacy, they are unlikely to become a vade mecum of anticoagulation to palliative care teams (Kundu et al. 2016).

Until recently, there has been limited data to inform the role of DOACs in the management of CAT, with the exception of the small proportion of cancer patients in the original DOAC VTE studies. A meta-analysis of all the cancer patient data from RE-COVER I and II, EINSTEIN DVT, and PE and Hokusai (but not AMPLIFY) demonstrated superiority of DOACs over warfarin, concluding they may offer an alternative to warfarin in CAT patients intolerant of LMWH (Schulman et al. 2009; Prins et al. 2014; EINSTEIN Investigators et al. 2010; Agnelli et al. 2013; Hokusai et al. 2013).

The pooled incidence rates of recurrent VTE were 4.1% (95% confidence interval [CI] 2.6–6.0) in cancer patients treated with DOACs and 6.1% (95% CI 4.1–8.5) in patients treated with warfarin (RR 0.66, 95% CI 0.38–1.2). The pooled incidence rates of major or nonmajor clinically relevant bleeding were 15% (95% CI 12–18) in cancer patients treated with DOACs and 16% (95% CI 9.9–22) in patients treated with warfarin (RR 0.94, 95% CI 0.70–1.3) (van der Hulle et al. 2014). However, it is important to note that VTE recurrence rates in both arms are low in comparison to other studies. A VTE recurrence rate of 6.1% in the warfarin arm is lower than the VTE rates in the LMWH arm of CLOT (9% LMWH vs 17% warfarin) (Lee et al. 2003), LITE (7% LMWH vs 16% warfarin) (Hull et al. 2006), and CATCH (7.2% LMWH vs 10.% warfarin) (Lee et al. 2015). However, this is not to infer that DOACs are as (or even more) efficacious than the LMWHs, since closer analysis of the data will reveal that the cancer patients in the DOAC vs warfarin studies are different to those in the LMWH vs warfarin ones. Table 9 summarizes the percentage of patients with metastatic disease in each arm of the LMWH vs warfarin CAT studies. Percentages of patients in each arm with metastatic disease, an independent risk factor for VTE, ranged from 47% to 66% in the LMWH arms and 36–69% in the warfarin arms. A subgroup analysis of the EINSTEIN studies has recently been published pooling data of 651 cancer patients (Prins et al. 2014). Recurrent VTE occurred in 16 (5%) of 354 patients allocated to rivaroxaban and 20 (7%) of 301 patients allocated to warfarin (hazard ratio [HR] 0·67, 95% CI 0·35–1·30). However, only 19% of patients in the rivaroxaban arm and 26% of those allocated to warfarin had metastatic disease. It is clear that the proportion of patients with metastatic disease were considerably less in the DOAC studies than the original LMWH studies. It would therefore be premature to infer that any of the DOACs have sufficient evidence to justify the first-line treatment of CAT. In particular, this current data is lacking in patients with advanced cancer and poorer performance status. Nevertheless, some

Table 10 Common drug-drug interactions with Direct Acting Oral Anticoagulants, based on (Lee and Peterson 2013)

	Dabigatran	Rivaroxaban	Apixaban	Edoxaban
Interaction effect	P-glycoprotein	P-glycoprotein CYP3A4	P-glycoprotein CYP3A4	P-glycoprotein
Increases DOAC plasma levels[a]	Cyclosporine	Cyclosporine	Cyclosporine	Cyclosporine
	Tacrolimus	Tacrolimus	Tacrolimus	Tacrolimus
	Tamoxifen	Tamoxifen	Tamoxifen	Tamoxifen
	Lapatinib	Lapatinib	Lapatinib	Lapatinib
	Nilotinib	Nilotinib	Nilotinib	Nilotinib
	Sunitinib	Sunitinib	Sunitinib	Sunitinib
		Imatinib	Imatinib	
Reduces DOAC plasma levels[b]	Dexamethasone	Dexamethasone	Dexamethasone	Dexamethasone
	Doxorubicin	Doxorubicin	Doxorubicin	Doxorubicin
	Vinblastine	Vinblastine	Vinblastine	Vinblastine

[a]Drugs that inhibit P-GP or CYP3A4 can increase DOAC levels
[b]Drugs that induce P-GP or CYP3A4 can lower DOAC levels

clinicians use DOACs first-line for CAT, contrary to the recommendations of guidelines (Noble et al. 2015a).

At the time of writing, two RCTs have been reported, comparing a DOAC with LMWH in the treatment of CAT (Raskob et al. 2018; Young et al. 2018). The SELECT-D pilot study, comparing rivaroxaban with dalteparin for the treatment of CAT, has been presented at the 59th American Society for Hematology meeting in Atlanta. Over 400 patients were recruited with over 90% having locally advanced or metastatic disease and 83% receiving chemotherapy. The VTE recurrence rate at 6 months was 11% (95% CI 7–17%) for patients on dalteparin and 4% (95% CI 2–9%) for patients on rivaroxaban. Major bleeds were similar across trial arms [six bleeds from six patients (3%; 95% CI 1–6%) on the dalteparin arm and nine bleeds from eight patients (4%; 95% CI 2–8%) on the rivaroxaban arm]. There were more clinically relevant nonmajor bleeds (CRNMBs) on the rivaroxaban arm and 5 bleeds from 5 patients (2%; 95% CI 1–6%) on dalteparin compared with 28 bleeds from 27 patients (13%; 95% CI 9–19%) on rivaroxaban. In total, 11 patients (5%; 95% CI 3–9%) on the dalteparin arm had bleeds categorized as either major bleeds or CRNMBs compared to 34 patients (17%; 95% CI 12–22%) on the rivaroxaban arm.

The HOKUSAI VTE Cancer study was an open label non-inferiority trial, comparing 5 days LMWH followed by edoxaban 60 mg once daily with dalteparin at a dose of 200 IU/kg for 1 month followed by dalteparin 150 IU/kg in cancer patients with VTE. Treatment was given for at least 6 months with a primary outcome being a composite of recurrent VTE and major bleeding (Raskob et al. 2018). One thousand forty-six patients were included in the modified intention to treat analysis. Edoxaban demonstrated non-inferiority with dalteparin with a primary outcome event in 67 of the 522 patients (12.8%) in the edoxaban group with 71 of the 524 patients (13.5%) in the dalteparin group (hazard ratio, 0.97; 95% confidence interval [CI], 0.70–1.36; $P = 0.006$ for non-inferiority; $P = 0.87$ for superiority). Reviewing recurrent VTE and major bleeding events separately, it appears that edoxaban results in fewer recurrent VTE events, at the expense of more major bleeding episodes. Recurrent VTE occurred in 41 patients (7.9%) in the edoxaban group and in 59 patients (11.3%) in the dalteparin group (difference in risk, −3.4 percentage points; 95% CI, −7.0 to 0.2). Major bleeding occurred in 36 patients (6.9%) in the edoxaban group and in 21 patients (4.0%) in the dalteparin group and was predominantly due to gastrointestinal (GI) bleeding. Major bleeding was also higher in particular cancers, namely, gastrointestinal (13.1%) and urothelial (7.9%). Based on this, it would seem unreasonable to use DOACs to manage CAT in these untreated/ active GI or urothelial cancers.

A final issue worthy of consideration lies with the potential for drug-drug interactions (Lee and Peterson 2013). DOACs, while subject to fewer interactions than warfarin, are particularly sensitive to medicines which inhibit P-glycoprotein or cytochrome P450 3A4 (CYP3A4). These are by no means insignificant, particularly in those receiving palliative chemotherapy, and are summarized in Table 10. Nevertheless, if patients are unable to take a LMWH, DOACs may be a better choice than warfarin. However, patients need to be aware of the limitations of data and the possible risks should they choose to take DOACs for the treatment of CAT.

6 Conclusion

Cancer-associated thrombosis remains a significant yet under-recognized issue for palliative patients, with the majority of practice based on low-quality evidence or data extrapolated from nonrepresentative populations. It is a problem that will become more prevalent over time, especially in those with metastatic disease. In an era of personalized medicine, where chemotherapy options are considered on the base of biomarkers and genetic mutations, it makes sense that an individualized approach to VTE management is also embraced by those clinicians caring for patients at the fringes of research-based data.

At present, the data supports LMWH first-line for the treatment of CAT. However, at the time of writing, non-inferiority randomized-controlled trials are being conducted to compare DOACs with LMWH, with first results expected in 2018. As with previous CAT studies, it is unlikely that these will reflect the patient population served by palliative care teams, but it may herald a change in clinical practice for the larger cancer population and consequently inform our practice.

Likewise, research is ongoing to define the true prevalence of VTE in hospice inpatients and the associated symptom burden. As such, the next 5 years are likely to see answers to several fundamental challenges in CAT management which will not only inform but also change the management of this underappreciated condition.

References

A Medical Research Council (MRC) randomised trial of palliative radiotherapy with two fractions or a single fraction in patients with inoperable non-small-cell lung cancer (NSCLC) and poor performance status. Medical Research Council Lung Cancer Working Party. Br J Cancer. 1992;65(6):934–41.

Abt D, Bywater M, Engeler DS, Schmid HP. Therapeutic options for intractable hematuria in advanced bladder cancer. Int J Urol. 2013;20(7):651–60.

Agnelli G, Buller HR, Cohen A, Curto M, Gallus AS, Johnson M, et al. Oral apixaban for the treatment of acute venous thromboembolism. N Engl J Med. 2013;369(9):799–808.

Ambrus JL, Ambrus CM, Mink IB, Pickren JW. Causes of death in cancer patients. J Med. 1975;6(1):61–4.

Bennett P, Patterson K, Noble S. Predicting post-traumatic stress and health anxiety following a venous thrombotic embolism. J Health Psychol. 2016;21(5):863–71.

Broadley KE, Kurowska A, Dick R, Platts A, Tookman A. The role of embolization in palliative care. Palliat Med. 1995;9(4):331–5.

Cameron MG, Kersten C, Vistad I, Fossa S, Guren MG. Palliative pelvic radiotherapy of symptomatic incurable rectal cancer – a systematic review. Acta Oncol. 2014;53(2):164–73.

Carrier M, Khorana AA, Zwicker JI, Noble S, Lee AY, Subcommittee on Haemostasis, et al. Management of challenging cases of patients with cancer-associated thrombosis including recurrent thrombosis and bleeding: guidance from the SSC of the ISTH: a reply to a rebuttal. J Thromb Haemost: JTH. 2014;12(1):116–7.

Carrier M, Lazo-Langner A, Shivakumar S, Tagalakis V, Zarychanski R, Solymoss S, et al. Screening for occult cancer in unprovoked venous thromboembolism. N Engl J Med. 2015;373(8):697–704.

Chee CE, Ashrani AA, Marks RS, Petterson TM, Bailey KR, Melton LJ 3rd, et al. Predictors of venous thromboembolism recurrence and bleeding among active cancer patients: a population-based cohort study. Blood. 2014;123(25):3972–8.

Cohen AT, Agnelli G, Anderson FA, Arcelus JI, Bergqvist D, Brecht JG, et al. Venous thromboembolism (VTE) in Europe. The number of VTE events and associated morbidity and mortality. Thromb Haemost. 2007;98(4):756–64.

Dequanter D, Shahla M, Paulus P, Aubert C, Lothaire P. Transarterial endovascular treatment in the management of life-threatening carotid blowout syndrome in head and neck cancer patients: review of the literature. J Mal Vasc. 2013;38(6):341–4.

EINSTEIN Investigators, Bauersachs R, Berkowitz SD, Brenner B, Buller HR, Decousus H, et al. Oral rivaroxaban for symptomatic venous thromboembolism. N Engl J Med. 2010;363(26):2499–510.

Eleje GU, Eke AC, Igberase GO, Igwegbe AO, Eleje LI. Palliative interventions for controlling vaginal bleeding in advanced cervical cancer. Cochrane Database Syst Rev. 2015;(5):CD011000.

Eriksson LG, Ljungdahl M, Sundbom M, Nyman R. Transcatheter arterial embolization versus surgery in the treatment of upper gastrointestinal bleeding after therapeutic endoscopy failure. J Vasc Interv Radiol. 2008;19(10):1413–8.

Gando S. The utility of a diagnostic scoring system for disseminated intravascular coagulation. Crit Care Clin. 2012;28(3):373–88, vi

Harper P, Young L, Merriman E. Bleeding risk with dabigatran in the frail elderly. N Engl J Med. 2012;366(9):864–6.

Harrington DJ, Western H, Seton-Jones C, Rangarajan S, Beynon T, Shearer MJ. A study of the prevalence of vitamin K deficiency in patients with cancer referred to a hospital palliative care team and its association with abnormal haemostasis. J Clin Pathol. 2008;61(4):537–40.

Harris DG, Finlay IG, Flowers S, Noble SI. The use of crisis medication in the management of terminal haemorrhage due to incurable cancer: a qualitative study. Palliat Med. 2011;25(7):691–700.

Havig O. Deep vein thrombosis and pulmonary embolism. An autopsy study with multiple regression analysis of possible risk factors. Acta Chir Scand Suppl. 1977;478:1–120.

Hokusai VTEI, Buller HR, Decousus H, Grosso MA, Mercuri M, Middeldorp S, et al. Edoxaban versus warfarin for the treatment of symptomatic venous thromboembolism. N Engl J Med. 2013;369(15):1406–15.

Hull RD, Pineo GF, Brant RF, Mah AF, Burke N, Dear R, et al. Long-term low-molecular-weight heparin versus usual care in proximal-vein thrombosis patients with cancer. Am J Med. 2006;119(12):1062–72.

Hunt BJ. The current place of tranexamic acid in the management of bleeding. Anaesthesia. 2015;70(Suppl 1):50–3, e18

Johnson MJ, Sherry K. How do palliative physicians manage venous thromboembolism? Palliat Med. 1997;11(6):462–8.

Johnson MJ, Sproule MW, Paul J. The prevalence and associated variables of deep venous thrombosis in patients with advanced cancer. Clin Oncol (R Coll Radiol). 1999;11(2):105–10.

Johnson MJ, Sheard L, Maraveyas A, Noble S, Prout H, Watt I, et al. Diagnosis and management of people with venous thromboembolism and advanced cancer: how do doctors decide? A qualitative study. BMC Med Inform Decis Mak. 2012;12:75.

Johnson MJ, McMillan B, Fairhurst C, Gabe R, Ward J, Wiseman J, et al. Primary thromboprophylaxis in hospices: the association between risk of venous thromboembolism and development of symptoms. J Pain Symptom Manag. 2014;48(1):56–64.

Kakkar VV, Howe CT, Flanc C, Clarke MB. Natural history of postoperative deep-vein thrombosis. Lancet. 1969;2(7614):230–2.

Kawaguchi T, Tanaka M, Itano S, Ono N, Shimauchi Y, Nagamatsu H, et al. Successful treatment for bronchial bleeding from invasive pulmonary metastasis of hepatocellular carcinoma: a case report. Hepato-Gastroenterology. 2001;48(39):851–3.

Khorana AA, Francis CW, Culakova E, Kuderer NM, Lyman GH. Thromboembolism is a leading cause of death in cancer patients receiving outpatient chemotherapy. J Thromb Haemost: JTH. 2007a;5(3):632–4.

Khorana AA, Francis CW, Culakova E, Kuderer NM, Lyman GH. Frequency, risk factors, and trends for venous thromboembolism among hospitalized cancer patients. Cancer. 2007b;110(10):2339–46.

Kundu A, Sardar P, Chatterjee S, Aronow WS, Owan T, Ryan JJ. Minimizing the risk of bleeding with NOACs in the elderly. Drugs Aging. 2016;33:491–500.

Langendijk JA, ten Velde GP, Aaronson NK, de Jong JM, Muller MJ, Wouters EF. Quality of life after palliative radiotherapy in non-small cell lung cancer: a prospective study. Int J Radiat Oncol Biol Phys. 2000;47(1): 149–55.

Lee AY, Peterson EA. Treatment of cancer-associated thrombosis. Blood. 2013;122(14):2310–7.

Lee AY, Levine MN, Baker RI, Bowden C, Kakkar AK, Prins M, et al. Low-molecular-weight heparin versus a coumarin for the prevention of recurrent venous thromboembolism in patients with cancer. N Engl J Med. 2003;349(2):146–53.

Lee AY, Kamphuisen PW, Meyer G, Bauersachs R, Janas MS, Jarner MF, et al. Tinzaparin vs warfarin for treatment of acute venous thromboembolism in patients with active cancer: a randomized clinical trial. JAMA. 2015;314(7):677–86.

Louzada ML, Carrier M, Lazo-Langner A, Dao V, Kovacs MJ, Ramsay TO, et al. Development of a clinical prediction rule for risk stratification of recurrent venous thromboembolism in patients with cancer-associated venous thromboembolism. Circulation. 2012;126(4):448–54.

Martins BC, Wodak S, Gusmon CC, Safatle-Ribeiro AV, Kawaguti FS, Baba ER, et al. Argon plasma coagulation for the endoscopic treatment of gastrointestinal tumor bleeding: a retrospective comparison with a non-treated historical cohort. United European Gastroenterol J. 2016;4(1):49–54.

Meignan M, Rosso J, Gauthier H, Brunengo F, Claudel S, Sagnard L, et al. Systematic lung scans reveal a high frequency of silent pulmonary embolism in patients with proximal deep venous thrombosis. Arch Intern Med. 2000;160(2):159–64.

Meyer G, Marjanovic Z, Valcke J, Lorcerie B, Gruel Y, Solal-Celigny P, et al. Comparison of low-molecular-weight heparin and warfarin for the secondary prevention of venous thromboembolism in patients with cancer: a randomized controlled study. Arch Intern Med. 2002;162(15):1729–35.

Nabi G, Sheikh N, Greene D, Marsh R. Therapeutic transcatheter arterial embolization in the management of intractable haemorrhage from pelvic urological malignancies: preliminary experience and long-term follow-up. BJU Int. 2003;92(3):245–7.

National Institute for Health and Care Excellence (NICE). Venous thromboembolism in over 16s: reducing the risk of hospital-acquired deep vein thrombosis or pulmonary embolism. NICE Guideline (NG89). NICE publishing, London; 2018.

Noble SF, Finlay IG. Is long-term low-molecular-weight heparin acceptable to palliative care patients in the treatment of cancer related venous thromboembolism? A qualitative study. Palliat Med. 2005;19(3):197–201.

Noble SI, Finlay IG. Have palliative care teams' attitudes toward venous thromboembolism changed? A survey of thromboprophylaxis practice across British specialist palliative care units in the years 2000 and 2005. J Pain Symptom Manag. 2006;32(1):38–43.

Noble S, Johnson M. Finding the evidence for thromboprophylaxis in palliative care: first let us agree on the question. Palliat Med. 2010;24(4):359–61.

Noble SI, Nelson A, Turner C, Finlay IG. Acceptability of low molecular weight heparin thromboprophylaxis for inpatients receiving palliative care: qualitative study. BMJ. 2006;332(7541):577–80.

Noble SI, Nelson A, Finlay IG. Factors influencing hospice thromboprophylaxis policy: a qualitative study. Palliat Med. 2008;22(7):808–13.

Noble S, Lewis R, Whithers J, Lewis S, Bennett P. Long-term psychological consequences of symptomatic pulmonary embolism: a qualitative study. BMJ Open. 2014;4(4):e004561.

Noble S, Matzdorff A, Maraveyas A, Holm MV, Pisa G. Assessing patients' anticoagulation preferences for the treatment of cancer-associated thrombosis using conjoint methodology. Haematologica. 2015a;100(11):1486–92.

Noble S, Prout H, Nelson A. Patients' Experiences of LIving with CANcer-associated thrombosis: the PELICAN study. Patient Prefer Adherence. 2015b;9:337–45.

Noble S, Pease N, Sui J, Davies J, Lewis S, Malik U, et al. Impact of a dedicated cancer-associated thrombosis service on clinical outcomes: a mixed-methods evaluation of a clinical improvement exercise. BMJ Open. 2016;6(11):e013321.

O'Shaughnessy DF, Atterbury C, Bolton Maggs P, Murphy M, Thomas D, Yates S, et al. Guidelines for the use of fresh-frozen plasma cryoprecipitate and cryosupernatant. Br J Haematol. 2004;126(1):11–28.

Pace V, Hall E, Bailey C. Prophylactic heparin in palliative care: a cautious welcome. BMJ. 2006;332(7543):728–9.

Pereira J, Phan T. Management of bleeding in patients with advanced cancer. Oncologist. 2004;9(5):561–70.

Preston NJ, Hurlow A, Brine J, Bennett MI. Blood transfusions for anaemia in patients with advanced cancer. Cochrane Database Syst Rev. 2012;(2):CD009007.

Prins MLA, Brighton T, Lyons R, Rehm J, Trajanovic M, Davidson B, Beyer-Westendorf J, Pap A, Berkowitz S, Cohen A, Kovacs M, Wells P, Prandoni P. Oral rivaroxaban versus enoxaparin with vitamin K antagonist for the treatment of symptomatic venous thromboembolism in patients with cancer (EINSTEIN-DVT and EINSTEIN-PE): a pooled subgroup analysis of two randomised controlled trials. Lancet Haematol. 2014;1(1):e37–e46A.

Raskob GE, van Es N, Verhamme P, Carrier M, Di Nisio M, Garcia D, Grosso MA, Kakkar AK, Kovacs MJ, Mercuri MF, Meyer G, Segers A, Shi M, Wang TF, Yeo E, Zhang G, Zwicker JI, Weitz JI, Büller HR; Hokusai VTE Cancer Investigators. Edoxaban for the treatment of cancer-associated venous thromboembolism. N Engl J Med. 2018;378(7):615–24.

Rickles FR, Falanga A. Activation of clotting factors in cancer. Cancer Treat Res. 2009;148:31–41.

Roberts I, Shakur H, Coats T, Hunt B, Balogun E, Barnetson L, et al. The CRASH-2 trial: a randomised controlled trial and economic evaluation of the effects of tranexamic acid on death, vascular occlusive events and transfusion requirement in bleeding trauma patients. Health Technol Assess. 2013;17(10):1–79.

Rodrigues G, Videtic GM, Sur R, Bezjak A, Bradley J, Hahn CA, et al. Palliative thoracic radiotherapy in lung cancer: an American Society for Radiation Oncology evidence-based clinical practice guideline. Pract Radiat Oncol. 2011;1(2):60–71.

Sakr L, Dutau H. Massive hemoptysis: an update on the role of bronchoscopy in diagnosis and management. Respiration. 2010;80(1):38–58.

Schiffer CA, Anderson KC, Bennett CL, Bernstein S, Elting LS, Goldsmith M, et al. Platelet transfusion for patients with cancer: clinical practice guidelines of the American Society of Clinical Oncology. J Clin Oncol. 2001;19(5):1519–38.

Schulman S, Kearon C, Kakkar AK, Mismetti P, Schellong S, Eriksson H, et al. Dabigatran versus warfarin in the treatment of acute venous thromboembolism. N Engl J Med. 2009;361(24):2342–52.

Seaman S, Nelson A, Noble S. Cancer-associated thrombosis, low-molecular-weight heparin, and the patient experience: a qualitative study. Patient Prefer Adherence. 2014;8:453–61.

Sheard L, Prout H, Dowding D, Noble S, Watt I, Maraveyas A, et al. Barriers to the diagnosis and treatment of venous thromboembolism in advanced cancer patients: a qualitative study. Palliat Med. 2013;27(4):339–48.

Tardy B, Picard S, Guirimand F, Chapelle C, Danel Delerue M, Celarier T, et al. Bleeding risk of terminally ill patients hospitalized in palliative care units: the RHESO study. J Thromb Haemost: JTH. 2017;15(3): 420–8.

Torbicki A, Perrier A, Konstantinides S, Agnelli G, Galie N, Pruszczyk P, et al. Guidelines on the diagnosis and management of acute pulmonary embolism: the Task Force for the Diagnosis and Management of Acute Pulmonary Embolism of the European Society of Cardiology (ESC). Eur Heart J. 2008;29(18): 2276–315.

van der Hulle T, den Exter PL, Kooiman J, van der Hoeven JJ, Huisman MV, Klok FA. Meta-analysis of the efficacy and safety of new oral anticoagulants in patients with cancer-associated acute venous thromboembolism. J Thromb Haemost: JTH. 2014;12(7): 1116–20.

Wells PS, Forgie MA, Rodger MA. Treatment of venous thromboembolism. JAMA. 2014;311(7):717–28.

Young AM, Marshall A, Thirlwall J, Chapman O, Lokare A, Hill C, Hale D, Dunn JA, Lyman GH, Hutchinson C, MacCallum P, Kakkar A, Hobbs FDR, Petrou S, Dale J, Poole CJ, Maraveyas A, Levine M. Comparison of an oral factor Xa inhibitor with low molecular weight heparin in patients with cancer with venous thromboembolism: results of a randomized trial (SELECT-D). J Clin Oncol. 2018.

Spinal Cord Compression

74

Kathy Pope, Catherine Mandel, and Damien Tange

Contents

K. Pope (✉)
Department of Radiation Oncology and Cancer Imaging, Peter MacCallum Cancer Centre, Melbourne, VIC, Australia
e-mail: Kathy.pope@petermac.org

C. Mandel
Swinburne Neuroimaging, Swinburne University of Technology, Melbourne, VIC, Australia
e-mail: cmandel@swin.edu.au

D. Tange
Department of Cancer Surgery, Peter MacCallum Cancer Centre, Melbourne, VIC, Australia
e-mail: Damien.Tange@petermac.org

R. D. MacLeod, L. Van den Block (eds.), *Textbook of Palliative Care*,
https://doi.org/10.1007/978-3-319-77740-5_72

Abstract

Spinal cord compression, one of the most dreaded complications of malignancy, is usually caused by metastatic bone disease compressing the spinal cord and/or nerve roots. If not recognized and treated promptly, it can have potentially catastrophic outcomes. As patients live longer due to newer treatments, the incidence of malignant spinal cord compression may increase, and the types of presentation or behavior of tumors may change. Spinal cord compression must be considered in all patients who have a cancer diagnosis presenting with back or neck pain and/or neurological symptoms or signs. In this chapter, the terminology used in the diagnosis and treatment of spinal cord compression will be defined and the epidemiology and pathophysiology described. Given that spinal cord compression is a true emergency, it must be diagnosed and managed promptly by a multidisciplinary team. Early detection and effective treatment can make the difference between independent living and being bed bound. This chapter will explore the many factors that should be considered in determining the most appropriate care plan and highlight how the ultimate goals of care and care plan need to be continually reassessed to ensure the best outcome for the patient. Surgical intervention and radiotherapy treatment decisions are complex and will be explained in detail, within the context of these above considerations. Technical aspects and illustrations to clarify treatment options will be provided. Predicted outcomes will be discussed; however it is important to note that the best outcomes occur when the degree of premorbid neurological deficit is minimal and the diagnosis and treatment initiated within 24–48 h of presentation.

1 Introduction

Spinal cord compression is one of the most dreaded complications of malignancy usually caused by metastatic bone disease compressing the spinal cord and/or nerve roots, with potentially catastrophic outcomes. It affects up to 14% of patients with cancer and is a true emergency, which must be diagnosed and managed promptly by a multidisciplinary team, taking into account many factors to instigate the most appropriate care plan for that individual patient. Best outcomes occur when the degree of premorbid neurological deficit is minimal and the diagnosis and treatment initiated within 24–48 h of presentation.

2 Definitions

Within this chapter, it is necessary to define the common interpretation of the terms used. The term "spinal cord compression" in degenerative terms is just that; compression of the spinal cord alone by a structure such as bone or disc. In malignant parlance, it has a much broader definition, and it usually refers to compression of the spinal cord or cauda equina either directly from a malignancy or compression by a pathological fracture caused by a malignancy and its associated clinical findings. Malignant spinal cord compression also commonly involves the compression of nerve roots in the intervertebral foramina and is an integral part of the clinical picture in the symptom pattern (Fig. 1) (Cole and Patchell 2008).

It is best to maintain strict clinical and radiological definitions. "Malignant spinal cord compression" should only include compression of the spinal cord and conus, whereas "malignant cauda equina compression" is the compression of the lumbar nerve roots in the lumbar vertebral canal. "Malignant nerve root compression" is the involvement of the nerve roots, including within the intervertebral foramina. It is important to distinguish between the use of the term compression in relation to clinical syndromes. Compression is the mechanical compression of the spinal cord or nerve roots as defined radiologically. Therefore cauda equina compression is a radiological definition and should not be confused with "cauda equina syndrome," which is the clinical picture of nerve root signs, perianal sensory loss, and double incontinence. It is important to remember that a patient can have radiological compression without symptoms. This is termed "subclinical cord compression."

"Impending cord compression" is a loose term that should be avoided. It is used frequently to indicate a radiological finding that may progress to definite cord compression, either from tumor growth or bone fracture. Instead the term "at risk of spinal cord compression" should be used.

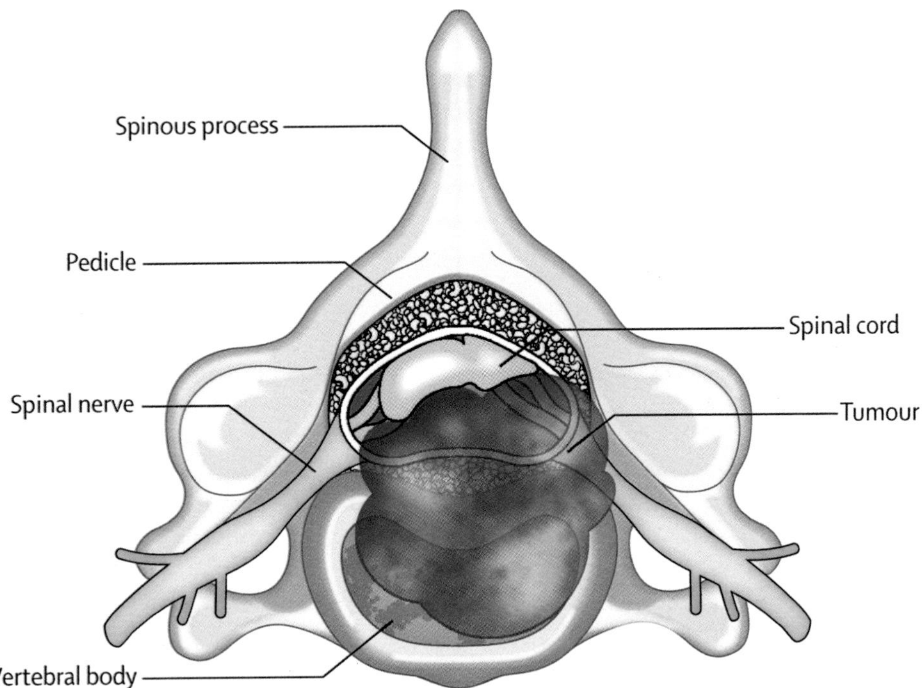

Fig. 1 Example of a tumor within a vertebral body, anterior to the spinal cord which is growing posteriorly into the vertebral canal to compress the spinal cord and/or nerve roots

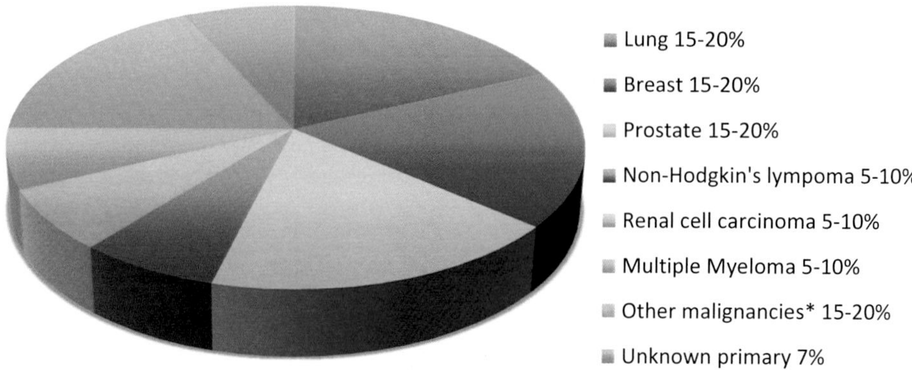

Fig. 2 Approximate proportion of primary tumors causing malignant spinal cord compression. *Other malignancies include colorectal carcinomas, sarcomas, melanomas, etc.

"Unstable fracture" in relation to malignancy indicates a vertebra that has developed a fracture and may possibly collapse further from loss of supportive elements. A "potentially unstable vertebra" is one that has lost a significant amount of its supportive elements and may go on to fracture.

3 Epidemiology and Pathophysiology

Estimates of the incidence of spinal cord compression from malignancy are variously quoted as between 5% and 14% of people with cancer (National Institute for Health and Clinical Excellence (NICE) 2008). In patients with bone metastases, approximately 60% will have metastases within the spine, and up to 10% of these patients will develop spinal cord compression (Spratt et al. 2017). With new treatments, patients with cancer are living longer, and it is likely that the incidence of spinal cord compression may increase. Of patients presenting with spinal cord compression, 77% have a known pre-existing malignancy. The remaining 23% have spinal cord compression as their first presentation of their malignancy (Levack et al. 2002).

Lung, breast, and prostate cancers are the commonest malignancies causing spinal cord compression and together account for over 50% of cases. Non-Hodgkin's lymphoma, renal cell cancer, and multiple myeloma each account for 5–10%, and most of the remainder of cases of malignant spinal cord compression are due to colorectal cancers, sarcomas, and melanomas (Cole and Patchell 2008). In 7% of patients, the site of primary tumor may remain unidentified (Fig. 2) (Levack et al. 2002).

The thoracic spine is most commonly affected with up to 70% of lesions. About 30% of lesions are within the lumbosacral spine and under 10% within the cervical spine (Helwig-Larsen and Sorensen 1994) (Fig. 3). Seventeen percent of patients have two or more levels of spinal cord compression (Levack et al. 2002).

Spinal cord and cauda equina compression can result from several different mechanisms. Direct growth of tumor (either from a vertebra or from paraspinal tissues) into the vertebral canal or intervertebral foramina is one mechanism. A pathological fracture with displacement of bone fragments is another. Often it is a combination of both. Malignant cells within the subarachnoid space may also result in neurological deficits caused by tumor deposits growing on the nerves or surface of the spinal cord within the vertebral canal. From a clinical perspective, it is helpful to consider any tumor in the subdural and subarachnoid space or within the spinal cord itself (compromising the spinal cord) as a cause of a patient's symptoms and signs and as lesions where a patient may benefit from treatment. Leptomeningeal disease is most commonly seen in patients with small cell lung cancer, melanoma, lymphoma, and tumors of the central nervous system, most commonly medulloblastoma.

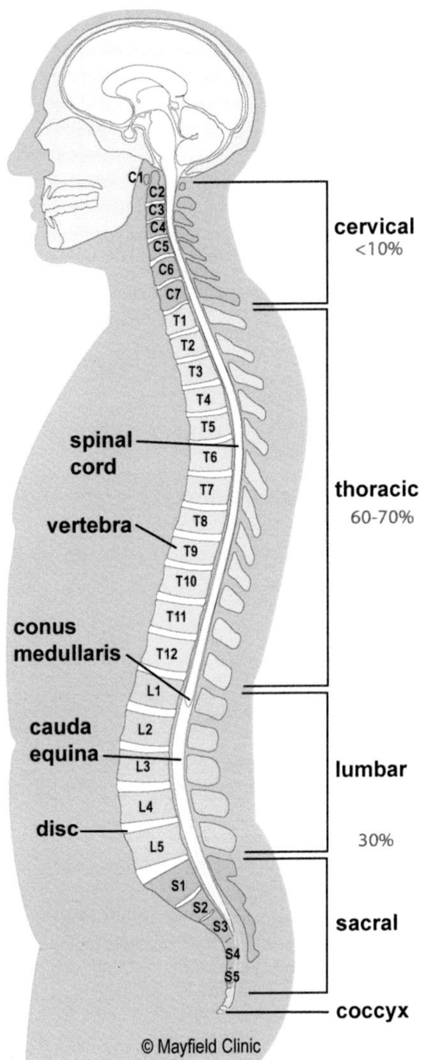

Fig. 3 Approximate distribution of the location of malignant spinal cord compression presentations. Percentages are given in red. 17% of patients have two or more levels of cord compression. (Illustration by Martha Headworth, printed with permission © 2016 Mayfield Clinic)

4 Clinical Features

Malignant spinal cord compression is one of the most dreaded complications of metastatic cancer. Its natural history, if untreated, is usually one of relentless and progressive pain, paralysis, sensory loss, and sphincter dysfunction (Loblaw and Perry 2005). These symptoms and signs can vary significantly between patients (Fig. 4), and therefore a detailed history and full neurological examination need to be performed and documented.

Back pain, the most common presenting problem in patients with spinal cord compression, may be sharp, shooting, deep, or burning. The pain can be localized to the back or may radiate in a band-like dermatomal distribution, if tumor compresses the nerve roots in or near the intervertebral foramina. Mechanical back pain is important to recognize, as it can be associated with spinal instability. An acute exacerbation of chronic back pain may be caused by a recent compression fracture.

In addition to pain, other common symptoms of spinal cord compression include motor dysfunction (weakness with associated reduction in mobility and/or sphincter disturbance with incontinence), sensory changes (paresthesia and loss of sensation), and autonomic dysfunction (urinary hesitancy and retention). At presentation patients tend to be more paraparetic than paralyzed and tend to be less aware of the sensory changes. Sphincter disturbance is usually a poor prognostic sign with regard to preservation or improvement of ambulatory status.

Patients with cauda equina syndrome usually present differently, with change in or loss of sensation over the buttock region, posterior-superior thighs, and perineal region. This is described as a "saddle distribution." Reduced anal tone and urinary retention, with overflow incontinence, are typically present.

A study (Husband 1998) of patients with malignant spinal cord compression found that more than half of the patients had lost further neurological function between the onset of symptoms and start of treatment. The majority of delays were attributed to lack of symptom recognition by the patient and diagnostic delay by the primary health provider or at the general hospital.

To prevent further deterioration and maximize the chances of neurological recovery, any new back pain or abnormal neurology that develops in a patient with a known malignancy needs to be investigated immediately, as the diagnosis of spinal cord compression warrants strong consideration.

Clinical symptom	Incidence in patients with spinal cord compression	Features
Back pain	83-95%	Localised or radicular Unilateral or bilateral Often worse at night Can be mechanical (worse with movement)
Motor deficits & difficulty ambulating	35-75%	Often described as 'heaviness or clumsiness' by patient Weakness on examination Can involve upper or lower motor neuron signs depending on level involved
Sensory deficts	50-70%	Change/loss of sensation typically begins distally and ascends as the disease advances
Autonomic dysfunction	50-60%	Bowel or bladder symptoms tend to occur late Rarely a presenting symtom

Fig. 4 Summary of the different clinical presentations of patients with malignant spinal cord compression (Cole and Patchell 2008)

Several studies have shown that patients with the slowest development of motor deficits before treatment had the best functional outcome compared with patients with faster development of motor deficits and that a greater interval from cancer diagnosis to the spinal cord compression independently predicted improved survival (Rades et al. 2002). Each of these factors probably reflects the presence of less aggressive tumors. Subclinical spinal cord compression (radiological evidence of cord compression in the absence of neurological deficits or pain) is also important to recognize as it represents a window for treatment with potentially the best clinical outcomes.

5 Radiological Diagnosis

5.1 Referral to Radiology

A low index of suspicion in a patient with a known malignancy is important. In a patient with the new onset of a neurological deficit, including bowel and bladder dysfunction or limb weakness, where malignant spinal cord compression or cauda equina syndrome is suspected, same-day magnetic resonance imaging (MRI) is important if the patient is deemed fit for treatment and this will be carried out in the same time frame. If a patient is not fit for treatment or would refuse any treatments offered, there is a little benefit in putting the patient through an MRI scan. The MRI scan can take up to an hour and can be an unpleasant experience for a patient, especially one who is in pain. Therefore if an MRI scan will not alter management, consider not referring the patient.

As a suspected spinal cord or cauda equina compression in a patient who is fit for treatment is a medical emergency, a personal phone call to the radiologist to expedite the radiological investigation is helpful. Discussion of the patient's underlying malignancy, symptoms, and signs assists the radiologist in determining the most appropriate imaging techniques and dedicated sequences, including extra sequences through the area of the spine that could be responsible for the neurological abnormality, to answer the clinical question and to look for other causes of the patient's presentation. It is critical to good radiological investigation that the patient is examined thoroughly. While imaging should include the whole spine, a radiologist who is aware of the neurological findings may detect smaller lesions on the extra, dedicated sequences that would not necessarily be seen on standard sequences.

The referral (or request) should include information about:

- Nature of the known malignancy
- Neurological findings
- Allergies
- Renal function
- Contraindications to MRI (detailed below)

5.2 Patient Care and Optimization of Image Quality

These patients are often in pain and usually anxious. The MRI scanner table is hard and uncomfortable. An examination of the whole spine can take 1 h, and it is imperative that the patient does not move during the examination. Some MRI sequences can take over 8 min, and any movement during this time can result in nondiagnostic images. It is helpful for patients to understand what to expect: radiographers are good at explaining the technical side of MRI to patients but do not have the training or knowledge of the clinical situation to be able to provide a more holistic explanation. For patient comfort and better diagnostic results, it is helpful for patients to be prescribed an appropriate dose of a suitable analgesic prior to the scan, such as morphine. This should be administered when the radiographers call the ward to arrange transport of the patient to MRI.

5.3 Radiological Techniques

Magnetic resonance imaging (MRI) is the imaging technique of choice (Baur et al. 2002; Jung et al. 2003) (Figs. 5, 6, and 7). Its advantages include:

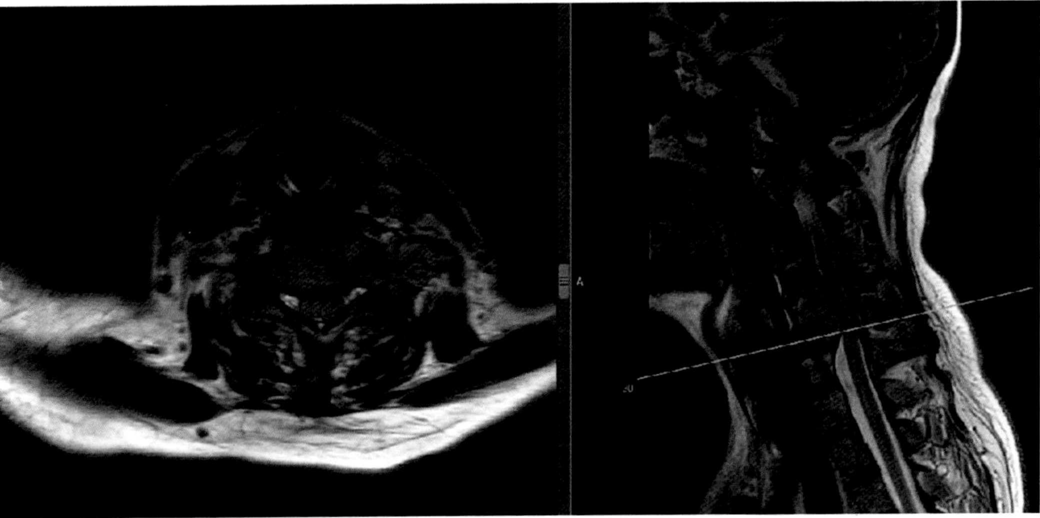

Fig. 5 A 50-year-old female with metastatic breast cancer to the bone only presented with neck pain/tenderness, increased upper limb reflexes, and urinary incontinence. Tenderness over the T5 level with associated bilateral radiating pain was also noted. An axial T2-weighted MR image (on left) through the C6 vertebra and a sagittal T2-weighted MR image of the cervical spine and upper thoracic spine (on right, with blue line demonstrating the level of the corresponding axial image). Confluent tumor at C5 and C6 levels replaces the vertebral bodies, with extension posteriorly into the vertebral canal, resulting in spinal cord compression. The signal return from the spinal cord is within normal limits

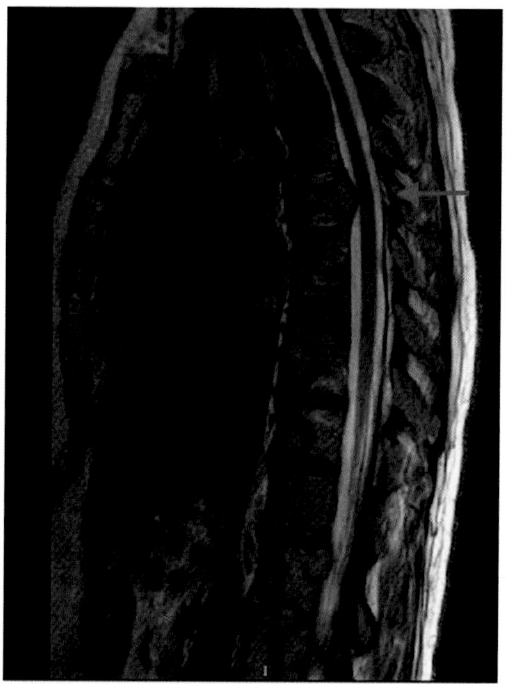

Fig. 6 A T2-weighted sagittal image of the thoracic spine of the same patient demonstrating a lesion in the T5 vertebral body extending into the anterior extradural space and abutting the ventral surface of the spinal cord (red arrow), without signal change within the cord. Numerous metastases involving the entire vertebral column were found on the whole spine images

- The ability to obtain images in any plane: usually at least two perpendicular planes and often three planes
- Good contrast between the relevant tissues including the spinal cord, nerve roots, cerebrospinal fluid, vertebrae, surrounding tissues, and tumor
- Good spatial resolution when the appropriate sequences are obtained and the patient is able to stay very still

There are, however, some disadvantages of MRI. These include:

- A long time required to acquire the imaging
- Patient discomfort if not adequately managed in advance
- Lack of access to MRI, especially for patients in rural locations or in departments where the MRI scanner is heavily booked (there are few opportunities to add in an extra patient with potential spinal cord compression, not least because of the long scanning time required for a full spine MRI)
- Difficulty monitoring patients when in the MRI scanner

MRI has a number of *absolute* contraindications. These include:

- Pacemakers: There are now some pacemakers that are MRI-compatible, but the majority are potentially lethal and without firm evidence of MRI compatibility; a pacemaker is an absolute contraindication.
- Defibrillators and other implanted stimulators.
- Aneurysm clips: The clips currently used by neurosurgeons are MRI-compatible, but many older clips are not. Placing a patient with an incompatible aneurysm clip in the MRI scanner can result in the clip twisting and tearing off the artery with fatal consequences. Unless there is definite proof that the clip type is safe, a patient with an aneurysm clip cannot be placed in the MRI scanner.
- Metal in the eye: Those who weld and grind metal can get metal fragments in the eye. If these have not been removed, then it is not safe to place the patient in the MRI scanner as the metal fragment may move, causing blindness.
- Some heart valves and intravascular stents are absolute contraindications. Definite proof of the nature of MRI-compatible devices is required prior to a patient being allowed in the MRI scanner.

Relative contraindications include:

- Being confused and/or unable to follow instructions. Communication problems can pose a risk with safety screening and an inability to understand the need to stay still for sufficient time to get diagnostic-quality images.
- Claustrophobia can result in a patient being unable to stay still in the MRI scanner or to stay in the scanner at all. Premedication with an anxiolytic can be helpful. The same effect may

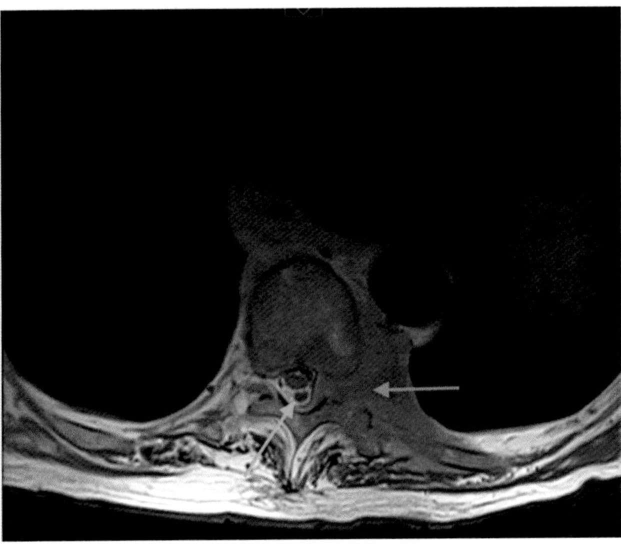

Fig. 7 This 93-year-old patient had metastatic angiosarcoma and presented with mid-lower thoracic radicular pain, radiating in a left T9–T10 dermatomal distribution. An axial T2-weighted MR image of the patient through the T9 level. There is nerve root compression from a left-sided paravertebral mass extending into the vertebral canal through the intervertebral foramen. The spinal cord is displaced to the right. Signal return within the spinal cord is normal (Orange arrow: tumor in the intervertebral foramen. Green arrow: tumor in the vertebral canal)

also be achieved by adequate analgesia with opiates.

- Recent operations with metal implants or clips. These items are problematic with recent operations (due to potential movement) and are considered safe after 6 weeks. Although it is safe to perform MRI after this period, as the prosthesis is fixed and stable, local tissue heating can occur. Patients are asked to let the radiographer know if they start to feel an area of heat. Metal in tattoo pigments can cause a similar effect.
- There is long checklist of other potential contraindications about which the radiographer and radiologist will need to be aware. The radiographer will complete this before an MRI scan can be performed. If the patient cannot speak English (or the language spoken in the country where he or she is being treated), an interpreter will be needed to complete the safety checklist.

If a patient is unable to undergo an MRI scan, then a CT scan and CT myelogram are appropriate imaging techniques. CT myelography is preferred as this more clearly demonstrates the effect of vertebral metastases on the spinal cord and intrathecal nerve roots. This is particularly helpful in the cervical and thoracic spine where a combination of artifacts from surrounding structures and little CSF surrounding the spinal cord can make it technically challenging to interpret a standard CT scan of the spine. Imaging patients with cauda equina syndrome can often be achieved with a CT scan alone. Myelography without a CT scan is no longer the standard of care. The lack of spatial and contrast resolution compromises clinical decision-making. On occasion a CT scan may assist a spine surgeon in planning treatment due to the better delineation of bony structures when compared with MRI. In this instance, the CT scan should be restricted to the region being treated.

The radiology report should always include a description of the extent and location of metastases, the effect (if any) on the spinal cord and nerve roots, any deformities of the spine, and any disease noted in adjacent tissues.

6 Goals of Treatment

The management options and decisions involved are complex for the team treating patients with malignant spinal cord compression. Perhaps the most fundamental question that must first be answered is as follows: *What are the goals of treatment*? The next question that follows is: *Are these goals actually achievable*? For example, the ultimate goal might be to regain the ability to walk, but the achievable goal may be to retain bed mobility and improve the patient's pain levels to enable easier transfers (from bed to chair). These treatment goals should be revisited at each decision point during a patient's management, ensuring that futile treatment is not recommended, and the "bigger picture" is kept in mind. Patients, their carers, and treating teams need to be open and honest about treatment goals.

To answer these questions relating to treatment goals, the key factors to consider are mobility, continence, analgesia, estimated prognosis of the patient, and patient preferences. Active treatments should be explored if ambulatory or sphincter function can be potentially preserved or recovered, or pain levels improved. These treatments include surgical interventions and/or radiotherapy. Best supportive care is imperative for all patients. The overarching treatment aim is always to improve the patient's quality of life.

7 Management Overview and Decision Process

Prompt diagnosis and instigation of appropriate treatment strongly affect the patient's ultimate outcome. The strongest prognostic factor for overall survival and the ability to ambulate after treatment is pretreatment neurological status and specifically motor function (Talcott et al. 1999). Therefore in a patient with known cancer, new back pain or abnormal neurological symptoms or signs should be investigated immediately. If the diagnosis of spinal cord compression is not consistent with the patient's known cancer biology, consideration should be given to arranging a biopsy. This will assist in excluding differential diagnoses, such as osteomyelitis.

Once the diagnosis of malignant spinal cord compression is confirmed, the treatment decisions need to be made quickly by the multidisciplinary team, comprising of the neurosurgeon, oncologists (both radiation and medical), palliative care physician, and community teams including the primary care provider. Urgent neurosurgical opinion should be considered for patients with symptomatic spinal cord compression, as evidence suggests that in selected patients, outcomes are better with decompressive surgery prior to radiotherapy (Patchell et al. 2005). Several national treatment guidelines and protocols suggest that treatment with surgery or radiotherapy ideally should be commenced within 24 h of *radiological diagnosis* for best functional outcome (National Institute for Health and Care Excellence (NICE) 2014; eviQ Cancer Treatments Online (Cancer Institute NSW) 2012), together with other studies confirming better outcomes if surgery is performed within 48 h of *initial presentation of symptoms* (Quraishi et al. 2013).

This initial multidisciplinary decision process may be performed utilizing a "virtual consultation" via telephone or the Internet, especially if the neurosurgical and oncology specialists are geographically distant from the patient. The treatment options can be divided into four categories (surgery, radiotherapy, systemic and supportive care) and will be detailed further in the next sections. Most patients require a combination of these treatments; however the decisions regarding sequencing can be complex.

There are many factors that the multidisciplinary team considers in developing a suitable treatment plan for each patient with malignant spinal cord compression. These can be divided into patient, tumor, and treatment factors (Fig. 8).

All of these factors are then synthesized together to choose the most appropriate treatment recommendation. For instance, for a patient with surgically appropriate disease, who has never received radiotherapy to the spine, with minimal burden of disease, and an excellent expected long-term prognosis, both surgical management and adjuvant radiotherapy would be recommended,

PATIENT FACTORS	Functional impact of symptoms (mobility & continence) Performance status (often measured as EGOG status) (Oken M 1982) prior to onset of syptoms/signs Pain levels Patient preferences Time elapsed since developing symptoms/signs Physical location of patient (distance to travel to hospital for surgery &/or radiotherapy delivery)) Any improvement with dexamethasone
TUMOUR FACTORS	Structural impact of disease (e.g. presence of bony compression and spinal instability) Levels within the spine involved Estimated prognosis • Bone only +/- visceral metastases • True 'oligo-metastatic' disease • Underlying cancer biology/progression
TREATMENT FACTORS	Predicted outcome from active treatments (i.e. potentially reverse or preserve function, or improve pain) Estimated length of time to achieve potential benefit from treatments Technical surgical factors Radio-responsiveness of tumour Response to systemic treatment options Previous treatments (neurosurgical interventions and radiotherapy in particular) Toxicities expected from treatments

Fig. 8 Factors to be considered by the multidisciplinary team in formulating a care plan for patients with malignant spinal cord compression

in addition to exploring aggressive systemic treatment with the best supportive care. For a patient with a poor performance status, previously treated spinal cord compression, who has a short prognosis and has exhausted systemic options, further surgery and/or radiotherapy may not be able to provide any potential benefit, and instead best supportive care alone is probably the best option. These factors will be explored further in the following section with respect to each treatment intervention, but it is important to further elaborate on a few general factors.

Given that the overall aim is to improve the patient's quality of life, it is extremely important to consider the premorbid level of function of the patient and what improvements are achievable. At best, interventions are able to reverse neurological abnormalities back to the patient's baseline level and eradicate pain. In practice this can be difficult to achieve, and therefore an honest and accurate estimation of "possible" versus "likely" benefit needs to be discussed with the patient and carers. Pain can be temporarily improved with steroid medication and analgesia, together with pressure care, insertion of indwelling urinary catheters, and other important supportive care measures. For more durable analgesia benefit, surgery and/or radiotherapy are the best options.

Estimated overall disease prognosis can be very difficult to predict accurately, despite many tools being developed (Krishnan et al. 2013), and probably deserves its own separate chapter. Essentially, if a patient has had a long disease-free interval (from diagnosis or last episode of disease progression to the development of spinal cord compression), has promising systemic options, or has oligo-metastatic disease, then they are likely to have a longer prognosis. Patients with particular tumor biologies (e.g., metastatic prostate cancer or receptor-positive breast cancer with bone-only disease) may also have better prognoses. The oncologist and palliative care physician who know the patient most closely are best placed to make this prognosis estimation.

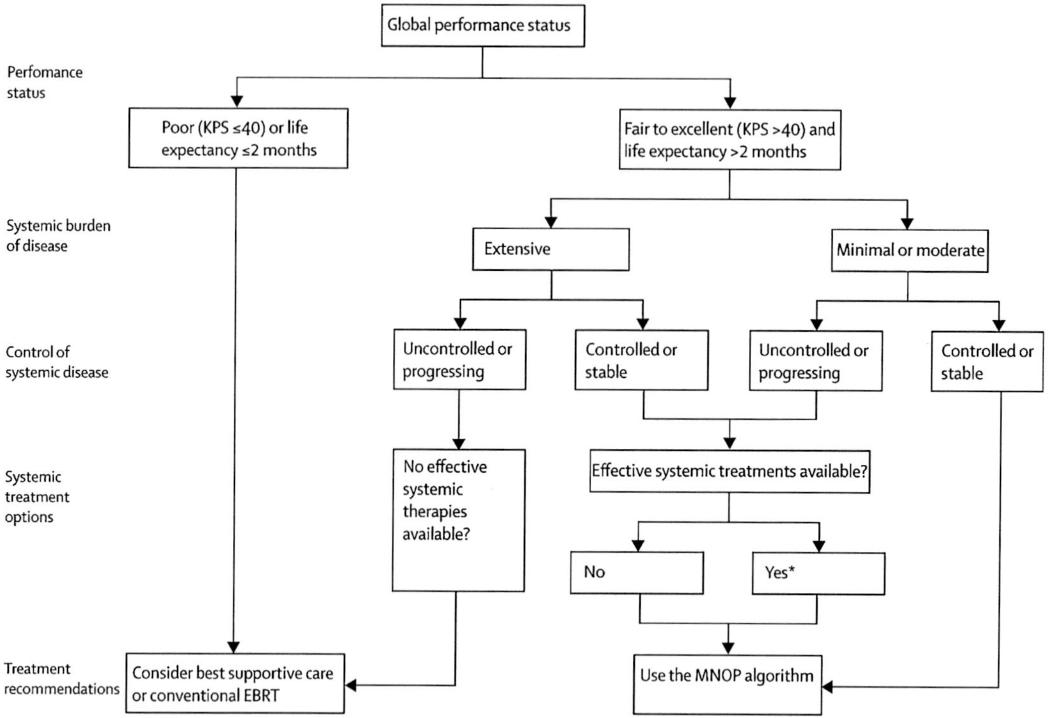

Fig. 9 Algorithm 1: initial assessment algorithm for patients with spinal metastases. *KPS* Karnofsky Performance status, *EBRT* external beam radiotherapy, *MNOP* mechanical, neurological, oncological, preferred treatment. *For selected patients with effective systemic therapy treatment options, systemic therapy without the use of radiotherapy might be most appropriate

For surgery and/or radiotherapy to achieve potential overall benefit, the predicted prognosis must be long enough to allow these treatments to be delivered, the toxicities managed, the patient to recover, and the best possible treatment outcomes realized. In the case of combined surgery and radiotherapy, a good rule of thumb is that if overall prognosis is less than 3 months, the patient may not live long enough to recover from the operation and anesthetic, proceed to radiotherapy (often five daily treatments over 1 week), heal from side effects, and await the 4–6 weeks it usually takes for maximal analgesia response and the initial consolidation of the structural benefit from radiotherapy. This has to be balanced by the patient's wishes and acceptance of potentially spending a prolonged period of time either in hospital or away from their usual place of residence, to receive these treatments.

Essentially the long-term benefits of an invasive, timely, or costly procedure might not manifest in patients with a short life expectancy. Furthermore, an overly aggressive treatment approach might cause more harm than benefit in patients who are frail and neurologically debilitated, or who are dying (Spratt et al. 2017). A number of algorithms have been developed to assist management teams in deciding appropriate treatment. The recent Lancet oncology review by Spratt et al. summarizes one such approach in patients with spinal metastases (Figs. 9 and 10) (Spratt et al. 2017). Spinal cord compression is detailed in the far-right portion (red box) of the MNOP (mechanical, neurological, oncological, preferred treatment) algorithm (Fig. 10).

8 Neurosurgical Intervention Overview

Surgical treatment in the management of malignant spinal cord or cauda equina compression remains controversial and difficult. It is not always an available option. The commonest treatment options are decompression, stabilization, or

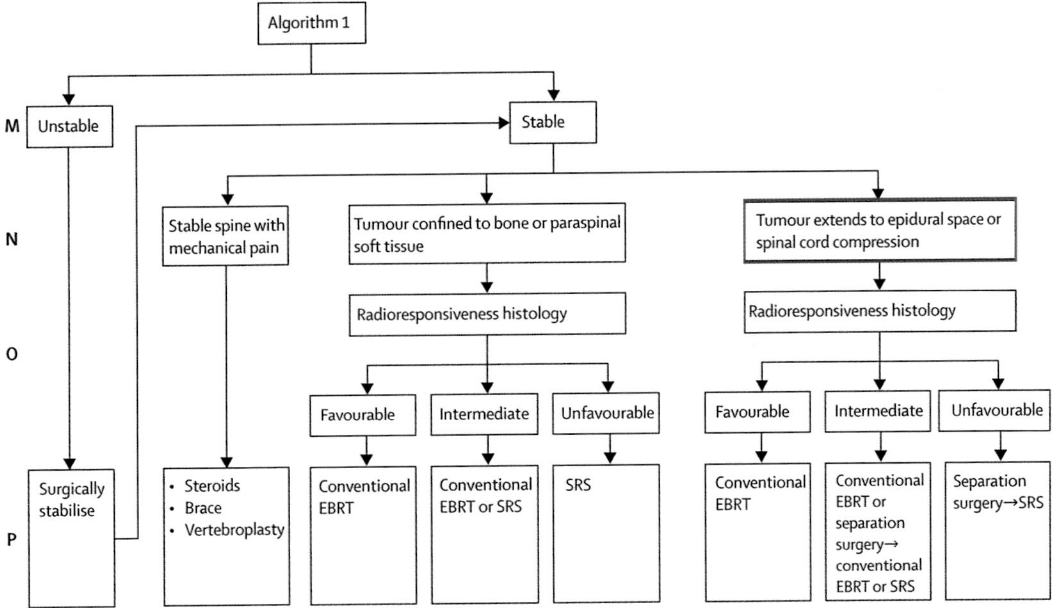

Fig. 10 MNOP algorithm for management of spinal metastases. Spinal cord compression is detailed in the far-right portion (red box). *MNOP* mechanical, neurological, oncological, preferred treatment, *EBRT* external beam radiotherapy, *SRS* stereotactic radiosurgery

both. The best-known studies showed that decompression alone produced a similar or worse outcome when compared with radiotherapy alone for malignant spinal cord compression, due to the destabilizing influence of the operation (George et al. 2015). For this reason, the majority of patients who now have surgery for spinal cord compression will have decompression combined with a form of stabilization. The preferred option is to make the decision and enact it, *prior* to the onset of major symptoms and signs. Prolonged paraplegia in a patient from malignant compression will generally not resolve with surgery.

The typical goals of surgery are:

1. Prevention of neurological deterioration
2. Restoration of neurological function
3. Treatment of pain from compression
4. Fracture stabilization for pain control and prevention of progressive deformity

The decision to operate needs to be based on the assessment of the value to the patient from the procedure. The questions that need to be asked are:

What does the patient want?

Patients will usually have an opinion in regard to what they are prepared to go through. This will depend on their expectations of the outcome. The potential outcomes must not be overstated. Surgery is going to be associated with a period of convalescence and likely rehabilitation, and the patient may not want to go through this.

Is surgery technically possible and what are the risks?

A surgical opinion with review of the radiology prior to discussion with the patient is invaluable, as many patients are not technically suitable for surgical intervention or the procedure will be too large considering the patient's condition.

Is the patient fit for any operation planned?

Surgery is precluded if the patient cannot have a prolonged anesthetic, is unable to stop any blood thinner medications, or is neutropenic or thrombocytopenic.

Is there a significant benefit to the patient from the surgery?

If the patient cannot walk prior to the surgery and has a predicted survival of less than 3 months, they are unlikely to walk again. If a patient has severe pain and has an unstable crush fracture, then stabilization should reduce the pain substantially which will significantly decrease medication requirements and hopefully supportive care measures, thereby improving quality of life.

What is the patient's life expectancy?

The only surgery that should be entertained in patients with short life expectancy is for the treatment of pain. If there is a long life expectancy, then it is appropriate to consider treatment early, as prevention of fractures and subsequent pain, kyphosis, and neurological deficit is ideal.

Rate of growth of the tumor and alternative treatment options?

In the palliative treatment of metastatic cancer involving the spine, it must be remembered that surgery is a temporary option, as the tumor will recur. If the lesion is radioresistant and there are no medical options, then even with surgical treatment, there is likely to be residual disease, and hence regrowth will occur at the known existing disease progression rate.

Should radiotherapy/radiosurgery be used perioperatively?

Conventional radiotherapy will affect tissue healing. If the patient has already had radiotherapy and subsequent surgery is planned, postoperative wound breakdown and infection will be much more likely. If stereotactic surgery to the tumor bed is planned, insertion of metal hardware may cause scatter of the radiation and affect the ability to plan the radiotherapy accurately. Preoperative radiosurgery, if time permits, may be a better and simpler option. If postoperative radiotherapy is planned, a period of at least 2 weeks is usually required for surgical healing, prior to fractionated radiotherapy.

9 Neurosurgical Procedures

9.1 Laminectomy

This involves the removal of a lamina from the back of the spine, thereby exposing the vertebral canal and allowing access to the spinal cord and any tumor around it. This is only suitable for patients who do not have any instability and predominately posterior and lateral extradural compression.

9.2 Stabilization Alone

This is usually a posterior procedure in the thoracic and lumbar spine. It involves the insertion of screws into the pedicles of the vertebral bodies and the linking of the screws to a rod that will cross an unstable segment of fracture. It can be imagined as an internal fixture or scaffolding. These are now usually constructed from titanium and, if done without other procedures, will be performed by a minimally invasive or percutaneous technique. Stabilization can be used in combination with external beam or stereotactic radiotherapy where tumor control would be adequate with radiation alone, but there is a risk of vertebral collapse.

9.3 Laminectomy with Posterior Stabilization

This is a combination of the above two procedures and allows for a more extensive bone removal and hence a wider decompression. In this combined procedure, the decompression may extend to involve the pedicles and part of the vertebra, which may then cause instability that needs to be treated with the stabilization. It may be a completely open procedure or combined with a minimally invasive technique.

9.4 Vertebrectomy with Stabilization

If the vertebra needs to be removed, this usually involves an anterior approach, but some surgeons will do certain levels from a posterior approach. The complexity and size of the operation increases from less complex in the cervical spine to much more complex in the lumbar spine. At most levels in the cervical spine, vertebrectomy with stabilization is relatively uncomplicated. Anterior surgery at vertebral levels C1 and C2 is not indicated in the palliative setting because of its complexity and risks. Similarly anterior surgery at vertebral levels T3–T5 is best avoided in the palliative setting. These levels are best treated from behind. If there is a high degree of instability either from the tumor or the operation, then an anterior decompression will be combined with posterior stabilization. Anterior surgical procedures in the lumbar and thoracic spine are less likely to be entertained in the palliative setting because of the risks.

10 Surgical Recovery and Length of Hospital Stay

Recovery from an operation will depend on the scale of the procedure undertaken and the preoperative state of the patient. An elective straightforward minimally invasive procedure over five thoracic vertebral levels with no preoperative deficit will typically involve a hospital stay of between 3 and 5 days in this patient group. A cervical vertebrectomy with anterior stabilization alone will be closer to 2 days.

11 Interventional Radiological Procedures

11.1 Vertebroplasty

Vertebroplasty is the fluoroscopically guided, percutaneous injection of bone cement into a vertebral body. Vertebroplasty will not relieve spinal cord compression; however, it can be helpful in relieving mechanical pain and stabilizing a vertebra at risk of fracture, particularly if the disease is within the vertebral body. As vertebroplasty is minimally invasive, it does not require a prolonged healing time before other treatments can be started.

11.2 Tumor Embolization

Very vascular tumors, such as renal carcinoma, may be rendered easier to treat surgically if embolized by a neuroradiologist and thereby made less vascular, prior to operation. Embolization can be performed using particles, coils, glue, or ethylene vinyl alcohol and may also contribute to reduction in a pain and neurological symptoms.

11.3 Image-Guided Tumor Ablation

There are a variety of radiological ablative techniques available, such as radiofrequency ablation, microwave ablation, thermal ablation, and cryoablation. These are typically used to treat painful metastases or as further treatment to areas previously irradiated. They are not used to treat acute spinal cord compression.

12 Radiotherapy

Radiotherapy is the mainstay of treatment for spinal cord compression and is given in combination with surgery, when appropriate. The main aims of radiotherapy are to reduce tumor bulk and pressure on the spinal cord and/or nerve roots, consolidate the mechanical benefit from surgery, and hopefully provide durable tumor control. Therefore, in a similar way to surgery, the overall goals with radiotherapy are to:

1. Prevent further neurological deterioration.
2. Restore neurological function.
3. Reduce pain.

It is important to note that even in the situation where any neurological improvement is unlikely, radiotherapy can still potentially palliate symptoms of pain and improve quality of life. The maximal benefits from radiotherapy usually takes 4–6 weeks to occur, so this needs to be considered in making decisions.

There are two main types of radiotherapy: conventional external beam radiotherapy and stereotactic radiotherapy, which will be discussed in more detail below. Radiotherapy can be given as a single dose or fractionated into several smaller doses. Prior to starting radiotherapy, all patients should be considered for a full spine MRI, and commenced on corticosteroids (up to 16 mg dexamethasone a day in divided doses) as soon as the diagnosis is suspected. There is little evidence that higher doses are more effective (George et al. 2015; Loblaw and Mitera 2012), but serious adverse events are frequently higher with high-dose steroids, as expected. If the patient is receiving concurrent cytotoxic chemotherapy or immunotherapy, the potential increased risk of side effects with the radiotherapy needs to be considered and discussed with the patient and medical oncologist. Early radiotherapy-associated toxicities (e.g., esophagitis or erythematous skin reaction) tend to peak approximately 7–10 days after radiotherapy is completed and are specific to the area treated. They should be monitored and managed until resolution occurs. Late radiation reactions are rare in this setting.

12.1 Radiotherapy Simulation (Set-Up Position and Planning)

For radiotherapy to be effective, it needs to deliver the prescribed dose to the correct location within the body, with an accuracy of millimeters. This is achieved by ensuring the patient has adequate analgesia prior to simulation and each treatment and is able to lie in a comfortable and reproducible position. Often a patient-specific molded vacuum bag is used to help keep the patient immobilized in a comfortable position, together with small tattoo marks that are used to line the patient up in the correct position via laser beams on the treatment machine (Fig. 11a, b). A CT simulation image is usually acquired prior to starting treatment, and the radiotherapy is planned from this. In an emergency this process is simplified and often condensed to a single step.

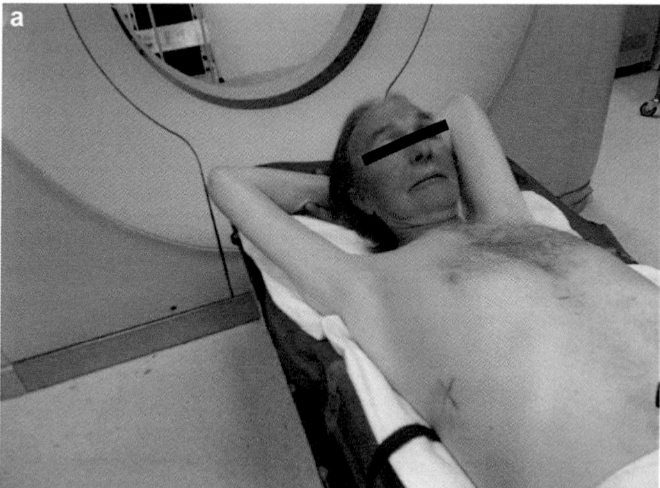

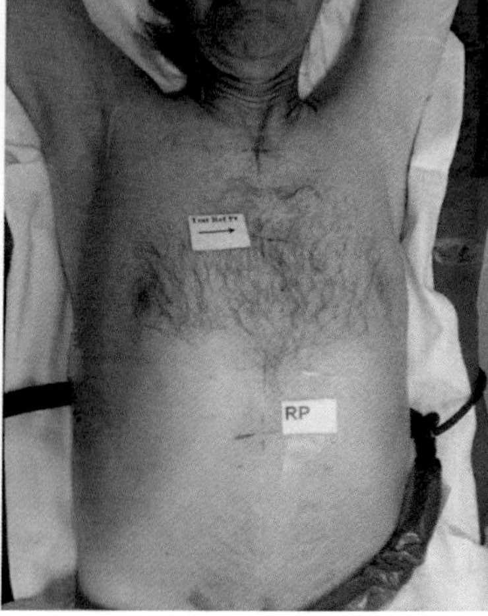

Fig. 11 (**a**) Patient lying supine on radiotherapy CT simulation couch for planning purposes. Blue vacuum bag is under patient. (**b**) Close-up photograph of treatment reference points (to be tattooed). This will assist with repositioning patient in the same position for radiotherapy treatment

12.2 Types of Radiotherapy

Conventional external beam radiotherapy is the most common technique used to treat spinal cord compression. It is a noninvasive method of delivering radiation to the tumor and surrounding structures (often the vertebral body above and below the level of concern) and is usually delivered using one to three radiotherapy beams (Fig. 12), depending on the location of the spinal cord or cauda equina compression. The radiation beams are shaped as they come out of the linear accelerator before they reach the patient to ensure they are directed at the tumor.

Stereotactic radiotherapy is another noninvasive technique but is more conformal using many smaller beams entering the body from a number of different angles. This means the radiotherapy dose distribution more closely matches the tumor and vertebral body (Fig. 13), avoiding nearby structures (particular organs at risk) compared with conventional external beam

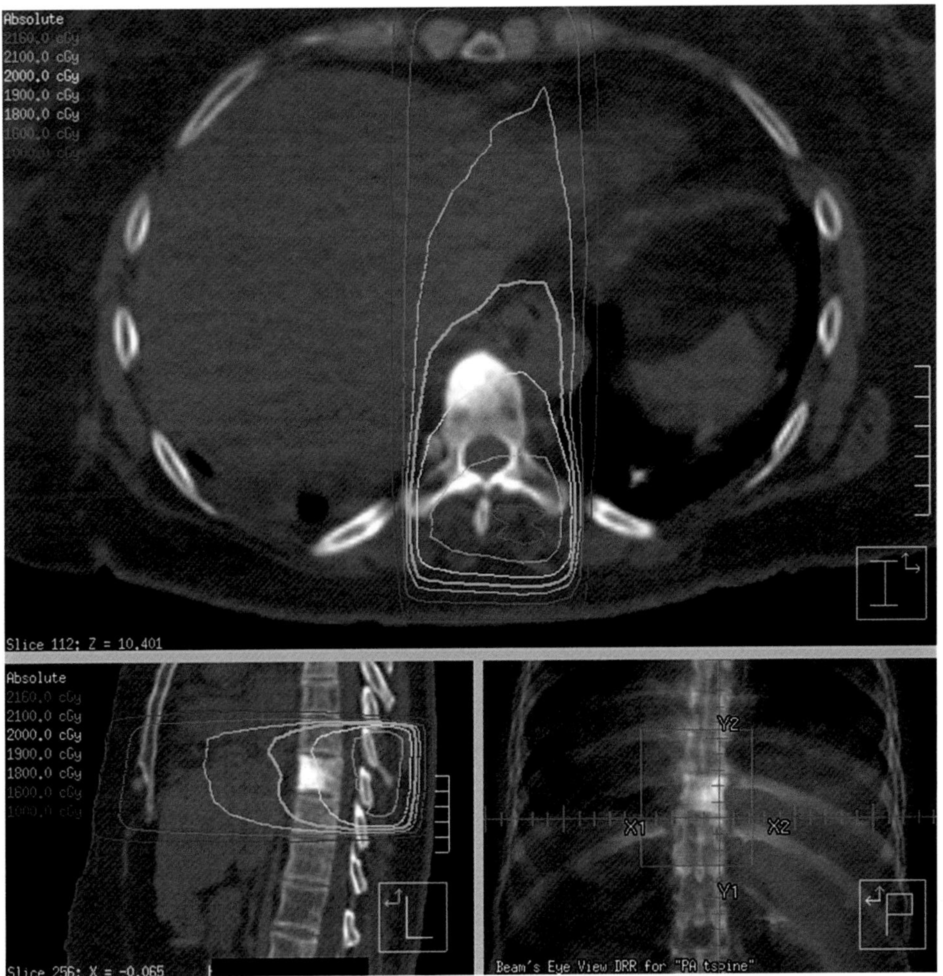

Fig. 12 Dosimetry of a conventional external beam radiotherapy plan for a patient with a single bone metastasis at T9 level. A single posterior beam is delivered, to a total dose of 20 Gy in five daily fractions. The green line is 95% of the prescribed dose. There is exit dose through the liver and stomach, potentially causing some mild temporary nausea

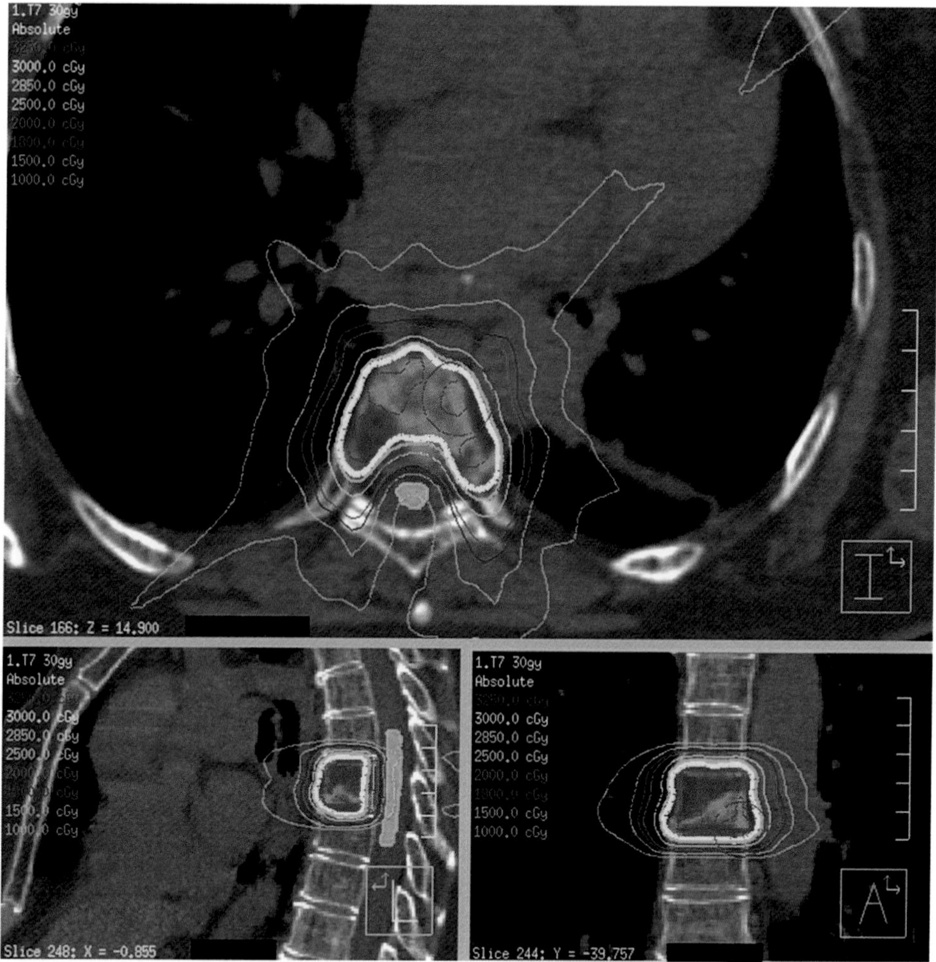

Fig. 13 Dosimetry of a stereotactic radiotherapy plan for a patient with a single bone metastasis at T7 level. Nine beams are delivered, to create a total dose of 30 Gy in four daily fractions. The yellow line is 100% of the prescribed dose and can be seen wrapping around (and therefore sparing) the spinal cord. There is minimal exit dose as the dose is highly conformal, therefore less toxicity to nearby organs

radiotherapy (Faculty of Radiation Oncology, The Royal Australian and New Zealand College of Radiologists 2017). Stereotactic radiotherapy is able to deliver a higher biological dose because it is better able to avoid normal healthy tissues and therefore requires tighter margins, a stricter set-up, and the patient to be very compliant and immobile during treatment planning and delivery. This higher biological dose may be particularly beneficial for tumor histologies (e. g., sarcoma, renal cell carcinoma, and melanoma) that have traditionally been regarded as relatively radioresistant.

While conventional external beam radiotherapy is widely available and easily delivered, stereotactic radiotherapy is more complex and may not be available in all situations. Stereotactic radiotherapy is unlikely to be used in an emergency situation because of the additional time required for planning and treatment verification. There are however two main advantages with stereotactic radiotherapy. Firstly, in a non-emergency situation for a patient with good prognosis disease, who has limited spinal metastases, the radiation oncologist may want to increase the radiotherapy dose to hopefully improve local control in the longer term (Loblaw and Mitera 2012). This may be given preoperatively (prior to insertion of surgical hardware) so that the radiotherapy dosimetry and treatment verification are more accurate. The second benefit of stereotactic radiotherapy is for patients who have had previous external beam radiotherapy to the same spinal level and have a good performance status and a malignancy with a good prognosis. In this situation there may be an opportunity to offer re-treatment with stereotactic radiotherapy, with the advantage of sparing the spinal cord (avoid dose being deposited there) and a reduction in the treatment volume (therefore avoiding other normal tissues receiving additional dose). These are complex decisions and treatments requiring multidisciplinary discussion. Currently in the United States, the RTOG 0631 trial is comparing stereotactic radiotherapy with conventional external beam radiotherapy and includes patients with a limited (one to three) number of spine metastases, with or without minimal extradural compression (RTOG Foundation Inc 2016).

12.3 Dose Fractionation

The radiation oncologist chooses the "best-fit" radiotherapy dose and fractionation schedule, depending on the factors that were listed earlier in Fig. 8. The total dose and the number of radiotherapy treatment fractions (#s) vary widely (George et al. 2015). Various doses are acceptable for conventional external beam radiotherapy, including a single 8 Gy #, 16 Gy in 2 × 8 Gy#s delivered 1 week apart, 20 Gy in five daily #s delivered over a week, or 30 Gy in 8#s delivered over 2 weeks (4 days break in the middle of split course). Consideration should also be given to weekend treatment, especially early on in a fractionated course, or with the single doses. Higher doses may be considered for patients who are of excellent performance status, have limited disease, and have a long disease natural history. Stereotactic spine radiotherapy dose schedules also vary widely and include single 8–24 Gy fractions and multi-fraction dose schedules of 27–30 Gy in 3–5#s (Huo et al. 2017).

12.4 Efficacy and Outcomes

Radiotherapy is the most widely used treatment in the management of malignant spinal cord compression. A Cochrane Review (George et al. 2015) included six randomized trials ($n = 544$) of which Patchell et al. (2005) was the only trial to compare surgery with radiotherapy (RT) versus radiotherapy alone. This trial reported the following outcomes:

- Overall ability to walk after treatment was 84% (surgery + RT, RR 0.67, CI 0.53–0.86) vs. 57% (RT alone) (Patchell et al. 2005).
- Ability to walk was maintained by 94% (surgery + RT) vs. 74% (RT alone) ($p = 0.024$), with the median length of time able to walk being 153 days (surgery + RT) vs. 54 days (RT alone) ($p = 0.024$).
- Regaining ability to walk after treatment was achieved by 62% (surgery + RT) vs. 19% (RT alone) ($p = 0.01$), with non-ambulant surgical patients walking for a median of 59 days vs. 0 days (RT alone) ($p = 0.04$)
- Median survival was 126 days (surgery + RT) vs. 100 days (RT alone) ($p = 0.033$).
- Serious adverse effects (perforated gastric ulcer, psychosis, and death due to infection) were reported in 17% of patients receiving high-dose corticosteroid (96–100 mg dexamethasone) vs. 0% in moderate-to-low-dose (10–16 mg dexamethasone) patients (George et al. 2015).

This Patchell study excluded patients with poor prognosis (<3 months survival), multiple levels of spinal cord compression, and radiosensitive tumors (lymphomas, leukemia, multiple myeloma, and germ-cell tumors). It is important to note that patients with pathological fractures and spinal instability were included in the randomization, a situation which radiotherapy alone would not be expected to reverse and may have contributed to the poorer ambulatory outcomes in the radiotherapy-alone arm. A requirement of the trial was neurosurgical anterior decompression within 24 h of diagnosis, which may not be achievable in many settings. Again it is important to note that even in patients with poor-prognosis disease, not suitable for surgery, or where neurological deficit reversal is unlikely, radiotherapy alone may still improve pain control and hence overall quality of life.

In terms of radiotherapy dose fractionation, the evidence suggests that single-fraction radiotherapy 8 Gy is just as effective as multiple fractions in patients with poor prognosis (<6 months survival) and no indication for primary surgery (diagnostic doubt, vertebral instability, bony impingement as the cause of spinal cord compression, or previous radiotherapy of the same area). No significant differences in overall survival, ambulation, duration of ambulation, pain response, and bladder control were reported in the two randomized controlled trials (Maranzano and Bellaviat 2005; Maranzano and Trippa 2009) comparing dose schedules (single versus multiple fractions) in these poor-prognosis patients.

For patients with a good prognosis, the use of surgery and radiotherapy should be considered where appropriate. Local tumor recurrence (within the radiotherapy field) may be more common, and consequently re-treatment rates higher, with a single dose, compared with higher-dose short-course radiotherapy schedules. Hence in patients who are expected to live longer, higher doses of radiotherapy are often prescribed, despite minimal evidence comparing radiotherapy schedules in patients with spinal cord compression and a good prognosis (George et al. 2015).

12.5 Early and Late Toxicities

Early radiotherapy toxicities are usually temporary, occurring midway during the radiotherapy course, peaking within 7–10 days of finishing, and usually resolving within approximately 4 weeks of radiotherapy course completion. These side effects will vary depending on the level of the spinal cord compression being treated (other organs/tissues within the RT field) and the dose delivered and may include:

- Esophagitis
- Nausea and vomiting (if the stomach in the radiotherapy field)
- Diarrhea (if bowel in the radiotherapy field)
- Alopecia (within the radiotherapy field only)
- Pneumonitis (if a significant volume of the lung is within the radiotherapy field)
- Skin reaction (includes itch, erythema, dry desquamation, but rarely moist desquamation at these lower doses) where the radiotherapy enters or exits the body
- Fatigue which is *independent* of the radiotherapy site and instead related presumably to cytokine release

Late radiotherapy toxicities are rare at these low palliative doses but may be permanent, usually occurring months to years after radiotherapy. Chronic progressive myelopathy is the main late side effect that must be considered. The estimated risk of myelopathy is low (<1%) for the conventional external beam radiotherapy dose schedules described above but may increase with dose-escalated stereotactic radiotherapy schedules (if spinal cord dose is not appropriately avoided) or in re-treatment settings (Kirkpatrick et al. 2010).

12.6 Re-treatment for Recurrent Spinal Cord Compression

Patients should be followed up clinically and/or radiographically to determine whether a local relapse develops. As with the first spinal cord compression diagnosis, prognosis, the probability of neurological recovery, and time to neurological recovery are highly dependent on pretreatment neurological status (Loblaw and Perry 2005). Patients should be considered for surgical decom pression with or without radiotherapy first, because salvage rates seem to be better despite higher complication rates (Patchell et al. 2005). If a patient is not medically and surgically operable, radiotherapy with or without steroids should be given. Consideration needs to be given to the cumulative dosage of the combined radiotherapy courses, and therefore technique of radiotherapy should be chosen to keep the cumulative dose of radiotherapy as low as possible to reduce the risk of myelopathy. Newer radiotherapy techniques such as stereotactic radiotherapy can be used to minimize cord dose (Loblaw and Mitera 2012; Ryu et al. 2010).

13 Systemic Treatments

A detailed explanation of all systemic agents that may be beneficial in patients with malignant spinal cord compression is beyond the scope of this chapter. Systemic agents include cytotoxic chemotherapy, immunotherapy, biological targets, hormonal therapy, and bisphosphonates. Each of these may have a role in different tumor subtypes, depending on the background performance status of the patient, burden of disease, previous systemic therapies received, and likelihood of benefit versus expected toxicities. However, these systemic agents are usually not suitable as primary treatment in the emergency setting for acute malignant spinal cord compression. Instead radiotherapy, surgery, or a combination of both is required.

For certain tumor biologies, the inclusion of systemic agents is of greater importance. In the case of multiple myeloma, although surgery and radiotherapy remain the primary approaches to treat malignant spinal cord compression, systemic therapy such as chemotherapy agents with steroids and either proteasome inhibitors or immunomodulatory drugs, with or without high-dose chemotherapy and stem cell transplantation, works rapidly and can be used instead of radiation in selected patients if there is minimal neurological deficit (Sen and Yavas 2016).

14 Supportive Care

Supportive care of all patients presenting with spinal cord compression is of utmost importance. This includes commencing corticosteroids, appropriate analgesia and aperients, exclusion/management of hypercalcemia, consideration of insertion of an indwelling urinary catheter, attention to pressure care, thromboprophylaxis, and referral to allied health and palliative care services if not already in place. The option of "best supportive care" without the active intervention of surgery and/or radiotherapy should always be considered and discussed with the patient and family if appropriate. Anxiety and depression are common in patients with cancer, and a referral to a psychosocial practitioner should be considered (eviQ Cancer Treatments Online (Cancer Institute NSW) 2012).

15 Conclusion

Spinal cord compression needs to be considered in all patients who have a malignancy and present with new or escalating back pain and/or abnormal neurology. Spinal cord compression is an emergency that must be diagnosed quickly, ideally with an MRI of the whole spine, urgent multidisciplinary input, and management instigated promptly. The best outcomes occur when the degree of premorbid neurological deficit is minimal and the diagnosis and treatment initiated within 24–48 h of presentation. Decompressive surgery with stabilization, followed by radiotherapy, in appropriately selected patients should be considered for best outcomes. Short courses or single fractions of radiotherapy (without surgery) are appropriate for patients with a predicted survival of less than 3 months, particularly if they are ambulant and have radiosensitive disease. Radiotherapy given to patients with very poor prognosis may still improve pain levels and quality of life, despite minimal improvement in neurological function.

References

Baur A, Stabler A, et al. Acute osteoporotic and neoplastic vertebral compression fractures: fluid sign at MR imaging. Radiology. 2002;225:730–5.

Cole J, Patchell R. Review: metastatic epidural spinal cord compression. Lancet Neurol. 2008;7:459–66.

eviQ Cancer Treatments Online (Cancer Institute NSW). Palliative spinal cord compression (SCC) EBRT.

Sydney; 5 July 2012. https://www.eviq.org.au/radiation-oncology/palliative/296-palliative-spinal-cord-compression-scc-ebrt

Faculty of Radiation Oncology. The royal Australian and New Zealand College of Radiologists. "Radiation Oncology – Targeting Cancer." Sydney; 1 Jan 2017. https://www.targetingcancer.com.au/radiation-therapy/ebrt/

George R, Jeba J, Ramkumar G, Chacko A, Tharyan P. Interventions for the treatment of metastatic extradural spinal cord compression in adults. Cochrane Database Syst Rev [1361–6137]. 2015; (9): CD006716–CD006716. https://www.ncbi.nlm.nih.gov/pubmed/26337716

Helwig-Larsen S, Sorensen P. Symptoms and signs in metastatic spinal cord compression: a study from first symptom until diagnosis in 153 patients. Eur J Cancer. 1994;30(A):396–8.

Huo M, Sahgal A, Pryor D, Redmond K, Lo S, Foote M. Stereotactic spine radiosurgery; review of safety and efficacy with respect to dose and fractionation. Surg Neurol Int. 2017;8:30.

Husband D. Malignant spinal cord compression: prospective study of delays in referral and treatment. Br Med J. 1998;317:18–21.

Jung H, Jee W, et al. Discrimination of metastatic from acute osteoporotic compression fractures with MR imaging. Radiographics. 2003;23:179–87.

Kirkpatrick J, van der Kogel A, Schulthesiss T. Radiation dose-volume effects in the spinal cord. Int J Radiat Oncol Biol Phys. 2010;76(3 (Suppl)):S42–9.

Krishnan M, Temel JS, Wright AA, Bernacki R, Selvaggi K, Balboni T. Predicting life expectancy in patients with advanced incurable cancer: a review. J Support Oncol. 2013;11(2):68–74.

Levack P, Graham J, et al. Don't wait for a sensory level – listen to the symptoms: a prospective audit of the delays in diagnosis of malignant cord compression. Clin Oncol. 2002;14:472–80.

Loblaw D, Laperriere N, Mackillop W. A population based study of malignant spinal cord compression in Ontario. Clin Oncol. 2003;14:472–80.

Loblaw A, Perry J, Chambers A, Laperriere N. Systematic review of the diagnosis and management of malignant extradural spinal cord compression: the Cancer Care Ontario Practice Guidelines Initiative's Neuro-Oncology Disease Site Group. J Clin Oncol. 2005; 23(9):2028–37.

Loblaw A, Mitera G, Ford M, Laperriere N. A 2011 updated systematic review and clinical practice guideline for the management of malignant extradural spinal cord compression. Int J Radiat Oncol Biol Phys. 2012;84(2):312–7.

Maranzano E, Bellaviat R, Rossi R, De Angelis V, Frattegiani A, Bagnoli R, et al. Short-course versus split-course radiotherapy in metastatic spinal cord compression: results of a phase III, randomized, multi-centre trial. J Clin Oncol. 2005;23(15):3358–65.

Maranzano E, Trippa F, Casale M, Costantini S, Lupattelli M, Bellavita R, et al. 8Gy single-dose radiotherapy is effective in metastatic spinal cord compression; results of a phase III randomized multicentre Italian trial. Radiother Oncol. 2009;93(2):174–9.

National Institute for Health and Care Excellence (NICE). Metastatic spinal cord compression in adults – quality standard (QS56). London; 1 Feb 2014. https://www.nice.org.uk/guidance/qs56/chapter/quality-statement-3-imaging-and-treatment-plans-for-adults-with-suspected-metastatic-spinal-cord#quality-statement-3-imaging-and-treatment-plans-for-adults-with-suspected-metastatic-spinal-cord

National Institute for Health and Clinical Excellence (NICE). Metastatic spinal cord compression: diagnosis and management of patients at risk of or with metastatic spinal cord compression. Clinical guideline 75. London: NICE; 2008.

Oken M, Creech R, Tormey D, et al. Toxicity and response criteria of the Eastern Cooperative Oncology Group. Am J Clin Oncol. 1982;5:649–55.

Patchell R, Tibbs P, Regine W. Direct decompressive surgical resection in the treatment of spinal cord compression caused by metastatic cancer: a randomised trial. Lancet. 2005;366(9486):643–8.

Quraishi A, Rajagopal T, Manoharan S, Elsayed S, Edwards K, Boszczyk B. Effect of timing of surgery on neurological outcomes and survival in metastatic spinal cord compression. Eur Spine J. 2013;22:1383–8.

Rades D, Heidenreich F, Karstens J. Final results of a prospective study of the prognostic value of the time to develop motor deficits before irradiation in metastatic spinal cord compression. Int J Radiat Oncol Biol Phys. 2002;53:975–9.

RTOG Foundation Inc. Clinical trials RTOG 0631 protocol information. Philadelphia; 2016. https://www.rtog.org/ClinicalTrials/ProtocolTable/StudyDetails.aspx?study=0631

Ryu S, Rock J, Jain R, et al. Radiosurgical decompression of metastatic epidural compression. Cancer. 2010; 116:2250–7.

Sen E, Yavas G. The management of spinal cord compression in multiple myeloma. Ann Hematol Oncol. 2016; 3(5):1090.

Spratt D, Beeler W, de Moraes F, Rhines L, Gemmete J, Chaudhary N, Shultz D, Smith S, Berlin A, Dahele M, Slotman B, Younge K, Bilsky M, Park P, Szerlip N. An integrated multidisciplinary algorithm for the management of spinal metastases: an International Spine Oncology Consortium report. Lancet Oncol. 2017;18:e720–30.

Talcott JA, Stomper PC, Drislane FW, et al. Assessing suspected spinal cord compression: a multidisciplinary outcomes analysis of 342 episodes. Support Care Cancer. 1999;7:31–18.

Superior Vena Cava Obstruction 75

Belinda A. Campbell, John M. Troupis, and Jonathan Langton

Contents

Abstract

In the current era of increased availability and frequency of surveillance imaging for oncology patients, superior vena caval obstruction (SVCO) is often an incidental finding in asymptomatic patients. Less commonly, SVCO may present with advanced symptomatology, and in these cases the SVCO may represent rapid disease progression and/or the first presentation of malignancy. Contrast enhanced computed tomography (CT) is exceptionally useful for the diagnosis of SVCO, and often reveals extrinsic compression by mediastinal lymphadenopathy as the

B. A. Campbell (✉)
Department of Radiation Oncology and Cancer Imaging, Peter MacCallum Cancer Centre, Melbourne, Australia
e-mail: belinda.campbell@petermac.org

J. M. Troupis
Department of Diagnostic Imaging, Monash Health, Clayton, Australia
e-mail: john.troupis@monashhealth.org

J. Langton
Department of Interventional and Diagnostic Imaging, Monash Health, Clayton, Australia
e-mail: jonathan.langton@monashhealth.org

R. D. MacLeod, L. Van den Block (eds.), *Textbook of Palliative Care*,
https://doi.org/10.1007/978-3-319-77740-5_73

more common mechanism for malignant SVCO. Non-small cell and small cell lung cancers constitute the more common histologies, with metastatic mediastinal lymphadenopathy or direct mediastinal invasion causing the SVCO. Radiotherapy is the traditional treatment of choice for patients with SVCO. For patients with severe symptoms, treatment of SVCO constitutes a medical emergency and requires urgent treatment with endovascular stenting to restore patency and produce rapid relief of potentially life-threatening symptoms.

1 Introduction

Superior vena caval obstruction (SVCO) is a changing entity in palliative care and oncology practice. The advent of improved radiological imaging, and its more widespread availability for the follow-up of cancer patients, has meant that SVCO is more frequently detected early while it is still asymptomatic. As such, the severe symptomatology that was not infrequently seen in the past is now a less common phenomenon in modern clinical practice. Nonetheless, left untreated, SVCO has the potential to cause significant symptomatology, undermining quality of life and potentially impacting on patient survival. In this chapter, the etiology, clinical features, radiological features, and management options of SVCO are discussed. For the purposes of this book, this chapter will focus on malignant etiologies of SVCO in the setting of palliative care.

2 Pathophysiology and Etiology

The superior vena cava is the major route for venous return to the heart from the head, arms, and upper torso. Despite the high flow volume, the superior vena cava is a relatively low pressure and thin walled structure that is readily compressible by adjacent masses arising in the superior or middle mediastinum. Slowly progressive SVCO allows for the development of a collateral bloodflow network, with enlargement of alternative draining pathways via the azygous, hemiazygous, intercostal, mediastinal, paravertebral, thoracoepigastric, internal mammary, thoracoacromioclavicular, and anterior chest wall veins. Therefore, in slowly progressive SVCO, this collateral venous network can alleviate the symptom development related to the venous congestion that is seen in more rapid onset SVCO.

SVCO may result from extrinsic or intrinsic luminal narrowing of the superior vena cava. In the current medical era, the most common cause of SVCO is due to luminal occlusion from malignant mediastinal masses (60–85% of cases of SVCO) (Lepper et al. 2011; Straka et al. 2016). However, as the utility of intravascular devices (e.g., catheters, pacemakers) increases, thrombus is an increasingly common, nonmalignant cause of SVCO. Infectious causes (e.g., tertiary syphilis) of SVCO are now rarely seen since the advent of antibiotic therapy.

The more common malignant causes for SVCO include non-small cell lung cancer (22–57%), small cell lung cancer (10–39%), and lymphoma (1–27%) (Straka et al. 2016). In these cases, obstruction may arise from extrinsic compression of the SVC by enlarged mediastinal lymph nodes or by direct invasion into the SVC. Of note, SVCO is the first presentation of malignancy in up to 60% of patients with a malignant SVCO (Lepper et al. 2011).

3 Symptoms and Clinical Features

The clinical features of SVCO are determined by the degree of increased venous pressure in the upper body. Typically, patients present with dyspnea and swelling of the upper body. Elevated venous pressure results in interstitial edema of the head, neck, arms, and upper thorax, and edema of the larynx or pharynx can cause hoarseness, cough, dyspnea, dysphagia, and stridor. On further examination, the jugular veins appear distended. Characteristically, visibly dilated veins are seen on the anterior chest wall, and are noncollapsing above the level of the heart, consistent with the venous distension of collateral

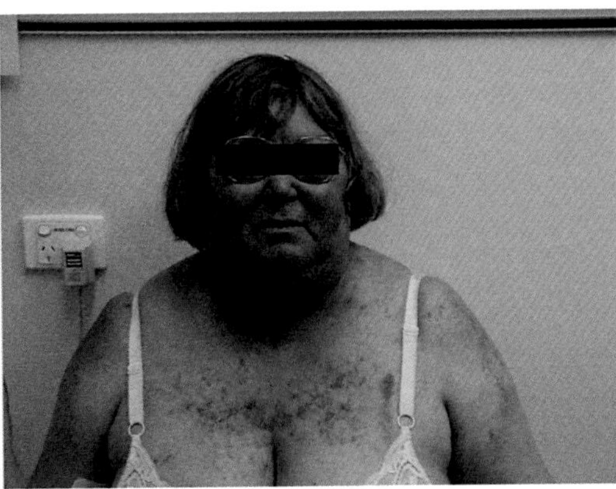

Fig. 1 Clinical photograph of a patient presenting with superior vena cava syndrome secondary to lung cancer with mediastinal lymph node metastases. Note the presence of visibly dilated veins on the anterior chest wall and upper arms, edema of the upper body, facial plethora, and cyanosis (Photograph kindly provided with permission to print by Professor David L. Ball, Peter MacCallum Cancer Centre, Australia)

vessels (Fig. 1). Facial plethora and cyanosis are less commonly presenting signs. Rarely, the patient may present with symptoms of cerebral edema, a serious and life-threatening consequence of SVCO, with headache, confusion, dizziness, and altered conscious state.

As previously mentioned, the severity of symptomatology depends not only on the degree of SVC compression, but also the rate of onset. Slowly progressive SVCO allows for the development of collateral venous channels, and thus the classically recognized symptomatology of SVCO may not be seen. A classification scheme for the grading of SVCO symptomatology was proposed by Yu et al. in 2008 (Table 1), patterned after the Common Terminology Criteria for Adverse Events (CTCAE) v3.0 of the National Institutes of Health (Yu et al. 2008). In this proposed grading system for SVCO, a grade of 0 to 5 is defined based on the severity of signs and symptoms attributable directly or indirectly to the underlying SVCO. An important distinction is the acknowledgment and differentiation of nonsevere, severe, and life-threatening situations. The majority of patients with SVCO are likely to present with mild or moderate symptomatology (75%); the remaining patients are likely to be asymptomatic (10%) or experience severe (10%) life-threatening (5%) or fatal (<1%) symptoms (Yu et al. 2008).

4 Radiological Features

4.1 Anatomy

The superior vena cava (SVC) is responsible for returning blood to the right heart from the upper limbs, neck, and head. It is formed from the confluence of the right and left brachiocephalic veins and drains into the right atrium and courses along the right side of the middle mediastinum, adjacent to the trachea and ascending aorta, which are both to the left. In healthy adults, free of cardiopulmonary disease, it has been assessed with high-resolution electrocardiography (ECG) – gated computed tomography (CT) angiography as measuring between 1.08 and 4.42 cm in cross-sectional area (Lin et al. 2009).

Inferiorly, the azygos vein, which extends from the abdomen, right and anterior to the thoracic vertebrae, inserts into the SVC after passing over the right tracheobronchial angle at the level of the carina. The azygous vein connects with the distal SVC from the posterior aspect.

Further smaller tributaries include esophageal, pericardial, and mediastinal veins (Gray 1918). Most draining veins are connected by smaller plexuses that are normally not well appreciated on routine cross-sectional imaging.

When the SVC is obstructed, the brachiocephalic veins, mediastinal venous plexus, and the tributaries dilate as a means of creating collateral venous circulation.

4.2 Imaging Modalities and Features of SVCO

Imaging modalities vary considerably in their clinical utility for sensitivity and specificity in the diagnosis of SVCO.

4.2.1 Chest X-ray

Chest radiography may demonstrate widening of the upper right mediastinal border suggesting

Table 1 Proposed grading system for superior vena cava syndrome (Yu et al. 2008) (Permission to reprint kindly provided by Elsevier and Dr. Frank Detterbeck, Yale Cancer Center, USA)

Grade	Category	Estimated incidence (%)	Definition[a]
0	Asymptomatic	10	Radiographic superior vena cava obstruction in the absence of symptoms
1	Mild	25	Edema in head or neck (vascular distention), cyanosis, plethora
2	Moderate	50	Edema in head or neck with functional impairment (mild dysphagia, cough, mild or moderate impairment of head, jaw or eyelid movements, visual disturbances caused by ocular edema)
3	Severe	10	Mild or moderate cerebral edema (headache, dizziness) or mild/moderate laryngeal edema or diminished cardiac reserve (syncope after bending)
4	Life-threatening	5	Significant cerebral edema (confusion, obtundation) or significant laryngeal edema (stridor) or significant hemodynamic compromise (syncope without precipitating factors, hypotension, renal insufficiency)
5	Fatal	<1	Death

[a]Each sign or symptom must be thought due to superior vena cava obstruction and the effects of cerebral or laryngeal edema or effects on cardiac function. Symptoms caused by other factors (e.g., vocal cord paralysis, compromise of the tracheobronchial tree, or heart as a result of mass effect) should not be considered as they are due to mass effect on other organs and not superior vena cava obstruction

SVC dilatation or a mediastinal mass. In the setting of a peripherally inserted central catheter (PICC), frontal and lateral radiographs are the primary imaging tools for assessment of the position of the catheter, with the tip expected to be either 85% of the distance from the sternoclavicular junction to the carina or 9 mm above the carina (Dulce et al. 2014).

4.2.2 Ultrasound

Ultrasound (US) may offer indirect evidence of central venous obstruction as direct visualization of the SVC is challenging due to both adjacent lung and bone overlay. Monophasic waveforms or lack of normal respiratory phasicity in the brachiocephalic, internal jugular, or subclavian veins at Doppler US and echocardiography are considered useful indicators for SVCO. Although direct visualization of the SVC is limited, there has been a recognized limited role in the assessment of the proximal SVC by utilizing the suprasternal and right supraclavicular windows (Khouzam et al. 2005).

4.2.3 Computed Tomography (CT)

Computed tomography (CT) imaging without contrast enhancement may demonstrate indirect findings of SVCO such as abnormal PICC or central venous catheter (CVC) position, or calcifications along the SVC that could be caused by calcified thrombi, fibrin sheaths, or retained lead fragments.

Contrast enhanced CT is considered exceptionally useful for the diagnosis of SVCO (Fig. 2). Although dedicated protocols have been developed (Lin et al. 2009; Bae et al. 2008; Kim et al. 2003), the SVC can be assessed both with and without dedicated protocols. Using diluted contrast material combined with optimal vascular window settings may minimize streak artifact. Additional delayed imaging beyond 50 s may be useful when thrombus is a possibility.

There is a high correlation between the CT imaging appearances of SVCO and the presenting clinical symptoms and signs (Plekker et al. 2008). The most commonly visible collateral venous circulation includes the azygous-hemiazygous-accessory hemiazygous system, the vertebral and subscapular plexuses, the mediastinal venous plexus, esophageal venous plexus, diaphragmatic venous plexus, lateral thoracic plexus, and superficial thoracoabdominal venous plexus (Gosselin and Rubin 1997). The appearance on contrast enhanced CT can vary depending on the exact location of the SVCO. If the obstruction is above the azygous arch, antegrade flow from the azygous to the right atrium will be demonstrated. However, if the obstruction is below the arch,

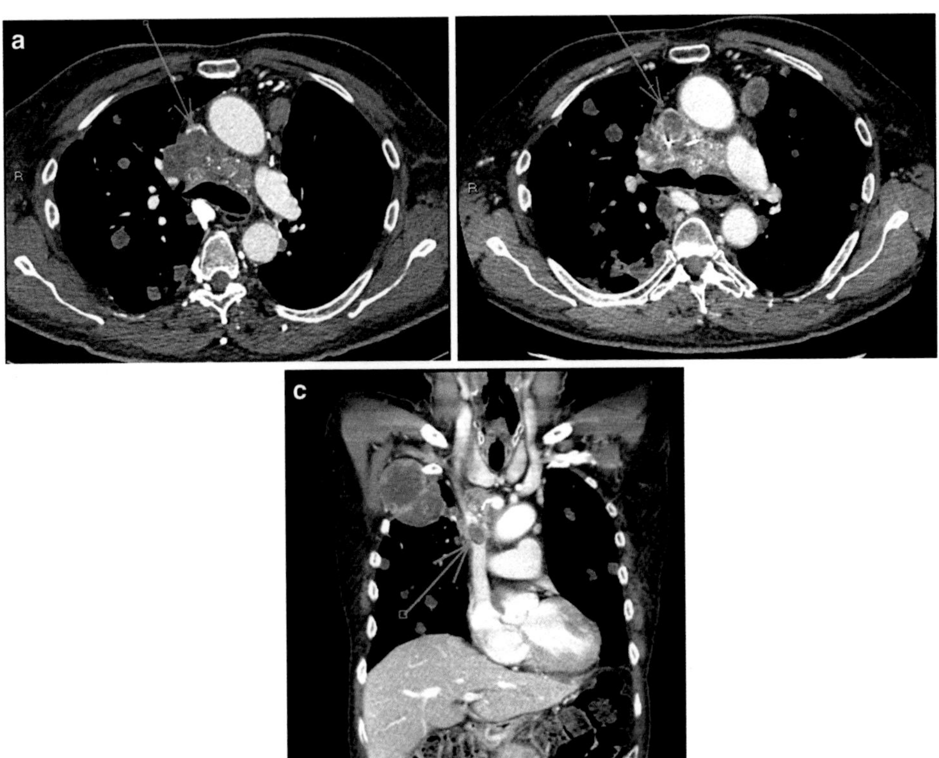

Fig. 2 A 63-year-old male with colorectal carcinoma metastases and SVCO secondary to malignant mediastinal nodal mass. (**a**) Axial image with purple arrow demonstrating an intrinsic filling defect within the central and posterior superior vena cava. (**b**) Axial image slightly more inferiorly than (**a**) with purple arrow demonstrating/highlighting the contrast outlining the tumor. (**c**) Coronal image with purple arrow highlighting the well-demonstrated tumor mass occupying the lumen of the superior vena cava

the entire azygous and hemiazygous veins will be heavily opacified due to the blood re-routing via this pathway to the inferior vena cava (IVC). Further variations may include demonstration of the paravertebral, intervertebral, and epidural veins where blood extends via the ascending lumbar veins to the azygous system. Chest wall and breast collateral veins may also dilate and intensely enhance (Lawler and Fishman 2001), as might abdominal venous collaterals in the abdominal wall or in the liver manifesting as perfusion anomalies.

4.2.4 Magnetic Resonance Venography

MR venography, utilizing Gadolinium-enhanced MR venography (gadobenate deglumine [MultiHance; Bracco Diagnostics, Milan, Italy], 0.1–0.2 mmol/kg), can include static high-resolution first-pass, time-resolved, or steady-state acquisitions (Kim and Merkle 2008). Furthermore, nonenhanced MR venography with three-dimensional (3D) steady-state free precession (SSFP) has been shown to be a useful tool for evaluation of the SVC (Tomasian et al. 2008) .

4.2.5 Radiographic Venography

Venography with the assistance of dynamic radiographic imaging (conventional venography) has numerous advantages for demonstrating strictures including extent and location, with further assessment of collateral pathways, thrombus, and relative functional (partial or complete) obstruction. Conventional venography has the advantage of allowing the procedure to extend into intervention to assist with either alleviation or resolution of the obstruction.

5 Management Options

Management is aimed at alleviating symptoms caused by the SVCO, and also at treating the malignant tumor that is causing the obstruction. Therefore, deciding on the optimal management pathway for SVCO will depend on the severity of the symptoms, the diagnosis of the underlying obstructing tumor, the stage of the malignancy, and the likely responsiveness of the tumor to treatment. Yu et al. published a proposed management algorithm based on these factors (Fig. 3) (Yu et al. 2008). Also to be considered are the previous treatments, comorbidities, and overall prognosis of the patient. Early involvement of the multidisciplinary team is strongly advisable for optimal patient care.

Life-threatening SVCO is uncommon, but notably requires emergency medical management. Positioning the patient in a seated position may help to reduce some of the pressure in the upper half of the body and may provide some degree of symptom relief. Oxygen, diuretics, and corticosteroids are traditional medical treatments that may also be helpful in providing some symptomatic relief in this situation, although there is a paucity of published evidence to support or quantify the benefit of these interventions. In the uncommon situation of stridor and airway compromise, intubation and airway management is required. Radiological imaging, including venogram, is performed to confirm the SVCO, and followed by urgent intravascular stenting that is aimed to achieve rapid relief of the obstruction. If there is associated thrombosis, then anticoagulation and/or direct thrombolysis should also be considered. Of note, SVCO slows venous return from the upper body, and therefore intravenous and intramuscular administration of drugs into the upper limbs should be avoided.

In patients with undiagnosed malignancy and nonemergency SVCO, it is advisable to first organize for prompt tissue biopsy and staging

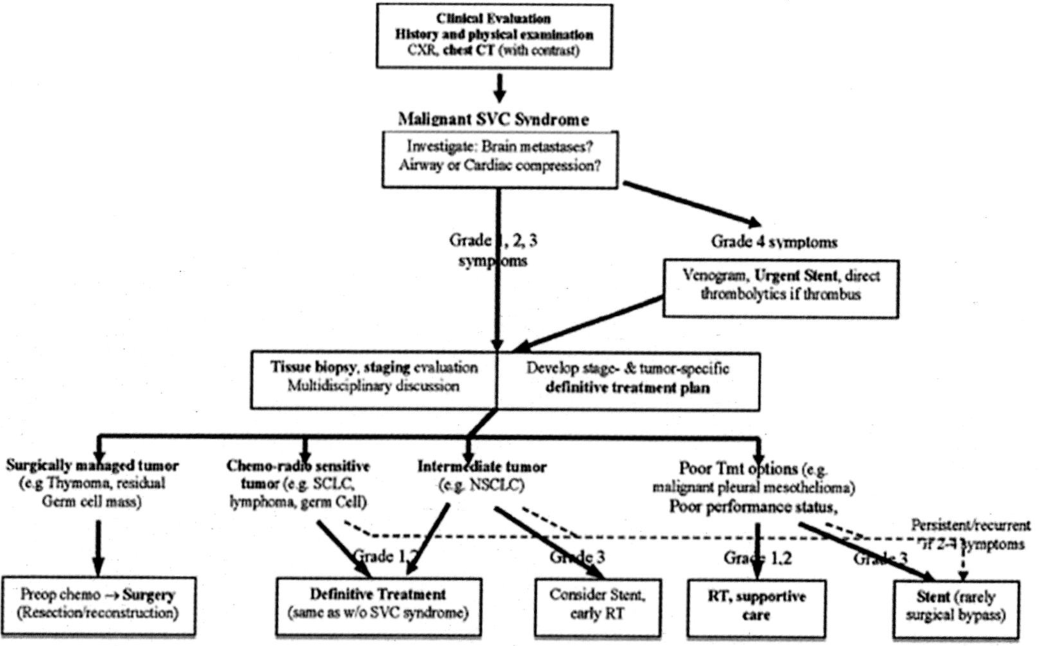

Fig. 3 Proposed management algorithm (Yu et al. 2008) (Permission to reprint kindly provided by Elsevier and Dr. Frank Detterbeck, Yale Cancer Center, USA)

evaluation, as this will allow for optimal management of the underlying tumor. These investigations will be important to determine if the patient is to be treated with curative- or palliative-intent, and will influence the choice of treatment modalities based on the expected responsiveness of the tumor (Fig. 3). Tissue biopsy may be obtained by endoscopic bronchial ultrasound of the mediastinal mass and offers a less invasive alternative to mediastinoscopy. Alternatively, in patients with more disseminated disease, a disease site that is more readily accessible to biopsy may be identified on the staging investigations.

5.1 Choice of Treatment Modality

For malignant causes of SVCO, the two most commonly practiced treatments are endovascular stenting and external beam radiotherapy. Less commonly, chemotherapy may be considered for chemo-sensitive tumors, or surgery may be considered for resectable tumors.

There are several factors to be considered in the choice of treatment modalities for SVCO. For patients with SVCO caused by malignancy, it is generally accepted that radiotherapy achieves a slower onset of response than stenting. Thus, stenting is often considered the treatment of choice for symptomatic patients requiring urgent intervention. For patients with severe SVCO, stenting offers an effective and rapid treatment for the relief of symptoms, with relief of headache occurring virtually immediately, resolution of facial edema within 24 h, and edema of arms and trunk within 72 h (Rowell and Gleeson 2002). Whereas in patients receiving radiotherapy for SVCO, the rapidity of response can generally be expected to take up to 1–2 weeks following treatment. On the other hand, the main advantage of external beam radiotherapy over stenting is that radiotherapy is a noninvasive technique. Unfortunately, there are no published randomized data to reliably compare quality of life outcomes or durability of response, and nonrandomized reports are subject to potential selection bias between the cohorts.

5.2 Role of Endovascular Stenting

5.2.1 Endovascular Stenting: Indications

Acute SVCO secondary to malignancy often responds to external radiation and steroids. However, if the SVCO is complicated by life-threatening symptoms, extensive thrombus, or is refractory to radiotherapy, then catheter-based treatments or surgery should be considered as the treatment of choice. Furthermore, the rapid relief of symptoms achieved by endovascular techniques makes SVCO extremely rewarding to treat. Whenever possible, stent placement should be considered at the onset of clinical symptoms, before the development of a tight stenosis, occlusion, or extensive chronic thrombus (Mauro et al. 2014).

5.2.2 Endovascular Stenting: Technique and Technical Considerations

The primary aim of treatment is to ensure relief of symptoms, which can usually be achieved by restoring inline drainage from one jugular vein to the right atrium (Kaufman and Lee 2004) (Fig. 4). A secondary consideration is the preservation of venous access sites, by minimizing the number of large caval tributaries occluded by stents, preventing future catheterization.

First, thrombus has to be cleared prior to stenting. Techniques to achieve this include the use of local thrombolysis or pharmachomechanical thrombectomy. A plasminogen activator (for example, tPA, rtPA, urokinase) is infused directly into the thrombus (Tzifa et al. 2007). Aspiration techniques and mechanical adjuncts accelerate the process. Low dose anticoagulation therapy is always given simultaneously, usually through a peripheral line.

Stenoses can usually be crossed with relative ease by an interventional radiologist, but more advanced techniques may have to be applied in the setting of occlusion and transmural invasion of the SVC. Combined femoral axillary or bilateral axillary approaches may be required to cross an occlusion (Massmann et al. 2016). The use of stiff

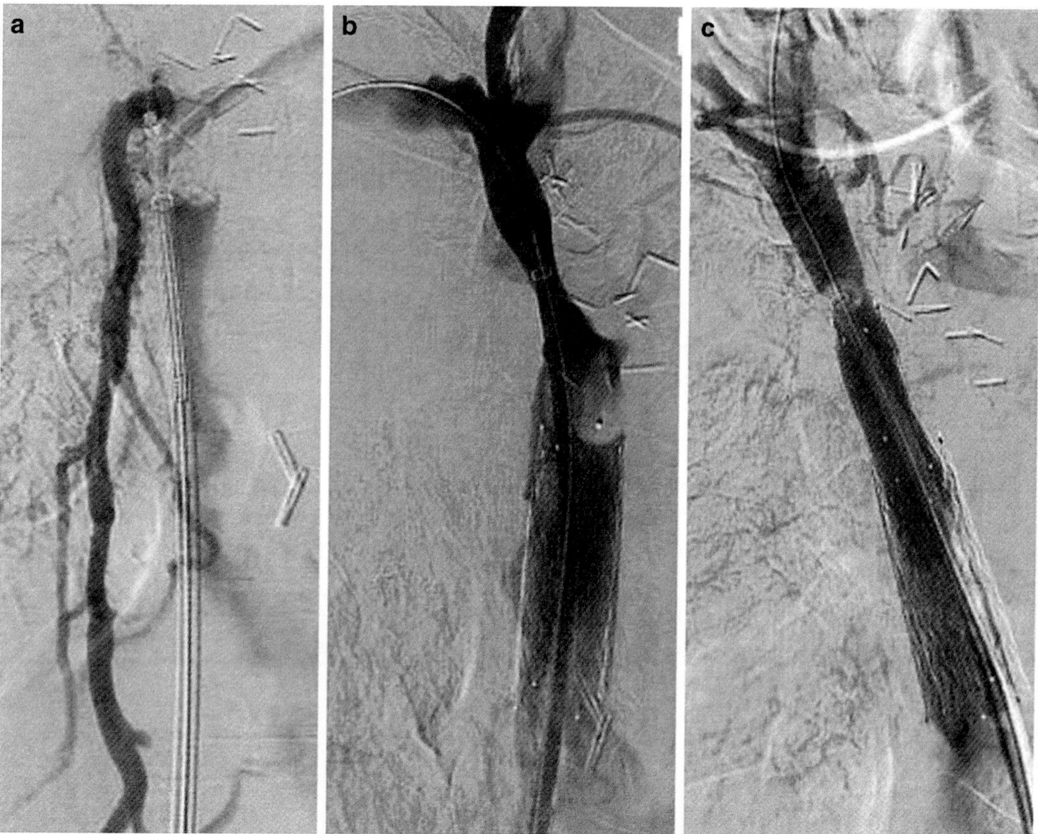

Fig. 4 Sequential stenting of the SVC. (**a**) SVC stenosis with alternate drainage of contrast via the azygos system. (**b**) Initial stent deployed in the distal portion of the SVC, residual filling defects requiring further stenting. (**c**) Inline stenting of the right innominate vein, restoring return of blood from the ipsilateral jugular vein to the right atrium

catheters, and even transjugular intrahepatic portosystemic shunt (TIPS) needles to cross tumor and regain access to the caval system, increases the likelihood of complications and requires careful intraoperative monitoring for cardiac tamponade.

Stent selection is an important aspect of the procedure. Large diameter (10–14 mm) bare metal stents are typically used, except in venous perforation or transmural tumor invasion, where covered stents would be deemed more appropriate (Fig. 5). If stent thrombosis occurs rapidly after placement, then the cause must be determined and treated appropriately with balloon plasty or additional stent placement (Fig. 4), after local thrombolytic therapy.

In cases where immediate and full restoration of flow is achieved across an SVC stenosis, in the absence of thrombus, then heparinization may not be required. Local thrombolysis should be considered in patients with residual thrombi adherent to the stent or vessel wall. It is usual practice to follow heparin therapy with oral anticoagulants for several months, to allow neo-endothelium to cover the stent (Mauro et al. 2014).

5.2.3 Endovascular Stenting: Patient Selection

Patient cooperation during any interventional procedure is imperative. Some patients with severe SVCO syndrome may have difficulty lying flat. If this is the case, then the procedure should be performed under a general anesthetic (Kaufman and Lee 2004).

Stenting of the airway should always precede management of caval obstruction in patients who

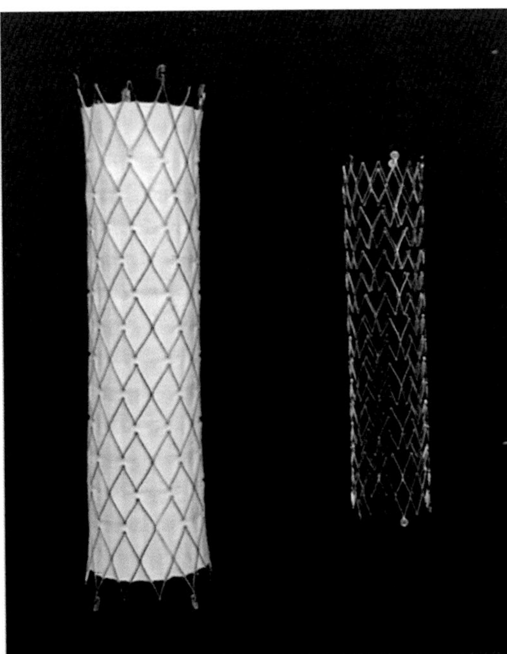

Fig. 5 Covered and uncovered stents. Covered stents are comprised of a fabric, such as polytetrafluoroethylene (PTFE), covering a metal stent (left). Applications for covered stents included sealing iatrogenic perforations or ruptures and exclusion of aneurysms

present with synchronous tracheobronchial narrowing secondary to mediastinal disease burden.

Contraindications to the use of thrombolytic agents include: active bleeding, brain metastases, and intracranial or intraspinal trauma within 2 months. These factors would preclude venous stenting in the setting of extensive venous thrombosis. Other relative contraindications, such as anatomy predisposing to severe technical difficulties, transmural tumor invasion, and advanced disease in preterminal patients, are important to consider. It is also important to note that transmural invasion is not an absolute contraindication, but would require the use of a covered stent.

5.2.4 Endovascular Stenting: Complication Risk

Complications related to venous stenting are relatively few and only seen in 5–7% of procedures (Ganeshan et al. 2009). Usual puncture site complications apply and include: venous thrombosis, arteriovenous fistula, venous pseudoaneurysm, and pneumothorax (jugular punctures). Stent related complications include misplacement or migration, fracture or fragmentation, especially if the stent inadvertently crosses the thoracic outlet. Misplaced stents crossing the thoracic outlet fracture from repeated compression between the clavicle and first rib. Rates of stent infection, bacteremia, and septicemia are minimized with strict aseptic technique. Extremely rare complications include caval perforation and pericardial tamponade.

5.2.5 Endovascular Stenting: Outcomes

In malignant SVC obstruction, the main aim of endovascular stenting is to achieve immediate relief of symptoms. About 68–100% of successful SVC stent deployments result in almost instant complete or significant improvement of symptoms, sustained to a follow-up of 16 months (Mauro et al. 2014). Patients report relief of tension in the face and neck within minutes of stent expansion and restoration of flow in the SVC. Edema in the face and neck resolves after 1–2 days and by day three in the scapula region and upper limbs. There is limited data on long-term patency, but in survivors re-occlusion of the SVC occurs in up to 40% (Mauro et al. 2014; Ganeshan et al. 2009). Previous thrombosis and smaller final stent diameters are associated with the highest rates of re-occlusion (Fagedet et al. 2013).

In conclusion, percutaneous, endovascular stenting of malignant SVCO syndrome offers a high initial success rate and rapid relief of symptoms, avoiding the morbidity associated with invasive surgery. Early detection and endoluminal treatment, before the full symptoms of SVC occlusion develop, are key in facilitating the best patient outcome.

5.3 Role of Palliative Radiotherapy

5.3.1 Radiotherapy: Principles of Treatment

Historically, radiotherapy was the mainstay of management of SVCO due to malignancy, and today remains an important component in the management of nonsevere or asymptomatic SVCO (Yu et al. 2008). Depending on the underlying tumor type and stage, radiotherapy may be delivered with either palliative or curative intent. The primary principles of palliative radiotherapy are to (i) deliver a dose of radiotherapy that is sufficient to adequately de-bulk the tumor to allow for un-occlusion of the SVC and therefore alleviate the symptoms of the SVCO, while (ii) minimizing the potential morbidity from radiotherapy-induced side effects that are more commonly associated with higher doses of radiotherapy. On the other hand, curative-intent radiotherapy involves delivering a higher dose of radiotherapy with the aim of achieving long-term sterilization of the tumor cells, and in this scenario, it is often reasonable to accept a higher risk of acute side-effects as a trade-off for more durable tumor control. In making this decision, it is vital for the clinician to pay careful attention to the relevant patient factors (i.e., comorbidities, performance state, patient wishes) and tumor factors (i.e., histological diagnosis, stage, alternative treatment options). Discussion in a multidisciplinary tumor board meeting is strongly recommended.

5.3.2 Radiotherapy: Efficacy of Treatment

The use of palliative radiotherapy to relieve SVCO has evolved over the preceding decades and is now an established treatment in clinical practice; however, the true efficacy of radiotherapy is not well reported in the literature. Rowell and Gleeson conducted a Cochrane systematic review of the effectiveness of SVCO treatments in patients with lung cancer (Rowell and Gleeson 2002). The investigators discovered that, in general, the included studies failed to define objective criteria for relief of SVCO, had variable definitions of treatment response, and lacked measurements of symptoms or quality of life (Rowell and Gleeson 2002). Considering these limitations, the authors of the systematic review reported that the response rate to radiotherapy was 94% in patients with no prior treatment for lung cancer, versus 74% in patients who had previously received treatment for lung cancer (Rowell and Gleeson 2002). The effectiveness of radiotherapy for SVCO did not appear to be related to any particular radiotherapy fractionation regimen (Rowell and Gleeson 2002).

5.3.3 Radiotherapy: Treatment Dose and Delivery

For palliative patients, external beam radiotherapy offers a noninvasive treatment option for the management of SVCO caused by malignancy (Fig. 6a and b). Depending on the patient's symptoms and performance state, radiotherapy may be delivered as an outpatient or an inpatient. In general, palliative courses of hypofractionated radiotherapy are delivered in daily fractions, 5 days per week, over 1–3 weeks. Standard fractionation schedules for the palliative treatment of SVCO include 20 Gy in five fractions (20Gy/5F) delivered over 1 week, 30 Gy in 10 fractions (30Gy/10F) delivered over 2 weeks, or 36 Gy in 12 fractions (36Gy/12F) delivered over 2½ weeks. Higher dose radiotherapy fractionation schedules may be considered for patients who are expected to have longer life expectancies, as it is thought that higher dose of radiotherapy may achieve more durable local disease control and reduce the risk of SVCO recurrence. This includes patients with good performance state, limited burden of disease, and with tumor histologies that are known to have a more indolent pattern of behavior. For patients who are suitable for curative-intent treatment, high doses of radiotherapy are often required for disease eradication; for example, for patients with non-small lung cancer who are suitable for curative-intent radiotherapy are usually treated to 60Gy in 30 fractions over 6 weeks, with concurrent radiosensitizing chemotherapy to further improve tumor control.

5.3.4 Radiotherapy: Side Effects of Treatment

As a noninvasive and localized treatment modality, external beam radiotherapy offers a generally well-tolerated treatment for palliative patients with SVCO. Common, acute side effects include localized esophagitis, localized skin erythema, and fatigue. In patients receiving higher dose

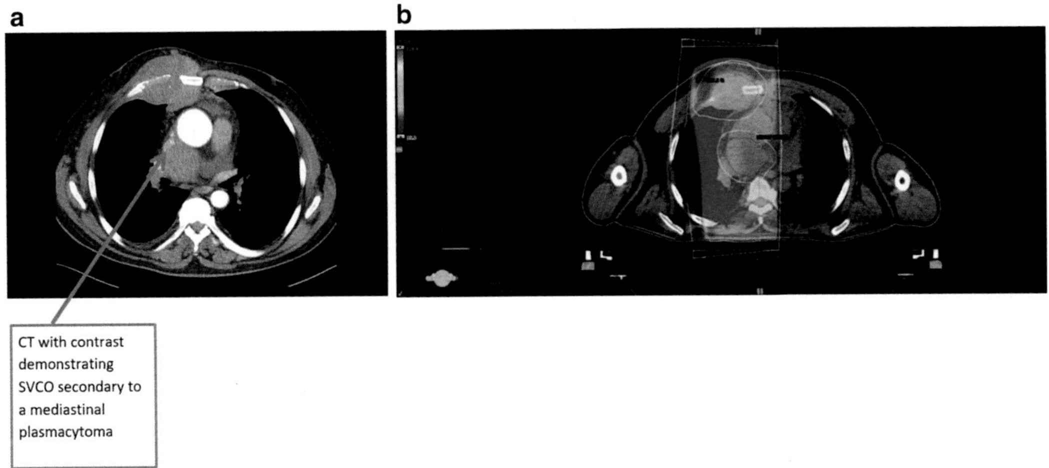

Fig. 6 Palliative radiotherapy to treat an asymptomatic SVCO caused by a mediastinal, extraosseous plasmacytoma in a patient with known chemo-refractory multiple myeloma (a rare cause of SVCO). Durable symptom control was obtained in these sites following radiotherapy; the patient succumbed to multiple myeloma 5 months later. (**a**) CT with contrast demonstrated the incidental finding of the asymptomatic SVCO, secondary to an extraosseous plasmacytoma in the mediastinum. This CT scan was originally performed to investigate the patient's anterior chest wall pain and deformity, caused by a large osseous plasmacytoma of the rib. (**b**) Dosimetry for the palliative radiotherapy plan to treat the symptomatic rib plasmacytoma and the asymptomatic mediastinal plasmacytoma causing the SVCO. The gross tumor volume is marked in red, and the planning target volume is marked in pale blue. The patient was treated with parallel-opposed 6MV photon beams, to a total dose of 20 Gy in 5 fractions, delivered over 5 consecutive days

fractionation schedules, the severity of these symptoms increases and patients may require analgesia and a soft food diet to manage the esophagitis. These acute side effects frequently peak in intensity approximately 10 days after completion of treatment.

For patients being treated with curative-intent radiotherapy, the longer-term toxicity profile must also be considered. Subacute side effects include risk of radiation pneumonitis, which characteristically presents approximately 3–6 months after radiotherapy, with symptoms of cough, fever, and breathlessness, and is best managed via early intervention with a short course of oral steroid therapy. Radiation pericarditis is a less commonly seen subacute side effect following radiotherapy for upper mediastinal tumors, but is also best treated early with oral steroid therapy. In cancer patients treated with curative-intent radiotherapy, long-term toxicity risks from thoracic radiotherapy may also include pulmonary fibrosis, esophageal stricture, spinal cord myelopathy (rare), and radiation-induced second malignancy (rare).

5.4 Role of Chemotherapy

Less commonly, SVCO may be caused by chemosensitive malignancies. These include small-cell lung cancer, mediastinal lymphomas, and mediastinal germ-cell tumors. These tumors usually respond well to appropriate chemotherapy regimens and symptoms of SVCO are quickly relieved. Depending on both patient and tumor factors, chemotherapy may be delivered with either curative or palliative intent; therefore, careful tumor staging and discussion in a multidisciplinary meeting is recommended prior to embarking on treatment.

6 Conclusion

SVCO is a changing entity in modern medical practice. In the current era, malignancy is the most common cause of SVCO; however, it is often detected while the patient is still asymptomatic. This is due to the increasing availability and sensitivity of medical imaging modalities and the increasing frequency of imaging in the follow-up of oncology patients; as such, patients rarely present with life-threatening symptoms of SVCO. It is recommended that all oncology patients with SVCO are discussed in a multidisciplinary meeting with review of the available imaging and pathology, prior to treatment. The optimal selection of medical treatment will depend on the severity of symptoms caused by the SVCO, the etiology of the obstructing lesion, the histology of the underlying malignant process, the stage of the disease, response to previous treatments, and patient comorbidities and performance state. The more frequently used treatment modalities include endovascular stenting and external beam radiotherapy, with chemotherapy and surgery having less common roles. In the uncommon scenario of severe or life-threatening SVCO, urgent endovascular stenting is the treatment of choice for rapid relief of symptoms from obstructing lesions.

References

Bae KT, et al. Contrast enhancement in cardiovascular MDCT: effect of body weight, height, body surface area, body mass index, and obesity. AJR Am J Roentgenol. 2008;190(3):777–84.

Dulce M, et al. Topographic analysis and evaluation of anatomical landmarks for placement of central venous catheters based on conventional chest X-ray and computed tomography. Br J Anaesth. 2014;112(2):265–71.

Fagedet D, et al. Endovascular treatment of malignant superior vena cava syndrome: results and predictive factors of clinical efficacy. Cardiovasc Intervent Radiol. 2013;36(1):140–9.

Ganeshan A, et al. Superior vena caval stenting for SVC obstruction: current status. Eur J Radiol. 2009; 71(2):343–9.

Gosselin MV, Rubin GD. Altered intravascular contrast material flow dynamics: clues for refining thoracic CT diagnosis. AJR Am J Roentgenol. 1997;169(6):1597–603.

Gray H. Gray's anatomy of the human body. Philadelphia: Lea & Febiger; 1918.

Kaufman J, Lee M. Vascular and Interventional Radiology: The Requisites. Requisites series. 2nd ed. Philadelphia: Elsevier Saunders; 2014.

Khouzam RN, Minderman D, D'Cruz IA. Echocardiography of the superior vena cava. Clin Cardiol. 2005; 28(8):362–6.

Kim CY, Merkle EM. Time-resolved MR angiography of the central veins of the chest. AJR Am J Roentgenol. 2008;191(5):1581–8.

Kim H, et al. Role of CT venography in the diagnosis and treatment of benign thoracic central venous obstruction. Korean J Radiol. 2003;4(3):146–52.

Lawler LP, Fishman EK. Pericardial varices: depiction on three-dimensional CT angiography. AJR Am J Roentgenol. 2001;177(1):202–4.

Lepper PM, et al. Superior vena cava syndrome in thoracic malignancies. Respir Care. 2011;56(5):653–66.

Lin FY, et al. The right sided great vessels by cardiac multidetector computed tomography: normative reference values among healthy adults free of cardiopulmonary disease, hypertension, and obesity. Acad Radiol. 2009;16(8):981–7.

Massmann A, et al. A wire transposition technique for recanalization of chronic complex central venous occlusions. Phlebology. 2016;31(1):57–60.

Mauro M, et al. Image-guided interventions. Expert radiology series. 2nd ed. Philadelphia: Elsevier Saunders; 2014.

Plekker D, et al. Clinical and radiological grading of superior vena cava obstruction. Respiration. 2008; 76(1):69–75.

Rowell NP, Gleeson FV. Steroids, radiotherapy, chemotherapy and stents for superior vena caval obstruction in carcinoma of the bronchus: a systematic review. Clin Oncol (R Coll Radiol). 2002;14(5):338–51.

Straka C, et al. Review of evolving etiologies, implications and treatment strategies for the superior vena cava syndrome. Spring. 2016;5:229.

Tomasian A, et al. Noncontrast 3D steady state free precession magnetic resonance angiography of the thoracic central veins using nonselective radiofrequency excitation over a large field of view: initial experience. Investig Radiol. 2008;43(5):306–13.

Tzifa A, et al. Endovascular treatment for superior vena cava occlusion or obstruction in a pediatric and young adult population: a 22-year experience. J Am Coll Cardiol. 2007;49(9):1003–9.

Yu JB, Wilson LD, Detterbeck FC. Superior vena cava syndrome–a proposed classification system and algorithm for management. J Thorac Oncol. 2008; 3(8):811–4.

Acute Cancer Pain Syndromes in Palliative Care Emergencies

76

Sophia Lam, Leeroy William, and Peter Poon

Contents

Abstract

Acute pain syndromes in palliative care are predominantly malignant in origin. These are often emergencies due to the severity of the pain, its meaning to the patient, the disruption of ongoing curative treatment, and the resultant erosion of quality of life. A prompt accurate pain assessment is a vital component of clinical management, followed by analgesic intervention and attention to the physical, psychological, social, and spiritual aspects of pain. Clinicians should develop excellent communication skills to support patients,

S. Lam (✉)
Department of Medicine, Cairns and Hinterland Hospital and Health Service, Cairns, QLD, Australia
e-mail: sophia.lam@health.qld.gov.au

L. William
Palliative Medicine, Monash Health, Eastern Health, Monash University, Melbourne, VIC, Australia
e-mail: leeroy.william@monash.edu

P. Poon
Supportive and Palliative Medicine, Monash Health, Eastern Palliative Care, Monash University, Clayton, VIC, Australia
e-mail: peter.poon@monash.edu

R. D. MacLeod, L. Van den Block (eds.), *Textbook of Palliative Care*,
https://doi.org/10.1007/978-3-319-77740-5_79

their families, and also other healthcare professionals in the delivery of optimal care. Pain will not always be managed according to the expectations of others, and so how we deliver care and explain the limitations of treatment is important.

Acute cancer pain that is not managed well can become chronic in nature. The development of chronic pain can greatly reduce the functional ability and mood of patients over time. As with all symptoms, managing the acute presentation should lead to an investigation of causative factors, mechanism of pain, and potential therapeutic interventions. Acute pain syndromes can be approached via two causative mechanisms: treatment-related pain and pain directly related to the cancer process. A multimodal and multidisciplinary approach to treatment is often required to not only help the patient, but also to support the family during an uncertain and unsettling period of care.

1 Introduction

The symptom of pain is likely to occur in 20–50% of people with cancer (Fischer et al. 2010), at multiple sites (Gutgsell et al. 2003), and for those with advanced disease about 80% will have moderate to severe pain (Bruera and Kim 2003). The negative impact of pain on functional status and quality of life (Kroenke et al. 2010; Porter and Keefe 2011) has driven efforts to improve pain management over a number of decades. A systemic review of the literature, covering the period between September 2005 and January 2014, aimed to look at pain prevalence and pain severity. Unfortunately, it revealed that cancer pain is still poorly controlled with a prevalence of 39.3% following curative treatment; 55% in people undergoing anticancer treatment; and 66.4% in people with advanced, metastatic, or terminal disease. Moderate to severe pain scores were also found in 38.0% of all patients (van den Beuken-van and Hochstenbach 2016).

Even the promotion of "pain as the fifth vital sign" by the American Pain Society in 1995 and its focus upon the numerical pain scale (NRS) has been questioned. The idea was to raise the awareness of pain as a priority healthcare issue; however, the campaign may have inadvertently contributed to the current opioid epidemic in the USA (Levy et al. 2018). Pain therefore remains a feared symptom by patients and their families, and adequate pain management is affected by barriers that are patient-related (e.g., reluctance to report pain and poor compliance to analgesics); clinician-related (e.g., insufficient knowledge of cancer pain management, and inadequate pain assessment skills); and societal-related (e.g., opiophobia and the stigma of opioid addiction) (Cipta et al. 2015; Pargeon and Hailey 1999).

The particular significance of pain, and the fear that accompanies it, in people with cancer should not be underestimated. Increasing pain is often perceived to be associated with progressive disease, or a shorter prognosis. Many patients choose to defer the use of regular opioids for a time in the future when they believe the pain will become more severe, or when they are closer to death. They also fear addiction to opioids and how opioids will affect their lives. Importantly, the resistance to adequate analgesia can be a barrier to ongoing curative treatment, causing breaks in therapy. Treatment breaks are common in cancer therapy, due to disease progression or toxicity from therapy, e.g., mucositis, radiation enteritis, or neutropenic sepsis. Pain may also coexist, adding to the picture of a more debilitated patient. Without the adequate assessment and treatment of pain, clinicians may assume that disease progression or treatment toxicity is responsible for functional deterioration and reduced quality of life. Hence, treatment may be modified in strength or even ceased under a false perception of deterioration. On the other hand, explaining this possible curtailment of oncological treatment can often motivate patients to accept and comply with prescribed analgesia.

Palliative care utilizes the concept of total pain, i.e., that pain is comprised of physical, psychological, social, and spiritual components. Therefore, the optimal management of pain addresses all these domains and promotes a multidisciplinary team approach. It is also important to plan for potential pain crises, via the use of breakthrough pain medications and supportive care plans. These considerations allow patients to have control and manage their pain while living their lives.

In this chapter, we aim to cover the management of acute cancer pain syndromes from the perspective of a palliative care emergency. Acute noncancer pain syndromes and chronic pain syndromes are not discussed here, as they would usually be managed by acute pain and chronic pain services, respectively. Palliative care services still predominantly see cancer patients, who invariably present with cancer pain. We will discuss the rapid assessment of patients and timely interventions for stabilization, alongside the holistic approach to care. Acute cancer pain syndromes will then be discussed considering the underlying cause of the pain. Firstly, pain caused by the treatment of the cancer, and then secondly the pain caused directly by the cancer itself.

2 Acute Cancer Pain Syndromes

2.1 Definitions

The classification of acute pain was recently reviewed by an expert panel involving the Analgesic, Anesthetic, and Addiction Clinical Trial Translations, Innovations, Opportunities, and Networks (ACTTION), American Pain Society (APS), and American Academy of Pain Medicine (AAPM). A multidimensional approach has now been adopted to the new definition (Kent et al. 2017):

"Acute pain is the physiological response to and experience of noxious stimuli that can become pathological, is normally sudden in onset, time limited, and motivates behaviours to avoid potential or actual tissue injury."

Acute pain can last up to 7 days, but may be prolonged to 30 days, and the duration is indicative of the mechanisms and severity of the causative process. Subacute pain has been defined by acute pain prolonged beyond 30 days, but less than 90 days (Kent et al. 2017). Although acute pain plays an important protective role in our recovery from an insult, it should be managed promptly to prevent neuronal remodeling and sensitization that commonly occurs in cancer and lead to chronic pain (Carr and Goudas 1999).

Chronic pain usually persists for more than 3–6 months and involves permanent or persistent tissue damage, alongside potential behavioral changes in coping with the pain and daily activities. There may be acute episodes of pain on a background of chronic pain, but treatment targeted at the underlying disease process can help both acute flares of pain as well as the baseline chronic pain.

Cancer pain has become more chronic in nature due to the successes of cancer therapies. Patients are living longer with their malignancies, contributing to an increasing chronicity of pain due to the cancer itself or as part of survivorship. However, acute events may increase pain, e.g., fractures, hemorrhages, and plexopathies. Furthermore, acute pain may occur from treatment of the cancer, e.g., peripheral neuropathy, mucositis, and radiotherapy.

3 General Cancer Pain Management

The World Health Organization (WHO) Analgesic Ladder has underpinned cancer pain management since 1986, and involves three steps in dealing with mild, moderate, and severe pain. Using the visual analogue scale (VAS), a mild pain equates to a score of 1–2/10, a moderate pain 3–6/10, and a severe pain 7–10/10. The first step involves the use of nonopioids, e.g., paracetamol and NSAIDs; the second step adds in weak opioids if the pain is not controlled, e.g., codeine, dihydrocodeine, and tramadol; and similarly, the third step involves the addition of strong opioids, e.g., morphine, fentanyl, and methadone. Adjuvant analgesics may be used at any time (WHO 1987). Over the years, the WHO ladder has been found to provide adequate analgesia for 45–100% of people with cancer pain (Azevedo et al. 2006). However, criticisms of the WHO ladder do exist, e.g. the second step is perhaps redundant due to the severity of cancer pain (Vadalouca et al. 2008);

the approach used does not evaluate the cause of the pain to guide analgesia (Ashby et al. 1992); and a modified version has included a fourth step to redress the omission of interventional analgesia (Vadalouca et al. 2008; Vargas-Schaffer 2010). Finally, the total pain approach promotes the nonpharmacological and multidisciplinary benefits to managing pain, in addition to the WHO ladder. These options should not be forgotten, even in the trying to control acute pain. Reassurance and support for patients in a pain crisis, as well as their families, can help until the analgesia becomes effective.

A pain assessment should include a review of the pain to explore the following: intensity, location, quality, interference on quality of life, emotional component of the pain, temporal pattern, treatments, duration, pain beliefs, pain history, exacerbating, and relieving factors (Hølen et al. 2006). Consideration of the mechanism of pain, as per Ashby et al., is essential and if used to determine the choice of first line analgesia may also prevent a delay of adequate pain control (Ashby et al. 1992). Nociceptive pain involves injury to somatic and visceral structures. Somatic pain affects the skin (superficial or cutaneous somatic pain) and other deeper structures, e.g., bone, muscle, and tendons (deep somatic pain). Visceral pain is seen in internal organs, e.g., lungs, liver, bowel, and heart). Neuropathic pain may be due to nerve compression or nerve injury (affecting central nerves, peripheral nerves, or sympathetically maintained nerves). Although pain may be nociceptive or neuropathic, in many malignant cases, a mixed picture with moderate to severe pain is common in clinical practice. Hence, the use of the WHO ladder in cancer pain may result in a delay in adequate pain control, due to the sequential step process (Maltoni et al. 2005; Forbes 2011).

Acute pain in the emergency setting, outside of palliative care, may involve intravenous morphine or fentanyl protocols that use small doses of opioid titrated to the pain, with frequent reviews to monitor for toxicity. Sedation and respiratory rate are carefully reviewed during the titration process, with the use of naloxone to counter opioid overdose. However, in a palliative care setting, subcutaneous opioids are usually titrated to effect as they provide a lower peak concentration and longer duration of action compared with intravenous delivery. Subsequently, naloxone is rarely required, but if needed small doses are used to avoid reversing analgesia. The appropriate team should manage nonmalignant causes of the acute pain, e.g., a nonmalignant fracture may require orthopedic surgery, and the perioperative analgesia would be best managed by the acute pain service. In these instances, a collaborative working relationship facilitates a smooth transition between acute interventions and palliative care for the patient. Postoperatively, the acute pain team can handover care to palliative care services where appropriate.

If patients are opioid-naïve on presentation with acute pain, opioids can be titrated using regular small doses as required. In some instances, the pain may be unresponsive to opioids, or partially opioid responsive, e.g., colicky abdominal pain from malignant bowel obstruction, or pathological fractures, hence the importance to consider the mechanism of pain. In these cases, adjuvants may be useful to achieve pain control, e.g., hyoscine butylbromide for colicky abdominal pain, and steroids or NSAIDs for pathological fractures. Interventional adjuvants may also be appropriate, and sometimes the optimal management, but require time to organize, e.g., orthopedic management of pathological fractures, stenting of mechanical bowel obstructions, or radiotherapy for bone metastases. For patients who are not opioid-naïve, the management requires a different approach. There are few consensus guidelines for acute cancer pain management in this scenario; however, a recent eight-step approach has been suggested (Fadul and Elsayem 2016):

1. Assessment of the pain syndrome, including pain location, severity, onset, and exacerbating and relieving factors
2. Holistic assessment of factors potentially affecting the pain
3. Calculate the total morphine-equivalent daily dose (MEDD)

4. Prescribe 10–15% of the MEDD as the rescue dose
5. Assessment of the pain response within 15 min of giving the first analgesic rescue dose. Dose can be repeated if pain relief is not satisfactory
6. Assessment of the functional ability of the patient, correlated with pain
7. Adjustment of the basal opioid dose either by adding the rescue doses needed over the past 24 h or an incremental increase by 30%
8. For patients whose pain is refractory to these initial steps, prompt consultation with pain or palliative care experts, if available, is recommended

There are further options in management provided by the expertise of the specialists involved in step 8. These may include the commencement of patient-controlled analgesia (PCA), continuous subcutaneous infusions (CSCI), or opioid rotations with the introduction of co-analgesics specific to the pain mechanism, as discussed above. In an older study, Mercadante et al. used the titration of morphine 2 mg intravenously every 2 min to effectively manage acute, severe cancer pain in less than 10 min for palliative care patients. Once control was achieved, conversion to oral morphine was possible (Mercadante et al. 2002). For patients with large background opioid doses, the use of ketamine may be useful due to its antiinflammatory effects and reduction of central sensitization (Matthews et al. 2018). As mentioned earlier, the other elements of multidisciplinary care should not be forgotten, as the patient-centered approach is likely to provide most benefit to the patient (Luckett et al. 2013).

There are well-described cancer pain syndromes that can cause acute pain. These can be divided into those induced by treatment and those related to disease (Portenoy and Lesage 1999).

4 Treatment-Induced Acute Pain Syndromes

Treatment-induced acute pain syndromes can be broadly divided into those arising from:

1. Diagnostic and therapeutic procedures
2. Surgical management
3. Chemotherapy, hormonal therapy, and immunotherapy
4. Radiation therapy
5. Mucositis

4.1 Acute Pain due to Diagnostic and Therapeutic Procedures

(a) Thoracocentesis and pleurodesis are therapeutic procedures for the palliative management of breathlessness due to malignant pleural effusion. Thoracocentesis can also be a diagnostic and recurrent procedure. Access to the pleural space is gained via a large bore tube to remove fluid. Pleurodesis involves the chemical or mechanical induction of pleural inflammation to adhere the visceral and parietal pleura, thereby eliminating the space for air of fluid to accumulate. The procedure is better for recurrent malignant pleural effusions and is attempted days after a thoracocentesis has completely drained the effusion. Talc is the most common agent used in pleurodesis. Both tube insertion and pleurodesis are acutely painful processes due to surgical skin incision and pleural irritation but involve local anesthetic during the procedure. Such pain can subsequently be managed with opioid and NSAIDs analgesics (Rahman et al. 2015).

(b) Lumbar punctures are frequently performed for diagnostic purposes and as a means of delivering therapeutic treatment. Headache is a common post procedural occurrence. Supine position, hydration, simple analgesia, opioids and antiemetics are used for management of mild to moderate symptoms. Rarer and with more severe consequences are spinal subdural hematomas, presenting with severe low back pain, radicular pain, sensory loss, or paraparesis in the hours or days post-lumbar puncture. Management options include blood patch, epidural saline, epidural dextra 40, and oral and intravenous caffeine. Decompressive laminectomy may be required (Ahmed et al. 2006).

(c) Embolization is an endoluminal procedure used to occlude a vessel for therapeutic benefit. There is a plethora of possible sites for intervention and a number of agents used; consequently, a wide spectrum of side effects and complications exist (Bilbao et al. 2006). Transarterial chemo embolization (TACE) is useful in the palliative management of primary hepatocellular cancer and less commonly in hepatic metastases from neuroendocrine or gastrointestinal malignancies. A common (up to 86%) Post-embolization Syndrome (PES) of fever, right hypochondrium pain, nausea, vomiting, and a rise in transaminases can occur 48–72 h post procedure and is felt to be due to a combination of liver capsule distension and parenchymal necrosis. Treatment is symptomatic, with steroids reserved for severe cases (Rammohan et al. 2012).

(d) Percutaneous nephrostomy tube insertion is a frequently performed procedure to relieve urinary obstruction. Major complication rates are low but vary depending on size of catheter introduced (large is 28F–30F), approach (subcostal vs. intercostal), and amount of intrarenal manipulation required (Hart and Ryu 2002). Mild peritube insertion nociceptive pain is to be expected in the immediate postoperative period with use of anxiolytics and local anesthesia at time of insertion, and simple opioid analgesia post insertion. Occurrence of more severe complications such as periorgan (bowel, spleen, liver) damage, infection, and abscess formation can result in more intense pain, requiring surgical intervention, intravenous antibiotics, and strong opioids.

4.2 Surgical Management: Acute Postoperative Pain

Curative and diagnostic surgical intervention is common in the management of cancer. Acute pain is an expected part of the postoperative experience in these procedures that remove affected primary sites of malignancy. Untreated or undertreated pain can lead to persistent pain in up to 50% of individuals, up to 20% of whom will have severe chronic pain or development of chronic postsurgical pain syndromes (Wu and Raja 2011). Acute postsurgical pain is nociceptive in nature from skin, soft tissue, and muscle interruption and/or neuropathic from nerve damage. Severity and presentation depends on location and extent of surgery. Effective management to prevent the long-term sequelae of a chronic pain syndrome usually requires a multimodal, multidisciplinary approach in the perioperative period.

(a) Acute postmastectomy pain

Acute postmastectomy pain is usually due to intercostal brachial nerve injury. Injury to this nerve is almost unavoidable if axillary dissection is required, although some approaches can minimize the sensory symptoms. Pain can present acutely or up to 6 months post procedure, as a neuropathic pain distributed across the medial upper arm, axilla, and anterior chest wall. A combination of intra- and perioperative analgesic interventions can minimize progression to a chronic pain syndrome. Intraoperative techniques which result in better pain outcomes are: minimizing surgical trauma, nerve preservation, and minimally invasive staging techniques leading to less axillary dissection. Perioperative pain management that reduces severity and duration of acute pain involves use of multireceptor analgesic agents (NSAIDs, neuropathic agents, opioids, and NMDA receptor antagonists) as well as recognizing and addressing psychological distress earlier.

(b) Thoracotomy pain

Thoracotomy is associated with a high risk of severe and long-lasting acute postoperative pain. Pain is due to intercostal nerve injury during rib separation with or without rib resection. It presents as an aching sensation along the incision and can be associated with sensory and autonomic changes. Persistence of this pain beyond 2 months is termed the Post-thoracotomy Pain Syndrome (PTPS). Multimodal peri- and intraoperative analgesia is recommended for acute pain management. This includes the use of regional anesthesia and intravenous ketamine postoperatively. Regional anesthesia techniques employed are mostly thoracic epidural anesthesia (TEA), thoracic paravertebral block, and secondarily, pleural infusion or intercostal nerves block. A mixture of opioids and local anesthetic agents are used. Ketamine preoperatively as an epidural and intravenous intra- and postoperatively appears to lessen the nociceptive process causing severe pain (Della Corte et al. 2012).

(c) Acute postnephrectomy pain

Acute postnephrectomy pain is primarily nociceptive from tissue damage with some contribution from parietal and nerve damage. The symptoms are aching deep back pain and incision pain on mobility, which relate to the pathophysiology is of tissue inflammation, spinal pain mechanism activation, and reflexive muscle spasm. Laparoscopic approaches can cause neuropathic pain due to trochar injury to neural structures. Severe postoperative pain and neuropathic pain are associated with the development of a chronic postoperative pain syndrome (Oefelein and Bayazit 2003).

(d) Limb amputation pain

Limb amputation is always followed phenomena associated with the missing body part. Two of the well-described syndromes can present with acute pain; stump pain and phantom pain. Both are common, arising in over 50% of cases. Stump pain occurs in the immediate postsurgery phase and is the acute nociceptive pain arising from the site of tissue injury. It usually resolves within a few weeks and is managed with simple analgesia and opioids. Phantom pain most commonly presents within a few weeks of amputation, but onset can be delayed for up to years. It is described in multiple terms such as shooting, burning, cramping, and aching, characteristically located at the distal end of the affected limb. The precise pathophysiology is unknown, but postulated theories all describe abnormal sensory processing although at different levels. In the absence of well-studied effective management, a multidisciplinary, multimodal approach to treatment is advisable. There is some evidence but not enough to support the use of preoperative epidural pain relief. Short-term postoperative pain control has been shown to be achievable with the use of strong opioids, sciatic, or posterior tibial nerve blocks intra- or postoperatively; intravenous salmon calcitonin; and transcutaneous electrical nerve stimulation TENS. No trials were able to show improvement in the long-term outcome of preventing phantom limb pain (Jackson and Simpson 2004).

4.3 Acute Pain due to Chemotherapy, Immunotherapy, and Hormonal Therapy

There are numerous acute pain syndromes caused by treatment with chemotherapy, immunotherapy, hormonal therapy, and growth factors. There are those associated with infusion technique; those due to specific drugs; and those due to drug toxicity. Most are self-limiting and ameliorated with slowing infusion rates, dose reductions, or drug cessation. Patient education prior to initiation of the causative cytoreductive agent allows early recognition of the acute pain syndrome and prompt initiation of the appropriate symptomatic therapy.

4.3.1 Acute Pain Syndromes Associated with Infusion Technique

(a) Intravenous infusion pain

Venous spasm, chemical phlebitis, vesicant extravasation causing extreme pain, anthracycline-associated localized skin flare reaction (Portenoy and Conn 2009).

(b) Hepatic artery infusion pain

While the portal vein contributes 70% of the hepatic blood supply and the hepatic artery delivers 30%, almost 100% of the blood supply to primary and metastatic cancer is delivered via the hepatic artery. Taking advantage of this anatomy, direct infusion of chemotherapy such as floxuridine with dexamethasone, or with mitomycin, into the hepatic artery via an implanted pump is sometimes utilized. Side effects include generalized abdominal pain, gastric ulceration, and cholangitis. Pain usually resolves with cessation of infusion (Cohen and Kemeny 2003).

(c) Pain from intraperitoneal chemotherapy

Administration of chemotherapy directly into the intraperitoneal space is used to treat cancers of the abdominal region. Intraperitoneal chemotherapy is given either as Hyperthermic Intraperitoneal Chemotherapy (HIPEC) as an intraoperative procedure, or as a course of up to six cycles delivered via a port. Abdominal pain during and after administration is a common side effect that can limit the ability to tolerate a full course of chemotherapy. This pain can be improved by adjusting the fill volumes in line with the individual patient's physique (Zeimet et al. 2009). Catheter-associated problems such as positioning, kinking, and infection can also cause pain. The repeated dose regimen is associated with a higher likelihood of all side effects including pain (Blinman et al. 2013).

(d) Intrathecal chemotherapy

The central nervous system is a unique location of malignant disease due to the inability of many standard oral and intravenous chemotherapeutic drugs to penetrate the blood-brain barrier. Administration of therapy directly into the leptomeninges via intrathecal infusion is therefore employed. An Ommaya reservoir is an intraventricular catheter system which can deliver drugs or be used for aspiration of cerebrospinal fluid. It is placed to facilitate intrathecal chemotherapy and improve flow. Along with the side effects associated with lumbar puncture already mentioned, there are additional potential neurotoxicities from the drugs more commonly used which can cause pain (Kerr et al. 2001). Methotrexate and cytarabine can both cause an acute chemical arachnoiditis, presenting with symptoms of headache, nuchal rigidity, back pain, vomiting, fever, and CSF pleocytosis. This is usually self-limiting (Jacob et al. 2015).

4.3.2 Acute Pain due to Specific Drug Reaction Syndrome

(a) Paclitaxel

Paclitaxel, most commonly used in treatment of breast cancer, is associated with a particular set of symptoms known as the Paclitaxel Acute Pain Syndrome (P-APS). Onset of symptoms is 24–96 h after dosing, most commonly with a diffuse aching discomfort, most often in the legs, hips, and lower back, although it can be widespread. Resolution of symptoms is over 24–96 h. Symptoms can recur at greater or less intensity with repeated dosing and can evolve to develop into a sensory peripheral neuropathy, with greater initial intensity a predictor for this (Loprinzi et al. 2011). P-APS can be managed with dose reduction and analgesics, but no methods of prevention are known. Aggressive treatment of P-APS may prevent development of the chronic sensory neuropathy.

(b) 5-Fluorouracil

5-Fluorouracil, commonly used in the treatment of gastrointestinal malignancies, has well-described potential cardiotoxicity mediated by coronary vasospasm. The cardiotoxicity manifestation ranges across a wide spectrum from ECG changes to angina pain to cardiogenic shock. Treatment of angina is in accordance with standard cardiac pain protocols.

(c) All-Trans-Retinoic Acid

All-Trans-Retinoic Acid is used in the treatment of acute promyelocytic leukemia. Headache is a common side effect. A less common side effect is development of pseudotumor cerebri with severe headache (Tallman et al. 1997).

(d) Hormonal therapies

Hormonal therapies are used to suppress tumor progression in malignancies which are hormone responsive. The use of estrogens, antiestrogens, androgens, and gonadotrophin-releasing hormone (GnRH) agonists is associated with a tumor flare syndrome and thus has implications in the management of breast and prostate cancer. Initiation of these agents in the treatment of breast cancer can be accompanied by one or more of the manifestations; acute bony pain; hypercalcemia; or rapid increase in size of tumor foci causing pain and swelling. Onset of these symptoms within days to weeks of initiation and spontaneous resolution differentiates the symptoms of tumor flare syndrome from disease progression (Margolese et al. 2003). Treatment is symptomatic. Tumor flare after initiation of GnRH agonists in prostate cancer can be biochemical and/or clinical with potential significant adverse effects. Onset is within 1–2 weeks of commencing androgen deprivation therapy and the most common manifestation is bony pain although ureteral obstruction, urinary retention, spinal cord compression, lymphedema, and death have been reported. Tumor flare from a GnRH agonist can be prevented or minimized with antiandrogenic agents such as cyproterone acetate, diethylstilbestrol, flutamide, nilutamide, or ketoconazole (Thompson 2001).

(e) Colony-stimulating factors

Colony-stimulating factors are associated with a range of constitutional symptoms and a diffuse aching bone pain is the most frequently reported adverse effect (Vial and Descotes 1995).

(f) Intravenous steroid

Acute perineal pain due to intravenous steroid has been described in the literature. It is immediate, brief (seconds to minutes), and self-resolving. Pain is burning and shooting in nature, localized to the perineal area and severe in intensity. Pathophysiology is unknown (Neff et al. 2002).

4.3.3 Acute Pain due to Chemotherapy Toxicity

(a) Many chemotherapy agents are neurotoxic and thus associated with peripheral neuropathy sequelae which are usually a polyneuropathy and rarely mononeuropathic. Agents with a higher incidence of polyneuropathy are vinca alkaloids, platinum drugs, taxanes, thalidomide, and bortezomib (Wolf et al. 2008). Presentation can be acute, with paresthesias and dysesthesias commonly in the fingers and toes. Other sites are also described such as the pharygolarnygeal spasm of oxaliplatin. More commonly, the onset is gradual, with increasing pain intensity with repeated administrations. Dose reductions and cessation of the agent can resolve the symptoms, but a chronic residual neuropathy can develop. Vincristine is associated with a rare mononeuropathy causing acute orofacial pain due to trigeminal or glossopharyngeal nerve toxicity (McCarthy and Skillings 1992). Several preventative and ameliorating approaches are used, including dose modification and delays. Symptomatic treatment is with neuropathic agents and behavioral modifications.
(b) Palmar-plantar erythrodysesthesia syndrome is a well-described toxicity reaction to a number of chemotherapy drugs. Most commonly implicated are capecitabine, doxorubicin, cytarabine, and fluorouracil. Symptoms include erythema, swelling, pain, paresthesia, dysesthesia, and desquamation. Onset, extent, and severity of symptoms are variable, but appear to increase with prolonged exposure or high dose exposure to the causative agent. Management is supportive with emollients, analgesia, and limiting exposure to noxious environments. The reaction is essentially self-limiting and responds to dose modification and drug cessation (Lokich and Moore 1984).
(c) Gastrointestinal Mucositis (see below)

4.4 Acute Pain due to Radiation Therapy

(a) Radiation therapy (nonmucosal)

Radiation therapy to breast, lung, and head and neck cancers pose a risk to proximate critical structures such as the brachial plexus. The syndrome of radiation-induced brachial plexopathy (RIBP) is one of the possible late effects of radiation. It most commonly presents months after the radiation but can occur years later, making diagnosis difficult (Amini et al. 2012). A rare, early transient RIBP syndrome has also been described, presenting during or within 3 months of treatment (Metcalfe and Etiz 2016). There is a spectrum of symptoms with pain, numbness, paresthesia, and motor deficits that can be extremely debilitating. RIBP is thought to be due to demyelination leading to irreversible axon loss and symptomatic treatment is difficult. Balancing the tolerance of the brachial plexus with the risk of treatment failure during radiation planning is complex.

(b) Oral Mucositis (see below)

4.5 Mucositis

Mucositis may cause acute pain via a number of modalities: chemotherapy, radiation, or hemopoietic stem cell transplant-induced oral and gastrointestinal (GI) mucositis.

Oral and gastrointestinal mucositis is the most common side effect causing pain in the treatment of malignancies. Up to 100% of patients undergoing high dose chemotherapy and hemopoietic stem cell transplant (HSCT) suffer from oral and GI mucositis. Up to 80% of patients receiving radiation therapy for head and neck cancers suffer from oral mucositis. Between 5% and 15% of patients receiving chemotherapy agents are affected by GI mucositis although 5-fluorouracil treatment has a 40% incidence rate with doxorubicin and methotrexate, the other most common causes of oral mucositis (Sonis et al. 2004).

Oral mucositis is the result of injury to the submucosal tissue by radiation or chemotherapy. This damage initiates a cascade of events beginning with free radical generation causing DNA damage, followed by an inflammatory state, then an ulceration phase, and finally a healing phase. Full thickness mucosal damage is present during the ulcerative phase that often occurs at the same time as neutropenia and is exacerbated by bacterial colonization. This phase is most likely associated with the pain of mucositis.

Gastrointestinal (GI) mucositis has a similar pathophysiology, with differences in function accounting for the differences in symptoms and morbidity when compared to oral mucositis. GI mucositis is more common in chemotherapy due to the large numbers of rapidly dividing cells.

Symptoms of oral mucositis are of oral pain, swelling, difficulty eating, speaking, and swallowing, with onset 2–5 days after radiation or chemotherapy and lasting 7–14 days. Symptoms of GI mucositis are abdominal pain, bloating, and diarrhea between days 3 and 7 following chemotherapy. Morbidity can be severe with significant treatment limiting and delay implications, although mucositis is a self-limiting process (Rubenstein et al. 2004).

Management of oral mucositis consists of prevention strategies, educating patients on basic oral care, and pain control with systemic opioids, coating agents, and topical anesthetic/analgesics. Patient-controlled analgesia for oral mucositis in HSCT has level 1 evidence (Pillitteri and Clark 1998).

5 Disease-Related Acute Pain Syndromes

Most acute cancer pain syndromes occur in relation to investigations and treatment, i.e., iatrogenic causes. Acute pain syndromes due to the cancer itself are limited by comparison, e.g., pathological fractures, spasms, or perforations due to malignant bowel obstructions, and bleeding into tumors. Cancer pain due to disease usually has a more chronic duration with acute exacerbations and encompasses invasion into visceral, somatic, and neural tissue. The most common presentation of cancer pain is of a mixed nature, where a number of tissues may have been affected, e.g., spinal cord compression in relation to malignant invasion of bone and neuropathic tissues.

Management of the underlying disease process can provide analgesia via controlling the disease and its complications. Hence the consideration of the pathology and disease biology of cancers is important in optimizing analgesic interventions. As treatment for the underlying malignancy continues, it can be easier to recognize more chronic pain states that develop over time.

In this section, we discuss the tumor-specific causes of acute cancer pain syndromes.

5.1 Tumor-Specific Acute Pain Syndromes

Acute pain syndromes that are directly related to the tumor necessitate urgent treatment of the underlying lesion, in addition to aggressive pain control. The degree to which the lesion is treated often depends upon the goals of care for the patient in question, i.e., curative, restorative, palliative, or terminal goals of care.

(a) Pathological fracture

Bone pain is the commonest type of pain caused by cancer, with skeletal metastases in 30–69% of cancer patients, especially from advanced breast, lung, and prostate cancers (Li et al. 2014). Malignant bone disease may be asymptomatic, but growth within the bone may cause moderate to severe pain and lead to acute pathological fractures (Zhu et al. 2015). Patients describe the sudden onset of back or limb pain, with or without any particular trauma of note. There may be pain that worsens on movement, i.e., incident pain, with a background of localized bone pain which is tender on palpation.

Incident pain can be a marker of vertebral instability and is often poorly managed due to the lack of attention to the temporal nature of the pain. It has a quick onset with movement, a high intensity and a short duration of seconds to minutes. Immediate-release opioids take 20–30 min to act and therefore may not be ideal for incident pain. Vertebral pain is often only partial opioid responsive, i.e., opioids alone will not provide adequate analgesia. Baseline long-acting opioids should first be optimized, in conjunction with the use of analgesic adjuncts such as nonsteroidal or steroidal antiinflammatories and a holistic approach. The incident pain may resolve enough to be tolerable and nonpharmacological approaches, e.g., a brace to support the back, may allow adequate analgesia. Where pain continues to be problematic, then rapid-onset opioids (ROOs) can be used, e.g., fentanyl lozenges and fentanyl sublingual/buccal tablets. When ROOs are used, they are titrated to efficacy using the recommended dosing regimen, and not dosed according to a proportion of the baseline opioid.

In severe cases of vertebral instability, urgent neurosurgery may be warranted in order to provide rapid stabilization and reduce the risk of associated neurological impairment. Surgical stabilization of long bone fractures, if feasible and consistent with the overall goals of care, may relieve pain and should be considered. In addition, a femoral nerve block can provide regional anesthesia, e.g., for a neck of femur fracture or osteosarcoma (Pacenta et al. 2010) Similarly, sacral bone pain from metastatic disease can be aided by a sciatic nerve block (Fujiwara et al. 2015). Surgery should also be considered if there is no fracture, but the cortex of the bone is at risk of being breached from malignancy.

Radiation therapy is usually considered for all pathological fractures post surgery and often augments pain control over a maximal period of 6–8 weeks. If surgery is not part of the management of the fracture, and pain cannot be managed adequately with medications, then radiotherapy is also warranted. A pain flare may occur during or post radiotherapy, where the addition or increase of steroids is likely to be of benefit.

Vertebral collapse may be treated conservatively with analgesics, e.g., opioids, NSAIDs, and/or steroids. As discussed, radiotherapy may be considered but another option is vertebral augmentation, i.e., vertebroplasty or kyphoplasty, especially in osteolytic lesions. These techniques are best performed for fractures that are less than 6 weeks old. They may also avoid the potential deterioration of the fracture post radiotherapy if the cancer is so radiosensitive that it causes vertebral instability after responding to the radiotherapy. Vertebroplasty involves the infiltration of the vertebral body with cement, to strengthen the bone, ablate the cancer deposit, and reduce the pain. Kyphoplasty involves the same injection of cement, except a balloon is inflated into the vertebral body to create the space for the cement. These are usually day case procedures, with local anesthetic and minimal sedation, with rapid resolution of pain and functional ability (Chandra et al. 2018).

Vertebral augmentation requires careful selection of patients, with absolute contraindications listed as: spinal column infection or other active systemic infection; uncontrollable bleeding; inability to tolerate a prone procedure with sedation or general anesthesia; significant myelopathy due to cord compromise at the site under consideration, because of epidural tumor extension or fracture retropulsion; and known bone cement allergy. For sacroplasty patients, i.e., sacral augmentation, sacral decubitus ulcers are an absolute contraindication to avoid osteomyelitis and implant infection. The main complications of these procedures are: subcutaneous and/or paraspinal hematoma; fractures (of rib, pedicle, vertebral body, or sacrum depending on treatment level); infection (osteomyelitis, epidural abscess); cement leakage; nerve or spinal cord damage resulting in paralysis or bowel/bladder dysfunction; pulmonary embolus (secondary to cement or fat emboli); hypotension or depressed myocardial function (secondary to free methyl methacrylate monomer or fat emboli); pneumothorax (for thoracic vertebroplasty and kyphoplasty); and worsened pain or failure to treat (Chandra et al. 2018).

(b) Hemorrhage into a tumor

A sudden hemorrhage into a tumor can lead to acute pain, e.g., bleeding into tumors of the brain and liver, in both primary and metastatic disease. The hemorrhage may be due to clotting abnormalities, erosion into blood vessels, or rupture of vasculature of the tumor. Opioids are the mainstay of treatment. In cases of bleeding into organs with a capsule, e.g., the liver or spleen, distension of the capsule leads to acute pain. NSAIDs and steroids can provide analgesia in conjunction with opioids in such capsular pain. Hemorrhages can be a life-threatening complication of cancer and clinical interventions may include transfusions, analgesia, and sedation, according to the goals of care. In some cases, if appropriate, more urgent action to control the bleeding may be needed, e.g., trans-arterial embolization, but if unsuccessful, emergency surgery may be required.

(c) Obstruction/perforation of a hollow viscus

Acute pain can occur when a hollow viscus is obstructed, increasing the risk of a potentially fatal perforation. Pancreatic cancers may cause right upper quadrant pain from biliary duct obstruction. In patients with a poor prognosis, stenting of the biliary tree or the duodenum may provide symptomatic relief. The options of bypass surgery require careful consideration, given the median survival of 6.5 months for those eligible for surgery (Sohn et al. 1999).

Prostate, bladder, and pelvic cancers can cause ureteric obstruction, as can lymphadenopathy and retroperitoneal fibrosis via direct invasion or extrinsic compression. In patients with a good prognosis, retrograde stenting of the ureter or percutaneous nephrostomy can be considered. The acute pain may be relieved, but these procedures can also cause pain. One-third of patients will have a failed stent within 6 months, and coupled with the risk of infection or displacement, the management can be frustrating for patients and their families. For patients in whom retrograde stenting is impossible, the option of percutaneous nephrostomy and/or anterograde stent insertion is available but carries the same management problems.

Malignant bowel obstruction can be managed conservatively, via a syringe driver and in some instances a nasogastric tube. Hyoscine butylbromide can help with colicky abdominal pain and the reduction of large bowel fluid. Octreotide has an antisecretory effect on the upper small bowel, and therefore has usually been reserved for multilevel or malignant small bowel obstructions. Constipation is a common dilemma in the management of patients with malignant bowel obstruction. Hyoscine butylbromide can relieve colicky abdominal pain, to spare opioid uses and reduce somnolence. Steroids can also help to reduce peritumoural edema, at a dose of 4–8 mg daily. These patients may also benefit from decompressive procedures, stenting, or occasionally surgery.

Bowel perforations are generally fatal, but may also be small and become walled off, to allow for some repair of the injury and better prognosis. The presentation of an acute abdomen usually warrants a review for urgent surgical intervention, but in palliative care, this is invariably inappropriate. The goal of care becomes symptom management and preparation for a potential death. Opioids, benzodiazepines, and antipsychotics may all be used, according to the agitation and distress that exists. Often a syringe driver will be needed with appropriate breakthrough medications. The need for review is important, to ensure that adequate symptom control is being achieved and that the syringe driver can be changed if needed.

(d) Spinal cord compression

The urgent management of spinal cord compression is discussed in the relevant chapter of the Palliative Care Emergencies section.

(e) Thrombosis and acute pulmonary embolism

The urgent management of venous thromboembolism is discussed in the relevant chapter of the Palliative Care Emergencies section.

6 Summary

Acute pain in palliative care is always an emergency to assess and manage the pain appropriately and in a timely fashion. This may involve leading the care or collaborating with other healthcare professionals in the management. Acute interventions may be required, e.g., with fractures, but the patient needs review to determine if the emergency treatment is appropriate for the goals of care. Acute pain management may also require the involvement of acute pain services.

We have discussed common acute cancer pain syndromes to highlight the diagnosis and consider management accordingly. Acute pain can occur independently, or as an episode of pain on a background of chronic pain. The development or worsening of chronic pain states drives the urgency for treatment, which invariably is best provided in a multimodal fashion, via a multidisciplinary team.

References

Ahmed SV, Jayawarna C, Jude E. Post lumbar puncture headache: diagnosis and management. Postgrad Med J. 2006;82(973):713–6.

Amini A, Yang J, Williamson R, McBurney ML, Erasmus J, Allen PK, Karhade M, Komaki R, Liao Z, Gomez D, Cox J. Dose constraints to prevent radiation-induced brachial plexopathy in patients treated for lung cancer. Int J Radiat Oncol Biol Phys. 2012;82(3):e391–8.

Ashby MA, Fleming BG, Brooksbank M, et al. Description of a mechanistic approach to pain management in advanced cancer: preliminary report. Pain. 1992;51:153–61.

Azevedo SLFK, Kimura M, Jacobsen-Teixeira M. The WHO analgesic ladder for cancer pain control, twenty years of use. How much pain relief does one get from using it? Support Care Cancer. 2006;14(11):1086–93. Epub 2006 Jun 8

Bilbao JI, Martínez-Cuesta A, Urtasun F, Cosín O. Complications of embolization. Semin Intervent Radiol. 2006;23(02):126–42.

Blinman P, Gainford C, Donoghoe M, Martyn J, Blomfield P, Grant P, Kichenadasse G, Vaughan M, Brand A, Shannon C, Gebski V. Feasibility, acceptability and preferences for intraperitoneal chemotherapy with paclitaxel and cisplatin after optimal debulking surgery for ovarian and related cancers: an ANZGOG study. J Gynecol Oncol. 2013;24(4):359–66.

Bruera E, Kim HN. Cancer pain. JAMA. 2003;290(18): 2476–9.

Carr DB, Goudas LC. Acute pain. Lancet. 1999;353:2051–8.

Chandra RV, Leslie-Mazwi T, Hirsch JA. Vertebroplasty, Kyphoplasty, and Sacroplasty. Essentials of interventional techniques in managing chronic pain. Cham: Springer; 2018. p. 431–42.

Cipta AM, Pietras CJ, Weiss TE, Strouse TB. Cancer-related pain management in clinical oncology. J Community Support Oncol. 2015;13:347–55.

Cohen AD, Kemeny NE. An update on hepatic arterial infusion chemotherapy for colorectal cancer. Oncologist. 2003;8(6):553–66.

Della Corte F, Messina A, Mendola C, Cammarota G. Post thoracotomy pain syndrome: InTech; Open Access Publisher; [online] from http://cdn.intechopen.com/pdfs/26930/InTech-Post_thoracotomy_pain_syndrome.pdf. 2012.

Fadul N, Elsayem A. Palliative Care in the Emergency Center. In: Manzullo EF, Gonzalez CE, Escalante CP, Yeung S-CJ, editors. Oncologic emergencies. New York: Springer; 2016. p. 273–85.

Fischer DJ, Villines D, Kim YO, et al. Anxiety, depression, and pain: differences by primary cancer. Support Care Cancer. 2010;18(7):801–10.

Forbes K. Pain in patients with cancer: the World Health Organization analgesic ladder and beyond. Clin Oncol. 2011;23:379–80.

Fujiwara S, Komasawa N, Hyoda A, Kuwamura A, Kido H, Minami T. Ultrasound-guided sciatic nerve block (pulsed radiofrequency) for intractable cancer pain caused by sacral bone metastasis. Masui. 2015;64:663–5.

Gutgsell T, Walsh D, Zhukovsky DS, et al. A prospective study of the pathophysiology and clinical characteristics of pain in a palliative medicine population. Am J Hosp Palliat Care. 2003;20(2):140–8.

Hart CYT, Ryu JH. Complications of percutaneous nephrostomy tube placement to treat nephrolithiasis. Hosp Physician. 2002;38(6):43–6.

Hølen JC, Hjermstad MJ, Loge JH, Fayers PM, Caraceni A, De Conno F, et al. Pain assessment tools: is the content appropriate for use in palliative care? J Pain Symptom Manag. 2006;32:567–80.

Jackson MA, Simpson KH. Pain after amputation. Continuing education in Anaesthesia. Critical Care & Pain. 2004;4(1):20–3.

Jacob LA, Sreevatsa A, Chinnagiriyappa LK, Dasappa L, Suresh TM, Babu G. Methotrexate-induced chemical meningitis in patients with acute lymphoblastic leukemia/lymphoma. Annals of Indian Academy of Neurology. 2015;18(2):206.

Kent ML, Tighe PJ, Belfer I, Brennan TJ, Bruehl S, Brummett CM, et al. The ACTTION–APS–AAPM pain taxonomy (AAAPT) multidimensional approach to classifying acute pain conditions. Pain med. Oxford University Press. 2017;18:947–58.

Kerr JZ, Berg S, Blaney SM. Intrathecal chemotherapy. Crit Rev Oncol Hematol. 2001;37(3):227–36.

Kroenke K, Theobald D, Wu J, et al. The association of depression and pain with health-related quality of life, disability, and healthcare use in cancer patients. J Pain Symptom Manag. 2010;40:327–41.

Levy N, Sturgess J, Mills P. "Pain as the fifth vital sign" and dependence on the "numerical pain scale" is being abandoned in the US: why? Br J Anaesth. 2018; 120(3):435–8. Available: https://www.sciencedirect.com/science/article/pii/S0007091217541823

Li BT, Wong MH, Pavlakis N. Treatment and prevention of bone metastases from breast Cancer: a comprehensive review of evidence for clinical practice. J Clin Med Res. 2014;3:1–24.

Lokich JJ, Moore C. Chemotherapy-associated palmar-plantar erythrodysesthesia syndrome. Ann Intern Med. 1984;101(6):798–800.

Loprinzi CL, Reeves BN, Dakhil SR, Sloan JA, Wolf SL, Burger KN, Kamal A, Le-Lindqwister NA, Soori GS, Jaslowski AJ, Novotny PJ. Natural history of paclitaxel-associated acute pain syndrome: prospective cohort study NCCTG N08C1. J Clin Oncol. 2011;29(11):1472–8.

Luckett T, Davidson PM, Green A, Boyle F, Stubbs J, Lovell M. Assessment and management of adult cancer pain: a systematic review and synthesis of recent qualitative studies aimed at developing insights for managing barriers and optimizing facilitators within a comprehensive framework of patient care. J Pain Symptom Manag. 2013;46:229–53.

Maltoni M, Scarpi E, Modonesi C, Passardi A, Calpona S, Turriziani A, et al. A validation study of the WHO analgesic ladder: a two-step vs three-step strategy. Support Care Cancer. 2005;13:888–94.

Margolese RG, Hortobagyi GN, Buchholz TA. Management of Metastatic Breast Cancer. In: Kufe DW, Pollock RE, Weichselbaum RR, et al., editors. Holland-Frei Cancer medicine. 6th ed. Hamilton: BC Decker; 2003.

Matthews ML, Melika R, Murray Y. Nonopioid and adjuvant analgesics for acute pain management. Clinical approaches to hospital medicine. Cham: Springer; 2018. p. 225–41.

McCarthy GM, Skillings JR. Jaw and other orofacial pain in patients receiving vincristine for the treatment of cancer. Oral surgery, oral medicine, oral pathology. 1992;74(3):299–304.

Mercadante S, Villari P, Ferrera P, Casuccio A, Fulfaro F. Rapid titration with intravenous morphine for severe cancer pain and immediate oral conversion. Cancer. 2002;95:203–8.

Metcalfe E, Etiz D. Early transient radiation-induced brachial plexopathy in locally advanced head and neck cancer. Contemp Oncol (Pozn). 2016;20(1):67–72.

Neff SP, Stapelberg F, Warmington A. Excruciating perineal pain after intravenous dexamethasone. Anaesth Intensive Care. 2002;30(3):370–1.

Oefelein MG, Bayazit Y. Chronic pain syndrome after laparoscopic radical nephrectomy. J Urol. 2003;170:1939–40.

Pacenta HL, Kaddoum RN, Pereiras LA, Chidiac EJ, Burgoyne LL. Continuous tunnelled femoral nerve block for palliative care of a patient with metastatic osteosarcoma. Anaesth Intensive Care. 2010;38(3):563–5.

Pargeon KL, Hailey BJ. Barriers to effective cancer pain management: a review of the literature. J Pain Symptom Manag. 1999;18:358–68.

Pillitteri LC, Clark RE. Comparison of a patient-controlled analgesia system with continuous infusion for administration of diamorphine for mucositis. Bone Marrow Transplant. 1998;22(5):495–8.

Portenoy RK, Conn M. Cancer pain syndromes. In: Bruera ED, Portenoy RK, editors. Cancer pain: assessment and management. 2nd ed; 2009.

Portenoy RK, Lesage P. Management of cancer pain. Lancet. 1999;353(9165):1695–700.

Porter LS, Keefe FJ. Psychosocial issues in cancer pain. Curr Pain Headache Rep. 2011;15:263–70.

Rahman NM, Pepperell J, Rehal S, Saba T, Tang A, Ali N, West A, Hettiarachchi G, Mukherjee D, Samuel J, Bentley A. Effect of opioids vs NSAIDs and larger vs smaller chest tube size on pain control and pleurodesis efficacy among patients with malignant pleural effusion: the TIME1 randomized clinical trial. JAMA. 2015;314(24):2641–53.

Rammohan A, Sathyanesan J, Ramaswami S, Lakshmanan A, Senthil-Kumar P, Srinivasan UP, et al. Embolization of liver tumors: past, present and future. World J Radiol. 2012;4:405–12.

Rubenstein EB, Peterson DE, Schubert M, Keefe D, McGuire D, Epstein J, Elting LS, Fox PC, Cooksley C, Sonis ST. Clinical practice guidelines for the prevention and treatment of cancer therapy–induced oral and gastrointestinal mucositis. Cancer. 2004;100(S9):2026–46.

Sohn TA, Lillemoe KD, Cameron JL, et al. Surgical palliation of unresectable periampullary adenocarcinoma in the 1990s. J Am Coll Surg. 1999;188:658.

Sonis ST, Elting LS, Keefe D, Peterson DE, Schubert M, Hauer-Jensen M, Bekele BN, Raber-Durlacher J, Donnelly JP, Rubenstein EB. Perspectives on cancer therapy-induced mucosal injury. Cancer. 2004;100(S9):1995–2025.

Tallman MS, Andersen JW, Schiffer CA, Appelbaum FR, Feusner JH, Ogden A, Shepherd L, Willman C, Bloomfield CD, Rowe JM, Wiernik PH. All-trans-retinoic acid in acute promyelocytic leukemia. N Engl J Med. 1997;337(15):1021–8.

Thompson IM. Flare associated with LHRH-agonist therapy. Reviews in urology. 2001;3(Suppl 3):S10.

Vadalouca A, Moka E, Argyra E, Sikioti P, Siafaka I. Opioid rotation in patients with cancer: a review of the current literature. J Opioid Manag. 2008;4:213–50.

van den Beuken-van M, Hochstenbach L. Update on prevalence of pain in patients with cancer: systematic review and meta-analysis. J Pain Symptom Manage: Elsevier; 2016. Available: http://www.sciencedirect.com/science/article/pii/S0885392416300483

Vargas-Schaffer G. Is the WHO analgesic ladder still valid? Twenty-four years of experience. Can Fam Physician. 2010;56:514–7. e202–5

Vial T, Descotes J. Clinical toxicity of cytokines used as haemopoietic growth factors. Drug Saf. 1995;13(6):371–406.

Wolf S, Barton D, Kottschade L, Grothey A, Loprinzi C. Chemotherapy-induced peripheral neuropathy: prevention and treatment strategies. Eur J Cancer. 2008;44(11):1507–15.

World Health Organization. Traitement de la douleur cancéreuse. Geneva: World Health Organization; 1987.

Wu CL, Raja SN. Treatment of acute postoperative pain. Lancet. 2011;377(9784):2215–25.

Zeimet AG, Reimer D, Radl AC, Reinthaller A, Schauer C, Petru E, Concin N, Braun S, Marth C. Pros and cons of intraperitoneal chemotherapy in the treatment of epithelial ovarian cancer. Anticancer Res. 2009;29(7):2803–8.

Zhu X-C, Zhang J-L, Ge C-T, Yu Y-Y, Wang P, Yuan T-F, et al. Advances in cancer pain from bone metastasis. Drug Des Devel Ther. 2015;9:4239–45.

Acute Dyspnoea

77

Rachel Wiseman

Contents

R. Wiseman (✉)
Canterbury District Health Board, Christchurch,
New Zealand
e-mail: Rachel.wiseman@cdhb.health.nz

R. D. MacLeod, L. Van den Block (eds.), *Textbook of Palliative Care*,
https://doi.org/10.1007/978-3-319-77740-5_80

Abstract

Acute (or episodic) dyspnoea is a debilitating symptom that induces fear and anxiety in patients and family/carers alike. Management focuses on addressing the underlying cause where this can be identified. In addition to addressing reversible causes, management of acute dyspnoea or a dyspnoea crisis will be discussed. Evidence for both pharmacological and non-pharmacological management strategies is outlined, with discussion of how these can be incorporated into a comprehensive, individualized management plan. Involvement and education of the wider interdisciplinary team across healthcare settings is essential. This chapter will also cover some of the more specific causes of acute dyspnoea such as anxiety or breathing pattern disorders, stridor or upper airway obstruction, bronchospasm, and the sensation of choking with a focus on neuromuscular diseases.

1 Introduction

This chapter will focus specifically on acute dyspnoea, more commonly described in the literature as episodic breathlessness. At times, episodic breathlessness may lead to a dyspnoea crisis, an important feature to recognize and actively manage. Information regarding chronic breathlessness syndrome is featured elsewhere in this textbook, as is the management of massive hemoptysis and superior vena cava obstruction. Specific information about palliative care in lung disease is detailed in a separate chapter.

Assessment and management of acute dyspnoea will depend on the stage of the patient's disease, their ability and willingness to undergo investigation, and the support available to them in their place of care. While this chapter covers some reversible causes of acute dyspnoea, the appropriateness of investigating and managing potentially reversible causes of decline need to be assessed on an individual basis. Many patients experience repeated episodes of acute dyspnoea, and this experience can be drawn upon to initiate and negotiate a care plan in advance – such as an advance care plan, advance directive, or breathlessness management plan – especially important since patients are usually unable to relate their wishes to healthcare professionals when acutely dyspnoeic. Many patients report feeling that their breathlessness is unrecognized by healthcare professionals (Gysels and Higginson 2011) despite the significant impact this symptom has on quality of life.

The aim of this chapter is to give health professionals an overview of:

- Acute (or episodic) dyspnoea and the recent research that is helping to define this symptom
- The assessment of an acutely dyspnoeic patient
- Investigations and treatments for certain clinical conditions or emergencies
- Non-pharmacological and pharmacological management strategies for a dyspnoea crisis
- Individualized dyspnoea crisis management plans

2 Episodic Breathlessness and Breathlessness Crises

Acute dyspnoea is a common, under-researched symptom that has a significant impact on both carers and patients. Retrospective studies have shown that in 3 months prior to death, 50% of patients referred to a palliative care service experienced no dyspnoea, falling to 35% at the time of death. Dyspnoea severity is higher in those with noncancer diagnoses (Currow et al. 2010). More recent research has focused on the type of dyspnoea, classifying breathlessness as continuous, episodic, or both. Episodic breathlessness has been further defined via a Delphi consensus method:

> Episodic breathlessness is one form of breathlessness characterised by a severe worsening of breathlessness intensity or unpleasantness beyond usual fluctuations in the patient's perception. Episodes are time-limited (seconds to hours) and occur intermittently, with or without underlying continuous breathlessness. (Simon et al. 2014)

Episodic breathlessness may occur without continuous breathlessness, but the opposite is rarely described (Simon et al. 2013a).

Episodic breathlessness was studied in 82 patients with chronic obstructive pulmonary disease (COPD) or lung cancer (Weingartner et al. 2015) and was reported in 71% of patient interviews, most often in COPD. The majority of episodes lasted less than 20 min. In other work, the duration of episodes has been described as 2–10 min (Reddy et al. 2009) and 1–5 min (Weingartner et al. 2013). Episodes could occur several times a day and are defined by a beginning and an end, with peak severity being worse in patients with a diagnosis of COPD (Weingartner et al. 2015). A systematic review found the prevalence of episodic breathlessness to be 81–85% in one lung cancer study (Simon et al. 2013b) or 61% in a second study (Reddy et al. 2009).

Simon et al. (2013c) has further described subtypes of episodic breathlessness in patients with lung cancer, COPD, heart failure, or motor neuron disease. These are detailed below. Types 3, 4, and 5 are less predictable and more likely to induce a panicked response.

1. Triggered episodes with normal levels of breathlessness (e.g., heavy exertion)
2. Triggered episodes with predictable response (e.g., talking, emotion)
3. Triggered episodes with unpredictable response (e.g., climbing stairs)
4. Non-triggered, unpredictable, attack-like episodes
5. Triggered or non-triggered wavelike episodes in COPD (more gradual onset, severe)

Episodic breathlessness is important to consider for two reasons. The first is that the sensation of breathlessness is intimately linked to panic and fear, more so when the dyspnoea becomes acutely worse for an unknown reason. However, even predictable episodes of breathlessness can have a significant impact on the individual due to the second reason – trigger avoidance. Breathlessness triggered by a known cause, such as exertion, leads to avoidance of that trigger and consequent deconditioning with a resultant increase in overall breathlessness (Janssens et al. 2011). High dyspnoea-related fear is associated with impaired quality of life and worse dyspnoea during exercise but also responds more positively to interventions such as pulmonary rehabilitation.

Episodic breathlessness, especially subtypes 3, 4, and 5 described above, may precipitate a "dyspnoea crisis." This has been defined as:

> sustained and severe resting breathing discomfort that occurs in patients with advanced, often life-limiting illness and overwhelms the patient and caregivers' ability to achieve symptom relief. (Mularski et al. 2013a)

Little is known about the incidence and prevalence of dyspnoea crises, the theoretical components of which were proposed during an American Thoracic Society Workshop. A survey of members of the American Thoracic Society performed prior to this workshop obtained 109 responders, 75% of whom had encountered outpatients in a palliative phase of their illness with acute crisis dyspnoea resulting in a 911 call or attendance at an emergency department (ED). Responders had encountered this situation weekly (19%), monthly (41%), or yearly (38%) (Mularski et al. 2013b).

The three required components for a dyspnoea crisis are:

- A worsening in dyspnoea
- A biopsychosocial/spiritual patient response
- An overwhelmed caregiver/environment

The workshop suggested that in order to manage the breathlessness crisis, all of the above components need to be assessed and actively managed on an individual basis. Only 9.6% of responders in the above survey indicated that their practice had any local policy or guideline on the management of acute crisis dyspnoea (Mularski et al. 2013b).

2.1 Impact on Patients

The impact of episodic breathlessness on patients is significant. Terms used by patients include frightening, panic (Gysels and Higginson 2011), smothering, choking, couldn't get air, deathly sick, fighting for breath (Parshall et al. 2001), fear of choking, drowning, and suffocating (Simon et al. 2013c). Many patients fear that they will die suddenly of suffocation or choking during an attack or when asleep (Giacomini et al. 2012). Bailey described the dyspnoea–anxiety–dyspnoea cycle, a circular relationship with ever-escalating symptoms until the cycle is somehow broken. However, patients also describe that heightened emotion is an indicator of increasing breathlessness and may be the first sign of an impending crisis (Bailey 2004). While it is possible for patients to develop their own strategies to deal with the panic that arises during episodes, in one qualitative study, only 8 of 51 patients described having learnt to do so (Simon et al. 2013c). Many patients describe having never received health professional advice on how best to manage their breathlessness (Gysels and Higginson 2011).

2.2 Impact on Families and Caregivers

The impact of episodic dyspnoea and breathlessness crises on families and lay caregivers cannot be underestimated. During episodes, caregivers express a sense of helplessness and fear. There is significant relief and a sense of security once help is sought (Bailey 2004). Heightened vigilance leads to disturbed sleep, due to the unpredictability of episodes and the need to "sleep with one eye open" (Hearson et al. 2011). In COPD, relatives are repeatedly called to the hospital to "say goodbye" during acute exacerbations, only for the patient to survive and the cycle to recur again at some undetermined point in the future. Many relatives of patients with COPD fear that the dying process will be as prolonged as the disease course itself. However, in retrospect these relatives described the death as peaceful and calm, as if sleeping, as opposed to what the patient had most feared (Ek et al. 2015).

As described above, the family/caregiver plays a pivotal role during a dyspnoea crisis. During this time, the patient may be unable to self-manage their increased breathlessness, and the assistance of a family member or lay carer is therefore essential. Management of acute dyspnoea not only requires impeccable assessment of the patient but also of the family members or lay caregivers concurrently.

3 Causes of Acute Dyspnoea

When an episode of dyspnoea does not resolve or return to baseline, this requires further assessment in order to optimize management. Even for those at the very end of life, this can be worthwhile as simple strategies may be effective. Patient and caregiver distress is likely to be heightened. Taking the time to explore with the patient and their carer the change in their dyspnoea is an important acknowledgment of this symptom and validation of their concerns.

When assessing acute dyspnoea, it is important to identify those causes with a potentially reversible component. Progression of the underlying disease tends to occur over weeks or months and is a less likely cause of an acute dyspnoea episode. Commonly, the cause of the acute episode is due to a new diagnosis or complication, e.g., aspiration pneumonia. While anxiety can cause a dyspnoea crisis, this is a diagnosis of exclusion. Table 1 outlines causes of dyspnoea that have a relatively rapid onset and relevant investigations.

The degree to which these investigations are pursued will depend on the patient, the stage of their disease, and their wishes around management. Conversations around this can be difficult to negotiate during a crisis and should ideally have been anticipated in advance. For some, a change in location of care may be appropriate if a more supported environment is required to manage the dyspnoea, even if further investigation of the underlying cause is not pursued.

4 Assessment

As always, a clinical history is a vital component of the assessment of acute dyspnoea. In patients with a background of continuous dyspnoea, specific qualities of the dyspnoea itself may be difficult to tease out. Despite this, patients (or carers) may be able to describe the degree of functional impairment compared to baseline (e.g., normally I can walk to the bathroom; today I can't get out of bed). The impact of the acute dyspnoea on the psychological state of the patient and their carers is an important component of the history. As outlined above, increasing anxiety may be either a consequence of acute dyspnoea or the initial symptom of an acute episode. The psychological state of the patient and carer will impact on their ability to cope with the acute episode and therefore the management strategy that is put in place. Specific questions may need to be directed at what happened immediately prior to the episode of acute dyspnoea, individual triggers, and management strategies that have or have not helped previously.

Dyspnoea has many components and subtypes, just as pain can be neuropathic or pleuritic in nature. Terms that have been consistently used by patients to describe their dyspnoea can be grouped under the headings "air hunger or unsatisfied inspiration," "work/effort," and "tightness" (Parshall et al. 2012). Other descriptors include heavy/fast, shallow, or suffocating. The term "tightness" when used by patients has been consistently associated with a diagnosis of asthma, but other qualities of dyspnoea are not reliably associated with a specific condition. In patients with high anxiety scores, terms such as frightening or awful are more frequent, as is the term "shallow" in patients with interstitial lung disease (Chang et al. 2015).

Associated symptoms may be present, such as cough, fever, production of purulent sputum, facial pain or postnasal drip relating to sinus infection, chest pain, peripheral edema, calf tenderness, paroxysmal nocturnal dyspnoea, or orthopnea.

In the respiratory system, clinical examination can help to narrow a differential diagnosis, is noninvasive, and easily performed at the patients' location of care. Many of the causes of acute dyspnoea in Table 1 have distinct clinical examination findings that can be picked up at the bedside. For example, abnormal pulse rate and rhythm can suggest arrhythmia, expiratory wheeze suggests bronchospasm, and stridor suggests upper airway obstruction.

Patient observations can be very helpful in refining the differential diagnosis, such as temperature, oxygen saturations, pulse, and blood pressure. However, a caveat is that in many patients with advanced lung disease, their baseline figures for these observations may be abnormal. For example, a patient with COPD may have a baseline oxygen saturation of 90% on room air and a heart rate of 100 beats per minute. It is therefore the *change* in the observation value that is most useful during assessment of an acute episode.

Table 1 Causes of acute dyspnoea and onset and investigations

Onset usually minutes or hours	Relevant investigations	Onset usually days	Relevant investigations
Acute MI	ECG, serial troponins	Cardiac tamponade	Echocardiogram
Diabetic ketoacidosis	Blood glucose, ABG	Congestive cardiac failure	BNP, CXR
Arrhythmia	ECG	Pneumonia	CXR
Sepsis	Blood culture	Exacerbation of COPD	FBC, CRP, CXR
Bronchospasm	Auscultation Peak expiratory flow in asthma	Upper airway obstruction	CXR, CT neck/chest or endoscopy
Pulmonary embolism	CTPA or V/Q scan	Anemia	FBC
Pneumothorax	CXR or USS chest	Pleural effusion	CXR or USS chest
Anxiety	ABG	Superior vena cava obstruction	CT chest with contrast

MI myocardial infarction, *ECG* electrocardiogram, *ABG* arterial blood gas, *CTPA* computed tomography pulmonary angiogram, *V/Q* ventilation perfusion scan, *CXR* chest x-ray, *USS* ultrasound scan, *BNP* brain natriuretic peptide, *FBC* full blood count, *CRP* C-reactive protein, *CT* computed tomography

5 Investigations

Whether or not to perform investigations for acute dyspnoea will depend on a number of factors, including the stage of the illness and patient's goals of care. Many of the investigations in Table 1 will require admission to a hospital or similar facility. Patients may have suffered many episodes of acute dyspnoea and will often be guided by previous experiences.

The clinical suspicion of a pulmonary embolism (PE) often brings difficult decision-making, as definitive diagnosis requires a computed tomography pulmonary angiogram (CTPA) or V/Q scan. The D-Dimer test is routinely used in ruling out a pulmonary embolism but has most utility in patients with a low probability of PE. The majority of cancer patients or those with advanced, life-limiting nonmalignant disease will not fall into a low probability group according to Wells' criteria, which makes the D-Dimer test less useful in this group. Consideration should be given to proceeding directly to definitive imaging in those where there is a high clinical suspicion of PE (Linkins and Takach Lapner 2017).

Pleural ultrasound is a relatively new, noninvasive technique that can be applied at the bedside to diagnose cardiogenic pulmonary edema, pleural effusion, pneumothorax, or consolidation in trained operators. It is increasingly being used by emergency physicians to aid in narrowing a differential diagnosis for patients presenting with breathlessness. While the interobserver and intra-observer variability has been reported as low in skilled operators, the main limitation of its use lies in operator training and experience (Wimalasena et al. 2017).

6 Management of Specific Conditions

The management of massive hemoptysis and superior vena cave obstruction is covered elsewhere in this textbook. Discussed below are management strategies for several causes of acute dyspnoea that commonly cause distress.

6.1 Anxiety or Breathing Pattern Disorders

Anxiety as a cause of acute dyspnoea or dyspnoea crisis is a diagnosis of exclusion, when organic causes have been ruled out. In some patients, a more chronic breathing pattern disorder can occur, such as hyperventilation syndrome or periodic deep sighing. These conditions are more common in those with underlying respiratory disorders, most commonly asthma. They are difficult to diagnose but should be suspected when chronic changes in breathing pattern result in dyspnoea, in excess of that expected for the underlying disease, plus non-respiratory symptoms resulting from hypocapnia such as dizziness or tingling of the extremities. The Nijmegen questionnaire is helpful in identifying individuals with this diagnosis, and evidence of hyperventilation on an arterial blood gas is also suggestive. Identification of a breathing pattern disorder is important as physiotherapy-directed breathing techniques can be effective in managing this condition. In the acute setting, rebreathing is no longer recommended; reassurance and time are usually sufficient to allow symptoms of an acute attack to settle (Boulding et al. 2016).

6.2 Stridor or Upper Airway Obstruction

Stridor can be defined as an "abnormal high-pitched musical sound caused by an obstruction in the trachea or larynx" (Harris et al. 2014). Stridor may be accompanied by drooling or inability to swallow secretions. Causes in the palliative setting are usually malignant, most commonly due to lung cancer (Guibert et al. 2016) but can include more benign causes such as foreign body aspiration. Rapid deterioration can occur if swelling, secretions, or bleeding narrows the airway lumen further. The management of stridor will depend greatly on the goals of care for the individual and range from emergency intubation or tracheostomy to palliative sedation in the last days of life.

For those patients not appropriate for intubation or surgical airway management, initial treatment will include supportive care with positioning (usually in the upright position), attention to secretion management with gentle suction as required, and oxygen for those who are hypoxemic. Nebulized adrenaline has been used in this setting with anecdotal benefit in case reports (Flockton et al. 2007). Doses recommended are adrenaline 1:1000 made up to 5 ml with 0.9% saline and delivered via nebulizer up to four times a day, though doses used for croup in the pediatric setting can be much higher than this. Reported side effects are tachycardia, tremor, hyperactivity, and hypertension.

Heliox, a mixture of helium and oxygen gas, has been reported as beneficial for patients with acute upper airway obstruction (Smith and Biros 1999). Room air is mainly a mixture of nitrogen and oxygen; when nitrogen is substituted for helium, the overall gas density is reduced, and laminar airflow is restored, a theoretical advantage in those patients with large airway obstruction causing turbulent airflow. Helium is inert, with an excellent safety profile in humans. There are no evidence-based guidelines around the use of heliox in acute upper airway obstruction, but a trial of therapy should be considered as a bridge to definitive treatment. Numerous case reports describe clinical improvement following heliox in patients with upper airway obstruction due to lymphoma, cancer, or radiation therapy (Smith and Biros 1999; Diehl et al. 2011).

Depending on the likely cause of the upper airway obstruction, steroids may be indicated. Dexamethasone is usually the drug of choice due to its potent anti-inflammatory effects. Due to the nature of action of dexamethasone, full benefit may not be seen for several days. Steroids should therefore be initiated early in conjunction with other management strategies as mentioned above.

Interventional bronchoscopy is a developing field and is available in many centers worldwide. For malignant tumors causing central airway obstruction in the trachea, main bronchus, or bronchus intermedius, interventional techniques may provide palliation of symptoms. Between 20% and 30% of lung cancers will cause central airway obstruction, either from endoluminal blockage, extrinsic compression, or a combination of both (Guibert et al. 2016). Bronchoscopic techniques that can allow rapid reversal of central airway obstruction include thermocoagulation with electrocautery, argon plasma coagulation or Nd–YAG (neodymium-doped yttrium aluminum garnet) laser. These techniques are contraindicated in patients requiring supplementary oxygen with a FiO_2 exceeding 0.4 due to the risk of combustion. Once the airway lumen has been enlarged, an endoluminal stent may be placed to prevent recurrence. For extrinsic compression, stenting may be the only bronchoscopic option available. A registry study of therapeutic bronchoscopic procedures quotes technical success rates of over 90% but with improvements in dyspnoea scores and quality-of-life (QoL) scores of 48% and 42%, respectively. It was noted that those patients with higher dyspnoea scores and lower QoL pre-procedure gained most benefit in terms of relief of symptoms. The overall complication rate was 3.9% with a 0.5% procedural mortality rate (Ost et al. 2015). In summary, interventional bronchoscopic techniques may be appropriate for selected patients with central airway obstruction, which is causing significant dyspnoea or impaired QoL and who do not require high-flow oxygen.

6.3 Bronchospasm

Bronchospasm can be defined as "an excessive and prolonged contraction of the smooth muscle of the bronchi and bronchioles, resulting in an acute narrowing and obstruction of the respiratory airway" (Harris et al. 2014). It is usually reversible. Precipitants include underlying asthma or COPD, allergic reactions such as anaphylaxis, or pseudoallergic reactions such as a drug reaction. Pseudoallergic reactions can occur on first exposure to a drug, such as the histamine release induced by morphine. This side effect of morphine is generally described when given intravenously, often during general anesthesia, but can cause itching, bronchospasm, and vasodilatation.

Other drugs such as aspirin, nonsteroidal anti-inflammatory drugs or beta blockers may cause bronchospasm, particularly in those with underlying diseases such as asthma.

Increasingly, nebulized therapy is being utilized in many areas of medicine, e.g., nebulized saline for troublesome secretions or nebulized lignocaine for intractable cough. Any nebulized treatment has the potential to cause bronchospasm, especially in those with risk factors such as asthma. In practice, if there is clinical concern that bronchospasm may occur, then serial spirometry performed before and after administration of the drug in question may be helpful; in many centers a 200 ml or 12% drop in FEV1 readings post-administration would be considered significant. In those patients unable to perform spirometry, premedication with a beta agonist may be required.

Treatment of acute bronchospasm involves the use of bronchodilator medication. This falls into two groups, beta agonists and muscarinic antagonists. In the acute setting, inhaled, short-acting beta-2 agonists are the drug of choice. Beta-2 agonists act on bronchial smooth muscle to affect rapid bronchodilation, acting within 3–5 min with a peak effect at 15–20 min. When short-acting beta-2 agonists such as salbutamol are delivered via metered dose inhaler (MDI) and spacer device by appropriately trained personnel, they can be as efficacious as a nebulizer device. However, nebulized short-acting beta-2 agonists may be appropriate for those who are unable to use an MDI (e.g., incoordination, poor technique, unable to activate device), and many patients express a preference for nebulized therapy. The increased risk of transmission of airborne infection limits the use of nebulizers in the hospital setting. Side effects of beta-2 agonists include tremor, nervousness, tachycardia, and rarely paradoxical bronchospasm (Cates et al. 2013).

Short-acting muscarinic antagonists such as ipratropium can be considered as additional treatment for those not responding to beta-2 agonists and are available in both MDI and nebulized forms. Side effects include dry mouth, nausea, headache, and rarely paradoxical bronchospasm.

Both beta-2 agonists and muscarinic antagonists are available in long-acting formulations, evidence for their use centers around chronic management of asthma or COPD. With the exception of formoterol, their onset of action is too long to be of use in the management of an acute dyspnoea crisis and should not be used in this setting. In asthmatics, use of a long-acting beta agonist without concurrent use of inhaled steroid should be avoided.

6.4 Choking Episodes

Choking episodes are uncommon in patients with life-limiting illness but cause significant anxiety and distress. They are particularly common in those with neurological disorders affecting swallow, such as motor neuron disease (MND). Choking episodes can also occur in those with malignancies affecting the upper airway or lower respiratory tract due to excessive secretions, particularly bronchoalveolar cell carcinoma of the lung which can occasionally produce a high volume of secretions (or bronchorrhea) (Remi et al. 2016).

Much of the evidence around choking episodes centers on MND, where bulbar dysfunction affects between 20% and 30% of patients (Banfi et al. 2015). While many patients with MND are worried about choking to death, retrospective studies have shown that this does not occur in reality (Neudert et al. 2001). In one review, 7% of patients experienced episodes of choking on saliva or mucous within the last 24 h prior to death, with 4% experiencing coughing. A further study comparing coughing or choking episodes in patients with MND to healthy controls revealed that the majority of MND patients experienced coughing or choking episodes, ranging between 1 and 50 episodes over a 3-day period. Twenty-seven percent of patients described the episodes as moderate or very distressing, and 32% described shortness of breath or inability to breathe during episodes (Hadjikoutis et al. 2000).

Much of the management of choking episodes focuses on chronic management of secretion production. Secretions may either be “thick” and cause problems with difficultly expectorating sputum or "thin" due to excessive saliva production and inability to swallow saliva or bronchorrhea. It is essential that the type of secretion problem be assessed carefully; in one study 40% of MND patients described thin secretions, 23% thick secretions, and 37% both. Overtreatment of thin secretions can cause thick secretions to become a problem (McGeachen et al. 2017a).

Chronic management of thin secretions includes the use of anticholinergics such as hyoscine butylbromide, tricyclic antidepressants, atropine (eye drops, used sublingually), glycopyrronium, and nasal anticholinergics such as propantheline or ipratropium (used sublingually). For thick secretions, medications such as carbocisteine or 0.9% saline via nebulizer may be of benefit, in addition to conservative measures such as fruit juices (e.g., grape or pineapple) and attention to hydration (McGeachen et al. 2017a).

Acute management of choking episodes is less evidence-based. These episodes should be anticipated in advance in those at risk, and an action plan developed with the patient and carer may reduce anxiety and distress. Attention should be paid to positioning (sitting upright, use of mechanical aids to allow easy change in position, or turning to the contralateral side if bed-bound). Gentle suction can be helpful, particularly for those with thin secretions. Carer education is essential, for example, in the use of devices such as suction machines and nebulizers or performing manually assisted cough in those with poor respiratory muscle function.

Thick secretions can be challenging to manage in an acute choking episode; saline nebulizers may be helpful as well as manually assisted cough (McGeachen et al. 2017b). For those with tracheostomies, suction is essential but is of more limited use for those with an intact oropharyngeal airway and gag reflex.

7 Management of the Dyspnoea Crisis

As described above, a dyspnoea crisis can be defined as:

> sustained and severe resting breathing discomfort that occurs in patients with advanced, often life-limiting illness and overwhelms the patient and caregivers' ability to achieve symptom relief. (Mularski et al. 2013a)

The majority of these episodes are short-lived, up to 10 min duration (Reddy et al. 2009) and mainly occur in the patients' place of care, such as their own home. Such a crisis may have an acute, reversible underlying cause, but many episodes resolve spontaneously or with measures targeted at relieving the dyspnoea itself. Despite this, acute on chronic breathlessness has been shown to be responsible for at least 5.2% of all presentations to the ED in one study. In this study population, only one in five patients had a GP or paramedic involved in the decision to attend the ED, with patients and family/friends most frequently initiating the decision to present. Although patients rated their shortness of breath as "severe" at the time of the decision to attend, the rating had reduced to "mild" by the time of assessment in the ED itself, supporting the fact that the episodes are generally short-lived (Hutchinson et al. 2017). For some patients, where a dyspnoea crisis is sustained or severe, it may be appropriate to seek medical assessment for consideration of investigation or treatment. This will depend on the patient and families' goals of care, which can be impossible to discuss during an acute episode.

7.1 Non-pharmacological Measures

Management of chronic refractory dyspnoea is detailed in ▶ Chap. 11, "Palliative Management of Breathlessness" and will not be reiterated here. Most of the measures described can be applied in some way to episodes of acute dyspnoea or a dyspnoea crisis. Non-pharmacological measures may provide simple, effective means of managing a dyspnoea crisis with little or no side effects; however evidence to support this is lacking, with most research focusing on chronic refractory dyspnoea. While many non-pharmacological measures can be easily put into practice during a crisis, such as switching on a handheld fan or adjusting position, others are less easily utilized.

Relaxation and breathing control techniques in particular cannot be learnt in a state of heightened anxiety and panic and must be taught when the patient is in a more stable condition. These techniques require practice and reinforcement to utilize them effectively, meaning that a degree of planning must take place before a dyspnoea crisis occurs.

7.2 Pharmacological Measures

More recently, research has focused on the utility of pharmacological measures to manage a breathlessness crisis or episode of acute dyspnoea. Because of the short duration of breathlessness episodes, an ideal drug is one which is absorbed swiftly, with a rapid onset of maximum effect and short duration of action. For this reason, the transmucosal, intranasal, or nebulized routes of drug administration are particularly attractive. Since a systematic review of opioids in the management of dyspnoea failed to show any beneficial effect of nebulized opioids over nebulized saline, this route has fallen out of use (Jennings et al. 2002), and with the advent of oral transmucosal drug delivery systems, such as fentanyl citrate, research has been focused on this area.

Depending on the preparation, the onset of action of oral transmucosal fentanyl citrate is between 5 and 10 min with a bioavailability of between 50% and 90% (Cabezon-Gutierrez et al. 2016). Similarly, intranasal medications such as midazolam have been reported to have a median time to maximum effect of 10–14 min with bioavailability of 50–83% (Hardy et al. 2016). Drugs with a short half-life, such as fentanyl or midazolam, would seem ideally suited to the management of an acute episode of dyspnoea to tailor the duration of effect as closely as possible to the duration of the crisis.

Fentanyl has been the most studied opioid for the management of an acute episode of dyspnoea or dyspnoea crisis. However, most trials to date have been small or nonrandomized; therefore evidence of significant benefit is currently lacking. A systematic review by Simon et al. in 2013 identified only two randomized controlled trials (one of which included only two patients), with several case studies and before–after studies, totalling 88 patients. A variety of routes of administration were described, including oral transmucosal and intranasal. All studies reported successful relief of breathlessness after fentanyl application, but the only randomized controlled trial failed to demonstrate a statistically significant difference compared with placebo (Simon et al. 2013d). A further non-systematic review by Cabezon-Gutirriez of opioids for the management of episodic breathlessness identified 4 clinical trials and several case series, totalling 204 patients. Drugs studied included oral transmucosal fentanyl, intranasal or subcutaneous fentanyl, morphine and/or midazolam, and oral or subcutaneous hydromorphone. While these studies reported an improvement in dyspnoea, the heterogeneity of the study design makes it difficult to ascertain efficacy of any one intervention. Side effect reporting was low and limited to somnolence and dizziness, suggesting that opioids for the treatment of episodic dyspnoea are safe in the majority of patients (Cabezon-Gutierrez et al. 2016). Further trials are underway at the time of writing.

Despite the lack of evidence for the use of benzodiazepines for managing chronic, refractory breathlessness, these medications are commonly used. As described above, a dyspnoea crisis overwhelms the ability of the patient and/or caregivers' ability to cope, often due to the anxiety and panic caused by severe shortness of breath. Intuitively, therefore, use of a short-acting anxiolytic agent, such as midazolam, could modify this anxiety and break the dyspnoea–anxiety–dyspnoea cycle. Evidence is limited however. A randomized, double-blind trial of intranasal midazolam for chronic refractory dyspnoea showed no benefit over placebo (Hardy et al. 2016). Evidence specifically in episodic dyspnoea is very limited, and to date no clear benefit has been shown (Simon et al. 2016). A pragmatic approach should be taken until further research can guide the use of benzodiazepines in this setting. Medications with more robust evidence for the palliation of dyspnoea should be used first-line, with reservation of benzodiazepines as second- or third-line therapy for those patients where there is a significant degree of anxiety or panic during dyspnoea crises. To minimize harms, an individualized (or n-of-1) trial should be undertaken, with a short-acting benzodiazepine initiated at low dose and titrated upward.

Oxygen is commonly used during episodes of breathlessness. Patients with chronic breathlessness or frequent episodes of acute dyspnoea requiring emergency medical assessment are often familiar with the use of oxygen during an emergency. High flows of oxygen are applied immediately on arrival of the paramedic or at the ED. While in reality multiple interventions are occurring for the patient during this time, many patients recall the initiation of oxygen as having a positive effect on reducing their breathlessness. Evidence for this is lacking, however, particularly in the group with maintained oxygen saturations of greater than 90% on room air. In chronic, refractory breathlessness, a large randomized double-blind trial showed no beneficial effect of oxygen over room air when delivered by gas concentrator for 16 h or more per day. A significant number of patients declined to continue therapy at the end of the trial, as the burdens were felt to outweigh the benefits by those individuals (Abernethy et al. 2010). Evidence for ambulatory oxygen, for those with exertional oxygen desaturation, is similarly lacking with a large trial in COPD showing no benefit on quality of life or walking distance (LOTT Group 2016). Domiciliary oxygen is not without harms and is contraindicated in active smokers. For this reason, oxygen should not be used first line as an intervention for breathlessness crises but trialed on an individual basis as part of a comprehensive management plan.

7.3 Palliative Sedation

For some patients with overwhelming distress, sedation may be required. The aim of sedation may vary from transient (for a period of hours until the current episode has resolved) to palliative sedation for a patient in the last days of life experiencing intolerable suffering due to dyspnoea. Where it is anticipated that sedation may be required, it is important to recognize, plan for, and discuss this with the patient and family prior to an event occurring. Many patients and families consent to transient sedation during a breathlessness crisis where symptoms cannot be controlled by other means. It is important to emphasize the goals around this and expectations regarding the duration and depth of sedation. This is usually delivered by bolus medications on an "as required" basis.

Palliative sedation in the last days of life involves continuous administration of sedating medications to render the patient unaware of the symptom that is causing intolerable suffering, i.e., dyspnoea. Palliative sedation in this setting has not been shown to hasten death (Godbout et al. 2016). The decision to commence palliative sedation can be difficult and ideally should involve engagement with the wider healthcare team as well as family/carers, with preemptive education and opportunity for discussion. This can be impossible to achieve in the setting of a dyspnoea crisis, where decision-making is usually rapid. Where possible, this option should be discussed in advance with patients at risk of requiring palliative sedation or who disclose fears about control of breathlessness in the last days of life.

7.4 Advance Care Planning

Advance discussions around the goals of care for an individual are imperative when managing a breathlessness crisis. During an episode, most patients are unable to communicate their wishes effectively; they are usually too breathless or too panicked to be able to engage in a complex discussion about their wishes for treatment. Similarly, most family members or carers will be focused on managing the distress of their loved one a rather than specific treatment options. It is therefore important to recognize discussions around the goals of care as essential to managing those at risk of a dyspnoea crisis and for these conversations to occur during a time of relative stability.

Repeatedly in the literature, patients express a wish to know their future prognosis but wait for their healthcare practitioner to initiate this conversation. Components of the discussion should focus on a shared understanding of the disease process, expected complications, and prognosis, with a strong focus on the goals of the individual in the time ahead. Once goals are established and agreed upon, treatments can be considered that may or may not achieve these goals, such as invasive ventilation or cardiopulmonary resuscitation. For some patients it can be difficult to make advance decisions, particularly in diseases where the course of events is less certain, such as COPD (MacPherson et al. 2012). For this group, advance conversations can still add value by identifying a surrogate decision-maker and preparing the patient for *how* decisions may be made in the event that a crisis occurs.

The value of these discussions lies in the conversations between the patient, their loved ones, and the treating healthcare practitioner. Many patients will choose to write down advance decisions to assist with transparency over multiple healthcare settings and to avoid future conflict or uncertainty. This can be done via an advance directive, advance care plan, or other format such as Physician Orders for Life-Sustaining Treatment (POLST) form.

7.5 Individualized Dyspnoea Crisis Management Plans

Since the majority of episodes of dyspnoea crisis occur outside of healthcare settings, self-management is essential. Despite this, few guidelines are available for either healthcare professionals or patients/carers with regard to self-management of breathlessness episodes. A review of internet-based guidelines for patient self-management of chronic breathlessness found multiple websites of varying quality. Specific guidance for breathlessness crises suggested attending the ED immediately, rather than subsequent to implementing incremental management strategies; none offered support for goal setting. Website content for carers was limited, and compliance with American Medical Association benchmarks for quality were low (Luckett et al. 2016).

An American Thoracic Society workshop in 2009 on the assessment and management of dyspnoea crisis proposed a customizable self-management patient/caregiver plan, incorporating the management strategies described above (Mularski et al. 2013a). While there is little evidence for the effectiveness of such plans as yet, such a multicomponent intervention is difficult to assess. Management plans for a dyspnoea crisis involve utilizing interventions that the patient and caregiver have previously found beneficial for their breathlessness, in a specified order. It is therefore imperative that specific techniques or medications, such as a fan or opioids, have been trialed individually before a comprehensive plan can be created. Individual components may be assessed by patient/caregiver report or a symptom control diary. Each plan should be individualized and may involve multiple members of the interdisciplinary team in its creation. Plans should be fluid enough to adapt to the patient experience; reviews should be scheduled regularly. Vital to the plan is identification of who to call for help should the end of the management cascade be reached, as well as transparency as to the goals of care and indications for transfer to an alternative place of care, such as the ED.

An example of a management plan cascade is below. The order of specific therapies will depend on the patient. In general, non-pharmacological therapies are used first, but in some patients with a significant anxiety component to their dyspnoea crises, medications may need to be administered early as panic limits the ability to engage with therapies such as relaxation techniques.

- Call or signal for help.
- Attend to positioning and environmental factors, e.g., switch on a fan or open a door.
- Distraction – music, TV. Reassurance. Relaxation techniques.
- Medications – include specific therapies that have worked previously, e.g., salbutamol.

Include dose and time interval for expected effect. Repeat doses if necessary.
- Oxygen if indicated.
- Who to call for help if above steps have failed.
- Ceiling of care or where documentation of this may be found.

Family or lay caregivers are integral to the success of a management plan for dyspnoea crisis. Family caregivers are deeply affected by a dyspnoea crisis which can cause feelings of anxiety, inadequacy, helplessness, and uncertainty. A qualitative interview of patients with lung cancer or COPD and their carers found that carers wished to know more about managing anxiety, panic, and breathlessness. More specifically, carers wish to know how to recognize panic and how to respond confidently in order to manage breathlessness. Carers acknowledged that their response was often unhelpful – e.g., asking the patient what they want during a time of crisis and that they themselves often felt anxious and panicked (Farquar et al. 2017). Mularski et al. suggest components for patient (and family/carer) education in dyspnoea crisis which include:

- Basic facts about triggers and causes
- Signs and symptoms that may indicate a crisis
- Measuring change in dyspnoea intensity and distress
- Breathing retraining
- Relaxation techniques
- Use of oxygen, ventilation, or fans
- Appropriate administration and dosing of medications

These facets of patient education should be delivered from diagnosis and reinforced at every encounter, not only with patients but also with those caregivers who are likely to be present at the time of a dyspnoea crisis.

One of the greatest challenges to healthcare currently is ensuring that such plans are visible and transferable across healthcare settings. Communication between patient, family/carers, and all healthcare professionals is key to successful implementation of an individualized dyspnoea crisis management plan and therefore control of a dyspnoea crisis. In some cases, it may be necessary to nominate a single family spokesperson to communicate with healthcare professionals. Many healthcare professionals are unfamiliar with the management of a dyspnoea crisis and will require targeted education within relevant local practice guidelines and continuing education programs (Mularski et al. 2013a).

8 Conclusion and Summary

Assessment of acute dyspnoea as well as management of specific conditions such as stridor, bronchospasm, and choking is essential knowledge for the palliative care practitioner.

Episodic breathlessness is a significant and distressing symptom for patients with advanced life-limiting illness, which at times may precipitate a dyspnoea crisis. Impeccable, holistic assessment of the patient presenting with an acute exacerbation of their dyspnoea is essential to reverse treatable causes. For those without an immediately reversible cause for their dyspnoea, or for whom investigation is inappropriate, management should focus on non-pharmacological and pharmacological approaches – which present unique challenges in this setting due to the short duration of episodic dyspnoea and lack of evidence in this area. Comprehensive management plans, including a stepwise approach to previously trialed interventions, should be individualized, shared, and reviewed on a regular basis. Carer engagement is key to successful implementation. Education and involvement of the interdisciplinary healthcare team across multiple settings is essential.

References

Abernethy AP, et al. Effect of palliative oxygen versus room air in relief of breathlessness in patients with refractory dyspnoea: a double-blind, randomised controlled trial. Lancet. 2010;376:784–93.

Bailey PH. The dyspnea-anxiety-dyspnea cycle- COPD patients' stories of breathlessness: "it's scary when you can't breathe". Qual Health Res. 2004;14(6): 760–78.

Banfi P, et al. A review of options for treating sialorrhea in amyotrophic lateral sclerosis. Respir Care. 2015; 60(3):446–54.

Boulding R, et al. Dysfunctional breathing: a review of the literature and proposal for classification. Eur Respir Rev. 2016;25:287–94.

Cabezon-Gutierrez L, et al. Opioids for management of episodic breathlessness or dyspnea in patients with advanced disease. Support Care Cancer. 2016; 24:4045–55.

Cates CJ, et al. Holding chambers (spacers) versus nebulisers for beta-agonist treatment of acute asthma. Cochrane Database Syst Rev. 2013;9:CD000052.

Chang AS, et al. Prospective use of descriptors of dyspnea to diagnose common respiratory diseases. Chest. 2015;148(4):895–902.

Currow DC, et al. Do the trajectories of dyspnea differ in prevalence and intensity by diagnosis at the end of life? A consecutive cohort study. J Pain Symptom Manage. 2010;39(4):680–90.

Diehl JL, et al. Helium in the adult critical care setting. Ann Intensive Care. 2011;1:24.

Ek K, et al. "The unpredictable death" – the last year of life for patients with advanced COPD: relatives stories. Palliat Support Care. 2015;13:1213–22.

Farquar M, et al. Six key topics informal carers of patients with breathlessness in advanced disease want to learn about and why: MRC phase 1 study to inform an educational intervention. PLoS One. 2017;12(5): e0177081.

Flockton RJ, et al. Use of nebulised adrenaline in the management of steroid resistant stridor. Palliat Med. 2007;21:723–4.

Giacomini M, et al. Experiences of living and dying with COPD: a systematic review and synthesis of the qualitative empirical literature. Ont Health Technol Assess Ser. 2012;12(13):1–47.

Godbout K, et al. A distress protocol for respiratory emergencies in terminally ill patients with lung cancer or chronic obstructive pulmonary disease. Am J Hosp Palliat Med. 2016;33(9):817–22.

Guibert N, et al. Techniques of endoscopic airway tumour treatment. J Thorac Dis. 2016;8(11):3343–60.

Gysels MH, Higginson IJ. The lived experience of breathlessness and its implications for care: a qualitative comparison in cancer, COPD, heart failure and MND. BMC Palliat Care. 2011;10:15.

Hadjikoutis S, et al. Coughing and choking in motor neuron disease. J Neurol Neurosurg Psychiatry. 2000; 68:601–4.

Hardy J, et al. A randomised, double-blind controlled trial of intranasal midazolam for the palliation of dyspnoea in patients with life-limiting disease. Support Care Cancer. 2016;24(7):3069–76.

Harris P, Nagy S, Vardaxis N. Mosby's dictionary of medicine, nursing and health professions. Marrickville: Elsevier; 2014.

Hearson, et al. Sleeping with one eye open: the sleep experience of family members providing palliative care at home. J Palliat Care. 2011;27(2):69–78.

Hutchinson A, et al. Breathlessness and presentation to the emergency department: a survey and clinical record review. BMC Pulm Med. 2017;17:53–9.

Janssens, et al. Dyspnoea perception in COPD: association between anxiety, dyspnoea-related fear and dyspnoea in a pulmonary rehabilitation program. Chest. 2011; 140(3):618–25.

Jennings AL, et al. A systematic review of the use of opioids in the management of dyspnoea. Thorax. 2002;57:939–44.

Linkins LA, Takach Lapner S. Review of D dimer testing: good, bad and ugly. Int J Lab Hematol. 2017; 39(Suppl 1):98–103.

LOTT Group. A randomised trial of long-term oxygen for COPD with moderate desaturation. N Engl J Med. 2016;375:1617–27.

Luckett T, et al. Content and quality of websites supporting self-management of chronic breathlessness in advanced illness: a systematic review. Prim Care Respir Med. 2016;26:16025.

MacPherson A, et al. The views of patients with severe chronic obstructive pulmonary disease on advance care planning: a qualitative study. Palliat Med. 2012; 27(3):265–72.

McGeachen AJ, et al. A multicentre evaluation of oropharyngeal secretion management practices in amyotrophic lateral sclerosis. Amyotroph Lateral Scler Frontotemporal Degener. 2017a;18:1–9.

McGeachen AJ, et al. Management of oral secretions in neurological disease. Pract Neurol. 2017b;17:96–103.

Mularski, et al. An official American thoracic society workshop report: assessment and palliative management of dyspnea crisis. Ann Am Thorac Soc. 2013a; 10(5):S98–S106.

Mularski, et al. ATS dyspnoea crisis supplementary methods document and evidence summary. Ann Am Thorac Soc. 2013b;10(5). Online supplement date of access 7th Feb 2017.

Neudert C, et al. The course of the terminal phase in patients with amyotrophic lateral sclerosis. J Neurol. 2001;248:612–6.

Ost DE, et al. Therapeutic bronchoscopy for malignant central airway obstruction. Chest. 2015;147(5): 1282–98.

Parshall MB, et al. Dyspnea duration, distress and intensity in emergency department visits for heart failure. Heart Lung. 2001;30(1):47–56.

Parshall MB, et al. An official ATS society statement: update on the mechanisms, assessment and management of dyspnea. Am J Respir Crit Care Med. 2012; 185(4):435–52.

Reddy SK, et al. Characteristics and correlates of dyspnoea in patients with advanced cancer. J Palliat Med. 2009;12(1):29–36.

Remi C, et al. Pharmacological management of bronchorrhea in malignant disease: a systematic literature review. J Pain Symptom Manage. 2016;51(5): 916–25.

Simon ST, et al. Episodic and continuous breathlessness: a new categorization of breathlessness. J Pain Symptom Manage. 2013a;45(6):1019–29.

Simon ST, et al. Episodic breathlessness in patients with advanced disease: a systematic review. J Pain Symptom Manage. 2013b;45(3):561–77.

Simon ST, et al. Episodes of breathlessness: types and patterns – a qualitative study exploring experiences of patients with advanced diseases. Palliat Med. 2013c;27(6):524–32.

Simon ST, et al. Fentanyl for the relief of refractory breathlessness: a systematic review. J Pain Symptom Manage. 2013d;46(6):874–86.

Simon ST, et al. Definition, categorization, and terminology of episodic breathlessness: consensus by and international Delphi survey. J Pain Symptom Manage. 2014;47(5):828–38.

Simon ST, et al. Benzodiazepines for the relief of breathlessness in advanced malignant and non-malignant diseases in adults. Cochrane Database Syst Rev. 2016; 10:Art no CD007354.

Smith SW, Biros M. Relief of imminent respiratory failure from upper airway obstruction by use of helium-oxygen: a case series and brief review. Acad Emerg Med. 1999;6(9):953–6.

Weingartner V, et al. Characterizing episodic breathlessness in patients with advanced disease. J Palliat Med. 2013;16(10):1275–9.

Weingartner V, et al. Characteristics of episodic breathlessness as reported by patients with advanced chronic obstructive pulmonary disease and lung cancer: results of a descriptive cohort study. Palliat Med. 2015; 29(5):420–8.

Wimalasena Y, et al. Lung ultrasound: a useful tool in the assessment of the dyspnoeic patient in the emergency department. Fact or fiction? Emerg Med J. 2017;0:1–9.

Neutropenic Sepsis

78

William Thompson, Rosalie Stephen, and Michelle K. Wilson

Contents

W. Thompson · R. Stephen · M. K. Wilson (✉)
Cancer and Blood Services, Auckland City Hospital, Auckland, New Zealand
e-mail: WThompson@adhb.govt.nz; RStephens@adhb.govt.nz; miwilson@adhb.govt.nz

R. D. MacLeod, L. Van den Block (eds.), *Textbook of Palliative Care*,
https://doi.org/10.1007/978-3-319-77740-5_81

Abstract

Febrile neutropenia is a common complication of cytotoxic therapies and can be potentially life threatening. Treatment for neutropenic fever has evolved with the advent of antibiotics with mortality rates falling as a consequence. Patterns of infection have changed from being predominantly related to gram-negative organisms to now being mostly caused by gram-positive organisms. However, in the majority of cases, no source is isolated.

Higher rates of febrile neutropenia are seen with cytotoxic treatments for hematological malignancies, compared to that for solid malignancies. Therapies to reduce the risk of febrile neutropenia should be considered in patients at high risk of prolonged (>7 days) and severe ($<1 \times 10^9$ cells/L) neutropenia and also in those who would poorly tolerate the complication. Risk factors for neutropenic fever include age >65, prior exposure to chemotherapy or radiation, persistent neutropenia, bone marrow involvement by tumor, recent surgery and/or open wounds, renal dysfunction, and liver dysfunction.

Management requires prompt commencement of antibiotics, careful investigations into a possible source, and supportive cares. Empiric antibiotics with an antipseudomonal cephalosporin or a carbopenem should be started early. Data around the synergism of aminoglycosides is unclear. Treatment should be modified dependent on the results of the investigations. In the setting of a persistent fever, the addition of vancomycin and/or an antifungal agent should be considered.

Patients should be well informed of this potential life-threatening complication. Mortality can vary from 1% in low-risk patients to 50% in those requiring ICU admission with septic shock.

1 Introduction

Febrile neutropenia is a potentially life-threatening complication of cytotoxic therapy in both oncology and hematology patients. Febrile neutropenia is defined as a temperature above 38.5 °C or consecutive temperatures above 38 degrees Celsius more than 1 h apart associated with a neutrophil count of less than 0.5×10^9 cells/L or one expected to fall below 0.5×10^9 cells/L (Table 1). The risk of febrile neutropenia is higher in patients receiving chemotherapy for hematological malignancies compared with those receiving treatment for solid organ cancers. In approximately 50% of cases, the cause of the fever is not found and

Table 1 Important definitions

	Definition
Febrile neutropenia	A temperature above 38.5 °C or consecutive temperatures above 38 °C more than 1 h apart associated with a neutrophil count of less than 0.5×10^9 cells/L or one expected to fall below 0.5×10^9 cells/L
Neutropenic sepsis	Severe sepsis in the context of febrile neutropenia
Severe sepsis	New evidence of organ dysfunction or decreased perfusion including lactic acidosis, oliguria (<0.5 mL/kg/hr), hypotension (<90 mmHg systolic blood pressure or a decrease of >40 mmHg), or delirium
Septic shock	A situation where severe sepsis and hypotension persist despite adequate fluid resuscitation and in the absence of other explanations for hypotension
Clinically unstable	The presence of severe sepsis or septic shock
Clinically stable	The absence of severe sepsis or septic shock
Complicated infection	One or more of the following: Persistent fever greater than 48 h despite treatment Evidence of secondary infection such as endocarditis, osteomyelitis, or abscess Development of a fungal infection Severe sepsis Septic shock Congestive heart failure, ECG changes, or arrhythmia Respiratory failure Renal failure Intensive care admission Bleeding requiring transfusion Allergic reaction
Uncomplicated infection	The absence of a complication as defined above

treatment is empiric. The prognosis for patients with neutropenic fever has improved with the advent of antibiotics. Prompt treatment with antibiotics and supportive care is critical. In this chapter, we will review the pathophysiology of neutropenic fever, causative organisms, treatment, and prognosis of febrile neutropenia.

2 History

Although previous studies had indicated a relationship between leukopenia and infection in patients with acute leukemia, it was not until 1966 that a *quantitative* relationship between leukocyte counts and infection was established (Bodey et al. 1966). Infection was the primary cause of death in these patients. Early efforts to treat infection were hampered by resistant organisms, with mortality from *Staphylococcus aureus* infections around 40%, predominantly due to high rates of penicillin resistance. This changed with the invention of methicillin with fatality falling to less than 5%, again by the 1960s (Bodey 1997). Over the last half century, patterns of infection associated with cancer treatments have continued to change.

A historic principle was that infection should not be treated until the causative organism had been identified. In 1971, this idea was challenged following the Schimpff et al. study, when it became recognized that empiric antibiotics should be used to treat patients with evidence of infection in leukemia (Bodey 1997). This principle was subsequently applied for all patients treated with myelosuppressive therapy presenting with this complication.

3 Pathophysiology

Chemotherapy-induced leukopenia can cause fever in the absence of infection, due to the release of cytokines such as interleukin-6 (IL-6) and tumor necrosis factor (TNF) (Bennett et al. 2013). However, fever in the context of chemotherapy-induced neutropenia is often the result of invasive infection and can be fatal. It is difficult to know the exact proportion of febrile neutropenia episodes resulting from invasive infection, as microbiological evidence of infection is found in less than 50% of cases of febrile neutropenia (Bucaneve et al. 2005).

Chemotherapy leads to impairment of the innate immune system in two ways. The first relates to impairment of the barrier function of the gut and to a lesser extent the skin. This is most commonly due to chemotherapeutic toxicity and mucositis allowing the transposition of bacteria into the bloodstream. In allogeneic hematopoietic stem cell transplant recipients, graft-versus-host disease (GVHD) may also affect this barrier function. In many cases, patients will also have long-term central venous catheters which can act as a route by which bacteria can bypass barriers and cause invasive infection. The second relates to chemotherapy-induced neutropenia. Neutrophils play a role in the non-specific phagocytic killing of bacteria and fungi as well as in the mediation of an inflammatory response, the absence of which allows infection to progress much faster.

3.1 Microbiology

Microbiological evidence of infection is found in less than 50% of cases of febrile neutropenia (Bucaneve et al. 2005). Bacteremia is found in only 20–30% of cases (Feld 2008). Over the last half century, patterns of infection have changed from a predominance of gram-negative organisms to now more commonly gram-positive organisms. One study found that the proportion of gram-negative and gram-positive organisms changed from 71% and 29%, respectively, in 1973–1975 to 33% and 67% in 1992–1994 (Klastersky 1998). This pattern has been less prominent in developing countries (Feld 2008). One possible explanation for this observation is the increasing use of prophylactic antibiotics and central venous catheters, particularly in developed nations. The use of prophylactic antibiotics can result in a reduced proportion of gram-negative to gram-positive bacteremia (from approximately 50% to 25%) (Feld 2008).

Patients with febrile neutropenia and gram-negative bacteremia have higher rates of mortality than those with gram-positive bacteremia (Feld 2008). Mortality in those with gram-negative bacteremia was found to be 18% in a population including both patients with hematological and solid organ malignancies treated in predominantly Western countries. This is compared with a mortality rate of 5% in those with gram-positive bacteremia from the same cohort. The most common gram-negative organisms included *E. coli*, *Klebsiella* species, and *P. aeruginosa*. The most common gram-positive organism was coagulase-negative staphylococci (in 50% of gram-positive bacteremia), followed by streptococcal species, and less commonly *S. aureus* and *Enterococcus*.

Fungal organisms are an important cause of mortality and morbidity in significantly immunosuppressed patients (Richardson 1998). The population primarily at risk are those patients with hematological malignancies undergoing hematopoietic stem cell transplant. The risk is increased in those with neutropenic periods longer than 7–10 days (Richardson 1998). In those receiving *allogeneic* transplants, the period of immunosuppression may be prolonged beyond the period of neutropenia, depending on the nature of the conditioning regimen and additionally on the use of immunosuppressives to reduce the risk of, or to treat, GVHD in the posttransplant period. The most common fungal organisms include *Aspergillus* and *Candida* species.

Candida are ubiquitous colonizers of mucosal surfaces, and breakdown of the skin and mucosa can lead to invasive infection (Freifeld et al. 2011). Azole prophylaxis has reduced their rates of invasive infection, but resistant forms of *Candida* such as *C. krusei* and *C. glabrata* are not uncommon and may be increasingly prevalent due to the use of prophylaxis (Freifeld et al. 2011). *Aspergillus* is an ubiquitous organism that is not usually pathogenic. Invasive aspergillosis is uncommon if neutropenia lasts less than 10 days, but beyond this time the incidence increases in proportion to the length of the neutropenic period (Gerson et al. 1984).

Finally, viral organisms can cause infections in the immunocompromised host. Herpes simplex virus (HSV) is common and can cause mucous membrane ulcers. Varicella zoster virus (VZV) is the cause of shingles, a vesicular skin rash typically in a dermatomal distribution. In those who are severely immunocompromised, VZV can present in a more widespread pattern. Both organisms can also cause encephalitis. These organisms typically become evident as a result of a deficiency in immune control, leading to reactivation of the latent virus. Other viral infections such as cytomegalovirus do not usually occur in the neutropenic period, but rather later as a result of other immunosuppressive agents used in the prevention of GVHD.

4 Incidence

It is difficult to estimate the true incidence of febrile neutropenia due to a number of factors, e.g., varying definitions of febrile neutropenia, the nature and extent of the underlying cancer, comorbidity in the studied population, the intensity of the chemotherapy, and the varying use of granulocyte colony-stimulating factor (G-CSF) prophylaxis. In addition, data often comes from trial patients who tend to be fitter and are treated with more rigorous adherence to regimen protocols.

As a general rule, chemotherapy for hematological malignancies is associated with a greater risk of febrile neutropenia than solid organ malignancies. Estimates range from a 10% to 40% risk of developing febrile neutropenia in those receiving chemotherapy for solid organ tumors to greater than 80% for those with hematological malignancies (Penack et al. 2014). The National Comprehensive Cancer Network (NCCN) guidelines provide a useful summary of approximate risks of febrile neutropenia with various chemotherapy regimens (NCCN 2017).

5 Prevention

A number of preventative strategies have been investigated to reduce the risk of febrile neutropenia. These include granulocyte colony-stimulating factor and antimicrobials. Current practice can vary significantly between centers. Typically prophylactic antibiotics are only recommended in patients expected to have prolonged (>7 days) and profound (<0.1 x 10^9 cells/L) neutropenia (Freifeld et al. 2011; Flowers et al. 2013). In this section, different preventative strategies will be reviewed.

5.1 Granulocyte Colony-Stimulating Factor (G-CSF) Prophylaxis

International guidelines suggest that if the estimated risk of febrile neutropenia is greater than 20% with a given regimen, primary prophylaxis with G-CSF should be used (Bennett et al. 2013). In those with an intermediate risk of 10–20% prophylaxis should be considered if other risk factors are present (Table 2).

Guidelines also propose that secondary prophylaxis should be considered if the previous cycle was complicated by an episode of febrile neutropenia (NCCN 2017), particularly if neutropenia *alone* would otherwise require a chemotherapy dose reduction. The occurrence of non-hematological toxicities from chemotherapy may necessitate a dose reduction in any case. It is important to consider the intent of chemotherapy in this decision. A lower threshold for a dose reduction may be appropriate in those being treated with palliative intent, in contrast to those treated with adjuvant or curative intent where maintaining maximum dose intensity is of key importance.

Table 2 Risk factors for febrile neutropenia

Patient risk factors for febrile neutropenia
Age > 65
Prior exposure to chemotherapy or radiation
Persistent neutropenia
Bone marrow involvement by tumor
Recent surgery and/or open wounds
Renal dysfunction (CrCl <50mLs/min)
Liver dysfunction

Adapted from NCCN guidelines (NCCN 2017)

5.2 Antibiotic Prophylaxis

One strategy postulated to reduce the risk of febrile neutropenia and associated mortality is antibiotic prophylaxis. Balanced against this are fears of increasing rates of antibiotic resistance by the selection of resistant organisms.

Many studies have explored antibiotic prophylaxis, but only the recent Cochrane systematic review has shown a mortality benefit. However, these studies involved a selected group at high risk of prolonged neutropenia (>7 days) (Gafter-Gvili et al. 2012). Most studies included in this systematic review investigated patients undergoing hematopoietic stem cell transplantation or intensive treatment for acute leukemia. The number needed to treat to prevent one death in this group was 33, with a reduction in all-cause mortality from 7.9% to 4.2% (Gafter-Gvili et al. 2012). Only a few of the studies included investigated patients with lymphoma and solid organ cancers receiving chemotherapy (but still only those receiving regimens with a high risk of prolonged neutropenia). A smaller mortality benefit was seen in this group with a number needed to treat to prevent one death of 50 and a reduction in all-cause mortality from 3.1% to 1.4% (Gafter-Gvili et al. 2012). Based on these studies, quinolones are the preferred prophylactic antibiotics, but no significant difference has been shown compared to cotrimoxazole. In the population at risk of *Pneumocystis jirovecii*, cotrimoxazole is the preferred option.

Two large trials published in *The New England Journal of Medicine* in 2005 also serve to guide the use of prophylactic antibiotics, the first assessing a population at high risk of febrile neutropenia and the second a low-risk population.

The first trial randomized 760 patients with either hematological or solid organ tumors where neutropenia (<1 × 10^9 cells/L) was expected to last at least 7 days but excluded those receiving *allogeneic* transplantation (Bucaneve et al. 2005). Levofloxacin was given continuously from up to 3 days prior to the commencement of chemotherapy or infusion of stem cells until the resolution of neutropenia. Although no mortality benefit was seen, there were significantly less febrile episodes (65% vs. 85%) and microbiologically documented infection (22% vs. 39%) in the levofloxacin group compared to placebo.

The second trial randomized 1565 patients with either lymphoma or solid organ tumors expected to have a neutrophil nadir of less than 0.5×10^9 cells/L with regimens not routinely given with G-CSF prophylaxis (Cullen et al. 2005). Levofloxacin was given for the 7 days of the expected neutropenic period. Although there were significantly less febrile episodes in the treated group (10.8% vs. 15.2%) and less hospitalizations (15.7% vs. 21.6%), there was no difference in severe infection defined as severe sepsis or death (1% vs. 2%).

Antibiotic resistance is difficult to assess and was not rigorously studied in these trials, although all groups acknowledged this as a potential issue. Multiple studies have been done in this area (Freifeld et al. 2011). For example, one hematology-oncology unit stopped fluoroquinolone prophylaxis in acute leukemia treatment for 6 months where it was previously routinely given. They showed that quinolone resistance in *E. coli* isolates reduced from >50% to 15% during this period, suggesting that antimicrobial resistance is an important consideration in the use of prophylactic antibiotics (Kern et al. 2005). In addition, there is thought to be a significantly increased risk of *Clostridium difficile*-associated diarrhea when using fluoroquinolones (Pépin et al. 2005).

Both the American Society of Clinical Oncology (ASCO) and the Infectious Disease Society of America (IDSA) guidelines recommend fluoroquinolone prophylaxis only for those expected to develop prolonged (>7 days) and profound ($<0.1 \times 10^9$ cells/L) neutropenia (Freifeld et al. 2011; Flowers et al. 2013).

5.2.1 Antifungal and Antiviral Prophylaxis

Antifungal and antiviral agents are only indicated in those at high risk of prolonged neutropenia, such as those receiving hematopoietic stem cell transplant and those with acute leukemia receiving intensive induction chemotherapy (Freifeld et al. 2011). ASCO practice guidelines recommend prophylactic use of antifungals in high-risk patient populations at risk of prolonged (>7 days) and profound ($<0.1 \times 10^9$ cells/L) neutropenia (Flowers et al. 2013).

6 Risk Assessment and Prognosis

There is a body of literature that seeks to stratify patients presenting with neutropenic fever into those at low or high risk of complication, for the purpose of identifying those who may be able to be treated with oral antibiotics or as an outpatient.

One such method which is recognized in international guidelines is the Multinational Association for Supportive Care in Cancer (MASCC) risk index (Table 3) (Klastersky et al. 2000). The derivation set included 756 patients, and independent factors predictive of complication were identified and weighted. Complications were defined as one or more of the following: hypotension, respiratory or renal failure, intensive care admission, confusion or altered mental status, congestive heart failure, bleeding requiring transfusion, ECG changes, arrhythmia, development of a fungal infection, or an allergic reaction.

In the initial validation cohort of 383 patients with febrile neutropenia, the index achieved a positive predictive value of 91% in identifying those who would not experience serious medical complications (Klastersky et al. 2000). The MASCC index was later validated in a prospective cohort including 80 episodes of febrile

Table 3 Multinational Association for Supportive Care in Cancer (MASCC) risk index

Prognostic factor	Score
Burden of illness (no or mild symptoms)	5
Burden of illness (moderate symptoms)	3
Burden of illness (severe symptoms)	0
No hypotension (systolic BP > 90 mmHg)	5
No chronic obstructive pulmonary disease	4
Solid tumor or lymphoma with no previous fungal infection	4
No dehydration	3
Outpatient (at onset of fever)	3
Age < 60 years	2

Scores ≥21 are at a low risk of complications. *MASCC Prognostic Index* (Klastersky et al. 2000)

neutropenia, all of whom received empiric intravenous antibiotics and inpatient management (Uys et al. 2004). It achieved a positive predictive value of 98.3%. Another study which utilized this index to identify low-risk cases, before management with initial oral antibiotics and a plan for early discharge (after at least 24 h), achieved a positive predictive value of 96.7% in identifying those who would not develop serious medical complication (Innes et al. 2008). The score's use has become widely accepted.

Alternative international guidelines specify characteristics of patients that place them in a group at high risk of complication in addition to those identified above (Freifeld et al. 2011; NCCN 2017). These recognize that low-risk patients are increasingly being managed with oral therapies or as outpatients after a period of observation. These include:

- Significant medical comorbidity or presence of clinical instability
- Hepatic (aminotransferases >5 times upper limit of normal) or renal insufficiency (CrCl <30 mL/min)
- Complex infection such as pneumonia or catheter-related infection
- Grade 3 or 4 mucositis
- Uncontrolled progressive cancer defined as a leukemic patient not in complete remission or any non-leukemic patient with evidence of disease progression after more than two courses of chemotherapy
- Alemtuzumab within the past 2 months
- Anticipated prolonged profound neutropenia ($< 0.1 \times 10^9$ cells/L expected to last >7 days)

6.1 Mortality from Febrile Neutropenia

The European Society of Medical Oncology (ESMO) guidelines suggest a mortality rate in febrile neutropenia of around 5% in those with solid tumors but as low as 1% in low-risk patients (de Naurois et al. 2010). Mortality rates may be as high as 11% in some hematological malignancies.

One population-based study assessed outcomes using a database of records from 115 university or community teaching hospitals across the USA between 1995 and 2000 (Kuderer et al. 2006). It included 41,779 patients hospitalized with febrile neutropenia. The overall inhospital mortality rate was 9.5%, 8.0% for solid tumors, and 14.3% for leukemia. The number of major comorbidities also significantly affected mortality rates. Those with no major comorbidities compared to one, and more than one major comorbidities had mortality rates of 2.6%, 10.3%, and >21.4%, respectively. Those with confirmed infection had higher mortality rates at 15.3% overall. The mortality rate was highest with invasive aspergillosis at 39.2%.

Using the MASCC prognostic index outlined above, in those with confirmed bacteremia, low-risk patients have a 3% mortality rate compared with up to 36% of those defined as particularly high risk (high risk in this instance was defined as a MASCC score of <15; high risk is normally defined as a score of <21 with low risk being a score of ≥21) (Feld 2008).

7 Management of Low-Risk Patients

A Cochrane systematic review has been conducted on the use of oral versus intravenous antibiotics for febrile neutropenia (Vidal et al. 2013). The typical oral regimen usually included a quinolone combined with ampicillin-clavulanic acid. All studies excluded those with severe sepsis or shock, most excluded those with acute leukemia, and about half excluded those with pneumonia, severe cellulitis, or intravascular infection. In this patient population (i.e., primarily patients with low-risk febrile neutropenia), there was no statistically significant difference in rates of treatment failure or mortality when treated with either oral or intravenous antibiotics.

Assuming, therefore, that oral antibiotics are a safe and effective alternative, further research has explored whether outpatient management of low-risk cases is feasible. There is some evidence to suggest that early discharge, after a minimum of 24 h observation during which time the fever resolves and no complications have developed, is safe and also cost-effective (Innes and Marshall 2007).

Full outpatient management does not currently have evidence to support its routine practice. The MD Anderson Cancer Center developed an outpatient pathway with stringent follow-up and published outcomes on a series of 712 patients with low-risk febrile neutropenia for whom this was utilized (Elting et al. 2008). Approximately 20% of eligible patients were treated as inpatients for psychosocial reasons. Although 20% of outpatients subsequently required admission, all ultimately responded to antibiotics. There were no deaths, but there were serious medical complications in approximately 1% of both inpatients and outpatients. However, this data is not necessarily generalizable as outcomes would depend heavily on local protocols and systems. Randomized evidence is lacking in this area.

8 Management of High-Risk Patients

High-risk patients should be admitted and commenced empirically on broad-spectrum intravenous antibiotics as soon as possible, although preferably after at least two sets of blood cultures have been sent including one from any indwelling central venous catheter.

Time to administration of antibiotics has been shown to be important. Delayed time to antibiotics was associated with increased mortality in a population of patients with septic shock, with an absolute increase in inhospital mortality of 7.6% for every hour of delay following recognition of hypotension (Kumar et al. 2006). Data is not as strong in the febrile neutropenic population, but it is thought that the same principle applies. One Brazilian study, evaluating inpatients with hematological malignancies receiving chemotherapy, found that increased time to antibiotic treatment after the development of febrile neutropenia was associated with increased 28-day mortality (Rosa and Goldani 2014).

8.1 Supportive Care

The management of severe sepsis and septic shock has been extensively studied; however, there is less data specific to those with neutropenic sepsis. Similar principles have been applied including adequate fluid resuscitation and treatment of respiratory failure (Penack et al. 2014). It should be noted that steroid supplementation has not been consistently shown to be helpful, with the exception of those who have previously been on long-term steroids. The benefit in these patients is due to the risk of adrenal suppression and therefore an inadequate stress response. This group of patients were not included in the trials of glucocorticoids in septic shock, as steroid use is mandatory in this group (Sprung et al. 2008).

Other adjunctive therapies such as intravenous immunoglobulin and granulocyte transfusions do not have evidence to recommend their use (Penack et al. 2014).

The management of severe sepsis and septic shock is complex (Angus and van der Poll 2013). In those with septic shock (hypotension not responding to fluid resuscitation), or respiratory failure not responding to ward-based oxygen supplementation, or noninvasive positive pressure ventilation (if available), intensive care unit involvement is indicated for consideration of vasopressor therapy and/or invasive ventilation. Unfortunately, in patients requiring an admission to the intensive care unit for neutropenia and severe sepsis, or septic shock, mortality is high. One analysis of this population in a French teaching hospital found a mortality rate of around 50% (Legrand et al. 2012).

8.2 Antibiotic Choice

Antibiotic choice will be heavily influenced by local resistance patterns, but typical regimens include an antipseudomonal cephalosporin or a carbopenem.

A Cochrane systematic review has been conducted to determine whether adding an aminoglycoside to a beta-lactam antibiotic improves outcomes, when compared to a beta-lactam antibiotic alone for empiric treatment of febrile neutropenic patients, primarily in a hematological population (Paul et al. 2013). Interestingly, the combination was not associated with a mortality benefit but was associated with a higher rate of nephrotoxicity and fungal superinfection. Theoretical benefits of the combination were not borne out in the data with no evidence of "synergism" improving patient outcomes. In addition, bacterial superinfection rates were similar with both monotherapy and the combination, suggesting that the combination did not reduce the development of resistant organisms. Limitations of the review largely stem from the contributing studies. The authors noted a paucity of data for some patient subgroups, such as those with microbiologically confirmed *Pseudomonas aeruginosa* and those with confirmed gram-negative bacteremia, making conclusions more difficult (Paul et al. 2013). It did not perform a subgroup analysis in those with severe sepsis or septic shock.

Most guidelines, therefore, suggest a broad spectrum antipseudomonal beta-lactam as first-line empiric therapy for febrile neutropenia (Fig. 1). However, due to the limitations in available evidence, some guidelines still suggest consideration of the addition of an aminoglycoside empirically in selected patients, such as those at a high risk of prolonged neutropenia (de Naurois et al. 2010), severe sepsis (Penack et al. 2014), septic shock (Penack et al. 2014), or radiologically confirmed pneumonia (Freifeld et al. 2011). In addition, an aminoglycoside may be added in unstable patients with complicated infections after confirmation of a gram-negative bacteremia (Freifeld et al. 2011; de Naurois et al. 2010). There is a lack of randomized data to support or refute this approach.

A regimen involving a beta-lactam with or without an aminoglycoside does not achieve good response rates for a number of gram-positive organisms. These primarily include less virulent organisms such as *Staphylococcus epidermidis* and corynebacteria. Therefore many guidelines recommend the commencement of vancomycin if fever fails to settle after 48 h. Introducing vancomycin at this stage rather than at presentation does not detrimentally impact mortality or complication rates (Paul et al. 2014). By using this approach, clinicians hope to minimize the rates of vancomycin-resistant organisms such as

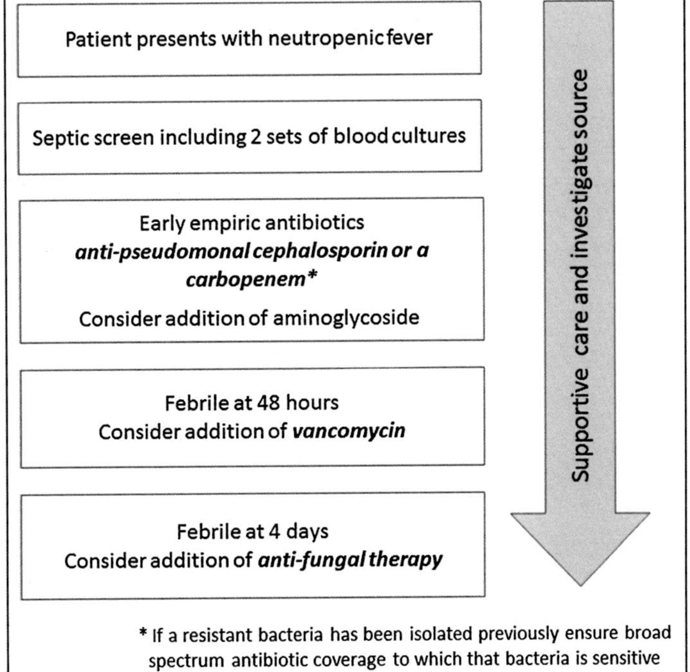

Fig. 1 Summary of empiric antimicrobial management for neutropenic fever

vancomycin-resistant enterococcus (VRE) which have emerged over the last decade or so. In centers with high rates of methicillin-resistant *Staphylococcus aureus* (MRSA), vancomycin might be appropriate as initial empiric therapy.

It remains uncertain whether the empirical use of vancomycin in all patients with persistent fevers of unknown origin is beneficial. One double-blind trial randomized 165 patients with persistent fever after 48–60 h on single agent piperacillin-tazobactam to additional vancomycin or placebo and found no significant difference in mortality or time to defervescence (Cometta et al. 2003). However, the power to detect a clinically significant difference was low. It should be noted that patients with septic shock, lung infiltrates, soft tissue or skin infection, catheter-related infection, microbiologically confirmed gram-negative infection, and microbiologically confirmed gram-positive infection resistant to piperacillin-tazobactam were excluded. In the absence of adequate evidence, delayed empiric vancomycin is a generally accepted practice.

Most guidelines suggest that patients who have previously had resistant bacteria isolated, causing either colonization or invasive infection, should receive a broad-spectrum antibiotic to which that bacteria is sensitive.

In addition, in those who have an evident focus of infection, or a high suspicion of this, targeted treatment should be commenced as summarized in Table 4. For example, in those with pneumonia, the addition of a macrolide antibiotic to cover for atypical infections is prudent.

Length of antibiotic course tends to depend on the organism and site of infection. Antibiotics are traditionally continued at least until the neutrophil count is increasing and above 0.5×10^9/L, although rationalization of antibiotics or a change to oral preparations may be considered before then, in stable patients with uncomplicated infection (Freifeld et al. 2011).

Table 4 Targeted treatment for cases with a focus of infection

Specific infection	Addition to empiric treatment
Pneumonia	Macrolide (to cover atypical organisms such as mycoplasma of legionella) Cotrimoxazole (if high suspicion of PJP pneumonia)
Diarrhea	Consider oral metronidazole (to cover *C. difficile*)
Intra-abdominal source	Metronidazole
Suspected meningitis (require lumbar puncture)	Amoxicillin or carbapenem (to cover *Listeria*)
Vesicular lesions	Acyclovir
Suspected invasive CMV	Ganciclovir
Viral encephalitis (require lumbar puncture)	High-dose acyclovir
Cellulitis	Consider addition of vancomycin

8.3 Role of Antifungal Agents

Rates of invasive fungal infection, particularly candida and aspergillosis, increase as the duration of neutropenia increases (Gerson et al. 1984). This is more relevant to the hematology setting. Therefore some guidelines suggest empiric antifungal therapy after 4–7 days of persistent fevers despite broad-spectrum antibiotics.

Traditionally amphotericin B, and more recently liposomal amphotericin B, which has less renal toxicity, has been used in this setting. However, even liposomal amphotericin B is associated with significant levels of renal dysfunction and hypokalemia, particularly when combined with aminoglycosides or calcineurin inhibitors (immunosuppressive agents used in allogeneic transplant patients). Alternatives include voriconazole, an azole which has activity against candida including the fluconazole-resistant *C. krusei* and *C. glabrata* as well as *Aspergillus*, and caspofungin, an echinocandin with a similar spectrum of activity to voriconazole (Freifeld et al. 2011).

Voriconazole is generally accepted as an alternative to liposomal amphotericin B in this setting, although it did not reach the defined threshold for non-inferiority in one randomized study (Walsh et al. 2002). A Cochrane review on the subject found some deficiencies in that study and concluded amphotericin B was significantly more effective (Jørgensen et al. 2014). It should be remembered that azoles are not without side effects. Voriconazole can cause visual disturbance. In addition, immunosuppression is a suspected class effect of the azoles as evidenced by increased rates of bacteremia in azole-treated neutropenic patients, compared with placebo in a number of trials (Gøtzsche and Johansen 2014).

The empiric addition of antifungals in those with persistent febrile neutropenia has been questioned, as a result of data suggesting that while around 30% of febrile neutropenic patients would receive antifungals based on this approach, only about 4% will actually have fungal infection (Freifeld et al. 2011). Therefore, studies have compared outcomes using empiric antifungals, versus so-called preemptive antifungals whereby a combination of clinical, radiological, and biochemical information is used to then start early broad-spectrum antifungal treatment if indicated (Freifeld et al. 2011). Radiological evidence involves features suggesting fungal infection on CT of the chest. Biochemical evidence includes assays of either B-(1-3)-D glucan or galactomannin. Both suffer from poor sensitivity and specificity when assayed in blood, and therefore serial testing is generally utilized if at all. In bronchoalveolar lavage specimens, galactomannin is very specific and approximately 80% sensitive and may have more utility in this setting. Polymerase chain reaction (PCR) assays are also being developed.

In summary, small studies suggest that the "preemptive" approach (as opposed to empiric use) could reduce antifungal use without adversely affecting outcomes, but there is not enough evidence yet to make this standard practice (Freifeld et al. 2011). In high-risk populations, such as those receiving hematopoietic stem cell transplants (especially allogeneic stem cell transplants) or those receiving chemotherapy for acute leukemia, there is evidence that the use of liposomal amphotericin B, either prophylactically or empirically, decreases overall mortality when compared with preemptive treatment of fungal infection. This suggests empiric antifungal use is appropriate for these high-risk populations (Gøtzsche and Johansen 2014).

Treatment recommendations change little in those who develop a suspected fungal infection on antifungal prophylaxis, although there is little evidence in this setting (Freifeld et al. 2011). Typically an azole is avoided if one has been used as prophylaxis. Prophylaxis is used for very high-risk populations such as those with acute leukemia receiving intensive remission induction chemotherapy regimens or allogeneic stem cell transplant recipients. Agents commonly used include oral preparations of fluconazole and posaconazole. Both have limitations. Fluconazole has a narrow spectrum of activity covering primarily *Candida albicans*. Posaconazole has a very broad spectrum of activity but can suffer from poor absorption and therefore inadequate levels in the blood. As such, in the absence of clear pathogen and sensitivity information, a switch to intravenous therapy with either liposomal amphotericin B, caspofungin, or voriconazole is reasonable.

8.4 Role of Antiviral Agents

These agents are only indicated if there is microbiological or laboratory evidence of active disease (Freifeld et al. 2011). There is no role for empiric therapy. The exception to this guidance might be the empiric addition of a neuraminidase inhibitor such as oseltamivir, if a neutropenic patient presents with flu-like symptoms in the context of an influenza outbreak.

In neutropenic patients, the typical viruses are either herpes simplex virus or varicella zoster virus. Acyclovir is the treatment of choice, with the dose dependent on the site of disease.

8.5 Use of Hematopoietic Stimulating Factors

Granulocyte-macrophage colony-stimulating factor (GM-CSF) supports the survival and differentiation of multiple cells including neutrophils, eosinophils, basophils, monocytes, and dendritic cells while granulocyte colony-stimulating factor (G-CSF) primarily affects neutrophils. As well as increasing numbers of neutrophils in circulation, it also enhances their functionality (Bennett et al. 2013).

As previously described, prophylactic G-CSF is generally recommended in those considered to have a greater than 20% chance of febrile neutropenia when exposed to chemotherapy.

However, G-CSF or GM-CSF is not recommended to *treat* episodes of febrile neutropenia together with antibiotics. While there is statistically significant evidence that their use can shorten the duration of hospitalization, shorten the duration of fever, and hasten neutrophil recovery, a mortality benefit has not been demonstrated (Mhaskar et al. 2014). Despite this, many still advocate its use in some cases, due to a suspicion that there is a subgroup within the febrile neutropenic population who do benefit.

9 Specific Clinical Scenarios

Based on the results of the investigations and clinical setting, a potential source of the fever may be identified. It is important that treatment is directed to these specific clinical scenarios (de Naurois et al. 2010).

9.1 Lung Infiltrates

Diffuse lung infiltrates should raise suspicion of either *Pneumocystis jirovecii* infection or fungal infection with organisms such as *Aspergillus*.

Aspergillus in particular has distinctive features on CT, such as nodules with haloes or ground-glass change. Occasionally, it can also cause an interstitial pneumonia. It is resistant to fluconazole which is often used as antifungal prophylaxis in high-risk patients. Treatment therefore involves either voriconazole, liposomal amphotericin B, or caspofungin.

Pneumocystis jirovecii tends to occur in patients who have been on a prolonged course of corticosteroids, in those who are on immunosuppression for previous organ transplantation, or in those with previous exposure to purine analogues such as fludarabine or azathioprine. Clinically they present with a high respiratory rate and rapid desaturation with minimal exertion. Treatment is with cotrimoxazole. In those at risk, prophylactic cotrimoxazole is usually recommended.

9.2 Central Venous Catheter-Associated Infections

Central venous catheters are commonly used in oncology and hematology but also can be a potential source of infection. Bacteria and occasionally mycotic organisms can colonize the hub of a catheter and then multiply under the cover of a biofilm, which can protect them from host defense mechanisms before gaining entry into the circulation with infusions or physical movement of the catheter. There is little data specific to neutropenic patients with catheter-related infections and so general principles of management are applied. Estimates based primarily on ICU environments with a wide variety of patients suggest an incidence of infection of around 5 per 1000 catheter days (Wolf et al. 2008). Port-a-caths, used most commonly in those receiving outpatient chemotherapy for solid organ tumors, have lower rates of infection than this. A large pediatric series demonstrated a low rate of port-a-cath-related infections at 0.11 episodes per 1000 port-a-cath days (Hengartner et al. 2004).

Local infection, such as localized redness, induration, tenderness, and purulent discharge, does not always indicate the presence of systemic infection. Even deeper (more than 2 cm from the entry site) tunnel or pocket infections do not always result in systemic infection. While the gold standard for diagnosis of catheter-related infection relies on identifying the same organism (with identical antibiotic sensitivities) in both culture of the catheter tip and peripheral blood cultures, diagnosis prior to catheter removal can allow preservation of the catheter in some cases. One reliable method to diagnose catheter-related systemic infections with high sensitivity and specificity, *without catheter removal*, is the differential time to positivity (DTTP) (Blot et al. 1999). This is defined as blood cultures from the catheter becoming positive at least 2 h before peripheral cultures taken at the same time. In the absence of this finding, other clinical factors can suggest the catheter as the source. These include local infection plus positive peripheral blood cultures; peripheral blood cultures growing an organism consistent with catheter-related infection; or the failure to identify another source, particularly in those with refractory fevers despite antibiotics (Wolf et al. 2008).

Organisms implicated in catheter-related infections tend to be commensal skin bacteria. By far the most common are the coagulase-negative staphylococci. Other common causes include the gram-positive organisms *Staphylococcus aureus*, corynebacteria, and enterococci. More rarely *Candida* species or gram-negative organisms, such as *Pseudomonas aeruginosa*, *Stenotrophomonas maltophilia*, and *Acinetobacter baumannii*, may be involved (Wolf et al. 2008).

Management depends on the organism identified, whether infections are uncomplicated or complicated (defined as persistent fever greater than 48 h or evidence of secondary infection such as endocarditis, abscess, or osteomyelitis) and whether the patient is clinically stable or unstable (defined as severe sepsis or septic shock) (Wolf et al. 2008). Antibiotic management is the same as that given above, although guidelines generally advocate the use of glycopeptides such as vancomycin in those highly suspected of having a catheter-related infection (de Naurois et al. 2010).

Another important consideration in management is whether catheters should be removed or preserved (Table 5). Catheter removal is associated with potential risk in patients with neutropenia, particularly those with associated thrombocytopenia. Additionally, many of these patients require a new central line to be placed for further treatment. *Staphylococcus aureus* infections generally require the immediate removal of the catheter as less than 20% of infections are resolved if the catheter remains in situ (Wolf et al. 2008). In addition, there are high rates of hematogenous spread of the organism, leading to invasive infections at other sites such as endocarditis or abscess. Candida infections are also resistant to treatment in the absence of catheter removal. However, one study identified the source of fungemia as the catheter in only 27% of cases, suggesting that a thorough search for another source is appropriate before removal of the catheter. Unstable patients or those with complicated infections should also have removal of the catheter. Local exit site infections can usually be managed with catheter preservation, but deeper tunnel or pocket infections require removal. Finally, in stable patients with fever of unknown origin and no microbiological evidence of catheter-related infection, catheter preservation is reasonable. This recommendation is based on a randomized study in non-neutropenic ICU patients demonstrating equivalent outcomes using either catheter removal or preservation (Wolf et al. 2008).

Table 5 Indications for catheter removal

Indications for catheter removal	Indications for trial of catheter preservation
Staphylococcus aureus infection Candidal infection (relative) Complicated infection (persistent fever or secondary infection) Unstable patients (severe sepsis or septic shock) Persistent fever despite antibiotics Recurrence of fever after antibiotic cessation Tunnel or pocket infections	Stable patient with uncomplicated infection by other organisms Stable patient with persistent fever of unknown origin Localized exit site infections *not* involving the tunnel or pocket

9.3 Diarrhea

Diarrhea in the context of chemotherapy can have multiple causes. Chemotherapeutic agents and particularly capecitabine, 5-fluorouracil, and irinotecan can cause grade 3 or 4 diarrhea (Common Terminology Criteria for Adverse Events (CTCAE) – grade 3 or above means hospitalization indicated) in patients at a rate of between 10% and 30% (Stein et al. 2010). Newer agents such as the immune checkpoint inhibitors and tyrosine kinase inhibitors can also cause enterocolitis. The management of enterocolitis may change depending on the cause, but this is outside the scope of this chapter. A key point is that the normal barrier function of the gut will be impaired increasing the risk of bacterial translocation. As such, patients with febrile neutropenia and diarrhea should have an agent active against anaerobic bacteria such as metronidazole added to their empiric regimen (de Naurois et al. 2010).

Differential diagnoses to consider include the development of an infective gastroenteritis, *Clostridium difficile* and associated toxin-mediated diarrhea, or neutropenic enterocolitis (usually only in those receiving treatment for leukemia or stem cell transplant recipients). Therefore patients need investigation at least with a stool specimen and appropriate targeted treatment commenced as appropriate.

10 Conclusion

Febrile neutropenia is a common complication of cytotoxic therapies used to treat cancer and can be fatal. The patient should be well informed of this potentially serious complication and have a management plan in place should this occur. Therapies to reduce the risk of febrile neutropenia should be considered in patients at high risk, and also in those who would poorly tolerate the complication such as those with major comorbidities. Management requires the prompt commencement of antibiotics, careful investigation into a possible source, and supportive cares as appropriate.

References

Angus DC , van der Poll T. Severe sepsis and septic shock. N Engl J Med. 2013;369(9):840–51. Available from: http://www.ncbi.nlm.nih.gov/pubmed/23984731

Bennett CL, Djulbegovic B, Norris LB, Armitage JO. Colony-stimulating factors for febrile neutropenia during cancer therapy. N Engl J Med. 2013;368(12):1131–9.

Blot F, Nitenberg GE, Chachaty E, Raynard B, Germann N, Antoun S, et al. Diagnosis of catheter-related bacteraemia: a prospective comparison of the time to positivity of hub-blood versus peripheral-blood cultures. Lancet. 1999;354(9184):1071–7. [cited 2017 Feb 24]. Available from: http://www.ncbi.nlm.nih.gov/pubmed/10509498

Bodey GP. The treatment of febrile neutropenia: from the dark ages to the present. Support Care Cancer. 1997;5:351–7.

Bodey GP, Buckley M, Sathe YS, Freireich EJ. Quantitative relationships between circulating leukocytes and infection in patients with acute leukemia. Ann Intern Med. 1966;64(2):328–40. [cited 2017 Feb 24]. Available from: http://www.ncbi.nlm.nih.gov/pubmed/5216294

Bucaneve G, Micozzi A, Menichetti F, Martino P, Dionisi MS, Martinelli G, et al. Levofloxacin to prevent bacterial infection in patients with cancer and neutropenia. N Engl J Med. 2005;353(10):977–87. Available from: http://www.nejm.org/doi/abs/10.1056/NEJMoa044097

Cometta A, Kern WV, De Bock R, Paesmans M, Vandenbergh M, Crokaert F, et al. Vancomycin versus placebo for treating persistent fever in patients with neutropenic cancer receiving piperacillin-tazobactam monotherapy. Clin Infect Dis. 2003;37(3):382–9.

Cullen M, Steven N, Billingham L, Gaunt C, Hastings M, Simmonds P, et al. Antibacterial prophylaxis after chemotherapy for solid tumors and lymphomas. N Engl J Med. 2005;353(10):988–98. [cited 2017 Feb 24]. Available from: http://www.nejm.org/doi/abs/10.1056/NEJMoa050078

de Naurois J, Novitzky-Basso I, Gill MJ, Marti FM, Cullen MH, Roila F. Management of febrile neutropenia: ESMO Clinical Practice Guidelines. Ann Oncol. 2010;21(Suppl 5):v252–6.

Elting LS, Lu C, Escalante CP, Giordano SH, Trent JC, Cooksley C, et al. Outcomes and cost of outpatient or inpatient management of 712 patients with febrile neutropenia. J Clin Oncol. 2008;26(4):606–11.

Feld R. Bloodstream infections in cancer patients with febrile neutropenia. Int J Antimicrob Agents. 2008;32(Suppl 1):S30–3.

Flowers CR, Seidenfeld J, Bow EJ, Karten C, Gleason C, Hawley DK, et al. Antimicrobial prophylaxis and outpatient management of fever and neutropenia in adults treated for malignancy: American society of clinical oncology clinical practice guideline. J Clin Oncol. 2013;31(6):794–810.

Freifeld AG, Bow EJ, Sepkowitz KA, Boeckh MJ, Ito JI, Mullen CA, et al. Clinical practice guideline for the use of antimicrobial agents in neutropenic patients with cancer: 2010 Update by the Infectious Diseases Society of America. Clin Infect Dis. 2011;52:427–31.

Gafter-Gvili A, Fraser A, Paul M, Vidal L, Lawrie TA, van de Wetering MD, et al. Antibiotic prophylaxis for bacterial infections in afebrile neutropenic patients following chemotherapy. Cochrane database Syst Rev. 2012;1(1):CD004386. [cited 2017 Feb 24]. Available from: http://doi.wiley.com/10.1002/14651858.CD004386.pub3

Gerson SL, Talbot GH, Hurwitz S, Strom BL, Lusk EJ, Cassileth PA. Prolonged granulocytopenia: The major risk factor for invasive pulmonary aspergillosis in patients with acute leukemia. Ann Intern Med. 1984;100(3):345–51. [cited 2017 Feb 24]. Available from: http://www.ncbi.nlm.nih.gov/pubmed/6696356

Gøtzsche PC, Johansen HK. Routine versus selective antifungal administration for control of fungal

infections in patients with cancer. Cochrane Database Syst Rev. 2014;9:CD000026.
Hengartner H, Berger C, Nadal D, Niggli FK, Grotzer MA. Port-A-Cath infections in children with cancer. Eur J Cancer. 2004;40(16):2452–8. [cited 2017 Feb 24];Available from: http://www.ncbi.nlm.nih.gov/pubmed/15519519
Innes H, Marshall E. Outpatient therapy for febrile neutropenia. Curr Opin Oncol. 2007;19(4):294–8. Available from: http://www.ncbi.nlm.nih.gov/pubmed/17545790
Innes H, Lim SL, Hall A, Chan SY, Bhalla N, Marshall E. Management of febrile neutropenia in solid tumours and lymphomas using the Multinational Association for Supportive Care in Cancer (MASCC) risk index: feasibility and safety in routine clinical practice. Support Care Cancer. 2008;16(5):485–91.
Kern WV, Klose K, Jellen-Ritter AS, Oethinger M, Bohnert J, Kern P, et al. Fluoroquinolone resistance of *Escherichia coli* at a cancer center: epidemiologic evolution and effects of discontinuing prophylactic fluoroquinolone use in neutropenic patients with leukemia. Eur J Clin Microbiol Infect Dis. 2005;24(2):111–8. [cited 2017 Feb 24]. Available from: http://link.springer.com/10.1007/s10096-005-1278-x
Jørgensen KJ, Gøtzsche PC, Dalbøge CS, Johansen HK, et al. Voriconazole versus amphotericin B or fluconazole in cancer patients with neutropenia (Review). Cochrane Database Syst Rev. 2014;24(2). [cited 2017 Feb 24]. Available from: http://doi.wiley.com/10.1002/14651858.CD004707.pub3
Klastersky J. Science and pragmatism in the treatment and prevention of neutropenic infection. J Antimicrob Chemother. 1998;41(Suppl D):13–24. [cited 2017 Feb 24]. Available from: http://www.ncbi.nlm.nih.gov/pubmed/9688448
Klastersky J, Paesmans M, Rubenstein EB, Boyer M, Elting L, Feld R, et al. The Multinational Association for Supportive Care in Cancer risk index: a multinational scoring system for identifying low-risk febrile neutropenic cancer patients. J Clin Oncol. 2000;18(16):3038–51. [cited 2017 Feb 24]Available from: http://www.ncbi.nlm.nih.gov/pubmed/10944139
Kuderer NM, Dale DC, Crawford J, Cosler LE, Lyman GH. Mortality, morbidity, and cost associated with febrile neutropenia in adult cancer patients. Cancer. 2006;106:2258–66.
Kumar A, Roberts D, Wood KE, Light B, Parrillo JE, Sharma S, et al. Duration of hypotension before initiation of effective antimicrobial therapy is the critical determinant of survival in human septic shock. Crit Care Med. 2006;34(6):1589–96. Available from: https://www.ncbi.nlm.nih.gov/pubmed/16625125
Legrand M, Max A, Peigne V, Mariotte E, Canet E, Debrumetz A, et al. Survival in neutropenic patients with severe sepsis or septic shock. Crit Care Med. 2012;40(1):43–9. Available from: https://www.ncbi.nlm.nih.gov/pubmed/21926615
Mhaskar R, Clark OA, Lyman G, Engel Ayer Botrel T, Morganti Paladini L, Djulbegovic B. Colony-stimulating factors for chemotherapy-induced febrile neutropenia. Cochrane Database Syst Rev. 2014;10: CD003039.
NCCN Clinical Practice Guidelines in Oncology™. [cited 2017 Feb 24]. Available from: https://www.nccn.org/professionals/physician_gls/f_guidelines.asp
Paul M, Dickstein Y, Schlesinger A, Grozinsky-Glasberg S, Soares-Weiser K, Leibovici L. Beta-lactam versus beta-lactam-aminoglycoside combination therapy in cancer patients with neutropenia. Cochrane database Syst Rev. 2013;6(6):CD003038. [cited 2017 Feb 24]. Available from: http://doi.wiley.com/10.1002/14651858.CD003038.pub2
Paul M, Dickstein Y, Borok S, Vidal L, Leibovici L. Empirical antibiotics targeting Gram-positive bacteria for the treatment of febrile neutropenic patients with cancer. Cochrane Database Syst Rev. 2014;1(1): CD003914. [cited 2017 Feb 24]. Available from: http://doi.wiley.com/10.1002/14651858.CD003914.pub3
Penack O, Becker C, Buchheidt D, Christopeit M, Kiehl M, von Lilienfeld-Toal M, et al. Management of sepsis in neutropenic patients: 2014 updated guidelines from the Infectious Diseases Working Party of the German Society of Hematology and Medical Oncology (AGIHO). Ann Hematol. 2014;93(7):1083–95. [cited 2017 Feb 24]. Available from: http://www.ncbi.nlm.nih.gov/pubmed/24777705
Pépin J, Saheb N, Coulombe M-A, Alary M-E, Corriveau M-P, Authier S, et al. Emergence of fluoroquinolones as the predominant risk factor for Clostridium difficile-associated diarrhea: a cohort study during an epidemic in Quebec. Clin Infect Dis. 2005;41(9):1254–60. Available from: http://www.ncbi.nlm.nih.gov/pubmed/16206099
Richardson MD. Antifungal therapy in "bone marrow failure". Br J Haematol. 1998;100:619–28.
Rosa RG, Goldani LZ. Cohort study of the impact of time to antibiotic administration on mortality in patients with febrile neutropenia. Antimicrob Agents Chemother. 2014;58:3799–803.
Sprung CL, Annane D, Keh D, Moreno R, Singer M, Freivogel KWY, Benbenishty J, Kalenka A, Forst H, Laterre PF, Reinhart K, Cuthbertson BH, Payen D, Briegel J, CORTICUS Study Group. Hydrocortisone therapy for patients with septic shock. N Engl J Med. 2008;358(2):111–24.
Stein A, Voigt W, Jordan K. Chemotherapy-induced diarrhea: pathophysiology, frequency and guideline-based management. Ther Adv Med Oncol. 2010;2(1):51–63. Available from: http://www.ncbi.nlm.nih.gov/pubmed/21789126, http://www.pubmedcentral.nih.gov/articlerender.fcgi?artid=PMC3126005
Uys A, Rapoport BL, Anderson R, Uys A, Rapoport BL, Anderson R. Febrile neutropenia: a prospective study to validate the Multinational Association of Supportive Care of Cancer (MASCC) risk-index score. Support Care Cancer. 2004;12:555–60.
Vidal L, Ben dor I, Paul M, Eliakim-Raz N, Pokroy E, Soares-Weiser K, et al. Oral versus intravenous antibiotic treatment for febrile neutropenia in cancer

patients. In: Vidal L, editor. Cochrane database of systematic reviews. Chichester: Wiley; 2013. [cited 2017 Feb 24]. Available from: http://doi.wiley.com/10.1002/14651858.CD003992.pub3.

Walsh TJ, Pappas P, Winston DJ, Lazarus HM, Petersen F, Raffalli J, et al. Voriconazole compared with liposomal amphotericin B for empirical antifungal therapy in patients with neutropenia and persistent fever. N Engl J Med. 2002;346(4):225–34.

Wolf H-H, Leithäuser M, Maschmeyer G, Salwender H, Klein U, Chaberny I, et al. Central venous catheter-related infections in hematology and oncology. Ann Hematol. 2008;87(11):863–76. [cited 2017 Jan 4]. Available from: http://www.ncbi.nlm.nih.gov/pubmed/18629501

Seizures

79

Eswaran Waran

Contents

E. Waran (✉)
Royal Darwin Hospital, Tiwi, NT, Australia

Territory Palliative Care, Tiwi, NT, Australia
e-mail: eswaran.waran@nt.gov.au

R. D. MacLeod, L. Van den Block (eds.), *Textbook of Palliative Care*,
https://doi.org/10.1007/978-3-319-77740-5_75

Abstract

Seizures are a common occurrence in patients with a life-limiting illness. The assessment and management of seizures in the palliative patient require the interplay of many factors, including patient and treatment goals, counterbalanced with the need to maintain quality of life. Throughout this chapter, the reader is provided with current evidence regarding definitions, classification, assessment, and management of seizures. Anti-epileptic medications are discussed in detail, with an emphasis on the administration routes, commonly used in the palliation population. Current concepts regarding status epilepticus are outlined, including pathophysiology and management. The chapter concludes with a comment on seizures, driving, and the palliative patient.

1 Introduction

Epilepsy and seizures are common neurological conditions and possibly among the few, true palliative emergencies. It has been estimated that up to 13% of patients with cancer will experience a seizure at some point of their illness (Grewal et al. 2008). The majority of these patients will have an underlying primary or secondary intracranial malignancy (Singh et al. 2007). Seizures can cause significant distress, to the patient and their family. Palliative patients with brain tumors, and their relatives, fear seizures at the end of life (Sizoo et al. 2014).

The management of a seizure, in the palliative patient with an advanced illness, requires the composite interplay of many different factors. Consideration needs to be given to the goals of care and the maintenance of quality of life. Reflection is provided throughout this chapter, on the need to consider these important factors in the assessment and management of the palliative patient presenting with a seizure.

Although the focus of this chapter is on seizures in the adult patient, the reader will be provided with additional references, where appropriate, for the pediatric population.

2 Definition and Etiology

In 2005, the International League Against Epilepsy (ILAE) provided a conceptual definition of seizures and epilepsy (Fisher et al. 2014). They defined an epileptic seizure as a "transient occurrence of signs and/or symptoms due to abnormal excessive or synchronous neuronal activity in the brain" (Fisher et al. 2014). Epilepsy was defined as "a disorder of the brain characterised by an enduring predisposition to generate epileptic seizures, and by the neuro-biologic, cognitive, psychological, and social consequences of this condition" (Fisher et al. 2014). Additionally, the diagnosis of epilepsy required the occurrence of two unprovoked epileptic seizures occurring at least 24 h apart.

In 2014, the ILAE expanded the definition of epilepsy, by providing an operational (more practical than the previous conceptual one) definition of epilepsy, that better reflected the practice of expert epileptologists (Fisher et al. 2014). It had long been recognized that for some patients, the risk of subsequent seizures after the first unprovoked seizure, when due to an underlying enduring predisposition, was comparable to individuals who had two unprovoked seizures. It was formally recognized by the ILAE, in their new operational definition, that these individuals, with one unprovoked seizure and a probability

Table 1 ILAE operational (practical) definition of epilepsy

Epilepsy is defined by the presence of any one of the following conditions
1. At least two unprovoked seizures occurring at least 24 h apart
2. One unprovoked seizure and a probability of further seizures similar to the general recurrence risk (at least 60%) after two unprovoked seizures, occurring over the next 10 years
3. Diagnosis of an epilepsy syndrome

of further seizures comparable to the general recurrence risk after two unprovoked seizures, should also be considered as having epilepsy. The current ILAE operational (practical) definition of epilepsy is summarized in Table 1. In this report, the ILAE definition of "unprovoked" "implies the absence of a temporary or reversible factor lowering the threshold and producing a seizure at that point in time" (Fisher et al. 2014). "Provoked" seizures are caused "by transient factor acting on an otherwise normal brain to temporarily lower the seizure threshold"(Fisher et al. 2014). Provoked seizures are not considered epilepsy. Table 2 outlines common list of such precipitating factors responsible for provoked seizures.

ILAE have provided recommendations in 2010, to enable the categorization of unprovoked seizures, based on underlying etiology (Berg et al. 2010). The previously used terms idiopathic, symptomatic, and cryptogenic were replaced by the terms "genetic," "structural/metabolic," and "unknown cause" to describe underlying causation. In the genetic category, the seizure(s) are the direct result of a known or presumed genetic defect(s) and are a core symptom of the condition. The structural, or metabolic group, includes various conditions associated with a significantly elevated risk of developing seizures. These structural or metabolic conditions may be congenital or acquired. The unknown category (previously cryptogenic) includes patients where the etiology is currently unknown. Seizures with unremarkable imaging and no chronicled genetic, metabolic, or immune etiology are included in this group.

The underlying etiology for epilepsy is undefined in more than half of cases. Table 3 outlines defined causes of epilepsy. The imprecise borders of the provoked and unprovoked seizure are recognized in that precipitating factors (Table 2) and may still be present in individuals with an underling enduring epileptogenic abnormality (Table 3). In the elderly, cerebrovascular disease, tumor, and degenerative etiologies predominate (Ropper et al. 2014). In children, congenital malformations are responsible for a significantly higher proportion of epilepsy (greater than 60% of seizures with a defined cause in the 0–14 age group), than in other age groups (Ropper et al. 2014).

Table 2 Causes of provoked seizures

Precipitating factors responsible for a temporary reduction in seizure threshold
Alcohol and drug withdrawal
Drug intoxication
Hyponatremia, hypernatremia
Hypomagnesemia
Hypocalcemia
Hypoglycemia
Non-ketotic hyperglycemia
Uremia
Hypoxia
Hyperthyroidism
Dialysis disequilibrium syndrome
Porphyria

Table 3 Epilepsy etiology

Epilepsy underlying etiology
1. Undefined
2. Head trauma
3. Stroke
4. Intracranial infection
5. Cerebral degeneration
6. Congenital brain malformations
7. Inborn errors of metabolism

3 Classification

The ILAE provided an opinion regarding the terminology and concepts with regard to seizure classification in 2010 (Table 4) (Berg et al. 2010). This new classification would allow an up-to-date arrangement, to better accommodate

Table 4 Classification of seizures

ILAE seizure classification 2010
Generalized seizures
Tonic-clonic
Absence
Typical
Atypical
Absence with special features
Myoclonic absence
Eyelid myoclonia
Myoclonic
Myoclonic
Myoclonic atonic
Myoclonic tonic
Clonic
Tonic
Atonic
Focal seizures
Unknown
Epileptic spasms

Table 5 Seizure history

Relevant details for seizure history
Associated features
Health at seizure onset
Precipitating events other than illness – examples include sleep deprivation, stress (physical and emotional), and alcohol
Symptoms during seizure
Aura
Pre-ictal symptoms
Motor features during seizure
Conscious state during seizure
Symptoms following seizure
Amnesia
Confusion
Transient focal weakness (Todd's paralysis)
Tongue biting

changes in neuroimaging, molecular biology, and genomic technologies. The principle subdivision of seizures, as currently defined by the ILAE, is by mode of onset into "generalized," "focal" (previously partial), and "unknown." Generalized seizures derive from some point within the brain and rapidly engage bilaterally distributed networks. Hence, for these seizures, the clinical and electroencephalographic (EEG) findings reflect bilateral hemispheric involvement at seizure onset. Focal seizures emanate from networks limited to a single hemisphere. Where the mode of onset is unknown as to whether generalized or focal, the seizure is classified as unknown. Important changes to the 1981 classification include seizures in neonates no longer being considered as a separate entity, a new group for spasms (epileptic spasms), and the elimination of the previously used terms simple and complex partial as well as secondary generalization. Instead of the terms simple or complex partial seizures, the use of clinical descriptors to delineate focal seizures is recommended. This can include statements reflecting states of consciousness/awareness, dyscognitive features, localization, and ictal progression.

4 Assessment

The initial assessment should take place after the emergency stabilization of the patient. This should include history, examination, and investigations to firstly exclude other significant disorders that may be differentials to the diagnosis of epilepsy and secondly to determine causation. The need to exclude other diagnoses is especially important in the elderly who may present with a first seizure-like event. The increased prevalence of cardiac and neurological differentials in this population is important to consider. The history should include a thorough review of the medical, past medical, and family history, not only from the patient but also from relevant witnesses. Table 5 outlines important relevant areas that need exploration in the history. The physical examination is often unremarkable but is necessary to evaluate the presence of lateralizing signs.

In a review paper, Krumholz et al. (2007) explored the utility of various imaging, electrophysiological, and laboratory tests in the evaluation of the first seizure in adults. With respect to the electrophysiological studies, they recommended that the EEG should be considered for all adults presenting with an apparent unprovoked first seizure. Its utility is because of its yield (29% of EEGs in the above context demonstrating significant abnormalities) and for defining the risk of seizure recurrence. With respect to neuroimaging, the authors have recommended either computed tomography (CT) or magnetic resonance imaging (MRI) as a core requirement for evaluation of the adult with a first seizure. The yield of imaging in the unprovoked first seizure in an adult was 10%. In the same population, Krumholz et al. (2007) found no evidence to support or refute a routine recommendation for the testing of blood glucose, blood counts, or electrolytes. The authors have suggested that such testing should be guided on an individual basis, according to the findings of the history and examination. The authors reached similar conclusions for lumbar puncture and routine toxicology. It is important to note here that Krumholz et al. (2007) excluded individuals who had "provoked seizures" (as earlier defined), in their analysis. Practitioners need to assess for "precipitating factors," as applicable for each individual concerned (Table 2), as part of their assessment of the adult who presents with a seizure. For the assessment of seizures in the pediatric population, the reader is encouraged to examine the review paper by Hirtz et al. (2000).

The above discussion provides an evidence-based framework for the assessment of seizures. In the context of a palliative patient faced with a life-limiting diagnosis, the health practitioner is faced with the need for possible compromise. The practitioner needs to carefully determine the treatment and patient goals. The benefits of a detailed history, examination, and additional investigations need to be balanced with the burden of undertaking these assessments. The variability of circumstances, and the paucity of research in this area, limits the ability to make generalizable or explicit recommendations for the assessment of seizures in palliative patients.

5 Overview of Management

The management goals for the patient with a life-limiting diagnosis that presents with a first seizure need to include the following: control of seizures, minimization of treatment adverse effects, and maintenance of quality of life.

For the palliative patient, who presents with a provoked seizure (Table 2), there is a need to treat the underlying precipitating factor that has caused a temporary reduction in the seizure threshold. The failure to manage the relevant precipitating factor may predispose the patient to continuing or further seizures. However, the need to undertake this treatment will, by necessity, be guided by the shared treatment goals agreed upon by the patient and their clinician. As an example, the assessment and reversal of underlying electrolyte abnormalities may be entirely appropriate for a patient with good pre-seizure quality of life, in the early stages of a life-limiting illness. Alternatively, in some circumstances, the underlying abnormalities are a reflection of advanced stage illness. In these circumstances, the assessment and management of provoking factors may be inappropriate. In the latter, the availability of advanced care directives and substitute decision-maker(s) can assist health practitioners in their decision-making.

For the palliative patient presenting with an unprovoked seizure, the role for antiepileptic medications needs consideration, in addition to discussions regarding shared treatment goals. The risk of seizure recurrence plays an important additional role in the decision to commence an antiepileptic drug (AED). Krumholz et al. (2015) have identified certain clinical factors associated with a heightened risk of seizure recurrence. These include an underlying brain lesion or insult, an EEG with epileptiform abnormalities, significant brain imaging abnormality, and nocturnal seizures. These patients may have up to twice the risk of seizure recurrence, when compared to patients with no defined underlying cause (Krumholz et al. 2015). Krumholz et al. (2015) additionally noted that the following features were not associated with recurrence after an unprovoked first seizure: age, sex, family history, type of seizure, and status epilepticus as presentation. The authors of this review also revealed that immediate AED therapy, when compared with no treatment, is likely to reduce the 2-year absolute risk of seizure recurrence by about 35%. The above conclusions from the review by Krumholz et al. (2015) should be considered alongside the new operational definition of epilepsy (see Table 1), to guide the health practitioner in decision-making. For an excellent review on the management of the pediatric patient with a first unprovoked seizure, the reader is encouraged to consult the paper by Hirtz et al. (2003).

The decision to treat a patient who presents with their first unprovoked seizure with an AED, or to defer treatment, will need consideration of the impact on quality of life. A large randomized trial in the UK examined this question of quality of life in patients with unprovoked seizures with respect to two treatment groups: immediate AED treatment vs deferred treatment (Jacoby et al. 2007). The authors found no significant differences in quality of life outcomes between these two treatment groups at 2 years. This included areas such as general health, cognitive function, psychological well-being, and social functioning. Their findings suggest a balance of impacts on quality of life, between taking AEDs and continuing of further seizures. The authors, however, add that the only area where there was a clear disadvantage with regard to quality of life was in the deferred treatment group, with respect to driving (Jacoby et al. 2007). Therefore, in the palliative patient, with a reasonable prognosis and for whom driving is still a valuable and important task, the balance may favor early AED treatment.

When deemed appropriate, guidelines recommend the use of a single AED (i.e., as monotherapy) (Glauser et al. 2013). Despite the rapid increase in the number of AEDs, no single agent has been deemed superior to another for all seizure types (Glauser et al. 2013). Treatment with an AED, hence, needs to be individualized to the patient. Therefore, in consideration of an agent, the palliative care practitioner needs to review the following: the effectiveness of the AED for the seizure type concerned, the potential adverse effect profile of the AED, the drug interaction profile of the AED, the patient age, and the presence of comorbidities.

In a recent review, Glauser et al. (2013) examined the evidence for various AEDs as monotherapy in relation to specific seizure types (see Table 4 for seizure types). For adults with focal seizures, levetiracetam, zonisamide, carbamazepine, and phenytoin, all have class A (established as effective) evidence, supporting their use for monotherapy. For the elderly (65 years and older), with focal seizures, gabapentin and lamotrigine, both have class A evidence, supporting their use. There is a lack of adequate trials examining AED monotherapy in both children and adults with generalized seizures (Glauser et al. 2013). Glauser et al. (2013) conclude that the following AED should be considered as first-line but have only class C (possibly effective) evidence backing their use in adults with generalized onset tonic-clonic seizures: carbamazepine, lamotrigine, oxcarbazepine, phenobarbital, phenytoin, topiramate, and valproate.

6 The Antiepileptic Drugs

Although structurally and functionally distinct, all the AEDs act by the inhibition of rapidly firing neurons, with the resultant effect on symptoms originating from this excessive neuronal action, in any component of the nervous system (Twycross et al. 2014). The mode of action of the AEDs commonly used in palliative care, as well as other AEDs that the palliative care health practitioner may frequently encounter, is detailed in Table 6. First-generation AEDs include carbamazepine, phenobarbital, phenytoin, and valproate. The other AEDs, discussed below, belong to the second generation (i.e., coming into use after the first-generation agents). The present section will discuss dosing (as monotherapy) and current evidence relating to subcutaneous route of administration in relation to specific AEDs. It is important to note that none of the AEDs discussed were developed to be used subcutaneously, and hence much of their use in palliative care is "off-label" (Leppik and Patel 2015). Health practitioners using these AEDs subcutaneously need to follow appropriate local guidelines with regard to "off-label" use of pharmaceuticals and inform the patient of this fact. The dose recommendations detailed below are as they apply to an adult. For recommendations regarding the pediatric population, the reader is

Table 6 Mode of action of antiepileptic drugs

Drug	Na+ channel blocker[a]	K+ channel activator[a]	Ca+ channel blocker[b] (N, P, Q type)	SV2A binding[c]	NMDA antagonist[d]	GABA receptor[e]	GABA metabolism[e]
Benzodiazepine						++	
Carbamazepine	++						
Gabapentin		+	++				
Lamotrigine	++		++				
Lacosamide	++						
Levetiracetam				++			
Oxcarbazepine	++	+					
Phenobarbital						++	
Phenytoin	++						
Pregabalin			++				
Topiramate	++					++	
Valproate	+				+		+
Zonisamide	++		++				

Adapted from Twycross et al. (2014)
++ = predominant mode of action, + = non-predominant mode of action
[a]Membrane stabilization action through blocking of sodium channels and/or opening potassium channels
[b]Ca channel blockade in pre-synaptic neurons reduces neurotransmitter release
[c]*SV2a* synaptic vesicle protein 2A. Binding to SV2A reduces neurotransmitter release from vesicles in the pre-synaptic neurons
[d]*NMDA* N-methyl-D-aspartate. Antagonism of the NMDA receptors in the post synaptic neurons alters neurotransmitter effect
[e]*GABA* Gamma aminobutyric acid. Action through augmented GABA receptor activation or altered GABA reuptake and breakdown

encouraged to review a local reference source for that population (e.g., the *Australian Medicines Handbook*, in Australia). The doses recommended will need appropriate adjustment for comorbid conditions and drug-drug interactions. The subsequent section will examine the adverse effects, drug interactions, and the impact of comorbid conditions on the AEDs.

6.1 Levetiracetam

The starting dose for this medication is 250–500 mg twice daily, with the therapeutic daily dose required being between 750 and 3000 mg (maximum recommended daily dose) (Twycross et al. 2014). Oral and parenteral doses are equivalent for levetiracetam (Twycross et al. 2014). Although not licensed for subcutaneous administration, the evidence for the use of levetiracetam through this route relies on case series (Remi et al. 2014; Wells et al. 2016; Murray-Brown and Stewart 2016). The PO:IV:SC ratio for levetiracetam is 1:1:1. Remi et al. (2014) undertook a retrospective chart review of 20 palliative patients who were commenced on continuous subcutaneous infusion of levetiracetam, due to the inability to swallow medications orally. The authors combined this AED with at least one other commonly used palliative care medication in 19 of the cases. These medications included midazolam, morphine, hyoscine butylbromide, hydromorphone, levomepromazine, metoclopramide, dexamethasone, and glycopyrrolate. Levetiracetam, through this route, was effective (80% of the patients had no further seizures) and well tolerated. The authors concluded that levetiracetam is an ideal AED for subcutaneous administration, in a palliative care patient who is unable to swallow, and where there is a need to avoid the adverse effects and drug interactions of the other AEDs that are commonly administered in such instances (phenytoin, valproate, phenobarbital, and benzodiazepines) (Remi et al. 2014).

The diluent that has been suggested for the infusion is water for injection or sodium chloride 0.9% (normal-saline) (Twycross et al. 2014).

6.2 Valproate

The starting dose for this medication is 200 mg twice daily, with the therapeutic daily dose required being between 1000 and 2500 mg (maximum recommended daily dose) (Twycross et al. 2014). The IV route is an alternative when the oral route cannot be used and is given as a continuous or intermittent infusion (Twycross et al. 2014). Although not licensed for the subcutaneous route, the *Palliative Care Formulary* (PCF) has outlined the use of this drug in a continuous subcutaneous infusion at a PO: SC dose ratio of 1:1, with water for injection as a diluent, resulting in seizure benefit and minimal infusion site reactions (Twycross et al. 2014). A recent case series of seven patients (personal communication) has demonstrated the safety and efficacy of sodium valproate, when administered subcutaneously, for seizure prophylaxis, at the end of life (O'Connor 2016).

6.3 Phenobarbital

The adverse effect (cognitive, behavioral, and sedation) profile of this drug limits its utilization as an AED even among those with a life-limiting diagnosis (Twycross et al. 2014). The exception is in the context of status epilepticus. When used as a maintenance antiepileptic, in the palliative patient who is unable to swallow, it should be second-line to valproate, levetiracetam, and midazolam (Twycross et al. 2014). Because of the irritant nature of parenteral phenobarbital, the loading dose (100 mg) should be given IV and only then followed by a continuous subcutaneous infusion (Twycross et al. 2014). The maximum daily dose via continuous subcutaneous infusion, for this indication (maintenance AED), is 400 mg over 24 h, although substantial higher doses have been used in the context of status epilepticus and terminal agitation (Twycross et al. 2014). With substantially higher doses, the volumes required to achieve the dilution recommended by the PCF are substantial (80 ml for a 24 h infusion dose of 1600 mg).

In the context of its irritant nature when administered subcutaneously, and the unlicensed nature of this route of administration, a recent study examined the injection site tolerability of phenobarbital (Hosgood et al. 2016). In this retrospective review that included 69 patients and 774 distinct subcutaneous injections, local reactions (maximum Grade 1 only) were seen in only 0.3% of injections. The patients in this study were being treated with this agent for refractory palliative symptoms and not exclusively as an AED; however, some patients received up to 35 injections. Importantly, in this study all doses were administered at a concentration of 65 mg/ml, with maximum volumes used for individual injections and continuous subcutaneous infusion rates, being 2 ml and 3 ml/h, respectively (i.e., at greater concentrations than that recommended by the PCF).

6.4 Benzodiazepines

Although benzodiazepines are the first-line treatment for the management of acute seizures (including status epilepticus), the development of tolerance and adverse effects (especially sedation) generally precludes their chronic use as an AED (Twycross et al. 2014). In this setting, their use is restricted to seizures refractory to other measures. The PCF recommends clonazepam in chronic treatment, 500 mcg to 1 mg as a nighttime dose to a maximum daily dose of usually no more than 4 mg (Twycross et al. 2014). In the end-of-life setting with loss of oral intake, midazolam is recommended at starting doses of 20–30 mg over 24 h as a continuous subcutaneous infusion for seizure prevention (Twycross et al. 2014). Alternatively, if the practitioner prefers to maintain the patient on the same benzodiazepine, clonazepam can be administered via continuous subcutaneous infusion with non-PVC tubing or as a single or twice daily subcutaneous dose. The use of PVC tubing results in adsorption of clonazepam onto syringe driver tubing with loss of medication. Schneider et al. (2006) demonstrated that with PVC tubing, at 2 and 4 mg of clonazepam administered over 24 h, the loss was 50% and 25%, respectively. This additionally suggests that clonazepam loss is concentration dependent. However, the loss was not dependent on the co-administered medication or diluent. Dickman and Schneider (2016) commented that although the clinical significance of this effect is undetermined, the use of non-PVC tubing is recommended.

6.5 Phenytoin

The initial dose recommended for this AED is 4–5 mg/kg daily in one to two divided doses, with the usual therapeutic daily dose recommended lying between 200 and 500 mg (Pharmaceutical Society of Australia 2014). There is a dearth of evidence examining the role of phenytoin in the palliative care population. In a recent study, Wallace et al. (2012) reviewed AED use in patients with high-grade central nervous system tumors; the authors demonstrated that phenytoin was the most commonly utilized AED. They criticized the inconsistent nature of seizure management, with the lack of expert neurologist involvement in AED selection. No studies have detailed the use of phenytoin sodium via the subcutaneous route.

6.6 Lacosamide

The initial dosing recommendation for lacosamide is 50 mg twice daily, increased gradually to the typical therapeutic daily dose of 200 mg (maximum daily dose is 400 mg) (Pharmaceutical Society of Australia 2014). Lacosamide is well tolerated, has low risk for drug interactions, and is available in a parenteral formulation. There is limited case report evidence for effectiveness of this agent through the subcutaneous route. As an adjunct to subcutaneous levetiracetam, Remi et al. (2016) used a PO:SC dose ratio of 1:1, undiluted solution, with an infusion rate of 20 mg/min. They did not mix the AED with any other drugs and reported no significant adverse effects. Remi et al. (2016) concluded, albeit based on single case experience, that lacosamide was an appropriate option for use as an AED via the subcutaneous route, in circumstances when the oral or intravenous routes were unavailable or inappropriate for palliative patients.

7 Antiepileptic Drugs Only Available Through the Oral Route

7.1 Carbamazepine

The *Australian Medicines Handbook* recommends a starting dose of 100 mg twice daily, with the therapeutic daily dose required for seizure control ranging from 400 to 2 g (maximum recommended daily dose) (Pharmaceutical Society of Australia 2014).

7.2 Gabapentin

The initial starting dose for gabapentin is 300 mg at bedtime, with the dose increased as tolerated to the therapeutic daily dose range of 1800–3600 mg (maximum total daily dose) (Pharmaceutical Society of Australia 2014).

7.3 Pregabalin

The initial starting dose for pregabalin is 75 mg twice daily, with the dose increased to the therapeutic daily dose range of 300–600 mg (maximum total daily dose) (Pharmaceutical Society of Australia 2014).

7.4 Oxcarbazepine

The initial starting dose for oxcarbazepine is 150 mg twice daily, with the dose increased to the therapeutic daily dose range of 900–2400 mg (maximum total daily dose) (Pharmaceutical Society of Australia 2014).

7.5 Lamotrigine

The initial starting dose for lamotrigine is 25 mg daily, with the dose increased to the therapeutic daily dose range between 100 and 400 mg (maximum daily dose is 700 mg) (Pharmaceutical Society of Australia 2014).

7.6 Zonisamide

The initial starting dose for zonisamide is 100 mg daily, with the dose increased to the therapeutic daily dose range between 200 and 600 mg (maximum daily dose is 600 mg) (Pharmaceutical Society of Australia 2014).

7.7 Topiramate

The initial starting dose for topiramate is 25 mg daily, with the dose increased to the therapeutic daily dose range between 75 and 200 mg (maximum daily dose is 500 mg) (Pharmaceutical Society of Australia 2014).

8 Adverse Effects of the Antiepileptic Drugs

All AEDs can produce adverse effects, and the side effect profiles play a significant role in individualized AED selection (Cramer et al. 2010; Perucca and Meador 2005; Perucca and Gilliam 2012). The frequency of AED adverse effects is dependent on the mode of assessment. Spontaneous patient reporting when compared to the systematic use of a checklist has been demonstrated to result in significant underreporting of adverse effects (Perucca and Gilliam 2012). The evidence from studies that have used screening methods and checklists suggests that adverse effects to AEDs are very common (65–90%) (Perucca and Gilliam 2012). Tolerability is best achieved by slow introduction and gradual titration to achieve the ideal balance between bearable side effects and seizure control (Cramer et al. 2010).

Perucca and Gilliam (2012) have recommended a classification of AED adverse effects into five groups.

Type A – related to the known mode of action of the AED, typically acute, and dose related.

Central nervous system (CNS) effects are shared by all the AEDs and include somnolence, dizziness, fatigue, ataxia, and cognitive impairment. Cognitive effects include impairment in attention, executive function, intelligence, language skills and memory. Perucca and Meador (2005) have outlined the impact of cognitive impairment on quality of life and work. CNS adverse effects are more pronounced in first-generation AEDs and with topiramate (Cramer et al. 2010).

Based on a large meta-analysis in 2008, the US Food and Drug Administration (FDA) issued a warning for suicidal ideation risk with all AEDs (Perucca and Gilliam 2012). In 2013, the ILAE released an expert consensus statement that raised concerns with regard to the meta-analysis underpinning the FDA decision (Mula et al. 2013). They concluded that suicidality in epilepsy was multifactorial (complex interplay of biological, constitutional, and psychosocial variables) and the benefits of seizure prevention will often exceed the potential risk of AED-induced suicidal ideation. Nevertheless, the ILAE recommended the screening of patients prior to AED commencement for underlying mood disorders (Mula et al. 2013). With reference to the AEDs discussed previously, phenobarbital, topiramate, and zonisamide have been associated with depressed mood. Levetiracetam and lamotrigine have been associated with irritability, hostility, and emotional lability (Mula et al. 2013).

Type B – not related to the known mode of action of the AED, related to individual vulnerability, and not usually dose related.

Severe mucocutaneous reactions, which are potentially fatal, have been associated with the AEDs (Perucca and Gilliam 2012). These include Stevens-Johnson syndrome, drug rash with eosinophilia and systemic symptoms (DRESS), and toxic epidermal necrolysis. Mortality rates associated with these conditions range from 10% to 40% (Yang et al. 2011). The most common associated AEDs are carbamazepine, phenytoin, phenobarbital, and lamotrigine (Yang et al. 2011). A genetic predisposition for severe mucocutaneous reactions has been suggested, through a study involving a Han Chinese population, by the presence of the HLA-B*1502 haplotype in 100% of patients with carbamazepine-induced Stevens-Johnson syndrome (Yang et al. 2011).

Other important Type B (idiosyncratic) reactions include aplastic anemia (carbamazepine, phenytoin, valproate, zonisamide), agranulocytosis (carbamazepine, phenytoin, valproate, zonisamide, lacosamide), prolonged PR interval-heart block (lacosamide), pancreatitis (carbamazepine, valproate), and hepatotoxicity (carbamazepine, phenytoin, valproate) (Perucca and Meador 2005).

Type C – longer term, related to cumulative exposure.

Type C adverse effects include changes in weight (Perucca and Gilliam 2012). This may be a gain (valproate, gabapentin, pregabalin) or loss (topiramate, zonisamide) of weight associated with AED use. Other important Type C reactions can include endocrine disturbances, gingival hyperplasia, hair loss, osteoporosis, hirsutism, kidney stones, visual field loss, and vitamin deficiencies (Perucca and Meador 2005).

Type C reactions may have decreased relevance in the patient facing a life-limiting diagnosis.

Type D – teratogenic and carcinogenic effects.

The use of certain AEDs (particularly first-generation agents) in the first trimester of pregnancy has been associated with an elevated risk of congenital malformations (Perucca and Gilliam 2012). The evidence for safety of second-generation agents is lacking due to sparse exposure data. The evidence from animal models suggests carcinogenic risk with the first-generation AED phenobarbital and phenytoin (Perucca and Meador 2005).

As with category C adverse effects, the palliative care health practitioner needs to make an individualized selection of the appropriate AED – Type D adverse effects may have limited relevance to the vast majority of palliative patients.

Type E – adverse drug interactions.

The most important pharmacokinetic drug interactions associated with the AEDs are related to metabolism. Carbamazepine, phenytoin, and phenobarbital are potent inducers of different isoforms of cytochrome P450 hepatic enzymes (Patsalos et al. 2002). The consequence of this is a reduced serum concentration of a wide range of co-administered medications (potentially including antibiotics and antineoplastics). Valproate is a potent inhibitor of cytochrome P450 enzymes; its co-administration may increase the serum concentrations of other medications and hence their potential for toxicity (Patsalos et al. 2002). Lamotrigine, levetiracetam, gabapentin, and pregabalin do not inhibit or induce enzymes involved in drug metabolism (Patsalos et al. 2002). Another important pharmacokinetic interaction relates to protein binding. The addition of a highly protein-bound drug will displace other protein-bound drugs, thereby increasing their free fraction and potential for toxicity. This is accentuated in the low-protein states seen in many patients with life-limiting illnesses. Gabapentin, pregabalin, topiramate, lamotrigine, and levetiracetam are not significantly protein bound and have lower risk for this pharmacokinetic interaction (Patsalos et al. 2002).

With regard to the adverse effects of the AEDs in the pediatric population, the reader is directed to excellent reviews by Perucca and Gilliam (2012) and Rosati et al. (2015).

9 Comorbid Medical Conditions

The palliative care patient population is likely to suffer from significant comorbid medical issues. Hepatic and renal impairment can act as precipitating factors in seizure causation, and their presence needs consideration in AED selection and dose determinations (Lacerda et al. 2006).

In the setting of renal impairment, the dose of the following drugs (from the list in Table 6) needs reduction (the degree is dependent on creatinine clearance): gabapentin, pregabalin, zonisamide, lacosamide, and levetiracetam (Lacerda et al. 2006). During hemodialysis, water-soluble and low protein-bound AEDs (from the list in Table 6, this includes gabapentin, pregabalin, topiramate, levetiracetam, lacosamide, and phenobarbital) are likely to be removed and require supplemental dosing following dialysis (Lacerda et al. 2006).

In hepatic impairment, there is a need to avoid valproate, which has the potential of causing further hepatotoxicity (Perucca and Gilliam 2012). Additionally, caution is required in the use of AEDs that are highly protein bound (includes the following from Table 6 – carbamazepine, valproate, phenytoin, and clonazepam) or that are predominantly metabolized by the liver (includes the following from Table 6 – carbamazepine, valproate, phenytoin, phenobarbital, oxcarbazepine, clonazepam, and lamotrigine) (Lacerda et al. 2006). Lacerda et al. (2006) have recommended the following AEDs in the setting of hepatic impairment: pregabalin, gabapentin, levetiracetam, or topiramate.

10 Special Populations

10.1 Poststroke Seizures

Strokes are the most commonly defined cause of seizures and account for 30% of newly diagnosed seizures in the elderly (Camilo and Goldstein 2004). A large, prospective, multicenter, cohort study carried out by Bladin et al. (2000) identified that seizures occurred in 8.9% of patients after a hemispheric stroke. This proportion of patients with seizures poststroke was higher for individuals who sustained a hemorrhagic stroke (10.6%) when compared with patients who sustained an ischemic (8.6%) stroke. Cortical location of insult was a risk factor for seizures (in both hemorrhagic and ischemic strokes). Seizures associated with both types of strokes were predominantly "partial" (note old classification) and usually occurred within 24 h post event. Recurrent seizures only occurred in 2.5% of the stroke patients in this study. The risks for recurrent seizures were higher for patients with later onset (more than 2 weeks post stroke) seizures. After adjusting for other variables, only late-onset ischemic (not hemorrhagic) strokes were associated with recurrent seizures. Camilo and Goldstein (2004) outlined the underlying pathophysiology in early seizure poststroke, as resulting from "cellular biochemical dysfunction leading to electrically irritable tissue," and in late seizure poststroke, as "gliosis ...[with] the development of a meningocerebral cicatrix."

A recent Cochrane review failed to show any benefits for AEDs for the primary or secondary prevention of seizures after stroke (Sykes et al. 2014). However, this review only included one trial, which utilized valproate, in primary prevention after hemorrhagic stroke. Sykes et al. (2014) concluded that despite the paucity of evidence with regard to this issue, recurrent unprovoked poststroke seizures probably warrant treatment. Given the typical focal onset of these seizures, Silverman et al. (2002) have suggested the use of agents typically utilized for seizures of this classification (levetiracetam, phenytoin, carbamazepine, zonisamide) in monotherapy. In selecting an AED, the palliative health practitioner additionally needs to consider the following issues, which are likely to be accentuated in this age group: adverse effects, interactions, and comorbid conditions.

10.2 Primary and Metastatic Brain Tumors

Seizures are a common problem in patients with brain tumors (Avila and Graber 2010). They may represent the initial manifestation (in up to 50%) or as a later complication (van Breemen et al. 2007). The palliative care health practitioner needs to be aware of precipitating factors (see Table 2), even in the brain tumor population, as they may be responsible for a reversible reduction in the seizure threshold. These precipitating factors have a higher prevalence in this population, resulting from the impact of metabolic encephalopathies (organ dysfunction, electrolyte abnormalities), chemotherapy, radiotherapy, other drugs, and opportunistic infections (van Breemen et al. 2007). Important factors that influence the risk for seizure in a patient with a brain tumor include the tumor type, grade, and location (Avila and Graber 2010). Low-grade primary tumors are more epileptogenic (low-grade astrocytoma 75% risk, high-grade astrocytoma 30–50% risk) (Rossetti and Stupp 2010). While Avila and Graber (2010) outlined that this may relate to the greater time to allow the formation of aberrant pathways, van Breemen et al. (2007) added that the longer survival in these patients might account for the higher frequency of seizures. Seizures are, in general, less common in patients with metastatic brain tumors, when compared to those with primary brain tumors, with the exception being melanomas (Oberndorfer et al. 2002). Primary and secondary brain tumors in the cortex (especially temporal, frontal, and parietal) are more epileptogenic, in comparison to tumors in other locations (Avila and Graber 2010).

The patient with a primary or secondary brain tumor that has a seizure should be classified as having epilepsy (see ILAE definition in Table 1), because of the significant risk of further unprovoked seizures, resulting from the persistent structural abnormality. In this context, treatment with an AED is justified to prevent recurrent seizures and the resultant impact on functional and emotional well-being (Avila and Graber 2010; van Breemen et al. 2007; Rossetti and Stupp 2010). Published evidence does not point to any single AED with superior efficacy in patients with primary or secondary brain tumors (Schiff et al. 2015). Previous reviews on this subject have recommended the use of a second-generation agent (lower impact on hepatic enzymes) in monotherapy, as they offer the best balance between effectiveness and toxicity (Rossetti and Stupp 2010; Schiff et al. 2015). Rossetti and Stupp (2010) suggested a choice between levetiracetam, gabapentin, pregabalin, and lamotrigine, while Schiff et al. (2015) recommended lacosamide, as an additional option. Rossetti et al. (2014) have recently completed a small, open-label randomized controlled trial (RCT), comparing the safety and efficacy of levetiracetam to pregabalin, in patients with primary brain tumors and at least one seizure. They concluded that both drugs were effective (65% seizure-free in levetiracetam group and 75% seizure-free in pregabalin group) and well tolerated. It is important that the palliative care health practitioner additionally considers the role of tumor-directed therapies (surgery, radiotherapy, and systemic therapy), for patients with primary and secondary brain tumors. Systemic therapy may include the use of steroids, such as dexamethasone for reduction of peritumoral edema (van Breemen et al. 2007). In the appropriately selected patients, these therapeutic options may ameliorate seizure activity (Avila and Graber 2010).

Previous reviews including one by the Cochrane collaboration have failed to demonstrate any benefit for AEDs in primary seizure prophylaxis for the patient with a primary or secondary brain tumor (Tremont-Lukats et al. 2008). The Cochrane review found no evidence for benefit but a greater risk for adverse events. However, they were clear that these conclusions were only applicable to the first-generation agents: phenytoin, phenobarbital, and valproate. A more recent review suggested a favorable role for levetiracetam for seizure prevention in brain tumor patients (Nasr et al. 2016). The authors included 21 studies including 3 RCTs. However, two of the RCTs were for patients post craniotomy, and the other was the Rossetti et al. (2014) RCT, which included patients who already had at least one seizure. Certainly the tolerability and reduced risk for drug interactions make the second-generation AEDs more suitable for primary seizure prophylaxis; however in the absence of more robust evidence, there can be no clear endorsement of this recommendation.

For the patient commenced on an AED, Rossetti and Stupp (2010) have recommended they remain on AED treatment as long as the underlying structural abnormality is present. For patients who have had successful operative clearance, the cessation of AEDs needs careful assessment, with consideration of the risk of local tumor recurrence (especially gliomas) and seizure return. Others have counseled long-term continuation of treatment, because of the impaired life expectancy, and quality-of-life concerns with seizure recurrence (including loss of driving) (van Breemen et al. 2007).

10.3 Preventing Seizures at the End of Life

Seizures at the end of life are not an uncommon occurrence in the palliative population and are an important consideration in patients with brain tumors. In one large retrospective study involving high-grade glioma patients, 36.9% of the patients had a seizure in the last 4 weeks of life (Pace et al. 2013). In the last week of life, when patients are less likely to have the ability to swallow oral AEDs, the proportion of high-grade glioma patients who had a seizure, in the retrospective cohort of Sizoo et al. (2014) was 29%. Therefore, proper control of seizures even at the end of life is warranted, and furthermore their occurrence has been associated with a non-peaceful death (Bausewein et al. 2003). An important determination in this context is the role of the AED in the end of life. A discussion regarding the appropriateness and timing of AED cessation needs to occur at an early stage, allowing patient participation and preferably included in an advanced care directive. At the very least, the nomination of a substitute decision-maker at early stage of illness may help ensure that the patient's wishes are followed where appropriate at the end of life. Where possible, if the patient was commenced on the AED for an unprovoked seizure, and especially if there is an underlying persistent structural abnormality, the patient should continue these medications while they can swallow (Krouwer et al. 2000). When the ability to swallow is lost, and the patient/family or treating palliative health practitioner believes continuing seizure prevention is important, alternative routes of administration need to be sought. There is insufficient data regarding the preferred drug or route in this situation (Pace et al. 2013). Pace et al. (2013) espouse the use of intramuscular phenobarbital, or intravenous levetiracetam, for seizure prevention at the end of life. Krouwer et al. (2000) have outlined options for the rectal route (parenteral solution of phenobarbital and oral carbamazepine solution) for seizure prevention in the context of patients at the end of life. Koekkoek et al. (2016) used the buccal route (clonazepam) to administer prophylactic antiseizure treatment. Finally, the author has earlier discussed the subcutaneous route (not licensed) for various AEDs. The treatment of the acute seizure and status epilepticus will be discussed in the following sections.

11 Status Epilepticus

The definition of status epilepticus has seen many revisions over the past few decades. In particular this has been related to the duration of continuous seizure activity. Lowenstein and Alldredge (1998), in a review paper, outline initial definitions that do not define a length of time, to later ones that specified 30 min of continuous seizure activity, as status epilepticus. The derivation for 30 min was from animal models that suggested that neuronal injury is likely in continuous seizure activity beyond this point (Trinka et al. 2015). Lowenstein and Alldredge (1998) suggested the need for a more "operational definition," as the need for treatment is imperative well before this period of time has elapsed. They suggested a definition for generalized convulsive status epilepticus of "either continuous seizures lasting at least 5 minutes or two or more discrete seizures between which there is incomplete recovery of consciousness" (p. 970). Chen and Wasterlain (2006) provided statistical argument for the 5 min threshold, documenting that this was 18–20 standard deviations away from the duration of generalized convulsive seizures (the isolated seizure).

In 2015, the ILAE proposed a broad definition that would encompass all types of status epilepticus (tonic-clonic, focal with impaired consciousness, absence) (Trinka et al. 2015). They defined status epilepticus as:

> A condition resulting either from the failure of mechanisms responsible for seizure termination or from the initiation of mechanisms which lead to abnormally prolonged seizures (after time point t1). It is a condition that can have long-term consequences (after time point t2), including neuronal death, neuronal injury, and alteration of neuronal networks, depending on the type and duration of seizures. (p. 1517)

The definition for t1 would guide clinicians as to the timing of when a seizure needs to be considered as status epilepticus. For tonic-clonic seizures, the ILAE has suggested this be set at 5 min (focal with impaired consciousness and absence set at 10 min). The definition for t2 would guide clinicians as to the time beyond which neurological sequela may be expected. For tonic-clonic status epilepticus, this has been set at 30 min (focal with impaired consciousness at greater than 60 min and undefined for absence).

Lowenstein and Alldredge (1998) have outlined that the fundamental pathophysiology involved in status epilepticus as a "failure of mechanisms that normally abort an isolated seizure" (p. 971). They delineate this as the result of the confluence of persistent, excitatory, and ineffective inhibitory mechanisms. Chen and Wasterlain (2006) have further detailed this interplay between loss of inhibition and promotion of excitation, in their hypothesis of "receptor trafficking." In the transition from isolated seizure to status epilepticus, they document animal models demonstrating a reduction in GABA (gamma aminobutyric acid) receptors (resultant loss of inhibition) and increased AMPA (α-amino-3-hydroxyl-5-methyl-4-isoxazole-propionate) and NMDA (N-methyl-d-aspartate) receptors (increased excitation), per synapse. Understanding of these mechanisms assists in elucidating the loss of potency of GABAergic drugs as status epilepticus becomes established (pharmacoresistance) and the potential for NMDA blocker effectiveness even in prolonged status (Chen and Wasterlain 2006). With persistent status epilepticus, there are, additionally, a depletion of inhibitory and increase in pro-convulsant neuropeptides in the hippocampus (Chen and Wasterlain 2006).

Chen et al. (Trinka et al. 2015) have suggested that the neuronal injury and death in status epilepticus is the result from "excessive neuronal firing, through excitotoxic mechanisms" (p. 249). The evidence for neuronal death in status is derived from the finding of elevated levels of markers of nerve cell death in the serum, and the demonstration on imaging of cerebral edema and atrophy, in patients post status (Trinka et al. 2015). Furthermore, Chen et al. (Trinka et al. 2015) elaborate that postmortem findings of reduced neuronal density in the hippocampi of patients deceased from status epilepticus are also consistent with the evidence for nerve cell death associated with status. Status epilepticus is therefore a neurological emergency.

Brophy et al. (2012) have outlined that the 30-day mortality for convulsive status epilepticus ranges from 19% to 27%, while that for nonconvulsive status epilepticus approaches 65%. These outcomes are likely to be poorer if status epilepticus occurs in association with an advanced life-limiting condition (Droney and Hall 2008). In such group of patients, status epilepticus may be the terminal event. In the survivors of an episode of status epilepticus, there is additional morbidity related to neurological or cognitive sequelae (up to 16%) and decline in functional status (up to 26%) (Brophy et al. 2012).

Factors associated with poorer outcomes in convulsive status epilepticus include underlying cause, advanced age, presence of comorbidities, duration of seizure, impaired conscious state at presentation, and the presence of focal neurological features at seizure onset (Brophy et al. 2012). It is the underlying etiology, however, that has the greatest importance as an outcome predictor for status epilepticus (Rosetti et al. 2006; Scholtes et al. 1994). As outlined by Rosetti et al. (2006), in patients with potentially fatal underlying conditions, it is the etiology "rather . . . [than] status epilepticus per se . . . [that] is the major determinant of outcome." Finally, Brophy et al. (2012) have outlined the role of both insufficient therapy or lack of adherence to treatment protocols as being associated with poorer outcomes. In a prospective study, Aranda et al. (2010) demonstrated that the key factor in predicting convulsive status epilepticus termination (with resultant reduced refractory status, length of stay, and complications) was adherence to protocol.

Factors associated with poorer outcome, in nonconvulsive status epilepticus, include underlying etiology and duration of seizures. Delayed diagnosis of nonconvulsive status epilepticus (more likely than convulsive status epilepticus, owing to lack of motor activity) is additionally an important factor in the poorer outcome associated with nonconvulsive, when compared to convulsive status epilepticus (Young et al. 1996). Young et al. (1996) have suggested that nonconvulsive status epilepticus is "often unsuspected in patients with comorbid conditions such as cancer or organ failure" (p. 89). In their cohort of intensive care patients, with continuous EEG monitoring, they outline a better outcome with respect to mortality for those patients whose seizures were identified within 30 min of onset (36%), when compared to those whose diagnosis was delayed by more than 24 h (75%) (Young et al. 1996). Lorenzl et al. (2008) have recommended the need for the palliative health practitioner to be aware of the possibility of nonconvulsive status epilepticus in the patient with an acute change in mental status or behavior. Important examination findings suggestive of this condition include mild myoclonic jerks of the facial muscles and epileptic nystagmus (Lorenzl et al. 2010). Given the common occurrence of myoclonic jerks in the patient with an advanced illness (opioid toxicity, metabolic derangement), the detection of nonconvulsive status epilepticus requires an acute awareness of this disorder and a thorough neurological assessment of the patient with a sudden altered conscious state or behavioral change.

The etiology of status epilepticus has classically been defined as acute symptomatic, remote symptomatic, and idiopathic (DeLorenzo et al. 1996). DeLorenzo et al. (1996) outlined that status epilepticus with an acute symptomatic etiology develops within 7 days of the onset of an acute event, while remote symptomatic status epilepticus has no acute trigger but instead has a remote history of central nervous system insult. With idiopathic etiologies, there is no acute or remote cause that can be identified as being responsible for the status epilepticus (DeLorenzo et al. 1996). Table 7 summarizes the common etiologies underlying status epilepticus. In practice, the underlying etiology for any individual patient may have a combination of acute and remote factors, for example, a previous insult with a superimposed acute trigger.

In their retrospective review of 204 status epilepticus events, DeLorenzo et al. (1996) identified that almost 50% of adult status epilepticus had a cerebrovascular disease (acute and remote) etiology. Additionally, they identified anoxia and hypoxia acute symptomatic etiologies, as having the highest mortality (71% and 53%, respectively). Cerebrovascular disease similarly was responsible for a significant proportion of acute and remote symptomatic status epilepticus in the 172 cases examined by Coeytaux et al. (2000). Acute symptomatic status, occurring in the context of anoxia/hypoxia and especially in older patients, is associated with the highest mortality (Lowenstein and Alldredge 1998).

12 Treatment of the Acute Seizure and Status Epilepticus

The treatment of the acute seizure in the patient with a life-limiting diagnosis needs to be guided by the goals of care, stage of illness, and prognosis. The management of the acute seizure in this setting needs therefore be considered in the context of the patient's clinical situation. For many patients a seizure event may be anticipated because of the pathophysiology and natural history of the underlying life-limiting condition. For these patients a preemptive discussion with the patient and family can delineate appropriate treatments that may be offered within the context of the patient's goals, stage of illness, and overall prognosis. However, anxiety in the patient and family may occur with such discussions, and it is important that these discussions occur judiciously. The outcome of such discussions should be recorded in advanced care directives.

Table 7 Etiology underlying status epilepticus (Brophy et al. 2012; DeLorenzo et al. 1996)

Status epilepticus etiology	
Acute symptomatic	
Anoxia	Acute deprival of oxygen to the central nervous system from prolonged cardiorespiratory arrest
Hypoxia	Respiratory insufficiency
Cerebrovascular disease	Includes occlusion, embolism, and infarct
Hemorrhage	Includes intracerebral and subarachnoid
Tumor	Primary and secondary
Sepsis	Systemic febrile illness
Central nervous system infection	Includes bacterial, viral, fungal, and other causes
Metabolic disturbances	Includes electrolyte abnormalities, hypoglycemia, hyponatremia, hypocalcemia, hypomagnesemia, hepatic encephalopathy, and uremia
Sub-therapeutic anticonvulsant medications	Includes non-compliance with medications
Drug toxicity	Includes overdose (drugs lowering seizure threshold) and intoxication
Drug withdrawal	Includes opioids, benzodiazepines, and alcohol
Head trauma	Includes closed head injuries
Autoimmune	Includes multiple sclerosis and anti-NMDA receptor encephalitis
Remote symptomatic	
Prior central nervous system insult	Includes cerebrovascular accidents, central nervous system infections, congenital pathologies (malformations, hydrocephalus, genetic diseases), trauma, hemorrhage, or tumor
Idiopathic	

Adapted from Brophy et al. (Chen and Wasterlain 2006) and DeLorenzo et al. (Lorenzl et al. 2010)

In the treatment of the acute seizure, the palliative health practitioner needs to consider the presence of precipitating factors (Table 2) and the appropriateness of investigation and treatment of these triggers. Importantly, the vast majority of seizures cease spontaneously within 2 min from onset, usually obviating the need of medications for seizure termination (Chen and Wasterlain 2006). However, as seizure time elapses, there is not only increased neuronal injury but also progressive development of pharmacoresistance to the commonly used anticonvulsants (Chen and Wasterlain 2006). Therefore, in the patient who has active treatment goals and an excellent prognosis, aggressive treatment needs to be commenced early as "time is brain" (Chen and Wasterlain 2006).

The Neurocritical Care Society has provided excellent consensus-based guidelines for the management of status epilepticus, which has been summarized in Table 8 (Brophy et al. 2012). The guidelines as per Table 8 are pertinent for the patient for whom intensive care unit (ICU), intubation, ventilation, and cardiopulmonary resuscitation are still considered appropriate. It is important to note that the notion of "time is brain" is reflected in the timing of interventions as outlined in Table 8, and therefore, the health practitioner needs to consider that any acute seizure may progress to status epilepticus. For additional pediatric guidelines, the reader is encouraged to review the manuscripts by Glauser et al. (2016) and Sofou et al. (2009).

Portions of the Neurocritical Care Society guidelines may have applicability for the palliative patient with less aggressive goals of treatment and care. While intubation, vasopressor support, and refractory status epilepticus require ICU level of care, the other components of care can be provided at the ward level in most tertiary hospitals. Furthermore, for others much of the guideline recommendations may be inappropriate if the prognosis is poor or if the patient is at the end of life.

Table 8 Status epilepticus treatment outline (convulsive and nonconvulsive)

Critical care treatment	Timing – minutes post onset
1. Noninvasive airway protection +O2	0–2
2. Intubation – if step (1) compromised	0–10
3. Vital signs	0–2
4. Vasopressor support of BP if required	5–15
5. Finger stick blood glucose	0–2
6. IV access	0–5
Emergent initial AED[a]	
Fluids	
Thiamine/dextrose	
7. Urgent SE control therapy[b]	5–10
8. Neurological examination	5–10
9. Lab tests[c]	5
10. Refractory SE therapy[d]	20–60

02 oxygen therapy, *BP* blood pressure, *IV* intravenous, *AED* antiepileptic drug, *SE* status epilepticus
[a]Emergent initial AED therapy: benzodiazepine – lorazepam IV is preferred. If not available, diazepam, clonazepam, or midazolam IV is secondary options
[b]Urgent SE control therapy: phenytoin, valproate, or levetiracetam as IV bolus dosing
[c]Lab tests: diagnostic studies should be tailored to the individual patient
[d]Refractory SE (RSE) therapy: midazolam, propofol, or pentobarbital continuous IV infusion, this will necessitate ICU support, assisted ventilation, and continuous EEG monitoring (determines cessation of RSE)
[e]Adapted from Brophy et al. (2012)

The PCF recommends lorazepam intravenously as first-line agents for acute seizure (Twycross et al. 2014). For the treatment of an acute seizure, there is a need to use a route that allows for the shortest time for that AED to reach maximum plasma concentration. Droney et al. (Droney and Hall 2008) urged for consideration of the intravenous route, even in the palliative patient, as the suffering from continuing or repetitive seizure activity needs to be weighed against the distress of obtaining intravenous access. In circumstances when an intravenous route is not possible, a recent review concluded that midazolam given intramuscularly and diazepam given per rectally have characteristics that allow rapid absorption and efficacy (Leppik and Patel 2015). In a review of pediatric status epilepticus, Brigo et al. (2015) demonstrated that buccal midazolam was more effective than rectal diazepam in seizure control (also more socially acceptable). The authors do caution that the generalizability of these findings is limited to the pediatric population. Kalviainen (2015) reported on a review of adult and pediatric studies examining the use of intranasal therapies for seizures and concluded that intranasal midazolam was more effective than rectal diazepam. These studies help provide the palliative care health practitioner with options for use in the abortion of seizures, for both the community and inpatient setting.

For prolonged seizures, the PCF demonstrates a preference for intravenous phenobarbital in preference to phenytoin, because of its more likely availability in palliative care units (Twycross et al. 2014). In the context of an end-of-life setting, the subcutaneous route may be used to treat seizures. The *Therapeutic Guidelines Palliative Care* outlines the use of clonazepam or midazolam bolus doses for the acute seizure, with phenobarbital as second-line agent (Palliative Care Expert Group 2010). Continuous subcutaneous infusions, with phenobarbital, midazolam, or clonazepam, may be considered to maintain seizure control (Palliative Care Expert Group 2010). In certain patients, where it is important to avoid the adverse effects of sedation (associated with phenobarbital, midazolam, and clonazepam), valproate, levetiracetam, and lacosamide may be considered for seizure prevention (Remi et al. 2014, 2016). However, it is important to note that in Remi et al. (2014) levetiracetam was administered with midazolam in 75% of their patients (i.e., not in monotherapy), and similarly, in Remi et al. (2016) lacosamide was not administered as the sole AED (administered with levetiracetam and midazolam). Valproate, being a potent inhibitor of cytochrome P450 hepatic enzymes, has risk of drug interactions and toxicity. Table 9 details the drugs commonly used in seizure management, including for status epilepticus. The reader is reminded that the use of AEDs via some of the routes detailed is “off-label” and based on limited evidence supporting efficacy and safety.

Table 9 Acute seizure and status epilepticus: agents commonly used, route[a], and dosing

Medication	Dose
Lorazepam	IV: 4 mg may repeat in 5–10 min
Diazepam	IV: 10 mg may repeat in 10–15 min
	Rectal solution: 10–20 mg may repeat in 10–15 min
Midazolam	IV/IM/SC[b]: 10 mg (acute seizure-bolus dose)
	Buccal/intranasal: 10 mg (parenteral soln) may repeat in 10–15 min
	IV (RSE)[c]: 0.2 mg/kg then 0.05–2 mg/kg/h CI
	CSCI[b]: 30–60 mg/24 h
Clonazepam	IV/SC[b]: 1 mg (acute seizure-bolus dose)
	CSCI[b, d]: 2–10 mg/24 h
Phenytoin	IV[e]: 20 mg/kg
Valproate	IV[e]: 20–40 mg/kg
	CSCI[b]: 400–1800 mg/24 h
Levetiracetam	IV[e]: 1000–3000 mg
	CSCI[3]: 1000–4000 mg/24 h
Lacosamide	CSCI[b]: 100–400 mg/24 h
Propofol	IV (RSE)[c]: 1–2 mg/kg then 30–200 mcg/kg/min CI
Pentobarbital	IV (RSE)[c]: 5–15 mg/kg then 0.5–5 mg/kg/h CI
Phenobarbital	IV/IM[b]: 100 mg
	CSCI[b]: 600–2400 mg/24 h

Adapted from Brophy et al. (2012), Twycross et al. (2014), Remi et al. (2014, 2016), Droney et al. (Droney and Hall 2008), Wells et al. (2016), and the Pharmaceutical Society of Australia (2014)
RSE refractory status epilepticus, *CI* continuous infusion, *CSCI* continuous subcutaneous infusion
[a]Where possible the IV route is always preferable, the subcutaneous route may be acceptable in the end-of-life setting
[b]These are options for seizure control in the palliative patient at the end of life
[c]Note these are instructions for RSE in the patient ventilated and managed in ICU (see Table 8)
[d]Non-pvc tube recommended
[e]Doses are for Table 8 status epilepticus IV bolus therapy

13 Seizures, Driving, and the Palliative Patient

Most countries have driving licensing authorities (DLAs), who are charged with the responsibility of deciding on an individual's safety to drive a motor vehicle. The relevant DLAs rely on appropriate health professional input in their decision-making process. As a result, there is often an interplay between patient, DLA, and health professional, which can create complex ethical and legal issues for the health practitioner. The health professional may find themselves entangled, between the importance of patient autonomy, confidentiality, and preservation of the doctor-patient relationship on one side and an obligation to public safety on the other. Furthermore, the failure to report the "at-risk" driver, who subsequently causes injury or death, additionally exposes the health practitioner to potential civil or criminal liability.

Previous research suggests inconsistent reporting to DLAs of the patient at increased risk of seizure, or with a history of seizures, from an underlying brain tumor. One such study was a large survey of neurosurgeons and oncologists, treating patients with brain tumors (primary and secondary), in the United States (Thomas et al. 2011). Over a quarter of the respondents acknowledged that they did not discuss any driving restrictions with their patients, and a similar proportion were unaware of their state regulations with respect to the need to inform DLAs of medically unfit drivers. A Canadian study found that only 57% of brain tumor patients with seizures were reported to the DLA, despite this being clearly mandated by the Canadian Medical Association (Louie et al. 2013). In an Irish study by Wallace et al. (Pharmaceutical Society of Australia 2014) of the medical records of patients with high-grade primary brain tumors, it was revealed that instructions with regard to driving were not documented in any of the 27 cases examined.

In circumstances where their patient continues to drive, the palliative care practitioner has a responsibility to discuss fitness to drive with their patients. Patients with advanced life-limiting illness are likely to be exposed to many factors that risk impairing their neurocognitive capabilities. Palliative health practitioners need to familiarize themselves with the standards and regulations that are applicable to their region of practice. In general, all patients with a seizure need a period of restricted driving, the duration of which is as regulated by their relevant national standards. As national standards define periods of restriction based on seizure history, a difficulty arises in the management of the patient who has not had a seizure but who has a brain tumor (and hence risk of seizure and progressive or sudden deficits). Every patient in this circumstance who is considering continuing to drive needs a thorough neurocognitive assessment to determine fitness for this task. In such circumstances, the assistance of allied health practitioners (occupational therapist) and other specialists (neurologists) may be necessary. An excellent algorithm (produced by the Cancer Institute NSW) is available, which helps illuminate the assessment of the brain tumor patient, with regard to fitness to drive (McDonald 2011; Cancer Institute NSW 2016).

14 Summary

It is important to recognize that there is no "standard" palliative patient. Therefore, the palliative care health practitioner is faced with the task of adapting the information provided here to their individual patient. The goals of care, stage of disease, and prognosis, all help guide the health practitioner, in determining how best to utilize the recommendations provided in this chapter, for their specific patient.

References

Aranda A, Foucart G, Ducasse J, Grolleau S, McGonigal A, Valton L. Generalized convulsive status epilepticus management in adults: a cohort study with evaluation of professional practice. Epilepsia. 2010; 51(10):2159–67.

Avila E, Graber J. Seizures and epilepsy in cancer patients. Curr Neurol Neurosci Rep. 2010;10(1):60–7.

Bausewein C, Hau P, Borasio G, Voltz R. How do patients with primary brain tumours die? Palliat Med. 2003; 17(6):558–9.

Berg A, Berkovic S, Brodie M, Buchhalter J, Cross J, van Emde Boas W, et al. Revised terminology and concepts for organization of seizures and epilepsies: report of the ILAE Commission on Classification and Terminology, 2005–2009. Epilepsia. 2010;51 (4):676–85.

Bladin C, Alexandrov A, Bellavance A, Bornstein N, Chambers B, Cote R, et al. Seizures after stroke: a prospective multicentre study. Arch Neurol. 2000; 57(11):1617–22.

Brigo F, Nardone R, Tezzon F, Trinka E. Nonintravenous midazolam versus intravenous or rectal diazepam for the treatment of early status epilepticus: a systematic review with meta-analysis. Epilepsy Behav. 2015; 49:325–36.

Brophy G, Bell R, Claassen J, Alldredge B, Bleck T, Glauser T, et al. Guidelines for the evaluation and management of status epilepticus. Neurocrit Care. 2012;17:3–23.

Camilo O, Goldstein L. Seizures and epilepsy after ischemic stroke. Stroke. 2004;35(7):1769–75.

Cancer Institute NSW. Brain tumours and driving: a guide for clinicians [Internet]. Cited 2016 Oct 15. Available from: https://www.nsa.org.au/documents/item/48.

Chen J, Wasterlain C. Status epilepticus: pathophysiology and management in adults. Lancet Neurol. 2006;5:246–56.

Coeytaux A, Jallon P, Galobardes B, Morabia A. Incidence of status epilepticus in French-speaking Switzerland: (EPISTAR). Neurology. 2000;55(5):693–7.

Cramer J, Mintzer S, Wheless J, Mattson R. Adverse effects of antiepileptic drugs: a brief overview of important issues. Expert Rev Neurother. 2010;10(6):885–91.

DeLorenzo R, Hauser W, Towne A, Boggs J, Pellock J, Penberthy L, et al. A prospective, population-based epidemiologic study of status epilepticus in Richmond, Virginia. Neurology. 1996;46(4):1029–35.

Dickman A, Schneider J. The syringe driver: continuous subcutaneous infusions in palliative care. 4th ed. Oxford: Oxford University Press; 2016.

Droney J, Hall E. Status epilepticus in a hospice inpatient setting. J Pain Symptom Manag. 2008;36(1):97–105.

Fisher R, Acevedo C, Arzimanoglou A, Bogacz A, Cross H, Elger C, et al. ILAE official report: a practical clinical definition of epilepsy. Epilepsia. 2014;55(4): 475–82.

Glauser T, Ben-Menachem E, Bourgeois B, Cnaan A, Guerreiro C, Kalviainen R, et al. Updated ILAE evidence review of antiepileptic drug efficacy and effectiveness as initial monotherapy for epileptic seizures and syndromes. Epilepsia. 2013;54(3):551–63.

Glauser T, Shinnar S, Gloss D, Alldredge B, Arya R, Bainbridge J, et al. Evidence-based guideline: treatment of convulsive status epilepticus in children and adults: report of the guideline Committee of the American Epilepsy Society. Epilepsy Curr. 2016; 16(1):48–61.

Grewal J, Grewal H, Forman A. Seizures and epilepsy in cancer: etiologies, evaluation, and management. Curr Oncol Rep. 2008;10(1):63–71.

Hirtz D, Ashwal S, Berg A, Bettis D, Camfield C, Camfield P, et al. Practice parameter: evaluating a first nonfebrile seizure in children: report of the quality standards subcommittee of the American Academy of Neurology, The Child Neurology Society, and The American Epilepsy Society. Neurology. 2000; 55(5):616–23.

Hirtz D, Berg A, Bettis D, Camfield C, Camfield P, Crumrine P, et al. Practice parameter: treatment of the child with a first unprovoked seizure: report of the Quality Standards Subcommittee of the American Academy of Neurology and the Practice Committee of the Child Neurology Society. Neurology. 2003; 60(2):166–75.

Hosgood J, Kimbrel J, Protus B, Grauer P. Evaluation of subcutaneous phenobarbital administration in hospice patients. Am J Hosp Palliat Med. 2016;33(3):209–13.

Jacoby A, Gamble C, Doughty J, Marson A, Chadwick D. Quality of life outcomes of immediate or delayed treatment of early epilepsy and single seizures. Neurology. 2007;68(15):1188–96.

Kalviainen R. Intranasal therapies for acute seizures. Epilepsy Behav. 2015;49:303–6.

Koekkoek J, Postma T, Heimans J, Reijneveld J, Taphoorn M. Antiepileptic drug treatment in the end-of-life phase of glioma patients: a feasibility study. Support Care Cancer. 2016;24(4):1633–8.

Krouwer H, Pallagi J, Graves N. Management of seizures in brain tumor patients at the end of life. J Palliat Med. 2000;3(4):465–75.

Krumholz A, Wiebe S, Gronseth G, Shinnar S, Levisohn P, Ting T, et al. Practice parameter: evaluating an apparent unprovoked first seizure in adults (an evidence-based review): report of the quality standards Subcommittee of the American Academy of Neurology and the American Epilepsy Society. Neurology. 2007;69(21): 1996–2007.

Krumholz A, Wiebe S, Gronseth G, Gloss D, Sanchez A, Kabir A, et al. Evidence-based guideline: management of an unprovoked first seizure in adults: report of the Guideline Development Subcommittee of the American Academy of Neurology and the American Epilepsy Society. Neurology. 2015;84(16):1705–13.

Lacerda G, Krummel T, Sabourdy C, Ryvlin P, Hirsch E. Optimizing therapy of seizures in patients with renal or hepatic dysfunction. Neurology. 2006; 67(12 Suppl 4):s28–33.

Leppik I, Patel S. Intramuscular and rectal therapies of acute seizures. Epilepsy Behav. 2015;49:307–12.

Lorenzl S, Mayer S, Noachtar S, Borasio G. Nonconvulsive status epilepticus in terminally ill patients-a diagnostic and therapeutic challenge. J Pain Symptom Manag. 2008;36(2):200–5.

Lorenzl S, Mayer S, Feddersen B, Jox R, Noachtar S, Borasio G. Nonconvulsive status epilepticus in palliative care patients. J Pain Symptom Manag. 2010; 40(3):460–5.

Louie A, Chan E, Hanna M, Bauman G, Fisher B, Palma D, et al. Assessing fitness to drive in brain tumour patients: a grey matter of law, ethics, and medicine. Curr Oncol. 2013;20(2):90–6.

Lowenstein D, Alldredge B. Status epilepticus. New Engl J Med J Med. 1998;338:970–6.

McDonald K. Brain tumors and driving. J Neuro-Oncol. 2011;104(1):399–400.

Mula M, Kanner A, Schmitz B, Schachter S. Antiepileptic drugs and suicidality: an expert consensus statement from the Task Force on Therapeutic Strategies of the ILAE Commission on Neuropsychobiology. Epilepsia. 2013;54(1):199–203.

Murray-Brown F, Stewart A. Remember Keppra: seizure control with subcutaneous levetiracetam infusion. BMJ Support Palliat Care. 2016;6(1):12–3.

Nasr Z, Paravattil B, Wilby K. Levetiracetam for seizure prevention in brain tumor patients: a systematic review. J Neuro-Oncol. 2016;129(1):1–13.

O'Connor N. Personal communication. 2016.

Oberndorfer S, Schmal T, Lahrmann H, Urbanits S, Lindner K, Grisold W. The frequency of seizures in patients with primary brain tumors or cerebral metastases. An evaluation from the Ludwig Boltzmann Institute of Neuro-Oncology and the Department of Neurology, Kaiser Franz Josef Hospital, Vienna. Wien Klin Wochenschr. 2002;114(21–22):911–6.

Pace A, Villani V, DiLorenzo C, Guariglia L, Maschio M, Pompili A, et al. Epilepsy in the end-of-life phase in patients with high-grade gliomas. J Neuro-Oncol. 2013;111(1):83–6.

Palliative Care Expert Group. Therapeutic guidelines: palliative care. 3rd ed. Melbourne: Therapeutic Guidelines Limited; 2010.

Patsalos P, Froscher W, Pisani F, van Rijn C. The importance of drug interactions in epilepsy therapy. Epilepsia. 2002;43(4):365–85.

Perucca P, Gilliam F. Adverse effects of antiepileptic drugs. Lancet Neurol. 2012;11:792–802.

Perucca E, Meador K. Adverse effects of antiepileptic drugs. Acta Neurol Scand Suppl. 2005;112(Suppl 181):30–5.

Pharmaceutical Society of Australia. Australian medicines handbook. Adelaide: Australian Medicines Handbook Pty Ltd; 2014.

Remi C, Lorenzl S, Vyhnalek B, Rastorfer K, Feddersen B. Continuous subcutaneous use of levetiracetam: a retrospective review of tolerability and clinical effects. J Pain Palliat Care Pharmacother. 2014;28(4):371–7.

Remi C, Zwanzig V, Feddersen B. Subcutaneous use of lacosamide. J Pain Symptom Manag. 2016;51(2):e2–4.

Ropper A, Samuels M, Klein J. Adam and Victor's principles of neurology. 10th ed. New York: McGraw-Hill; 2014.

Rosati A, De Masi S, Guerrini R. Antiepileptic drug treatment in children with epilepsy. CNS Drugs. 2015;29(10):847–63.

Rosetti A, Hurwitz S, Logroscino G, Bromfield E. Prognosis of status epilepticus: role of aetiology, age, and consciousness impairment at presentation. J Neurol Neurosurg Psychiatry. 2006;77(5):611–5.

Rossetti A, Stupp R. Epilepsy in brain tumor patients. Curr Opin Neurol. 2010;23(6):603–9.

Rossetti A, Jeckelmann S, Navy J, Weller M, Stupp R. Levetiracetam and pregabalin for antiepileptic monotherapy in patients with primary brain tumors. A phase II randomized study. Neuro-Oncology. 2014; 16(4):584–8.

Schiff D, Lee E, Nayak L, Norden A, Reardon D, Wen P. Medical management of brain tumors and the sequelae of treatment. Neuro-Oncology. 2015;17(4): 488–504.

Schneider J, Good P, Ravenscroft P. Effect of tubing on loss of clonazepam administered by continuous subcutaneous infusion. J Pain Symptom Manag. 2006;31(6):563–7.

Scholtes F, Renier W, Meinardi H. Non-convulsive status epilepticus: causes, treatment, and outcome in 65 patients. Epilepsia [Internet]. 1994;35(5):1104–12. Available from: https://www.ncbi.nlm.nih.gov/pmc/articles/PMC486466/

Silverman I, Restrepo L, Mathews G. Poststroke seizures. Arch Neurol. 2002;59(2):195–201.

Singh G, Rees J, Sander J. Seizures and epilepsy in oncological practice: causes, course, mechanisms and treatment. J Neurol Neurosurg Psychiatry. 2007; 78(4):342–9.

Sizoo E, Koekkoek J, Postma T, Heimans J, Pasman H, Deliens L, et al. Seizures in patients with high-grade glioma: a serious challenge in the end-of-life phase. BMJ Support Palliat Care. 2014;4:77–80.

Sofou K, Krisjansdottir R, Papachatzakis N, Ahmadzadeh A, Uvebrant P. Management of prolonged seizures and status epilepticus in childhood: a systematic review. J Child Neurol. 2009;24(8):918–26.

Sykes L, Wood E, Kwan J. Antiepileptic drugs for the primary and secondary prevention of seizures after stroke. Cochrane Database Syst Rev. 2014;(1): CD005398. https://doi.org/10.1002/14651858.CD005398.pub3.

Thomas S, Mehta M, Kuo J, Robins H, Khuntia D. Current practices of driving restriction implementation for patients with brain tumors. J Neuro-Oncol. 2011; 103(3):641–7.

Tremont-Lukats I, Ratilal B, Armstrong T, Gilbert M. Antiepileptic drugs for preventing seizures in people with brain tumors. Cochrane Database Syst Rev. 2008;16(2):CD004424.

Trinka E, Cock H, Hesdorffer D, Rossetti A, Scheffer I, Shinnar S, et al. A definition and classification of status epilepticus – report of the ILAE task force on classification of status epilepticus. Epilepsia. 2015; 56(10):1515–23.

Twycross R, Wilcock A, Howard P, editors. Palliative care formulary. 5th ed. Nottingham: Palliativedrugs.com Ltd; 2014.

van Breemen M, Wilms E, Vecht C. Epilepsy in patients with brain tumours: epidemiology, mechanisms, and management. Lancet Neurol. 2007;6(5):421–30.

Wallace E, O'Reilly M, Twomey M. A review of the use of antiepileptic drugs in high grade central nervous system tumors. Am J Hosp Palliat Med. 2012;29(8):618–21.

Wells G, Mason L, Foreman E, Chambers J. Continuous subcutaneous levetiracetam in the management of seizures at the end of life: a case report. Age Ageing. 2016;45(2):321–2.

Yang C, Dao R, Lee T, Lu C, Huang S, Chung W. Severe cutaneous adverse reactions to antiepileptic drugs in Asians. Neurology. 2011;77(23):2025–33.

Young B, Jordan K, Doig G. An assessment of nonconvulsive seizures in the intensive care unit using continuous EEG monitoring: an investigation of variables associated with mortality. Neurology. 1996;47:83–9.

Tumor Lysis Syndrome

80

Gareth P. Gregory and Jake Shortt

Contents

G. P. Gregory · J. Shortt (✉)
Monash Haematology, Monash Health, Clayton, VIC, Australia

School of Clinical Sciences at Monash Health, Monash University, Clayton, VIC, Australia
e-mail: gareth.gregory@monashhealth.org; jake.shortt@monash.edu

Abstract

Tumor lysis syndrome refers to the laboratory and clinical results of rapid breakdown of high volumes of malignant cells. Significant electrolyte disturbances, particularly hyperkalemia, hypocalcemia, and hyperphosphatemia, in

R. D. MacLeod, L. Van den Block (eds.), *Textbook of Palliative Care*,
https://doi.org/10.1007/978-3-319-77740-5_76

tandem with severe hyperuricemia, are disease hallmarks. The most significant clinical sequelae of these disturbances include life-threatening cardiac arrhythmias, sudden death, seizures, and renal failure due to precipitation of uric acid or calcium phosphate in the renal tubules.

With the advent of more potent targeted and biological therapies, tumor lysis syndrome is being encountered in diverse oncology patient settings, with increasing incidence, and in diseases previously not considered high risk. Failure to identify and apply preventative strategies to at-risk patients may result in life-threatening complications and premature death. Once established, tumor lysis syndrome is a medical emergency that requires acute intervention but is inherently reversible with appropriate supportive measures.

In the palliative care setting, cancer patients remain at risk of tumor lysis syndrome, and clinicians should be aware of its potential at all times, particularly as its onset may be iatrogenic. Clear communication between clinicians and patients is critical in order to ensure that appropriate interventions are delivered in a timely fashion while considering a patient's wishes delimiting ceilings of care.

This chapter provides an overview of the etiology, symptomatology, and standardized definitions of tumor lysis syndrome. We also discuss prevention, management, and special considerations in the palliative care setting.

1 Introduction

Tumor lysis syndrome (TLS) represents a medical emergency due to the potentially severe clinical sequelae of electrolyte disturbances resulting from rapid tumor cell breakdown. Following the first descriptions of renal complications of cancer by Frei in 1963 (Frei et al. 1963), the full clinical spectrum of TLS has now been defined, and guidelines for prevention and management are well annotated. Disease states such as acute leukemia or Burkitt lymphoma, hallmarked by a high tumor burden and rapid cell turnover (Swerdlow et al. 2008), exemplify the classical scenario in which a high TLS risk is usually cognizant to the treating clinician. However, the increasing deployment of more potent biological and targeted therapies has resulted in an increased potential for TLS and a broadening of the diseases considered at risk. This includes ambulatory patients being with diseases considered incurable by conventional therapies and thus being treated with "palliative intent."

While the complications of TLS can usually be successfully navigated, appropriate treatment may be both intensive and invasive, albeit for a short period of time until the underlying tumor breakdown subsides. In the palliative care setting, this may present a difficult clinical management scenario as acute interventions (e.g., hemofiltration or dialysis) may contradict advanced care directives in a patient where the presence of TLS may indicate that the underlying malignancy is actually susceptible to therapeutic intervention. Thus, short-term intensive management of the reversible complications of TLS may be warranted in the context of underlying cancer control and longer-term alleviation of symptomatology for the patient.

This chapter provides a contemporary overview of TLS with the aim of updating the knowledge of health providers and alerting them to the potential for TLS in patients with cancer. Special attention is given to the palliative setting, where awareness of the risk of TLS allows effective preventative strategies, and early recognition and intervention may alleviate morbidity. Indeed, TLS may be a "biomarker" of a tumor's responsiveness to therapeutic intervention, and with appropriate management this inherently reversible complication may herald improvements in both symptomatology and prognosis.

2 Etiology

Historically, TLS was usually associated with the administration of conventional cytotoxic therapy. However, spontaneous TLS is also observed in untreated patients with highly proliferative tumors, such as acute leukemia, Burkitt lymphoma, and small-cell lung carcinoma (Cohen et al. 1980; Kalemkerian et al. 1997; Agha-Razii et al. 2000;

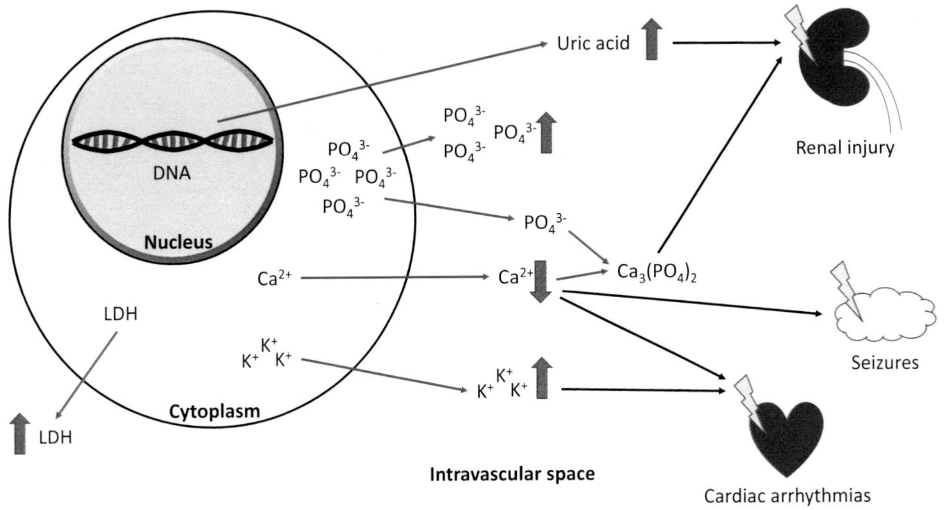

Fig. 1 Schematic overview of the etiology, key serum electrolyte aberrations, and resultant toxicities of tumor lysis syndrome. *DNA* deoxyribonucleic acid, *LDH* lactate dehydrogenase, PO_4^{3-} phosphate, Ca^{2+} calcium, $Ca_3(PO_4)_2$ tricalcium phosphate (representative of calcium phosphate family), and K^+ potassium. Red arrows denote shift of electrolytes; blue arrows denote laboratory assessable aberrations resulting from tumor lysis syndrome; black arrows denote severe clinical sequelae of tumor lysis syndrome

Riccio et al. 2006; Kanchustambham et al. 2017). Indeed TLS may be precipitated in chemo-refractory lymphoid malignancy simply by the addition of corticosteroids, which are frequently employed for symptom control in palliative care. Hallmarks of TLS are also observed in the absence of symptomatic end-organ dysfunction, the so called laboratory TLS. With the recent introduction of novel biological (noncytotoxic) therapies, both clinical and laboratory features of TLS may be observed in unanticipated disease contexts – particularly where conventional therapies did not usually result in rapid tumor destruction. These factors have led to a broadening in the use of the term to encompass any situation of laboratory or clinical TLS (as described below) attributable to active malignancy in the presence or absence of therapy.

3 Pathophysiology

TLS results from the rapid release of intracellular components from cancer cells into the extracellular and intravascular spaces. This rapid metabolic and electrolyte shift leads to the classical pattern of hyperuricemia, hyperphosphatemia, hypocalcemia, and hyperkalemia with resultant features of acute renal failure (Fig. 1).

3.1 Hyperuricemia

Breakdown of deoxyribonucleic acid (DNA) strands leads to the release of purine nucleotides, which may be even more abundant in tumor cells due to chromosomal aneuploidy. These nucleotides are initially catabolized to hypoxanthine, and then the enzyme, xanthine oxidase, sequentially catalyzes the generation of uric acid via a xanthine intermediary (Fig. 2). Uric acid is renally excreted though poorly soluble in urine, particularly at acid pH where it exists as urate (Klinenberg et al. 1965; Goldfinger et al. 1965). Uric acid precipitation is one of the mechanisms by which the metabolic derangement of TLS leads to acute renal dysfunction. Other mammalian species possess the enzyme, urate oxidase, which converts uric acid to the more soluble allantoin (Fig. 2). However, an evolutionary conserved nonsense mutation has led to absence of this enzyme in *Homo sapiens* and several other non-human primates (Yeldandi et al. 1991).

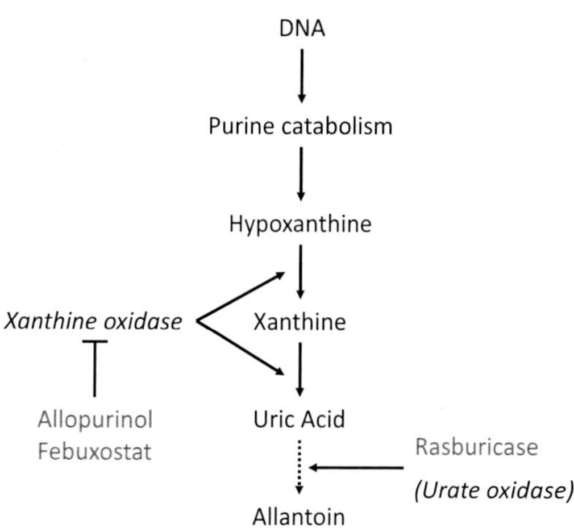

Fig. 2 Pathway leading to purine catabolism and uric acid generation. Italic font denotes enzymes with brackets indicating site of action of urate oxidase which is absent in humans. Red text denotes uricosuric agents and their sites of activity. (Modified with permission from Cairo and Bishop 2004).

3.2 Hyperphosphatemia

Intact cells contain a rich supply of organic and inorganic phosphate, which is a substrate for critical cellular functions including intracellular signaling and synthesis of DNA and phospholipid (Bergwitz and Jüppner 2011). Furthermore, malignant cells have been reported to contain significantly greater intracellular phosphate when compared to nonmalignant cells (Frei et al. 1963). Upon rapid release of intracellular phosphate, renal excretion increases and tubular resorption reduces until saturation occurs. This excess excretion of phosphate may also precipitate in the renal tubules as calcium phosphate, to further exacerbate renal dysfunction associated with TLS. Indeed, since introduction of allopurinol use to reduce uric acid formation (discussed later), nephrocalcinosis has become a more prevalent cause of renal dysfunction complicating TLS than precipitation of uric acid. The development of hyperphosphatemia (serum phosphate $\geq$1.45 mmol/L in adults or $\geq$2.1 mmol/L in children; Table 1) is typically indirectly symptomatic through induction of hypocalcemia (Cairo and Bishop 2004).

3.3 Hypocalcemia

Following the release of intracellular phosphate, calcium phosphate deposition in the renal tubules and other tissues leads to hypocalcemia. Symptomatic hypocalcemia may take the form of neuromuscular irritation with muscle weakness and cramping, tetany, paresthesia, and occasionally bronchospasm or dysphagia relating to smooth muscle spasm.

3.4 Hyperkalemia

The abrupt release of intracellular potassium can cause potentially fatal hyperkalemia, representing the most significant acute and life-threatening complication of TLS. Mild to moderate hyperkalemia is asymptomatic, so clinicians and nursing staff must be aware of this possibility in order to implement appropriate treatments. Hyperkalemia may induce arrhythmias, including loss of consciousness or cardiac arrest due to ventricular tachycardia (VT) or ventricular fibrillation (VF) as the first clinically evident sign. As such, many guidelines advocate the use of frequent electrocardiographic (ECG) monitoring to detect the development of arrhythmias including the classical sinusoidal tracing of the QRS complex through to frank VT/VF.

4 Diagnosis

The earliest formal classification of TLS was described by Hande and Garrow (1993). Almost a decade later, Cairo and Bishop provided an updated classification system which remains the standard to this day (Cairo and Bishop 2004). The Cairo-Bishop classification provides definitions of laboratory TLS (LTLS) and clinical TLS (CTLS), as shown in Tables 1 and 2.

4.1 Cairo-Bishop Classification

The Cairo-Bishop LTLS classification addresses aberrant biochemical results occurring within a

Table 1 Laboratory tumor lysis syndrome Cairo-Bishop definition (modified with permission from Cairo and Bishop 2004). The definition requires two or more of the listed criteria be met within the period from 3 days prior to 7 days post initiation of therapy. The definition assumes the use of hyperhydration and hypouricemic agent as preventative measures

Cairo-Bishop definition: laboratory tumor lysis syndrome	
Electrolyte	Criterion
Uric acid	$\geq$476 μmol/L or $\geq$25% increase from baseline
Potassium	$\geq$6.0 mmol/L or $\geq$25% increase from baseline
Phosphate	$\geq$1.45 mmol/L (adult) or $\geq$2.1 mmol/L (pediatric) or $\geq$25% increase from baseline
Calcium	$\leq$1.75 mmol/L or $\geq$25% decrease from baseline

L liter

Table 2 Clinical tumor lysis syndrome Cairo-Bishop definition (Modified with permission from Cairo and Bishop 2004). The definition requires the presence of one or more of the listed criteria and the presence of laboratory tumor lysis syndrome as per Table 1

Cairo-Bishop definition: clinical tumor lysis syndrome
Criterion
Creatinine $\geq$1.5 $\times$ laboratory ULN[ab] (age >12 or age adjusted)
Cardiac arrhythmia or sudden death[a]
Seizure[a]

[a]Definition requires the clinical criterion that is not otherwise attributable to another therapy such as nephrotoxic agent
[b]Definition does not specify guidance for interpretation of preexisting renal dysfunction due to comorbid illness or nephrotoxic agent. *ULN* laboratory upper limit of normal

window from 2 days prior to 7 days post-therapy (Cairo and Bishop 2004). It requires two or more derangements of serum uric acid, phosphate, calcium, and potassium according to predefined laboratory limits or 25% derangement from baseline in the expected direction for TLS (Table 1). Furthermore, this algorithm assumes the application of preventative measures such as adequate hydration and hypouricemic agent administration.

The Cairo-Bishop classification also provides criteria for clinical stigmata of TLS. This requires the patient meets the criteria for LTLS and also demonstrates one or more clinical sequelae including renal dysfunction (according to creatinine measurement), cardiac arrhythmia, sudden death, or seizure (Table 2). The definition concedes that intercurrent nephrotoxic therapies may contribute to renal dysfunction and allows for this to negate that criterion. Notably however, the criteria do not include reference to preexisting renal dysfunction due to comorbid illness. In such a situation, the clinician would not attribute such derangement to CTLS unless a significant worsening of the renal function were to occur. No arbitrary criteria have been included in the Cairo-Bishop classification to provide guidance as to what level of creatinine or glomerular filtration rate derangement is required in the setting of preexisting renal dysfunction for CTLS to be defined.

In order to quantitatively grade TLS, Cairo-Bishop also provides a grading classification beyond the qualitative assessment. This quantitative grading (Table 3) assesses the relative severity of the CTLS signs and renal dysfunction and provides a grading from 0 to V, whereby 0 is the absence of LTLS and CTLS and V is death attributable to TLS. This differs from the National Cancer Institute Common Terminology Criteria for Adverse Events (NCI-CTCAE) where the only applicable grades for TLS are 3 (present), 4 (life threatening with urgent intervention indicated), and 5 (death), as shown in Table 4 (National Cancer Institute 2009).

5 Risk Factors

Historically, at-risk diseases for TLS were those characterized by a high rate of proliferation and sensitivity to cytoreductive therapy. Aggressive hematological malignancies (e.g., acute leukemias and aggressive lymphomas) have previously been considered highest risk. However, with the identification of oncogenic dependencies of other malignancies and the advent of potent targeted therapies against these, other conditions previously considered low risk have had to be reclassified due to frequent observation of TLS at initiation of therapy.

Table 3 Severity grading classification of tumor lysis syndrome (Modified with permission from Cairo and Bishop 2004)

Cairo-Bishop definition: grading classification						
	0	I	II	III	IV	V
LTLS	Absent	Present	Present	Present	Present	Present
Creatinine[a, b]	≤1.5 × ULN	1.5 × ULN	1.5–3 × ULN	>3–6 × ULN	>6 × ULN	Death[c]
Cardiac arrhythmia[a]	Absent	No intervention required	Non-urgent medical intervention required	Symptomatic and incompletely controlled or requiring device	Life-threatening (symptomatic arrhythmia)	Death[c]
Seizure[a]	Absent	–	One brief seizure, seizure controlled by anticonvulsant or infrequent focal motor seizures not interfering with ADL	Complex seizure, poorly controlled seizure, breakthrough seizures despite intervention	Prolonged, repetitive, or difficult to control seizures such as status epilepticus and intractable epilepsy	Death[c]

[a]Definition requires the clinical criterion that is not otherwise attributable to another therapy such as nephrotoxic agent
[b]Definition does not specify guidance for interpretation of preexisting renal dysfunction due to comorbid illness or nephrotoxic agent
[c]Death is attributable to tumor lysis syndrome. *LTLS* laboratory tumor lysis syndrome, *ULN* laboratory upper limit of normal, *ADL* activities of daily living

Table 4 National Cancer Institute Common Terminology Criteria for Adverse Events (NCI-CTCAE) grading classification for tumor lysis syndrome (National Cancer Institute 2009)

NCI-CTCAE: grading classification for tumor lysis syndrome	
Grade	Description
1	–
2	–
3	Present
4	Life-threatening consequences, urgent intervention indicated
5	Death

5.1 Disease-Based Risk Stratification

In order to assist clinicians to identify patients at high risk for developing TLS, evidence-based guidelines have been published and subsequently updated (Coiffier et al. 2008; Cairo et al. 2010). These contemporary guidelines were based upon the disease type, tumor burden, therapeutic intervention, anticipated response to therapy, and the patient's baseline renal function. From these parameters, patients are stratified into three risk groups. High risk are those where the incidence of TLS exceeds 5%, intermediate risk are those where the incidence is 1–5%, and low risk captures the group with an incidence less than 1%. The stratification of risk in these guidelines is predominantly based on disease biology and stage (Table 5) (Cairo et al. 2010).

However, as discussed below, this risk stratification model requires amendment in the context of novel agents and chemo-immunotherapy combinations in diseases not previously considered high risk. In particular, low-grade leukemias and lymphomas such as chronic lymphocytic leukemia (CLL)/small lymphocytic lymphoma are an area of recognized hazard. Therefore, where emerging therapies have been recurrently linked to TLS, CLL patients with lymph node diameter ≥10 cm or 5–10 cm with peripheral blood lymphocytosis ≥25 × 10^9/L are now considered high risk (Goede et al. 2014).

Table 5 Evidence-based and disease-based risk stratification for TLS. *AML* acute myeloid leukemia, *WBC* white blood cell count, *ALL* acute lymphoblastic leukemia, *LDH* lactate dehydrogenase, *ULN* upper limit of normal for the laboratory, *CLL* chronic lymphocytic leukemia (Adapted with permission from Cairo et al. 2010)

Disease-based risk stratification
High-risk disease states (TLS >5%)
Burkitt leukemia/lymphoma
AML with WBC $\geq$100 × 10^9/L
ALL with WBC $\geq$100 × 10^9/L or LDH $\geq$ two times the ULN
Lymphoblastic lymphoma with advanced stage or LDH $\geq$ two times the ULN
Adult T-cell lymphoma, diffuse large B-cell lymphoma, peripheral T-cell
Lymphoma, transformed indolent lymphoma, and blastoid variant mantle cell lymphoma with
Adult: LDH > ULN and disease bulk
Pediatric: Ann Arbor stage III/IV and LDH $\geq$ two times the ULN
Intermediate-risk disease with baseline renal dysfunction or baseline LTLS parameters indicating TLS prior to initiation of therapy
Intermediate-risk disease states (TLS incidence 1–5%)
CLL treated with targeted or biological therapies
AML with WBC 25–100 × 10^9/L or <25 × 10^9/L with LDH $\geq$ two times the ULN
ALL with WBC <100 × 10^9/L and LDH < two times the ULN
Lymphoblastic lymphoma with early stage and LDH < two times the ULN
Pediatric patients with anaplastic large-cell lymphoma
Adult T-cell lymphoma, diffuse large B-cell lymphoma, peripheral T-cell lymphoma, transformed indolent lymphoma, and blastoid variant mantle cell lymphoma
Adult: LDH >ULN and non-bulk disease
Pediatric: Ann Arbor stage III/IV and LDH < two times the ULN
Otherwise low-risk lymphoma and leukemia with renal impairment
Solid tumors: neuroblastoma, small-cell lung cancer, and germ cell tumors
Low-risk disease states (TLS incidence <1%)
Solid tumors not listed in "intermediate-risk group" above
Multiple myeloma and associated plasma cell dyscrasias
Chronic myeloid leukemia
Hodgkin lymphoma
Indolent B-cell lymphomas including marginal zone lymphoma, follicular lymphoma, mucosa-associated lymphoid tissue, non-blastoid variant mantle cell lymphoma, and cutaneous T-cell lymphoma

5.2 Therapy-Related TLS Risk

The risk of TLS is not restricted to the disease type but also contingent of the treatment that is being delivered. The 2010 risk guidelines specifically addressed this for the first time by adapting the algorithm addressing CLL (Cairo et al. 2010). Here, CLL treated only with alkylating agents is classified as low risk, whereas treatment with biological or targeted therapies is classified as intermediate risk. Howard et al. recently performed a systematic contemporary review of TLS in hematological malignancies in the era of targeted and novel therapies and such ongoing updates are periodically required in order to maintain vigilance with risk stratification guiding TLS prevention (Howard et al. 2016).

5.2.1 Radiotherapy

Radiotherapy is frequently used due to its efficacy in symptom control of malignancy. Due to its direct DNA-damaging effects, purine catabolism rapidly ensues, and this may occur on a large scale in the setting of disease bulk. There have been a number of publications describing TLS attributable to radiotherapy, in both settings of hematological or solid organ cancer (Fleming et al. 1991; Schifter et al. 1999; Rostom et al. 2000; Yamazaki et al. 2004).

5.2.2 Chemotherapy

The highest-risk diseases for development of TLS include acute leukemia and Burkitt lymphoma (Cairo et al. 2010). These diseases share the properties of rapidly proliferative disease and often high tumor burden in the bone marrow or lymphoid compartments (in the case of acute lymphoblastic leukemia and Burkitt lymphoma). The mainstay of therapy for these diseases remains chemotherapy, incorporating the use of corticosteroids for lymphoid malignancies. Hence, clinicians have gained their greatest insight into the identification, prevention, and management of TLS through experience with cytotoxic chemotherapies and their use in these high-risk diseases.

5.2.3 Venetoclax

Venetoclax is a small molecule that directly antagonizes antiapoptotic cellular proteins to induce cell death. It has demonstrated unprecedented single-agent activity in CLL and mantle cell non-Hodgkin lymphoma. This includes patients with very poor-prognosis disease who would otherwise be managed with palliative intent. Indeed, the median progression-free survival of 18–24 months from early-phase venetoclax studies (Roberts et al. 2016) of heavily pre-treated individuals (median three prior lines of therapy) is comparable to historical age-matched cohorts treated with immunochemotherapy at first progression after just one prior line of fludarabine-containing regimen (Tam et al. 2014). Presently a number of phase II studies combining venetoclax with both conventional and novel agents further augment its capacity to induce rapid tumor lysis. Unfortunately, a failure to recognize this risk in the early stages of drug development led to TLS-related fatalities (Roberts et al. 2016). During the initial safety component of the phase I clinical trial in patients with relapsed and refractory CLL, an 18% incidence of TLS was reported, including one death (Roberts et al. 2016). This prompted an amendment requiring a dose-escalation schedule to be initiated and for frequent monitoring for LTLS. While the product information states that low-risk patients (lymph nodes <5 cm and blood lymphocyte count $<25 \times 10^9$/L) may have therapy initiated at home with 1.5–2 L oral hydration required, in practice many clinicians favor venetoclax initiation in an inpatient setting to assist timely diagnosis of TLS and acute intervention. Despite identification of this risk, two other early-phase clinical trials of venetoclax in CLL have each also reported one fatality attributable to TLS (Howard et al. 2016).

5.2.4 Cyclin-Dependent Kinase Inhibitors

Cyclin-dependent kinases (CDKs) regulate cell growth and proliferation and play a critical role in oncogenic transcription. For these reasons, a number of CDK inhibitors are in clinical development for both solid and liquid tumor indications. The risk of TLS is associated with drugs targeting transcriptional CDKs, rather than predominantly cell-cycle active drugs such as palbociclib, which was recently approved as a treatment for breast cancer. In particular, flavopiridol and dinaciclib, which rapidly reduce the cellular transcription of key antiapoptotic proteins, have been associated with high incidences of TLS when used either alone or in combination, although no associated deaths were reported (Flynn et al. 2015; Zeidner et al. 2015; Gregory et al. 2015).

5.2.5 Monoclonal Antibody Therapy

Therapeutic antibodies binding to antigens predominantly expressed on tumor cell populations also have the capacity to induce rapid cell death. The anti-CD20 antibody rituximab is widely used in B-cell malignancies and may induce TLS, particularly when used in combination with nucleoside analogues (Keating et al. 2005). Rituximab is an example of a "type 1" antibody with antineoplastic effects predominantly mediated by complement fixation and engagement of antibody-dependent cell cytotoxicity. More recently "type 2" antibodies such as obinutuzumab have been developed which demonstrate a different binding mode to target cells conveying a greater capacity to directly induce cell death (Mossner et al. 2010). The CLL11 clinical trial assessed the efficacy of obinutuzumab plus chlorambucil versus rituximab plus chlorambucil versus chlorambucil monotherapy in patients with previously untreated CLL (Goede et al. 2014). The incidence of TLS in the obinutuzumab arm was 4% as compared to less than 1% with chlorambucil monotherapy. This again highlights that the disease-related risk of TLS is much higher for CLL in the era of potent targeted therapies.

5.2.6 Other Agents

A recent systematic review (Howard et al. 2016) also identified several cases of TLS attributable to other biological agents in the form of ibrutinib or lenalidomide for CLL (Wendtner et al. 2012), carfilzomib for multiple myeloma (Berenson et al. 2014), panobinostat for acute leukemia (Kalff et al. 2008), and the drug-antibody conjugate, brentuximab vedotin, for anaplastic large cell lymphoma (Pro et al. 2012). TLS is also being increasingly described with biological therapies in solid organ malignancies (Saylor and Reid 2007; Huang and Yang 2009). The rapidity with which new classes of novel and biological agents are being introduced to the clinic makes it increasingly difficult to predict at-risk patients. A paradox of the palliative care setting is that patients considered to be in the terminal phases of their illness "without conventional treatment options" are often the exact population exposed to such drugs as part of clinical trials.

6 Prevention

Despite the inherent dangers and potentially fulminant onset of TLS, in practice it is readily managed so long as it is anticipated, simple preventive measures are put in place, and the patient is closely monitored. Timely intervention typically ensures that patients can safely negotiate the period of TLS, following which sufficient tumor is debulked and the risk of clinical sequelae soon abates. The reader is reminded that the information discussed in this chapter is not to be used in lieu of institutional guidelines when dealing with potentially life-threatening emergencies associated with this syndrome.

6.1 Monitoring

Although spontaneous TLS is well recognized in association with specific and rare disease entities, the vast majority of TLS cases occur immediately following the initiation of or re-exposure to an active therapeutic in a high-disease-burden setting. Patients identified as having a low risk of TLS may be safely managed in the outpatient setting, particularly where ambulatory laboratory testing and clinical monitoring are available. However, our practice is to admit all patients with high-risk features or those with intermediate risk in the context of comorbidities for initial inpatient management. This is particularly relevant for those patients with low baseline organ reserve (e.g., renal impairment) or an impaired capacity to maintain oral hydration due to active malignancy or on going toxicities from prior therapies.

6.1.1 Blood Sampling

A number of laboratory measurements can be readily performed to diagnose and monitor TLS. For high-risk patients, blood sampling immediately pretreatment then every 4–6 h for 48 h is adequate to allow early detection of LTLS. In addition to monitoring serum electrolytes, renal function, and uric acid levels (Fig. 1), lactate dehydrogenase (LDH) is a useful biomarker as this represents an intracellular enzyme present in malignant and normal cells of hematopoietic origin and a number of other tissues, which is released on cell lysis. For hematopoietic malignancies in leukemic phase, assessment of the peripheral blood cell counts provides another indication of tumor cell volume and response to therapy, which may correlate with risk for TLS development. It is critical that blood sampling for serum uric acid after rasburicase treatment (discussed below) be transported on ice and processed within 4 h to avoid ex vivo urate catabolism. In this context, delayed sample processing may provide a falsely reassuring low serum uric acid level to the treating clinician (Jones et al. 2015).

6.1.2 Clinical Review

The development of electrolyte disturbances such as hyperkalemia and hypocalcemia may be relatively asymptomatic, but their effects on cardiac conduction are readily measurable through ECG monitoring. If there is any suspicion for development of these electrolyte aberrations clinically or through laboratory evaluation, an ECG should be promptly performed and treatment initiated without delay. Evidence-based guidelines recommend continuous monitoring with cardiac telemetry if the serum potassium reaches $\geq$6.0 mmol/L (Jones et al. 2015). ECG signs of hyperkalemia include peaking of the T-waves and widening of the QRS complex through to VT or VF (Cairo and Bishop 2004).

Clinical review of the patient may also allow for detection of symptomatic hypocalcemia, as painful muscle cramping or tetany will be reported by the patient and readily assessed by clinical examination. Furthermore, clinical review will identify the rarer clinical manifestations of hypocalcemia such as bronchospasm/wheeze through auscultation, pulse oximetry, and changes of the respiratory rate.

While acute renal dysfunction may manifest clinically as uremia, associated symptoms, e.g., pruritus, are usually only evident with the development of chronic renal impairment. Careful clinical monitoring of volume status is required, particularly in patients receiving hyper-hydration as a means to mitigate renal damage. The concurrent management problem of acute electrolyte disturbances and aggressive hydration requirements is particularly difficult in patients with comorbidities that exacerbate volume overload, such as left ventricular failure or liver disease. Given the inherent reversibility of TLS as a complication, consideration of aggressive supportive measures remains appropriate in patients being treated with palliative intent. Specific considerations include the placement of a central venous catheter (for fluid and electrolyte replacement), indwelling urinary catheter insertion (to accurately quantify urine output), and transfer to a high-dependency or critical care environment.

6.2 Fluid Management

To prevent acute renal dysfunction due to TLS, the patient should be adequately hydrated to promote excretion of uric acid, potassium, and phosphate. Concurrent nephrotoxic agents such as nonsteroidal anti-inflammatory drugs ought to be withheld where possible. Intravenous hyperhydration (3 L/m^2 of body surface area per day inclusive of oral intake in adults) without potassium supplementation must be initiated prior to therapy (Cairo and Bishop 2004; Hochberg and Cairo 2008; Jones et al. 2015). Hartmann's solution is not favored due to its potassium content. The target urinary output is $\geq$100 mL/m^2/h (or $\geq$3 mL/kg/h for pediatric patients weighing less than 10 kg) (Coiffier et al. 2008). To maintain urinary output and further assist excretion of potassium and phosphate, diuresis is often assisted by a loop diuretic such as frusemide, with avoidance of potassium-sparing diuretics such as spironolactone. If required, diuresis may be further augmented by the administration of 0.5 mg/kg mannitol. Urinary alkalinization has previously been considered important as it promotes the solubilization and excretion of uric acid. However, alkaline conditions render hypoxanthine and xanthine less soluble and may precipitate xanthine crystals in the urinary tract to cause acute renal impairment. As such, urinary alkalinization is no longer recommended for the prevention or treatment of TLS (Jones et al. 2015).

6.3 Hypouricemic Agents

6.3.1 Allopurinol

Hypouricemic agents provide the mainstay of medical prevention of TLS. Allopurinol inhibits xanthine oxidase and leads to a reduced production of uric acid (Fig. 2). Its use is recommended for all patients at high or intermediate risk of TLS. As allopurinol prevents production but does not assist excretion of uric acid, it should be initiated up to 7 days prior to initiation of therapy in order to reduce baseline serum uric acid effectively and should be continued for at least 7 days post-therapy. The recommended adult dose is 200–400 mg/m^2/day in one to three divided oral doses, though often a flat dose of 300 mg daily (or 100 mg daily in moderate-severe renal impairment) is used. Intravenous allopurinol may be used at the same doses in situations where oral intake or retention of medications is not feasible (Smalley et al. 2000). In situations where hyperuricemia develops despite the 300 mg daily dose, the dose should be further increased and rasburicase considered (Jones et al. 2015). The recommended dose of allopurinol for children is 300–450 mg/m^2/day with a daily total up to 400 mg in three divided doses or 3.3 mg/kg three times daily for infants weighing less than 10 kg (Jones et al. 2015).

Hypersensitivity reactions are rare but may be severe, including Stevens-Johnson syndrome. As allopurinol also interferes with the metabolism of purine analogues, 6-mercaptopurine and azathioprine should be withheld or significantly dose reduced when commencing allopurinol. In the event of contraindication, hypersensitivity, or intolerance of allopurinol, the non-purine selective inhibitor of xanthine oxidase, febuxostat, may be considered as an alternative; however, clinical experience in TLS is limited.

6.3.2 Rasburicase

In the case of high-risk situations for development of TLS, the pharmacological urate oxidase, rasburicase, should be administered instead of allopurinol. Such situations include Burkitt lymphoma and acute leukemia according to tumor bulk and (WBC) blood cell count, patients with renal impairment and intermediate-risk diseases as shown in Table 5, and high-risk patients with CLL (lymph node $\geq$10 cm or 5–10 cm with lymphocytosis $\geq 25 \times 10^9$/L) starting treatments such as venetoclax (Cairo et al. 2010; Howard et al. 2016). Rasburicase is administered by the intravenous route, and the recommended dose is 0.2 mg/kg/day as a 30 min infusion for adults or children, though in practice many hematologists use the flat dose of 3 mg for adult patients and this is considered acceptable according to published guidelines (Jones et al. 2015). Repeated dosing for a total of 3–7 days should be considered pending the serum uric acid measurements following administration of therapy.

Rasburicase converts poorly soluble uric acid to the more soluble allantoin, which is readily renally excreted (Fig. 2). As rasburicase promotes removal of uric acid, it should be used instead of allopurinol when the patient already has baseline elevation in serum uric acid pretreatment ($\geq$0.45 mmol/L) or when manifestations of TLS are apparent despite allopurinol use (Jones et al. 2015). The use of rasburicase is contraindicated for patients with glucose-6-phosphate dehydrogenase (G6PD) deficiency due to the risk of acute hemolytic anemia and methemoglobinemia. As such, preemptive testing for G6PD deficiency is recommended and is usually readily performed in the diagnostic pathology laboratory.

The relative efficacy of allopurinol versus rasburicase for at-risk adult patients with hematological malignancies has been assessed in a phase III clinical trial comparing allopurinol versus allopurinol plus rasburicase versus rasburicase alone (Cortes et al. 2010). This trial found a statistically significant improvement in rates of normalization of serum uric acid in the group treated with rasburicase, and a trend toward improvement in the combination arm, when each were compared to allopurinol monotherapy. The time to normalization of serum uric acid was also significantly shorter for the rasburicase-containing arms, with a median time of 4 h compared with 27 h for those treated with allopurinol monotherapy. These changes led to a significant reduction in incidence of LTLS with rasburicase (21%) and a trend toward significant reduction for the combination arm (27%) when compared with allopurinol alone (41%). However, there was no benefit in terms of reduction in incidence of CTLS with the addition or rasburicase (3% for each of the rasburicase arms and 4% for allopurinol monotherapy). It must be noted that this study was not restricted to high-risk populations, and therefore caution must be used in extrapolating conclusions to specific risk groups.

6.3.3 Pre-phase Treatment

In some situations, debulking of tumor with other therapies such as "pre-phase corticosteroids" for lymphoid malignancies should be considered to prevent or minimize TLS severity. Such an approach has typically been utilized for elderly, frail patients with aggressive lymphoma as a means to reduce their overall disease burden and improve their performance status in order to allow delivery of definitive therapy (Pfreundschuh 2004; Chaganti et al. 2016). Specific guidance regarding emerging TLS inducing therapies (e.g., venetoclax and obinutuzumab) borne out of early clinical trial experience is likely to be agent specific.

7 Treatment

7.1 Hyperkalemia Management

The most dangerous acute complication of TLS is development of hyperkalemia. Hyperkalemia represents a medical emergency due to risk of potentially fatal cardiac arrhythmias, and prompt diagnosis and intervention are required. Many centers have institutional guidelines for the management of hyperkalemia, and these should be initiated without delay. The principles of hyperkalemia management are briefly discussed here, but the reader is advised to familiarize themselves with their own institutional guidelines for patient management.

Criteria as to what level of hyperkalemia grades as mild, moderate, or severe vary in their definition. One example used lists mild hyperkalemia as <6.0 mmol/L, moderate as 6.0–6.4 mmol/L, and severe as ≥6.5 mmol/L. Evidence-based guidelines provided by the British Committee for Standards in Haematology (BCSH) recommend that hyperkalemia ≥6.0 mmol/L or ≥25% increase from baseline should prompt continuous cardiac monitoring (Jones et al. 2015). At levels ≥7.0 mmol/L dialysis is indicated and indeed may also be at lower levels according to clinical assessment and local guidelines.

Hemodialysis represents the most rapid and effective method for correction of electrolyte abnormalities associated with severe TLS. As a temporizing measure, interventions to redistribute intravascular hyperkalemia to the intracellular space may be beneficial, including inhaled or intravenous salbutamol and the use of intravenous insulin and dextrose. Enteric calcium resonium (polystyrene sulfonate) is also commonly used for management of non-TLS hyperkalemia, though as the time to onset is prolonged it is of little to no benefit for acute TLS. Furthermore, in the setting of abundant intravascular phosphate, enteric or parenteral calcium should be kept to an absolute minimum in order to minimize calcium phosphate formation. Similarly, many centers include early use of intravenous calcium gluconate for prevention of cardiac arrhythmias in the setting of hyperkalemia. The benefit of this intervention must again be weighed against the risk of calcium phosphate development in the setting of TLS.

7.2 Hypocalcemia Management

Due to the risk of calcium phosphate formation described above, asymptomatic hypocalcemia should not prompt replacement. Should corrected serum calcium levels reach ≤1.75 mmol/L or fall 25% or more from baseline levels, the BCSH again recommend cardiac monitoring be initiated (Jones et al. 2015). Symptomatic hypocalcemia should be corrected with intravenous calcium gluconate as per institutional dosing instructions, though only for the purposes of abrogating symptoms and not with the intent of correcting the serum calcium to within the normal biochemical range.

7.3 Hyperphosphatemia Management

Asymptomatic hyperphosphatemia is not an indication for treatment. Previous guidelines have included use of phosphate binders, but the oral forms of these are delayed in their onset of action, and due to issues of poor tolerability, they are not recommended according to current guidelines (Jones et al. 2015). The most effective treatment for correction of symptomatic hyperphosphatemia is through hemodialysis.

7.4 Renal Replacement Therapy

Renal replacement therapy represents the single most definitive and rapid treatment through which to correct the biochemical aberrations caused by TLS. If any clinical concern exists or the trend is toward dangerous parameters with TLS, urgent arrangements for renal replacement therapy should be made. Indications for hemodialysis in TLS are non-responsive fluid overload, hyperuricemia, hyperkalemia, hypocalcemia, or hyperphosphatemia (Jones et al. 2015).

Hemodialysis is the form of renal replacement therapy recommended for TLS as it can be rapidly facilitated and provides the fastest correction of electrolyte abnormalities. Furthermore, hemodialysis allows for rapid removal of fluid for those patients already developing oliguric/anuric renal failure with signs of fluid overload. In terms of the optimal modality of renal replacement therapy, there are no reported trials that have assessed the efficacy of intermittent hemodialysis versus continuous hemofiltration. The decision of the intensivist and renal physician regarding preferred dialysis modality is typically contingent upon the hemodynamic stability of the patient and the need for continuous cardiac monitoring. Dialysis should be continued until correction of renal function, urine output, and severe electrolyte abnormalities occurs (Jones et al. 2015). Peritoneal dialysis is not indicated as the time to correction of electrolyte abnormalities is protracted. Furthermore, fluid is less readily removed in the setting of overload when compared with hemodialysis. Finally, a significant proportion of high-risk patients (ALL and Burkitt/high-grade lymphoma) may have intra-abdominal malignancy or hepatosplenomegaly, limiting the safety and utility of peritoneal dialysis.

While hemodialysis is clearly the gold standard treatment of emergencies associated with TLS, it is invasive and costly and requires extensive resources to implement. In the palliative setting, early or preemptive discussion with the patient is important in order to determine whether they wish hemodialysis to be performed if indicated. Open communication is key in this situation, as some staff may empirically consider the palliative patient to be inappropriate for renal replacement therapy. However, case-by-case discussion is warranted as hemodialysis for TLS is often limited in duration and indicative of responsive disease, which may improve the patient's overall symptomatology and prognosis.

7.5 Implications for Further Therapy

The onset of TLS indicates a potential for subsequent TLS episodes with retreatment, where tumor bulk in any compartment (i.e., solid organ, bone marrow, or blood) persists or recurs in the treatment-free interval. This phenomenon was highlighted by a recent study of the CDK inhibitor, dinaciclib, in relapsed and refractory acute leukemia (37). Here, dinaciclib was dosed every 3 weeks, including administration to patients with highly proliferative disease. Initial objective responses, as evidenced by a reduction in WBC count and LTLS, were unfortunately only transient, and LTLS recurred with subsequent doses in tandem with rebound of the underlying leukemia (Gojo et al. 2013). However, the onset of TLS is not an absolute contraindication to continuing or re-challenge with the precipitating agent, as the initial tumor debulking heralded by TLS is often protective against future episodes.

8 Conclusions

Tumor lysis syndrome represents a medical emergency that ought to be readily prevented and managed. With the advent of more potent biological and targeted cancer therapies, TLS is now observed more frequently and in diseases which were previously considered low or intermediate risk. These agents are often administered to frail, older, or otherwise comorbid patients in diverse healthcare settings, including patients being managed with palliative intent. While prevention and management usually allow resolution of TLS, it is appreciated that some patients will have documented directives precluding some of the interventions listed within this chapter. It is important to distinguish, for example, short-term hemodialysis support for TLS from long-term dialysis in irreversible chronic renal failure. This highlights the need for open and transparent communication between clinicians and patients as to the potential for development of TLS with initiation of a new therapy and the potential complications thereof. As TLS is readily managed, its development in the palliative setting should not necessarily be seen as a terminal event and indeed may herald significant tumor debulking and potential improvement in symptomatology.

References

Agha-Razii M, et al. Continuous veno-venous hemodiafiltration for the treatment of spontaneous tumor lysis syndrome complicated by acute renal failure and severe hyperuricemia. Clin Nephrol. 2000;54(1):59–63.

Berenson JR, et al. Replacement of bortezomib with carfilzomib for multiple myeloma patients progressing from bortezomib combination therapy. Leukemia. 2014;28(7):1529–36.

Bergwitz C, Jüppner H. Phosphate sensing. Adv Chronic Kidney Dis. 2011;18(2):132–44.

Cairo MS, Bishop M. Tumour lysis syndrome: new therapeutic strategies and classification. Br J Haematol. 2004;127(1):3–11.

Cairo MS, et al. Recommendations for the evaluation of risk and prophylaxis of tumour lysis syndrome (TLS) in adults and children with malignant diseases: an expert TLS panel consensus. Br J Haematol. 2010;149(4): 578–86.

Chaganti S, et al. Guidelines for the management of diffuse large B-cell lymphoma. Br J Haematol. 2016;174(1): 43–56.

Cohen LF, et al. Acute tumor lysis syndrome. A review of 37 patients with Burkitt's lymphoma. Am J Med. 1980;68(4):486–91.

Coiffier B, et al. Guidelines for the management of pediatric and adult tumor lysis syndrome: an evidence-based review. J Clin Oncol. 2008;26(16):2767–78.

Cortes J, et al. Control of plasma uric acid in adults at risk for tumor lysis syndrome: efficacy and safety of rasburicase alone and rasburicase followed by allopurinol compared with allopurinol alone–results of a multicenter phase III study. J Clin Oncol. 2010; 28(27):4207–13.

Fleming DR, Henslee-Downey PJ, Coffey CW. Radiation induced acute tumor lysis syndrome in the bone marrow transplant setting. Bone Marrow Transplant. 1991;8(3):235–6.

Flynn J, et al. Dinaciclib is a novel cyclin-dependent kinase inhibitor with significant clinical activity in relapsed and refractory chronic lymphocytic leukemia. Leukemia. 2015;29(7):1524–9.

Frei E, et al. Renal complications of neoplastic disease. J Chronic Dis. 1963;16(7):757–76.

Goede V, et al. Obinutuzumab plus chlorambucil in patients with CLL and coexisting conditions. N Engl J Med. 2014;370(12):1101–10.

Gojo I, et al. Clinical and laboratory studies of the novel cyclin-dependent kinase inhibitor dinaciclib (SCH 727965) in acute leukemias. Cancer Chemother Pharmacol. 2013;72(4):897–908.

Goldfinger S, Klinenberg JR, Seegmiller JE. The renal excretion of oxypurines. J Clin Investig. 1965; 44(4):623–8.

Gregory GP, et al. CDK9 inhibition by dinaciclib potently suppresses Mcl-1 to induce durable apoptotic responses in aggressive MYC-driven B-cell lymphoma in vivo. Leukemia. 2015;29(6):1437–41.

Hande KR, Garrow GC. Acute tumor lysis syndrome in patients with high-grade non-Hodgkin's lymphoma. Am J Med. 1993;94(2):133–9.

Hochberg J, Cairo MS. Tumor lysis syndrome: current perspective. Haematologica. 2008;93(1):9–13.

Howard SC, et al. Tumor lysis syndrome in the era of novel and targeted agents in patients with hematologic malignancies: a systematic review. Ann Hematol. 2016; 95(4):563–73.

Huang WS, Yang CH. Sorafenib induced tumor lysis syndrome in an advanced hepatocellular carcinoma patient. World J Gastroenterol. 2009;15(35):4464–6.

Jones GL, et al. Guidelines for the management of tumour lysis syndrome in adults and children with haematological malignancies on behalf of the British Committee for Standards in Haematology. Br J Haematol. 2015;169(5):661–71.

Kalemkerian GP, Darwish B, Varterasian ML. Tumor lysis syndrome in small cell carcinoma and other solid tumors. Am J Med. 1997;103(5):363–7.

Kalff A, et al. Laboratory tumor lysis syndrome complicating LBH589 therapy in a patient with acute myeloid leukaemia. Haematologica. 2008;93(1):e16–7.

Kanchustambham V, et al. Spontaneous tumor lysis syndrome in small cell lung cancer. Cureus. 2017;9(2):1–9.

Keating MJ, et al. Early results of a chemoimmunotherapy regimen of fludarabine, cyclophosphamide, and rituximab as initial therapy for chronic lymphocytic leukemia. J Clin Oncol. 2005;23(18):4079–88.

Klinenberg JR, Goldfinger SE, Seegmiller JE. The effectiveness of the xanthine oxidase inhibitor allopurinol in the treatment of gout. Ann Intern Med. 1965; 62:639–47.

Mossner E, et al. Increasing the efficacy of CD20 antibody therapy through the engineering of a new type II anti-CD20 antibody with enhanced direct and immune effector cell-mediated B-cell cytotoxicity. Blood. 2010;115(22):4393–402.

National Cancer Institute. Common terminology criteria for adverse events v4.0, NCI, NIH, DHHS. 2009. NIH publication # 09-7473.

Pfreundschuh M. Two-weekly or 3-weekly CHOP chemotherapy with or without etoposide for the treatment of elderly patients with aggressive lymphomas: results of the NHL-B2 trial of the DSHNHL. Blood. 2004; 104(3):634–41.

Pro B, et al. Brentuximab vedotin (SGN-35) in patients with relapsed or refractory systemic anaplastic large-cell lymphoma: results of a phase II study. J Clin Oncol. 2012;30(18):2190–6.

Riccio B, et al. Spontaneous tumor lysis syndrome in acute myeloid leukemia: two cases and a review of the literature. Cancer Biol Ther. 2006;5(12):1614–7.

Roberts AW, et al. Targeting BCL2 with venetoclax in relapsed chronic lymphocytic leukemia. N Engl J Med. 2016;374(4):311–22.

Rostom AY, et al. Tumor lysis syndrome following hemi-body irradiation for metastatic breast cancer. Ann Oncol: Off J Eur Soc Med Oncol. 2000;11(10): 1349–51.

Saylor PJ, Reid TR. Tumor lysis syndrome after treatment of a gastrointestinal stromal tumor with the oral tyrosine kinase inhibitor sunitinib. J Clin Oncol. 2007; 25(23):3544–6.

Schifter T, Cohen A, Lewinski UH. Severe tumor lysis syndrome following splenic irradiation. Am J Hematol. 1999;60(1):75–6.

Smalley RV, et al. Allopurinol: intravenous use for prevention and treatment of hyperuricemia. J Clin Oncol. 2000;18(8):1758–63.

Swerdlow SH, et al., editors. WHO classification of tumours of haematopoietic and lymphoid tissues. 4th ed. Lyon: IARC Press; 2008.

Tam CS, et al. Long-term results of first salvage treatment in CLL patients treated initially with FCR (fludarabine, cyclophosphamide, rituximab). Blood. 2014; 124(20):3059–64.

Wendtner C-M, et al. Final results of a multicenter phase 1 study of lenalidomide in patients with relapsed or refractory chronic lymphocytic leukemia. Leuk Lymphoma. 2012;53(3):417–23.

Yamazaki H, et al. Acute tumor lysis syndrome caused by palliative radiotherapy in patients with diffuse large B-cell lymphoma. Radiat Med. 2004;22(1):52–5.

Yeldandi AV, et al. Molecular evolution of the urate oxidase-encoding gene in hominoid primates: nonsense mutations. Gene. 1991;109(2):281–4.

Zeidner JF, et al. Randomized multicenter phase 2 study of flavopiridol (alvocidib), cytarabine, and mitoxantrone (FLAM) versus cytarabine/daunorubicin (7+3) in newly diagnosed acute myeloid leukemia. Haematologica. 2015;100(9):1172–9.

Suicide and Attempted Suicide

81

Akshay Ilango

Contents

A. Ilango (✉)
RANZCP, Melbourne, VIC, Australia

Monash Health, Melbourne, VIC, Australia

Austin Health, Melbourne, VIC, Australia
e-mail: Akshay.Ilango@monashhealth.org

R. D. MacLeod, L. Van den Block (eds.), *Textbook of Palliative Care*,
https://doi.org/10.1007/978-3-319-77740-5_84

Abstract

To provide a broader perspective on suicide, this chapter has drawn on knowledge from the areas of suicide risk assessment in general psychiatry and consultation liaison psychiatry. Epidemiology of suicide and contextual factors are mentioned briefly to set the scene. A framework to assess and manage the suicidal patient is described in some detail, to assist the palliative care clinician. This is followed by a description of the key issues involved in the care of a psychiatric patient within the palliative care context. The latter part of the chapter elaborates on the experiences of those bereaved after a suicide. The impact of suicide on clinicians is explored, as well as strategies to manage the distress that can ensue. The chapter ends with a discussion of the unspoken issue of physician suicide. Terms such as mental illness, psychiatric illness, and psychiatric disorder will be used interchangeably. Specific aspects of management of underlying psychiatric disorders are detailed in the Chap. 85, "Distinguishing and Managing Severe Psychological and Psychiatric Distress" (authored by Ms. Jane Fletcher and Dr. Di Clifton). Acute non-suicidal self-harm (previously termed para-suicide), chronic suicidal ideation, chronic self-harm, and suicide in special populations, e.g., adolescents, have been excluded from the chapter. Requests for a hastened death, physician-assisted suicide, and euthanasia have been detailed in the chapter 90, "Request for Assisted Suicide" (authored by Dr. Diamond, Dr. Khurana, and Prof Quill).

1 Introduction

The following points are of relevance to the palliative care clinician:

- Acute suicidal ideation is an emergency.
- The rates of suicide are higher in the medically unwell and in those with cancer.
- The palliative care physician has knowledge of the biological contributors to suicidal ideation (e.g., intractable pain) and biological mitigating factors (e.g., medical management of pain).
- The palliative care team may need to take the lead in the assessment and management when a patient refuses to engage with the mental health service or if an immediate referral to the mental health clinician is not feasible.
- Desire for hastened death statements may reflect underlying suicidal thoughts.
- A positive therapeutic relationship is associated with lower rates of suicidal ideation and may reduce future episodes.
- Knowledge of risk factors is key, and the palliative care clinician is an integral part of the global challenge to reduce suicide.

2 Definitions

- Suicidal ideation is defined as thinking about, considering, or planning suicide.
- A suicide attempt is defined as a nonfatal, self-directed, potentially injurious behavior with an intent to die as a result of the behavior.
- Suicide is defined as a death caused by self-directed injurious behavior with an intent to

die as a result of the behavior (Centers for Disease Control and Prevention 2016). Suicidal thoughts range from mild and transient to severe and persistent. The suicidal behavior may be impulsive, ambivalent, planned, or recurrent.

3 Background

Neither attempted suicide nor suicide is a diagnosis, and there is no known precise cause. They are both complex behaviors resulting from the interaction between an individual and the environment. Suicide is reported in three main populations: the general population, those with a mental illness, and the medically unwell (including those with cancer). There are some common risk factors and some that are specific to the palliative care population. Given the relative paucity of research in this area, this chapter draws on knowledge from the areas of suicide risk assessment in the general psychiatric practice, consultation liaison psychiatry, and palliative care setting. Suicidal ideation and behaviors are assessed on a spectrum from mild and transient to severe and persistent. Suicidal behavior is multi-determined, and mental illness, including depression and demoralization in the palliative care population, is risk factor for suicide. The chapter aims to provide a framework for clinicians who wish to perform a suicide risk assessment. It is anticipated that palliative care clinicians will refine their risk assessment skills and embed them into routine practice.

4 Epidemiology and Contextual Issues

Suicidal thoughts and behaviors are common in the general population. From a survey in 2013, 4% of the American population reported having suicidal thoughts in the preceding year, 1.1% had made plans to attempt suicide, and 0.6% had attempted suicide (Results from the 2013 2014a). It is difficult to determine true prevalence rates for attempted suicide because the available data relies on self-reporting, not all suicide attempts require medical intervention, and reporting practices vary. Suicide is also underreported but remains a leading cause of death worldwide (World Health Organisation 2012). Unless the person had expressed suicidal intent or left a suicide note, the coroner may not make a finding of suicide, and it is likely that many open and indeterminate findings represent deaths by suicide. Given the reporting constraints, true suicide figures are likely to be higher than the observed figures. In 2012, suicide accounted for an annual global suicide rate of 11.4 deaths per 100,000 population (males were twice as likely to suicide than females). More than 800,000 lives were lost through suicide that year, i.e., one suicide death every 40 seconds.

The rates of suicide vary greatly from one country to another, e.g., suicide rates in the USA were less than half the rates observed in Southeast Asia (World Health Organisation 2012). Inconsistency in suicide data collection methodology makes it difficult to draw any firm conclusions about the reasons for considerable regional variation. However, it is hypothesized that there exists a base rate of suicide worldwide (attributed to medical and psychiatric disorders) and the variation is attributed to local sociocultural, economic, and political factors (Goldney 2015). This finding has substantial implications for suicide prevention, in that sociocultural interventions may be necessary to reduce and prevent suicide.

A process described as a psychological autopsy has examined the association between suicide and mental illness. The process involves making retrospective assessments through speaking to informants, and gathering medical records of people who have completed suicide, to identify indicators of mental illness. There are studies reporting that 90% of those who completed suicide had a psychiatric disorder or substance use disorder (Cavanagh et al. 2003).

The rates of psychiatric disorders in the cancer population are reported to be higher than the general population. Half the proportion of patients with an advanced cancer meet the threshold for a psychiatric diagnosis, and 40% of patients in oncological, hematological, and palliative care settings had some form of a mood disorder (Mitchell et al. 2011). The most common diagnoses include adjustment disorder and major depression (Miovic and Block 2007). Serious mental illness is seen in 10–20% of cancer patients, with only half accessing mental health services (Kadan-Lottick et al. 2005). Palliative care frontline clinicians are well placed to identify psychiatric comorbidity and ensure access to care. It is generally accepted that suicide is twice as common in the cancer population (Misono et al. 2008).

People with a serious mental illness, such as schizophrenia, bipolar disorder, and personality disorder are almost twice as likely to die prematurely (between 10 and 20 years earlier than those without a mental illness) as a result of medical conditions including diabetes and heart disease (Kisely et al. 2005). Interestingly, persons with a serious mental illness have a lower incidence of cancer than the general population (male cancer incidence rate ratio = 0.86 and female cancer incidence rate ratio = 0.92) (Kisely et al. 2013). Patients with schizophrenia have lower rates of prostate and colorectal cancer (Tabarés-Seisdedos et al. 2011), in which genetic and immune mechanisms are implicated. Furthermore, despite high rates of tobacco smoking, patients with schizophrenia have a lower lung cancer incidence. However, the overall cancer-related mortality is higher in persons with a mental illness, for the following reasons: they are less likely to participate in screening measures, e.g., women with a serious mental illness are half as likely to have screening mammography than the general population (Mitchell et al. 2014); they are more likely to present late with metastases; and they are less likely to have specialist interventions like chemotherapy, radiotherapy, and surgical treatment (Kisely et al. 2015).

In summary, patients with a serious mental illness have higher rates of premature death, lower cancer incidence but higher cancer-related mortality, and increased rates of suicide.

5 Ethics and Related Issues

Suicide is confronting for the physician. Firstly, in the pursuit of relief from suffering, there needs to be a shared view on the path to wellness. It is this shared view that forms the basis of the therapeutic relationship; however suicide is a departure from this shared view. Secondly, the value of life as an end in itself is a fundamental value held by clinicians, but it is a value that is difficult to articulate. The clinician knows that life has value, but the suicide of a patient confronts this deeply held view. Despite our best efforts in healthcare, we have been unable to eliminate suicide, which in turn challenges our belief system around the value of life. Subsequently, we become aware that the drive to preserve life may succumb to a drive to end life. The clinician has to revisit personal attitudes and beliefs about suicide that inevitably evoke strong personal feelings that may impact on the care of the suicidal patient. When clinicians care for a suicidal patient, they are uncomfortably reminded of the fact that they too are at risk of suicide, and suicide rates are higher among physicians than the general population.

Clinicians may avoid asking about suicide, and their own fears can hinder their engagement with the suicidal patient. The language used to elicit suicidal ideation is vital. The question "You haven't had suicidal thoughts, have you?" is very different from "Have you ever felt that life had no meaning, or that you couldn't go on with life?" The former puts pressure on the patient to respond in the negative, and the latter is more likely to set the scene for a dialogue. Our patients ask us to prognosticate and expect us to respond to a question like "Doctor, how long do I have?" Managing this type of question requires experience and skill because the answer to this question will impact on the patient. The physician has to walk the fine line of responding to the patient's query with integrity while communicating a broader sense of hope, even when the prognosis is poor or uncertain. The refusal of lifesaving medical treatment raises questions of capacity to refuse such treatments, and this is particularly so in those with a known or suspected psychiatric disorder, especially depression.

A discourse on the relationship between various religions and suicide is beyond the scope of this chapter; however, religion has long been viewed as a protective factor against suicide. O'Reilly and Rosato (2015) examined the relationship between religion and suicide in one million residents of Northern Ireland, where 40% were Roman Catholic, 40% were Protestant, 7% were Conservative Christians, and only 13% did not identify with any religion. If church attendance is protective, then the rates of suicide should be lowest in Catholics and greatest in those with no religious affiliation; and if religiosity is important, then suicide rates should be lowest in conservatives and highest in those without religious affiliation. Younger Roman Catholics had higher suicide rates, but as a whole Roman Catholics, Protestants, and those who had no religious affiliation had similar suicide rates. Conservative Christians had a lower suicide rate, possibly attributable to lower alcohol consumption rather than church attendance or religiosity (O'Reilly and Rosato 2015). These findings challenge common societal perceptions; however, church attendance is a poor measure of religiosity. It remains unclear whether religiosity (religious salience) is associated with lower suicide rates.

In summary, in assessing the suicidal patient, the clinician needs to not only know what to ask but also how to ask exploratory questions. The clinician's preconceptions, values, and fears will impinge on the therapeutic relationship.

6 Risk Factors

There are some common risk factors observed in the general, psychiatric, nonmalignant palliative care, and cancer populations, e.g., male gender, single status, depression, hopelessness, etc. However, there are also some specific risk factors observed in the cancer population. The risk factors vary in their strength of association and temporal correlation with the suicide attempt.

6.1 Family History of Mental Illness and Family History of a Suicide Death

From family, twin, and adoption studies, it has been established that psychiatric illnesses and suicides cluster within families. It is plausible that suicides cluster within families because psychiatric illnesses cluster within families; however, there is evidence to suggest that the genetics of suicide may be independent of the genetics of psychiatric illness. Qin et al. (2002) examined suicide risk in relation to family history of completed suicide and psychiatric disorders (Qin et al. 2002). For a patient without a family history of suicide but with a family history of a psychiatric admission, the adjusted odds ratio (OR) for suicide was 1.31; and for a patient with a family history of a suicide but without a family history of a psychiatric admission, the adjusted odds ratio (OR) for suicide was 2.58. When the patient had both a family history of a psychiatric admission and a family history of suicide, the adjusted OR for suicide was 2.68. Genetic factors account for almost 50% of the variance in the familial transmission of suicide risk (Statham et al. 1998).

In summary, suicidal behavior runs in families, and half the vulnerability is attributed to genetics. A positive family history of suicide and a family history of psychiatric disorder "significantly and independently" increase suicide risk.

6.2 Past History of a Self-Harm or Suicide Attempt

After an episode of self-harm, the risk of suicide increases incrementally over the subsequent 15 years, especially in men and with increasing age at the time of self-harm (Hawton et al. 2003). Similarly, a past suicide attempt is a strong risk factor for future suicide, and the risk remains high for several decades (Suominen et al. 2004). Only 50% of suicide attempters receive intervention, which is typically only for a few weeks (Hunt et al. 2009).

In summary, it is clinically relevant to ask about past history of an attempted suicide and brief after-care does not address the high long-term suicide risk.

6.3 Substance Use and Comorbidity with Psychiatric Disorder as Risk Factors

In the general population, adults with a substance abuse or dependence diagnosis in the past year were more likely to have serious suicidal thoughts, to make suicidal plans, and to attempt suicide (Results from the 2013 2014b). There was substantial comorbidity between substance abuse disorders and mental disorders, and having one disorder more than doubled the risk of having the other. The OR for a suicide attempt seemed to follow a gradient (lowest in nonusers, followed by those with substance use history, followed by those with a substance abuse disorder, and highest in those with a substance dependence disorder). This gradient was particularly evident in alcohol users. The OR for alcohol nonusers was 1.0, for alcohol use (without abuse/dependence) was approximately 2.0, alcohol abuse (without dependence) was approximately 3.0, and for those with alcohol dependence was approximately 6.0, even after controlling for comorbid mental illness (Borges et al. 2000). The association between substance use and suicide revealed much higher odds ratios when mental illness was not controlled, suggesting that mental illness plus substance abuse may have cumulative effects on suicidal behavior. Substance use disorders are more prevalent in cancer, e.g., alcohol abuse and dependence are more prevalent in head and neck tumors (further details are in ▶ Chap. 85, "Distinguishing and Managing Severe Psychological and Psychiatric Distress").

6.4 Psychiatric Disorder

As stated in the chapter entitled ▶ Chap. 85, "Distinguishing and Managing Severe Psychological and Psychiatric Distress" the rates of psychological distress and psychiatric disorder are significantly elevated in the cancer population. The comorbidity confers greater vulnerability to suicide. Bipolar disorder, schizophrenia, substance use disorder, and borderline personality disorder have substantially higher rates of suicide (five- to tenfold) compared to the general population (Chesney et al. 2014). Depressive disorders confer the greatest suicide risk (20-fold risk) (Harris and Barraclough 1997). Therefore, an accurate psychiatric diagnosis and prompt treatment are central to suicide prevention.

In summary, substance use disorder and mental disorders are two independent risk factors for suicide. The risk of suicide is greatest with a substance dependence disorder and comorbid psychiatric disorder. This is of particular relevance because substance use disorders and psychiatric disorder are more prevalent in the cancer population.

6.5 Developmental Adversity

The experience of emotional neglect and abuse (physical, emotional, and sexual) is a risk factor for mental illness generally and suicide in particular, but not everyone with this history will develop a mental illness or attempt suicide. It is hypothesized that early adversity may induce long-term epigenetic changes in gene expression, resulting in an upregulation of the hypothalamo-pituitary-adrenal axis and an increased stress response. Adversity may also impact on the genes involved in the down-regulation of brain-derived neurotrophic factor (BDNF), which is central to neurogenesis and neuronal plasticity. Neglect and abuse also impact on the psychological development of the individual and are associated with low self-esteem, a risk factor for suicide. There are observable problem-solving deficits in those with a remote history of abuse in the context of adverse life events, and they are more likely to experience hopelessness, thus increasing suicide risk.

6.6 History of Medical Illness

Certain medical illnesses are more likely to be associated with mental illnesses and therefore suicide. There are studies suggesting an independent link between medical illness and suicide (even after controlling for mental illness) (Goodwin et al. 2003; Druss and Pincus 2000). Neurosurgical disorders increase suicide rates by 20-fold, renal disease confers a 14-fold increase, epilepsy confers a 5-fold increase, and malignant disease doubles the risk of suicide (Harris and Barraclough 1997; McGirr et al. 2008).

6.7 Cancer-Specific Suicide Risk Variables

The shared risk factors observed in the general population and in patients with a mental illness may also be observed in the cancer patient, such as male gender, age greater than 65, and social isolation. However, there are some cancer-specific risk factors. Depression is more common in the cancer population, and there are neurobiological causes to support this finding. Cancer activates a persistent humoral immune response leading to an upregulation of inflammatory cytokines such as IL-6 (Spoletini et al. 2011). Immune dysregulation and cytokines are associated with onset and progression of cancer and depression. Patients are more likely to attempt suicide within 1 year of a cancer diagnosis. Advanced stage at diagnosis, locally advanced cancer, and metastatic disease are also at risk. While the total number of deaths from suicide in cancer patients is relatively small in comparison to cancer-related deaths, suicide rates are higher in the cancer population in comparison to the general population (by a factor of 1.5–2.0) (Vyssoki et al. 2015). Certain cancer sites are particularly associated with suicide such as lung, biliary-pancreatic, head and neck, and CNS tumors. The risk of suicide was greater in those who underwent high-morbidity surgery. While surgery may offer renewed hope, there are postoperative outcomes that can increase suicidal behavior, e.g., physical disability, loss of bodily function, loss of autonomy, existential distress, poor pain control, and the use of disinhibiting drugs (e.g., opiates). Other risk factors include a past history of self-harm or suicide attempt and poor social support especially in advanced cancer (Chochinov et al. 1998). Patients with advanced disease are more likely to have a high symptom burden, functional impairment, pain, and depression. The perception of poor pain control, and associated hopelessness, was a more significant risk factor for attempted suicide than the intensity of pain (Passik et al. 2007).

In summary, certain types of cancer, a new diagnosis, and advanced cancers pose a greater risk of suicide. Suicide deaths in the cancer population constitute a small proportion of all-cause deaths; however, the rates of suicide are twice as high.

Palliative care patients not uncommonly express a desire for hastened death. Such statements may reflect an underlying request for physician-assisted suicide, euthanasia, and a communication of suicidal thoughts. Depression and hopelessness are two independent factors that contribute to a desire for hastened death. Depressed patients were four times more likely to have a high desire for hastened death than the non-depressed palliative care inpatients. Hopelessness is more strongly associated with suicidal behavior (and desire for hastened death) than depression in the terminally ill. Hopelessness is a pessimistic cognitive style rather than the patient's knowledge of a hopeless prognosis. It is the patient's appraisal of their situation that leads them to feel hopeless, and it may have little to do with the reality of their prognosis. Patients who had neither depression nor hopelessness were unlikely to desire a hastened death. Lack of social support and physical functioning also contributed to a desire for hastened death (Breitbart et al. 2000). These findings fundamentally change how we as a society should conceptualize the desire for a hastened death in a palliative care context, in that such a desire should not be dismissed as an understandable response to a cancer diagnosis.

In summary, the expressed desire for hastened death may represent underlying depression, hopelessness, and suicidal ideas.

6.8 Mediating Mental States that Increase the Desire to Die

Palliative care patients not uncommonly express a desire for hastened death. Such statements may reflect an underlying request for physician-assisted suicide, euthanasia, and a communication of suicidal thoughts. Depression and hopelessness are two independent factors that contribute to a desire for hastened death (Breitbart et al. 2000). Depressed patients were four times more likely to have a high desire for hastened death than the nondepressed palliative care inpatients. Hopelessness is more strongly associated with suicidal behavior (and desire for hastened death) than depression in the terminally ill. Hopelessness is a pessimistic cognitive style rather than the patient's knowledge of a hopeless prognosis. It is the patient's appraisal of their situation that leads them to feel hopeless, and it may have little to do with the reality of their prognosis. Patients who had neither depression nor hopelessness were unlikely to desire a hastened death. Lack of social support and physical functioning also contributed to a desire for hastened death (Breitbart et al. 2000). These findings fundamentally change how we as a society should conceptualize the desire for a hastened death in a palliative care context, in that such a desire should not be dismissed as an understandable response to a cancer diagnosis.

The key mental states that directly mediate an increase in suicidal thoughts are 1) a sense of the pointlessness or meaninglessness of life, 2) hopelessness or helplessness, 3) worthlessness, 4) loss of control, and 5) shame (Kissane 2014; Robinson et al. 2017). The intensity of these mental states is moderated by inadequate physical and mental symptom control, poor social support, increasing loss of pleasure (anhedonia) and growing frailty. On the other hand, religious beliefs, close relationships and improved quality of life prove protective. Demoralization is a clinical syndrome that captures much of the phenomenology present in these mediators of the desire to hasten death. Demoralization is a mental state of lowered morale and poor coping, which is characterized by feelings of hopelessness, helplessness, loss of meaning and purpose in life, and feeling trapped or stuck in a predicament. Demoralisation then interferes with a person's appreciation of the value of life and may adversely impact on medical treatment decision-making processes and treatment choices. This is a common clinical syndrome, with a prevalence of 13–18 percent of patients in palliative care and predictors include single status, female gender, physical symptom burden, reduced social support and the presence of severe psychiatric disorders (Robinson et al. 2015). Studies in cancer have shown that loss of meaning and demoralization contribute a 3-fold greater risk of developing suicidal thoughts than depressive symptoms (Fang et al. 2014; Robinson et al. 2017; Vehling et al. 2017). In summary, suicidal ideation may represent underlying hopelessness, demoralization and depression.

7 Management of the Suicidal Patient

7.1 Understanding the Suicidal Cancer Patient

Religious, sociological, and philosophical conceptualizations predate medical perspectives on suicide. It was only in the nineteenth century that the physician Esquirol viewed suicide as a medical problem (Berrios 1996). Psychiatry and psychoanalysts have since dominated the medical arena in the conceptualization of suicide. Freud (1856–1939) conceptualized mental life in terms of sexual and aggressive drives, at a time in history when the expression of aggression and sexuality was taboo. Freud understood suicide to be a consequence of aggressive drives turned inward (homicidal impulses are converted into suicidal impulses). Over the last decade, neurobiological research has led to a better understanding of the genetics of suicidal behaviors and biomarkers that indicate a predisposition to suicidal behavior. Juxtaposed with this emerging evidence, there are fundamental gaps in our understanding of suicide. For instance, suicidal behaviors are also observed in the absence of psychiatric disorders, and suicide is not a common outcome in those who have psychiatric disorders and cancer.

Contemporary models for suicide are based on a "stress-diathesis model" and are essentially biopsychosocial in approach (Turecki 2016) (Fig. 1). The model suggests that suicidal behavior is a consequence of the interaction between various risk factors (Turecki and Brent 2016). As we endeavor to move toward understanding

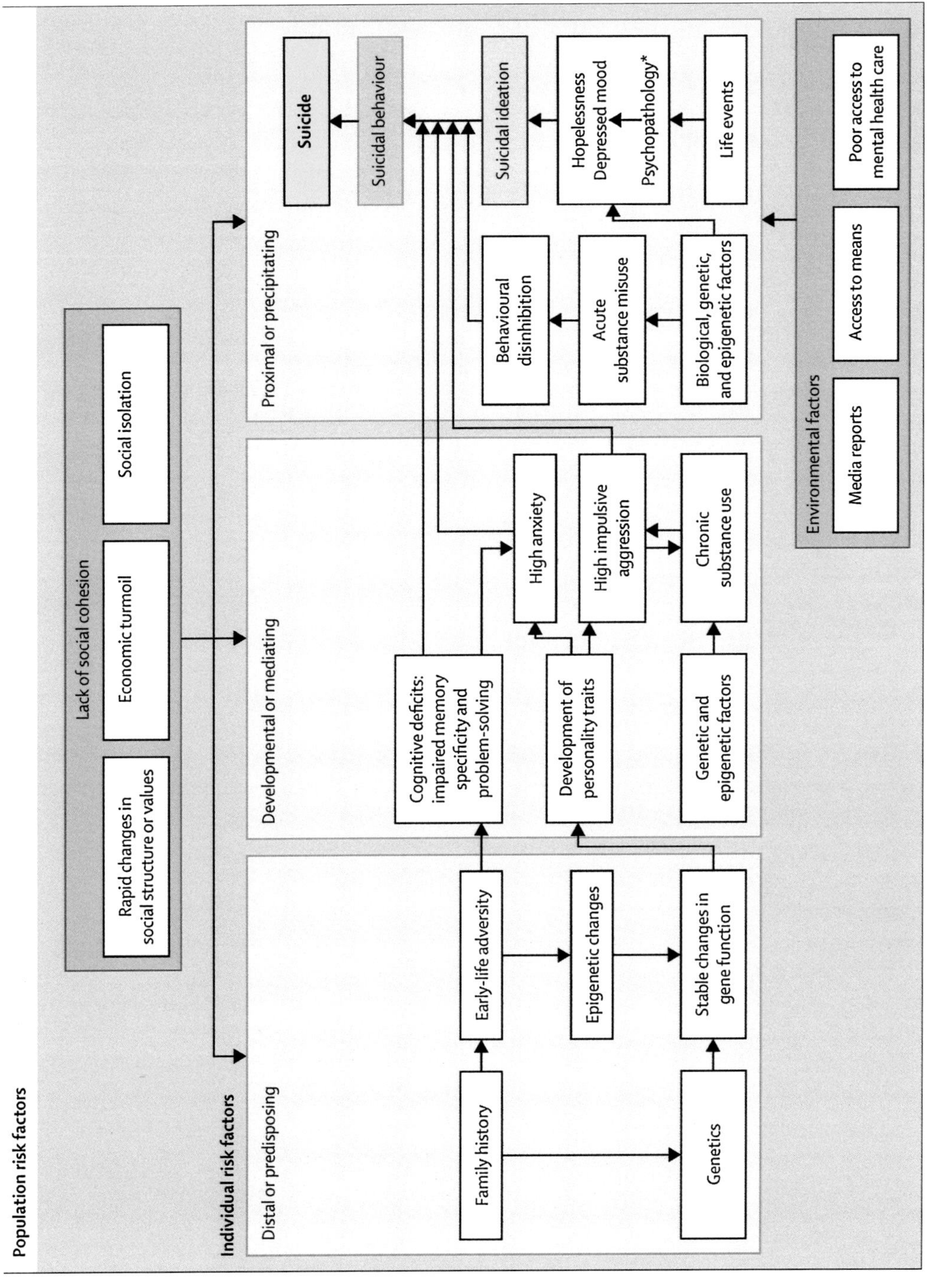

Fig. 1 Model for suicide risk. (Reprinted with permission from Turecki G, Suicide and suicidal behaviour. The Lancet 2016; 387:page 1229, Elsevier 2016)

the plight of our suicidal patient, we undertake a process of integrating information about interconnected factors; the process is described as a formulation (refer to Table 1). The formulation aims to answer a fundamental question: "Why does this patient suffer these problems, in this way, at this point of time?" (Selzer and Ellen 2014).

7.2 Approach to the Assessment of the Suicidal Patient

Most palliative care patients are assessed by a range of clinicians (medical, nursing, and allied health) at the point of entry to the service. The multidisciplinary approach can provide different perspectives and a deeper understanding of the whole patient through integrating the available information. Nurses are often the frontline staff responding to the concerns of family members, provide hands-on care, and respond to the emotional needs of the patient. Patients may open up when being nursed at vulnerable times or during intimate care. Junior medical staff should take a meticulous medical history enquiring about pre-existing medical illness, onset, duration, progression and associated treatments, and relevant negatives in the history and examination to provide the necessary details required in the biological column in the Table 1. A respectful and curious clinician can elicit the psychological factors. The social circumstances and how they have changed over time are often known to the team social worker. Social workers routinely ask about the family context and adjustment to illness, as well as provide counseling. Pastoral care service may explore the personal meaning attached to life and enquire about the spiritual and existential aspects of the patient's experience.

The multidisciplinary team should integrate the data obtained by various clinicians, from different sources, to provide a succinct formulation of the presenting problem for the patient and their family. Suicidal ideation is no different, and all members of the team should be vigilant for signs that suggest the patient may be suicidal. Breitbart provides sample questions that can be used to assess suicidal risk (refer to Table 2). Clear communication between team members, including clear documentation, well-defined roles, and mutual respect for one another, are prerequisites for a well-functioning multidisciplinary team and, as a consequence, effectively manage the suicidal patient.

The suicidal patient may be identified as at risk at the point of entry to the service or early in the admission. Early identification allows the clinicians time to prepare an approach to the patient. At other times, the patient may not be identified as at risk, and the patient may voice suicidal thoughts after a significant incident, e.g., after disclosure of a poor prognosis. Staff will intuitively check on the emotional state of the patient who has received bad news. Clinicians will need to be attentive to any verbal or nonverbal communication from the patient and be willing to explore further. For instance, the patient may say, "What's the point, I can't do it anymore!" which would need to be explored by the clinician to elicit suicidal ideation. The patient's refusal to shower or refusal to eat a meal may present the nurse with an opportunity to engage the patient in a discussion of their emotional state. A well-timed question such as "Are you are too tired to shower today?" can provide a point of engagement.

After a preliminary assessment conducted by the frontline staff, a decision may be made to perform a more detailed examination of the patient. The assessment should ideally be conducted by the clinician who is:

- able to understand the nature of the underlying medical condition and its impact on the brain and mind.
- curious about patient's psychological experience of cancer.
- willing to engage with the distressed, indifferent, uncooperative, or guarded patient.
- aware of their own fears and attitudes toward the suicidal patient. The clinician may experience anxiety, anger, denial, and helplessness or may view suicide as understandable or even justifiable.

There are at least three good reasons for the palliative care clinician to participate in the task of risk assessment:

Table 1 Formulation of suicide risk

	Biological factors	Psychological factors	Social/cultural/ spiritual factors
Predisposing factors confer vulnerability to suicide			
Predisposing factors	Male and increasing age (>65 years) **Family history of suicidal behavior and psychiatric disorder**[a,c] **Psychiatric disorder**[a,c] **Prior suicide attempts**[a,c] **Substance use disorder**[a,c] **Chronic medical illness**[c], especially brain disease/injury[b], delirium[a] Impulsivity – genetic contribution[c] Neuropsychological vulnerabilities; poor problem-solving skills; **Cancer-related variables**[a] (within 1 year of diagnosis, advanced stage, locally advanced or metastatic disease of the lung and pancreas and cancer-related pain and fatigue), treatments of cancer and drug interactions, e.g., role of steroids in mood disorders	Childhood maltreatment and developmental adversity[c] Modeling (knowing someone who attempted suicide) **Hopelessness**[a,b] as a cognitive style (rather than a hopeless prognosis) **Helplessness**[a] **Depression**[a] Low self-esteem Loss[c] (in relationships, employment, and leisure activities)	Single status Unemployment **Social isolation**[a,c] Homelessness or unstable housing Migration and displacement (indigenous people) Cultural and religious beliefs Local epidemics of suicide[c] Barriers to access to healthcare services, stigma, and barriers to receiving care[c]
Precipitating factors temporally correlate with the onset of suicidal ideation			
Precipitating factors	Identify a change in the trajectory of cancer that correlates with the onset of suicidal ideation, e.g., disease progression and increasing pain or fatigue Change in the trajectory of psychiatric illness, e.g., new onset/ relapse of depression Delirium Change in medications/treatments (e.g., radiotherapy to the brain or thyroid, steroids) and new drug interactions Drug dependence (withdrawal) or intoxication Nonadherence to interventions	Identify a change in experience of cancer. **Trigger points**: at initial diagnosis, initiation of curative treatment, side effects or intolerance of treatment, refusal or withdrawal of treatment, disease progression, relapse and recurrence, transition to palliative care where the focus may change from curative treatment to quality of life issues, and confronting issues of death and dying and survivorship Explore the following domains (**five Ds of cancer**): death, dependence, disfigurement, disruption in relationships, and disability Current suicidal ideation, plan, or intent [a]**Hopelessness and feeling a burden** **Demoralization** [a]**Loss of meaning** [a]**Loss of dignity and worthlessness** Depressive cognitions, e.g., "I am worthless"	Change to single status Recent unemployment Recent homelessness **Social isolation**[a,c] Financial strain Legal issues Child custody issues Cultural and religious issues Access to lethal means[c] (e.g., guns) Disasters Discrimination (LGBT) issues

(*continued*)

Table 1 (continued)

	Biological factors	Psychological factors	Social/cultural/ spiritual factors
Perpetuating factors are the persistent or ongoing risk factors that are known to increase risk			
Perpetuating factors	Ongoing biological factors (as listed above) that may contribute to persistent suicidal thoughts	Ongoing psychological factors (as listed above)	Ongoing social factors (as listed above)
Protective factors are often an absence of risk factors listed above			
Protective factors	*Absence* of psychiatric disorder[c] or substance use disorder[c] *Effective treatment of above risk factors*, e.g., effective treatment of pain	*Absence of above risk factors* Extroversion and optimism[b] Ability to identify their psychological experience (psychological mindedness) Problem-solving skills and conflict resolution skills[b,c] Motivation to improve their situation and willingness to seek help Strong reasons for living[b] Deeper sense of meaning and purpose	*Absence of above risk factors* Social connectedness[c] and family cohesion Stable employment and housing Responsibility for children[b] Positive therapeutic relationship[c] Access to mental healthcare[c]

Information extracted from the following sources: Alici et al. (2016) indicated with a, (Turecki and Brent 2016) indicated with b, and (Violence Prevention 2016) indicated with c

Table 2 Assessing suicidal thoughts, plan and intent

Assessing suicidal thoughts	
Suicidal ideation	Many patients have passing thoughts of suicide, such as "if my pain was bad enough, I might. . .." Have you had thoughts like that? Have you found yourself thinking that you do not want to live or that you would be better off dead? Have you stopped or wanted to stop caring for yourself?
Suicide plan	Have you thought about how you would end your life? Do you plan to hurt yourself?
Suicide intent	Do you intend to hurt yourself? What would you do? Do you think you would carry out these plans?

Reprinted with permission from Olden M, Pessin H, Lichtenthal W, and Breitbart W. Suicide and desire for hastened death in the terminally ill. In Chochinov HM and Breitbart W, editors. Handbook of psychiatry in palliative medicine. New York. Oxford University Press; 2012. p. 107

1. Data suggests that 45% of those who complete suicide see a physician in the month before their suicide and may not volunteer suicidal ideation unless specifically asked (Luoma et al. 2002).
2. Talking about suicide does not increase suicidal thoughts in the person who is being assessed (Law et al. 2015).
3. A strong therapeutic relationship with the treating oncologist is associated with lower rates of suicidal ideation and may reduce future suicidal ideation (Trevino et al. 2014).

The assessment of the suicidal patient may begin with the request from a team member or a family member, in which case begin with step 1. At other times, the patient will disclose suicidal thoughts during a routine consultation that will require further exploration: begin with step 3. A structured approach to the assessment of the suicidal patient is suggested.

Step 1: Speak to the "team" before assessing the patient.

- A team member, or a member of the family, may initiate the request for an assessment. Enquire about the event that has triggered the need for further assessment and be specific about the enquiry: "Has the patient said or done something to suggest that the patient is suicidal; have they made a suicide attempt?"

- Enquire about the patient's past history including that gathered by the other members of the team:
  - Past psychiatric history, the specific prescribed treatment, and last known mental state examination, including a cognitive assessment.
  - Past suicide attempts.
  - Be aware of the nature and impact of the medical condition, pain, and the results of blood tests and imaging.
  - Drug and alcohol history – intoxication/dependence/withdrawal.
  - Family history of psychiatric illness, suicide, and substance use.
  - Current medications (medical and psychiatric).
  - Social history – next of kin details; is there an advance care directive?
  - Premorbid values and goals and attitudes toward treatment.

Step 2: Thinking time.

- Ask yourself "Why might the patient be suicidal at this time (consider the biopsychosocial vulnerabilities/predisposing factors listed in Table 1) and what has changed for the patient of late (precipitating or perpetuating factors)?"
- Consider differential diagnoses before examining the patient (e.g., dementia, delirium, depressive disorder, or other).
- What are the gaps in your knowledge of the patient and who can help fill in the gaps? Often collateral history from informants helps.
- Consider consulting a senior colleague or a psychiatrist before seeing the patient as this may help in planning an approach to the assessment, particularly if the assessment is likely to occur in the patient's home. It is important to be aware of the local legislation that pertains to the treatment of those with a mental illness.

Step 3. Speak to and examine the patient.

- Introduce yourself to the patient and explain your role in the team; it is important to be explicit with the patient about the purpose of the review, e.g., "I am here because your nurse mentioned that you were feeling hopeless about your situation and had been thinking that life was not worth living. If it is okay with you, I am here to understand what you are going through and then to suggest a way forward." Inform the patient of the limitations of the right to confidentiality and that you may need to consult the duty psychiatrist. Take a confident but curious stance. Respect and empathy go a long way in managing the patient's distress as they tell their story. Interview in a quiet space and be clear about the time available to address this issue.
- Obtain a full psychiatric history:
  - Ask about the current cancer and the impact on the person.
  - Ask about the current psychiatric symptoms to exclude a major mental illness (such as dementia, delirium, depression) and current suicidal thoughts and plans and ask about access to firearms.
  - Ask about the current psychiatric and physical health medication history and elicit information regarding any recent medication changes.
  - Ask about the current drug and alcohol use to elicit a change in the pattern of drug use, intoxication, and withdrawal states.
  - Ask about the current social context and stressors. Asking the patient: "How do you understand the factors that led you to feel suicidal?" is a reasonable question. Enquiry about the meaning of the suicidal thoughts for the patient is helpful. Suicidal comments may represent a mere communication of their suffering, a wish to be relieved of intolerable suffering, a fear of a painful death, a wish to be reunited with a deceased person, or a statement to reassert their autonomy on life and death. In the context of a cancer diagnosis, loss and threat emerge as recurring themes. Understand that for the patient, there is a threat to their physical and psychological integrity as a result of the cancer diagnosis and a loss of previous good health and loss of future possibilities. The nature and quality of

relationships also change as a consequence of ill health. The spouse may become the carer. Patients may be physically debilitated and may be more dependent on others for basic activities of daily living, and this may be intolerable for them.

- Identify risk factors conferring vulnerability to suicide. Ask the patient about prior adverse life events and challenges and how the person coped with the challenge. Ask about how the person maintains a sense of dignity, and a deeper sense of meaning.
- Ask about past psychiatric history with specific treatment details and previous suicide attempts. For example, the patient may have had a past history of depression with previous suicide attempts that required electroconvulsive therapy (ECT) and psychiatric medications to achieve remission.
- A general physical examination is usually documented in the records at the point of entry to the service; however, focus on biological factors known to precipitate suicidal ideation. If the patient has attempted suicide, a targeted physical examination will be necessary, for instance, examination after a laceration or an overdose.
- Mental state examination (MSE):

  A typical mental state examination includes an assessment of cognition (to exclude delirium or dementia), appearance and behavior, speech, mood, affect, thought stream, form, and content. Specific and detailed inquiry into suicidal ideation, intent, and plan is important. It is also important to exclude psychotic symptoms, to assess insight and the patient's capacity to make medical and psychiatric treatment decisions.

  The following features suggest high acute suicide risk: agitation, disturbance in the affect (which is the emotional tone during the interview). Elicit despondency, despair, suicidal preoccupation with intent or plan, and access to lethal means. Perception of being a burden on others and feelings of hopelessness are potent risk factors. Command auditory hallucinations and nihilistic delusions also increase suicide risk. Insight and judgment also need to be assessed because they influence management. Ask the patient: "What is the medical condition you suffer from? How does it affect you? What are your treatment options? What is your understanding of your prognosis? Help me understand how suicide is the best option for you at the moment?"

Step 4: Construct a "formulation" to understand the patient and guide management.

The focus is on the patient and their unique circumstances and not on a collection of risk factors. The assessment needs to be contextualized in the formulation wherein risk factors are juxtaposed with protective factors. The formulation requires a process of integration and prioritization of the information obtained by the team which in turn informs management (Simon 2009).

In formulating a case, the first task is to identify the **predisposing factors** (refer to Table 1), which are remotely implicated in the presentation of the person. The information is elicited during the process of history taking, examination, investigations, and information obtained from collateral sources, often at the point of entry into the service. These factors are historical, such as family history of mental illness. For instance, when a patient reports that a parent suffered a mental illness, the clinician may speculate that the patient has a genetic vulnerability to mental illness (and possibly suicide). It would also be important to consider the impact of parental mental illness on the nature and quality of the parenting, parent-child relationship, and the patient's personality development. It would be reasonable to ask the patient: "How did your father's mental illness impact on the way he raised you and your relationship with him?" If the patient reports that a parent committed suicide, the clinician may speculate that the family history of suicide suggests genetic loading for mental illness and suicide. Suicide is a powerful behavioral incentive for others to suicide, a process described as modeling, and family members who attempt suicide provide powerful maladaptive messages to the living about the challenges of life and how to overcome them. The patient is more likely to attempt suicide within 1 year of a cancer diagnosis, especially in the context of a locally advanced pancreatic cancer or if the patient has had a high-morbidity surgical procedure, often with substantial psychological consequences. The social (cultural and spiritual) predisposing factors are often elicited by the social worker and pastoral care worker on the team.

The next task is to identify the **precipitating factors**. Reflect on "Why is this person suicidal now?" and temporally correlate onset of suicidal ideation with changes in the patient's biopsychosocial situation. For instance, if the patient says that (s)he began contemplating suicide 1 month ago, the clinician should search for a change in the patient's context that corresponds to that timeframe. Note however, that there can be a time lag between a change in the situation and the onset of suicidal ideation. Gene-environment interaction may explain the apparent time lag.

There are key *trigger points* in the illness trajectory that may cause substantial emotional distress. These trigger points correspond to the time when the patient first notices a symptom, the time of a new diagnosis, initiation of curative treatment, side effects or intolerance of treatment, refusal or withdrawal of treatment, relapse and recurrence, survival, advancing disease, transition to palliative care, and dying. As the patient transitions from one stage to another, the clinician should explore the psychological experience of a change in their circumstances and explore the **five Ds of cancer** (Hodgkiss and Mascarenhas 2012):

- **D**eath anxiety and fear of what dying entails (e.g., "With all that has happened to you lately, have you been thinking about death?")
- **D**ependence on others, which may be distressing (e.g., "How has your situation impacted on your capacity for independence?")
- **D**isfigurement as a result of the cancer or treatments (e.g., "How has the cancer and the treatment impacted on how you see yourself?")
- **D**isruption in relationships and changed dynamics (e.g., "How has the cancer changed the quality of your relationship with…?")
- **D**isability associated with the cancer (e.g., "How has the cancer changed what you can do for yourself or what you would like to do for yourself?")

The loss of **D**ignity, **D**emoralisation and **D**epression may also lead the person to contemplate suicide. Dignity is defined as the state of being worthy of honor or respect. There are three factors that impact upon the sense of dignity. Firstly, the cancer may cause distressing symptoms and may impact upon the person's level of independence and therefore their dignity. These are the illness-related concerns. Secondly, the person may maintain a sense of dignity through adhering to a set of personal values and attributes such as hopefulness, wish to maintain autonomy, or by doing things to preserve their dignity, termed dignity-conserving repertoire. Lastly, the dynamics within key relationships may either bolster or undermine the patient's sense of dignity, termed social dignity inventory.

Then aim to identify the **perpetuating factors**. Here the clinician aims to identify persistent or ongoing biopsychosocial risk factors that are known to increase risk. Advanced cancer, intractable symptoms (such as pain), side effects from the treatment, partially treated depression, nonadherence to antidepressants, fatigue, family conflict, perceived helplessness, hopelessness, loss of dignity and meaning, and a sense of being a burden are likely to render the person suicidal. Single status and social isolation are key social determinants for mental illness and suicide in particular.

Finally, identify the **protective factors** that will mitigate the risk. Often an absence of biopsychosocial factors that are known to precipitate or perpetuate the risk of suicide are seen as protective factors. The patient may need the clinician to identify protective factors at a time when all hope appears to have been lost. The patient may hold a deeper sense of meaning and purpose, have dependent children, and have a love of music, and the team can draw upon these factors to mitigate risk.

Step 5: Make a diagnosis and identify the imminent suicide risk.

Consider several differential diagnoses: dementia, delirium, psychiatric disorders secondary to general medical condition, substance-induced psychiatric disorders, and other psychiatric syndromes such as depression and demoralization. A high-suicide-risk patient is one with suicidal ideas, suicidal intent, and suicidal planning and has access to lethal means to commit suicide, including prescription medication.

Step 6: An approach for the management plan for the imminently suicidal patient.

The physician empathizes with the patient's suffering by saying something like "I can only imagine how you must feel looking at the scar across your chest" for a patient with a mastectomy scar. Even a well-intentioned statement like "The scar does not look too bad" may be experienced by the patient as being invalidating. The physician puts himself in the patient's shoes and views the situation, as perceived by the patient, as a means to understand the patient's distress to demonstrate empathy.

Early in the interview, the physician says something like "It is very common for people with cancer to think about death, dying, and suicide, often when they feel alone and have lost all hope." This lifts the veil of secrecy. The patient is then invited to elaborate on their suicidal thoughts and distress as a tangible sign of physician's concern for the patient. As the physician actively listens and makes an attempt to understand the patient's predicament, the patient feels understood. A curious stance goes a long way in creating a therapeutic space wherein the patient articulates their distress without fear of judgment.

The physician provides a clinician's formulation to the patient, and this facilitates rapport, and the formulation serves a road map for intervention. There are various factors that the clinician needs to take in to account in deciding how much to share with the patient. For instance, the clinician needs to be aware of the patient's general level of intelligence, their proficiency with language, their capacity to process and understand information, and their psychological mindedness in determining how much of the clinician's formulation is communicated to the patient. The biological, psychological, and social factors contributing to the patient's distress and suicidal thoughts are actively managed. Collaboratively working toward symptom relief instills hope. As stated previously, the physician-patient relationship is a key determinant in suicide risk. Drawing upon the patient's social support systems in the ongoing management may prove helpful in managing the suicidal patient. The physician challenges unhelpful thought patterns (e.g., thoughts like "There's no point"), provides information, problem solves, offers reassurance, and instills hope. The clinician obtains consent to contact family for collateral information and reviews the patient frequently. If the patient is assessed as a high risk of suicide, an immediate psychiatric consultation should be sought. The palliative care team will need to manage the patient in the interim.

The social worker may provide a formulation based on the patient's narrative or family systems theory, assess, and manage unhelpful family dynamics with a view to help the patient make sense of their situation. Interventions offered range from supportive psychotherapy to family therapy. Pastoral care workers bring to light the religious conflicts faced by the patient, for instance, suicidal thoughts may be in conflict with the patient's conservative Christian ideology. Pastoral care discusses themes of guilt, shame, and punishment in the patient's narrative with respect to religion. Involving the patient's family is a vital component of the treatment plan because they are often a source of collateral information, support for the patient, and an ally to the team.

Based on the individualized formulation, a management plan is constructed by remediating factors known to precipitate and perpetuate suicidal thoughts and building upon protective factors to mitigate risk. For the acutely suicidal patient, creating a safe environment is the immediate priority. This invariably involves treatment in an inpatient palliative care unit, if specialist palliative care is necessary. It would be uncommon to transfer a patient with suicidal thoughts and palliative care needs from a palliative care unit to a psychiatric ward.

Management decisions need to be made by the multidisciplinary team because each member of the team may have a specific role in the ongoing management. Nursing staff may be able to provide direct supervision of the patient, administer medication, and clear the surrounds of dangerous items (e.g., belts and kitchen knives). There may be circumstances when it may be necessary to arrange a psychiatrically trained nursing staff member to engage with the suicidal patient and provide constant visual observation.

Consider the role of **psychotropic medication** in the context of a broader biopsychosocial management plan for the cancer patient (refer to Table 3 below). Pharmacological management of specific underlying psychiatric syndromes is described in the chapter entitled ▶ Chap. 85, "Distinguishing and Managing Severe Psychological and Psychiatric Distress."

The consultation liaison psychiatry service will assess the suicidal patient as a matter of urgency and suggest a **psychological therapy** depending on the individualized formulation. The ▶ Chap. 85, "Distinguishing and Managing Severe Psychological and Psychiatric Distress" details a range of psychotherapeutic approaches used in palliative care. The therapy is targeted to address the key aspects of psychological distress, which may in turn drive suicidal ideation.

When demoralization is seen to be mediating suicidal ideation, existentially-oriented and meaning-centered therapies restore much needed hope and morale (Kissane 2011, 2017). Recent randomized-controlled trials have confirmed the efficacy of meaning-centered therapies, whether using a group (Breitbart et al. 2015) or individual approach (Breitbart et al. 2018). Clinicians should pay attention to sources of continued meaning in a person's life: focus on their role within a family and the quality of their relationships; recognise the value of their life and accomplishments, making an active choice to embrace meaning and enjoy life through sources of creativity (arts, music and literature). These key areas of significance for patients all foster a deeper investment in life, despite infirmity (Lethborg et al. 2018). It remains unclear whether the above therapies directly reduce suicide rates, although there is clear evidence that there are evidence-based therapies to reduce distress and demoralization in palliative care.

7.3 Additional Issues to Consider in the Management of a Patient with a Serious Mental Illness

Societal marginalization and rejection lead the psychiatric patient to expect being rejected by their healthcare team, and staff may be anxious when admitting a person with a history of a serious mental illness. Not uncommonly, psychiatric patients have endured neglect and abuse up until they recieve holistic care during the hospice admission. Patients feel cared for and are grateful for the care. The patient with a psychiatric illness is more likely to have multiple medical comorbidities, a life-span 20 years less than the general population, and a higher cancer mortality. Howard et al. (2010) highlight issues arising in the treatment of those with a psychiatric disorder (Howard et al. 2010). Patients with schizophrenia may have thought disorder, rendering them unable to communicate their cancer-related symptoms clearly, or have auditory hallucinations that tell them to refuse treatment, or they may be amotivated leading them to miss medical appointments. The patient with schizophrenia may have disrupted frontolimbic circuits (involved in pain perception) leading to an apparent under-reporting of pain. It is important to anticipate the potential challenges when planning treatment with patients with mental illness. The refusal of lifesaving medical treatment in the context of active psychiatric disorder should prompt a referral to the liaison psychiatry service.

Assertive management of the medical and psychiatric illness is vital. Consider drug interactions between psychiatric medications and anticancer treatments. In terms of the *pharmacodynamic drug interactions*, it is important to note that

Table 3 Role of psychotropics in the suicidal patient

	Advantages	Disadvantages
Psychotropic medications may be prescribed for (Grassi et al. 2014). • The treatment of emotional distress without psychiatric disorder • A pre-existing/underlying psychiatric disorder • For nonpsychiatric disorders such as pain disorders • Cancer-related symptoms such as anorexia, nausea, etc. • Non-cancer symptoms such as sleep disturbance		
Other considerations before prescribing psychotropic medications. • Constellation of psychiatric symptoms • Comorbid medical conditions • Efficacy data • Safety profile • Drug interactions and • Cancer stage and goals of care (curative vs. end-of-life care)		
Antidepressants	Reduce impulsivity, treat underlying depression, and anxiety. Management of cancer-related symptoms such as pain (dual-acting antidepressants), fatigue (modafinil, bupropion, and reboxetine), anorexia, and insomnia (mirtazapine) may indirectly reduce suicide risk	Can cause restlessness, increase suicidal ideation, and lead to an instability in mood especially early in the treatment and with dose increments. Regular monitoring of suicidal ideation is advised
Benzodiazepines	Benzodiazepines do not reduce suicide per se but alleviate emotional distress and treat anxiety disorders. Other indications are insomnia, non-specific agitation, dyspnea, and terminal restlessness, as adjuncts to antiemetics and as antiepileptics which again may have indirect effects on suicide risk	Can rarely lead to "disinhibition or paradoxical excitement" and increase impulsivity. If prescribed with other sedative agents can be lethal in overdose. Managing the access may mitigate risk
Antipsychotics	Efficacious in the treatment of psychotic disorders and mood disorders, thereby reducing suicidality through treatment of the underlying disorder. Antipsychotics may be used in the management of behavioral disturbance in the setting of a dementia, delirium, and paraneoplastic syndromes. Haloperidol is commonly used antipsychotic in palliative care as a hypnotic, antiemetic, augmenting agent for analgesia, and in delirium	Concomitant use of antiemetics can infrequently prolong QTc. Can be subject to drug interactions. An anticholinergic delirium is a rare side effect at low doses but common in an overdose context
Ketamine	Acute antidepressant like action with rapid-onset anti-suicide properties with few side effects in the short term, in cancer patients (Reinstatler and Youssef 2015; Fan et al. 2016). Ketamine treatment was associated with a reduction in suicidal ideation independent of depression (Murrough et al. 2013).	Longer-term safety and efficacy data is lacking
Psychostimulants	Can be activating, improve attention and have a rapid onset of antidepressant activity, and are used to alleviate cancer-related fatigue, anorexia (in low doses), and poor quality of life in terminal cancer and to manage sedation secondary to opiates	Rarely used and no evidence in the suicidal patient. Often a regulated drug. Inhibit cytochrome system. Can precipitate psychosis and cause arrhythmias

(*continued*)

Table 3 (continued)

Lithium and clozapine	*Level 1 evidence for the treatment of bipolar disorder and schizophrenia but also have independent "anti-suicide" effects*	*Prescribed under the supervision of a psychiatrist. Rarely used in the palliative care context and therefore rarely studied*
Electroconvulsive therapy	*ECT has been shown to rapidly alleviate suicidal intent in almost 40% of acutely suicidal depressed patients within 1 week, and 60% by the end of the second week were no longer acutely suicidal* (Kellner et al. 2005). "*ECT is recommended as first-line treatment in extremely severe melancholic depression, particularly when the patient refuses to eat or drink and/or is a very high suicide risk, or when the patient has very high levels of distress, has psychotic depression, catatonia or has previously responded to ECT*" (Malhi et al. 2015). *There is level 1 evidence in support of ECT as an efficacious treatment option in the depressed patient with medical comorbidities and cancer is not a contraindication* (Zwil and Pelchat 1994)	

psychiatric medications and anticancer therapies impact on a range of organ systems, e.g., the liver. Concurrent medications that affect bone marrow functioning need to be considered, e.g., agranulocytosis is a known side effect of clozapine, carbamazepine, clonazepam, and a range of chemotherapy agents. Furthermore, antipsychotics, chemotherapy agents, and antiemetics (metoclopramide) can cause prolongation of the QTc, as seen on the electrocardiogram (ECG) which can increase the risk of Torsades de pointes (TdP), a fatal arrhythmia. Hepatotoxicity and renal impairment with concurrent medication usage should be anticipated, and close monitoring is advised. In terms of *pharmacokinetic drug interactions*, consider the impact of a medication on the metabolism of another. Medications may be metabolized through the cytochrome P 450 system, such as CYP 1A2, 2D6, and 3A4. Inhibitors of this system may lead to an accumulation of the substrate and consequent toxicity. Fluoxetine and fluvoxamine are potent inhibitors of CYP 2D6. Tamoxifen is a prodrug metabolized by CYP 2D6 to the active metabolite, endoxifen. Hence, inhibition of CYP 2D6 leads to an accumulation of the prodrug rather than the active metabolite, rendering treatment ineffective (Andersohn and Willich 2010). There are innumerable drug interactions, and it is prudent to check before prescribing.

7.4 Experience of Those Bereaved Through Suicide

Suicide does not occur in a vacuum. It occurs within a family and social system, and in palliative care, a suicide will also impact the treating team. Suicide is ubiquitous, and therefore, it is not uncommon to know a person bereaved after suicide: a suicide survivor. When suicide occurs in the physically well, the suicide survivors are more likely to report perplexity ("Why did he do it?"), guilt about not being able to prevent the suicide ("I couldn't prevent it."), guilt about missing the early signs ("I should have seen it coming."), a sense of rejection by the deceased ("Why did he do it to me?"), and stigma from society (people might think "What in the family caused it?") (Sveen and Walby 2008).

When a suicide occurs in the context of a terminal illness, the survivor may experience emotions similar to the ones described above. However, survivors may view the cancer suicide as an understandable response to pain and suffering, a noble act in the face of an inevitable death, and the survivor may not feel guilty because the patient would have died from the cancer in time. The suicidal patient may have the covert permission from the survivor, and in this scenario, relief may be mixed with guilt. The experience of a suicide survivor is impacted upon by their personality, genetic predisposition, developmental stage, capacity to "make sense of the suicide," as well as the shared environmental factors such as family and social supports for the survivor (Andriessen et al. 2015). The nature and quality of the relationship and meaning of the relationship have a bearing on the experiences of the suicide survivor. In the general psychiatric literature, suicide survivors were not at an increased risk of suicide when compared to those bereaved by sudden unnatural causes, but suicide survivors were at higher risk of suicide than those bereaved by sudden natural causes (Pitman et al. 2016). Spouses bereaved by suicide were at a greatly increased risk of suicide (Agerbo 2003). It is unclear whether spouses of cancer suicide are at increased risk of suicide and whether there are differences in terminal cancer suicide versus suicides early in the cancer trajectory.

7.5 Management After a Suicide

After a suicide, the responsibility of the clinician shifts to the care of those left in the aftermath of the suicide. A designated staff member will make early contact with the family, may attend the funeral if possible, advise on what to expect in the bereavement process, suggest a grieving ritual, provide information on local suicide bereavement groups, and consider a referral to specialist services (Alici et al. 2016). The physician should take advice from a senior colleague and the medicolegal unit before speaking to the family, in order to provide accurate information and express regret at the loss of a life.

There will often be two distinct staff meetings with two distinct agendas within days of the incident. Firstly, a staff support meeting would offer informal comfort within days of the event. When attending to the emotional needs of the staff, it is suggested that staff express their feelings toward the deceased (sorrow, relief, anger, etc.) and express their feelings about their own role in the care of the patient (guilt, shame, relief, etc.) (Grad 1996). The convener of the group educates staff about the signs of emotional distress and strategies to cope with the loss while also maintaining a high standard of care for staff and other patients. Secondly, a psychological autopsy meeting is convened to ascertain accurate information regarding the deceased. This second meeting has a different membership, including senior clinical staff and operations managers. They adopt a detailed approach to examine processes and systems of care and deal with any immediate systemic issues that may compromise the care of other patients. The meetings should remain focused on the events and processes rather than people or feelings. Undue focus on people or feelings can exacerbate feelings of guilt or shame. There may be formal reporting processes within organizations involving the Quality Assurance Unit (QAU). There may be a fear that the QAU will abandon the physician so as to protect the institution and its reputation (Misch 2003). The clinician may be mandatorily required to notify systems outside the institution, such as the Coroner's Office and/or the Office of the Chief Psychiatrist. A suicide should go through multiple levels of scrutiny as part of the overall local suicide prevention strategy. The inquiry process itself is stressful for the clinician.

8 The Professional Carer

8.1 The Clinician Survivor: Physician's Experience After a Patient Suicide

Given the paucity of literature on the physician's experience on this matter, physicians may benefit from the reflections of psychiatrist survivors. The personality style (e.g., perfectionism and obsessional personality traits confer vulnerability) and their emotional state at the time of the suicide will impact on the experience of a patient suicide (International Association 2016). The quality and duration of the therapeutic alliance, professional skill base, whether there were other clinicians involved in patient care, and finally the physician's career developmental stage have a bearing on the clinician's experience (Gitlin 1999).

The quality of the doctor-patient relationship varies from one patient to another, and so the suicide of one patient may affect the clinician differently from another. In the dyad, one has unconscious and conscious feelings toward the other, which are activated at various times in the course of the therapeutic relationship. The quality of the therapeutic relationship is often changing and is dynamic. Therefore, the timing of the suicide in the context of the prevailing therapeutic relationship will have a bearing on the clinician's experience of the suicide. For example, the suicide at a time when the therapeutic relationship was strong may be experienced differently from the suicide which occurs in the context of an estranged relationship.

The suicide reactivates deep emotions from the physician's private life, often based on unconscious conflicts within the physician's past relationships. Unconscious conflicts are out of the conscious awareness, and the physician may not be able to readily articulate these deeper emotions (Misch 2003). In simple terms, the suicide death of a patient may resurrect internal emotional conflicts from the physician's past. It follows then that there is no one set pattern of how a suicide will impact upon the physician. After the suicide, a range of painful unconscious feelings may torment the physician. In the first week, the physician may experience disbelief and denial, followed by emotional turmoil that can last a couple of months. The physician experiences heightened anxiety and surreal feelings such as depersonalization and numbness. Physicians may experience a sense of shame for failing an internally set standard of care (Tillman 2003). He/she may become angry with the deceased. The doctor may experience excessive guilt, as if responsible for killing the patient. Perceived guilt may be disguised or concealed, manifesting as over-conscientiousness and excessive care of other patients. Internal conflict may lead to poorly planned discharges or overly restrictive practices so as to prevent another suicide (Little 1992). There may be an internal sense of relief disguising itself in thoughts such as the recognition that the patient is now at peace. Unconsciously, the physician could be relieved at not having to manage this once challenging patient or experience denial manifesting as forgetting vital information about the patient. The physician is likely to keep these ambivalent and painful feelings private.

The physician will also have a range of emotions that are subject to conscious awareness and can be articulated. The suicide of a patient may activate a sense of threat and/or loss.

In the short term, the doctor may experience:

- Feelings of shame and incompetence manifesting as self-doubt: "Am I good enough?", "Will I identify the next suicidal patient?"
- Fears of being exposed as incompetent or fears of persecution by the patient's family and "Will I lose my job over this?"
- A changed view of oneself and a loss of the competent self which may manifest as "I am not good enough and my colleagues no longer respect my clinical skill and I am the topic of hushed conversations."
- Loss of support from colleagues, a sense of failing to meet the standards set by one's colleagues, and meeting colleagues who no longer want to associate themselves with the management of this patient.

At this lonely hour, grieving staff may turn to literature to seek closure and meticulously read the case notes to see what could have been done differently. Speaking up can be painful and may be taboo within the unit. Staff will avoid breaking down at work because it may be misunderstood as a sign of weakness or an admission of incompetence. Staff will continue with their duties with a brave professional façade. In the longer term, burnout, depression, post-traumatic stress disorder, and substance abuse may ensue.

Gitlin (1999) suggests a few strategies to assist the clinician survivor (Gitlin 1999). Firstly, the physician should manage the sense of isolation by talking to a senior colleague, friends, or family. If appropriate, speaking to the bereaved family may be appropriate and may also reduce the sense of isolation. Secondly, the physician could educate colleagues about the management of this type of scenario. Consider a case presentation or writing up as a case report for a journal. Writing about yourself, in third person, helps in distancing yourself from the case. Next, remind yourself that suicide is a preventable outcome in many but not all cases. Suicide rates in inpatient psychiatric units have remained fairly constant over the last 75 years, despite advances in interventions such as antidepressants, antipsychotics, lithium, and ECT (Cotton et al. 1983). From this knowledge, the physician may conclude that despite evidence-based treatments, suicide remains an undeniable reality in those with a serious mental illness. The physician can remind himself that the cancer patient is at greater risk of suicide and again suicide may be a possible outcome despite treatment. Note that suicide may be a failure of the treatment (not a failure of the physician). Suicide prediction is a flawed science with low positive predictive value and high false positives (Pokorny 1983). Little suggests a departmental review and case presentation of the incident after 2 months but before 6 months (to describe what happened) with the aim of staff education (to see what can be learnt) (Little 1992). Finally, the physician can take the lessons learned from one suicide and use it in the management of the next. Notwithstanding the turmoil experienced by the clinician, there is opportunity for emotional growth.

In summary, there is no one predictable trajectory after a patient suicide. Several factors impact on the clinician's experience of a suicide. Some of the factors are accessible to one's conscious awareness while others are not. However, there are tangible steps a clinician can take to regain a sense of mastery and control.

8.2 Physician Suicide

The physician is more vulnerable to depression and substance use; suicide rates are consistently higher among physicians than among the general population. Even though the absolute numbers of suicides among physicians is small, it would not be unusual to know of a physician who committed suicide. There are about 300 physician suicides in the USA each year (American Foundation 2016). A meta-analysis found that male and female physicians in the USA were at greater risk of suicide (suicide rate ratios of 1.41 and 2.27, respectively) than the general population (Schernhammer and Colditz 2004). More recent Australian data (Milner et al. 2016) found that suicide rates were significantly higher in females who worked in healthcare professions (doctors, nurses, psychologists, and allied health staff) in comparison to females working in non-healthcare professions. Suicide rates followed a gradient, being highest in female nurses, followed by female doctors (two and a half times more likely to suicide than females working in non-healthcare professions), followed by male nurses (who were one and a half times more likely to suicide than males in non-healthcare professions). Ease of access to prescription medication was a key risk factor and one which is of particular relevance in palliative care. The rates of suicide were comparable for male doctors and males in non-healthcare professions (Milner et al. 2016). Higher rates of suicide are attributed to two sets of vulnerability factors. Firstly, general suicide risk factors such as depression and substance misuse. Secondly, risk factors are associated with being a clinician such as personality attributes (e.g., perfectionism), gender role conflict, stress of work, workplace bullying, and harassment. There are substantial expectations of their role, their personal identity may be defined by the work, and staff may experience vicarious traumatization. Male nurses may experience stigmatization as a result of career choice, and female healthcare professionals may feel conflicted about their responsibilities at home and work. For the abovementioned reasons, the palliative care clinician is at risk. There are organizational barriers, such as rising insurance costs and restrictions on scope of practice following disclosure of mental illness, thereby reducing the likelihood of a disclosure of mental illness (Lindeman et al. 1999).

Middleton (2008), a family physician and a suicide survivor, wrote an essay on her experience of losing a colleague to suicide (Middleton 2008). She reminds us that, firstly, the issue of a physician suicide is an unacknowledged problem and, secondly, stigma prevents our profession from managing it. The suicidal physician is under pressure to remain silent or risk being labeled as an impaired physician, a label that threatens his professional identity and dignity, right to practice, and livelihood.

After a physician suicide, colleagues are left grappling with questions like "Why didn't you ask for help…did I fail you?" The survivor is also under pressure to grieve in silence. Center et al. (2003) prepared a consensus statement with recommendations for physicians to address the issue of physician suicide. Center recommends ensuring healthcare for the physician, recognizing the symptoms of depression in oneself and colleagues, seeking treatment of mood disorder and substance abuse, being aware of the local services available for the mental health of doctors, and having working knowledge of the local laws regarding confidentiality and the statutory obligation to inform regulatory authorities (Center et al. 2003).

9 Conclusion and Summary

Suicidal behavior, much like an acute abdomen, is a medical emergency. The general perception in the community is that suicide in the cancer patient is an understandable response to the illness and that it is somehow different from suicide in other populations. Arising from this misperception is the notion of rational suicide in cancer. The desire for hastened death is not uncommon in palliative care and may reflect underlying suicidal thoughts. There are known general risk factors and cancer-specific risk factors. Suicide in this population represents a desperate attempt to escape internal or external stressors, and these stressors can be conceptualized via biological, psychological, and social factors or a combination of the above. Patients with cancer are more likely to have a comorbid psychiatric disorder and are at greater risk of suicide; however, death through suicide in a cancer patient is a relatively rare outcome. Suicide is a multi-determined behavior, and correspondingly, interventions also need to be multimodal to address issues such as symptom control, emotional distress, and social isolation. An individualized formulation of the suicidal patient aims to alleviate distress. The palliative care clinician, in the context of an established therapeutic relationship, is ideally placed to undertake the task of a suicide risk assessment and then arrange a psychiatric consultation if needed. As public opinion shifts, physician-assisted suicide has gained traction in palliative care. In the context of this cultural change, there is a risk that society may revert to thinking of suicide as a legitimate means to end intolerable suffering, and it is conceivable that family may assist the patient in ending their own life. Suicide prevention is a global challenge, and ongoing medical education is vital if we are to have any chance of preventing suicide at an individual level. As we focus our attention to the care of our patient, it is also important that clinicians care for themselves and each other.

References

Agerbo E. Risk of suicide and spouse's psychiatric illness or suicide: nested case-control study. BMJ. 2003; 327(7422):1025–6.

Alici Y, Jaiswal R, Pessin H, Breitbart W. Suicide. In: Bruera E, Higginson I, von Gunten CF, Morita T, editors. Textbook of palliative medicine and supportive care. 2nd ed. Boca Raton: CRC Press; 2016. p. 887–95.

American Foundation for Suicide Prevention [Internet]. New York: American Foundation for Suicide Prevention; 2016. Ten facts about physician suicide and mental health; 2016 [2016 December 2]. Available from: http://afsp.org/wp-content/uploads/2016/11/ten-facts-about-physician-suicide.pdf

Andersohn F, Willich S. Interaction of serotonin reuptake inhibitors with tamoxifen. BMJ. 2010;340:c783.

Andriessen K, Draper B, Dudley M, Mitchell P. Bereavement after suicide. Crisis. 2015;36(5):299–303. https://doi.org/10.1027/0227-5910/a000339.

Breitbart W, Rosenfeld B, Pessin H, Applebaum A, Kulikowski J, Lichtenthal WG. Meaning-centered group psychotherapy: an effective intervention for improving psychological well-being in patients with advanced cancer. J Clini Oncol. 2015;33:749–54.

Breitbart W, Pessin H, Rosenfeld B, Applebaum AJ, Lichtenthal WG, Li Y, et al. Individual meaning-centered psychotherapy for the treatment of psychological and existential distress: a randomized controlled trial in patients with advanced cancer. Cancer. 2018. https://doi.org/10.1002/cncr.31539

Berrios GE. The history of mental symptoms; descriptive psychopathology since the nineteenth century. Cambridge: Cambridge University Press; 1996. p. 443.

Borges G, Walters EE, Kessler RC. Associations of substance use, abuse, and dependence with subsequent suicidal behaviour. Am J Epidemiol. 2000;151(8):781–9.

Breitbart W, Rosenfeld B, Pessin H, Kaim M, Funesti-Esch J, Galietta M, Nelson CJ, Brescia R. Depression, hopelessness, and desire for hastened death in terminally ill patients with cancer. JAMA. 2000;284(22):2907–11.

Cavanagh JT, Carson AJ, Sharpe M, Lawrie SM. Psychological autopsy studies of suicide: a systematic review. Psychol Med. 2003;33(03):395–405.

Center C, Davis M, Detre T, Ford DE, Hansbrough W, Hendin H, Laszlo J, Litts DA, Mann J, Mansky PA, Michels R. Confronting depression and suicide in physicians: a consensus statement. JAMA. 2003; 289(23):3161–6.

Centers for Disease Control and Prevention. Definitions: self-directed violence [Internet]. Georgia: Centers for Disease Control and Prevention; 2016. [updated 2016 August 15; cited 2016 October 14]. Available from: http://www.cdc.gov/violenceprevention/suicide/definitions.html

Chesney E, Goodwin GM, Fazel S. Risks of all-cause and suicide mortality in mental disorders: a meta-review. World Psychiatry. 2014;13(2):153–60.

Chochinov HM, Wilson KG, Enns M, Lander S. Depression, hopelessness, and suicidal ideation in the terminally ill. Psychosomatics. 1998;39(4):366–70.

Cotton PG, Drake RE Jr, Whitaker A, Potter J. Dealing with suicide on a psychiatric inpatient unit. Psychiatr Serv. 1983;34(1):55–9.

Druss B, Pincus H. Suicidal ideation and suicide attempts in general medical illnesses. Arch Intern Med. 2000;160(10):1522–6.

Fan W, Yang H, Sun Y, Zhang J, Li G, Zheng Y, Liu Y. Ketamine rapidly relieves acute suicidal ideation in cancer patients: a randomized controlled clinical trial. Oncotarget. 2016;8(2):2356–60.

Fang CK, Chang MC, Chen PJ, Lin CC, Chen GS, Lin J, et al. A correlational study of suicidal ideation with psychological distress, depression, and demoralization in patients with cancer. Support Care Cancer. 2014;22:3165–74. https://doi.org/10.1007/s00520-014-2290-4

Gitlin MJ. A psychiatrist's reaction to a patient's suicide. Am J Psychiatr. 1999;156(10):1630–4.

Goldney R. The importance of mental disorders in suicide. Aust N Z J Psychiatry. 2015;49(1):21–3. https://doi.org/10.1177/0004867414549200.

Goodwin RD, Marusic A, Hoven CW. Suicide attempts in the United States: the role of physical illness. Soc Sci Med. 2003;56(8):1783–8.

Grad OT. Suicide: how to survive as a survivor? Crisis. 1996;17(3):136–42.

Grassi L, Caruso R, Hammelef K, Nanni MG, Riba M. Efficacy and safety of pharmacotherapy in cancer-related psychiatric disorders across the trajectory of cancer care: a review. Int Rev Psychiatry. 2014; 26(1):44–62.

Harris EC, Barraclough B. Suicide as an outcome for mental disorders. A meta-analysis. Br J Psychiatry. 1997;170(3):205–28.

Hawton K, Zahl D, Weatherall R. Suicide following deliberate self-harm: long-term follow-up of patients who presented to a general hospital. Br J Psychiatry. 2003;182(6):537–42.

Hodgkiss A, Mascarenhas S. Psycho-oncology. In: Guthrie E, Rao S, Temple M, editors. Seminars in liaison psychiatry. Glasgow: Bell and Bain Limited; 2012. p. 190.

Howard LM, Barley EA, Davies E, Rigg A, Lempp H, Rose D, Taylor D, Thornicroft G. Cancer diagnosis in people with severe mental illness: practical and ethical issues. Lancet Oncol. 2010;11(8):797–804.

Hunt IM, Kapur N, Webb R, Robinson J, Burns J, Shaw J, Appleby L. Suicide in recently discharged psychiatric patients: a case-control study. Psychol Med. 2009; 39(03):443–9.

International Association for Suicide Prevention IASP (Internet). Washington, D.C.: Grad O; Guidelines to assist clinical staff after the suicide of a patient; [cited 2016 October 11]. Available from: https://www.iasp.info/pdf/postvention/guidelines_to_assist_clinical_staff_after_suicide_patient_grad.pdf

Kadan-Lottick NS, Vanderwerker LC, Block SD, Zhang B, Prigerson HG. Psychiatric disorders and mental health service use in patients with advanced cancer. Cancer. 2005;104(12):2872–81.

Kellner CH, Fink M, Knapp R, Petrides G, Husain M, Rummans T, Mueller M, Bernstein H, Rasmussen K, O'Connor K, Smith G. Relief of expressed suicidal intent by ECT: a consortium for research in ECT study. Am J Psychiatr. 2005;162(5):977–82.

Kisely S, Smith M, Lawrence D, Maaten S. Mortality in individuals who have had psychiatric treatment. Population-based study in Nova Scotia. Br J Psychiatry. 2005;187(6):552–8.

Kisely S, Crowe E, Lawrence D. Cancer-related mortality in people with mental illness. JAMA Psychiat. 2013;70(2):209–17.

Kisely S, Forsyth S, Lawrence D. Why do psychiatric patients have higher cancer mortality rates when cancer incidence is the same or lower? Aust N Z J Psychiatry. 2015;50(3):254–63.

Kissane DW, Levin T, Hales S, Lo C, Rodin G. Psychotherapy for depression in cancer and palliative care. In: Kissane DW, Maj M, Sartorius N, editors. Cancer and depression. Wiley: Chichester; 2011.

Kissane DW. Demoralization – a life-preserving diagnosis to make in the severely medically ill. J Palliat Care. 2014;30(4):255–8.

Kissane DW, Bobevski I, Gaitanis P, Brooker J, Michael N, Lethborg C, et al. Exploratory examination of the utility of demoralization as a specifier for adjustment disorder and major depression. Gen Hosp Psychiatry. 2017;46:20–4. https://doi.org/10.1016/j.genhosppsych.2017.01.007

Law MK, Furr RM, Arnold EM, Mneimne M, Jaquett C, Fleeson W. Does assessing suicidality frequently and repeatedly cause harm? A randomized control study. Psychol Assess. 2015;27(4):1171–81.

Lethborg C, Kissane DW, Schofield, P. Meaning and Purpose (MAP) Therapy I: therapeutic processes and paradox in how it helps patients with advanced cancer. Palliat Support Care. 2018 (in press).

Lindeman S, Henriksson M, Isometsä E, Lönnqvist J. Treatment of mental disorders in seven physicians committing suicide. Crisis. 1999;20(2):86–9.

Little JD. Staff response to inpatient and outpatient suicide: what happened and what do we do? Aust N Z J Psychiatry. 1992;26(2):162–7.

Luoma JB, Martin CE, Pearson JL. Contact with mental health and primary care providers before suicide: a review of the evidence. Am J Psychiatr. 2002;159(6):909–16.

Malhi GS, Bassett D, Boyce P, Bryant R, Fitzgerald PB, Fritz K, Hopwood M, Lyndon B, Mulder R, Murray G, Porter R. Royal Australian and New Zealand College of Psychiatrists clinical practice guidelines for mood disorders. Aust N Z J Psychiatry. 2015; 49(12):1087–206.

McGirr A, Renaud J, Seguin M, Alda M, Turecki G. Course of major depressive disorder and suicide outcome: a psychological autopsy study. J Clin Psychiatry. 2008;69(6):966–70.

Middleton JL. Today I'm grieving a physician suicide. Ann Fam Med. 2008;6(3):267–9.

Milner AJ, Maheen H, Bismark MM, Spittal MJ. Suicide by health professionals: a retrospective mortality study in Australia, 2001–2012. Med J Aust. 2016;205(6):260–5.

Miovic M, Block S. Psychiatric disorders in advanced cancer. Cancer. 2007;110(8):1665–76.

Misch DA. When a psychiatry resident's patient commits suicide: transference trials and tribulations. J Am Acad Psychoanal Dyn Psychiatry. 2003;31(3):459–75.

Misono S, Weiss NS, Fann JR, Redman M, Yueh B. Incidence of suicide in persons with cancer. J Clin Oncol. 2008;26(29):4731–8.

Mitchell AJ, Chan M, Bhatti H, Halton M, Grassi L, Johansen C, Meader N. Prevalence of depression, anxiety, and adjustment disorder in oncological, haematological, and palliative-care settings: a meta-analysis of 94 interview-based studies. Lancet Oncol. 2011;12(2):160–74.

Mitchell AJ, Santo Pereira IE, Yadegarfar M, Pepereke S, Mugadza V, Stubbs B. Breast cancer screening in women with mental illness: comparative meta-analysis of mammography uptake. Br J Psychiatry. 2014;205(6):428–35.

Murrough JW, Iosifescu DV, Chang LC, Al Jurdi RK, Green CE, Perez AM, Iqbal S, Pillemer S, Foulkes A, Shah A, Charney DS. Antidepressant efficacy of ketamine in treatment-resistant major depression: a two-site randomized controlled trial. Am J Psychiatr. 2013;170(10):1134–42.

O'Reilly D, Rosato M. Religion and the risk of suicide: longitudinal study of over 1 million people. Br J Psychiatry. 2015;206(6):466–70.

Passik SD, Gibson C, Breitbart W, Rotta ML. Psychiatric issues in cancer pain management. In: Fisch M, Burton AW, editors. Cancer pain management. New York: McGraw-Hill; 2007. p. 140.

Pitman AL, Osborn DP, Rantell K, King MB. Bereavement by suicide as a risk factor for suicide attempt: a cross-sectional national UK-wide study of 3432 young bereaved adults. BMJ Open. 2016;6(1):e009948.

Pokorny AD. Prediction of suicide in psychiatric patients: report of a prospective study. Arch Gen Psychiatry. 1983;40(3):249–57.

Qin P, Agerbo E, Mortensen PB. Suicide risk in relation to family history of completed suicide and psychiatric disorders: a nested case-control study based on longitudinal registers. Lancet. 2002;360(9340):1126–30.

Reinstatler L, Youssef NA. Ketamine as a potential treatment for suicidal ideation: a systematic review of the literature. Drugs R&D. 2015;15(1):37–43.

Results from the 2013 National survey on Drug Use and Health: Mental Health Findings [Internet]. Rockville: Substance Abuse and Mental Health Services Administration; November 2014a. Suicidal thoughts and behaviour; November 2014 [cited 2016 September 21]; p. 29. Available from: http://www.samhsa.gov/data/sites/default/files/NSDUHmhfr2013/NSDUHmhfr2013.pdf

Results from the 2013 National Survey on Drug Use and Health: Mental Health Findings [Internet]. Rockville: Substance Abuse and Mental Health Services Administration; November 2014b. Substance use among adults with mental illness; November 2014 [cited 2016 September 21]; pp. 48–49. Available from: http://www.samhsa.gov/data/sites/default/files/NSDUHmhfr2013/NSDUHmhfr2013.pdf

Robinson S, Kissane, DW, Brooker, J, Burney, S. A systematic review of the demoralization syndrome in individuals with progressive disease and cancer: a decade of research. J Pain and Symptom Manage. 2015;49 (3):595–610. https://doi.org/10.1016/j.jpainsymman

Robinson S, Kissane DW, Brooker J, Burney S. A review of the construct of demoralization: history, definitions, and future directions for palliative care. Am J Hosp Palliat Med. 2016;33(1):93–101. https://doi.org/10.1177/1049909114553461

Robinson S, Kissane DW, Brooker J, Hempton C, Burney S. The relationship between poor quality of life and desire to hasten death: a multiple mediation model examining the contributions of depression, demoralization, loss of control, and low self-worth. J Pain Symptom Manage. 2017;53(2). https://doi.org/10.1016/j.jpainsymman.2016.08.013

Schernhammer ES, Colditz GA. Suicide rates among physicians: a quantitative and gender assessment (meta-analysis). Am J Psychiatr. 2004;161(12):2295–302.

Selzer R, Ellen S. Formulation for beginners. Australas Psychiatry. 2014;22(4):397–401.

Simon RI. Suicide risk assessment forms: form over substance? J Am Acad Psychiatry Law. 2009;37(3):290–3.
Spoletini I, Gianni W, Caltagirone C, Madaio R, Repetto L, Spalletta G. Suicide and cancer: where do we go from here? Crit Rev Oncol Hematol. 2011;78(3):206–19.
Statham DJ, Heath AC, Madden PA, Bucholz KK, Bierut L, Dinwiddie SH, Slutske WS, Dunne MP, Martin NG. Suicidal behaviour: an epidemiological and genetic study. Psychol Med. 1998;28(04):839–55.
Suominen K, Isometsä E, Suokas J, Haukka J, Achte K, Lönnqvist J. Completed suicide after a suicide attempt: a 37-year follow-up study. Am J Psychiatr. 2004;161(3):562–3.
Sveen CA, Walby FA. Suicide survivors' mental health and grief reactions: a systematic review of controlled studies. Suicide Life Threat Behav. 2008;38(1):13–29.
Tabarés-Seisdedos R, Dumont N, Baudot A, Valderas JM, Climent J, Valencia A, Crespo-Facorro B, Vieta E, Gómez-Beneyto M, Martínez S, Rubenstein JL. No paradox, no progress: inverse cancer comorbidity in people with other complex diseases. Lancet Oncol. 2011;12(6):604–8.
Tillman J. The suicide of patients and the quiet voice of the therapist. J Am Acad Psychoanal Dyn Psychiatry. 2003;31(3):425–7.
Trevino KM, Abbott CH, Fisch MJ, Friedlander RJ, Duberstein PR, Prigerson HG. Patient-oncologist alliance as protection against suicidal ideation in young adults with advanced cancer. Cancer. 2014;120(15):2272–81.
Turecki G, Brent DA. Suicide and suicidal behaviour. Lancet. 2016;387(10024):1227–39. Panel 1, page 1233
Vehling S, Kissane DW, Lo C, Glaesmer H, Hartung TJ, Rodin G, Mehnert A. The association of demoralization with mental disorders and suicidal ideation in patients with cancer. Cancer. 2017;123(17):3394–401. https://doi.org/10.1002/cncr.30749
Violence Prevention (Internet). Atlanta: Centers for Disease Control and Prevention; 2016. Suicide: risk and protective factors; 2016 (date cited 2016 February 24). Available from http://www.cdc.gov/violence prevention/suicide/riskprotectivefactors.html
Vyssoki B, Gleiss A, Rockett IR, Hackl M, Leitner B, Sonneck G, Kapusta ND. Suicide among 915,303 Austrian cancer patients: who is at risk? J Affect Disord. 2015;175:287–91.
World Health Organisation. Global Health Observatory data [Internet]. Geneva: World Health Organization; 2012. [cited 2016 November 13]. Available from: http://www.who.int/gho/mental_health/suicide_rates/en/
Zwil AS, Pelchat RJ. ECT in the treatment of patients with neurological and somatic disease. Int J Psychiatry Med. 1994;24(1):1–29.

Transfer to a Preferred Place of Death 82

Leeroy William

Contents

Abstract

The preferred place of death is an important consideration in end-of-life care, especially when the dying person is definite about their choice. The preferred place of care may well be the same location, but this is not always the case. When the two venues are different, and the patient's prognosis is poor, a decision has to be made whether to move the patient or not. The expectation to not only transfer the dying person in a timely fashion but also to minimize the time in the current setting often makes the situation a palliative care emergency. However, should the move occur at all? The risk of dying in transit may be high. Furthermore, respecting the wishes of the dying person needs to be balanced with the practicalities of

L. William (✉)
Palliative Medicine, Monash Health, Eastern Health, Monash University, Melbourne, VIC, Australia
e-mail: leeroy.william@monash.edu

R. D. MacLeod, L. Van den Block (eds.), *Textbook of Palliative Care*,
https://doi.org/10.1007/978-3-319-77740-5_85

safe ongoing care. These are practical and ethical decisions that should be made as early as possible.

How do we facilitate the smooth transfer from one location to another? Coordination and communication are vital in planning the process and supporting the discharge. The provision of the right medications and equipment, relevant information, and strategies for managing future problems should increase the chance of a successful transfer. Sometimes a smooth transfer will not be possible, but patients and family members will usually be happy with a successful one.

1 Introduction

The request to die in an alternative setting to the current venue of care is often stressful, until transfer to the preferred place of death has been achieved. It is not a singular decision but rather a process of considering and reviewing the relevant factors at various points in time. It is important to remember that views may change over time, e.g., due to clinical deterioration or psychosocial issues. Therefore, a careful review of any request is critical.

In order to fulfill the wish of the dying person, the process of transfer is usually deemed an emergency by palliative care teams. The aim of this chapter is to provide a systematic and practical approach for such transfers, considering the needs of all those involved. A multidisciplinary team approach will be beneficial, especially if the prognosis is limited. Last minute requests are complicated by the lack of time but are not uncommon. It may be impossible to fulfill the request of the patient/family in a limited timeframe and provides another reason for earlier referral to palliative care teams for appropriate assistance.

2 The Preferred Place of Death

Most people report that they want to die at home, and 80% do not change their mind as death approaches, although the preference to die at home varies between patients (31–87%), caregivers (25–64%), and members of the public (49–70%) (Gomes et al. 2013). Other research suggests that the views of patients and their carers do change over time, and we need to carefully distinguish between the preferred place of death and the preferred place of care (the venue in which people would like to receive most of their care) (Agar et al. 2008). In planning for end-of-life care (EOLC), healthcare professionals should be encouraged to ask and identify these venues of care; failure to do so is more likely to lead to a hospital admission (Ali et al. 2015).

Despite the desire to die at home, most people actually die in hospitals in the western world. Internationally, comparing 14 countries across 4 continents, we have found that 12–57% of cancer patients die at home and 26–87% die in hospital. The authors attribute these differences to the healthcare resources of the countries and their specific EOLC strategies for cancer patients (Cohen et al. 2015). Many healthcare services have been organized to meet the perceived demand for home deaths, especially in cancer patients, but these figures demonstrate limited success. In people with nonmalignant disease, it is likely that their preferred and actual place of death will differ, due to poor recognition of the terminal phase of disease, not establishing a preference in venue of death, and an inadequate provision of available supportive and palliative care (Billingham and Billingham 2013). Cohen et al. compared people with lung cancer and people with chronic obstructive pulmonary disease (COPD), across 14 countries, and highlighted that those with COPD were overall more likely to die in hospital or in a nursing home (Cohen et al. 2017). Similarly, people with end-stage renal disease are more likely to die in hospital, unless they are not receiving dialysis (Lovell et al. 2017).

Dying at home can be more peaceful for patients and provide less traumatic grieving for families, when compared with hospital deaths, providing the following have occurred: a discussion of the patient's preferences, the involvement of a general practitioner (GP) who can provide home visits, and the ability for the family to be given time off work to support care at home

(Gomes et al. 2015). These findings provide some insight into the challenges of dying well at home.

Furthermore, societies have changed over the years, e.g., families are more dispersed around the globe than previously. Patients may not have family nearby to care for them, but even if they do, they may not want to be a burden to them. Similarly, some immigrant communities may not have the cultural and supportive networks to remain at home. Societies have also entrusted their health in a predominantly biomedical model and believe in the "rescue culture" of medicine (Poppito 2013). These changes influence the choices about the venue of care and venue of death between the primary decision-makers, i.e., patients, carers, and healthcare professionals. The decisions may favor home, aged care facilities, hospital, or hospice settings at different times; however the impact of family wishes, cultural, and religious beliefs should not be underestimated (Lin et al. 2017; Gott et al. 2013).

From a population perspective, two studies delineate a change in where people are dying. There has been a drop in the number of people dying in hospitals in England and Wales (2004–2014) and in Norway (1987–2011). However, both studies report (during their respective periods) and predict a rise of deaths in aged care facilities (Bone et al. 2017; Kalseth and Theisen 2017). Given the aging population in modern societies, not only will the number of facilities require review, but there will also be a challenge to the provision of optimal EOLC in this sector.

As healthcare professionals, we should plan ongoing care with the preferred place of care in mind. The preferred place of death will be more difficult to determine, due to the changing views and circumstances of dying people and their families over time (Agar et al. 2008). As a result, sometimes transfers will occur more rapidly than expected. There are excellent patient transfer guides online that may be useful to review, e.g., the "National Rapid Discharge Guidance for Patients Who Wish to Die at Home" (Ireland) and the "Accelerated Discharge to Die at Home" (New South Wales, Australia). In healthcare settings, the transfer destination should provide more appropriate care for the needs of the patient. Implied in the statement is also a view that the setting from which the transfer occurs cannot provide the necessary care to the individual. A further expectation is that the person is likely to improve at the destination venue. In an end-of-life context, we need to reconsider these statements, but there is often an ethical dilemma that exists for all parties concerned.

3 Dealing with the Request to Be Transferred

Palliative care teams frequently receive requests for transfers to another setting. These patients may or may not be dying, but when the reason is to die in a desired destination, the sense of urgency increases. The first response is usually to find out more about the referral, and a phone call may be the first means of triage.

The triage process aims to determine the urgency of the referral. A written referral may not include all the relevant information, and so discussing the case with either the referrer or caregiver will help. The tone of the discussion may be enough to decide that the case is an emergency, but we need to know about the patient, their family, and any other reasons relevant to their decision. Perhaps the most common scenario involves a patient wanting to return home to die from the acute hospital ward. In this case, the referral will have been made by a junior medical officer who may, or may not, know the case well. Calling the nurse in charge of the ward may be helpful, as they may have more knowledge of the multidisciplinary team approach to the care thus far.

A similar case may involve a dying person at home, where the family prefer the death to occur in an institution, e.g., they may not want to live with the memory of the death at home, or they may not be coping with caring at home. The person may be conscious, semicomatose, or unconscious. Furthermore, the decision may be in keeping with their wishes or contrary to them. The referral may have come from the GP, or the community palliative care (CPC) team, but once again speaking to the person with the best overall knowledge of the case will be most helpful.

So, when do these scenarios become a palliative care emergency? There are three main reasons to urgently review the case, assuming the transfer is desired:

- Firstly, if the person has a poor prognosis, e.g., days, then a greater need for action will be required. A delay could lead to death in the current venue of care, which does not meet the patient wishes and may anger the family.
- Secondly, the presence of significant distress in the current setting, from any of the relevant parties, would also increase the acuity for intervention.
- Finally, assuming the dying person wishes to be moved and/or the family are agreeable, then the referring healthcare professionals may be strongly advocating for urgent action.

Ultimately, there is a balance between meeting expectations, minimizing the time in the current venue of care, and maximizing the time in the desired venue of care. In terms of the patient and family, we therefore have a duty of care to ensure the discharge would be feasible, safe, supported, and beneficial. Modern healthcare systems can challenge the decisions we make in these scenarios, e.g., moving someone because of acute hospital bed pressures or requiring the patient to meet the specialist palliative care requirements for a hospice bed (Bergenholtz et al. 2016; Love and Liversage 2014). Overall, palliative care teams aim to respect the wishes of people who are dying as much as possible and support their families through whatever decision is made.

4 Patient Review and Family Discussions

The transition to palliative care should be a process over time, integral to the clinical handover of the patient's care. However, referrals to palliative care teams are often later than desired, despite evidence of less aggressive EOLC, improved quality of life, and reduced healthcare costs (Scibetta et al. 2016; Smith et al. 2014). The referral marks a move from living with a disease to dying from it. We need to recognize that a palliative care referral often marks a significant psychological step toward death. Patients and families may be at different stages of dealing with the illness, irrespective of the actual clinical status. It is important to establish who is the main spokesperson for the family as early as possible, in order to save time and repetition of information. How these conversations are managed, at such an emotional time, may have lasting repercussions in bereavement (Stajduhar et al. 2017). Late palliative care referrals mark an altered course in the condition and care of the patient, which requires a more rapid adjustment from previous beliefs. Hence, allowing time for people to express their concerns and wishes regarding future care is necessary (Romo et al. 2016; Smith et al. 2016).

The coping mechanisms of the family and staff at the site of care should be considered when deciding upon possible transfers. As discussed above, it is important to understand the situation we will encounter when we review the patient in person. The priority of care should be focused on the patient, and therefore any distressing symptoms should be managed urgently. Advice may have been given over the phone, so a review of the efficacy of the suggested interventions is possible when the patient is assessed in person. The family are more likely to concentrate on their conversation with the clinician, if they see attentive and effective care being given to their loved one first.

Once the patient is settled, we need to consider what information the family has been given and their current understanding of the situation. Determining the goals of care, e.g., curative/restorative, palliative, or terminal (Thomas et al. 2014), for the patient provides an excellent starting point to plan an ongoing management, as medically the parameters of care should be defined. In consultation with the patient and/or their family, the next step would be to ascertain the preferred place of death and an idea of their advance care plans. Finally, these elements should be considered in discussion with the family and the treating team, to achieve a shared decision about the planned management.

The necessary conversations may have occurred previously, but a quick review of the relevant views establishes current priorities.

The condition of the patient informs the feasibility of any transfer. Hence, clinical examination and obtaining a history of deterioration are important to estimate prognosis. In some cases, the person may not be dying, and the consultation provides an opportunity to listen to their wishes. There may be an underlying reversible cause for their deterioration, e.g., infection, opioid toxicity, or hypercalcemia, that requires discussion about potential treatment. In such cases, even though treatment is possible, a decision should be made regarding the appropriateness of prolonging life, according to the individual circumstances.

Prognostication is one of the three important skills in clinical medicine; we have honed our skills in the first two, diagnosis and treatment, but neglected prognostication by comparison (Glare et al. 2008). There may be prognostic tools to help, but in our given situation, reviewing the patient with a corroborative history is key. The family and treating team should provide a trajectory of the deterioration to make a quick assessment of prognosis. Remember that the family knows the patient better than anyone and is a valuable source of information about who the patient is and their life narrative. If there are no reversible causes and the deterioration has occurred day by day, it would be reasonable to assume a prognosis of days. However, if the deterioration has occurred in hours, then a shorter prognosis of hours is likely. Any decisions made in regard to an imminent death should be supported by clinical evidence, e.g., comatose, Cheyne-Stokes breathing, and thready erratic pulse. Hui et al. determined some useful bedside clinical signs in cancer patients, to predict impending death within 3 days, i.e., nonreactive pupils, reduced response to verbal and visual stimuli, inability to close the eyelids, drooping of nasolabial fold, hyperextension of the neck, grunting of the vocal cords, and upper gastrointestinal bleeding (Hui et al. 2015).

Should the prognosis permit a possible transfer home, we need to evaluate the stability of the patient for transfer. A useful way to approach the decision is to review the last routine clinical observations, i.e., temperature, pulse, blood pressure, and respiratory rate. If these measures, or any other clinical concerns under normal circumstances, would prompt a medical emergency team (MET) review, then clinical instability for transfer exists. Review if they have symptoms that need to be managed to facilitate a smooth transfer, e.g., pain, dyspnea, or agitation. Without addressing these symptoms, the patient suffers in transit, and their care may be viewed as suboptimal. The transfer reflects the care we provide to the patient and family; therefore how stable the patient is in transit and on arrival at the destination is a testament of that care. Hence, the decision to transfer a person who is imminently dying is a difficult balance between respecting the views of others and maintaining our professional and personal standards of care.

5 No Transfer Due to Imminent Death

Transfers are unlikely when the prognosis is estimated in hours. In the context of respecting the wishes of a patient and/or their family, delivering such a short prognosis may lead to a volatile situation. There may also be anger about the inability to fulfill the dying wishes of the patient. The clinician should be prepared to encounter and manage any reaction from the family, including potentially violent or abusive behavior. Although we may understand the grief and anger in certain situations, personal safety measures should be implemented as a priority if deemed necessary. Preempting how families may react, after assessment of the situation, may change the approach to the consultation.

The prognosis may be a relief to the family, or at least some of them, but an explanation of the reasoning behind the timeframe and the reluctance to transfer must be clear. Going through some symptoms and signs of dying may be helpful, if appropriate, supported by leaving the family a pamphlet with this information that can be reviewed as needed. Be prepared, and offer, to repeat any information to the family. Where possible, consultations accompanied by another healthcare professional (e.g., nurse, social worker, pastoral care worker) can help with safety issues, as well as respond to the emotions of family members.

The potential of deterioration in transit should be emphasized and can act as a sobering reminder of the inherent risks of the transfer. Instances do occur where families refuse the advice to remain in the current venue of care. In a community setting, an ambulance may have been called, and the decision rests with the ambulance crew. Without prior warning, the scenario is difficult for ambulance staff that will invariably try and adopt the best approach for the patient and the family. In ward settings, the family may carry the person to their vehicle and request the help of staff to aid them. As traumatic as these events are for staff, keeping the focus on the family can sometimes diffuse the situation. Should a hospital discharge occur against medical advice, then liaison with the GP, community services, the CPC team, and other family members may provide the required support in the community.

We do have a primary duty of care to the patient, and so emphasizing that ongoing care will be provided to support family can be helpful. It may be useful to point out how comfortable the patient is at present and that moving them is likely to disrupt their stability. If possible, allay any feelings of guilt or failure in the family, and positively reinforce the efforts they have already made. Emphasize that the patient will be less aware of their actual location but may be more responsive to family around the bedside. It is a time for the family to come together and be present for the patient, as well as each other. It is perhaps more a time for them to be family, rather than adopting the additional roles of nurses, doctors, and pharmacists. Reassure them that it will be our responsibility as healthcare professionals to ensure the patient's comfort and to support their grief. Enquire how we may best support them spiritually or culturally, and do not make any assumptions. Be present, be human, and be kind – many situations will be diffused with this approach.

There are some instances when the clinical needs of the patient would automatically preclude the possibility of transfer. Examples include patients who would die soon after extubation, patients requiring high-flow oxygenation, and patients who require ionotropic support to remain clinically stable. Often these patients would be on intensive care units, and weaning or ceasing life-supporting measures occurs after a consensus decision. A period of 24h usually provides some evidence of stability for transfer if still desired. Practically, the options for venue of care/death would be, in order of clinical preference, a ward in the hospital, the palliative care unit (PCU), or home. However, there are cases where patients have been extubated at home (Unger 2016; Mann et al. 2004). The extent to which services are prepared to help home deaths can often be admirable, especially in pediatric cases (Needle 2010). However, many more cases miss the opportunity to facilitate a home death due to late discussions, referrals, and coordination of care.

6 Transfer Options

Once the decision to transfer a patient has been agreed upon, the organization of the transfer can begin. The palliative care team is often required to coordinate efforts to ensure the smooth transition from one care setting to another. A checklist can ensure that nothing is forgotten but also streamline the process and reduce the time for transfer, especially when busy. These checklists can be sent to community teams, to ensure all tasks have been completed and education continues. The Liverpool Care Pathway for the Rapid Discharge Home of the Dying Patient provided effective guidance in EOLC (Murphy et al. 2004; Ahearn et al. 2013) and has been incorporated in other EOLC guidelines, e.g., Te Ara Whakapiri: Principles and guidance for the last days of life (the New Zealand EOLC guide).

Ambulance crews can be very helpful and flexible with transfers to the preferred place of death. Importantly, a "do not resuscitate order" is vital for the transfer. They will usually need to know about access to the house, if the venue is home, in case they need an extra person to assist in the transfer. If any charges are incurred for ambulance trips, then families should be notified of the cost. It is also important to notify the ambulance crew and the family of what should happen if death occurs in transit. The standard advice is that they should continue to the final destination, alerting those who may be awaiting their arrival. Here the family can be supported and the necessary arrangements made to manage the deceased.

Once a discharge to the community has occurred, some palliative care services have a rapid response team, allowing the enhancement of care alongside existing services. They may provide a short period of care until the CPC team can takeover or provide support for EOLC at home or in aged care facilities (Gage and Holdsworth 2015). It may also be possible to optimize EOLC in aged care facilities post-discharge using hospital subacute services that visit them. A collaborative and educational approach between palliative care, elderly care, and aged care staff can ensure patient wishes are respected.

In the following sections, we consider each possible transfer and the role of the palliative care team in facilitating the urgent relocation.

7 Transfer from Ward Facility to Designated Home Setting

A meta-synthesis of qualitative studies over 25 years (1990–2015) provides seven themes that patients viewed as important for EOLC in acute hospitals. These are expert care, effective communication and shared decision-making, respectful and compassionate care, adequate environment for care, family involvement, financial affairs, and maintaining a sense of self. Apart from the last theme, family members shared the previous six perspectives. However, the same study also found four themes specific to the views of family members. They believed that maintaining patient safety, preparation for death, bereavement care, and enabling patient choice at the end of life were important to EOLC in acute hospitals (Virdun et al. 2016). These findings perhaps give an idea of what needs to be achieved in acute hospitals to optimize EOLC. They also provide an insight into why patients and families may want to leave hospitals at the end of life.

If a transfer is deemed appropriate from a ward setting, then a hospital palliative care team (HPCT) can assist in the discharge. As stated earlier, the timing of the referral can affect the urgency and the ability of the HPCT to meet expectations. The lead clinical team on the ward should be guided in the tasks needed to transfer care to the community. Liaising with the CPC team or the district nursing team, as well as the GP, will be critical in ongoing care at home. Discharging someone home without the support in the community to continue care only increases the chances of readmission and burdens the family with unwanted stress. Early notification to the relevant community nursing services will allow the service to better prepare for the transfer home. It is often reassuring for families to know when these services will be visiting. A GP who can visit, as mentioned earlier, is integral to the network of healthcare professionals who will contribute to the EOLC at home and fulfill the lead medical role in the community.

The lead team on the ward may have notified members of the allied health team appropriately, but the HPCT should ensure that the right individuals remain involved in EOLC. These may include:

- Case managers (with essential knowledge of the patient, family, and clinicians involved in the patient's care in particular conditions, e.g., motor neurone disease patients)
- Pharmacists (both hospital and community pharmacists – to ensure appropriate medications are in place)
- Occupational therapists (to maintain daily activities as much as possible for both patients and carers, e.g., via equipment/aids to facilitate ongoing care).
- Physiotherapists (for mobility reviews if needed, soft tissue and therapeutic massage, and advice on passive movements and positioning)

- CPC teams (especially the nurse that will visit the home post-discharge)
- Music therapists (to provide support and symptom relief)
- Home-based care programs (either to cease or increase their involvement)
- Social workers (for patient and family advocacy, counseling, loss and grief support, family support, and social services support)

The involvement of these allied health professionals contributes to the holistic goals we aim to achieve in palliative and EOLC. Furthermore, there may be some continuity of care provided by these members of the healthcare team who have supported a patient and family over a number of previous hospital admissions. Their support and knowledge of the patient and family, and how they have coped with the episodic deteriorations, can provide valuable insights into EOLC.

The physical needs of the patient may require several pieces of equipment for home care. For example, a hospital bed and air mattress will aid EOLC for patients and their families; an oxygen concentrator will be required for hypoxic patients, where dyspnea is distressing. During the coordination of the transfer home, the delivery of equipment will require a family member to take responsibility to permit entry into the house and inform of access and location for the equipment. Occasionally, families may be so keen to get home that they may not wait for equipment, e.g., hospital bed, and prefer to let the person sleep in their own bed. It may be a small detail, but hospital beds are not invariably double beds that may allow the intimacy of a couple sharing their last few nights together. A pragmatic approach should be adopted, where advice should be documented, but we work to facilitate the transfer home as the main objective. Waiting for the safest transfer, at such a critical time, may jeopardize the goal – most families will wait for deliveries or pick equipment up once the patient gets home.

The family should be aware of the care that will be required at home. Although nursing a bedbound patient is often deemed easier in practical terms, performing personal care for their loved one may still cause distress. An early family meeting, involving a social worker, can clarify and inform the family of the undertaking ahead and determine if a transfer will occur. It can be helpful to highlight the shifts of professional carers involved on the ward each day, so that family and friends can be prepared for what is required once at home. The discussion should not aim to dissuade the family but to provide an informed decision about the transfer.

While on the ward, families should be given the opportunity to learn and participate in the nursing care. Pressure injury prevention, with associated safe positioning of the patient, e.g., tilt and turns, should be taught by the nursing staff, and the family should be observed in their practical involvement. Mouth cares, hygiene cares, and feeding will all be areas for education. For some families, these tasks may deter them from going ahead with the transfer. By contrast, larger families may accept and share the tasks to facilitate their planned move. Equipment for hygiene care will need to be provided, and urinary retention should be excluded. The consideration of an indwelling urethral catheter may prevent distress, readmission, and inappropriate medication usage.

There may be times when the coping mechanisms of the family, or their social supports, are not sufficient to provide optimal care from our professional caregiver perspective. At these times, the multidisciplinary team involved need to make a decision about pursuing the transfer, especially if the patient is deteriorating. Families may be adamant that they will cope, either out of a sense of duty or determination to respect the wishes of the patient. In these circumstances, challenging their decision may not be helpful. It may be better to document that there are professional concerns, which the family has been advised of, but they remain steadfast in their views. Planning for the failure of the discharge may also help the family, e.g., to know that they can return to the ward or have a direct admission to the PCU, should the care become too problematic at home is reassuring. Community teams and other services, e.g., PCUs, should be advised of all important discussions, in order to support the discharge as much as possible and coordinate care as needed in a crisis.

Syringe driver orders, breakthrough medications, and emergency medications are all likely to be required via the lead medical team. Often, junior doctors will be unsure of the right medications and lack confidence in prescribing the right doses. In such instances, the HPCT can educate and support junior doctors, either via their usual practice or in conjunction with EOLC guidelines. It is also important to instill and demonstrate an ethos of holistic care, and the provision of EOLC provides an opportunity to highlight the necessity for an individualized approach. Discussions about artificial hydration and nutrition will need to be completed, also explaining the rationalization of medications due to reduced oral intake. Some deaths will need to be reported to the coroner. It is the lead medical team's responsibility to ensure that this information is conveyed to the family, as well as the process involved. However, the HPCT should check the completion of this task and also ensure the GP and community teams are advised.

Pastoral care and cultural liaison workers, if available, should address spiritual and cultural needs, respectively. There may be instances when these considerations are critical to the transfer. For example, there may be a desire for a blessing or cultural ritual prior to the transfer to ensure a safe passage or accommodate for a death in transit. Bereavement support should also be highlighted as a future service, so that families know who will be contacting them and when. Hence, as in all care, the holistic approach can be a powerful factor in demonstrating a respectful approach to the patient and the family if the right conversations are undertaken.

Patients returning to aged care facilities may require a higher level of care than they had previously. In some countries, there may be a requirement to reassess the current level of care required before the patient can return to the facility. Here, allied health assessments are essential if the diagnosis of dying is not so clear. Even under these circumstances, many facilities will need support from GPs and CPC services. Usually staff from these facilities are eager to continue the care of their patient and keen to learn about palliative care skills to help them. As with families caring for a loved one at home, the symptoms and signs of dying may need to be reiterated, with instructions to call the GP or CPC team if needed.

8 Transfer from Hospital Ward to Palliative Care Unit

The transfer to a PCU is often managed by a HPCT. However, in the absence of such a team, admissions are arranged directly with the PCU using admission criteria. PCUs vary between those that accommodate more acute cases and those that operate solely for the imminently dying. In the USA, the latter PCU is termed a "hospice." Although PCUs differ in practice across the world, the common grounds for admission may restrict some patient transfers. For example, a family may want to continue intravenous fluids and antibiotics due to preferences for their loved one, but some hospices may not facilitate such treatment. Admission to the PCU may be dependent upon the cessation of the intravenous management and appropriate conversations with the family, hence delaying the transfer.

There are many issues to consider in these transfers. The lead clinical team on the ward will value a transfer based on their assessment of the patient, their confidence in caring for a dying patient, the family expectations, the acute bed status of the ward, and the empty beds available in the PCU. These are all valid considerations, but often the acute hospital is unaware of the demands on the PCU from community patients, as well as other hospital campuses.

PCUs should provide specialist palliative care services to those patients admitted to its care. Hence, the question often raised by the PCU staff is whether the admission from the acute hospital requires specialist palliative care management. EOLC guidelines, such as the Liverpool Care Pathway (LCP), were developed to help manage the nonspecialist palliative care deaths occurring in acute hospitals or in the community. However, misuse and media interpretation of the implementation of these guidelines has undermined the intention to improve the standard of EOLC outside PCUs. In services where a HPCT exists, many patients can be supported in the acute hospital setting via the collaboration with acute teams. For many clinicians, the ability to continue caring for patients and families familiar to them is both personally and professionally rewarding.

Organizational imperatives, such as patient flow, are more prominent when the PCU is part of the acute hospital system. Within such organizations, the movement of patients to the most appropriate ward is a priority, and PCUs are often considered the best site for EOLC. Tensions can arise when seemingly all deaths are referred to the PCU, irrespective of their need for specialist palliative care. Determining the urgency for transfer on the basis of patient or family need should be the PCUs objective, but it can often be challenging. The organizational need for an acute bed may be the main factor behind a referral and can be difficult to defer when PCU beds are empty. Once again, a HPCT can clarify the need for transfer and ensure supportive care until the move can occur. When PCUs are not governed by the acute hospital organization, referrals can be reviewed without the same pressures and therefore ensure the appropriate patient cohort for the PCU.

Another important factor in transfers from acute hospitals to PCUs is the distance between the two facilities. The movement of a patient in the terminal phase of their illness is affected by the transit mode and duration of the transfer. The HPCT will need to decide if the person is likely to survive the trip, whether by ambulance, helicopter, or airplane. The same issues apply with regard to the comfort of the patient during transit, as discussed earlier. The balance between the stabilization of symptoms and the goal of preferred place of death often means a compromise. Pre-transfer medications are usually given to ensure comfort, but the longer the trip the riskier the transfer becomes in terms of comfort or death in transit. Hence longer trips may not be sanctioned by HPCTs.

A family meeting, led by the social worker, is the best initial process to ensure all parties understand what is happening. A member of the HPCT should attend the meeting not only to hear the discussions and meet the family but also to demonstrate a clinical handover of care. The HPCT can clarify the workings of the PCU and arrange the transfer at the most appropriate time. Some family members may not accept that death is imminent for their loved one. Acute care interventions, delayed decisions, and the fear of the PCU may all delay the transfer. Many family meetings may be required to gain a consensus plan, but transfer without such agreement will only cause more problems on the PCU.

9 Transfer from Designated Home Setting to Ward Facility

If most people want to die at home, then community services are tasked with the challenge to keep people at home, under difficult circumstances. A recent review of the essential components of quality community palliative care reports six vital requirements: integrated teamwork; management of pain and physical symptoms; holistic care; caring, compassionate, and skilled providers; timely and responsive care; and patient and family preparedness (Seow and Bainbridge 2018). These are the elements that all healthcare organizations strive toward, but the aging population remains a challenge that will increase demands and place community healthcare under immense strain.

There are two major settings to consider as a designated home for people. The first is the usual private residence, recognized as home, and the second is an aged care facility. Each has their problems in the transfer of patients into a ward, whether acute or subacute in nature. Subsequently, we shall consider them separately in the following discussion.

9.1 Transfers from Home

People dying at home may, or may not, be known to a CPC service. GPs and district nurses can usually provide support to carers at home and obtain advice from CPC services as needed. Dying at home remains difficult in the cities of the western world, as discussed earlier. In many cases the social networks are less prominent than in former years, prompting a movement for "compassionate communities" and EOLC as a focus for public health reform (Kellehear 2013; Sallnow et al. 2017). The concept is growing from a public health perspective, to better support carers in the community and recreate links within our societies based upon compassion. Many rural and traditional communities have operated in a similar fashion for years, due to the close-knit relationships and traditions over many generations (Sallnow et al. 2010).

CPC services vary around the world in terms of personnel, provision of care, and funding. The aim may have been to facilitate dying at home, but more modern services are aware of the changing needs of the population. People may want to be admitted to a hospital or PCU for a number of reasons, and CPC teams should recognize the choices made regarding the venue of death. Early recognition of deterioration can trigger discussions about transfer from the home environment. Usually, CPC teams liaise with PCUs for an admission as early as possible. However, a PCU bed may not be available when required and hence an urgent admission via the hospital system is necessary. The emergency department (ED) should preferably be avoided, but families usually value being rescued from a crisis situation at home even if an admission must occur via the ED. There is still merit in these admissions, e.g., there may be continuity of care with the lead treating team, reversible causes of deterioration can be reversed, and patients who refuse a PCU admission can be reviewed and followed-up by the HPCT if they get admitted.

Once again, the assessment of the dying patient is critical. Home visits often encounter families who have been struggling for days to maintain the level of care required. These later reviews may find an imminently dying patient, who is too unwell to transfer. However, community teams facing such a scenario need to act calmly and quickly to deal with the situation. Families who are keen for a transfer to occur may pressurize the visiting clinician for an admission; similarly the clinician may also feel the least risky decision is to admit. Both the needs of the patient and the family can underpin these decisions, but invariably a PCU bed will be sought if possible. It should be noted that community palliative care staff might walk into unexpected scenarios of despair and distress. The consultation may be the first with the family about the seriousness of the situation, and establishing a quick rapport can be difficult. Subsequently, the clinician receiving the call from the CPC nurse should recognize the predicament the patient, family, and CPC nurse is facing.

There are times when some admissions to a PCU do not match the specialist palliative care criteria for entry. These referrals may emanate from the community, where the home option is no longer viable due to the level of care and support that are required. Recognizing this fact, PCUs prioritize community referrals above hospital referrals, where the clinical teams are available and can be supported in delivering palliative care. Clinicians triaging these referrals often understand the community situation and accept the referral, even though it may be deemed "inappropriate" for a specialist unit. The quicker the decision is made, the sooner the referring clinician can inform the family and organize transfer.

9.2 Transfers from Aged Care Facilities

Aged care facilities are the homes for many frail people in our population. In many countries they may be divided into high-level (nursing homes) and low-level (residential homes) care facilities. People with higher nursing care needs are more likely to require palliative care services; however not all facilities are served by CPC teams. CPC support may be provided for the staff at aged care facilities but may not be as "hands-on" as desired. Staff would certainly benefit from, and appreciate, the clinical experiential learning from CPC teams.

Medical support is also required. GPs may be associated with the patients by virtue of the facility or via an ongoing relationship that began before admission to the facility. Patients who want to die in the facility should be known to the GP and linked in with the CPC team. Out-of-hours care may involve locum medical staff, where acute decisions may not be underpinned by patient or family wishes. Here again the importance of advance care planning is highlighted for those out-of-hours visits. Locums will refer people to hospital, if they are unsure of the clinical plan for the patient or the wishes of the patient/family under certain circumstances.

Ideally, patients admitted to aged care facilities should be asked about their wishes at the time of their admission to the facility. Conversations at this time, involving substitute decision-makers, will inform future care planning. Although these conversations may seem straightforward, how they are performed and updated require careful consideration. Firstly, the circumstances of the admission to the facility should highlight the more vulnerable and frail nature of the patient. A review of their deterioration can give an idea of their disease trajectory, but their comorbidities also factor into the prognosis. The GP has a major role in these conversations, to guide and coordinate the views of patients, families, and specialists in an advance care plan. How these conversations occur will determine the effectiveness of the plan created. Medically the goals of care need to be clear, and the patient's wishes need to be woven into the management plan. Conversations about death and dying may need to occur, at a time when functional change is traumatic for both the patient and members of their family. However, these conversations cannot be delayed.

Once an advance care plan is achieved, there should be accompanying medication changes to deal with the immediate care and future care. De-prescribing allows a streamlining of medications, but planning for emergencies may prevent an unnecessary admission. An awareness of potential modes of deterioration should be in the forefront of the clinician's mind when reviewing the patient. Are they likely to have a catastrophic event, e.g., massive gastrointestinal hemorrhage, or massive hemoptysis? Is a clinical deterioration in condition likely sooner or later? If so, these are further conversations that should occur with the family and staff of the facility.

A completed advance care plan will need to be reviewed and appropriately updated. When should this occur to remain up to date? Certainly, after an acute admission to hospital, there should be a review of the plan. However, it may be prudent for the staff of the facility, the family, and the GP to meet periodically to review the patient's progress and to plan for any deterioration. There may be a presumption that the patient and/or the family will prefer conservative management in the aged care facility. Once again, assumptions should not be made, and possible transfer options should be discussed. If the patient and family wishes are clear that a hospital admission should be made, then staff can respond appropriately if deterioration occurs.

Another option may be the admission to a PCU. Often, these admissions are firstly discussed with the CPC teams. Support may be provided to the facility staff and GP, but two triggers may change this approach. Firstly, the patient may display specialist palliative care needs, e.g., uncontrolled pain, dyspnea, or terminal delirium. Secondly, the family or staff may decide that care needs are not being adequately met in the facility. In the latter cases, an admission to either an acute hospital or a palliative care unit may rescue the situation sufficiently to minimize suffering and potential bereavement complications. Once again, the timeframe to plan the transfer to another venue of care can be limited.

Generally, the ambulance transfer can occur rapidly once the decision has been made. The hope is that the decision is a well-informed one and reflects the wishes, values, and expectations of the dying person concerned.

10 Transfers from a Palliative Care Unit to the Acute Hospital

Admissions to a PCU usually have a specific goal of care in mind. End-of-life care is often the main goal of care, but in the modern hospice setting, other goals may exist. For example, the admission could be for symptom management and then discharge home. For some patients, a period of assessment may be required. In such cases, the patient may eventually go home, require placement in an aged care facility, or enter the terminal phase of their disease. Time often allows the inpatient palliative care team the ability to review the prognosis and plan care accordingly.

However, in modern PCUs there may be a need to transfer the patient back to the acute hospital. A family meeting, led by a social worker, is often the best forum to discuss the transfer and prepare appropriately, if possible. There may always be the potential for the patient to die before the transfer, but the team should prepare and advise according to the discussion above. Further coordination is required with the hospital teams, in order to facilitate the best support for the patient and family.

Families may be keen for a transfer, as they may have not understood the philosophy of the PCU. Hope can be maintained by a transfer, as "more can be done" in the hospital. Some family members will find it difficult to leave the PCU, especially if they believe the decision to leave is wrong. Families often struggle with the emotions between the devotion to the dying person and their wishes, the practical issues of coping with the decisions, and the safe haven of the PCU.

Another factor to consider is the relationship the patient and family may have with their treating team in the acute setting. Many patients with chronic diseases will have developed a strong bond with the multi-professional team on the acute ward. Examples include patients with end-stage renal disease or end-stage chronic obstructive pulmonary disease. The relationship may also be reciprocal with the acute care staff, as often displayed by their willingness to care for these patients at the end of life (Gott et al. 2013).

In the current healthcare system, patients and families often have a misperception of palliative care. Without time to process the need for palliative care, it is not difficult to understand the reluctance of some patients and families to stay in the PCU. The familiarity with the acute hospital team and the environment is one factor, but the kind of medicalized care provided is another. The mismatch of expectations and experiences can prompt a request for a transfer back to the acute hospital. Sometimes the transfer may be difficult to facilitate, due to organizational systems, but invariably an understanding can be reached from a patient-centered approach.

Once in the acute hospital, the HPCT may be able to monitor the progress of the patient, collaborate with the lead clinical team, and support the family as required. Abandonment of the patient and their family can be an important factor in the delivery of care, during the terminal phase of an illness (Smith et al. 2016). Even if the HPCT is not required, the supportive role can remain significant for all concerned. The lead clinical team will require a handover, due to the complexities of care. In both scenarios, the HCPT should be involved and relevant to the supportive processes.

11 Conclusion

Transfers to a chosen venue of death require planning, clear goals of care, and empathic communication in order to facilitate a smooth transition of care. The knowledge of the patient and family wishes, as early as possible, is critical to allow the coordination of required services. The introduction of more systematized advance care planning in our communities, and increasing societal conversations about death and dying, provides useful opportunities to plan care. Ultimately, under difficult circumstances, we are trying to honor the wishes of a dying person. For those people whose goal we achieve, there is much satisfaction and gratitude. There may be instances where the goal was achieved, but how we were successful was less satisfactory. Finally, there will be times when we failed to achieve the goal and there is disappointment and anger. In each case there is an uncertainty to accept and a reflection to learn from, but how we fought to realize someone's preferred place of care and then death will live with families as a memory of our respect for their departed.

12 Summary

The preferred place of death remains an important factor in good EOLC but may not always be the home setting we are led to believe. Many people prefer other venues of death, for many reasons including societal, cultural, and psychological considerations. A recent systematic review of the barriers and facilitators to dying at home provides a succinct overview to facilitating the preferred place of death. The facilitators include coordinated care, skilled staff, effective communication, and support for patients and HCPs. On the other hand, the barriers included a lack of knowledge, skills, and support among informal caregivers and HCPs; informal caregiver and family burden; recognizing death; unfavorable social circumstances; inadequate discharge processes; condition-specific discrepancies, e.g., the inequity of access to palliative care for people with nonmalignant conditions; and poor planning (Wahid et al. 2017).

Whatever the setting of care, the early knowledge about the wishes of the patient is important. Only then can we plan and realistically obtain a smooth transition to the venue of death. Prognostication adds to the complexity of the situation, amidst the current standards of healthcare communication. These decisions cannot be made lightly but are often made in emergency situations. Taking the time to understand the decisions of patients and the families can ensure the right choices are made in the timeframe available. The coordination of services, reduction of adverse risks, and compassionate communication help achieve the best outcomes in these situations.

References

Agar M, Currow DC, Shelby-James TM, Plummer J, Sanderson C, Abernethy AP. Preference for place of care and place of death in palliative care: are these different questions? Palliat Med. 2008;22:787–95. https://journals.sagepub.com

Ahearn DJ, Nidh N, Kallat A, Adenwala Y, Varman S. Offering older hospitalised patients the choice to die in their preferred place. Postgrad Med J. 2013;89:20–4.

Ali M, Capel M, Jones G, Gazi T. The importance of identifying preferred place of death. BMJ Suppor Palliat Care. 2015:bmjspcare-2015.

Bergenholtz H, Jarlbaek L, Hølge-Hazelton B. Generalist palliative care in hospital – cultural and organisational interactions. Results of a mixed-methods study. Palliat Med. 2016;30:558–66.

Billingham MJ, Billingham S-J. Congruence between preferred and actual place of death according to the presence of malignant or non-malignant disease: a systematic review and meta-analysis. BMJ Support Palliat Care. 2013;3:144–54. https://spcare.bmj.com

Bone AE, Gomes B, Etkind SN, Verne J, Murtagh FE, Evans CJ, et al. What is the impact of population ageing on the future provision of end-of-life care? Population-based projections of place of death. Palliat Med. 2017; 269216317734435. https://journals.sagepub.com.

Cohen J, Pivodic L, Miccinesi G, Onwuteaka-Philipsen BD, Naylor WA, Wilson DM, et al. International study of the place of death of people with cancer: a population-level comparison of 14 countries across 4 continents using death certificate data. Br J Cancer. 2015;113:1397–404. https://nature.com

Cohen J, Beernaert K, Van den Block L, Morin L, Hunt K, Miccinesi G, et al. Differences in place of death between lung cancer and COPD patients: a 14-country study using death certificate data. NPJ Prim Care Respir Med. 2017;27:14. https://ncbi.nlm.nih.gov

Gage H, Holdsworth LM. Impact of a hospice rapid response service on preferred place of death, and costs. Biomed Chromatogr. 2015. bmcpalliatcare.biomedcentral.com. Available: https://bmcpalliatcare.biomedcentral.com/articles/10.1186/s12904-015-0065-4.

Glare P, Sinclair C, Downing M, Stone P, Maltoni M, Vigano A. Predicting survival in patients with advanced disease. Eur J Cancer. 2008;44:1146–56. Elsevier.

Gomes B, Calanzani N, Gysels M, Hall S, Higginson IJ. Heterogeneity and changes in preferences for dying at home: a systematic review. BMC Palliat Care. 2013;12:7. https://bmcpalliatcare.biomedcentral.com

Gomes B, Calanzani N, Koffman J, Higginson IJ. Is dying in hospital better than home in incurable cancer and what factors influence this? A population-based study. BMC Med. 2015;13:235. https://bmcmedicine.biomedcentral.com

Gott M, Frey R, Robinson J, Boyd M, O'Callaghan A, Richards N, et al. The nature of, and reasons for, "inappropriate" hospitalisations among patients with palliative care needs: a qualitative exploration of the views of generalist palliative care providers. Palliat Med. 2013;27:747–56.

Hui D, Dos Santos R, Chisholm G, Bansal S, Souza Crovador C, Bruera E. Bedside clinical signs associated with impending death in patients with advanced cancer: preliminary findings of a prospective, longitudinal cohort study. Cancer. 2015;121:960–7.

Kalseth J, Theisen OM. Trends in place of death: the role of demographic and epidemiological shifts in end-of-life care policy. Palliat Med. 2017;31:964–74. https://journals.sagepub.com

Kellehear A. Compassionate communities: end-of-life care as everyone's responsibility. QJM. 2013;106:1071–5. https://academic.oup.com

Lin Y, Myall M, Jarrett N. Uncovering the decision-making work of transferring dying patients home from critical care units: an integrative review. J Adv Nurs. 2017. Wiley Online Library; Available: http://onlinelibrary.wiley.com/doi/10.1111/jan.13368/full.

Love AW, Liversage LM. Barriers to accessing palliative care: a review of the literature. Prog Palliat Care. 2014;22:9–19.

Lovell N, Jones C, Baynes D, Dinning S, Vinen K, Murtagh FE. Understanding patterns and factors associated with place of death in patients with end-stage kidney disease: a retrospective cohort study. Palliat Med. 2017;31:283–8. https://journals.sagepub.com

Mann S, Galler D, Williams P, Frost P. Caring for patients and families at the end of life: withdrawal of intensive care in the patient's home. N Z Med J. 2004;117:U935. https://search.proquest.com

Murphy D, Ellershaw JE, Jack B, Gambles M, Saltmarsh P. The Liverpool care pathway for the rapid discharge home of the dying patient. J Integr Care Pathways. 2004;8:127–8. Sage Publications.

Needle JS. Home extubation by a pediatric critical care team: providing a compassionate death outside the pediatric intensive care unit. Pediatr Crit Care Med. 2010;11:401–3. https://journals.lww.com

Poppito SR. Advancing Medical Education in Existential. Psychooncology. American Psychiatric Pub; 2013; 201.

Romo RD, Wallhagen MI, Smith AK. Viewing hospice decision making as a process. Am J Hosp Palliat Care. 2016;33:503–10.

Sallnow L, Kumar S, Numpeli M. Home-based palliative care in Kerala, India: the neighbourhood network in palliative care. Prog Palliat Care. 2010;18:14–7. Taylor & Francis.

Sallnow L, Richardson H, Murray S, Kellehear A. Understanding the impact of a new public health approach to end-of-life care: a qualitative study of a community led intervention. Lancet. 2017;389:S88. Elsevier.

Scibetta C, Kerr K, Mcguire J, Rabow MW. The costs of waiting: implications of the timing of palliative care consultation among a cohort of decedents at a comprehensive cancer center. J Palliat Med. 2016;19:69–75. https://online.liebertpub.com

Seow H, Bainbridge D. A Review of the Essential Components of Quality Palliative Care in the Home. J Palliat Med. Mary Ann Liebert Inc.; 2018;21:S37–S44.

Smith S, Brick A, O'Hara S, Normand C. Evidence on the cost and cost-effectiveness of palliative care: a literature review. Palliat Med. 2014;28:130–50. https://journals.sagepub.com

Smith C, Bosanquet N, Riley J, Koffman J. Loss, transition and trust: perspectives of terminally ill patients and their oncologists when transferring care from the hospital into the community at the end of life. BMJ Support Palliat Care. 2016. https://doi.org/10.1136/bmjspcare-2015-001075. https://spcare.bmj.com

Stajduhar K, Sawatzky R, Robin Cohen S, Heyland DK, Allan D, Bidgood D, et al. Bereaved family members' perceptions of the quality of end-of-life care across four types of inpatient care settings. BMC Palliat Care. 2017;16:59. https://bmcpalliatcare.biomedcentral.com

Thomas RL, Zubair MY, Hayes B, Ashby MA. Goals of care: a clinical framework for limitation of medical treatment. Med J Aust. 2014;201:452–5.

Unger KM. Withdrawal of ventilatory support at home on hospice. J Pain Symptom Manage. 2016;52:305–12. Elsevier.

Virdun C, Luckett T, Lorenz K, Davidson PM, Phillips J. Dying in the hospital setting: a meta-synthesis identifying the elements of end-of-life care that patients and their families describe as being important. Palliat Med. 2016. https://doi.org/10.1177/0269216316673547. https://pmj.sagepub.com

Wahid AS, Sayma M, Jamshaid S, Kerwat D'A, Oyewole F, Saleh D, et al. Barriers and facilitators influencing death at home: a meta-ethnography. Palliat Med. 2017; 269216317713427. https://journals.sagepub.com.

Challenging Family Dynamics

83

Dianne Clifton and Margaret Ross

Contents

D. Clifton (✉)
RANZCP, St Vincent's Hospital Melbourne, Cabrini Hospital, Albert Road Clinic, Hawthorn Road Consulting Suites, International Psycho-oncology Society, University of Melbourne, Fitzroy, VIC, Australia

Psychosocial Cancer Care, St Vincent's Hospital Melbourne, Fitzroy, VIC, Australia
e-mail: cliftondiannealice@gmail.com

M. Ross
Department of Psychosocial Cancer Care, St Vincent's Hospital, Melbourne, VIC, Australia
e-mail: margaret.ross@svha.org.au

R. D. MacLeod, L. Van den Block (eds.), *Textbook of Palliative Care*,
https://doi.org/10.1007/978-3-319-77740-5_86

Abstract

At a time when palliative care guidelines are advocating greater respect for patient autonomy and the inclusion of patients and families in decision-making with clinicians, families themselves have become increasingly complex and more broadly defined. Some families bond internally with one another and with the clinicians to best meet the needs of the patient despite the significant stress of facing the death of one of their members; others become more obstructively dysfunctional, jeopardizing patient care and creating stress in the healthcare system. Conflict may arise from the interaction between the nature and circumstance of the patient's care and contextual family factors reflecting structure, dynamics, and prior history. Thorough family assessment can provide a basis for interventions to avert a crisis. Early recognition and management of potentially damaging family conflict is illustrated throughout this chapter by clinical vignettes. The published literature and the clinical experience of the authors are drawn upon to illustrate the management of situations that threaten to escalate out of control. The need for communication skills training for all staff involved in palliative care is highlighted.

1 Introduction

Care of the dying person has involved the family from the inception of the hospice movement (Saunders 1978). The term "family" cannot be regarded as a unitary entity (Wellisch and Kissane 2009). Families may include not only the traditional model of parents, children, extended family, but also same-sex couples, former partners, stepfamilies and blended families, adopted or fostered children, friends, partners, and caregivers who are regarded by the patient as "family." Cultural and religious factors also influence not only who is identified as family, but also the function and role of its members (Baider and Goldzweig 2012). A broad understanding of the many subsystems under the rubric of "family" that are thrust together into the physical, psychological, existential, and spiritual space of a person suffering from terminal illness is needed. Without this, health professionals will miss the opportunity to optimally ease the patient through the dying process and assist the family into the bereavement phase.

Very few families are perfectly cohesive; even "healthy" families can become temporarily dysfunctional during a normal process of adaptation when catapulted into the intensely emotional, confronting, and unchartered world of a dying family member. Family conflict is not a unidimensional construct and can become quite complex (Kramer et al. 2006). Long-standing, entrenched, and maladaptive patterns of coping, communicating, and relating (often trans-generational in origin) are brought into high relief in the complexity of palliative care settings (Lichtenthal and Kissane 2008). Family context includes the historical issues, family structure, involvement with care and other demands and resources, as well as the presence of substance abuse, religion, culture, and belief systems and the extent to which plans or promises have been made in relation to the dying patient (Boelk and Kramer 2012; Kramer and Boelk 2015).

This chapter will discuss different palliative care service sites, setting the scene for emergencies involving families that may be more likely to arise, or more difficult to manage, in these settings. It will describe assessment of families, family typologies, attachment styles, and different models of family conflict and will present a series of clinical cases dealing with aspects of the family context, the circumstances and location of the conflict, the contributing factors, and the consequences of the conflict for patient, family, and staff. Management of these individual challenging situations will be described, and general principles of dealing with difficult family situations will be presented. Throughout these discussions, the importance of training in communication skills for all palliative care workers will be emphasized.

2 The Palliative Care Inpatient Setting

The inpatient palliative care unit can be an intense crucible where staff and families are thrown together for prolonged periods of time in situations of heightened emotional and physical suffering, disparate expectations, intimate spectacles, and little privacy. The goal of the admission may be symptom management, assessment, respite, end-of-life care, or stabilization prior to transfer to more appropriate longer-term accommodation. Whatever the circumstances of admission, patients and their families find themselves in an unfamiliar environment devoid of the comforts and routines of home and may feel unsettled, even when they are relieved that the burden of care will shift to the multidisciplinary team. Exhausted and distressed family caregivers may feel guilt and have difficulty in relinquishing their role. On the other hand, they may be more able to be present as supportive family members instead of having time and energy consumed by the practical and emotional demands of caring. The patient can experience even greater loss of dignity, autonomy, and independence in a hospital environment, which impacts on the family's perception of care. Pre-existing family conflict escapes from the privacy of family life into the public arena and draws staff members into a complex drama.

3 Community Palliative Care

Palliative care administered in the patient's home can avoid some of the disruptive elements of admission to a palliative care unit and is more often the preferred choice of patient's and family (Gomes et al. 2015). It allows the maintenance of normal family routines; the nurturing presence of family pets; a neighborly or community support network; the comfort of familiar objects; reminders of the life lived; and favorite views, cushions, and positions. Community palliative care staff enjoy the privilege of entering the patient's world, gaining insights into the needs and functioning of the family and an understanding of how best to engage them to provide optimal care. There are additional challenges, however, as staff do not have the same degree of control or certainty about the care the patient is receiving and lack the backup of a multidisciplinary team when difficulties arise. Considering the family, they have no real respite from caring, even when they have a roster of availability – they cannot "go home" after an emotionally and physically exhausting day. In rural and remote areas, community teams may have to travel vast distances to provide services. Some teams supplement their visits with Skype or FaceTime connection on mobile devices, providing a reassuring virtual presence. Specialist palliative physicians provide regular consultancy visits to regional areas and have an on-call consultant to provide telephone advice in some countries. People requiring palliative services who belong to indigenous communities may want to be cared for by their extended family, in their own familiar landscape. It is therefore important to liaise with indigenous workers who are able to sensitively interpret the needs and wishes of the patient and family (McGrath et al. 2005).

4 Palliative Care Consultation Teams

As the concept of palliative care has become increasingly integrated into general medical and surgical units, a specialized consultation team has been developed in some of the larger health facilities. These teams assess and recommend treatment for patients with malignant or nonmalignant disease who have palliative care needs. The patient remains under the care of the admitting unit, and conflicts can arise where the treating team pursues treatments that are at odds with the palliative care team's goals of care. The palliative care consultation team has a culture of holistic care of the patient and family, which contrasts with the more medical focus of the treating team. Subsequently, the palliative care consultant becomes an important link in the medicalized hospital environment. Communication about clinical information can be inadequate between teams, unless the palliative care consultant is able to participate in the multidisciplinary team meetings of each unit. There is considerable variability in the respect shown for the palliative care consultant's perspectives and recommendations, both between the senior doctors of the same unit and between units. The stable nature of the palliative care consultation team contrasts with the rotating junior medical staff and in complex cases may provide the only source of continuity and "holding of the story" for patients and families. Medical and surgical teams are often reluctant to acknowledge that a patient is dying and generally lack the specialist communication skills training of their palliative care colleagues. As a consequence, there is often poor preparation of patients and families for death and a retreat from time-consuming interactions with families. Even when the treating team is on-board with the person- and family-centered approach to clinical care, arranging a full family meeting with members of the treating team and the palliative care consultation team can be logistically difficult; in a general hospital setting, there is often less space and fewer resources to deal with the needs of the family.

5 Assessing Families

Assessment of family structure and functioning needs to begin from the earliest contact with a patient entering palliative care. It may begin with the construction of a genogram, which notes not only the members of the family of origin and generative family of the patient (as well as others considered by the patient to be family) but also significant information about their relationships, occupation, closeness or estrangement, role in decision-making, mental and physical health, previous loss and trauma, substance abuse problems, beliefs and values, and potential sources of conflict. Having some foreknowledge of family dynamics helps the clinician to understand what might be happening when crises arise with families at a time of heightened distress and guides effective communication strategies.

Further understanding of the family functioning develops over time with skillful observation of interactions between patient and family, family members, and family and staff. Evidence of particular strengths, vulnerabilities, coping styles, and issues not initially apparent may emerge in the process of engagement with the family. These observations should be shared at team meetings so that a comprehensive picture of the patient's world can be created. Well-conducted family meetings, which are encouraged in palliative care settings (Hudson et al. 2009), allow further opportunities for observation of family dynamics. They are not only useful for discussion of goals of care, treatment options, and care planning with the patient and family but can be optimized through circular

Table 1 Strategies for conducting a family meeting in palliative care (Lichtenthal and Kissane 2008)

Strategies for conducting a family meeting[a]
Planning and prior setup to arrange the family meeting
Welcome and orientation of the family to the goals of the family meeting
Check that each family member understands the illness and the patient's prognosis
Check for consensus about the current goals of care
Identify family concerns about their management of key symptoms or care needs
Clarify the family's view of what the future holds
Clarify how family members are coping and feeling emotionally
Identify family strengths and affirm their level of commitment and mutual support for each other
Close the family meeting by final review of agreed goals of care and future plans

[a]Content reproduced with permission from Lichtenthal and Kissane (2008)

Table 2 Practical elements of the family-focused grief therapy model (Kissane and Bloch 2002)

Practical elements of the family-focused grief therapy model[a]
Build rapport with each family member to create a therapeutic alliance
Elicit concerns
Acknowledge and foster family strengths
Focus first on improving teamwork and communication and then target conflict
Remain neutral
Reframe by shifting attention away from content of arguments to underlying meaning (i.e., why they feel so heated, what the difference represents)
Pose questions that invite reflections and curiosity
Invite storytelling
Generate hypotheses about family dynamics related to cohesiveness, expressiveness, and conflict resolution
Summarize hypotheses for consideration and modification

[a]Content reproduced with permission from Kissane and Bloch (2002)

questioning to reveal how the family members relate to each other, if there are any possible conflicts or misunderstandings, and their perceptions, hopes, and fears. Good communication skills are essential for conducting a family meeting so that each member feels supported and heard. Table 1 sets out strategies for conducting a family meeting in palliative care (Lichtenthal and Kissane 2008). Practical strategies from family-focused grief therapy (FFGT) (Kissane and Bloch 2002) are outlined in Table 2 and can be used to explore family dynamics, communication patterns, and areas of conflicting views. The styles of questioning used by therapists in FFGT are presented in Table 3 and may be useful in family meetings (Kissane and Zaider 2011).

6 Typologies of Family Functioning

Four fundamental interactional concepts in families dealing with a terminally ill member described by Wellisch and Kissane (Wellisch and Kissane 2009) are:

- *Homeostasis* (the relative constancy of the family internal emotional environment when dealing severe stresses)
- *Bonding* (the ability of the family to maintain its own territory by regulating the incoming and outgoing people, objects, and ideas)
- *The family system* (whether open, closed, or random)
- *Resilience*

Kissane and Bloch (2002) introduced a different way of describing family types in their extensive study of grief and psychosocial morbidity in bereaved family members. The patterns of emotional functioning have been characterized as supportive, conflict-resolving, intermediate, sullen, and hostile. Using the Family Relationship Index, they derived scores on three key dimensions of family competence – cohesiveness, communication, and conflict resolution. The dysfunctional families in this framework are the hostile families, who show high conflict, low cohesiveness, and poor expressiveness and sullen families who had more moderate limitations in these domains. Families with moderate to high levels of cohesiveness and expressiveness and lower levels of conflict were better able to adapt to the challenges associated with a terminally ill family member.

Although not typologies of family functioning, there are other concepts of family relationship and

Table 3 Styles of questioning used by therapists in family-focused grief therapy (Kissane and Zaider 2011)

Styles of orientating and influencing questions asked by therapists in FFGT[a]		
Complementary types of questions	Description of the function and purpose of each questioning style	Typical examples use in FFGT
Linear (generally orientating and informative about individuals)	These generate a one-to-one conversation between the therapist and each individual, help to obtain information, join with and support individuals, prove useful when open-ended to take a history but are conservative in promoting family interaction.	What job do you have?What grade are you in at school?What sports do you like to play?
Circular (orientating and informative about family as a whole dynamics)	These seek observations from one family member about others, asking each iteratively to step into the shoes of one another and share diverse views that stimulate family discussion and reveal relational dynamics.	How are your spouse and children coping? Who talks to whom? Who are you most worried about?
Reflexive (generally influencing without being directive)	These encourage mutual understanding and support via greater insight and awareness of the meaning of any individual responses, can include hypotheses about dynamics inserted into the wording of the question, and seek to promote reflection upon solutions and consideration of acceptance or change.	What are your expectations about the future? How might things look difference in one year? If X were still alive, what would they ask of you? Why do you think they are becoming more irritable?
Strategic (both influencing and potentially more directive in intent)	These invite a search for a solution and aim to build consensus about future directions, including options for acceptance or change; if too directive, they may be constraining rather than generative.	How helpful might it be for Dad to reach out to old friends? What benefits would come from talking about end-of-life care? Might more open sharing of feelings which increase your sense of family connection?

[a]Content reproduced with permission from Kissane and Zaider (2011)

communication that are helpful in formulating the challenges faced in dealing with families in distress. The concept of **death awareness** is the subject of a seminal work by Glaser and Strauss half a century ago. They described types of awareness of dying between patients and caregivers:

- *Open* (where both patient and family are aware the patient is dying and are open to talking about it)
- *Suspected* (where the patient suspects, but dying is not openly discussed)
- *Mutual pretense* (where one or both parties of the dyad pretend that they do not know)
- *Closed* (where the caregiver is aware that the patient is dying, but this knowledge is kept from the patient) (Glaser and Strauss 1966)

Death awareness is a complex issue influenced by culture, spiritual and religious beliefs, family history, and the perception of the patient's or caregiver's ability to cope with the knowledge of impending death (Strada 2009).

The second important concept is **attachment theory** and its application to patient and family in terminal illness. In the 1950s, British psychoanalyst John Bowlby proposed that attachment of infants and children to caregivers was the expression of an innate drive to secure care and protection and hence survival (Bowlby 1969). He introduced the concepts of a *secure base* formed through attachment to a sensitive and responsive caregiver, a *safe haven* to go to in times of need, and *separation distress* when the attachment figure is unavailable. Individuals form an internal representation of their relationship with caregivers that endures in expectations, beliefs, and patterns of future relationships that are relevant to their experience of security.

In the 1960s, developmental psychologist Mary Ainsworth explored patterns of attachment through her strange situation research (Ainsworth et al. 1978). She described three basic types of attachment – secure, insecure anxious/ambivalent, and insecure anxious/avoidant – to which a fourth pattern disorganized/disoriented was added by a colleague Mary Main (Main and Solomon 1990). The attachment system is inevitably activated in the situation of a dying family member, where the impending separation is irrevocable. In the decades of research on attachment theory, increasing attention has been paid to how attachment styles manifest within families and in the patient-clinician relationship. Petersen and Koehler (2006) use their observations of attachment style, evident in the first encounter with the patient and family with the powerful activator of impending separation, to inform psychotherapeutic intervention during the terminal phase. They note that even patients who have a disorganized attachment style can, with sensitive care, come to experience a secure and stable attachment for their remaining lifetime.

Milberg and Friedrichsen (2017) interviewed families during the delivery of palliative home care to patients. They found that family, friends, health practitioners, pets, and for some people God were described by patients as a source of security and trust. The comforting contact could be of a physical or nonphysical nature (e.g., by telephone). When strong, these attachments could provide a sense of security in the threat of progressive illness, and they could then focus on everyday life in the knowledge that they were being competently cared for. Some family members however experienced a fading sense of security as the ravages of illness altered the patient's personality and behavior, and this loss was accompanied by a deep loneliness. These authors recommended that each patient and close family member be assessed in relation to attachment by asking: "When you are afraid or feel insecure, who or what is a potential source of comfort to you?"

Recognizing that attachment styles affect both help-seeking behavior and the capacity to be soothed by, or accept help from, healthcare professionals, Tan et al. (2005) explored the empathic responsiveness of clinicians to specific attachment needs and fears which might significantly influence the success of the therapeutic relationship. Patients with *disturbed attachments* may find the vulnerability associated with dependency on others so intolerable that they wish to escape through death, and a tailored therapeutic response is essential. Patients with *dismissive attachment* styles may close off their feelings and maintain contradictory needs for autonomy and support. An approach allowing active participation in treatment or care decisions can enable an acceptance of emotional support on these patients' terms. Patients with *fearful attachment* styles have difficulty acknowledging their emotions, dependent needs, and feelings of vulnerability because they find them threatening and may appear to reject help. Facilitating awareness of these factors may initially be met with anger but can pave the way for a new equilibrium with family members and clinicians. The extreme anxiety that characterizes patients with *preoccupied attachment* styles can exhaust staff and family members who find these patients excessively needy, demanding, and unable to be reassured. Providing structured, reliable, and consistent time with staff and setting clear limits can reduce anxiety and fears of abandonment and lessen caregiver burden. It is important to acknowledge that clinicians bring to the relationship with the patient and family their own attachment history and need to be sensitively attuned to how this may contribute to the interpersonal dynamics.

7 Ethical Considerations in Relation to Families

When family members take on the role of "caregiver" of their terminally ill loved one, enormous stress is placed on the relational dynamic as they cope with increasingly complex care needs (Given et al. 2001). The World Health Organization (WHO) definition of palliative care states that the palliative care aims to improve "...the quality of life of patients *and their families* facing the problems associated with life-threatening illness. . ." (Alliance WPC et al. 2014).

The well-being of family members and caregivers has significance for the overall well-being of the patient, with a meta-analysis suggesting that a reciprocal caregiver-patient dyad occurs whereby the patient is significantly influenced by the distress of the caregiver and vice versa in an "emotional system" (Hodges et al. 2005). This consideration holds even greater importance when working with challenging family dynamics, as the focus of care can become so overshadowed by conflict that failure to consider family member well-being and relational dynamics could further aggravate existing issues and distress.

The ethics of providing care for both patient and family brings up questions about boundaries of provision of support in challenging situations and the way forward can be unclear. The four general principles of medical ethics are:

- Respect for autonomy/persons (accepting the right of a person to decide what is done to them)
- Non-maleficence (do no harm)
- Beneficence (acting in the best interests of the patient and family)
- Justice (duty to treat all patients with the same dedication)

These are useful to consider in light of challenging situations. For example, a family member with a personality disorder who provokes punitive or evasive reactions in staff can cause team members to fail to observe the principles of non-maleficence and justice. Respect for autonomy can also be extremely problematic when a family member is in strong denial about the gravity of the patient's medical condition, when family members are in conflict with the patient's wishes, and where substitute decision makers are indifferent, incapable, or opposed to what the patient would have wanted if competent.

Clinicians are faced with questions such as: "How much time and service provision should be given to dependent and distressed family members?," "Should I prescribe for a family member if they are distressed and needing pharmacotherapy?," and "How much should I protect the patient if the family is obstructing treatment?" Lederberg (2010) provides clear ideas and practical guidance for navigating "ethical stalemates" when dealing with patients and family members in oncology settings which could be extrapolated to palliative situations.

The identified family of concern in these issues may include the primary carer, a recipient of supportive care from the palliative care team, proxy decision-makers, and, very occasionally, a litigator.

Ashby and Mendelson (2008) argue that instead of ethical discussion being considered only when there is an "ethical dilemma," ethical awareness should be well integrated into day-to-day discussions and embedded in clinical practice. The authors argue that while the primary clinical responsibility is to that of the patient, the family is also embraced in the palliative care model. However, they caution that not all family members wish to be the recipients of care themselves. As such, the provision of service or support to family members must only be provided with explicit consent (Ashby and Mendelson 2008).

The difficulty facing many palliative care staff in highly complex situations is that the "true" nature of problems can be hidden under layers of strong emotional reactions to cases, resulting in intransigent clinical positions. Discussions discriminating facts from beliefs or values held by staff can be beneficial in assisting staff to step back from the clinical situation to gain a more objective view. Where negotiation with all parties fails to move beyond an impasse, the patient's well-being and comfort remain at the fore, and medicolegal advice may need to be sought (Ashby and Mendelson 2008). Where the needs of a family member go beyond what palliative care teams are resourced to provide, or clearly require specialist assistance, the team need to refer the family member to the appropriate service outside of the team (Hudson et al. 2009).

8 Culture, Religion, and Belief Systems Impacting on Work with Families

In Western cultures, emphasis is placed on fulfilling the patient's wishes with secondary consideration given to the minimization of family distress. This contrasts with collectivist cultures, where decisions are deferred to the

Table 4 Cultural diversity (Baider and Goldzweig 2012)

Cultural diversity[a]
Emphasis on individualism versus collectivism
Definition of family (extended, nuclear, nonblood, kinship)
Common views of gender roles, child-rearing practices, and care of older adults
Views of marriage and relationships
Communication patterns (direct and indirect; relative emphasis on nonverbal communication; meanings of nonverbal gestures)
Common religious and spiritual-belief systems.
Views of physicians
Views of suffering
Views of afterlife

[a]Content reproduced with permission from Baider and Goldzweig (2012)

family unit as a collective rather than promotion of patient autonomy (Lederberg 2010). For instance, most Asian cultures have family-based decision-making processes; conflict within these families can impede these processes and lead to hostility among members (Lichtenthal and Kissane 2008). Muslim families believe that the ultimate decision-maker is Allah; they believe in predestination and attribute the occurrence of disease as the will of Allah. No one but Allah knows the future, which makes discussions about prognosis from a Western perspective difficult, although it is permissible to explain the natural history of a terminal illness in general terms. Decisions are made about care by the male family leader and females are unable to influence his decisions. The authority of the family overrules the patient's autonomy (Baider and Goldzweig 2012). It is important to respect the rituals of prayer that need to be accommodated into the treatment plan. In different cultures, physical and existential pain may be experienced differently; some cultures may value suffering; others may see it as God testing their faith, a divine punishment, or a mark of shame or guilt that must be hidden (Surbone and Kagawa-Singer 2013). Culture, religion, and belief systems also influence the way illness is expressed, the extent to which people seek or accept psychological help, truth-telling, and coping style. It is important not to make assumptions based on stereotypes of different groups, as there are wide variations in adherence to lore and intergenerational differences that are determined by the degree of acculturation of immigrants from another background. Table 4 demonstrates the different aspects of cultural diversity (Baider and Goldzweig 2012).

9 Context of Challenging Issues with Families

9.1 Families in Conflict with One Another

All happy families are alike; each unhappy family is unhappy in its own way (Tolstoy 1980).

With this famous philosophical line, Leo Tolstoy opens his epic novel of love and tortured family relationships, *Anna Karenina.* Families who are unhappy often exhibit conflict, defined as "interpersonal tension or struggle among two or more persons whose opinions, values, needs or expectations are opposing or incompatible" (Kramer et al. 2006), and family conflict is commonly encountered in a palliative setting. Preexisting conflict may become exacerbated by the intensity of emotions and uncomfortable propinquity around the dying family member's bedside. For all families, there are potential disagreements around aspects of the patient's care, e.g., which caregivers should be involved, the location of care, the needs of the patient, the appropriate medications to be used, who the decision-makers should be, how actively treatments should be pursued, what the patient or other family members should be told, funeral planning, and legacy issues.

Boelk and Kramer (2012) developed an explanatory matrix of family conflict at the end of life, based on their earlier qualitative research with families in different cancer and palliative care settings (Kramer et al. 2006). The matrix includes the conditions which may increase the risk of escalation of conflict; contributing factors; whether the conflict is between family members, between patient and family, or between family/patient and staff; and the consequences of the

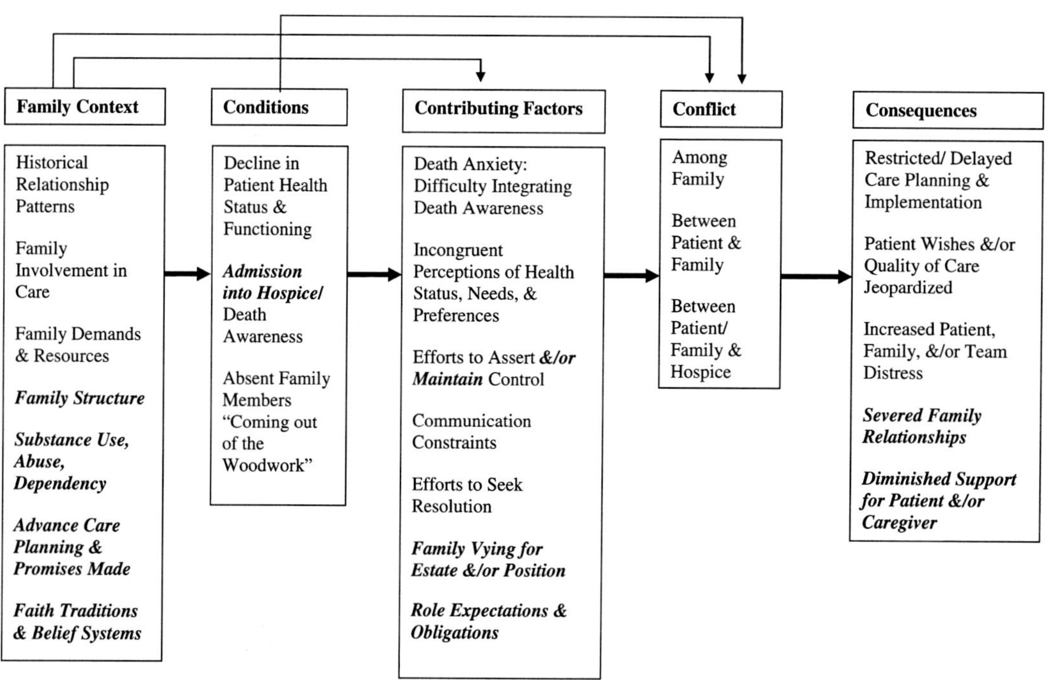

Fig. 1 Explanatory matrix of family conflict at the end of life (Boelk and Kramer 2012)

conflict. This model provides a useful way of examining the many contributing factors to family conflict (see Fig. 1) (Boelk and Kramer 2012).

Johanna, an 85-year-old woman born in Greece, was admitted for end-of-life care with several medical problems, including advanced transformed leukaemia, renal failure and diabetes. Each of her children had varying expectations and understandings of her medical state and very strong, but different views about how her treatment should be managed. The eldest child, who had medical power of attorney, became focused on the history of the diagnosis and treatments and preoccupied with which illness was causing her deterioration. Another one of her children became fixated on the dose, indication and type of medication proposed. One of her daughters wanted to ensure that everything was done, and that medical staff and the rest of the family didn't just "give up" on her too early. She was reluctant for her mother to be administered opioids, which she thought would hasten death, and wanted her to have blood transfusions, despite their no longer providing therapeutic benefit. Initially, individual children would have separate lengthy discussions with the medical staff and nursing staff but they had not formed a common view about her care.

Intervention: Medical and nursing staff held a family meeting with all the children present to provide support and education around Johanna's disease status, medications, symptom management and end-of-life care. Common ground was identified in that all children wanted to ensure that Johanna did not suffer if she was dying. Ongoing support was provided and the gentle realignment of goals were communicated consistently with clear handover among staff. The family came to understand that with the goal of care being alleviation of distress, medications would be required to achieve this. Johanna was eventually commenced on a syringe driver and died comfortably with the children by her bedside. In this case, family functioning premorbidly had not been particularly conflictual, highlighting how the stress of imminent loss of a loved one can forge divisions in any family system.

9.2 Families in Conflict with the Patient

Brochure images of a dying patient surrounded by loving family members gloss over an unpleasant reality for many families: that the end of life can be punctuated by unresolved conflicts. The dying patient may not be a "loved one." Indeed, the patient may have acted toward family members in ways that were less than loving, even abusive, creating long-standing resentment. Family members may feel angered by the neediness of the patient, and the expectation that they should now provide care and support, when they had never felt cared for or loved by the patient.

Edward was a 78-year-old married man, with no children, and was living at home with end-stage cardiac failure. He was known to a community palliative care team for symptom management in the context of increasing shortness of breath, fatigue and general functional decline. He struggled to acknowledge his increasing care needs to the team and became angry and anxious when his wife Jean was not by his side, though he denied any such emotions. His breathlessness was exacerbated by his anxiety, but he could not acknowledge any psychological component to his symptoms. Edward asserted that he did not need further assistance, despite the obvious progressive decline of his mobility, and he stated that he could 'easily' get along with the sole assistance of Jean. The team noticed that Jean was rarely present when they visited Edward, but when she was present, he would berate her for leaving his side and generally complain about his treatment. He would also criticise her housekeeping and make statements that indicated her absence was having a negative impact on the practical day to day running of the household.

Intervention: A family support worker spoke with Jean who described assuming a passive role in a "dull, lifeless marriage," in which she felt subordinated and criticised. Her current pattern of leaving the house allowed her to achieve some respite from Edward's increasingly burdensome care needs, and to "feel free of him" for several hours at a time while she played bingo. It also emerged that Jean felt a sense of triumph when leaving the house after being criticised by Edward. The support worker attempted to facilitate a couple session, which quickly broke down when Edward started to blame his wife for being unable to do "what a good wife should." Jean walked out. She phoned the support worker shortly after the attempted mediation, and stated that she could no longer care for Edward as he could no longer toilet himself and he was deteriorating. Edward was admitted to inpatient hospice care where he became belligerent and angry towards Jean, demanding to return home. The team attempted to enlist the assistance of Edward's younger brother and sister but they were "busy with work." It became clear that Edward had alienated many family members. Jean told staff that she would like Edward to be placed in a nursing home, but could not articulate this in front of him for fear of his anger. Further attempts were made to try and mediate the situation, but both Edward and Jean refused psychological support or input from the psychosocial team. Edward died in hospice care a few weeks afterwards. Jean was not present at the time of death.

9.3 The Family at Odds with the Team

Challenging situations can arise with families where the views of the family about the most appropriate care are at odds with those of the team. Such scenarios include pursuit of futile treatments (e.g., blood transfusions, repeated ascitic taps, intravenous fluids, tube feeding, or force-feeding), insistence on "natural" therapies (e.g., high-dose vitamin C infusions, homeopathy, strict exclusion diets) or alternative therapies (e.g., ozone therapy), misunderstandings about the purpose of medication, refusal to acknowledge that the patient is dying, and clashes of cultural expectations.

Anthea was a 32-year-old single woman who had returned home to live with her parents. She had been diagnosed with uterine cancer 2 years earlier, but now had metastatic lung involvement which was causing pain, dyspnoea and anxiety. These symptoms were requiring several admissions to the palliative care unit for symptom management. During her last admission to the unit she was found to have liver metastases and it was evident that her disease was progressing rapidly. A meeting was held with Anthea's parents and three siblings, to discuss the likelihood that Anthea would die within a week. The family members were distressed and shocked because they had all seen Anthea rally on many occasions after being very ill, and they had not expected her to die so soon. Anthea's pain and anxiety were difficult to control and she was beginning to become jaundiced over the first few days of admission. The family wanted to take her home by ambulance to die at home, which was her expressed wish.

Intervention: Long discussions were held with the family during the day, allowing them to process their grief and recognise the obvious signs of deterioration, e.g. worsening hepatic encephalopathy. The loving and caring nature of the family was acknowledged, and their courage to fulfil her wishes was commended. However, they were also advised of the distress from hepatic encephalopathy when adequate and responsive titration of medication was unavailable. Anthea was requiring the addition of phenobarbitone to her syringe driver to settle her. Staff emphasised that a ride in an ambulance, across the city in peak hour traffic, would cause her additional unnecessary suffering. Since she was too ill to be taken home, the most loving thing they could do for her was to bring a sense of home to her bedside with her favourite things and the people she loved. The family came around to accepting the advice of the staff and they kept a vigil at her bedside for the next two days until she died peacefully. The consultants involved in her care met with members of the family to answer questions that had arisen for them during her care, and this helped to bring some closure to lingering fears that they may have failed her in some way.

Fardin was a 40-year-old Muslim man from the Indian subcontinent who had suffered a cerebral bleed from metastatic adenocarcinoma of the lung. His wife (Safina) was a highly educated and articulate advocate for his end-of-life care, which included caring for him at home after he became unconscious. She had hoped that he would recover enough to be able to say the prayers for the dead, a prerequisite for a better life. She not only believed she would not be forgiven, or be able to forgive herself, but also had pressure from overseas relatives and the local Muslim community in which she was culturally and spiritually ensconced. Safina believed that Allah had allowed Fardin to live before and may do so again, if it were His wish. Her role was to keep Fardin alive until Allah decided.

Intervention: The community team attempted to work with the cultural beliefs and expectations of the family, in spite of their concerns about the patient's optimal care. They understood that what they might, in Western terms, call denial of an inevitable death, was rather a manifestation of the belief that Fardin's life should be continued until Allah had called him. The team felt mandated by their own professional ethics and found it difficult to reconcile cultural awareness with their professional obligations. They accommodated some of the wishes of the family, but had difficulty dealing with suboptimal palliative care. Safina wanted to cease his subcutaneous delivery of anticonvulsants and morphine, because she believed they were making him unconscious. She told staff that suffering in their faith was an affirmation of life and that it should not be seen as a negative thing. Safina believed hydration would reverse Fardin's unconscious state and she enlisted a community doctor to set up a subcutaneous infusion of fluid. Fardin died after several days, but the circumstances of his terminal care left the community team feeling distressed and powerless.

9.4 The Return of the Former Spouse

It is not an uncommon experience in a palliative care unit to have former spouses or partners return to be involved in the care of a patient. They are often the other parent of the patient's children who are involved in the care of, or at least visiting, their terminally ill parent. This may create difficulties for a new partner who may experience a power-play with the former partner in relation to who "really knows" the patient and who has the right to have input into treatment decisions. Alliances are usually formed between the children and their parent, so that the new partner feels "pushed out" and may even be excluded from discussions with the team. Issues of rights to inheritance may also arise, particularly if the new partner has been in the relationship with the patient for a short time. The patient may feel torn and too fatigued to deal with the conflicting emotions and allegiances.

Paul was a 75-year-old man of considerable wealth, with metastatic pancreatic cancer. He was admitted to inpatient palliative care for symptom management and end-of-life care. He was in a "complicated" relationship with his second wife (Zoe), who had moved to another place of residence, but had not officially separated from Paul, telling people they were still married. Zoe left most of her husband's increasing care needs and details to his three children from his first marriage. Zoe barely acknowledged the children from the first marriage and felt that they were "just hanging out for his money," but as next of kin she allowed them to facilitate care arrangements. All three children felt Zoe was a "gold-digger" and were suspicious of her motives. Upon learning that Paul had altered his will to leave most/all of his inheritance for his children some time earlier, Zoe appeared at the inpatient unit with two solicitors. She wished to amend the will which had, according to Zoe, been Paul's wish before he entered the hospice. When Zoe came to amend the will with the solicitors, Paul was bed-bound, fluctuating in and out of conscious state, and while rousable, could not muster more than a few words, but was agreeable and cooperative to requests. A member of the nursing staff witnessed the interaction between Paul, Zoe and the two solicitors, and quickly alerted the medical team. The interaction was ceased, and a private discussion took place with the trio and medical staff. Zoe was extremely unhappy with the medical opinion that Paul no longer had capacity to sign a will, and threatened the doctor with legal action. Two of Paul's children returned, found Zoe engaged in discussion with the doctors and became angered when they were aware of the solicitors' presence and intent behind the visit. A heated argument ensued on the inpatient ward.

Intervention: The family were asked to leave the ward environment, social work engaged with the solicitors, and Paul died soon after amidst ongoing conflict.

9.5 The Distant Relative Syndrome

(Also known as the family member who "comes out of the woodwork" (Kramer and Boelk 2015) and described in the literature as "The daughter from California syndrome" (Molloy et al. 1991)).

This situation of family conflict arises when a member of the family, not involved with the patient's care, "flies in" during the late stages of a patient's illness. They are critical of the primary caregiver, undermining of the treatment plans, challenging of medical and nursing staff, and impeding of progress.

Carole was the youngest daughter of Mary, a 77-year-old woman with advanced Alzheimer's Disease and renal failure. Sue, Mary's oldest daughter, had never married and had always lived with her mother, being her primary carer for 10 years since the onset of Mary's dementia. She had left her employment as a receptionist in a medical practice to devote herself to her mother. Carole, on the other hand, had gone to university to study law, had married a wealthy man and led an active social life in a distant state. Her only contact with her mother since Mary's seventieth birthday had been monthly phone calls until her mother became too demented to respond appropriately to the calls. Mary had been diagnosed with an invasive basal cell carcinoma on her cheek a few months previously, but Sue had agreed with the doctors that in view of her dementia and renal failure she would not be a suitable candidate for the invasive surgery required. Sue said her mother had talked to her about her wishes if she became too unwell to make decisions for herself, while she was still competent, and would not have wanted to have facial surgery. Mary was admitted to a palliative care unit for symptom control of pain and possible end-of-life care. When Carole heard of her mother's cancer she arrived within days, demanding to know why her mother's cancer was not being treated. She was aghast at the disfiguration of her mother's face and her general deterioration. She had not seen her mother for 7 years and accused Sue of neglect. She threatened medical staff with legal action if they did not surgically remove the cancer and challenged them about the opiate medication being given to Mary for pain, blaming it for her cognitive decline.

Intervention: It was evident to staff that Carole was feeling guilt about her own neglect of her mother and projected this as blame onto Sue and the treating team. She was in denial about the gravity of her mother's health and disrupted the care plan by her interference. Staff had to be aware of their countertransference feelings of anger and spend time with Carole to bring her into the clinical reality. Other staff members supported Sue and ultimately it was possible for both daughters to meet with the psychologist to speak of their very different experiences of grief over the loss of their mother. During this session Carole was able to tearfully thank Sue for the care of their mother.

9.6 The Angry Family

Patients and families bring their worlds into the treating team dynamic. Pre-existing conflicts can be augmented under the stress of forced reunions with estranged family members. Deeply buried guilt, shame, helplessness, loss of control, or emotionally charged states can bubble to the surface creating a situation ripe for misdirected discharges of anger toward staff members, who are often a "safer" target than the patient or other family members. Lifelong maladaptive relational patterns of family members can be repeated with the treating team, and the recipients of these intense interactions can experience strong countertransference reactions. In heightened angry states, family members may experience any attempts by staff to explain or clarify their concerns as an affront and can further agitate the situation. The physiological arousal of intense anger can interfere with information processing, and misinterpretation is common. Staff often find it difficult to not take it personally, and a space outside the clinical interaction is often useful to gain perspective and understand the "true" cause of the family members' anger.

Agnes was a widowed, 79-year-old lady with metastatic oesophageal carcinoma, admitted to inpatient palliative care for symptom management which turned into end-of-life care. One of her five daughters Eleanor (who was her main carer) was noted to be anxious, irritable, verbally aggressive and frequently criticised the care given by all staff in an accusatory and angry way. Barraged by angry, critical comments and a daily litany of complaints, staff become avoidant, fearful, and angry. Eleanor seemed to have an inexhaustible list of problems and had begun documenting all clinical interactions in a notebook kept by the bedside. A family meeting was held to address Eleanor's concerns. Unfortunately, any attempt to clarify or address Eleanor's concerns only seemed to fuel her rage, despite many overtures by staff to listen to and address her issues.

She continued to say, "No-one is listening to me! You're all just trying to cover yourselves!." Following the meeting, a referral to the psychosocial team was made. The psychologist engaged the daughter following the meeting. Eleanor proceeded to explain that throughout her mother's illness, treating clinicians had not paid enough attention to her mother, and "...that's why she's dying! Because no-one listened to me!." She continued to rail against "inexperienced" and "incompetent" staff she had encountered, and blamed them all for her mother's illness and decline.

Intervention: The psychologist allowed her to speak, resisting any temptation to clarify, explain, "fix" or challenge her concerns. As she continued, the psychologist noted that Eleanor began to slow her speech, sigh heavily, her volume lowered, and the content began to shift from complaints towards themes of sadness at losing her mother. Gradually her anger began to soften into a well-protected grief, cordoned off by anger and blame. The psychologist offered empathic support and enquired how the daughter was coping through all of this. Eleanor immediately burst into tears. She began to talk of her sadness at losing the "rock" in her life, her own role as a "protector" in the family, and described her propensity to accept an inordinate amount of responsibility for "fixing" everyone in the family. Yet she could not "fix" her mother's terminal illness and felt guilty, ashamed, helpless and useless – that she had "failed" her mother. After some time, the psychologist then reflected back and empathized with Eleanor's situation and role in the family, in light of the current circumstances. Once this had been offered, the psychologist then addressed the issues raised, stating that there seemed to be misunderstandings that had occurred between the treating team, and clarified some of the concerns highlighted by Eleanor. With her anger defused and a feeling of alliance with the psychologist, Eleanor was more able to engage in productive dialogue with the team.

Warren was the 35-year-old husband of Cheryl, who was transferred from a country hospital to a metropolitan palliative inpatient unit for management of pain related to her ovarian cancer. He worked in a small town as a self-employed carpenter and had not been able to complete jobs because of the need to care for his ill wife and two young sons. The couple had high hopes that the major centre would fix Cheryl's problems and they could get back to a normal life. Scans performed at the country hospital had revealed extensive peritoneal and retroperitoneal metastasis of Cheryl's disease, but this information had not been conveyed to the couple prior to transfer. The palliative care team were unaware of the couple's ignorance of her devastating rapidly progressive disease, and it was only during a bedside ward round that this became apparent. The discussion with the consultant gently moved from plans for alleviating pain to the implications of the scan findings for her prognosis. Warren watched on in shock and disbelief as his wife started to sob uncontrollably. He started to scream at the consultant, "What's the matter with you people? We came here believing you were going to make her well again and now you tell us she is going to die!" He clenched his fists as if about to punch the consultant, then abruptly left the room, yelling loudly and punched the walls of the corridor.

Intervention: The team psychiatrist was passing the room at the time these events occurred and witnessed Warren's uncontrolled rage. She had met Warren on Cheryl's admission and noted that he was highly stressed. She had some inkling about what may have triggered this display of anger from the multidisciplinary team meeting, held just prior to the ward round. She guided Warren to a quiet room and invited him to sit down, but he refused and paced around the room smashing his fist into the palm of his hand. The psychiatrist pulled two chairs into a comfortable distance from one another, without impeding Warren's space, sat down and talked in a soothing manner, speculating in general terms about what might have transpired as Warren was unable to speak. Gradually Warren took over the story and described how cruelly his hopes and dreams had been blown apart, how angry he was that no-one had prepared them for this. He was angered by both Cheryl's oncologist in the country hospital and the heartless way the palliative care consultant had broken the news. These feelings were not challenged, but empathic statements were made about the shock he must have experienced when he had come with such different expectations. He sat down and put his head in his hands and sobbed. "Cheryl knew she was sick – she had lost 20 kg and was having these severe pains in her back which hadn't been there before. She said something bad was happening, but I wouldn't hear of it – I told her she had to be positive, that the doctors in the city would sort it out," he explained. Ultimately Warren became more composed, although he looked shattered and exhausted. "I'd better go back in to Cheryl. Thanks," he said as he left the consultation. Warren was seen on a daily basis where he continued to express his grief, and was able to start to make plans for his wife's end-of-life care and the care of his sons. Liaison with the country oncologist revealed that Warren had blocked frank discussions of the scan results – "we don't want to hear anything bad" prior to transfer. The rift in the relationship between the palliative care consultant and the couple was healed after they sat together and talked about the experience, which had been highly distressing for both of them.

A summary of the approaches that can be used to manage challenging communication is provided in Table 5 (Philip and Kissane 2017).

Table 5 Strategies for the difficult communication encounter (Philip and Kissane 2017)

Sequence of strategies for the difficult communication encounter[a]
1. Preparation – Be clear about clinical details and investigation results prior to meeting the patient. Make time
2. Listen – Using open-ended questions, allow the narrative to unfold. Develop a shared understanding of the experience, and develop shared goals from this point
3. Offer an empathic acknowledgment of the emotions expressed
4. Provide symptom relief
5. Involve experienced clinicians
6. If anger persists, reconsider approach. Important role for senior staff to guide this approach
7. and model appropriate behavior
8. Consider limit setting to the expression of emotion, where behavios present danger or disruption to care
9. Support of the team
10. Consider a second opinion or the involvement of an independent broker

[a]Content reproduced with permission from Philip and Kissane (2017)

9.7 The "Special" Family

Problems can arise in the palliative care of patients who are members of families that are famous, have celebrity status, are narcissistic, or contain healthcare professionals, important figures in public life, or religious leaders. Main wrote a classic paper on "the special patient" in "The Ailment" (Main 1957), which outlines how such a patient causes an unhealthy deviation from usual practices of staff on a psychiatric unit, with deleterious outcomes for both patient and staff. These observations are apt for "special" family members in the palliative setting.

Barbara was a 52-year-old woman diagnosed with lung cancer some years ago; a recent subacute cognitive change and subsequent MRI revealed that she had developed leptomeningeal metastases. Treatment was unable to halt progression of the disease and her care needs escalated to the point of requiring 24-h care. Barbara was in a long term, same sex relationship with a dermatologist, Nadia, and they lived together with their four children. Upon admission, Nadia made it perfectly clear to the staff that she was medically trained and able to assist with much of the care for Barbara as she "knew her needs better than anyone." The staff were very moved by the plight of the young family and the staff accommodated the wishes of the family as much as possible. It quickly became apparent that allowing the leeway of Nadia to determine care created major problems. Nadia had little to no understanding of palliative treatments and began to accuse staff of inappropriate treatments that "bordered on inhumane." Barbara's family had indicated that Nadia was not on good terms with them, and that Barbara had separated from Nadia some years previously before returning when she became ill, but things were "less than harmonious" prior to her deterioration. Nadia refused to speak with junior doctors and only allowed specific nurses to interact with the family. When Barbara was able to voice her requests, Nadia would override them by stating that she was "confused" and she knew what Barbara "really wanted." This included attempting to withhold pain relief and rousing Barbara in order to perform physiotherapy movements (not indicated by the palliative physiotherapist). Staff were extremely distressed by Nadia's care which was causing unnecessary pain and discomfort to Barbara. When medical staff explained that her disease had progressed and the need to rationalise medications in favour of comfort care, Nadia was enraged. She demanded that Barbara be given intravenous fluids despite medical staff explaining that this would overload her lungs. Nadia again accused medical staff of "inhumane" treatment, threatened legal action and going to the media. She frequently made comments that "no-one would treat their dog this way" and berated the medical team for their "so-called expertise."

Intervention: Unfortunately, attempts at trying to address concerns with Nadia resulted in family meetings being cancelled at the last minute, outright refusal to engage with any supports (including psycho-oncology, pastoral care and social work), splitting behaviours, and increasingly entitled demands directed at younger, less experienced staff who were more likely to give in to her demands. An urgent meeting was called with the head of department, senior consultant, nurse unit manager and social worker. Nadia laughed at attempts to clarify boundaries, offers of support for her, the offer to move Barbara to another inpatient facility if she felt the inpatient care was not adequate, and agreed mockingly to the new treatment plan whereby Nadia was to have less involvement in the medical care. She would appear to agree to new arrangements, only to later question and again belittle staff, attempting to override treatment plans and take matters into her own hands.

Intervention: The staff required multiple debriefings to discuss their anger about Nadia. Many felt highly distressed that Nadia was dictating Barbara's care in a "cruel" way, and were angry at how such a situation had come to be in the first place. Reflection and unpacking revealed that the standard manner of providing care had come to be exploited and taken advantage of in this instance. Staff realised that the family-centered approach of allowing family members to participate in care, "going above and beyond" to allow the family some control, in this case served only to feed the entitled and inappropriate demands of Nadia. Senior staff were allocated to Barbara's care and the tighter boundaries seemed to contain Nadia's problematic behaviours, but she continued to denigrate staff and the quality of care. Barbara died 12 weeks after admission. Staff continued to be affected by this situation for some time and required multiple staff support sessions.

9.8 The Family with a Member Who Has Mental Illness or Severe Personality Disorder

Family members who suffer from mental illness or severe personality disorder may relapse or decompensate, under the stress of having a close relative nearing the end of life. The dying patient may have been an important part of the family member's support network and may have played a role in monitoring symptoms of relapse or medication compliance. It is important to check that the family member has support from their psychiatrist, psychologist, case manager, or GP during this stressful time. For family members who have a history of unstable mental health, it is important to have a contingency plan in place to deal with any disturbed mental state that arises in the palliative setting. It is equally important not to fearfully anticipate difficulties with family members who have a mental illness and to afford them the same respect and opportunities for involvement in medical updates and planning meetings.

Anastasija was a 94-year-old widowed woman with end-stage heart failure. She had lived with her son Frank, who had experienced significant mental health issues for many years. Her other children had maintained a relationship with their mother Anastasija, but did not have a relationship with Frank, as he was reclusive, extremely avoidant, could become verbally aggressive, and was "peculiar" according to Anastasija's daughter, Marianne. Anastasija had survived the Holocaust in a concentration camp along with her husband, and they emigrated to Australia and raised their family. As part of her post-traumatic stress from her time in the forced labour camp, Anastasija had a long history of anxiety and hypervigilant behaviours. Prior to admission to the palliative care inpatient unit, she was admitted to hospital after phoning Marianne when she had fallen at home after a fainting episode. Frank had refused to call an ambulance at the time. Upon admission it was apparent that Anastasija was deteriorating in health, and would remain in palliative care until her death. Her children were very concerned that Frank would not cope with the idea that their mother was dying, and could decompensate or become violent.

Intervention: All efforts to make contact with Frank were unfruitful. Attempts to include him in family meetings were met with unanswered calls or letters and a failure to turn up. Staff had been informed about the possibility of Frank experiencing a relapse, and a management plan was given to staff should Frank become psychotic or distressed on the ward. Frank eventually accepted notes left at the doorstep by his sister Marianne. Given the treating team had not actually met Frank and were not aware of any current risks, it was difficult to initiate mental health crisis team involvement. His siblings reported that he had been non-compliant with mental health services previously, and had been discharged by his psychiatrist and case manager. Eventually Anastasija entered a terminal phase of illness. The treating team and Anastasija's other children remained aware of possible outbursts when Frank eventually came to say his goodbyes. He refused to engage with any staff or family, and returned to living a reclusive life at his home. The team felt quite powerless to assist or provide support to Frank; they could only provide a management plan, and offer crisis numbers to him and his family, in the hope that he would make contact if assistance was required.

9.9 The Family with a Member Who Has Drug or Alcohol Problems

Drug and alcohol abuse in the family network of a terminally ill patient can impact in a variety of ways. It can preoccupy the patient with concerns about the drug abuser, make a potential source of support emotionally unavailable and even a burden, create circumstances for abuse or diversion of medication supplied for the patient's symptom control, and create escalation of abuse through threat of loss; and the behavior of these family members in a palliative care setting may cause disruption of care delivery and increase staff anxiety.

Louise was aged 72 years and lived in a high-rise apartment with her methamphetamine-addicted 40-year-old son, Sam. She was attended by the community palliative care team, who noted that she had no food in the refrigerator and the patient's cat was not being fed. Sam was diverting her pain medication and as a result, Louise was experiencing poor pain control.

Intervention: Staff attempted to make alternative arrangements for pain medication delivery via her GP, but Louise resisted attempts that might result in causing her son to become displeased and violent. She would not initiate police intervention in the elder abuse that was obviously occurring. The community team attempted to deal with this situation of extreme compromise by providing ongoing support for Louise. They visited Louise in pairs during this conflicted period of dependency, and attempted to engage (unsuccessfully) drug and alcohol services. Louise received no helpful advice from an online self-help group, where other contributors were not experiencing life-limiting illness.

9.10 The Abusive Family

Abuse of a patient by family members may be a long-standing pattern of behavior or may arise out of frustration with the demands and burden of caregiving by vulnerable individuals. It may take the form of neglect, rough handling, outright physical abuse, withholding of medication, over-sedation, or verbal abuse. On rare occasions, sexual abuse can occur. Situations which heighten risk of abuse include personality change or cognitive decline in the patient (due to cerebral pathology, comorbid dementia, or undiagnosed psychiatric disorder), pre-existing conflict with the caregiver, substance abuse, and poor internal resources and social supports of the caregiver. When the patient is cared for at home, community workers may suspect abuse if the patient shows signs of unexplained injuries, appears neglected, or seems frightened in the presence of the carer. The community workers may not be allowed to speak to the patient alone to explore their concerns. In an inpatient setting, a patient who is being abused at home may exhibit fear at the prospect of discharge after stabilization of symptoms but be reluctant to divulge abuse because of compromising dependency on the caregiver. Sometimes it is the patient who has been abusive in the family system, and the dependency needs of progressive illness can elicit different reactions from individual family members.

Rinehart was an 83-year-old man with advanced dementia who was transferred to the palliative care unit via the emergency department, when he suddenly became unresponsive according to family members. He lived with his divorced son, and a daughter who lived close by also identified herself as one of Rinehart's main carers. Upon admission, he was found to be emaciated, dehydrated and had several pressure wounds that caused severe pain. The family would not elaborate on questions regarding the days leading up to his presentation and would not accept that he had dementia, saying he had become more forgetful as "he's an old man now." Moreover, when staff attempted to provide pain relief to Rinehart, they insisted that he would need only paracetamol. Staff were able to obtain records from a previous admission to another hospital, which indicated that the social worker had suspicions that Rinehart was a victim of elder abuse, with belongings being sold off and serious neglect of his physical health. A staff member observed Rinehart's son shaking him roughly and when they intervened, he stated that this was how he roused him.

Intervention: A family meeting was held and Rinehart's son became verbally abusive and threatening. Security was called and rules were put in place regarding the son's behaviour on the ward. He was not to handle Rinehart roughly, and he would be asked to leave if there were outbursts of anger or obstruction of treatment. Social work investigated further and found evidence of elder abuse. They were mandated to apply for a guardianship order to stop finances being drained and to appoint a third party to manage power of attorney matters. While Rinehart's son continued to be angry, he did abide by the rules and boundaries set in place by the team. Nonetheless, staff continued to feel unsafe because of his threats and unpredictability, and required regular staff support and guidance. Rinehart deteriorated and died before arrangements could be carried out regarding placement. Staff were distressed about Rinehart's condition on arrival, but were comforted that they were able to provide him with a safe place in which to die. They were concerned that Rinehart's son would return and become violent as he had threatened, but this did not eventuate.

Helen was the 42-year-old daughter of a 68-year-old man with lung cancer admitted for end-of-life care. Her father had been an alcoholic all his life and had been sexually and physically abusive to his three daughters. Her mother had been passively collusive in the abuse and left the family, leaving the girls abandoned, unprotected and homeless at a young age. Two of the daughters went on to have chaotic lives with failed relationships, children from different partners and drug abuse; but Helen, although a single mother, had become a health care worker. Helen had been estranged from her father for many years, but when she learned of his cancer, she made contact with him and visited him daily after work. During his admission to hospital, she continued her vigil to the neglect of her work and her children. Her sisters were furious with Helen for showing compassion to "this animal" and came to the ward to upbraid her and scream abuse at their father, saying he had ruined their lives and was now getting his "just deserts."

Intervention: A meeting was held with the three sisters to help defuse and contain the intense emotions expressed on the ward. It was evident that Helen still held a fantasy of finding the "good father" and had not addressed her history of traumatic attachments, becoming a "wounded healer" in the service of others. She was encouraged to seek individual psychotherapy.

9.11 The Family Contesting Inheritance

There are many circumstances that lead to arguments about the potential inheritors of the estate of the dying patient. These can begin even before the patient's death and can be played out distastefully in a palliative setting and extend into the legal arena. They may occur around warring factions in the family, former and new partners, conflict between families of origin of the patient and partner, rejection of the patient's choice of partner by the family, and disappointment that the will is made out to charities rather than family members. The team may receive requests for evaluation of competency and other information for which motives are unclear. Staff may feel distressed by the discordance between their focus on the patient's care and the extended family's preoccupation with material issues beyond the patient's death.

Benjamin was a 50-year-old interior designer with stage IV glioblastoma multiforme. He was a divorced father of three children, and was described by his few friends as someone who was extremely "self-absorbed." He had a lifelong history of ruptured relationships and punitive gestures towards those he believed had slighted him. His former wife Rachel, had supported Benjamin by bringing their children to the hospital to visit him during his dying weeks, so that meaningful legacy work could take place. During this time, Benjamin was amiable and pleasant. However, Rachel had previously received a barrage of angry, abusive letters in the 3 years between their divorce and his admission to palliative care. The final "punishment," according to Rachel, was the "deliberately" impractical will instructions whereby Benjamin had bequeathed his superannuation death payouts to his young children in manner that precluded access to the finances. Distribution of these finances were to be legally and meticulously determined and approved by Benjamin's sister (Jane). Jane despised Rachel and had not spoken to her since the birth of Rachel and Benjamin's first child. The children had no relationship with Benjamin's family, and Rachel's attempts to contact Jane to discuss the situation were met with unreturned phone calls, blocked emails, and silence. Rachel, who had existing Power of Attorney as Benjamin had forgotten to change this, contacted the palliative care unit requesting release of records of cognitive assessment around the period of his admission date. She had mistakenly thought that he had made his will while incompetent. However, he was in fact an inpatient at another facility at the time of making the will (which stipulated strict conditions on the inheritance for his children) and had undergone formal neuropsychological assessment, which had deemed him competent.

Intervention: Rachel was allowed to ventilate her feelings and concerns. The ongoing barrage of abuse and "punishment" of Rachel by Benjamin had continued post-death and Rachel felt distressed by the fact that "even now, he won't give me peace." Due to confidentiality and privacy laws, Rachel was provided with the information to apply for access to Benjamin's case notes via the federal Freedom of Information Act (which would indicate that neuropsychological assessment had taken place elsewhere, and that he was indeed competent at the time of writing his will). Benjamin's behaviour in spelling out his final wishes were in keeping with a lifelong narcissistic personality structure. Rachel was advised to seek legal aid, and obtain psychological support for the resurfacing of traumatic experiences in her relationship with Benjamin.

Simon, a 45-year-old stockbroker with stage IV colorectal cancer and brain metastases, was partnered to Mike, a 43-year-old physiotherapist. Simon and Mike had been in a same sex relationship for over 10 years and had lived together for over 7 years. Simon was admitted to an inpatient palliative care unit after a significant functional decline at home, and Mike's difficulty in managing Simon's care needs. During this admission, conflicts between Simon's family and Mike began to emerge. Simon's family had long expressed dissatisfaction with their relationship, trying on several occasions to force Simon to end the relationship. They had even told Simon that Mike was having an affair, and that Mike would end up "taking him to the cleaners." Simon told the psychosocial team member that he did not want his sister and nephew to visit, as they "only want to cause trouble." Mike described a telephone conversation he had with Simon's sister, where he was threatened with being thrown out of "Simon's house" when Simon died, and that he "wouldn't get a cent" of Simon's money. Mike and Simon had always had shared finances and despite Mike's name being on the title of their home, he was very distressed by the situation. Mike was unable to tell Simon exactly what his sister was saying, as he did not want to upset him further. Mike approached the psychosocial team member for advice as he was now not sleeping and struggling at work. He was afraid that every time his mobile rang it might be Simon's sister with another demand.

Intervention: The psychosocial team member encouraged Mike to obtain legal advice. Accurate information would likely reduce his anxiety, and give him space to be with his partner as he approached end of life. Simon died a few weeks later and the psychiatrist on team was approached by Simon's sister. She requested a report of Simon's competency assessment, because the will was made after diagnosis and she was planning to contest it.

9.12 Culture Clashes Within the Families of the Patient and Caregiver

Culture clashes are not only seen between the treating team and the patient's family but within the family system itself. This may arise when there are different levels of acculturation to the host culture, and it is not always the older members of the family who strictly adhere to the values and practices of their culture. Younger members who have been educated, even born, in the country of the treating culture, may be more fervent about keeping the traditions of their culture of origin.

It may also arise when there is intermarriage between different cultures, each group wanting to claim the right to determine information-sharing, decision-making, truth-telling, and rituals at the end of life.

Hanh was a 70-year-old man from Indo-China, who had arrived in the country as a boat refugee from his mainland during major conflict. His children had been born in his new country of refuge, but still held traditional beliefs about truth-telling. Hanh was admitted to an inpatient palliative care unit with a newly diagnosed, but very advanced, neuroendocrine tumour. His son, who had achieved high qualifications in his country of birth, insisted that the medical team not divulge to his father the nature of his terminal illness. He made sure he was present for every consultation with medical teams, to enforce the withholding of information about his prognosis. On one occasion, a medical student from his culture of origin reported that he was mis-translating the guarded words from the oncologist, to provide a more benign interpretation of his illness. The issue came to a head when the patient, in great distress, asked a nurse directly (in English) "Am I dying?"

Intervention: A meeting with the son and other members of the family was convened. It was explained that Hanh had an instinctive knowledge about his condition and was more distressed by the uncertainty, rather than the reality, of his short prognosis. It was emphasised that he wanted and needed to say his good-byes and prepare a legacy for his family.

Oliver was a 40-year-old man of south Asian descent with lung cancer and brain metastases admitted for end-of-life care. He was married with no children, and his wife (Sofia), was of African descent. Upon admission, it was evident that the young man's family did not approve of Sofia as an appropriate wife for their son and brother. The pre-existing conflict had become so intense in recent times that Oliver's siblings and parents had sought legal advice, with the intent of challenging Sofia's role as medical power of attorney. The family had repeatedly accused Sofia of delaying Oliver's treatment and keeping them away from him; it was evident that they were unaware of, or in denial about, the gravity of his condition. His family's anger towards Sofia was vocalized strongly, and their repeated attempts to inform staff about his "wicked wife," in order to collude with the family against Sofia, annoyed staff. Despite wishing to appear "neutral," most were quite obviously siding with Sofia. Conflicts escalated in the ward environment and then, unexpectedly, Sofia started to become verbally aggressive and accusatory towards any staff she saw speaking with Oliver's family, and requested that they should not provide care and treatment for him. The team began to realise that the family's "denial" was due more to a lack of awareness of his condition, as they had been allowed limited access to Oliver. His father struggled with the idea of losing his only son. Not being privy to the particulars of his son's disease and illness trajectory, only fueled his anger and suspicion that Sofia had contributed to Oliver's deterioration due to neglect and improper care. As time progressed, Sofia became increasingly restrictive of the family's time with Oliver, despite their pleas for a number of bedside rituals in keeping with their cultural traditions. Sofia would only allow them to see Oliver if they promised to drop their legal demands. She set visitation restrictions and insisted Oliver could only be seen in her presence. She also requested that staff cease engagement with certain family members.

Intervention: Family meetings were stilted and uncomfortable, but all agreed that Oliver's comfort was paramount. Staff implored the family to leave conflict outside of Oliver's room, as he was quite obviously affected by the distress and arguments that took place at his bedside. All agreed that this behaviour was not in the best interests of Oliver's care, and temporary visiting arrangements were agreed upon. Psychological support was accepted by most parties. The majority of them could acknowledge that anger was "easier" than being overwhelmed by the grief of losing Oliver, but they continued to feel anger towards one another. All parties were discouraged from using existing time with Oliver to ask him questions about who he preferred in the room with him (sometimes recording his responses to be used in argument, despite his worsening cognitive impairment). They were encouraged instead to think about how they could spend their time with him in a meaningful way. The last few days of his life were more peaceful as Sofia became exhausted and her absences meant that the family of origin could visit. Each family member devised personal ways to engage Oliver (with a favourite song, stories to recall), that allowed them to engage without conflict as the focus. Oliver's death reignited tensions however, as Sofia notified Oliver's extended family first, instead of his siblings and parents. The family were again extremely angry and felt this was Sofia's final punishment towards them. All family members and Sofia were offered post-bereavement support, but their grief was soon overshadowed by re-emerging anger as the legal threats resurfaced.

9.13 The Refugee/Asylum Seeker

Refugees and asylum seekers who are diagnosed with life-threatening illness are a particularly disadvantaged group. Often having fled war or persecution, they are separated from extended family who may have been tortured or killed. They may have poor language skills in the country to which they have fled and may have difficulty practicing the rituals related to their country of origin, particularly in relation to illness and the role of the family in provision of care.

Hasib was a 40-year-old man from the Middle East who had arrived by boat as an illegal immigrant, 18 years previously. He spent some time in a detention centre and ultimately worked in a catering business, before being diagnosed with a slow-growing brain tumour as an incidental finding following brain imaging after an accident. Neurosurgery was proposed but declined, until he developed neurological symptoms from the tumour a year later. He subsequently had four neurosurgical operations and brain irradiation over the ensuing 8 years. His admission to palliative care occurred after a gradual decline in his functional abilities. His illness course had been characterized by difficult behaviours, particularly towards women, and non-compliance with treatments and appointments. Many representations were made on his behalf to bring over his mother and brother to care for him, and to establish accommodation and community support. It was difficult to establish over this period whether the difficulties in his interpersonal interactions were related to his brain tumour, his post-surgical deficits, the steroids used to reduce intracranial pressure, his background of trauma, or amplification of symptoms to achieve the goal of bringing out his family. The only relative of Hasib lived in a distant state and he became an advocate in the latter months of his illness.

Intervention: The social worker spent an inordinate amount of time dealing with various advocacy agencies, government, and legal departments negotiating the most humane and culturally sensitive way of dealing with his end-of-life care. Hasib had a fluctuating mental state with intermittent seizures over 8 months of acute palliative inpatient care. The length of stay is indicative of the complexity of the case and the "bending over backwards" to provide care in a situation of uncertain prognosis. Although there were times over the previous months that staff thought he was deteriorating, there were no current indications that dying was imminent. He was unable to walk, almost blind and required full nursing care. Efforts to fund a medical air transport to a hospice near his only relative in the distant state were unsuccessful. Ultimately the local Muslim community gathered together to provide care in the grounds of a nearby mosque, and some members of this community came to the inpatient unit to learn how to perform his care needs. They believed that all things are determined by Allah, including whatever may eventuate from this courageous decision.

9.14 The Criminal "Family"

Everyone, from whatever background, ultimately dies – sometimes from a terminal illness, rather than a gunshot wound as in the case of many with a criminal background. If the patient is a prisoner at the time of need for palliative services, there are protocols and procedures for management, however deficient these might be. Some patients are associated with the "underworld" without a recorded criminal history, and "the Family" visitors to the patient in a palliative care setting can cause feelings of anxiety and menace in staff.

Leo was in his 70's and dying of lung cancer. A former gangster, he had reformed and was a negotiator between warring factions of the local Mafia. He had been in the process of negotiation with these factions, when a prominent member of one of the gangs was shot in a public restaurant where the negotiations were taking place. He had been called as a witness in court proceedings and was therefore a threat to the perpetrators. The hearing had been delayed until he recovered. Captive in his hospital bed, he was a perfect target for anyone who wanted to silence him. Most of this information was unknown to staff before they started to feel uneasy in the presence of "strange" visitors and tensions in the room during the visits.

Intervention: A referral to the psychosocial team resulted in obtaining a full history of Leo's background and revealed the circumstances of his predicament. He was provided with psychotherapeutic support which allowed him to provide his life narrative, including his transformation to the "good guy," trusted by all gang members, with a secret mission of bringing an end to gangland killings. Extra security measures were introduced to protect Leo, staff and other patients, including searching of visitors and presence of security staff during any visit.

10 Principles of Management of Challenging Family Situations

- Understand as much as possible about the patient and family before contact with palliative services in all circumstances.
- Be aware of potential problems.
- Take care not to judge prematurely, despite the forewarnings – family dynamics change in the face of life-threatening illness.
- Be alert to issues that arise for the first time in the face of impending death of a family member.
- Take into consideration family dynamics, the member most trusted with decision-making, unresolved issues, and cultural/religious/belief systems in planning care.
- Discuss the approach to care with other team members/supervisors.
- Ensure clear goals of care are established with the family, and where there are different points of view, arrive at a consensus early in the contact.
- Support family members by utilizing family meetings to discuss discordant points of view and establish common goals.
- Be prepared to adapt the treatment plan according to emerging perspectives and understandings of the family as the clinical situation evolves.
- Remember that this is a process, things will change, and usually for the better.

11 Staff Support

The case scenarios described above emphasize the need for a space in which staff can "step back" from the clinical situation to consider the complex interplay of influences of a challenging family dynamic. These include the personal histories of family members, the family system including alliances and conflicts, interpersonal patterns of relating, how families express emotionality, and how the staff themselves may have been triggered emotionally.

Many studies have indicated that repeated exposure to dying patients and grieving families can leave staff vulnerable to compassion fatigue and burnout (Slocum-Gori et al. 2013; Sansó et al. 2015). When interacting with challenging patients and families in emotionally charged encounters, staff may be more vulnerable to being themselves triggered emotionally. The ensuing cascade of countertransference reactions can easily pull staff into an intense dynamic that is not fully recognized or understood (Katz and Johnson 2016). Even the use of the "difficult" patient/family label cues the need for staff to carefully consider their own reactions as a "diagnostic barometer" and to acquire a deeper understanding of what the patient and family members bring to the clinical interaction (Philip and Kissane 2017). While some staff may happily reside in the idea that it is merely a "difficult" family, the clinical moment holds a complex, inter-relational dynamic where all parties bring their own histories, biases, patterns of relationship, communication skill level, and attunement. As staff, the need to develop greater awareness of our own emotional reactions, personal histories, biases, experiences, and personal triggers that can unwittingly eclipse our professional objectivity and clinical interactions cannot be overstated (Katz and Johnson 2016). Creating a culture of encouraged reflective practice where staff can consider personal or triggered responses can increase awareness of unexamined punitive reactions, over-involvement, helplessness, avoidance, intellectual distancing, or other defenses that staff may experience (Sansó et al. 2015; Katz and Johnson 2016; Turner et al. 2011).

11.1 Types of Support

While staff burnout can be attributed to many factors both personal, inter-relational, or organizational, higher burnout scores have been found to be associated with perceived lack of psychological support in one's place of work (Wenzel et al. 2011). Palliative care teams need to be especially mindful of provision of regular staff support, as compacted grief and other unexplored emotional consequences of palliative care work can be discharged in heightened interactions (Katz and Johnson 2016).

Staff support is multifaceted and includes discussion and education around psychological issues of patients and family members, a forum for staff to offer their "thoughts and feelings about their work," and an opportunity to provide peer support (Parkes 2000). One such model, the "Schwartz Rounds" has been increasingly adapted internationally across a range of clinical settings. The model features regularly scheduled sessions around particular cases where health providers can openly and honestly discuss the social and emotional issues they face in caring for patients and families. The focus is on the human dimension of medicine, and testimonies of the benefit of this approach can be accessed on the Schwartz Center website (www.theschwartzcentre.org).

A review of staff support in oncology health professionals indicated that promotion of staff "resilience" required a multipronged approach of both informal and formal interventions including skill development, communication skills training, provision of staff support (using expert facilitation to manage complex reactions and dynamics), reflective practice, mentorship, and supervision, as key strategies to support and educate staff (Turner et al. 2011).

12 Education and Management Strategies

Education remains a key requirement, as staff often find themselves in highly charged situations with little or no formal training regarding management of such scenarios (Turner et al. 2011; Aycock and Boyle 2009). In particularly challenging interactions, Philip and Kissane (2017) discuss important, but often overlooked, components of good communication. The importance of "staying present" with the distress of a patient and family member, even when it feels difficult or unjustified, cannot be underestimated. The subtle avoidance that staff can unconsciously promote by switching focus during an emotional discussion, to addressing physical concerns, can augment patients' and families' anger and experience of feeling misheard and disregarded (Philip and Kissane 2017).

However, while good communication skills may go a long way in defusing challenging interactions with family members, there are many times when anger or other strong emotion persists. These emotions may occur despite all reasonable attempts to defuse and calm a heightened dynamic with family members. The focus should then shift to supporting the staff directly involved, as the intense emotional impact of dealing with challenging families can be devastating for the morale of treating teams (Philip et al. 2007; Feely et al. 2013).

Education and staff support is particularly necessary in situations where a family member has personality disorder (particularly borderline and narcissistic personality disorders). One of the most well-known defense mechanisms of an individual with borderline personality disorder is "splitting." In such cases, the family member will "split" clinicians into "all good" or "all bad," due to the inability of the individual to hold ambivalent feelings toward others (based on early caregiver attachment experiences) (Gabbard and Wilkinson 2000). This can be most commonly identified in situations where staff experience strong reactions in apparent polarity to each other. For example, anger, anxiety, punitive impulses, exist at one end of the spectrum, compared with over-involvement, wish to rescue, and feeling that the staff member is the only one who really understands the individual (Feely et al. 2013; Hay and Passik 2000). Splitting has been well documented and can create havoc within treating teams. Educating staff about the individual with borderline personality disorder includes understanding the defenses exhibited by someone with borderline personality disorder; how to set boundaries in a respectful, nonpunitive manner; providing consistency in response across the team and operating as a unified front; not colluding with attempts to downgrade other staff and not getting caught in the hubris of idealization; not taking devaluation personally; understanding that the person with a personality disorder is genuinely distressed and doing their best to navigate their suffering in their own way; acknowledging that intense reactions are likely in staff and providing a space to explore these in staff support; and where possible, enlisting the assistance of a psychiatrist or psychologist to help formulate a management plan (via the psychosocial team, consultation/liaison service, or the person's own mental health professional) (Feely et al. 2013; Hay and Passik 2000; McLafferty and Childers 2012).

13 Self-Care

In addition to promotion of personal self-care strategies (Swetz et al. 2009; Kearney et al. 2009), other interventions facilitating emotional processing of staff include "letting go" of the day's concerns using "release rituals"; (Keene et al. 2010) semi-structured staff bereavement debriefing; (Keene et al. 2010) clinical supervision; (Edmonds et al. 2015); and work environments that encourage expressions of meaning and spirituality (e.g., memorial services, rituals, etc.), which can promote staff resilience and reduce burnout (Holland and Neimeyer 2005).

14 Conclusions

The public image of a palliative care setting is a place of hushed tranquility, soft-shoed steps of compassionate nurses administering gentle care, whispered voices and sounds of birdsong, glimpses of nature through sheer-curtained windows, and delicate strains of music drifting in the background. The reality is that while it can be all these things, it is also a stage where the last drama of life is played out. The audience to this drama can experience the most intense emotions and profound moments of their lives. Staff working in this setting see people behaving at their very best and their very worst (even when the worst is the best they can be in the circumstances). In a sense, the staff and the setting have to serve as the wise and containing parent, a trusted attachment figure who provides a safe haven for those who are frightened, angry, or wretched with emotional pain. While staff are immersed in a particularly difficult family situation, they may feel hurt, incompetent, angry, and exhausted during the experience. However, with the opportunity to share with colleagues and reflect on what forces were at play in the interaction, they can emerge with a sense of privilege from bearing witness to raw, authentic human emotion. There are many ways in which professionals can ease the pain of the family, and it is in the spirit of palliative care that we employ our expertise to this end. Not only does this help the patient to die more peacefully, but the ripple effect of poorly managed crises on surviving family members and generations to come is well known. Not only do staff develop greater self-confidence when they have managed a difficult situation well, but families too can grow from the experience. The greatest reward for staff after a particularly torrid time with a family is the family's acknowledgment of their good work.

15 Summary

This chapter has examined ways of looking at families to provide a framework for understanding what is going on in family dynamics that are experienced as challenging. It has discussed the importance of addressing family needs and assessing all families early in the palliative care context to prepare for potential problems. Apart from taking a comprehensive family history (including intergenerational issues) and being aware of the family context, culture, religious and belief systems, other concepts are important. For example, family competence and attachment styles may assist in the understanding of why some families are particularly challenging and how they may best be managed. Clinical cases illustrate a range of difficult family contexts, with interventions specific for the case outlined briefly and general management principles summarized. The importance of good communication skills training has been emphasized. Each patient and family brings their histories to the treatment setting, and there are established roles and expectations within each culture. In a situation of intense suffering and loss, staff may find it difficult to juggle and make sense of the clash of cultures between the treating system and individual families. Staff support, self-reflection, and supervision are critical components of self-care in this setting.

References

Ainsworth MDS, Blehar MC, Waters E, Wall S, et al. Patterns of attachment: assessed in the strange situation and at home. Hillsdale: Erlbaum; 1978.

Alliance WPC , Organization WH, et al. Global atlas of palliative care at the end of life. London: Worldwide Palliative Care Alliance; 2014.

Ashby M, Mendelson D. Family carers: ethical and legal issues. In: Family carers in palliative care. Oxford: Oxford University Press; 2008.

Aycock N, Boyle D. Interventions to manage compassion fatigue in oncology nursing. Clin J Oncol Nurs. 2009;13(2):183–91.

Baider L, Goldzweig G. Exploration of family care: a multicultural approach. In: Grassi L, Riba M, editors. Clinical psycho-oncology: an international perspective. Chichester: Wiley; 2012. p. 187–96.

Boelk AZ, Kramer BJ. Advancing theory of family conflict at the end of life: a hospice case study. J Pain Symptom Manag. 2012;44(5):655–70.

Bowlby J. Attachment, vol. 1 of attachment and loss. New York: Basic Books; 1969.

Edmonds KP, Yeung HN, Onderdonk C, Mitchell W, Thornberry K. Clinical supervision in the palliative care team setting: a concrete approach to team wellness. J Palliat Med. 2015;18(3):274–7.

Feely MA, Havyer RDA, Lapid MI, Swetz KM. Management of end-of-life care and of difficult behaviors associated with borderline personality disorder. J Pain Symptom Manag. 2013;45(5):934–8.

Gabbard GO, Wilkinson SM. Management of Countertransference with borderline patients. Northvale: Jason Aronson; 2000. 254 p

Given BA, Given CW, Kozachik S. Family support in advanced cancer. CA Cancer J Clin. 2001;51 (4):213–31.

Glaser BG, Strauss AL. Awareness of dying. Piscataway: Transaction Publishers; 1966. 305 p

Gomes B, Calanzani N, Koffman J, Higginson IJ. Is dying in hospital better than home in incurable cancer and what factors influence this? A population-based study. BMC Med. 2015;13:235.

Hay JL, Passik SD. The cancer patient with borderline personality disorder: suggestions for symptom-focused management in the medical setting. Psychooncology. 2000;9(2):91–100.

Hodges LJ, Humphris GM, Macfarlane G. A meta-analytic investigation of the relationship between the psychological distress of cancer patients and their carers. Soc Sci Med. 2005;60(1):1–12.

Holland JM, Neimeyer RA. Reducing the risk of burnout in end-of-life care settings: the role of daily spiritual experiences and training. Palliat Support Care. 2005;3(3):173–81.

Hudson P, Thomas T, Quinn K, Aranda S. Family meetings in palliative care: are they effective? Palliat Med. 2009;23(2):150–7.

Katz RS, Johnson TA. When professionals weep: emotional and countertransference responses in palliative and end-of-life care. New York: Routledge; 2016. 262 p

Kearney MK, Weininger RB, MLS V, Harrison RL, Mount BM. Self-care of physicians caring for patients at the end of life: "Being connected ... a key to my survival". JAMA. 2009;301(11):1155–64.

Keene EA, Hutton N, Hall B, Rushton C. Bereavement debriefing sessions: an intervention to support health care professionals in managing their grief after the

death of a patient. Pediatr Nurs. 2010;36(4):185–9. quiz 190
Kissane DW, Bloch S. Family focused grief therapy: a model of family-centered care during palliative care and bereavement. Buckingham: Open University Press; 2002.
Kissane DW, Zaider TI. Focused family therapy in palliative care and bereavement. In: Handbook of psychotherapy in cancer care. Hoboken: Wiley; 2011. p. 185–97.
Kramer BJ, Boelk AZ. Managing family conflict: providing responsive family care at the end of life. In: Christ GH, Behar LC, Messner C, Behar L, editors. Handbook of oncology social work: psychosocial care for people with cancer. New York: Oxford University Press; 2015. (Ambuel, Back, Boelk, Fineberg, Fisher, Hansen, et al., editors. Handbook of oncology social work: Psychosocial care for people with cancer.).
Kramer BJ, Boelk AZ, Auer C. Family conflict at the end of life: lessons learned in a model program for vulnerable older adults. J Palliat Med. 2006;9(3):791–801.
Lederberg MS. Negotiating the Interface of psycho-oncology and ethics. In: Holland JC, Breitbart WS, Jacobsen PB, Lederberg MS, Loscalzo MJ, McCorkle R, editors. Psycho-oncology. New York: Oxford University Press; 2010. p. 625–9.
Lichtenthal WG, Kissane DW. The management of family conflict in palliative care. Prog Palliat Care. 2008; 16(1):39–45.
Main TF. The ailment. Br J Med Psychol. 1957; 30(3):129–45.
Main M, Solomon J. Procedures for identifying infants as disorganized/disoriented during the Ainsworth strange situation. In: Greenberg MT, Cicchetti D, Cummings EM, editors. Attachment in the preschool years: theory, research, and intervention; 1990. 1, p. 121–60. The University of Chicago Press, Chicago.
McGrath P, Ogilvie KF, Rayner RD, Holewa HF, Patton MAS. The "right story" to the "right person": communication issues in end-of-life care for indigenous people. Aust Health Rev. 2005;29(3):306–16.
McLafferty L, Childers JW. Borderline personality disorder in palliative care #252. J Palliat Med. 2012;15(4):485–6.
Milberg A, Friedrichsen M. Attachment figures when death is approaching: a study applying attachment theory to adult patients' and family members' experiences during palliative home care. Support Care Cancer. 2017;25(7):2267–74.
Molloy DW, Clarnette RM, Braun EA, Eisemann MR, Sneiderman B. Decision making in the incompetent elderly: "The Daughter from California Syndrome". J Am Geriatr Soc. 1991;39(4):396–9.
Parkes CM. Hospice: a psychiatric perspective. In: Handbook of psychiatry in palliative medicine. New York: Oxford University Press; 2000. p. 3–11.
Petersen Y, Koehler L. Application of attachment theory for psychological support in palliative medicine during the terminal phase. Gerontology. 2006;52(2):111–23.
Philip J, Kissane DW. Responding to difficult emotions. In: Oxford textbook of communication in oncology and palliative care. Oxford University Press: Oxford; 2017. p. 91.
Philip J, Gold M, Schwarz M, Komesaroff P. Anger in palliative care: a clinical approach. Intern Med J. 2007;37(1):49–55.
Sansó N, Galiana L, Oliver A, Pascual A. Palliative care professionals' inner life: exploring the relationships among awareness, self-care, and compassion satisfaction and fatigue, burnout, and coping with death. J Pain Symptom Manag. 2015;50:200–7. Available from http://www.sciencedirect.com/science/article/pii/S088539241500086X
Saunders C. The philosophy of terminal care: first published in the management of terminal disease. In: Saunders C, editor. . 1st ed. London: Edward Arnold; 1978. p. 193–202. In: Cicely Saunders. Oxford: Oxford University Press; 2006.
Slocum-Gori S, Hemsworth D, Chan WWY, Carson A, Kazanjian A. Understanding compassion satisfaction, compassion fatigue and burnout: a survey of the hospice palliative care workforce. Palliat Med. 2013;27(2):172–8.
Strada EA. Grief, demoralization, and depression: diagnostic challenges and treatment modalities. Prim Psychiatry. 2009;16(5):49–55.
Surbone A, Kagawa-Singer M. Culture matters as well. J Clin Oncol. 2013;31(22):2832–3.
Swetz KM, Harrington SE, Matsuyama RK, Shanafelt TD, Lyckholm LJ. Strategies for avoiding burnout in hospice and palliative medicine: peer advice for physicians on achieving longevity and fulfillment. J Palliat Med. 2009;12(9):773–7.
Tan A, Zimmermann C, Rodin G. Interpersonal processes in palliative care: an attachment perspective on the patient-clinician relationship. Palliat Med. 2005;19(2):143–50.
Tolstoy L. Anna Karenina. Oxford: Oxford University Press; 1980.
Turner J, Kelly B, Girgis A. Supporting oncology health professionals: a review. Psycho Oncologie. 2011;5(2):77–82.
Wellisch DK, Kissane DW. Family issues and palliative care. In: Handbook of psychiatry in palliative medicine. New York: Oxford University Press; 2009. p. 275–89.
Wenzel J, Shaha M, Klimmek R, Krumm S. Working through grief and loss: oncology nurses' perspectives on professional bereavement. Oncol Nurs Forum. 2011;38(4):E272–82.

Delirium as a Palliative Care Emergency

84

Shirley H. Bush

Contents

S. H. Bush (✉)
Department of Medicine, Division of Palliative Care,
University of Ottawa, Ottawa, ON, Canada

Bruyère Research Institute, Ottawa, ON, Canada

Ottawa Hospital Research Institute, Ottawa, ON, Canada
e-mail: sbush@bruyere.org

R. D. MacLeod, L. Van den Block (eds.), *Textbook of Palliative Care*,
https://doi.org/10.1007/978-3-319-77740-5_87

Abstract
This chapter considers delirium in the context of a palliative care emergency. It reviews screening for delirium, tools to confirm the clinical diagnosis of delirium, and diagnostic challenges. It describes both the nonpharmacological and pharmacological management of delirium. It also reviews the delirium experience and associated distress. It concludes with a brief discussion of the role of palliative sedation for refractory delirium at the end of life.

1 Introduction

Delirium is a complex and often distressing neurocognitive syndrome which commonly occurs in patients with advanced life-threatening illness. Delirium is an index of a serious change reflecting major underlying pathology and homeostatic destabilization, such as acute worsening of an existing or acute emergence of a new medical condition, medication, toxic substance, etc. (American Psychiatric Association [APA] 2000).

Delirium is often considered a medical or clinical emergency. Its sudden onset requires the clinical healthcare team to take urgent action in order to not only minimize many potentially serious negative outcomes including increased risk of falls and risk of harm to patients themselves, their families, and staff due to aggressive behavior, but also because untreated delirium is life-threatening. There is a need to identify and promptly treat reversible delirium precipitants if consistent with a patient's goals of care.

The online English Oxford dictionary defines medical emergency as "a serious and *unexpected* situation involving illness or injury and requiring immediate action" (Oxford University Press 2017). However, delirium can often be *anticipated* as it is known that certain people are at higher risk of developing delirium. This includes people with pre-existing dementia or advanced illness such as cancer, a past history of a previous delirium episode, and who are over the age of 65 years. Patients with a pre-existing "vulnerable" brain only require a comparatively small precipitating insult to develop full syndromal delirium (Inouye et al. 2014a).

Both patients and families can become extremely distressed during an episode of delirium, requiring urgent intervention, support, and education. Patients may experience psychological distress due to vivid perceptual and delusional disturbances (Partridge et al. 2013). Families may continue to have ongoing distress in their bereavement. Delirium challenges the clinical assessment of other symptoms, and often leads to patients being unable to participate in decision-making and goals of care discussion, thus potentially adding to family burden. A delirious patient can be particularly challenging to manage in the home setting, even with the availability of an "emergency kit" of medications. Family members are often exhausted due to sleep deprivation if the delirious patient is not sleeping at night. While extra homecare support will often be required, potential referral for urgent inpatient care may be needed.

The aim of this chapter is to highlight the importance of considering delirium as a clinical emergency, requiring planning for its occurrence, and immediate action at its onset to reduce morbidity and mortality. It outlines the impact and potentially ominous outcomes of this very common neurocognitive syndrome. An overview of delirium screening and diagnostic tools to assist in the clinical diagnosis of delirium is presented, as well as diagnostic challenges. A patient- and family-centered approach to delirium management which incorporates the patient's goals of care, while avoiding an inappropriately pessimistic approach to investigation and management, is discussed. Nonpharmacological strategies used in the prevention and management of delirium are emphasized. Pharmacological management for symptom relief is reviewed in the context of recent research. Finally, the chapter discusses the importance of providing emotional and practical support to patients experiencing delirium and their families, including when a patient requires palliative sedation for refractory delirium at the end of life. The interested reader is also referred to ▶ Chap. 26, "Delirium" which provides a comprehensive description of delirium in palliative care patients, including pathophysiology.

2 Epidemiology

Delirium affects 20% of patients admitted to acute general medical care settings (Pendlebury et al. 2015), with delirium incidence increasing up to almost 29% in older patients ($\geq$ 65 years old) (Bellelli et al. 2016), 35% if >80 years (Ryan et al. 2013), and 56% in patients with dementia (Inouye et al. 2014a). Up to 20% of older persons presenting to the emergency department have delirium (Inouye et al. 2014a). Delirium is also common in palliative care patients. The prevalence of delirium on admission to a specialist palliative care inpatient setting ranges from 13.3–42.3% and increases to 88% in the last hours to weeks of life (Hosie et al. 2013). Most significantly for palliative care patients, delirium is a poor prognostic feature with an association with increase in mortality (Caraceni et al. 2000; Hui et al. 2015). In fact, delirium has even been called "a harbinger of death" in terminally ill patients, with death occurring within days to weeks of its onset (Breitbart and Alici 2008).

Delirium also causes an increase in patient morbidity, with a heightened risk of falls, longer hospital stays and associated increase in health care costs, and significant patient and family distress (see Fig. 1). In the increasingly recognized syndrome of "persistent delirium," delirium symptoms frequently continue and recovery rates are often poor in the elderly (Dasgupta and Hillier 2010). Cognitive decline after an episode of delirium is common. Delirium appears to worsen pre-existing dementia as well as increasing the risk of new-onset dementia (Fong et al. 2015). Functional decline and permanent institutionalization are also common outcomes after delirium.

3 Clinical Features of Delirium

The essential clinical feature of a delirium syndrome is impaired attention, with a change having occurred in a patient's baseline attention and awareness over a short period of time (APA 2013). Delirium usually fluctuates in severity within a 24-h period. Patients also develop disturbances in cognition, including perceptual

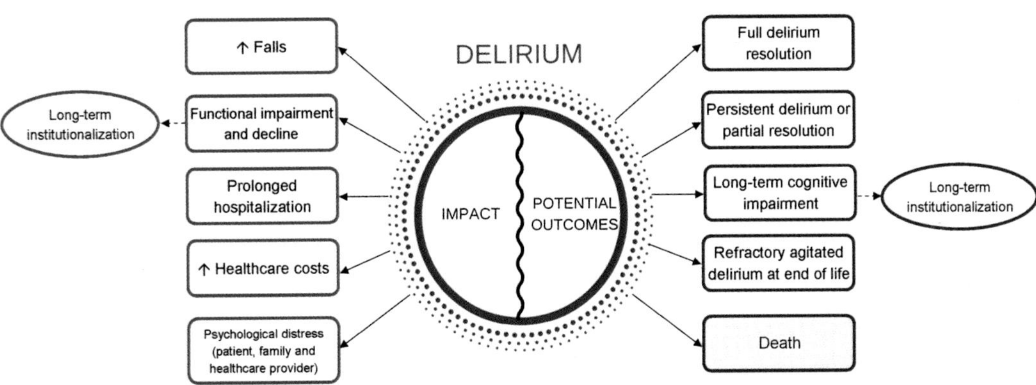

Fig. 1 Impact and potential outcomes of delirium

disturbances such as misinterpretations, illusions, and hallucinations. Other clinical features which may occur (but are not required features for a delirium diagnosis) include sleep-wake cycle disturbance, emotional lability, disorganized thinking, incoherent speech, and altered psychomotor activity (Breitbart and Alici 2012). Although not performed routinely, generalized slowing on an electroencephalogram (EEG) is a characteristic feature of delirium (Engel and Romano 1959).

Delirium is categorized into three subtypes according to the level of psychomotor activity: hyperactive, hypoactive, and mixed (with alternating features of both hyperactive and hypoactive subtypes). In a study of 100 palliative care unit inpatients with delirium whose motor activity was assessed with the Delirium Motor Subtype Scale (DMSS), almost a quarter of assessments were categorized as "no-subtype," as they did not meet criteria for the other defined subtypes (Meagher et al. 2012). The hypoactive and mixed subtypes are the most common in palliative care populations. Motor agitation is a feature of the hyperactive subtype and purposeless repetitive movements (such as plucking at bed sheets or pulling off clothes) may be observed. A patient with hyperactive delirium may be deemed to be in need of more urgent attention by the healthcare team due to visible motor agitation, but in fact patients with the hypoactive delirium subtype have a poorer overall prognosis with increased mortality (Kim et al. 2015).

After a positive result for possible delirium from routine screening or the onset of clinical signs, the diagnosis needs to be formally confirmed. Defined diagnostic criteria for delirium are codified in the *Diagnostic and Statistical Manual of Mental Disorders* (DSM-5) (APA 2013), and in the International Classification of Diseases (ICD-10) (World Health Organization 1992). The earlier that delirium is recognized, the sooner proactive management strategies can be put in place if previously implemented nonpharmacological strategies did not prevent its onset (see also ▶ Chap. 26, "Delirium").

4 Screening for Delirium

Back in 1959, Engel and Romano declared that: "Most delirious patients are considered either dull, stupid, ignorant, *or* uncooperative. It is only when their behaviour and content of thought *are* grossly deviant that an abnormal mental state is recognized, although [ids] not always correctly identified as delirium" (Engel and Romano 1959). Unfortunately, delirium remains under-recognized and is repeatedly missed or misdiagnosed (Clegg et al. 2011; Inouye et al. 2014a; de la Cruz et al. 2015a). Routine screening for delirium by all members of the health care team may improve its detection.

The Confusion Assessment Method (CAM) is a widely used instrument (Inouye et al. 1990). The rating of the CAM requires the co-administration of a brief cognitive assessment tool. The CAM has been validated in palliative care patients and raters require a moderate level of training to ensure reliability. Two nursing observational delirium screening tools rated at the end of each shift are the Nursing Delirium Screening Scale (Nu-DESC) and Delirium Observational Screening (DOS) Scale (Gaudreau et al. 2005; Schuurmans et al. 2003). The recently developed brief 4A Test (4AT) (available at: www.the4at.com) is designed to be used by a healthcare professional when first meeting a patient, or when delirium is suspected, as opposed to daily monitoring. It assesses for both cognitive impairment and delirium and has been validated in older hospitalized patients (Bellelli et al. 2014).

The prodromal features of delirium may provide an early warning to the healthcare team of the impending onset of a delirium episode. These early features include disruption of the sleep-wake cycle with reduced sleep at night, increased somnolence in the daytime, and also irritability, anxiety, and motor restlessness (Kerr et al. 2013). These features may occur before cognitive changes or perceptual disturbances such as hallucinations are observed. As part of the circle of care, the patient's family is also uniquely placed to identify the occurrence of subtle changes in a patient's behavior and/or cognition and should be encouraged to report this immediately to any member of the healthcare team. The Single Question in Delirium (SQiD) asks a family member or friend "Do you think [*name of patient*] has been more confused lately?" (Sands et al. 2010).

5 Making a Diagnosis of Delirium

Delirium is listed as a "neurocognitive disorder" in the *Diagnostic and Statistical Manual of Mental Disorders* (DSM-5) which lists formal diagnostic criteria for delirium (APA 2013). It is a complex syndrome with varying clinical features and deleterious effects. As per the DSM-5 criteria, an essential feature for the diagnosis of delirium is a disturbance in attention and awareness, accompanied by a change in baseline cognition which cannot be better explained by a preexisting, established, or evolving neurocognitive disorder. Delirium usually develops over hours to days, and its severity tends to fluctuate within a 24-h period. Patients may also be classified as having subsyndromal delirium (SSD) if they meet some but not all the criteria for full syndromal delirium (Leonard et al. 2014).

Although the CAM was designed as a screening tool, in clinical practice the CAM diagnostic algorithm is often utilized as a "diagnostic" tool. The recent 3D–CAM, which operationalizes the CAM using a 3-min assessment, was validated in 201 general medicine inpatients ($\geq$ 75 years) in a single center (Marcantonio et al. 2014). More lengthy delirium-specific assessment tools include the Delirium Rating Scale-revised-98 (DRS-R-98) (Trzepacz et al. 2001) and Memorial Delirium Assessment Scale (MDAS) (Breitbart et al. 1997).

5.1 Potential Diagnostic Challenges

Delirium impairs patient communication. It is often challenging to diagnose delirium in a patient with reduced communication or a reduced level of consciousness, due to delirium itself or the dying phase as a result of disease progression, employing many of the currently available delirium assessment tools. Differentiating dementia, depression, and hypoactive delirium can be problematic for healthcare providers. Dementia, where a change in cognition occurs with little or no clouding of consciousness, has an insidious onset over months. Notably, patients with dementia with Lewy bodies have *fluctuating* cognitive impairment with variations in attention and alertness, complex visual hallucinations, and parkinsonism. Delusions may also be a feature (Pealing and Iliffe 2011). Delirium is also commonly superimposed on dementia, making clinical evaluation more problematic compounded by a current lack of suitable assessment tools (Morandi et al. 2017). Hypoactive delirium may present as depression or fatigue.

Hyperactive delirium may be misdiagnosed as anxiety, akathisia, or mania. With akathisia, the subjective symptoms of feeling nervous or restless and the observed movements of the body may be misinterpreted as increasing agitation due to delirium, hence the necessity that health care providers should monitor for potential medication-induced akathisia and other adverse extrapyramidal side effects (EPS) of antipsychotic medications administered to a distressed delirious patient. Agitation is not specific to delirium, so possible other causes for a patient's agitation should be considered. Urinary retention, severe constipation, or fecal impaction may aggravate patient agitation, especially in the elderly. This is often overlooked and may require urgent intervention, e.g., insertion of a urinary catheter, or rectal suppositories/microenema. Uncontrolled pain may also cause patient agitation. Valid, reliable tools to assess pain in older cancer patients with delirium are needed (Gagliese et al. 2016).

Agitation may also be the presenting feature of two distinct syndromes, neuroleptic (antipsychotic) malignant syndrome (NMS) and serotonin syndrome, where it is a more typical clinical feature in the latter (Buckley et al. 2014; Katus and Frucht 2016). Timely recognition of these potentially life-threatening syndromes is critical as urgent management is required. NMS is an infrequent, idiosyncratic, and potentially fatal

Table 1 Comparing clinical features of neuroleptic malignant syndrome (NMS) and serotonin syndrome (Buckley et al. 2014; Katus and Frucht 2016)

Neuroleptic (antipsychotic) malignant syndrome	Serotonin syndrome
Precipitated by dopamine antagonists Clinical features: Severe rigidity Hyperthermia Altered mental status Autonomic dysfunction Develops over days to weeks, and includes hyporeflexia	Precipitated by serotonin agonists Classically a triad of: (i) Altered mental status, e.g., confusion, agitation (ii) Neuromuscular excitation, e.g., clonus, rigidity, hyperreflexia (iii) Autonomic excitation, e.g., tachycardia, hyperthermia Rapid in onset, <24 h

syndrome which develops over days to weeks and is precipitated by dopamine antagonists. Some features of NMS are similar to serotonin syndrome which is precipitated by serotonin agonists with a more rapid onset of less than 24 h (see Table 1).

In palliative care settings, any sudden change in patient behavior, such as anxiety and psychological distress, should be used as a trigger for patient reevaluation to exclude delirium. A delirious patient may show signs of moaning, groaning, and facial grimacing as a result of delirium, not pain. In addition, a delirious patient may have an increased expression of pain as a result of disinhibition. If these signs in a delirious patient are misinterpreted as an increase in pain production due to activation of nociceptors, the resulting administration of extra unnecessary doses of opioids may potentially increase the delirium severity.

6 Risk Factors for Delirium

Delirium is usually multifactorial and risk factors can be broadly divided into predisposing (baseline vulnerability) and acute precipitating factors with each delirium episode having a range of 1–6 superimposed precipitants (median 3) (Lawlor et al. 2000). The development of delirium arises from the interplay of these factors: patients with a pre-existing "vulnerable" or "fragile" brain need a smaller noxious precipitating insult in order to trigger full syndromal delirium, as compared to those with a "healthy" brain (Inouye et al. 2014a). (See ► Chap. 26, "Delirium," Fig. 1)

The most common predisposing factors for delirium are advanced age (>70 years) and pre-existing dementia or cognitive impairment. Others include: history of delirium, depression or alcohol abuse, reduced mobility, visual and auditory impairment, fracture or trauma, malnutrition, multiple co-morbidities, and advanced life-threatening illness (Laurila et al. 2008; Inouye et al. 2014a). Studies in palliative care patients have reported the elucidation of risk factors in around 50% of delirium episodes, with rates of up to 90% also reported (Lawlor et al. 2000; Morita et al. 2001). Multiple causes for a delirium episode frequently occur at the same time (for example, opioid-induced neurotoxicity, dehydration, and hypercalcemia), so a detailed clinical assessment is fundamental, provided it is in keeping with the established goals of care.

The identification of precipitating risk factors is dependent on the extent of possible laboratory and radiological investigations which in turn is influenced by a patient's location, as well as goals of care. The precipitating factors identified in observational studies in palliative care populations depend on the clinical setting and case mix with a few consistently identified risk factors, i.e., infection, organ failure, psychoactive medication, electrolyte abnormalities, and acute illness.

Figure 2 shows common causes of delirium and Table 2 shows etiologies that are less common or potentially missed by the healthcare team.

7 Decision-Making in the Management Approach

For palliative care patients, the management of delirium should be guided by the agreed goals of care. Goals of care can be defined as "the intended purposes of healthcare interventions and support as recognized by both a patient or substitute decision-maker and the healthcare team" (Winnipeg Regional Health Authority 2011). Discussing goals of care requires clear and sensitive communication with the substitute decision-maker

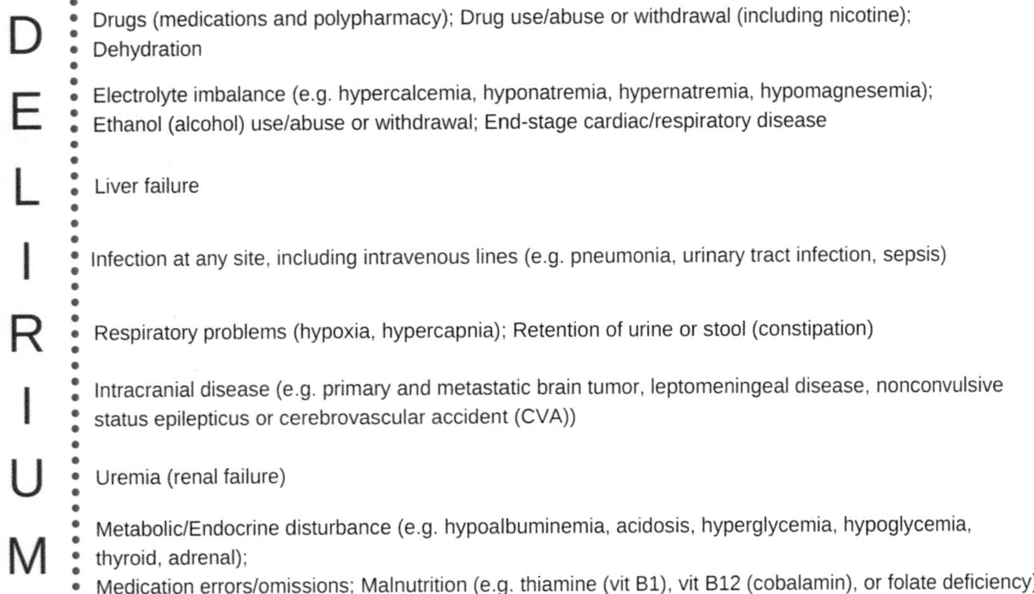

Fig. 2 Common causes of delirium

(which is usually a family member) as the delirious patient usually lacks decisional capacity, as well as an individualized approach. There is a risk of being unduly fatalistic by assuming that a palliative care patient has an irreversible delirium and subsequently failing not to investigate clinically, thereby missing potentially reversible precipitants. In such cases, death becomes a self-fulfilling prophecy and the opportunity for a period of meaningful communication between a patient and their family is lost.

It is advantageous to clarify what the patient's illness trajectory and functional status was like before the onset of delirium, to help confirm whether the patient has had a sudden precipitous change in condition, or if their condition has been steadily declining and they are in actual fact approaching the dying phase. Discussions should include the probable or suspected delirium precipitants, the potential for reversal or likelihood of nonreversal, in conjunction with ascertaining the patient's prior expressed goals of care and their possible desire to proceed or not proceed with further investigations and treatment. The burden and possible risk of inappropriate investigation and treatment should be taken into account. The conclusion of an informed decision-making process should reach an agreed management plan. As such, a timed trial of antibiotics for infection may be considered, for example. If the management plan does not aim for both delirium reversal (by way of investigation and treatment of precipitants) and symptom treatment, then symptom-directed treatment (nonpharmacological and potentially pharmacological) solely to control delirium symptoms should continue with the aim of ensuring comfort.

8 Clinical Assessment

Even with a detailed clinical assessment, delirium etiology in palliative care patients may remain unclear in approximately 50% of episodes.

8.1 Detailed History

The patient may be aware of feeling confused and report perceptual disturbances (visual or tactile hallucinations and illusions), or delusions. As part of a comprehensive past medical history assessment, an alcohol and substance abuse history should be obtained to identify delirium associated with withdrawal. A collateral history may be required from a family member or friend to

Table 2 Potentially missed and less common etiologies of delirium

Etiology
Hypercalcemia Reported calcium level within normal range, but hypoalbuminemia About 40% of the total serum calcium is bound to plasma proteins, mainly albumin "Total" calcium is reported by laboratories, and a "correction" is needed for the albumin level Measure *ionized* calcium if specific value needed
Hyperglycemia New finding in person with no preexisting history of diabetes mellitus Monitor glucose level of patients on high dose corticosteroids
Hypoglycemia
Hypoxia
Hypercapnia
Medication or substance withdrawal
Post-ictal phase
Nonconvulsive status epilepticus
Cerebrovascular accident (CVA)
Reversible posterior leukoencephalopathy syndrome (RPLS)
Paraneoplastic syndromes, e.g., paraneoplastic encephalomyelitis
Hematological, e.g., anemia, disseminated intravascular coagulation
Cytotoxic chemotherapy
Acute cerebral edema after brain irradiation
Cognitive deficits/impairment after radiation treatment/chemotherapy?

confirm the fluctuating nature and recent onset of delirium symptoms, as well as baseline mental status. Medication lists should be reviewed, not only for new medications, but also for long-standing medications and recent increases in doses. Opioid-induced neurotoxicity (OIN) is a syndrome of neuropsychiatric side effects that may occur with opioid therapy, especially if the opioid is administered in a large or rapidly increasing dose. OIN is exacerbated by dehydration.

8.2 Physical Assessment

In addition to a formal cognitive assessment and evaluation of attention, a physical examination should be conducted to look for potential underlying causes of delirium, such as infection, dehydration, and OIN. In addition to delirium and cognitive impairment, the clinical features of OIN are severe sedation, hallucinations, myoclonus, seizures, allodynia, and hyperalgesia. A patient may exhibit increased or decreased psychomotor activity. A further neurological examination of the patient may reveal abnormal movements such as asterixis, or cranial nerve deficits. In diffuse encephalopathies, signs of bifrontal dysfunction may be elicited, e.g., palmomental, snout, and grasp reflexes.

8.3 Investigations

It is less appropriate to extensively investigate for underlying causes of delirium in patients in the last hours of life. Laboratory investigations should be aimed at identifying potentially reversible causes and may include complete blood count, sodium, potassium, urea, creatinine, calcium, albumin, magnesium, random blood glucose, bilirubin, liver enzymes, ammonia levels (if severe liver impairment suspected), urinalysis, and urine culture. If suspected, tests for vitamin deficiencies such as Vitamin B1 (thiamine), B12 (cobalamin), and folate may be indicated. The patient's level of oxygen saturation should be assessed. A chest X-ray may confirm the presence of pneumonia. If in keeping with a patient's goals of care, radiological cerebral imaging may be appropriate, such as a computed tomography (CT) or magnetic resonance imaging (MRI) scan of the brain.

8.4 Management of Potentially Reversible Delirium Participants

Approximately, 50% of delirium episodes in advanced cancer patients are reversible (Lawlor et al. 2000). The decision to investigate for potentially reversible precipitants will depend on a patient's goals of care and assessment of burden of investigation and treatment, in addition to the type of care setting and availability of resources locally.

Delirium in palliative care patients is significantly more reversible if the precipitating factor is opioids and other psychoactive drugs, infection, and hypercalcemia (Lawlor et al. 2000; Morita et al. 2001). See Table 3 for the management of underlying causes of delirium. As part of good "deprescribing" practice to reduce polypharmacy, all patients' medication lists should undergo a systematic review, with a drug profile review by a pharmacist if possible, to reduce or discontinue medications, especially psychoactive drugs. Opioid rotation and discontinuation of other medications results in resolution of approximately 75–80% of episodes of drug-induced delirium. Reversal of delirium takes 2–7 days to occur. Conversely, delirium is less likely to improve in patients with an underlying dementia (Inouye et al. 2006), or if the delirium is related to hypoxic or global metabolic encephalopathy, or disseminated intravascular coagulation (Lawlor et al. 2000; Morita et al. 2001).

As delirium is often less reversible at the end of life, the challenge is discerning when attempts to reverse it are appropriate. Healthcare professionals are often inaccurate in their predictions of life expectancy, either under- or over-estimating the time left. Thus, it is important to try and identify if the person is imminently dying in order to establish the appropriateness of treating the precipitating causes of the delirium episode. However, diagnosing when a patient is entering the terminal phase can be especially challenging when viewed through the lens of fluctuating delirium signs and symptoms. Further development and research on predictive models of delirium reversibility in palliative care would assist in clinical decision-making.

9 Management of Delirium Symptoms in Palliative Care Patients

Delirium should be viewed as an acute clinical emergency requiring urgent evaluation by the interprofessional health care team. The seriousness and urgency of management to minimize its adverse effects is perhaps more pronounced if it is considered as a type of "acute brain dysfunction" (Morandi et al. 2008). The interprofessional team should work collaboratively to proactively manage patients with delirium, reduce its harmful effects, and support family members. As part of this endeavor, clear and consistent communication from the healthcare team with patients, families, and other team members is paramount. Consultation with Psychiatry or Psychogeriatrics is recommended for cases that are challenging to manage.

9.1 Nonpharmacological Management

Nonpharmacological strategies play a key role in the management of delirium, potentially preventing about 30% of delirium episodes in acute care settings (Siddiqi et al. 2016) (see Table 4). Delirious patients should be supported by frequent reorientation to who and where they are, and the names and roles of their healthcare team. Many components of existing nonpharmacological strategies constitute fundamental patient care and can be easily implemented into everyday clinical practice by the healthcare team, as well as family members with the support of the team. While evidence-based multicomponent nonpharmacological approaches have been shown to be effective in reducing delirium incidence and preventing falls in older persons $\geq$65 years (Hshieh et al. 2015), the efficacy of these approaches in palliative care populations across the illness trajectory is not known at this time (Gagnon et al. 2012).

It is important to be aware that an agitated patient with delirium is probably extremely scared. They may be experiencing frightening delusional beliefs, such as that the health care team is trying to harm them. Patients who have recovered from delirium commonly report that they feel they are not being listened to or understood, in addition to not being able to understand what staff are wanting (Partridge et al. 2013; Lawlor and Bush 2015). The healthcare team should communicate to delirious patients face to face with simple, concise, and clear sentences,

Table 3 Management of underlying causes of delirium

Underlying cause of delirium	Management approach
Opioid-induced neurotoxicity (OIN)	Reduction of opioid dose: if pain well controlled Rotate or switch opioid: with a decrease in the equianalgesic dose of the new opioid by at least 1/3 because of incomplete cross-tolerance between opioids (Indelicato and Portenoy 2002). With severe OIN, the equianalgesic dose may need to be reduced by up to 50%
Delirium caused by other medications	Consider discontinuing deliriogenic medication/s (note: this may require dose taper), or at least decreasing the dose
Dehydration	Medically-assisted hydration can be given via the intravenous or subcutaneous route (also known as hypodermoclysis – HDC) HDC can be provided with normal saline at 40–100 mL/h up to 1000 ml/day, or alternatively by giving subcutaneous boluses of 250 mL administered over 1 h, three or four times daily At this time, there is limited evidence for improving delirium with medically-assisted hydration (Nakajima et al. 2014). Hydration may be *inappropriate* for a patient who is imminently dying The risks, benefits and the values, culture, and goals of care for each person and his/her family need to be considered in each situation
Infection	For example, pneumonia, urinary tract infection, sepsis If in concordance with goals of care, consider time-limited trial of treatment with appropriate antibiotic (according to site of infection) after discussing treatment options with the patient and/or substitute decision maker
Hypercalcemia	Hypercalcemia occurs in about 8–10% of patients with cancer and is defined as a corrected calcium level of ≥2.65 mmol/L. Levels above 3.0 mmol/L usually cause significant problems Management (depending on the severity of symptoms, patient's wishes and estimated life expectancy) includes hydration, using saline, and additional treatment with a bisphosphonate or calcitonin (Stewart 2005) Subcutaneous denosumab, a RANK (receptor activator of nuclear factor kappa-B) ligand inhibitor, has been used to treat bisphosphonate-refractory hypercalcemia in advanced cancer patients (Hu et al. 2014). Patients should be monitored posttreatment as they may require calcium and vitamin D supplementation due to a risk of hypocalcemia after denosumab treatment (Body et al. 2017). Longer-term evaluation studies are needed
Hyponatremia	*Mild hyponatremia* (sodium levels of 126–130 mmol/L) is a common phenomenon in patients with advanced cancer and usually asymptomatic. This does not require treatment, especially in patients with very advanced disease. However, if the sodium level falls very low, then confusion and other symptoms may occur If *severe hyponatremia* (<126 mmol/L) occurs in a patient who potentially still has many weeks and months of life remaining, the syndrome of inappropriate antidiuretic hormone (SIADH) should be considered and confirmed or excluded with blood tests for sodium level and plasma osmolality, and also a urine specimen analyzed for urine osmolality. Management of SIADH is usually with fluid restriction, which would need to be reviewed in the context of the person's goals of care
Brain tumor or metastasis	Consider treatment with corticosteroids, e.g., dexamethasone 4–8 mg daily, in divided doses. (Higher doses of corticosteroids may be required in some patients with primary brain tumors, e.g., in patients with progressive symptoms from intracranial glioblastoma multiforme (GBM).) Depending on patient's overall condition, burden of treatment and goals of care, palliative radiotherapy may also be a treatment option
Hypoxia	Consider oxygen therapy and treat the underlying cause

using a calm voice and reassuring approach at all times. A delirious patient may misinterpret a reassuring touch from a family or team member as an act of aggression, so avoid using touch as a strategy to redirect. If delusional beliefs occur, use verbal distraction to shift the attention of a delirious patient to another topic. Rapid movements should be avoided at all times. Delirious patients

Table 4 Nonpharmacological strategies used in the management of delirium (Zimberg and Berenson 1990; Canadian Coalition for Seniors' Mental Health 2010; NICE 2010; Breitbart and Alici 2012; Inouye et al. 2014b)

Delirium management strategies	Details
Orientation: Environment	
Devices, e.g., visible clock, calendar, orientation board with name/date/location of setting	Simplify and organize patient's environment (call bell, water, telephone, and other essential items within sight and reach)
Familiar objects from home, photographs in patients rooms	
Familiar staff (continuity of care)	
Avoid frequent room changes	Single room if possible
Orientation: Verbal	
Reminders of time, day, place, who they are, who you are	Identify self every time, e.g., "I'm your nurse" – visible name badge
Family/close friends may be able to assist	Instruct family to interact in a simple, clear, and concise manner with patient
Communication:	
Face-to-face with patient Maintain a calm and supportive approach Evaluate need for language interpreters	Communication should be clear, slow-paced, short, simple, and repeated as necessary Present one task or stimulus at a time If delusional beliefs, use distraction to shift attention to another topic Explain each clinical intervention prior to instituting care or administering medication: avoid rapid movements or touching/grabbing that might be misinterpreted as aggressive
Ensure visual/hearing aids are accessible and used, and dentures where needed	Exclude and resolve impacted wax
Sleep Hygiene:	
Facilitate a normal sleep-wake pattern	For example, relaxation music at bedtime, warm noncaffeinated drinks, familiar sleepwear, minimize disruptions through the night Encourage exposure to bright natural light during the day Discourage napping during day, where possible
Environment: Avoid sensory deprivation	
Ensure appropriate lighting	For example, windowless room, excessive darkness Day-time: Shades/curtains open as much as possible during day hours Night-time: Utilize night light
Provide eyeglasses, magnifying lenses, hearing aids	
Environment: Avoid sensory overload	
Avoid excessive noise	For example, excess noise and activityImplement unit-wide noise reduction strategies, especially at night
Avoid patient over-stimulation (by staff and family)	Educate family regarding use of simple explanations and interactions with patient
Mobility:	Mobilize as patient's energy and performance status allows If unable to walk, encourage active range-of-motion exercises as tolerated Sit out of bed for meals whenever possible Minimize use of immobilizing urinary catheters, intravenous lines
Patient/staff safety: Restraint-free care as standard of care	Remove potentially harmful objects Implement a fall prevention protocol Designated sitter may be required Use of physical restraints should be avoided

(*continued*)

Table 4 (continued)

Delirium management strategies	Details
General:	
Monitor hydration and nutrition	Encourage patient to drink, if able to swallow safely Consider subcutaneous or intravenous hydration Assist patient at mealtimes Use patient's dentures, ensure diet consistency appropriate to patient's swallowing ability
Monitor bladder and bowel function	Assess for urinary retention, constipation and fecal impaction Implement interventions as needed Avoid unnecessary catheterization
Assess and monitor pain	Ensure analgesia is adequate
Consider referral to complementary services to reduce anxiety	For example, music therapy

are also hypersensitive to noise. In inpatient settings, unit-wide noise reduction strategies should be implemented (Darbyshire and Young 2013).

9.2 Pharmacological Management

(See also ▶ Chap. 26, "Delirium")

The Role for Antipsychotics

The "off-license" use of antipsychotics to treat delirium symptoms in palliative care patients has been a mainstay of clinical practice despite limited clinical evidence. Haloperidol has been the "practice standard" for many years. As one of the putative pathophysiological mechanisms for delirium development, the "cholinergic hypothesis" (with a deficit of acetylcholine and excess of dopamine) supports the dominant role of haloperidol as a potent dopamine-receptor antagonist in delirium management.

Back in 1996, Breitbart et al. reported a randomized, double-blind comparison trial in 30 adult AIDS patients (Breitbart et al. 1996). Patients who received low-dose haloperidol or chlorpromazine were reported to have an improvement in delirium symptoms as measured on the Delirium Rating Scale. Over the years, published literature has supported the use of antipsychotics in delirium management (Casarett and Inouye 2001; Michaud et al. 2007; Leentjens et al. 2012; Breitbart and Alici 2012). The National Institute for Health and Clinical Excellence (NICE) Clinical Guideline made the recommendation: "if a person with delirium is distressed or considered a risk to themselves or others...consider giving short-term haloperidol or olanzapine" (NICE 2010). It should be noted that this comprehensive guideline excluded "people receiving end-of-life care." In 2012, a Cochrane review found insufficient evidence for drug therapy for delirium management in terminally ill adult patients (Candy et al. 2012). Increasingly, recent systematic reviews have demonstrated a lack of evidence for antipsychotic efficacy, in addition to concerns regarding their harmful effects, especially in patients with pre-existing dementia (Flaherty et al. 2011; Inouye et al. 2014b; Maust et al. 2015; Neufeld et al. 2016).

An Australian multisite, double-blind, parallel-arm, dose-titrated randomized clinical trial of oral risperidone, haloperidol, or placebo solution over a 72-h period in adult inpatients with confirmed delirium and receiving hospice or palliative care has been recently published (Agar et al. 2017). The dosing schedule for antipsychotics (i.e., risperidone or haloperidol) was age-adjusted. In the two antipsychotic arms, participants $\leq$65 years received 0.5 mg as a loading dose, followed by 0.5 mg orally every 12 h. The dose of antipsychotic was titrated by 0.25 mg on day 1, then by 0.5 mg up to a maximum of 4 mg/day. Participants $>$65 years received half the loading, initial and maximum doses of antipsychotic. All participants could receive "rescue" midazolam in a dose of 2.5 mg subcutaneously every 2 h as needed for severe distress or safety. (The dose of midazolam was not age-adjusted.) Of the 247 participants included in the intention-to-treat (ITT) analysis, 65.6% were male with a mean age of 74.9 years, and the majority had cancer (88.3%). The baseline Australia-modified Karnofsky performance status (AKPS) ranged from 30% to 50%. Participants had mild to moderate delirium, as evidenced by median baseline Memorial Delirium Assessment Scale (MDAS) scores ranging from 13.7 to 15.1. For this study, delirium precipitants were also treated "where clinically indicated" and all participants received nonpharmacological approaches as part of delirium care. For the purposes of this study, three items on the Nu-DESC tool (assessing inappropriate behavior, inappropriate communication, and illusions and hallucinations) were combined to produce a delirium symptom score. In the ITT analysis, participants in the risperidone and haloperidol arms had significantly higher delirium symptom scores ($p = 0.02$ and $p = 0.009$, respectively) and received more "rescue" midazolam, as compared to the placebo arm. Median survival was 26 days in the placebo arm, 17 days in the risperidone arm, and 16 days in the haloperidol arm. From a post hoc analysis, the authors stated that participants "receiving an antipsychotic drug were approximately 1.5 times more likely to die." At the present time, it is not clear how to integrate the research findings from the study by Agar et al. (2017) into delirium care across the disease trajectory, in particular for palliative care patients with severe delirium, or frailer patients with a very poor performance status.

Antipsychotics are usually used to relieve perceptual disturbances (such as hallucinations or illusions) or agitation. A practical approach at this time is to maximize supportive nonpharmacological strategies for all patients, with identification and appropriate management of delirium precipitating factors where their reversal is in alignment with established goals of care. Pharmacological management approaches should be reserved for patients with severe agitation at risk of harm to themselves or if safety concerns, or to target psychotic symptoms causing severe distress. In these situations, the short-term use of antipsychotics in the lowest clinically effective dose may be indicated. This is in keeping with the pharmacological recommendation of the 2010 NICE Delirium Guideline (NICE 2010). Small starting doses of haloperidol (e.g., 0.5–1 mg PO or subcut q1hr p.r.n.) may suffice. In elderly or frail patients, lower doses should be used, e.g., haloperidol 0.25–0.5 mg, and titrated gradually. The efficacy of haloperidol should be evaluated 30–60 min after administration. Patients should also have routine assessments for akathisia and other extrapyramidal side effects (EPS). First-generation antipsychotics (e.g., haloperidol) should be avoided in patients with Parkinson's Disease or dementia with Lewy bodies (DLB), because of the risks of EPS and disease exacerbation. If treatment with an antipsychotic is required in these patients, then the second-generation antipsychotic quetiapine may be considered.

The Role for Benzodiazepines

Benzodiazepines are known to be deliriogenic, especially in higher doses, and are a risk factor for falls (Clegg and Young 2011; Stone et al. 2012). In view of this, it has been recommended that benzodiazepines are not used as first-line medications for the management of delirium that may be reversible (Irwin et al. 2013). However, benzodiazepines do have a role as first-line agents in managing agitation due to alcohol or benzodiazepine withdrawal.

Returning to the seminal trial in AIDS patients by Breitbart et al. mentioned above, only 6 of 30 patients received lorazepam, as the researchers stopped the lorazepam arm early due to concerns of treatment-limiting side effects (Breitbart et al. 1996). These included not only increased confusion, but also excess sedation, disinhibition, and ataxia. A recent study in 49 CAM-positive patients with agitation reported that a combination protocol of haloperidol and midazolam was more effective than haloperidol alone (Ferraz Gonçalves et al. 2016). The onset of action for a subcutaneous injection of midazolam is only 5–10 min. The optimal role of "rescue" doses of midazolam and other benzodiazepines such as lorazepam in the crisis management of a severely agitated and distressed delirious patient, who has not responded to nonpharmacological strategies or an antipsychotic as first-line management, requires further study.

10 The Delirium Experience and Support

Delirium causes significant distress for patients as well as their families, countering the oft-heard description of the "pleasantly confused" patient (Breitbart et al. 2002; Bruera et al. 2009). In two studies using the Delirium Experience Questionnaire (DEQ) in hospitalized cancer patients, 54–74% of patients recalled their own symptoms after delirium resolution, and had significant associated distress (Breitbart et al. 2002; Bruera et al. 2009). Of note, patients having no recall of their delirium episode were also significantly distressed, and that hypoactive delirium was just as distressing for patients as hyperactive delirium. Patients report feeling anxious, threatened, and a lack of control, as well as feeling that they are not being listened to or understood by the healthcare team. (See also Sect. 9.1 for communication strategies with delirious patients.) As part of their delirium experience, patients also experience visual hallucinations, misperceptions, and delusions which are frequently of staff, other patients, and deceased family members (Partridge et al. 2013). Patients who have recovered from delirium may require formal debriefing to alleviate their fears.

While the presence of a reassuring family member appears to be beneficial to delirious patients, family members experience distress when observing delirium in their loved one. Spouses and nonprofessional caregivers report higher distress rating scores on the DEQ than patients (Breitbart et al. 2002). Family members often feel helpless and describe negative emotions, include anxiety and caregiver burden (Buss et al. 2007; Finucane et al. 2017). Family distress may be ameliorated if they are expecting delirium as part of the patient's illness (Partridge et al. 2013). Families have previously described a need for more informational support about delirium (Namba et al. 2007; Toye et al. 2014). Communication must be clear and consistent from all members of the interprofessional healthcare team, and tailored to the family's needs. Family members report delirium information leaflets to be a useful strategy in supporting their needs (Otani et al. 2013).

The distress of family members increases with a patient's symptom severity, terminal illness progression and declining performance status (Dumont et al. 2006). The fact that delirium can deprive patients and family members of effective communication becomes even more poignant in the face of approaching death. As delirious patients are often psychologically absent although their body is still physically present, family members may experience "ambiguous" loss (Day and Higgins 2016). In turn, this may later lead to difficulties in an individual's grief journey. The healthcare team has a pivotal role in supporting families at this time, and legitimizing their feelings of loss.

Delirium also impacts on members of the healthcare team. Nursing staff report "stress due to the unpredictability of delirium and workload," as well as safety concerns (Partridge et al. 2013). The behaviors of patients with hyperactive delirium who appear to be uncooperative or pulling at tubes and lines can be particularly challenging to care for, especially at night (Mc Donnell and Timmins 2012). Effective educational training interventions in the management of patients with delirium are required for all members of the interprofessional healthcare team, with the aim of increasing knowledge, skills, and self-efficacy, as well as providing a unified and consistent approach to care. Unit-level debriefing sessions may be required following difficult cases as part of institutional support.

11 Refractory Delirium at the End of Life

A symptom is defined as *refractory* if it cannot be adequately controlled and continues to cause distress despite the use of all other possible and tolerable symptomatic treatments that do not compromise consciousness (Cherny and Portenoy 1994). The occurrence of an irreversible refractory delirium in a physically declining palliative care patient is a poor prognostic sign, indicating that death may occur in days or even hours, rather than weeks (Leonard et al. 2008; de la Cruz et al. 2015b). This information should be sensitively explained to the family, and patient where possible, and support provided to prepare for the dying phase.

Severe refractory delirium at the end of life may also necessitate "emergency" management by the interprofessional healthcare team. Critical action is warranted to reduce not only potential patient distress, but also importantly family distress at witnessing severe agitation in a loved one approaching the end of life which may subsequently negatively impact on their bereavement (Morita et al. 2007; Cohen et al. 2009). In the words of Dame Cicely Saunders who founded St. Christopher's Hospice in Sydenham, London in 1967: "How people die remains in the memory of those who live on." Dying patients with refractory delirium, who remain very agitated and distressed despite antipsychotics, may require additional pharmacological management in the form of palliative sedation.

12 Palliative Sedation for Refractory Agitated Delirium at the End of Life

Over the years, authors and guidelines have provided many definitions for palliative sedation, or sedation in the terminal phase (usually referring to the last days up to the last 2 weeks of life) (Bush et al. 2014). As part of a 10-point framework in 2009, the European Association of Palliative Care (EAPC) defined "therapeutic sedation" or "palliative sedation" as "the monitored use of medications intended to induce a state of decreased or absent awareness (unconsciousness) in order to relieve the burden of otherwise intractable suffering in a manner that is ethically acceptable to the patient, family and health care providers" (Cherny and Radbruch 2009). Proportionate palliative sedation is an ethically accepted intervention and does not hasten death. Palliative sedation can be administered intermittently, as temporary "respite" sedation for an uncontrolled symptom, or continuously. Midazolam is the medication most frequently used for palliative sedation and refractory delirium is the most common indication (Maltoni et al. 2012).

See ▶ Chap. 87, "Palliative Sedation: A Medical-Ethical Exploration."

More evidence is needed on the efficacy of palliative sedation for the management of refractory delirium, as well as other refractory symptoms at the end of life (Beller et al. 2015). In addition, it is important that palliative sedation guideline implementation is supported by comprehensive staff training and education strategies.

Family members require ongoing support at this time. While often feeling relief at seeing their loved one's comfort, family members may also experience distress due to patient's lack of communication, guilt over the decision-making process, in addition to anticipatory grief (Cherny and ESMO Guidelines Working Group 2014). Family members have also reported receiving insufficient or unclear information regarding palliative sedation (Bruinsma et al. 2013). Clear healthcare team communication with family members and other team members should be a priority, especially before and during palliative sedation. Families often have mixed feelings between wanting relief of the patient's suffering, but also wanting consciousness maintained (Finucane et al. 2017). As a practice point, if a patient has become increasingly agitated over the course of a day, it can be advantageous for the health care team to brief the family in advance (as well as the patient if possible) if the team anticipates that the patient is likely to require sedation overnight for their comfort. This preparation may help to mitigate some of the distress of family members if the sedated patient is not able to have meaningful conversations with them the next day.

13 Conclusion and Summary

Delirium is a clinical emergency requiring prompt assessment and management according to a patient's goals of care by all members of the interprofessional healthcare team. Delirium can be anticipated by the healthcare team if the patient is assessed to be in a high risk group, or approaching the last hours to weeks of life. The development of validated models (specific to palliative care populations) to predict delirium development and to predict response to treatment of delirium precipitants according to a patient's goals of care will assist in this endeavor. Further research is required to ascertain the optimal management strategies of delirium, according to underlying pathophysiology and across the palliative care patient's illness trajectory. Planning for the occurrence of delirium is of immense benefit to the patient, their family, and healthcare team and, in turn, has the potential to reduce the distress associated with this common deleterious neurocognitive syndrome.

References

Agar MR, Lawlor PG, Quinn S, Draper B, Caplan G, Rowett D, et al. Efficacy of oral risperidone, haloperidol, or placebo for symptoms of delirium among patients in palliative care: a randomized clinical trial. JAMA Intern Med. 2017;177:34–42. https://doi.org/10.1001/jamainternmed.2016.7491.

American Psychiatric Association. Diagnostic and statistical manual of mental disorders, text revision. 4th ed. Washington, DC: American Psychiatric Association; 2000.

American Psychiatric Association. Diagnostic and statistical manual of mental disorders. 5th ed. Washington, DC: American Psychiatric Association; 2013.

Bellelli G, Morandi A, Davis DHJ, Mazzola P, Turco R, Gentile S, et al. Validation of the 4AT, a new instrument for rapid delirium screening: a study in 234 hospitalised older people. Age Ageing. 2014;43:496–502. https://doi.org/10.1093/ageing/afu021.

Bellelli G, Morandi A, Di Santo SG, Mazzone A, Cherubini A, Mossello E, et al. "Delirium day": a nationwide point prevalence study of delirium in older hospitalized patients using an easy standardized diagnostic tool. BMC Med. 2016;14:106. https://doi.org/10.1186/s12916-016-0649-8.

Beller EM, van Driel ML, McGregor L, Truong S, Mitchell G. Palliative pharmacological sedation for terminally ill adults. Cochrane Database Syst Rev. 2015;CD010206. https://doi.org/10.1002/14651858.CD010206.pub2

Body JJ, Niepel D, Tonini G. Hypercalcaemia and hypocalcaemia: finding the balance. Support Care Cancer. 2017;25:1639–49. https://doi.org/10.1007/s00520-016-3543-1.

Breitbart W, Alici Y. Agitation and delirium at the end of life: "we couldn't manage him". JAMA. 2008;300:2898–910. https://doi.org/10.1001/jama.2008.885.

Breitbart W, Alici Y. Evidence-based treatment of delirium in patients with cancer. J Clin Oncol. 2012;30:1206–14. https://doi.org/10.1200/JCO.2011.39.8784.

Breitbart W, Marotta R, Platt MM, Weisman H, Derevenco M, Grau C, et al. A double-blind trial of haloperidol, chlorpromazine, and lorazepam in the treatment of delirium in hospitalized AIDS patients. Am J Psychiatry. 1996;153:231–7. https://doi.org/10.1176/ajp.153.2.231.

Breitbart W, Rosenfeld B, Roth A, Smith MJ, Cohen K, Passik S. The memorial delirium assessment scale. J Pain Symptom Manag. 1997;13:128–37. https://doi.org/10.1016/S0885-3924(96)00316-8.

Breitbart W, Gibson C, Tremblay A. The delirium experience: delirium recall and delirium-related distress in hospitalized patients with cancer, their spouses/caregivers, and their nurses. Psychosomatics. 2002;43:183–94.

Bruera E, Bush SH, Willey J, Paraskevopoulos T, Li Z, Palmer JL, et al. Impact of delirium and recall on the level of distress in patients with advanced cancer and their family caregivers. Cancer. 2009;115:2004–12. https://doi.org/10.1002/cncr.24215.

Bruinsma S, Rietjens J, van der Heide A. Palliative sedation: a focus group study on the experiences of relatives. J Palliat Med. 2013;16:349–55. https://doi.org/10.1089/jpm.2012.0410.

Buckley NA, Dawson AH, Isbister GK. Serotonin syndrome. BMJ. 2014;348:g1626.

Bush SH, Leonard MM, Agar M, Spiller JA, Hosie A, Wright DK, et al. End-of-life delirium: issues regarding recognition, optimal management, and the role of sedation in the dying phase. J Pain Symptom Manag. 2014;48:215–30. https://doi.org/10.1016/j.jpainsymman.2014.05.009.

Buss M, Vanderwerker L, Inouye SK, Zhang B, Block S, Prigerson H. Associations between caregiver-perceived delirium in patients with cancer and generalized anxiety in their caregivers. J Palliat Med. 2007;10:1083–92.

Canadian Coalition for Seniors' Mental Health. Guideline on the assessment and treatment of delirium in older adults at the end of life. Toronto: Canadian Coalition for Seniors' Mental Health; 2010.

Candy B, Jackson Kenneth C, Jones L, Leurent B, Tookman A, King M. Drug therapy for delirium in terminally ill adult patients. Cochrane Database Syst Rev. 2012;CD004770. https://doi.org/10.1002/14651858.CD004770.pub2

Caraceni A, Nanni O, Maltoni M, Piva L, Indelli M, Arnoldi E, et al. Impact of delirium on the short term prognosis of advanced cancer patients. Cancer. 2000;89:1145–9.

Casarett D, Inouye SK. American College of Physicans-American Society of internal medicine end-of-life care consensus panel. Diagnosis and management of delirium near the end of life. Ann Intern Med. 2001;135:32–40.

Cherny N, ESMO Guidelines Working Group. ESMO Clinical Practice Guidelines for the management of refractory symptoms at the end of life and the use of palliative sedation. Ann Oncol. 2014;25(Suppl 3): iii143–52. https://doi.org/10.1093/annonc/mdu238.

Cherny N, Portenoy R. Sedation in the management of refractory symptoms: guidelines for evaluation and treatment. J Palliat Care. 1994;10:31–8.

Cherny N, Radbruch L. European Association for Palliative Care (EAPC) recommended framework for the use of sedation in palliative care. Palliat Med. 2009;23:581–93. https://doi.org/10.1177/0269216309107024.

Clegg A, Young JB. Which medications to avoid in people at risk of delirium: a systematic review. Age Ageing. 2011;40:23–9. https://doi.org/10.1093/ageing/afq140.

Clegg A, Westby M, Young JB. Under-reporting of delirium in the NHS. Age Aging. 2011;40:283–6. https://doi.org/10.1093/ageing/afq157.

Cohen MZ, Pace EA, Kaur G, Bruera E. Delirium in advanced cancer leading to distress in patients and family caregivers. J Palliat Care. 2009;25:164–71.

Darbyshire JL, Young JD. An investigation of sound levels on intensive care units with reference to the WHO guidelines. Crit Care. 2013;17:R187. https://doi.org/10.1186/cc12870.

Dasgupta M, Hillier LM. Factors associated with prolonged delirium: a systematic review. Int Psychogeriatr. 2010;22:373–94. https://doi.org/10.1017/S1041610209991517.

Day J, Higgins I. Mum's absence(s): conceptual insights into absence as loss during a loved one's delirium. J Clin Nurs. 2016;25:2066–73. https://doi.org/10.1111/jocn.13268.

de la Cruz M, Fan J, Yennu S, Tanco K, Shin S, Wu J, et al. The frequency of missed delirium in patients referred to palliative care in a comprehensive cancer center. Support Care Cancer. 2015a;23:2427–33. https://doi.org/10.1007/s00520-015-2610-3.

de la Cruz M, Ransing V, Yennu S, Wu J, Liu D, Reddy A, et al. The frequency, characteristics, and outcomes among cancer patients with delirium admitted to an acute palliative care unit. Oncologist. 2015b;20:1425–31. https://doi.org/10.1634/theoncologist.2015-0115.

Dumont S, Turgeon J, Allard P, Gagnon P, Charbonneau C, Vézina L. Caring for a loved one with advanced cancer: determinants of psychological distress in family caregivers. J Palliat Med. 2006;9:912–21. https://doi.org/10.1089/jpm.2006.9.912.

Engel G, Romano J. Delirium, a syndrome of cerebral insufficiency. J Chronic Dis. 1959;9:260–77.

Ferraz Gonçalves JA, Almeida A, Costa I, Silva P, Carneiro R. Comparison of haloperidol alone and in combination with midazolam for the treatment of acute agitation in an inpatient palliative care service. J Pain Palliat Care Pharmacother. 2016;30:284–8.

Finucane AM, Lugton J, Kennedy C, Spiller JA. The experiences of caregivers of patients with delirium, and their role in its management in palliative care settings: an integrative literature review. Psychooncology. 2017;26:291–300. https://doi.org/10.1002/pon.4140.

Flaherty J, Gonzales J, Dong B. Antipsychotics in the treatment of delirium in older hospitalized adults: a systematic review. J Am Geriatr Soc. 2011;59(Suppl 2):S269–76. https://doi.org/10.1111/j.1532-5415.2011.03675.x.

Fong TG, Davis D, Growdon ME, Albuquerque A, Inouye SK. The interface between delirium and dementia in elderly adults. Lancet Neurol. 2015;14:823–32.

Gagliese L, Rodin R, Chan V, Stevens B, Zimmermann C. How do healthcare workers judge pain in older palliative care patients with delirium near the end of life? Palliat Support Care. 2016;14:151–8. https://doi.org/10.1017/S1478951515000929.

Gagnon P, Allard P, Gagnon B, Mérette C, Tardif F. Delirium prevention in terminal cancer: assessment of a multicomponent intervention. Psychooncology. 2012;21:187–94. https://doi.org/10.1002/pon.1881.

Gaudreau JD, Gagnon P, Harel F, Roy MA. Impact on delirium detection of using a sensitive instrument integrated into clinical practice. Gen Hosp Psychiatry. 2005;27:194–9. https://doi.org/10.1016/j.genhosppsych.2005.01.002.

Hosie A, Davidson PM, Agar M, Sanderson CR, Phillips J. Delirium prevalence, incidence, and implications for screening in specialist palliative care inpatient settings: a systematic review. Palliat Med. 2013;27:486–98. https://doi.org/10.1177/0269216312457214.

Hshieh TT, Yue J, Oh E, Puelle M, Dowal S, Travison T, et al. Effectiveness of multicomponent nonpharmacological delirium interventions: a meta-analysis. JAMA Intern Med. 2015;175:512–20. https://doi.org/10.1001/jamainternmed.2014.7779.

Hu MI, Glezerman IG, Leboulleux S, Insogna K, Gucalp R, Misiorowski W, Yu B, Zorsky P, Tosi D, Bessudo A, Jaccard A, Tonini G, Ying W, Braun A, Jain RK. Denosumab for treatment of hypercalcemia of malignancy. J Clin Endocrinol Metab. 2014;99:3144–52. https://doi.org/10.1210/jc.2014-1001.

Hui D, dos Santos R, Reddy S, Nascimento M, Zhukovsky DS, Paiva CE, et al. Acute symptomatic complications among patients with advanced cancer admitted to acute palliative care units: a prospective observational study. Palliat Med. 2015;29:826–33. https://doi.org/10.1177/0269216315583031.

Indelicato R, Portenoy RK. Opioid rotation in the management of refractory cancer pain. J Clin Oncol. 2002;20:348–52. https://doi.org/10.1200/JCO.2002.20.1.348.

Inouye SK, Van Dyck CH, Alessi CA, Balkin S, Siegal AP, Horwitz RI. Clarifying confusion: the confusion assessment method: a new method for detection of delirium. Ann Intern Med. 1990;113:941–8. https://doi.org/10.7326/0003-4819-113-12-941.

Inouye SK, Baker DI, Fugal P, Bradley EH. Dissemination of the hospital elder life program: implementation, adaptation, and successes. J Am Geriatr Soc. 2006;54:1492–9.

Inouye SK, Westendorp R, Saczynski J. Delirium in elderly people. Lancet. 2014a;383:911–22. https://doi.org/10.1016/S0140-6736(13)60688-1.

Inouye SK, Marcantonio E, Metzger E. Doing damage in delirium: the hazards of antipsychotic treatment in elderly persons. Lancet Psychiatr. 2014b;1:312–5.

Irwin S, Pirrello R, Hirst J, Buckholz G, Ferris F. Clarifying delirium management: practical, evidence-based, expert recommendations for clinical practice. J

Palliat Med. 2013;16:423–35. https://doi.org/10.1089/jpm.2012.0319.

Katus L, Frucht S. Management of serotonin syndrome and neuroleptic malignant syndrome. Curr Treat Options Neurol. 2016;18:39. https://doi.org/10.1007/s11940-016-0423-4.

Kerr CW, Donnelly JP, Wright ST, Luczkiewicz DL, McKenzie KJ, Hang PC, et al. Progression of delirium in advanced illness: a multivariate model of caregiver and clinician perspectives. J Palliat Med. 2013;16:768–73. https://doi.org/10.1089/jpm.2012.0561.

Kim S-Y, Kim S-W, Kim J-M, Shin I-S, Bae K-Y, Shim H-J, et al. Differential associations between delirium and mortality according to delirium subtype and age: a prospective cohort study. Psychosom Med. 2015; 77:903–10.

Laurila JV, Laakkonen ML, Laurila JV, Timo SE, Reijo TS. Predisposing and precipitating factors for delirium in a frail geriatric population. J Psychosom Res. 2008;65:249–54. https://doi.org/10.1016/j.jpsychores.2008.05.026.

Lawlor PG, Bush SH. Delirium in patients with cancer: assessment, impact, mechanisms and management. Nat Rev Clin Oncol. 2015;12:77–92. https://doi.org/10.1038/nrclinonc.2014.147.

Lawlor P, Gagnon B, Mancini I, Pereira J, Hanson J, Suarez-Almazor M, et al. Occurrence, causes, and outcome of delirium in patients with advanced cancer: a prospective study. Arch Intern Med. 2000;160:786–94.

Leentjens AFG, Rundell J, Rummans T, Shim JJ, Oldham R, Peterson L, et al. Delirium: an evidence-based medicine (EBM) monograph for psychosomatic medicine practice, commissioned by the Academy of Psychosomatic Medicine (APM) and the European Association of Consultation Liaison Psychiatry and Psychosomatics (EACLPP). J Psychosom Res. 2012; 73:149–52. https://doi.org/10.1016/j.jpsychores.2012.05.009.

Leonard MM, Raju B, Conroy M, Donnelly S, Trzepacz PT, Saunders J, et al. Reversibility of delirium in terminally ill patients and predictors of mortality. Palliat Med. 2008;22:848–54. https://doi.org/10.1177/0269216308094520.

Leonard MM, Agar M, Spiller JA, Davis B, Mohamad MM, Meagher DJ, et al. Delirium diagnostic and classification challenges in palliative care: subsyndromal delirium, comorbid delirium-dementia, and psychomotor subtypes. J Pain Symptom Manag. 2014; 48:199–214.

Maltoni M, Scarpi E, Rosati M, Derni S, Fabbri L, Martini F, et al. Palliative sedation in end-of-life care and survival: a systematic review. J Clin Oncol. 2012;30:1378–83. https://doi.org/10.1200/JCO.2011.37.3795.

Marcantonio ER, Ngo LH, O'Connor M, Jones RN, Crane PK, Metzger ED, et al. 3D-CAM: derivation and validation of a 3-minute diagnostic interview for CAM-defined delirium: a cross-sectional diagnostic test study. Ann Intern Med. 2014;161:554–61. https://doi.org/10.7326/M14-0865.

Maust DT, Kim HM, Seyfried LS, Chiang C, Kavanagh J, Schneider LS, et al. Antipsychotics, other psychotropics, and the risk of death in patients with dementia: number needed to harm. JAMA Psychiat. 2015;72:438–45. https://doi.org/10.1001/jamapsychiatry.2014.3018.

Mc Donnell S, Timmins F. A quantitative exploration of the subjective burden experienced by nurses when caring for patients with delirium. J Clin Nurs. 2012;21:2488–98. https://doi.org/10.1111/j.1365-2702.2012.04130.x.

Meagher DJ, Leonard M, Donnelly S, Conroy M, Adamis D, Trzepacz PT. A longitudinal study of motor subtypes in delirium: frequency and stability during episodes. J Psychosom Res. 2012;72:236–41. https://doi.org/10.1016/j.jpsychores.2011.11.013.

Michaud L, Büla C, Berney A, Camus V, Voellinger R, Stiefel F, et al. Delirium: guidelines for general hospitals. J Psychosom Res. 2007;62:371–83.

Morandi A, Pandharipande P, Trabucchi M, Rozzini R, Mistraletti G, Trompeo AC, et al. Understanding international differences in terminology for delirium and other types of acute brain dysfunction in critically ill patients. Intensive Care Med. 2008;34:1907–15. https://doi.org/10.1007/s00134-008-1177-6.

Morandi A, Davis D, Bellelli G, Arora RC, Caplan GA, Kamholz B, et al. The diagnosis of delirium superimposed on dementia: an emerging challenge. J Am Med Dir Assoc. 2017;18:12–8. https://doi.org/10.1016/j.jamda.2016.07.014.

Morita T, Tei Y, Tsunoda J, Inoue S, Chihara S. Underlying pathologies and their associations with clinical features in terminal delirium of cancer patients. J Pain Symptom Manag. 2001;22:997–1006.

Morita T, Akechi T, Ikenaga M, Inoue S, Kohara H, Matsubara T, et al. Terminal delirium: recommendations from bereaved families' experiences. J Pain Symptom Manag. 2007;34:579–89. https://doi.org/10.1016/j.jpainsymman.2007.01.012.

Nakajima N, Satake N, Nakaho T. Indications and practice of artificial hydration for terminal ill cancer patients. Curr Opin Support Palliat Care. 2014;8:358–63. https://doi.org/10.1097/SPC.0000000000000089.

Namba M, Morita T, Imura C, Kiyohara E, Ishikawa S, Hirai K. Terminal delirium: families' experience. Palliat Med. 2007;21:587–94.

National Institute for Health and Care Excellence. Delirium: diagnosis, prevention and management. Clinical guideline 103. 2010. http://www.nice.org.uk/CG103. Accessed 2 May 2017.

Neufeld K, Yue J, Robinson T, Inouye SK, Needham D. Antipsychotic medication for prevention and treatment of delirium in hospitalized adults: a systematic review and meta-analysis. J Am Geriatr Soc. 2016;64:705–14. https://doi.org/10.1111/jgs.14076.

Otani H, Morita T, Uno S, Yamamoto R, Hirose H, Matsubara T, et al. Usefulness of the leaflet-based intervention for family members of terminally ill cancer patients with delirium. J Palliat Med. 2013; 16:419–22. https://doi.org/10.1089/jpm.2012.0401.

Oxford University Press. Oxford dictionary. 2017. https://en.oxforddictionaries.com/definition/medical_emergency. Accessed 22 Mar 2017.

Partridge JS, Martin FC, Harari D, Dhesi JK. The delirium experience: what is the effect on patients, relatives and staff and what can be done to modify this? Int J Geriatr Psychiatry. 2013;28:804–12. https://doi.org/10.1002/gps.3900.

Pealing L, Iliffe S. A woman with forgetfulness and falls. BMJ. 2011;24:d7412. https://doi.org/10.1136/bmj.d7412.

Pendlebury S, Lovett N, Smith S, Dutta N, Bendon C, Lloyd-Lavery A, et al. Observational, longitudinal study of delirium in consecutive unselected acute medical admissions: age-specific rates and associated factors, mortality and re-admission. BMJ Open. 2015;5:e007808. https://doi.org/10.1136/bmjopen-2015-007808.

Ryan DJ, O'Regan NA, Caoimh RÓ, Clare J, O'Connor M, Leonard M, et al. Delirium in an adult acute hospital population: predictors, prevalence and detection. BMJ Open. 2013;3:e001772. https://doi.org/10.1136/bmjopen-2012-001772.

Sands MB, Dantoc BP, Hartshorn A, Ryan C, Lujic S. Single question in delirium (SQiD): testing its efficacy against psychiatrist interview, the confusion assessment method and the memorial delirium assessment scale. Palliat Med. 2010;24:561–5. https://doi.org/10.1177/0269216310371556.

Schuurmans MJ, Shortridge-Baggett LM, Duursma SA. The delirium observation screening scale: a screening instrument for delirium. Res Theory Nurs Pr. 2003;17:31–50.

Siddiqi N, Harrison JK, Clegg A, Teale EA, Young J, Taylor J, et al. Interventions for preventing delirium in hospitalised non-ICU patients. Cochrane Database Syst Rev. 2016;CD005563. https://doi.org/10.1002/14651858.CD005563.pub3

Stewart AF. Clinical practice. Hypercalcemia associated with cancer. N Engl J Med. 2005;352:373–9. https://doi.org/10.1056/NEJMcp042806.

Stone C, Lawlor P, Savva G, Bennett K, Kenny R. Prospective study of falls and risk factors for falls in adults with advanced cancer. J Clin Oncol. 2012;30:2128–33. https://doi.org/10.1200/JCO.2011.40.7791.

Toye C, Matthews A, Hill A, Maher S. Experiences, understandings and support needs of family carers of older patients with delirium: a descriptive mixed methods study in a hospital delirium unit. Int J Older People Nursing. 2014;9:200–8. https://doi.org/10.1111/opn.12019.

Trzepacz PT, Mittal D, Torres R, Kanary K, Norton J, Jimerson N. Validation of the delirium rating scale-revised-98: comparison with the delirium rating scale and the cognitive test for delirium [internet]. J Neuropsychiatry Clin Neurosci. 2001;13:229–42.

Winnipeg Regional Health Authority. WRHA policy number: 110.000.200: advance care planning – goals of care. 2011. http://www.wrha.mb.ca/index.php. Accessed 2 May 2017.

World Health Organization. The ICD-10 classification of mental and behavioural disorders: clinical descriptions and diagnostic guidelines. 1992. http://www.who.int/classifications/icd/en/bluebook.pdf. Accessed 3 May 2017.

Zimberg M, Berenson S. Delirium in patients with cancer: nursing assessment and intervention. Oncol Nurs Forum. 1990;17:529–38.

Distinguishing and Managing Severe Psychological and Psychiatric Distress

85

Dianne Clifton and Jane Fletcher

Contents

D. Clifton
RANZCP, St Vincent's Hospital Melbourne, Cabrini Hospital, Albert Road Clinic, Hawthorn Road Consulting Suites, International Psycho-oncology Society, University of Melbourne, Fitzroy, VIC, Australia

Psychosocial Cancer Care, St Vincent's Hospital Melbourne, Fitzroy, VIC, Australia
e-mail: cliftondiannealice@gmail.com; di.clifton@svha.org.au

J. Fletcher (✉)
Melbourne Psycho-oncology Service, Cabrini Health, Epworth Hospital, Monash University, Melbourne, VIC, Australia
e-mail: Jane.Fletcher@monash.edu

R. D. MacLeod, L. Van den Block (eds.), *Textbook of Palliative Care*,
https://doi.org/10.1007/978-3-319-77740-5_88

Abstract

Severe psychological distress in palliative care patients is not uncommonly encountered by healthcare professionals. It is a manifestation of suffering requiring appropriate intervention, every bit as important as unrelieved pain or nausea. Such distress may range from transient "normal" sadness and grief to more disturbed psychological states such as severe anxiety, depression, demoralization, manifestations of serious mental illness, decompensation of personality disorder, and post-trauma syndromes. At times, the underlying cause may be organic – a reaction to corticosteroids, manifestations of cerebral pathology, or delirium.

The first section of this chapter focuses on how the clinician can recognize and distinguish different forms of psychological and psychiatric disorder which manifest as distress in palliative care patients. The discriminating features are presented in comparative tables and highlighted by clinical cases. One case is described in detail at the end of this section, where the patient suffered severe distress from different clinical syndromes over the last 8 months of his life, illustrating the need for continuing vigilance and assessment. The second section introduces therapeutic responses to patients in severe distress that every clinician can develop to reduce suffering in the moment. In so doing, the need for "emergency management" of clinical scenarios can be reduced and treatment can pave the way for specialist intervention when required. It describes the various therapies which have a demonstrated evidence base for efficacy in this population and summarizes in table form the recommended approaches for easing suffering in different forms of distress.

1 Introduction

People dealing with life-limiting disease have cumulative stress throughout the course of their illness. From the early symptoms leading to diagnosis with cancer or nonmalignant terminal disease, they undergo a series of investigative procedures and treatments, e.g., surgery, chemotherapy, radiotherapy, hormone manipulation, immunotherapies, and corticosteroids. Their lives become an emotional rollercoaster of hope and disappointment, adaptation, and crisis. Patients no longer feel authors of their own lives; they struggle to redefine their identity and role, to find new purpose and meaning in a body that is letting them down. By the time they are receiving palliative care services, the focus has moved from seeking cure to maximizing quality of life in the time remaining for the patient and family.

While some patients negotiate this journey relatively smoothly and show a remarkable degree of acceptance and stoicism, many can experience high levels of distress. Rather than being viewed as a diagnosis, distress should be considered an umbrella term, a signifier of an underlying mental state, much as fever is an indicator of underlying infection. It is a signal of patient suffering and needs to be recognized and understood. The National Comprehensive Cancer Network (NCCN) has defined distress as:

> . . .an unpleasant emotional experience of a psychological, social and/or spiritual nature which extends on a normal continuum, from common normal feelings to those of vulnerable sadness and fears, to problems that are more disabling, such as true depression, anxiety, panic, (demoralization*), and feeling isolated or in a spiritual crisis. [*author's addition]

They added "no patient's distress should go unrecognised and untreated" (National Comprehensive Cancer Network 2003).

Clinicians may not recognize the significance of distress, believing it to be an understandable and appropriate reaction to the patient's predicament. They find it difficult to distinguish between sadness and more serious clinical states of depression and demoralization. They may consider that treatment with medications will only add to the patient's burden or stigmatize them. Many clinicians may be unaware of, or unskilled in, the various psychotherapies that are available. They may feel uncomfortable about probing into the patient's psychological experience for fear of making them worse. Some clinicians do not like to get too close to the patient's pain because of their own vulnerabilities. The patient may also be reluctant to divulge emotional states for fear of appearing "weak" or burdening family or staff. Any or all of these factors may contribute to a failure in exploring the patient's distress, leading to underdiagnosis and undertreatment of psychological or psychiatric disorders causing suffering.

The consequences for the patient include impaired pleasure, meaning, and connectedness; a reduced quality of life; amplification of physical symptoms; and distraction from the emotional work of separating from loved ones, who in turn may be suffering as witnesses to the distress. Severe distress may lead to a request for a hastened death and is a risk factor for suicide, especially if the patient is depressed (Block 2000) or demoralized (Kissane et al. 2004).

2 Section 1: Distinguishing Different Forms of Severe Distress

2.1 Recognizing Distress

The clinician may recognize signs of distress through the patient's demeanor and the nature of spontaneous talk, but many patients mask or minimize their emotional stress from fear of being seen as "not coping." The importance of recognizing distress as "the 6th vital sign" (after pain) was championed in Canada and endorsed internationally in 2010 (Bultz and Johansen 2011). The NCCN recommended screening for distress in all cancer patients and developed a visual "distress thermometer" and accompanying problem list (National Comprehensive Cancer Network 2003).

The distress thermometer indicates the presence or absence of distress, as well as its intensity, and the problem list shows the domains seen by the patient as the cause of the distress, only some of which are emotional or spiritual. A second stage of screening (e.g., the Hospital Anxiety and Depression Scale (Zigmond and Snaith 1983)) and a good clinical interview with a comprehensive history are required to identify possible psychiatric disorders (Widera and Block 2012).

2.2 Distinguishing Different Forms of Distress

It is one thing to recognize that a patient is distressed, but the clinician is often unsure of the following: origin of the distress, its clinical significance in representing underlying disorders, and the appropriate intervention indicated. Responses may range from "in the moment" empathic listening, attending to social issues, involving pastoral care, or referring to more specialized clinicians for further assessment and "diagnosis." Subsequently, different forms of staff supervision, psychotherapy, family work, and/or pharmacotherapy approaches may occur.

The clinician will need to be able to distinguish:

- Sadness
- Grief
- Anxiety and panic
- Depression
- Demoralization
- Post-trauma syndromes
- Decompensation of underlying personality disorder
- Manifestations of underlying serious mental illness (bipolar affective disorder, schizophrenia)
- Substance abuse and withdrawal
- Organic mental states

The clinical features of each of these states will be described, including how they may be distinguished from other psychological states and psychiatric disorder. Some of the distinguishing features will be summarized in comparative tables.

2.3 Sadness

Sadness is a common human emotion occasioned when a person reflects on his/her situation of disadvantage, limitation, losses of future prospects, and experiences sorrow or disappointment. Everyone experiences sadness at times, and although the person may become quiet, lethargic, and withdraw themselves from others, it is a normal response. In its more severe and pervasive form, it can be a symptom of depression (see Table 1).

Belinda, aged 56 years, a married mother of two teenage daughters and a former schoolteacher, was admitted into a palliative care unit for symptom management of breathlessness and increasing weakness related to Motor Neurone Disease (MND), diagnosed six months previously. She was referred to psycho-oncology because she appeared flat and at times tearful. Belinda described herself as feeling sad rather than depressed. She would look at her daughters and think about the children they would have, that she would never see. She missed working in her garden and the joy of bringing fresh flowers and vegetables into the home. She still derived great pleasure from the company of others and music was of great solace to her. She worked with the music therapist to compile a CD of her favourite pieces, which she used not only to soothe herself 'during this dreadful waiting period while I slowly die', but also as a focus point in reliving memories with her family and planning music for her funeral. (O'Callaghan et al. 2015)

Table 1 Core features of sadness and depression[a]

Sadness	Depression
Able to feel intimately connected with others	Feels outcast and alone
Feels someday this will end	Feeling of permanence
Able to enjoy happy memories	Regretful, rumination on irredeemable mistakes
Sense of self-worth	Extreme self-deprecation/ self-loathing
Comes in waves	Constant and unremitting
Looks forward to things	No hope/interest in future
Retains capacity for pleasure	Enjoys few activities
Will to live	Suicidal thoughts/behavior

[a]Content adapted from Rayner et al. (2011)

2.4 Grief

Grief is natural response to any experience of loss that restricts people by taking away possibilities and potential. In a palliative care setting, a patient's grief may be engendered by loss of autonomy, body function, social role, familiar body image, sense of dignity, and identity. The family's grief may begin well before the death of the loved one. Grief is a multidimensional phenomenon with physical, emotional, behavioral, spiritual, and social manifestations (see Table 2).

2.4.1 Grief over Loss of Aspects of Self (Clarke et al. 2005)

Muriel, aged 65 years, had been prominent in the fashion industry and had been very conscious of her physical appearance. She was inconsolable because an oral cavity tumour had disfigured her face and made it difficult for her to speak clearly. She wished for an early death and would not permit visits from people who knew her from her more glamorous days. She gradually warmed to a psychologist who 'saw' her beyond her face, and delighted in regaling her with stories of her colourful past in her last weeks of life.

Preparatory Grief

This refers to grief "that the terminally ill patient must undergo in order to prepare himself for his final separation from this world" (Lindemann 1944). While Kubler-Ross (1970) saw this as a normal process in response to the perceived losses experienced by people who are dying, Mystakidou and colleagues (2008) found associations between preparatory grief, hopelessness, and psychological distress.

Malcolm, a 73-year-old former businessman and child Holocaust survivor had been distressed and ruminating about things he had failed to achieve for

Table 2 Comparison of grief and depression[a]

	Grief	Depression
Nature of response	Adaptive	Maladaptive
Focus of distress	Relates to a particular loss	Pervasive
Stability of symptoms	Comes in waves Generally improves over time	Constant Unremitting
Mood	Sadness and dysphoria Lability	Protracted depression Flatness
Anger	Often expressed	Self-directed
Interest	Maybe lessened due to preoccupation	Markedly diminished
Pleasure	Capacity in certain activities	Anhedonia
Cognition	Confusion	Problems with concentration Indecisiveness
Guilt	May feel regret over specific things	Excessive feelings of guilt
Hope	Episodic and focal loss of hope Change over time to more positive orientation	Persistent and pervasive hopelessness
Self-worth	Maintained though helplessness common	Worthlessness Feeling one's life has no value
Suicidal ideation	Passive fleeting desire for death	Preoccupation with desire to die
Imagery	Vivid Fantasy	Self-punitive
Sleep	Difficulties falling asleep Episode of wakefulness Vivid dreams	Early morning wakening
Responsiveness	Responds to warmth, reassurance, and support	Limited

[a]Content adapted from Widera and Block (2012)

his family before his death from advanced renal failure. In a reparative narrative review of his life (Freadman 2015) he was able to balance some of his regrets with pride over his achievements and make plans for handing over the business more formally to his sons.

Susie, a young mother of three children, all under the age of twelve years, had metastatic melanoma and was noted by community palliative care staff to be disengaged from her children. This caused the staff considerable distress, because they had wanted her to spend as much quality time with the children as she could before she became too ill. In supervision they came to realise that, at an unconscious level, Susie was beginning to psychologically withdraw from her children (decathect) as a manifestation of her preparatory grief and protection from overwhelming psychological pain.

Anticipatory Grief

Anticipatory grief relates to the anticipated loss of a loved one (Lindemann 1944). Although originally viewed as a potential coping mechanism for a prospective loss, Fulton and Gottesman (1980) reviewed the research literature on the topic and found many methodological flaws. Whether anticipatory grief is functional or dysfunctional for a family depends upon many complex and interacting factors, including psychological, interpersonal, and sociocultural considerations.

Harry, a 75-year-old retired butcher from a country town had suffered with metastatic prostate cancer with widespread bone secondaries for twelve years, and was admitted for management of his pain. It was noticed by staff that his family would come to visit occasionally, but rarely engaged with him in conversation and occupied themselves with their phones or magazines. Harry tearfully told a nurse after a visit from his wife – "It's like I'm dead already for her. She probably looks at me and thinks – 'he's not the bloke I married'. She used to be warm and caring, but it's like she's switched off, I've been sick that long."

Complicated Grief

Although a term mostly used in the description of bereaved caregivers, complicated grief may also be experienced by the terminally ill patient. The double effect of unprocessed losses before and during their illness can cause patients grief about the imminent loss of their own life (Alessandra Strada 2013).

2.5 Anxiety

Most individuals with advanced disease will experience some level of anxiety as they adapt to changes in their disease status. Symptoms of anxiety in a palliative setting may include feelings of foreboding, apprehension, and dread (Roth and Massie 2007) and may be experienced as emotional distress or may be somatic (Hinshaw et al. 2002) or cognitive (Roth and Massie 2007) in nature. At the end of life, these symptoms can be profoundly distressing for the patient, family, and staff.

In a palliative setting, low levels of anxiety as a response to a physical or psychological stressor are often short lived (Valentine 2014). More persistent anxiety can interfere with the individual's ability to function, significantly reduce quality of life, and lead to the development of an anxiety disorder. Individuals most at risk of developing an anxiety disorder in a palliative setting are those with a past history of anxiety disorder (NHMRC National Breast Cancer Centre (Australia) 2003), poorly controlled physical symptoms, a lack of social support or social isolation, and poor communication with their healthcare professionals (Lloyd-Williams and Hughes 2008). Higher rates of anxiety disorder have also been reported in younger patients (Austin et al. 2011).

> Kelly, a 37-year-old women diagnosed with stage 4 colorectal cancer, presented with overwhelming feelings of dread and fear soon after being diagnosed. Her symptomatology included a range of physical manifestations of anxiety, including nausea, loss of appetite and sleep dysfunction. She was well supported by her husband, and had three children under four years old. However, she lacked family support as her parents were interstate and her parents-in-law lived in a regional centre. She had a past history of anxiety, but had never seen a mental health professional. She was referred by her oncologist because she was 'not coming to terms with the news' and was seen on the ward with her husband present. Kelly described constant nausea, and presented with an acute grief reaction with high levels of anxiety around her prognosis. She focused on her mortality and her catastrophic thought processes drove her fear and exacerbated her anxiety. She interpreted her physical symptoms as a sign that her disease had progressed further, and experienced multiple panic attacks with significant shortness of breath at rest. Her physical symptoms of anxiety escalated her death anxiety.

Estimated probable cases of anxiety in advanced cancer inpatients measured using the Hospital Anxiety and Depression Scale (HADS) (Zigmond and Snaith 1983) range from 34% (Teunissen et al. 2007) to 44% (Delgado-Guay et al. 2009), with up to 16% of requests for psychiatric consultation based on the assessment of symptoms of anxiety (Massie and Holland 1987).

There is limited data on the prevalence of anxiety in those with non-oncological disease. In a retrospective study of stroke deaths, Ntlholang et al. (2016) reported low rates of psychological distress (1.9%) but marked levels of agitation (25.9%). Gore et al. (2000) in a comparison study of those with non-small cell lung cancer (NSCLC) and those with chronic obstructive pulmonary disease (COPD) reported higher rates of anxiety and depression (90%) in those with COPD compared to those with NSCLC (52%). While chronicity of the disease and symptom burden may explain these differences, Sorenson (2013) suggests that poorer access to quality palliation may be factor. In individuals with congestive heart failure (CHF), rates of anxiety have been stated to be as high as 63% (Moser et al. 2016).

Anxiety is often a manifestation of other psychiatric disorders, and in a palliative population, differential diagnoses include depression, delirium, and medication or treatment side effects (Roth et al. 2009). Roth and Massie postulate that depression and anxiety can be viewed as syndromes that exist on a continuum with overlap in symptomatology (Roth and Massie 2007). While depression and anxiety may coexist (Wilson et al. 2007), key distinguishing features include the hopelessness, worthlessness, and anhedonia (loss of pleasure) associated with depression, compared with the feelings of worry, dread, and fear associated with anxiety (American Psychiatric Association 2013). When distinguishing anxiety and delirium, the key features of delirium which differentiates it from anxiety disorders include the presence of disorientation; impaired memory, attention, and concentration; fluctuating level of consciousness; and altered perceptions including hallucinations, delusions, and illusions (Wise and Rieck 1993).

It is important to remember the significant overlap between the somatic symptoms of anxiety and the side effects of treatment, illness, and the disease process (Zweers et al. 2016). A significant level of distress, anxiety, and depressive symptomatology may be attributable to the high level of physical symptom burden experienced by patients with advanced disease (Zweers et al. 2016). Uncontrolled pain is seen as a common cause of anxiety and agitation (Hinshaw et al. 2002), and suicidal ideation is common in those with uncontrolled pain (Roth and Massie 2007). In those with respiratory disease, dyspnea can cause significant distress and anxiety.

Table 3 summarizes the underlying medical causes of anxiety in a palliative setting and highlights the need to exclude other causes and manage physical symptoms such as pain, dyspnea, nausea, and sleep disturbance, in order to alleviate psychological distress (Andersen et al. 2014). While discussed in detail elsewhere, issues such as steroid psychosis and delirium should be treated as a medical/psychiatric emergency in order to reduce distress for the patient, family, and staff. Metabolic and physiological abnormalities (e.g., severe constipation and electrolyte and glucose imbalance) can lead to episodes of delirium with agitation, disturbances of consciousness, and changes in cognition. These clinical scenarios highlight that in medically compromised patients, symptoms of anxiety may be an early warning sign in relation to development of delirium (Hinshaw et al. 2002). Alcohol, nicotine, opioid, and benzodiazepine withdrawal has also been noted to cause anxiety that can lead to agitation and delirium (Irwin et al. 2005; Ginige 2016). Existential concerns such as death anxiety, fear of pain, loss of independence, being a burden, and unfinished business can lead to increased levels of anxiety in this population (Hinshaw et al. 2002).

Anxiety experienced by carers, friends, and family members can also have a profound impact on the patient's level of distress. Assessment of family distress and appropriate intervention is important, as is the provision of accurate information. Teaching the family how to manage their emotional reactions is likely to have a positive impact on the patient's ability to cope.

2.5.1 Anxiety Disorders

It is important to remember that anxiety is a symptom which may form part of several anxiety disorders, each with specific diagnostic criteria and symptomatology (American Psychiatric Association 2013). These include adjustment

Table 3 Medical causes of anxiety[a]

Uncontrolled pain	Respiratory disease/distress
Metabolic and physiologic issues	Drug induced
Hypoxia	Corticosteroids, dexamethasone, prednisolone
Delirium – hyperactive	Antiemetics
Sepsis	Bronchodilators
Blood loss	Psychostimulants
Pulmonary embolus	Caffeine
Hypocalcemia	
Hypoglycemia	
Electrolyte imbalance	Substances or withdrawal from substances
Undiagnosed hyperthyroidism	(alcohol, opioids, benzodiazepines)
Nutrition failure	Hormone secreting tumors – thyrotropic
Severe constipation	(TSH) – secreting adenomas

[a]Content adapted from Hinshaw et al. (2002); Roth and Massie (2007)

Table 4 Symptoms of anxiety[a]

Hyperarousal Restlessness Irritability	Thinking style Worry and foreboding Apprehension and dread
Panic Palpitations, tachycardia, tremor Diaphoresis (sweating) Dyspnea (shortness of breath) Gastrointestinal distress or nausea Feelings of impending doom	Recurrent unpleasant thoughts Fear of pain Fear of death Fear of dependency on others Fear of unfinished business
Sleep disturbance Initial insomnia (difficulty falling asleep) Less restorative sleep Nightmares Middle of the night or early morning waking	Negative thought patterns Catastrophization Overgeneralization Inevitability of negative outcome Helpless in hopeless situation
Changes in appetite Loss of appetite – may lead to wasting Increase appetite (mania)	Sexual dysfunction Reduced libido Erectile and orgasmic dysfunction

[a]Content adapted from Roth and Massie (2007)

disorder with anxiety, generalized anxiety disorder (GAD), panic disorder, phobic disorder, and obsessive compulsive disorder (OCD). Table 4 highlights the clinical signs and symptoms associated with each anxiety disorder. In a palliative setting, relying on rigid diagnostic criteria may lead to underidentification of disorders and has the potential to increase suffering in an already vulnerable population.

Wilson et al. (2007) in a Canadian study with palliative cancer patients reported 13.9% of respondents having an anxiety disorder, 5.5% panic disorder, 5.8% a GAD, 4.7% an anxiety disorder not otherwise specified, and 1.8% an anxiety disorder secondary to a medical condition.

Phobias

Phobic disorders should be considered especially in those who have had long episodes of illness with painful or traumatic interventions. Needle phobia is common and may have a negative impact on treatment decisions. Claustrophobia may be present in patients who are non-ambulatory or those who have extended admissions to hospital or inpatient palliative care services. Similarly, those with MND or degenerative neurological disorders may experience a phobic response associated with the fear of being "locked in" to their body. This may manifest as panic as their condition deteriorates. Individuals with end-stage lung disease and those with intractable dyspnea may find small spaces difficult and may create high levels of distress, e.g., showering may become problematic and lead to avoidant behavior. These phobias are difficult to overcome as they relate to physical symptoms that are profoundly distressing and often result in panic attacks.

Judy, a 68-year-old women, with end-stage respiratory disease lives alone after the death of her husband, Ben two years before, and the suicide of her only son, Michael five years earlier. Judy is on continuous oxygen therapy and is supported with mobile oxygen when out. She had become fearful of leaving the house and while still able to drive her car, now had to drive with the windows down. She had difficulty going into shopping centres and avoided small spaces such as change rooms and public toilets. She was admitted to an inpatient palliative care unit for symptom management and a member of the psychosocial team was asked to see her. She presented with marked dyspnoea and was hunched forward in the chair. In spite of the door being open, she asked that it not be closed and that the curtain not be pulled around her. She was struggling with her admission as she described feeling like she might suffocate if she did not get fresh air. She had not showered for days and was toileting using a bedpan, as she could not face going into the small bathroom.

Generalized Anxiety Disorder

The excessive worriers who come to palliative care may have an exacerbation of anxiety but paradoxically, now there is a real threat to contend with, may have a reduction in anxiety symptoms.

Panic Disorder

Panic attacks are characterized by periods of intense fear or discomfort. Symptoms develop abruptly and include palpitations and shortness of breath dizziness and derealization (feeling estranged or detached from one's environment) and depersonalization (altered and unreal perception of self, feelings, and situation) and fear of dying. As a combination of both physical and affective symptoms is used to diagnose panic, this can pose an issue for diagnosis in a palliative setting. The symptoms of depersonalization and derealization are more suitable for diagnosing panic disorder in those with life-limiting illness. For those with underlying shortness of breath, the fear of suffocating to death can drive panic attacks in this already vulnerable subgroup.

Death Anxiety

Death anxiety, often defined as the anxiety related to death awareness (Sussman and Liu 2014), has been described as the most profound fear and to be a driver of all anxiety. In his landmark book *The Denial of Death* (Becker 1974), the anthropologist Ernest Becker writes:

> …the fear (or terror) of death must be present in all our normal functioning, in order for the organism to be armed toward self-preservation. But the fear of death cannot be present constantly in one's mental functioning, else the organism could not function…. And so we can understand what seems like an impossible paradox: the ever-present fear of death in the normal biological functioning of our instinct of self-preservation, as well as our utter obliviousness to this fear in our conscious life.

As end of life approaches, death is no longer a distant prospect but part of rapidly approaching reality. The fear may relate to the dying process and the potential for poor symptom control especially in relation to pain or may relate to the existential nothingness and feelings of missing out that can be associated with death. A full assessment of the fears associated with end of life is important.

2.5.2 Depression

Depression is common among patients receiving palliative care but interestingly not more common than during the early stages of diagnosis and treatment and not an invariable outcome of advanced disease. A review by Hotopf et al. (2002) in 2002 and a later meta-analysis by Mitchell et al. (2011) estimated a prevalence of *Diagnostic and Statistical Manual of Mental Disorders* (DSM), defined major depressive disorder (MDD) of 15% and 14.3%, respectively (see Table 5 for summary of symptoms for DSM 5 MDD). The prevalence of DSM-defined minor depression was 9.6% and of adjustment disorder alone 15.4%. However the total prevalence of clinically significant mood disorder is estimated to be 30–40% (Mitchell et al. 2011). Many clinicians fail to recognize significant depression because of a tendency to "normalize" human responses to catastrophic situations such as life-threatening illness, leading to underdetection and therefore undertreatment (Rayner et al. 2010). The failure to recognize depression or enquire about mood is compounded by the observation that depressed patients are reluctant to volunteer symptoms (Hotopf et al. 2002).

Table 5 Summary of symptoms for DSM 5 MDD[a]

Five or more of the following, including at least one of items 1 and 2
1. Depressed mood
2. Loss of pleasure
3. Weight loss/weight gain or decreased appetite/ increased appetite
4. Insomnia/hypersomnia
5. Psychomotor agitation/retardation
6. Fatigue/loss of energy
7. Worthlessness/guilt
8. Decreased concentration/indecisiveness
9. Recurrent thoughts of death/suicidal ideation/plans/ attempts

[a]Content adapted from American Psychiatric Association (2013)

Adherence to strict DSM (American Psychiatric Association 2013) criteria of MDD is difficult in the palliative care context because of the overlap in symptoms of MDD and those of advanced medical illness (see Fig. 1). Greater emphasis needs to be placed on the patient's cognition and ability to experience pleasure than the somatic symptoms of depression. Some screening tools for depression omit somatic items and are more useful in the palliative care context. Two of the more commonly used assessment scales are the Hospital Anxiety and Depression Scale (HADS) (Zigmond and Snaith 1983; Mitchell et al. 2010), which has seven items relating to anxiety and six related to depression, and the Brief Edinburgh Depression Scale (BEDS) which has six items

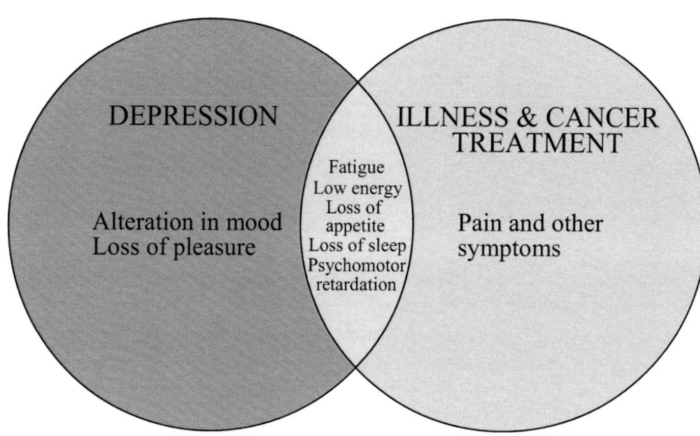

Fig. 1 Overlap between the somatic symptoms of depression and the side effects of treatment, illness, and the disease process

(Lloyd-Williams et al. 2007). Simply asking the patient "are you depressed?" (Chochinov et al. 1997) may accurately identify many depressed patients, but a two-item screen, which includes a question about loss of interest and pleasure in addition to mood and hopelessness has greater sensitivity and will pick up more cases (Mitchell 2008).

Early detection and treatment of depression is important, not only to relieve the suffering of the patient but also because depression exacerbates the physical effects of advanced disease, such as pain. Depression hinders adherence to treatment, obstructs the work of separating from the family and preparing for death, is a risk factor for high health service costs, and is associated with increased disability, poor prognosis, a higher mortality and higher risk of suicide or desire for hastened death (Widera and Block 2012; Rayner et al. 2010).

Table 6 Core features of demoralization and depression

Demoralization	Depression
Loss of meaning	Loss of pleasure
Loss of purpose	Loss of interest
Hopelessness	Hopelessness may be a feature
Helplessness	Withdrawal, isolation
Existential distress	Pervasively lowered mood
Shame	Guilt
Loss of anticipatory pleasure	
Feelings of failure or pointlessness, giving up[a]	Worthlessness
Difficulties coping and meeting expectations of self and others leading to lowered self-esteem[a]	
	Neurovegetative symptoms

[a]Proposed by Kissane as criteria for the revision of the Demoralization Scale-II and for establishment of demoralization in future editions of diagnostic systems such as DSM; Robinson et al. (2015)

2.6 Demoralization

The syndrome of demoralization, as a distinct clinical entity separate from depression and grief (Clarke et al. 2000), requiring recognition and treatment in the palliative care context and was first advanced by Kissane et al. in 2001 (2001), following the earlier work of Jerome Frank, as described by Clarke (2012). The core features of this syndrome are existential distress, loss of meaning and purpose, hopelessness, and helplessness (see Table 6). Demoralized individuals suffer immensely, lose self-esteem and a sense of mastery, see the future as pointless, and often yearn for release through death. This may lead to requests for a hastened death or suicide. Even when clinicians recognize the existential distress of the patient, they may see it as a totally understandable response to the circumstances and be unaware that the patient can, and should, receive appropriate intervention.

Although depression and demoralization share some common features, major depression is characterized by anhedonia and demoralization by loss of meaning and purpose. Patients who are demoralized can show a full range of affect and can experience pleasure in engaging in meaningful activities, although they may have difficulty in feeling anticipatory pleasure for things that are not in the here and now because they find it difficult to imagine a future without suffering. Demoralization can occur in the absence of clinical depression but when unattended can lead to depression; similarly, demoralization can become a secondary co-morbid disorder to unrelenting depression.

In a review of the literature pertaining to research of demoralization in progressive illness and cancer over the previous decade, Robinson et al. (2015) reported a prevalence of demoralization of 13–18%. It is interesting to note that, as for depression, the prevalence of demoralization is independent of time since diagnosis and stage of disease. Factors contributing to the development of demoralization include having poorly controlled medical symptoms, untreated depression or anxiety, poor social supports and social functioning, and having no partner.

The two measures of demoralization most often used in the studies reviewed were the categorically oriented Diagnostic Criteria for Psychosomatic Research (DCPR) (Fava et al. 1995), administered by structured interview and the dimensionally directed Demoralization Scale (DS), a 24 item self-report questionnaire (Kissane et al. 2004). The authors noted that the DCPR held the traditional psychosomatic notion that the mind directly causes the illness. However, in the development of the DS, Kissane viewed demoralization as a state of maladaptive coping in response to a stressor. Recently the DS was refined using classical test theory and Rasch's item response theory. The resulting 16-item, 2-component scale with 3 response options, the DS-II (see Fig. 2), has demonstrated internal and external validity; it is likely to be a useful tool in detecting demoralization and in tracking responses to meaning-centered therapies (Robinson et al. 2016a, b).

2.7 Post-trauma Syndromes

Post-traumatic stress disorder (PTSD) and other post-trauma syndromes may predate the onset of a terminal illness, be activated for the first time by the illness, or develop as a result of the experience of diagnosis and treatment of life-limiting disease itself. At times the distress manifested by the patient can be difficult to differentiate from grief, particularly if losses have been sustained in traumatic circumstances. Table 7 sets out the distinguishing features of grief and trauma. The significance of this for the patient is that there are many triggers in a palliative care context that create severe distress. The patient with pre-existing PTSD may have suffered childhood sexual and/or physical abuse, may be a refugee from a war-torn country, may have been held hostage, or may have developed the disorder from any number of traumatic experiences. People who have experienced trauma inflicted by other human beings rather than victims of natural disasters suffer more damaging consequences. Basic trust in others and the perceived safety of the world is severely challenged. The patient with PTSD experiences a cluster of symptoms:

Intrusive (memories, dissociative flashbacks, dreams, nightmares, symbolic associations)
Avoidant (efforts to avoid elements of the traumatic experience, including thoughts, feelings, memories, places, people)
Alterations in mood and cognition (dissociative amnesia, negative beliefs, negative emotions, emotional numbing, self-judgment, sense of foreshortened future, inability to feel happiness)
Hyperarousal (irritability, anger, hypervigilance, exaggerated startle response, recklessness, poor sleep and concentration)

All of these symptoms impact on the capacity to engage with staff in the setting of dependency and intimacy that characterizes palliative care. Pain, personal care, procedures, smells, and the death of other patients – a myriad of potent

For each statement below, please indicate how much (or how strongly) you have felt this way ***over the last two weeks*** *by circling the corresponding number.*

		Never	Sometimes	Often
1	There is little value in what I can offer others.	0	1	2
2	My life seems to be pointless.	0	1	2
3	My role in life has been lost.	0	1	2
4	I no longer feel emotionally in control.	0	1	2
5	No one can help me.	0	1	2
6	I feel that I cannot help myself.	0	1	2
7	I feel hopeless.	0	1	2
8	I feel irritable.	0	1	2
9	I do not cope well with life.	0	1	2
10	I have a lot of regret about my life.	0	1	2
11	I tend to feel hurt easily.	0	1	2
12	I feel distressed about what is happening to me.	0	1	2
13	I am not a worthwhile person.	0	1	2
14	I would rather not be alive.	0	1	2
15	I feel quite isolated or alone.	0	1	2
16	I feel trapped by what is happening to me.	0	1	2

Scoring Instructions:

Total score demoralization: Sum all 16 items.

Meaning and Purpose subscale: Sum items 1, 2, 3, 5, 6, 7, 13, and 14.

Distress and Coping Ability subscale: Sum items 4, 8, 9, 10, 11, 12, 15, and 16.

Fig. 2 Demoralization scale – II

Table 7 Comparison of grief and trauma[a]

Grief	Trauma
Sorrow (sadness) most prominent	Anxiety most prominent affect
Anxiety relates to separation	Anxiety is to the event and exposure to it
Preoccupations, intrusive memories, and images relate to the loss	Preoccupations, intrusive memories, and images relate to the traumatic event
Pining and yearning; seeks opportunity for contact: behavior is toward	Behavior is avoidant and withdrawing

[a]Content adapted from Raphael et al. (2004)

activators of PTSD in the palliative care setting – can interact with the patient's powerlessness and experience of being "done to" and activate post-traumatic stress. Delirium is common in the palliative care setting, and it is not uncommon for past traumatic experience to be relived during a delirium. This is distressing not only for the patient if it is remembered but for the family and staff who witness the event (Breitbart et al. 2002).

2.8 Decompensation of Underlying Personality Disorder

People who have an enduring pattern of inner experience and behavior that is maladaptive and causes significant impairment in interpersonal and social functioning are described as having personality disorder. During times of personal threat, the demand on coping strategies and need for adaptation are high. Those with personality disorder are not well-resourced internally and generally regress, with accentuation of the maladaptive emotions and behaviors. Although many types of personality disorders are described in DSM 5 (American Psychiatric Association 2013), this section will limit discussion and case examples to three types of personality disorders patients that are most likely to experience (and cause) severe distress in a palliative setting.

2.8.1 Borderline Personality Disorder

The core feature of borderline personality disorder (BPD) is the disturbed attachments in early life, through early loss, unpredictability or unavailability of caretaking figures, or outright emotional, physical, or sexual abuse. Their vulnerabilities make them exquisitely sensitive to real or imagined abandonment, and they experience intense fears of annihilation. The distress, powerlessness, and dependency that are almost inevitable in life-limiting illness and invasive or intimate treatments and care cause severe regression and the emergence of very primitive defense mechanisms. Patients may behave in ways that are experienced as manipulative and become self-destructive in a desperate effort to gain some measure of control and channel intense, aggressive drives, and dependent needs. Their interactions with staff can cause confusion, anger, and rejection or avoidance of the patient. The BPD patient at times idealizes and at other times devalues individual staff members; sometimes certain staff are experienced as "good," while others are dismissed contemptuously as "bad." This is known as "splitting" and the dynamic becomes apparent when different members of the team have opposing views of the patient, "taking sides" for or against the patient. The BPD patient is prone not only to project feelings (such as anger) onto staff (accusing them of being angry), but also in a more subtle process, unwanted affect is taken on by the staff member unconsciously in an intrapsychic process termed "projective identification." This latter process results in the clinician leaving a patient encounter feeling unaccountably powerless, enraged, or harboring punitive impulses toward the patient (Hay and Passik 2000).

Pauline, a 37-year-old divorced woman with three children from different relationships was admitted for pain management of peritoneal metastases from ovarian cancer. She had experienced childhood sexual abuse from her father from the age of 8–13 and had not been believed by her mother when she disclosed the abuse. Although she had received counselling from a sexual abuse agency in her 20's, after the birth of her first two children, her lifestyle had already developed a chaotic pattern, with unstable relationships and employment, alcohol abuse and self-harming episodes. Pauline was demanding, uncooperative and untrusting of staff. She insisted that all her care be delivered by one particular nurse who reminded her of an auntie who took her in when she ran away from home at sixteen years of age. She challenged nurses and doctors about every aspect of her care, to the degree that many staff were actively avoiding her and taking sick leave.

2.8.2 Narcissistic Personality Disorder

Patients with narcissistic personality disorder (NPD) can rankle staff because of their sense of entitlement, grandiosity, lack of empathy toward others, and contemptuous manner. They may invoke counterattack from staff whose own narcissism is challenged. The outward show of self-importance is a defense against core feelings of low self-esteem, shame, and self-doubt, and it is this vulnerability that makes NPD individuals at risk of experiencing a narcissistic wound under severe stress, sometimes with catastrophic consequences.

Sam was a 48-year-old musician with metastatic colorectal cancer, estranged from his wife and children because they could no longer tolerate his self-centredness. He was angry about his illness and expressed the feeling that he would be 'better off dead' than have to rely on the incompetence of others. Although efforts were made to safely secure his environment from potential means of suicide, he was found dead in the toilet following an overdose of barbiturates which had presumably been brought to him by a visitor.

2.8.3 Paranoid Personality Disorder

The mental life of a person with paranoid personality disorder (PPD) is characterized by suspicion and mistrust of others, hypervigilance, and lack of emotional warmth. The early background is often defined by harsh, critical, and humiliating treatment by caregivers. These individuals struggle with anger, resentment, vindictiveness, and fear, and the defense mechanisms of denial and projection make them difficult to engage. They may appear grandiose at times as everything is self-referential, and they are constantly scanning the environment to work out "what is really going on." In circumstances of life-threatening illness, the patient with PPD is precipitated into an unfamiliar situation of dependency on others and is likely to be highly critical and make angry accusations to unsuspecting staff, who are more accustomed to expressions of gratitude from the patients they care for.

Tom was a 74-year-old single man with Parkinson's Disease who was admitted to the inpatient palliative care unit for assessment, when the community palliative care team reported that he was becoming increasingly breathless. He had refused to go to his GP or a hospital for examination, but ultimately agreed to be admitted to a palliative care unit provided he could have his own room and no-one would bother him. His community care workers said that he had been very difficult to engage and would only relate to one worker provided that she kept a distance from him. He had lived alone all of his adult life and had no friends. An estranged sister told the team he was a 'difficult man, very much a loner and a bit on the paranoid side'. He had never been treated at a psychiatric hospital and community staff were not aware of any delusional thinking. From the moment of his arrival, Tom stated he was going to leave. Physical examination was not possible, nor any investigations, but he was noted to have swollen ankles and it was speculated that he may have cardiac failure. He became increasingly distressed with so many patients and staff around him that he abruptly left the unit in great distress on the third day. There were concerns for his safety as he had no medications at home for his Parkinson's Disease, so the community team called on him that evening only to find he had changed the locks and would not answer the door. Consideration was given to involving police to gain access to the house to perform a welfare check, but it was ultimately decided that such an intervention would be too distressing for him in view of his paranoid tendencies. The community team visited the following morning and were able to talk to him through the window, successfully winning back his trust over the following week.

2.9 Symptoms of Serious Mental Illness

Approximately 1% of the population suffers from schizophrenia: a further 1% from bipolar affective disorder (manic-depressive illness) (Miovic and Block 2007). As a group, people with serious mental illness are known to receive poor primary care, have inadequate screening for medical problems, have a high rate of medical comorbidities, lead lifestyles that may contribute to poor health (smoking, lack of exercise, alcohol abuse, use of marijuana and other illicit substances), and present later with cancer diagnoses, so that palliative rather than curative treatment is the only option. Other medical conditions related to serious mental illness that may lead to terminal illness include the metabolic syndrome, cardiomyopathy from antipsychotic medications, and lung or liver disease from smoking or alcohol abuse, respectively. In addition to these factors, the person with serious mental illness may have poor insight, difficulties in communication, cognitive disturbance, disturbed abstract reasoning and troubling or traumatic experiences of the world, and others during psychotic episodes and mental health treatments. They frequently experience disruptions in family relationships and social connectedness, homelessness, and interruption of the "normal" developmental trajectory with consequent deficits in sense of self. The entry of a person with serious mental illness into an unfamiliar healthcare system with a different language, culture, and technology creates a particularly acute vulnerability for the individual and anxiety and fear in professionals who often feel out of their depth. When such a patient shows evidence of severe distress, it can be difficult to determine whether it is related to these factors, relapse of the mental illness or the disease and/or the treatments.

Ray, aged 77 years, had been a loner all of his life, but had no previous psychiatric history. He presented with symptoms of breathlessness and was found to have lung cancer with metastatic disease to his brain. Radiotherapy could palliate his symptoms, but there was a question of his capacity to consent. Although Ray had delusional explanations of his illness (which revealed a long-standing and undiagnosed paranoid psychosis) and could not give informed consent, he expressed a desire to have available treatment for his disease. An empathic interview with a psychiatrist included the communication 'I can see what a hard-working man you are, and how you have always tried to do the right thing by other people. To be here with little sense of the reason why, and not to be in control must be unbearable. I will tell the team about you and make sure they are able to think about you when decisions are being considered'. Treatment proceeded after an application under the relevant act for procedures or interventions when the patient is not mentally competent.

Erica aged 27 years, suffered from Bipolar Affective Disorder (BAD). She rejected her diagnosis of lymphoma, became manic and was difficult to engage in treatment for a potentially curable disease. When she was stable enough to commence chemotherapy, she was administered steroids to reduce the swelling around the lymph nodes in her mediastinum which were causing breathlessness and had an acute steroid-induced mania. She subsequently developed a delirium secondary to toxicity from her mood-stabilizing lithium medication. Her compliance with treatment was erratic and her disease progressed, ultimately involving the central nervous system. Her palliative care management was complicated by the diagnostic challenges of multiple aetiologies of her fluctuating mental state.

Cyril was a 74-year-old single man with a long history of paranoid schizophrenia managed successfully by his GP for thirty years without relapse of his symptoms. He was admitted with end-stage renal failure for end-of-life care after ceasing dialysis, and in the second week became aggressive and paranoid towards staff. He was initially thought to have a delirium secondary to the accumulation of toxins that his kidneys were failing to excrete, but there was no disturbance of attention and orientation. Further investigation revealed that his GP had ceased his long-term depot antipsychotic injection when he withdrew from dialysis and as a result Cyril had been unmedicated for his psychosis for six weeks.

2.10 Substance Abuse and Withdrawal

Estimates of the prevalence of alcoholism in different palliative care settings range from 7% to 27%. Over one third of head and neck cancer patients meet criteria for alcohol dependence, and a further 6.5% meet criteria for abuse. Lung cancer patients have a prevalence of alcohol dependence of 6.5%. Point prevalence for other substance use disorders in the general population is 0.5–1% each for benzodiazepines, opioids, amphetamines, cocaine, and marijuana (Reisfield et al. 2009). Palliative care staff may neglect to enquire about alcohol and drug use, and the appearance of withdrawal symptoms may be unrecognized or misinterpreted (Irwin et al. 2005). The most dramatic of these is delirium tremens, which characteristically appears 3–5 days following abrupt withdrawal from heavy alcohol use. It can present as a psychiatric emergency, with physiological hyperarousal, agitation, paranoia, visual and auditory hallucinations, disorientation, and impulsive behavior that is driven by fear. It carries a high risk of mortality and requires prompt attention with a combination of diazepam, haloperidol, and thiamine and adaptations in the environment to secure the patient's safety.

Family members may also have alcohol and drug abuse problems. Methamphetamine (ICE) abuse is an increasingly encountered problem in health settings. These may lead to problem behaviors on the ward and abuse or neglect of the patient in the home environment. A particular issue for community palliative care workers is the potential for diversion of opiate medication by drug-abusing family members. This problem will be discussed in the ▶ Chap. 83, "Challenging Family Dynamics."

2.11 Organic Mental Disorders

It is imperative that healthcare professionals are mindful of possible organic causes of severe distress. In a palliative care context, these include delirium, drug-induced states (steroids, ketamine), and cerebral disease (primary or secondary cancer, leptomeningeal involvement, paraneoplastic syndromes). In delirium, the onset is usually rapid, the course fluctuating, and the symptoms worsen in the late afternoon and evening. A "quiet" or hypoactive delirium may go unrecognized, and the patient's distress about abnormal experiences may therefore not be addressed. This state may rapidly change to a hyperactive or mixed state. Attentional deficits, disorientation, mood disturbances, and perceptual abnormalities may become more apparent in agitated patients. In a drug-induced abnormal mental state, there is a clear relationship to the administration of the medication and a resolution when the drug is ceased. Corticosteroids (e.g., dexamethasone, prednisolone) can induce mania, depression, anxiety, paranoid psychosis, delirium, agitation, and wakefulness, while ketamine can cause unpleasant dissociative experiences in the doses used for refractory pain, and opiates can trigger a delirium. Mental state changes indicative of cerebral or meningeal involvement can be subtle and include odd behaviors, speech disturbance, and confabulation to cover up deficits. The essence to diagnosing these developments is alertness to changes in the usual mental state and a preparedness to listen to family members' observations of change.

2.12 Suicide

Ideas of suicide, suicide attempts, and completed suicide can occur in severely distressed patients who see no other way of ending their suffering. As we have noted, the demoralized, the depressed, and the narcissistically wounded are at special risk. The topics of suicide, suicide attempts, and requests for assisted suicide are discussed in separate chapters in this textbook, but Fig. 3 summarizes pathways to suicidal ideation and suicide.

What follows is a detailed description of one patient's changes in mental state during the last 8 months of life, illustrating features many of the disorders discussed above and concluding with the development of symptoms and signs of cerebral disease.

2.13 The Story of Arno

Arno was a 75-year-old man with recurrence of lymphoma, first treated 15 years previously. At the time he came to be assessed for severe distress, he had been receiving a targeted therapy in regular intravenous infusions for 2 months.

Arno had come to Australia from Holland with his family as a teenager in the early 1950s. As a child during World War II, he had witnessed his village being occupied by the Nazis and the disappearance of a lot of his Jewish neighbors, including his special friend. He did not understand the significance of these events until after the war. The atmosphere in the home was always very tense and volatile – father could be violent and mother was anxious and rarely left the house, spending long periods in bed. It fell to Arno as the eldest child to care for the five younger siblings. Both parents were communists, and although nominally protestant, religious practices were not observed in the home. Arno learned as

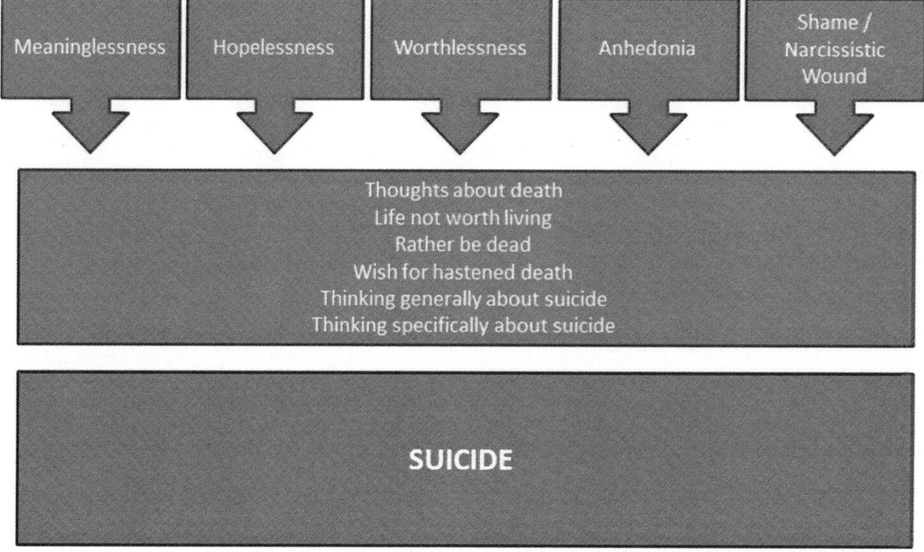

Fig. 3 Pathways to suicide

an adult that his maternal grandmother was Jewish and that he too would have been considered Jewish through the matriarchal lineage. With this knowledge came an understanding of the unspoken terror in the family relating to the fear of discovery and their relative isolation from the outside world. It also helped to make sense of his identification with Jewish people, to the degree that his school mates bullied him and called him "Levi the Jew-lover." He stood up to his bullies on one occasion and was never bothered again.

In Australia, Arno studied hard and obtained several degrees and diplomas. He worked as an engineer on a hydroelectric development that had created employment for many postwar European migrants. He had a traumatic experience of discovering bodies with their feet encased in concrete at the bottom of one of the dams but had never spoken about this to anyone. He married an Australian woman and had two children to whom he gave "old testament" names. He had one granddaughter whom he adored – "the light of my life."

Arno left engineering to become a shop steward and union man for a family business, a job he held until his retirement some years after his early illness. He was well-respected at work and had a reputation for being able to settle an argument "with a certain look I have." He had never been physically violent to others. He was known for his compassion; he and his wife would regularly take in and care for drug addicts, prostitutes, and homeless people. This was very much part of Arno's identity and he saw his actions as a way of reparation for the ugliness he had witnessed in human behavior. He considered his own life as fortunate. He had never been a smoker and drank alcohol only rarely.

2.13.1 Different Manifestations of Distress During the Last 8 Months of Arno's Life

Arno was referred as an urgent assessment after he had abruptly fled the chemotherapy unit, knocking staff and equipment in his path. He had been commenced on the monoclonal antibody rituximab because his lymphoma had progressed and was not responding to standard chemotherapy. Arno described classic features of a **panic attack** and felt he had to get out of the unit or he would die. He had already received three treatments without incident, but significant **death anxiety** was emerging since the news of his recurrence.

Over subsequent sessions a picture emerged of an underlying **major depression** somewhat masked by his stoic mien, with loss of pleasure and interest, irritability, tearfulness – "like a blubber-baby" – and poor appetite. He also described a long history of nightmares and flashbacks of his traumatic wartime experiences and episodes of cruelty and violence he had witnessed in his life. He avoided anything related to war, violence, or "bad things" happening to people and was always hypervigilant, "on the lookout" for people mistreating others. His wife complained of his emotional numbness in their marriage. He had a comorbid **post-traumatic stress disorder** which he had long managed through avoidant behaviors.

Arno responded very well to **mirtazapine** with improvement in mood, sleep, and appetite, but a month later he started to appear slumped and dejected in his sessions and conveyed a sense of shame. He said: "I just can't be the man I used to be. I feel useless. The men I used to look out for hardly call me anymore – they used to ask me for advice or just have a yarn or a whinge…I'm not well enough to look after the street people. I used to stand tall – have a certain presence…but now I feel invisible. I'm a waste of space. On the scrap heap." Arno had become **demoralized** even though his depression had improved, and the therapy started to focus more on a review of Arno's achievements and helping him to create new meaning and a sense of mastery.

Several months later, Arno developed pneumonia and became disoriented, agitated, and paranoid, while his intravenous antibiotics were being infused. Some of his post-traumatic experiences emerged in the **delirium,** and he misinterpreted messages over the public address system, believing that patients were being taken down to the basement to be shot or gassed. Medical staff in the private hospital did not recognize the delirium and contacted his psychiatrist to say that he had become psychotic. His delirium responded well over 24–48 h to parenteral haloperidol and the treatment of his pneumonia.

Six months into therapy, Arno came to a session in a highly distressed state, having canceled his session the previous week. His face was suffused; he was trying very hard to stifle his emotions, and he had great difficulty gaining composure enough to be able to speak. Eventually he began to sob and told the psychiatrist that his daughter's marriage had broken up. "Things will never be the same for little Essie – this isn't supposed to happen in my family – I won't be there to support them." Arno was displaying acute symptoms of **grief** over the loss of a secure future for his beloved granddaughter and although initially inconsolable, he became more soothed as the psychiatrist discussed with him the importance of his role in Essie's life right now.

Almost 8 months into therapy, Arno missed several sessions because of influenza. After a break of 5 weeks, he came to his session looking haggard and disheveled. He appeared wobbly and reached out for the walls and furniture to get his bearings and steady himself. His voice was thick and he had difficulty finding the right words. He said he had been sleeping more and not eating much, forgetting to take his medication. His thoughts were rambling. He said he thought he had "thrown in the towel" because he had been so unwell with the flu. The psychiatrist believed Arno was showing evidence of an **organic mental disorder** and arranged for an MRI, which revealed leptomeningeal infiltration of his lymphoma. Arno died in a private palliative care unit 3 weeks later.

2.13.2 Key Issues from the Story of Arno

- The underlying cause of severe distress can vary over time in the same patient.
- Demoralization is a distinct syndrome that can arise independently of depression.
- Accurate assessment and diagnosis are essential for the appropriate management of the underlying cause of distress.
- Not all distress is related to the illness – other life events occur.
- The clinician must always be mindful of organic causes of distress.

3 Section 2: Managing Different Forms of Severe Distress

3.1 General Approaches

The transition to palliative care can be a time of great distress for patients and families as they cope with a lack of information, communication issues, and feelings of abandonment associated with changes in their medical team. The establishment of a therapeutic relationship based on trust and dignity is important, and the healing power of this relationship should not be underplayed. While many of the psychological interventions specified further in this chapter require specialist training, it is important to recognize strategies that all members of the healthcare team can utilize to reduce distress. All members of the team should maintain a dignity-focused, patient-centered approach that fosters open communication. This includes the use of empathic engagement and a therapeutic presence (Chochinov et al. 2013) that goes beyond basic communication and counseling skills. It is the capacity to "sit with" suffering and "bear witness" to the narrative of the person's experience, pacing the encounter so as not to stifle or threaten. While open communication should be fostered in all clinical relationships, the need for honesty and compassion is ever present in a palliative setting. There is a need to acknowledge distress and engage in empathic, reflective listening practices. The clinician's task is to maintain the patient's trust and hold confidences, all the while working within individual competencies and referring as needed (see Table 8). While communication skills training is important in all areas of healthcare, the need for ongoing training for all members of the palliative care team is essential.

Concepts from mindfulness and dignity therapy can be used by all members of the treating team to reduce distress and existential suffering. Basic relaxation techniques should be

Table 8 When to refer to the psychosocial team

Diagnostic uncertainty or complexity Moderate-severe symptoms Preexisting serious mental illness Suicidal ideation or risk factors Desire for hastened death Failure of initial interventions Need for psychotherapy	Consultation for appropriate medication Assessment of competency to make decisions Evaluation of changes in mental state Need for specific skills, e.g., clinical hypnosis Need to understand difficult behaviors and interpersonal difficulties Complex or conflicted family dynamics

implemented for those with high levels of physiological arousal, and techniques such as focused breathing strategies will reduce distress and assist with emotional downregulation.

3.2 Treatments for Specific Disorders

The treatment of specific psychiatric disorders in palliative care generally involves a combination of psychotherapy, medication, family involvement, and a multidisciplinary approach to holistic care. Disorders may be mild, moderate, or severe; some general approaches to treatment apply at all levels of severity, but the type and level of specific interventions may change according to the degree of suffering. Table 9 summarizes the approaches used for anxiety, depression, and demoralization. Details about the different forms of psychotherapy that may be appropriate and guidelines for the choice of medication follow.

3.3 Psychotherapies

A range of psychotherapeutic interventions have been developed for use in a palliative setting (Kumar et al. 2012; Rodin 2009; Stagg and Lazenby 2012; Dunlop 2010; Freeman 2011; Kissane et al. 2010; Okuyama et al. 2017). Manualized interventions have been the focus of randomized controlled trials to demonstrate efficacy (Smith et al. 2012). In practice, therapists need to be highly skilled in a range of therapeutic modalities to meet the presenting needs of the patient group. These needs will determine the choice of therapy. Other factors to consider are the individual's personality style, performance status, and prognosis. In a palliative setting, in depth, long-term psychotherapy may not be appropriate, and those with shorter life expectancies will benefit from shorter interventions. The importance of single therapeutic encounters or therapeutic moments should also not be overlooked.

The therapist must adapt to the rapidly changing world in which the patient functions and meet the patient where they are, rather than coming in with a preconceived idea on what the therapeutic encounter will look like. Due to the high burden of disease, "homework" for patients in this setting is inappropriate and has the potential to increase feelings of hopelessness and worthlessness. Inexperienced therapists may further traumatize already vulnerable individuals, highlighting the need for those working in this area to undertake specialist training. Therapists must have knowledge of the illness process and treatment side effects, practice a non-purist approach, be flexible and holistic, and foster a dignity-conserving orientation.

While those with advanced disease (Kirk et al. 2004) and their carers (Hudson et al. 2004) need information in many areas, e.g., prognosis, likely symptoms, treatment and side effects, disease progression, grief and loss, as well as the dying process, it is important that the patient and their family drive the delivery of this information. This prevents the patient and family being overwhelmed by information and reduces the potential for a negative impact on well-being.

Individuals with life-limiting illness juggle the demands of treatment, and their physical capacity may make it difficult for them to be available for regular therapy sessions. The therapist needs to be flexible and may have to travel to the patient, rather than insisting that the patient attends consulting rooms. In a palliative setting, reducing distress may involve attending to practical concerns including helping patients sit up, fluff a

Table 9 Treatment of anxiety, depression, and demoralization

	Treatment of anxiety[a]	Treatment of depression[b]	Treatment of demoralization[c]
General	Exclude medical causes; attend to contributing discomfort, e.g., pain, nausea Engage the patient in an empathic discussion of how he/she is feeling Assess contributing factors, e.g., family, financial, or spiritual concerns – refer to social work, pastoral care according to these concerns Assess the nature and severity and intervene/refer as appropriate	Exclude organic disorder; attend to contributing discomfort, e.g., pain, nausea Engage the patient in an empathic discussion of how he/she is feeling	Foster a therapeutic presence and dignity focus to reduce shame, feelings of aloneness, and disconnection Use active listening to deepen the therapeutic relationship Reassure the patient in stressful situations to reduce apprehension, panic, and perception of threat Encourage active problem solving to reduce helplessness, increase mastery, and self-esteem Promote adaptive coping in times of uncertainty Encourage help seeking to reduce hopelessness Explore meaning and purpose to reduce existential despair and meaninglessness Assess and treat comorbid depression Monitor suicide risk and desire for hastened death
Mild	Provide psychosocial and/or family support Consider brief interventions, e.g., problem-solving, relaxation strategies, guided imagery, cognitive behavioral interventions, mindfulness, hypnosis Provide patient with self-help materials – apps, CDs Engage music therapist If persists, consider introducing anxiolytics	Provide psychosocial support Assess contributing factors, e.g., family, financial, or spiritual concerns – refer to social work, pastoral care according to these concerns Provide family support Consider brief interventions, e.g., problem-solving, life review, meaning or dignity therapy, cognitive behavioral therapies If persists, consider introducing antidepressants	Utilize empathic listening and supportive psychotherapy Acknowledge the patient's difficult situation in an empathic manner Normalize grief and distress as appropriate responses in a challenging situation Focus on the individual's strengths and sense of resilience Encourage adaptation Nurture a focus on living in the moment
Moderate	Observe the recommendations above Assess for comorbid depression Consider introducing appropriate antidepressant Continue anxiolytic, change dose and scheduling as needed Consider hypnotic if insomniac Engage patient in psychotherapy with a member of the psychosocial team If persists, consider change of antidepressant	Observe the recommendations above Introduce appropriate antidepressant Consider anxiolytic if anxiety prominent, hypnotic if insomniac Engage patient in psychotherapy with a member of the psychosocial team If persists, consider change of antidepressant or augmentation	Engage a combination of therapeutic frameworks including cognitive, existential, and meaning centered approaches Acknowledge unhelpful thinking styles and challenge/reframe where appropriate Foster a life focus rather than a mortality focus Encourage the individual to live in the moment Explore gratitude in the individual's life Encourage engagement in sources of meaning Encourage family

(*continued*)

Table 9 (continued)

	Treatment of anxiety[a]	Treatment of depression[b]	Treatment of demoralization[c]
			communication, teamwork, support, and adaptive coping Educate and support the family in relation to their caregiving role and the patient's expectations of care
Severe	Observe the recommendations above Ensure antidepressant is titrated to adequate dose Consider small dose antipsychotic if agitated Continue psychotherapeutic support Monitor closely for suicide risk If persists, review diagnosis – death anxiety, terminal restlessness, delirium, steroids	Observe the recommendations above Ensure antidepressant is titrated to adequate dose Introduce small dose antipsychotic if agitated Continue psychotherapeutic support Monitor closely for suicide risk Consider augmentation of antidepressant Electro-convulsive therapy (ECT) can be necessary for a severely agitated and tormented patient	Ensure adequate symptom control to reduce distress and suffering Use narrative approaches to establish hope and meaning Assist in therapeutic life review and legacy activities Foster realistic hope while acknowledging grief Support the patient in finding new purpose Assist the patient to redefine meaningful roles Encourage supportive relationships Reframe negative beliefs with cognitive behavioral techniques Use family meetings to promote family cohesion and protect against family demoralization

[a,b]Refer to pharmacotherapies section for guidance in choice of medication
[c]Content adapted from Clarke (2012); Watson and Kissane (2017)

pillow, or pour a glass of water. It may also involve bearing witness to existential distress and immense suffering. Somatic issues can be a cause of profound distress, and anxiety and panic associated with dyspnea, nausea, or pain require immediate attention. The role of the health professional may be to act as coach in relaxation and mindfulness interventions or as an advocate in family meetings for those who are marginalized. As suffering in this setting can take multiple forms, skills in a variety of interventional strategies are required.

Many psychotherapeutic approaches have been adapted for a palliative setting, and Table 10 contains a summary of the psychotherapeutic interventions most frequently used, with a focus on mindfulness, supportive, narrative, existential, and meaning-based interventions. Creative therapies such as music, art, and movement are also highlighted.

3.4 Pharmacotherapies

Good-quality research concerning the use and efficacy of psychotropic medications in palliative care settings is scarce. The population itself is very heterogeneous, time frames for treatment variable, and multiple interventions are often initiated at the one time in the provision of care, confounding outcomes. A 2017 Cochrane Review could find no studies about the efficacy of drugs used to treat anxiety in adult palliative care patients and only two that showed some promise for a future update (Salt et al. 2017). The European Palliative Care Research Collaborative published guidelines on the management of depression which included a section on the choice of antidepressant (Rayner et al. 2011b). A separate systematic review and meta-analysis were devoted to antidepressants in the treatment of depression in palliative care (Rayner et al.

Table 10 Psychotherapeutic interventions

Psychotherapeutic approaches used in palliative care[a]			
Supportive and supportive-expressive psychotherapy (incorporating active problem solving and information provision) (Rodin 2009; Lederberg and Holland 2011; Hinshaw et al. 2002)	Therapeutic approach • Described as a framework and the "single most important tool" of the therapist in palliative care • Validates individual experience and provides support • Encourages expression of emotion, self-understanding and reinforces strengths • Promotes adaptive coping and resolution of core conflicts	Therapeutic techniques • Establishment of the therapeutic relationship and building of rapport • Bearing witness to the patient's experience, life, and suffering • Empathic listening and encouragement • Development of narrative meaning as a way of managing distress and trauma • Provision of information in a format and language that is appropriate • Education and communication with patients and families • Focus on strengths • Encourage adaptive coping • Use active problem-solving in a structured, step-by-step way	Use in a palliative setting Anxiety, demoralization, depression, end of life, fear of dying, grief, guilt, legacy work, spirituality, transition to palliative care, and trauma
Mindfulness-based interventions (Sharplin et al. 2010; Bates and Bartley 2011; Hales et al. 2010; Beng et al. 2015)	Therapeutic approach • Nonjudgmental, focus attention in the present moment, increase awareness Therapies Mindfulness-based stress reduction (MBSR) • Focus on reduction of stress, pain, and other issues (manualized) Mindfulness-based cognitive therapy (MBCT) • Integrates elements of cognitive therapy into MBSR MBCT – Ca • Palliative adaptation of group-based intervention Managing cancer and living meaningfully (CALM) • Brief individual psychotherapy Mindfulness-based supportive therapy (MBST) • Palliative care specific intervention	Therapeutic techniques • Mindfulness meditation including body scan and breath awareness • Mindfulness movement, e.g., yoga, tai chi, qigong • Supplement with CDs and apps Mindfulness-based cognitive therapy (MBCT) • Helps the individual to gain distance from thoughts Mindfulness-based supportive therapy (MBST) • Uses five components: mindful presence, listening, empathy, compassion, and boundary awareness	Use in a palliative setting Anxiety, depression, grief, management of physical symptoms, e.g., pain and sleep, and reduce suffering

(*continued*)

Table 10 (continued)

Psychotherapeutic approaches used in palliative care[a]			
Existential and meaning-based approaches (Mount 1993; Breitbart et al. 2004; Breitbart and Poppito 2014a; Breitbart and Poppito 2014b; Rosenfeld et al. 2017; Lethborg et al. 2008)	Therapeutic approach • Based on Viktor Frankl's work • Therapeutic process is to challenge individuals to find meaning and purpose through suffering, work, and love Therapies Meaning-centered group psychotherapy • 8-Week intervention (manualized) Individual meaning-centered psychotherapy • 7-Week intervention (manualized) MaP therapy • A brief 4 session intervention (manualized) • Revised and extended to 8 session intervention with evaluation work currently in progress	Therapeutic techniques • Individual or group interventions • Acknowledge the importance of an orientation toward life • Encourage a focus on living in the moment as opposed to anticipating the future • Encourage connection with the patient's sources of meaning • Use paradoxical intention, dereflection, and diversion techniques • Reduce cognitive dissonance between the individual's pre-illness expectations of life and their current reality • Utilize positive reappraisal, benefit finding, and the revision of beliefs/goals	Use in a palliative setting Death anxiety, demoralization, depression, and grief
Cognitive and behavioral interventions (includes cognitive, cognitive behavioral, and behavioral therapies) *Cognitive and behavioral interventions* (Mallick 2009; Akechi et al. 2008; Moorey and Greer 2002; Freeman 2011) *Acceptance and commitment therapy* (Low et al. 2016; Sussman and Liu 2014)	Therapeutic approach • Present based • Teaches self-efficacy and a sense of personal control Therapies Cognitive behavioral therapy (CBT)[b] • Identifies and challenges maladaptive thoughts and behaviors Adjuvant psychological therapy (APT) • Brief, cognitive behavioral therapy designed for use in an oncological population that has utility in those with advanced disease Acceptance and commitment therapy (ACT)[c] • Tolerate problems, acceptance of what is out of the individual's personal control, and focus attention on the present rather than focusing on the future • Psychological skills such as mindfulness are used to effectively deal	Therapeutic techniques Cognitive behavioral therapy (CBT) • Acknowledge unhelpful thinking styles and challenge/reframe where appropriate • Use mental distraction – behavioral task distraction and inattention • Bring focus to the now • Use adaptive ways of coping with distress and anxiety, e.g., relaxation therapy or guided imagery • Encourage active problem solving when high levels of uncertainty and complex decisions Acceptance and commitment therapy (ACT) • Focus on what is in the individual's control • Observe uncomfortable thoughts Behavioral interventions • Behavioral activation and activity scheduling esp. for depression and demoralization	Use in a palliative setting *CBT useful for* anxiety, demoralization, depression, grief, an increased confidence in decision making, an increased sense of control and mastery, physical issues, e.g., pain, nausea, vomiting, sleep disturbance, and dyspnea ACT may be helpful for death anxiety Relaxation strategies used for anxiety and panic at end of life, distress, pain and physical symptoms and stressful situations, treatments or procedures

(*continued*)

Table 10 (continued)

Psychotherapeutic approaches used in palliative care[a]			
	with painful thoughts and feelings	• Focus on what can do rather than what cannot Relaxation techniques • Breathing techniques such as breath reregulation and pacing • Guided mental imagery and progressive muscle relaxation • Anchoring the person to keep them focused on the now • Role of the health professional as a coach is important in these situations	
Narrative approachesNarrative therapy (Mount 1993; Noble and Jones 2005)	Therapeutic approach • Through the individual's story, meaning is found during times of suffering • Therapeutic work is done by the patient "re-authoring" their story • Individual puts the experience of illness into the context of their whole life	Therapeutic techniques • Encourage patients to share their life stories, memories, and experiences and record them in way that is meaningful to them • Assist in life review and legacy activities	Use in a palliative setting Anxiety, demoralization, depression, grief, legacy, and preparation for death
Narrative approaches Dignity therapy (Chochinov 2012; Chochinov and McKeen 2011)	Therapeutic approach • Principle of bedside care in line with existential principle "To be known is to matter" • Reflects on how the individual wishes to be remembered by focusing on the patient's life story and memories • Uses dignity-conserving therapy question protocol to obtain information about the patient's life and what and who is important to them • The interview is recorded, transcribed, edited, and refined into a narrative document	Therapeutic techniques Dignity-conserving therapy question examples • Asks patients to talk about their life history and the parts they consider to be most important • When they felt most alive • What are their hopes and dreams for their loved ones • What have they learned about life that they would want to pass along to others	Use in a palliative setting Anxiety, demoralization, depression, existential distress, grief, and legacy
Narrative approaches Reminiscence and therapeutic life review (Keall et al. 2015; King et al. 2005; Stagg and Lazenby 2012)	Therapeutic approach • Provides a way of addressing existential and spiritual concerns Therapies Reminiscence • Descriptive and involves thinking about	Therapeutic techniques • Encourage participation in biography or life review programs, where available • Assist in the writing of biography as a form of legacy	Use in a palliative setting Reminiscence reduces depression, improves adaptation to life and quality of life Therapeutic life review reduces depression and improves quality of life at

(*continued*)

Table 10 (continued)

Psychotherapeutic approaches used in palliative care[a]			
	life and recalling memorable aspects • Biographical in nature Therapeutic life review • Evaluative with a focus on examination, addressing, and resolving or rectifying conflict • Helps the individual look for meaning in the events of their life • Utility when life expectancy is less than 6 months	• Individuals describe important life events • Use statements like "thinking of your life as a series of photographs, what ones would you choose to describe your life and why?" • Utilize activities such as the creation of scrapbooks, cookbooks, and family stories • Techniques can be incorporated into individualized psychotherapy • Provide individuals ways of addressing issues or starting conversations with family members	end of life and spiritual well-being Legacy activities reduce fear of being forgotten
Narrative approaches Expressive writing (Bruera et al. 2008; Freadman 2015)	Therapeutic approach • Focus on writing about thoughts and feelings associated with an event • Assists in trauma processing • Reparative writing involves encouraging the individual to develop, revise, and expand the writing of their illness story so that it becomes "less generic and more authentic"	Therapeutic techniques • Use journaling and more formalized interventions that can be conducted individually or in group settings	Use in a palliative setting Anxiety, depression, and trauma
Clinical hypnotherapy (Brann 2015; Brugnoli 2016; Willmarth 2017)	Therapeutic approach • Induces an altered state of consciousness with increased suggestibility • A state of deep relaxation can be achieved • Recognized by the National Institute of Clinical Excellence (NICE)	Therapeutic techniques • Engagement, induction, deepening, establishing response sets, introduction of metaphor according to the themes of the goal of hypnosis, checking in, posthypnotic suggestion, closure, and disengagement	Use in a palliative setting Anticipatory anxiety related to medical procedures, and the management of pain and phobias
Family-centered approaches (Kissane and Bloch 2002)	Therapeutic approach • Based on the family as a system and includes the needs of children • Interventions include family therapy and family-focused grief therapy	Therapeutic techniques • Encourage family communication, teamwork, and adaptive coping • Educate and support the family in relation to their caregiving role	Use in a palliative setting Improve communication, cohesion, and conflict resolution
Brief psychodynamic approaches[b] (Macleod 2009)	Therapeutic approach • Focus is on the individual's unconscious processes	Therapeutic techniques • Concepts such as transference, countertransference,	Use in a palliative setting Those already oriented to psychotherapy or where

(continued)

Table 10 (continued)

Psychotherapeutic approaches used in palliative care[a]			
	• Goals of therapy are client self-awareness and the influence of the past on present behavior	regression, and attachment used to understand the psychological processes involved in dying	psychodynamic issues have arisen
Other interventions *Music and art-based therapies* (McConnell et al. 2016; O'Callaghan et al. 2015) *Art therapy* (Fenton 2008) *Drama therapy* (Redhouse 2014) *Eye movement desensitization and reprocessing (EMDR)* (Udo and Gash 2012) *Sleep* (Hajjar 2008) *Physical activity and somatic therapies* (Lowe et al. 2016; Selman et al. 2012; MacDonald 2016; Falkensteiner et al. 2011)	Music therapy • Well established with reduction in depression and anxiety Art therapy • Assists those approaching end of life make meaning of their situation and helps to provide legacy Drama therapy • Used to create life story Eye movement desensitization and reprocessing (EMDR) • Recommended by National Institute of Clinical Excellence and the American Psychiatric Association for use in PTSD • Effectiveness in reducing hypervigilance, re-experiencing the experience and consequent avoidance associated with response to trauma, and may have relevance in those with life limiting disease Sleep • Important in the maintenance of mood is well established • Routine around sleep maintained even as end of life approaches • Structure sleep hygiene strategies important including maintaining sleep routine (arising and retiring at approximately the same time each night), techniques for thought dumping prior to bed, relaxation, or meditation techniques to get to sleep and to stay asleep. Physical activity and somatic therapies • The role of physical movement rather than exercise • Use of physical and somatic therapies such as dance, yoga, pilates, walking, and massage		

[a]Content adapted from Kissane et al. (2010) and Watson and Kissane (2017)
[b]Cognitive and behavioral interventions: Evidence for use in a palliative setting with cancer patients, Parkinson's disease, end stage respiratory and cardiac disease and dementia
[c]Limited evidence in a palliative setting, feasibility trial underway

2011a). They comment that in many studies they reviewed, people with poor physical health were excluded and that treatment decisions for depression at the end of life is guided by research in populations with better prognosis.

Farriols et al. (2012) reported an increase in prescription of benzodiazepines, antidepressants, and antipsychotics over a 7-year period from 2002 to 2009 in a palliative care unit in Barcelona. They noted that inclusion of a psychiatrist on the multidisciplinary team had probably improved recognition and treatment of psychiatric disorders and that new drugs and new routes of administration had become available during this period. The published literature on psychotropic drug use in palliative care inevitably lags behind the development and use of new drugs.

The choice of individual drugs is influenced by factors independent of efficacy. These include drug interactions, the presence of active metabolites, possible routes of administration, time to onset of action, adverse side effects, and beneficial effect profile which may be exploited to treat other symptoms such as nausea, anorexia, vomiting, insomnia, or neuropathic pain. In addition, the availability of drugs varies between countries, as does the different forms of preparation of the drug. Drug-regulating bodies determine which drugs are approved for a specific use and which qualify for pharmaceutical benefits schemes. Different centers have developed their own culture of prescribing practices, and individual clinicians often have their own "favorite" medications.

What follows below is a synthesis of the available literature and the current prescribing practices in major palliative care centers in Australia.

3.4.1 Anxiolytics

Anxiolytics are the most commonly prescribed psychotropic medications in palliative care. Farriols et al. (2012) reported that 84% of patients were prescribed a benzodiazepine (BZDP) in 2009, increased from 72.6% in 2002.

- ***Lorazepam*** is the most commonly prescribed BZDP. It has an intermediate half-life and provides good anxiolysis at low doses (0.5–1 mg) without excessive sedation.
- ***Oxazepam*** (7.5 mg, 15 mg, or 30 mg) is a little more sedative but is a useful alternative as it is cheaper and the patient may already have been prescribed it in the community.
- ***Midazolam*** is the second most commonly prescribed in a palliative care setting. It is very expensive and has a very short half-life. It is able to be administered parenterally and is commonly used with morphine in a syringe driver as a subcutaneous delivery in terminal sedation. It is also prescribed for catastrophic events, some distressing procedures, and with an antipsychotic in an agitated delirium.
- ***Diazepam*** has an active metabolite, nordiazepam which has a long half-life and can accumulate in frail patients with impaired metabolism. It should be reserved for management of delirium tremens, people with motor restlessness, and those who are BZDP-dependent with the objective of reducing the dose gradually. It has greater muscle-relaxant properties than the above BZDP and is more likely to cause amnestic effects.
- ***Clonazepam*** has a very long half-life and can accumulate in the body over days, causing ataxia. It is available in an oral solution (2.5 mg/ml, 0.1 mg/drop, 25 drops/ml), and some patients experience a greater sense of control over their anxiety by being able to titrate the number of drops according to need. It is also a powerful anticonvulsant and can be helpful in patients who have brain tumors in reducing agitation and seizures. Administration via PVC tubing has been shown to result in significant loss of drug. A syringe driver using non-PVC-based tubing should be used.
- ***Alprazolam*** is a very short-acting BZDP with a rapid onset of anxiolytic effect and a rapid offset; it creates a cycle of relief and exacerbation of anxiety which can lead to increasing doses, tolerance, dependence, and abuse. It can cause amnestic effects and disinhibited behaviors. Because of these factors, it has become a restricted drug in Australia. Patients already taking alprazolam when they come to palliative care should be changed over to a longer-acting BZDP.

3.4.2 Hypnotics

Insomnia is a common problem on a busy inpatient unit and is a symptom, not a diagnosis. Sleep hygiene factors need to be addressed and pain, nausea, or delirium managed accordingly. Where initial insomnia is the result of worry or noise levels, sleep tapes of hypnosis, guided imagery, or music may be a useful means of inducing sleep. If medication is required, a higher dose of the same BZDP used for the management of anxiety (e.g., **lorazepam** or **oxazepam**) may suffice. The short-acting **temazepam** commonly used in medical units is also used in palliative care units when no regular BZDP is prescribed for anxiety. It is important to avoid charting four or five different BZDP as the effects are cumulative. There is some benefit in initiating **mirtazapine** 7.5 mg or 15 mg in patients who are thought to be sleeping poorly because of depression. Some patients cannot sleep because of an agitated depression and may need a small dose of a sedative atypical antipsychotic (e.g., **quetiapine** 6.25–12.5 mg or **olanzapine** 2.5 mg) in addition to adequate doses of antidepressant medication. **Nitrazepam** is not used in most settings. Non-BZDP omega 1 hypnotics, **zolpidem** 10 mg, and **zopiclone** 7.5 mg are used in some centers, but there are reports of amnestic effects, dissociation, and unusual behaviors with these drugs, particularly with **zolpidem.** **(**Olsen 2008**)**

3.4.3 Antidepressants

In palliative care, time is short and antidepressants are increasingly being introduced early in the care of patients with depression, even when they may have syndromal depression rather that a DSM diagnosis of MDD. In part this is because some antidepressants have an effect profile that addresses other problematic symptoms. In a systematic review and meta-analysis (Rayner et al. 2010), antidepressants were superior to placebo at every time point measured and the difference increased over time.

- **Mirtazapine** is the most commonly prescribed antidepressant in palliative care (Farriols et al. 2012; Cipriani et al. 2009). It is classified as a NaSSA (noradrenaline and specific serotonergic agent) and is related to the tetracyclic mianserin but has a unique mechanism of action. It boosts both serotonin and noradrenaline neurotransmitters: it blocks alpha 2 presynaptic receptor, thereby increasing noradrenaline neurotransmission; blocks alpha 2 presynaptic receptor on serotonin neurons (heteroreceptors) thereby increasing serotonin – novel mechanisms independent of noradrenaline and serotonin reuptake blockade. It blocks 5HT2A, 5HT2C, and 5HT3 serotonin receptors as well as blocking H1 histamine receptors (Stahl 2014). It has a relatively rapid onset of action, improves sleep, reduces anxiety, acts as an antiemetic, reduces nausea, stimulates appetite, increases food intake and promotes weight gain, and acts as an adjuvant in pain control (Alam et al. 2013). It also alters serum inflammatory cytokines and has been studied in cancer related cachexia and anorexia (Riechelmann et al. 2010). Doses of 15–45 mg given at night lead to a rapid and sustained improvement in depressive symptoms. Vivid dreams are occasionally reported and liver enzymes may become mildly elevated, but mirtazapine is well-tolerated in patients with advanced disease.
- **SSRIs** (selective serotonin reuptake inhibitors) may be the first choice for the treatment of MDD in cancer (Li et al. 2017), but side effects of diarrhea, nausea, lowered seizure threshold, and insomnia, as well as their propensity for drug interactions through the cytochrome P450 (CYP450) enzyme system, make them less attractive in people who are on multiple medications and may be already struggling with these symptoms. The CYP450 metabolizing system has more than 50 enzymes, the most significant of these being CYP3A4 and CYP2D6; polymorphism is responsible for the variations in drug response among patients of different ethnic origin. Drugs can be inhibitors or inducers of enzymes, causing unanticipated drug interactions with severe adverse effects or therapeutic failure (Lynch and Price 2007). SSRIs in combination with other serotonergic drugs (e.g., ondansetron, metoclopramide, pregabalin, morphine, fentanyl, tramadol, methadone, warfarin, methylphenidate, and antidepressants – all common in palliative care) can cause potentially fatal serotonin toxicity, characterized by high body temperature, agitation, headache, increased reflexes, tremor, sweating, dilated pupils, and diarrhea (Sun-Edelstein et al. 2008). At normal doses, SSRIs can cause a distressing symptom of psychic and motor restlessness known as akathisia. They can also lower platelets, as well as cause a syndrome of inappropriate antidiuretic hormone (SIADH) resulting in hyponatremia. In addition, if doses are missed or reduced, SSRIs can cause an unpleasant discontinuation syndrome of flu-like symptoms, insomnia, nausea, imbalance, odd buzzing sensations in the head, and anxiety. Where they are prescribed or continued in palliative care, the most common SSRIs are **escitalopram** (10 mg), **citalopram** (20 mg), and **sertraline** (50 mg). **Paroxetine**, **fluvoxamine,** and **fluoxetine** should be avoided because of the high propensity for CYP450 drug interactions. The CYP450 system is very complex and the clinician is advised to check for possible interactions through drug information services or a reputable website (Flockhart 2007).
- **SNRIs** (selective serotonin and noradrenaline reuptake inhibitors) may be associated with higher remission rates for depression than SSRIs. Like the SSRIs, they are more

activating than mirtazapine and are commonly prescribed in the community. **Venlafaxine** (75–150 mg), its enantiomer and major metabolite **desvenlafaxine** (50–100 mg), and a third SNRI, **duloxetine** (30–60 mg), are among the most commonly prescribed of this group in the general population with MDD. **Venlafaxine** is metabolized by CYP2D6, unlike desvenlafaxine which is largely renally excreted. Both **venlafaxine** and **duloxetine** can increase blood pressure, and **duloxetine** may cause deranged liver function. **Venlafaxine** has been associated with an unpleasant discontinuation syndrome. **Duloxetine** has some benefit for neuropathic pain.

- **Tricyclic antidepressants** have no role in the treatment of depression in people with advanced disease. They have a strong anticholinergic profile which increases the risk for delirium (especially in patients on opiates), urinary retention, constipation, dry mouth, and blurred vision, and their alpha 1 adrenergic blocking activity causes postural hypotension. There is also a considerable time lag (4–6 weeks) before a therapeutic response in the treatment of depression. Small doses of **amitriptyline** (10–25 mg) or **doxepin** (10–25 mg) may be used at night as adjuvant treatment for neuropathic pain.
- **Others. Ketamine** is a N-methyl-D-aspartate (NMDA) receptor antagonist commonly used as an anesthetic agent. In addition to blocking NMDA receptor channels, it interacts with other calcium and sodium channels, cholinergic transmission, noradrenergic and serotonergic reuptake inhibition, glutamate transmission, synapse formation, and mu, delta, and kappa opioid-like effects. These other actions may contribute to its usefulness in pain and depression. **Ketamine** is inexpensive and well-tolerated and has a rapid onset of antidepressant action. Some people experience mild dissociative effects within an hour of receiving the drug, and blood pressure may spike. Concerns about long-term use in treatment-refractory patients with major depression are not an issue in a palliative care population. Several sites are investigating the use of daily oral ketamine for the treatment of depression and anxiety in patients receiving hospice care (Irwin et al. 2013). The results are promising and ketamine may prove to be a useful alternative to the treatment of depression with psychostimulants. This latter group of drugs, particularly methylphenidate, is used to achieve a rapid improvement in mood when the patient's prognosis is days to weeks (Hardy 2009). It is usually initiated at 2.5 mg in the morning and, if tolerated, may be titrated up to 5 mg morning and midday. However adverse effects such as restlessness, tachycardia, delirium, nausea, loss of appetite, and insomnia may occur.
- **Monoamine oxidase inhibitors** are contraindicated because of the likelihood of drug and food interactions. **Agomelatine**, **reboxetine,** and **vortioxetine** are not discussed because of the lack of evidence and clinical experience in this setting.

3.4.4 Antipsychotics

Haloperidol remains the drug of choice in the treatment of delirium because its properties are well-known and it is available in parenteral as well as oral form. As second-line treatment or where the patient has an agitated delirium, a more sedative atypical antipsychotic such as **quetiapine** or **olanzapine** may be preferred. **Risperidone** is favored in some units but can cause dyskinesias. **Levomepromazine** is a relatively weak antipsychotic but is popular in palliative care units as a third-line treatment for agitated delirium, terminal sedation, and in some very agitated patients with psychotic illness (Dietz et al. 2013). The management of delirium is discussed in a separate chapter. These atypical antipsychotics are also helpful in an agitated depression in combination with an antidepressant. If a patient suffers from a serious mental illness, it is best to continue the antipsychotic the patient has been treated with prior to admission. If a patient with schizophrenia has been treated with **clozapine**, weekly monitoring by the strict protocol must continue because of the risk of blood dyscrasias, myocarditis, and cardiomyopathy. Dose reduction or cessation may be required as the patient nears the terminal phase.

3.4.5 Mood Stabilizers

Mood stabilizers may be used in the palliative care setting where the patient is already receiving treatment for bipolar affective disorder or may be introduced to help manage manic effects induced by steroids or brain tumors. **Lithium carbonate** is difficult to manage in the medically ill, and the choice is usually made for **sodium valproate** over other drugs such as **carbamazepine** and **phenytoin** which have more problematic side effects. **Lamotrigine** is useful but may cause a Stevens-Johnson syndrome; it needs to be titrated up slowly and ceased immediately if a rash appears. **Gabapentin** and **pregabalin** have weak mood-stabilizing effects though they may have anxiolytic effects and are more often used in the treatment of neuropathic pain. **Levetiracetam** is commonly prescribed in patients with brain tumors but can cause anger, irritability, depression, and self-harm rather than stabilize mood (Thekdi et al. 2012).

3.5 Staff Education About Management of Patients with Personality Disorder

3.5.1 Borderline Personality Disorder

The scenario described in the case of Pauline in Sect. 2 can cause havoc on a ward and can be very destructive to a normally well-functioning team. Explanation of the origin of borderline dynamics and how regression and the primitive defenses mobilized under extreme stress impact on staff goes some way toward creating a framework for understanding the patient. In a team meeting, it is useful to have each staff member articulate their strong feelings about the patient and to understand that these feelings are useful data; it will become apparent then that each staff member carries a "fragment" of the disturbed inner world of the patient and a picture of the "whole" person can emerge. Patients with BPD find it hard to tolerate warmth, kindness, comfort, or intimacy. It is important to develop an empathic stance that is attuned to what the patient really needs and is able to tolerate, without loss of boundaries. Overly sympathetic responses may feel dangerous to the patient and promote withdrawal, further regression, or acting out. A few clearly defined and realistic limits may need to be set with the patient; it is important that the whole team participates in ensuring adherence to these limits because the patient will invariably test them to determine whether staff really care about them enough to contain them. While it is important for the clinician to have an understanding of the internal dynamics of the patient in order to form a collaborative and respectful relationship, it is equally important to avoid confronting and interpreting the patient's rage or entitlement, as this may lead to escalation of emotions. The primary focus of management of the BPD patient is education and support of staff who struggle with the rapid shifts in the patient's mental state and behaviors and may feel depleted, angry, incompetent, and sadistic or have personal vulnerabilities triggered by the encounters. Regular group supervision and reviews of management are necessary, and it should be recognized that some staff are unable to maintain their professional boundaries in working with BPD. It is worthwhile to remind staff that, while the behavior of BPD patients is dysfunctional, it is the best they can do under the circumstances.

While treatment of comorbid anxiety, depression, or substance abuse is indicated, psychotropic medication is not advised for the emotional dysregulation nor is psychotherapy for the traumatic early life helpful in a palliative care context unless requested. Enhancing self-regulation and self-control through techniques described later in Sect. 3 are of most benefit to the patient.

3.5.2 Narcissistic Personality Disorder

As the case of ***Sam*** in Sect. 2 demonstrates, any threat to the health and integrity of the body in individuals who place great store on how the outside world sees them can be experienced as a narcissistic wound. The person with NPD keeps others at a distance with displays of grandiosity and dismissiveness, hiding in shame the tenuous sense of self. The narcissistic rage that ensues when these defenses break down can turn against the fragile self and lead to suicide, often in dramatic circumstances. Nursing staff had learned, with supervision, to cope with his demanding behaviors by meeting his needs with prompt and efficient service while setting limits on his less reasonable expectations. Staff can be left with feelings of responsibility, guilt, challenged professional competence, emptiness, and low self-esteem, some of which mirror the patient's disavowed and projected inner sense of self. These impacts must be managed with great sensitivity in staff support sessions.

3.5.3 Paranoid Personality Disorder

In dealing with PPD, staff need to be aware that these patients have difficulty tolerating intrusions into their personal space. A formal, respectful, and courteous manner needs to be maintained in spite of a barrage of criticism and accusation. It is important to elicit the patient's understanding of what is happening and to explain any procedures and their rationale carefully, repeating explanations if necessary. Staff need to ensure that what they tell the patient will happen ("I will be back with your newspaper in an hour") does indeed happen. Keeping unnecessary interpersonal interaction to a minimum avoids pushing the patient into an overstimulated state which amplifies the defensive projections. In spite of these considerations, **Tom** could not withstand the ward environment and could not be adequately assessed. When the crisis of his abrupt departure arose, the senior members of the team had to make a decision based on non-maleficence and respect for his autonomy despite the potential risks.

3.6 Family Interventions

In the palliative setting, families are important collaborators in care and sources of information and observation for staff. Supporting family members who become distressed by the suffering they witness in their loved one is an important role of the team and can help to reduce the burden on the patient. Family meetings help to share information, establish goals of care, and plan care delivery (Hudson et al. 2009). They can also provide opportunities to explain the causes of the altered mental states families witness (e.g., delirium, cerebral irritation) and may reduce misunderstandings within the family. They provide a window through which the functioning of the family can be observed and may reveal deep conflict between members which requires more specific intervention. Challenging family dynamics are discussed in a separate chapter.

3.7 Staff Support

Working in a palliative setting places individuals at risk of empathy fatigue (compassion fatigue), burnout, and vicarious trauma. The incidence of each of these in this setting is unclear due to methodological differences between studies. Compassion fatigue has been cited as the cost of caring (Boyle 2015; Figley 1997; Sinclair et al. 2017). Remen (2002) states that:

> The expectation that we can be immersed in suffering and loss daily and not be touched by it is as unrealistic as expecting to be able to walk through water without getting wet. This sort of denial is no small matter. The way we deal with loss shapes our capacity to be present to life more than anything else. The way we protect ourselves from loss may be the way in which we distance ourselves from life and help. We burn out not because we don't care but because we don't grieve. We burn out because we've allowed our hearts to become so filled with loss that we have no room left to care.

The need for self-care strategies is well recognized as having a protective function for those working in a palliative setting (Mota Vargas et al. 2015). Supervision and skills training need to be embedded in the organizational structure, and staff support sessions around challenging clinical care should be available to staff on a regular and as needed basis.

4 Conclusions

Patients facing life-limiting illness are vulnerable to a vast array of psychological and psychiatric disturbances. These may be related to their existential plight, the impact of the illness on their life trajectory, the ravages of the disease process itself, or the interventions required to treat it. Unfortunately, many patients, families, and staff view suffering as inevitable and understandable – even "normalizing" severe distress given the patient's predicament. There is no place for therapeutic nihilism about our capacity to relieve suffering. There are powerful psychotherapeutic modalities that can be employed to help the patient to negotiate the challenges of living while dying. These may be employed on an ongoing basis by trained clinicians, but some of the concepts from different forms of psychotherapy can be introduced in the everyday interactions with patients and families. It is important to embrace the idea that every clinical encounter is potentially therapeutic, not only for the patient but also for the staff member who may feel helpless in the face of another's suffering. There are also psychotropic medications which have good efficacy in treating anxiety and depression along with a greater readiness to introduce medication early. An awareness that "something **can** be done" leads to better recognition of distress, more thorough assessment of the underlying cause, and more appropriate and timely treatment. The multidisciplinary nature of palliative care allows for whole person care, which includes attending to physical comfort and mobility, engagement with music and art therapies, and attention to spiritual and culture-specific needs.

5 Summary

This chapter has explored the various manifestations of severe distress in patients receiving palliative care for malignant and nonmalignant disease. It has demonstrated the distinction between the normal distress of sadness and grief and that associated with problematic anxiety, depression, demoralization, post-trauma syndromes, decompensating personality disorder, serious mental illness, drug and alcohol abuse and withdrawal, and organic mental states. It has endorsed the NCCN statement that "no patient's distress should go unrecognized and untreated" and has provided the clinician with ways of distinguishing the different psychological and psychiatric disorders that can manifest as severe distress. General and specific treatment approaches have been outlined, with descriptions of the most helpful psychotherapies in the palliative population. Guidelines for the use of various psychotropic medications have specifically focused on the rationale of choice for patients with advanced disease, rather than provide an exhaustive list of possibilities. The importance of all staff receiving communication skills training and becoming familiar with some of the concepts of psychotherapies for incorporation into everyday communication with patients has been emphasized. Engagement with the family and supervision and support of staff is stressed as an essential component of palliative care.

6 Key Points

- Distress is often unrecognized, underlying causes not assessed, and disorder untreated.
- Distress is often "normalized," causing unnecessary suffering.
- Acknowledging distress is an essential first step.
- Every clinical encounter with a patient has the potential to be therapeutic.
- Nonspecialist staff can provide very helpful "in the moment" interventions.
- Early intervention is essential.
- Refer according to recommendations.
- Provide supervision and support to reduce compassion fatigue and burnout.

References

Akechi T, Okuyama T, Onishi J, Morita T, Furukawa TA. Psychotherapy for depression among incurable cancer patients. Cochrane Libr [Internet]. 2008. https://doi.org/10.1002/14651858.CD005537.pub2.

Alam A, Voronovich Z, Carley JA. A review of therapeutic uses of mirtazapine in psychiatric and medical conditions. Prim Care Companion CNS Disord [Internet]. 2013;15(5). https://doi.org/10.4088/PCC.13r01525.

Alessandra Strada E. Grief and bereavement in the adult palliative care setting. New York: OUP; 2013. 126 p.

American Psychiatric Association. Diagnostic and statistical manual of mental disorders (DSM-5®). Washington DC: American Psychiatric Pub; 2013. 991 p.

Andersen BL, DeRubeis RJ, Berman BS, Gruman J, Champion VL, Massie MJ, et al. Screening, assessment, and care of anxiety and depressive symptoms in adults with cancer: an American Society of Clinical Oncology guideline adaptation. J Clin Oncol. 2014; 32(15):1605–19.

Austin P, Wiley S, McEvoy PM, Archer L. Depression and anxiety in palliative care inpatients compared with those receiving palliative care at home. Palliat Support Care. 2011;9(04):393–400.

Bates U, Bartley T. Mindfulness in palliative care. In: Mindfulness-based cognitive therapy for cancer. Wiley; 2011. p. 289–302.

Becker E. The denial of death. New York: The Free Press, New York; 1974.

Beng TS, Chin LE, Guan NC, Yee A, Wu C, Jane LE, et al. Mindfulness-based supportive therapy (MBST): proposing a palliative psychotherapy from a conceptual perspective to address suffering in palliative care. Am J Hosp Palliat Med. 2015;32(2):144–60.

Block SD. Assessing and managing depression in the terminally ill patient. Ann Intern Med. 2000;132(3): 209–18.

Boyle DA. Compassion fatigue: the cost of caring. Nursing. 2015;45(7):48–51.

Brann L. The handbook of contemporary clinical hypnosis: theory and practice. New York: Wiley; 2015. 652 p.

Breitbart WS, Poppito SR. Meaning-centered group psychotherapy for patients with advanced cancer: a treatment manual. New York: Oxford University Press; 2014a. (Albom, Andrykowski, Beals, Brady, Breitbart, Breitbart, et al., editors. Meaning-centered group psychotherapy for patients with advanced cancer: A treatment manual.)

Breitbart WS, Poppito SR. Individual meaning-centered psychotherapy for patients with advanced cancer: a treatment manual. Oxford: Oxford University Press; 2014b. 128 p.

Breitbart W, Gibson C, Tremblay A. The delirium experience: delirium recall and delirium-related distress in hospitalized patients with cancer, their spouses/caregivers, and their nurses. Psychosomatics. 2002; 43(3):183–94.

Breitbart W, Gibson C, Poppito SR, Berg A. Psychotherapeutic interventions at the end of life: a focus on meaning and spirituality. Can J Psychiatr. 2004;49(6):366–72.

Bruera E, Willey J, Cohen M, Palmer JL. Expressive writing in patients receiving palliative care: a feasibility study. J Palliat Med. 2008;11(1):15–9.

Brugnoli MP. Clinical hypnosis for palliative care in severe chronic diseases: a review and the procedures for relieving physical, psychological and spiritual symptoms. Ann Palliat Med. 2016;5(4):280–97.

Bultz BD, Johansen C. Screening for distress, the 6th vital sign: where are we, and where are we going? Psycho-Oncology. 2011;20(6):569–71.

Chochinov HM. Dignity therapy: final words for final days. New York: Oxford University Press; 2012. 199 p.

Chochinov HM, McKeen NA. Dignity therapy. In: Handbook of psychotherapy in cancer care. Wiley; 2011. p. 79–88.

Chochinov HM, Wilson KG, Enns M, Lander S. Are you depressed? Screening for depression in the terminally ill. Am J Psychiatry. 1997;154(5):674–6.

Chochinov HM, McClement SE, Hack TF, McKeen NA, Rach AM, Gagnon P, et al. Health care provider communication. Cancer. 2013;119(9):1706–13.

Cipriani A, Furukawa TA, Salanti G, Geddes JR, Higgins JP, Churchill R, et al. Comparative efficacy and acceptability of 12 new-generation antidepressants: a multiple-treatments meta-analysis. [Review] [151 refs]. Lancet. 2009;373(9665):746–58.

Clarke DM. Depression, demoralization, and psychotherapy in people who are medically ill, The Psychotherapy of Hope: The Legacy of Persuasion and Healing. Baltimore: Johns Hopkins University Press; 2012. p. 125–57.

Clarke DM, Mackinnon AJ, Smith GC, McKenzie DP, Herrman HE. Dimensions of psychopathology in the medically ill. A latent trait analysis. Psychosomatics. 2000;41(5):418–25.

Clarke DM, Kissane DW, Trauer T, Smith GC. Demoralization, anhedonia and grief in patients with severe physical illness. World Psychiatry. 2005; 4(2):96–105.

Delgado-Guay M, Parsons HA, Li Z, Palmer JL, Bruera E. Symptom distress in advanced cancer patients with anxiety and depression in the palliative care setting. Support Care Cancer. 2009;17(5):573–9.

Dietz I, Schmitz A, Lampey I, Schulz C. Evidence for the use of Levomepromazine for symptom control in the palliative care setting: a systematic review. BMC Palliat Care. 2013;12(1):2.

Dunlop S. Cognitive behavioural therapy in palliative and end-of-life car. J Soc Work End Life Palliat Care. 2010;4(1):38–44.

Falkensteiner M, Mantovan F, Müller I, Them C. The use of massage therapy for reducing pain, anxiety, and depression in oncological palliative care patients: a narrative review of the literature. ISRN Nurs. 2011;2011:929868.

Farriols C, Ferrández O, Planas J, Ortiz P, Mojal S, Ruiz AI. Changes in the prescription of psychotropic drugs in the palliative care of advanced cancer patients over a seven-year period. J Pain Symptom Manag. 2012; 43(5):945–52.

Fava GA, Freyberger HJ, Bech P, Christodoulou G, Sensky T, Theorell T, et al. Diagnostic criteria for use in psychosomatic research. Psychother Psychosom. 1995;63(1):1–8.

Fenton JF. "Finding one's way home": reflections on art therapy in palliative care. Art Therapy [Internet]. 2008;25:137. https://doi.org/10.1080/07421656.2008.10129598.

Figley CR. Burnout in families: the systemic costs of caring. Boca Raton: CRC Press; 1997. 240 p.

Flockhart DA. Drug interactions: cytochrome P450 drug interaction table. Indiana University School of Medicine. 2007;2010. https://drug-interactions.medicine.iu.edu/main.table.aspx

Freadman R. Spanning cancer: cancer as an episode in an individual life story. Society. 2015;52(5):490–7.

Freeman SM. Cognitive behavioral therapy within the palliative care setting. In: Sorocco KH, Lauderdale S, editors. Cognitive behavior therapy with older adults: innovations across care settings. New York: Springer Publishing Co; 2011. p. 367–89.

Fulton R, Gottesman DJ. Anticipatory grief: a psychosocial concept reconsidered. Br J Psychiatry. 1980;137:45–54.

Ginige S. Nicotine withdrawal: an under-recognised cause of terminal restlessness. Eur J Palliat Care. 2016; 23(3):128–9.

Gore JM, Brophy CJ, Greenstone MA. How well do we care for patients with end stage chronic obstructive pulmonary disease (COPD)? A comparison of palliative care and quality of life in COPD and lung cancer. Thorax. 2000;55(12):1000–6.

Hajjar RR. Sleep disturbance in palliative care. Clin Geriatr Med. 2008;24(1):83–91. vii.

Hales S, Lo C, Rodin G. Managing Cancer And Living Meaningfully (CALM) treatment manual: an individual psychotherapy for patients with advanced cancer. Toronto: Psychosocial Oncology and Palliative Care Princess Margaret Hospital, University Health Network; 2010.

Hardy SE. Methylphenidate for the treatment of depressive symptoms, including fatigue and apathy, in medically ill older adults and terminally ill adults. Am J Geriatr Pharmacother. 2009;7(1):34–59.

Hay JL, Passik SD. The cancer patient with borderline personality disorder: suggestions for symptom-focused management in the medical setting. [Review] [45 refs]. Psycho-Oncology. 2000;9(2):91–100.

Hinshaw DB, Carnahan JM, Johnson DL. Depression, anxiety, and asthenia in advanced illness. J Am Coll Surg. 2002;195(2):271–7. discussion 277–8.

Hotopf M, Chidgey J, Addington-Hall J, Ly KL. Depression in advanced disease: a systematic review part 1. Prevalence and case finding. [Review] [77 refs]. Palliat Med. 2002;16(2):81–97.

Hudson P, Aranda S, Kristjanson L. Information provision for palliative care families. Eur J Palliat Care. 2004; 11(4):153–7.

Hudson P, Thomas T, Quinn K, Aranda S. Family meetings in palliative care: are they effective? Palliat Med. 2009;23(2):150–7.

Irwin P, Murray S, Bilinski A, Chern B, Stafford B. Alcohol withdrawal as an underrated cause of agitated delirium and terminal restlessness in patients with advanced malignancy. J Pain Symptom Manag. 2005;29(1):104–8.

Irwin S, Hirst J, Fairman N, Prommer E. Ketamine for the management of depression in palliative care: an update on the science (FR413). J Pain Symptom Manag. 2013;45(2):371.

Keall RM, Clayton JM, Butow PN. Therapeutic life review in palliative care: a systematic review of quantitative evaluations. J Pain Symptom Manag. 2015; 49(4):747–61.

King DA, Heisel MJ, Lyness JM, et al. Clin Psychol Sci Pract. 2005;12(3):339–53.

Kirk P, Kirk I, Kristjanson LJ. What do patients receiving palliative care for cancer and their families want to be told? A Canadian and Australian qualitative study. BMJ. 2004;328(7452):1343.

Kissane DW, Bloch S. Family focused grief therapy. Philadelphia: OU Press; 2002.

Kissane DW, Clarke DM, Street AF. Demoralization syndrome – a relevant psychiatric diagnosis for palliative care. J Palliat Care. 2001;17(1):12–21.

Kissane DW, Wein S, Love A, Lee XQ, Kee PL, Clarke DM. The Demoralization Scale: a report of its development and preliminary validation. J Palliat Care. 2004;20(4):269–76.

Kissane DW, Levin T, Hales S, Lo C, Rodin G. Psychotherapy for depression in cancer and palliative care. In: Depression and cancer. Wiley; 2010. p. 177–206.

Kubler-Ross E. On death and dying. London: Tavistock Publications; 1970.

Kumar S, Morse M, Zemenides P, Jenkins R. Psychotherapies for psychological distress in the palliative care setting. Psychiatr Ann [Internet]. 2012;42:133. https://doi.org/10.3928/00485713-20120323-05.

Lederberg MS, Holland JC. Supportive psychotherapy in cancer care: an essential ingredient of all therapy. In: Handbook of psychotherapy in cancer care. Wiley; 2011. p. 1–14.

Lethborg C, Aranda S, Kissane D. Meaning in adjustment to cancer: a model of care. Palliat Support Care. 2008; 6(1):61–70.

Li M, Rosenblat J, Rodin G. Psychopharmacologic management of anxiety and depression. In: Kissane WA, editor. Management of clinical depression and anxiety. Washington, DC: American Psychological Association; 2017.

Lindemann E. Symptomatology and management of acute grief. AJP. 1944;101(2):141–8.

Lloyd-Williams M, Hughes JG. The management of anxiety in advanced disease. Prog Palliat Care. 2008; 16(1):47–50.

Lloyd-Williams M, Shiels C, Dowrick C. The development of the Brief Edinburgh Depression Scale (BEDS) to screen for depression in patients with advanced cancer. J Affect Disord. 2007;99(1–3):259–64.

Low J, Serfaty M, Davis S, Vickerstaff V, Gola A, Omar RZ, et al. Acceptance and commitment therapy for adults with advanced cancer (CanACT): study protocol for a feasibility randomised controlled trial. Trials. 2016;17:77.

Lowe SS, Tan M, Faily J, Watanabe SM, Courneya KS. Physical activity in advanced cancer patients: a systematic review protocol. Syst Rev. 2016;5(1):43.

Lynch T, Price A. The effect of cytochrome P450 metabolism on drug response, interactions, and adverse effects. Am Fam Physician. 2007;76(3):391–6.

MacDonald J. In: Chaiklin S, Wengrower H, editors. Amazon journeys: dance movement therapy interventions in palliative care. New York: Routledge/Taylor & Francis Group; 2016.

Macleod AD. Psychotherapy at the end of life: psychodynamic contributions. Prog Palliat Care. 2009;17(1):3–12.

Mallick S. Palliative care in Parkinson's disease: role of cognitive behavior therapy. Indian J Palliat Care. 2009;15(1):51–6.

Massie MJ, Holland JC. Consultation and liaison issues in cancer care. Psychiatr Med. 1987;5(4):343–59.

McConnell T, Scott D, Porter S. Music therapy for end-of-life care: an updated systematic review. Palliat Med. 2016;30(9):877–83.

Miovic M, Block S. Psychiatric disorders in advanced cancer. Cancer. 2007;110(8):1665–76.

Mitchell AJ. Are one or two simple questions sufficient to detect depression in cancer and palliative care? A Bayesian meta-analysis. Br J Cancer. 2008;98(12): 1934–43.

Mitchell AJ, Meader N, Symonds P. Diagnostic validity of the Hospital Anxiety and Depression Scale (HADS) in cancer and palliative settings: a meta-analysis. J Affect Disord. 2010;126(3):335–48.

Mitchell AJ, Chan M, Bhatti H, Halton M, Grassi L, Johansen C, et al. Prevalence of depression, anxiety, and adjustment disorder in oncological, haematological, and palliative-care settings: a meta-analysis of 94 interview-based studies. Lancet Oncol. 2011;12(2):160–74.

Moorey S, Greer S. Cognitive behaviour therapy for people with cancer. New York: Oxford University Press; 2002. 208 p.

Moser DK, Arslanian-Engoren C, Biddle MJ, Chung ML, Dekker RL, Hammash MH, et al. Psychological aspects of heart failure. Curr Cardiol Rep. 2016;18(12):119.

Mota Vargas R, Mahtani-Chugani V, Solano Pallero M, Rivero Jiménez B, Cabo Domínguez R, Robles Alonso V. The transformation process for palliative care professionals: the metamorphosis, a qualitative research study. Palliat Med. 2015;30(2):161–70.

Mount B. Whole person care: beyond psychosocial and physical needs. Am J Hosp Palliat Care. 1993; 10(1):28–37.

Mystakidou K, Parpa E, Tsilika E, Athanasouli P, Pathiaki M, Galanos A, et al. Preparatory grief, psychological distress and hopelessness in advanced cancer patients. Eur J Cancer Care. 2008;17(2):145–51.

National Comprehensive Cancer Network. Distress management. Clinical practice guidelines. J Natl Compr Cancer Netw. 2003;1(3):344–74.

NHMRC National Breast Cancer Centre (Australia). Clinical practice guidelines for the psychosocial care of adults with cancer. Sydney: National Breast Cancer Centre, National Cancer Control Initiative; 2003. 242 p.

Noble A, Jones C. Benefits of narrative therapy: holistic interventions at the end of life. Br J Nurs. 2005; 14(6):330–3.

Ntlholang O, Walsh S, Bradley D, Harbison J. Identifying palliative care issues in inpatients dying following stroke. Ir J Med Sci. 2016;185(3):741–4.

O'Callaghan C, Forrest L, Wen Y. Music therapy at the end of life. In: Wheeler BL, editor. Music therapy handbook. New York: Guilford Press; 2015. p. 468–80.

Okuyama T, Akechi T, Mackenzie L, Furukawa TA. Psychotherapy for depression among advanced, incurable cancer patients: a systematic review and meta-analysis. Cancer Treat Rev. 2017;56:16–27.

Olsen LG. Hypnotic hazards: adverse effects of zolpidem and other z-drugs. Aust Prescr. 2008;31(6):146–9.

Raphael B, Martinek N, Wooding S. In: Wilson JP, Keane TM, editors. Assessing traumatic bereavement. New York: Guilford Press; 2004.

Rayner L, Price A, Evans A, Valsraj K, Higginson IJ, Hotopf M. Antidepressants for depression in physically ill people. Cochrane Database Syst Rev. 2010;3: CD007503.

Rayner L, Price A, Evans A, Valsraj K, Hotopf M, Higginson IJ. Antidepressants for the treatment of depression in palliative care: systematic review and meta-analysis. Palliat Med. 2011a;25(1):36–51.

Rayner L, Price A, Hotopf M, Higginson IJ. The development of evidence-based European guidelines on the management of depression in palliative cancer care. Eur J Cancer. 2011b;47(5):702–12.

Redhouse R. Life-story; meaning making through dramatherapy in a palliative care context. Dramatherapy [Internet]. 2014;36:66. https://doi.org/10.1080/02630672.2014.996239.

Reisfield GM, Paulian GD, Wilson GR. Substance use disorders in the palliative care patient# 127. J Palliat Med. 2009;12(5):475–6.

Remen RN. Kitchen table wisdom: stories that heal. Pan Macmillan Australia; 2002. 336 p.

Riechelmann RP, Burman D, Tannock IF, Rodin G, Zimmermann C. Phase II trial of mirtazapine for cancer-related cachexia and anorexia. Am J Hosp Palliat Care. 2010;27(2):106–10.

Robinson S, Kissane DW, Brooker J, Burney S. A systematic review of the demoralization syndrome in individuals with progressive disease and cancer: a decade of research. J Pain Symptom Manag. 2015;49(3):595–610.

Robinson S, Kissane DW, Brooker J, Burney SA. Review of the construct of demoralization: history, definitions, and future directions for palliative care. Am J Hosp Palliat Med. 2016a;33(1):93–101.

Robinson S, Kissane DW, Brooker J, Michael N, Fischer J, Franco M, et al. Refinement and revalidation of the demoralization scale: the DS-II-internal validity. Cancer. 2016b;122(14):2251–9.

Rodin G. Individual psychotherapy for the patient with advanced disease. Handbook of psychiatry in palliative medicine. London: Oxford University; 2009. p. 443–53.

Rosenfeld B, Saracino R, Tobias K, Masterson M, Pessin H, Applebaum A, et al. Adapting meaning-centered psychotherapy for the palliative care setting: results of a pilot study. Palliat Med. 2017;31(2):140–6.

Roth AJ, Massie MJ. Anxiety and its management in advanced cancer. Curr Opin Support Palliat Care. 2007;1(1):50–6.

Roth AJ, Massie MJ, Chochinov HM, Breitbart W. Anxiety in palliative care. Handb Psychiatry Palliat Med. 2009;2:69–80.

Salt S, Mulvaney CA, Preston NJ. Drug therapy for symptoms associated with anxiety in adult palliative care patients. Cochrane Database Syst Rev. 2017;5: CD004596.

Selman LE, Williams J, Simms V. A mixed-methods evaluation of complementary therapy services in palliative care: yoga and dance therapy. Eur J Cancer Care. 2012;21(1):87–97.

Sharplin GR, Jones SBW, Hancock B, Knott VE, Bowden JA, Whitford HS. Mindfulness-based cognitive therapy: an efficacious community-based group intervention for depression and anxiety in a sample of cancer patients. Med J Aust. 2010;193(5 Suppl):S79–82.

Sinclair S, Raffin-Bouchal S, Venturato L, Mijovic-Kondejewski J, Smith-MacDonald L. Compassion fatigue: a meta-narrative review of the healthcare literature. Int J Nurs Stud. 2017;69:9–24.

Smith TJ, Temin S, Alesi ER, Abernethy AP, Balboni TA, Basch EM, et al. American Society of Clinical Oncology provisional clinical opinion: the integration of palliative care into standard oncology care. J Clin Oncol. 2012;30(8):880–7.

Sorenson HM. Improving end-of-life care for patients with chronic obstructive pulmonary disease. Ther Adv Respir Dis. 2013;7(6):320–6.

Stagg EK, Lazenby M. Best practices for the non-pharmacological treatment of depression at the end of life. Am J Hosp Palliat Care. 2012 May;29(3):183–94.

Stahl SM. Prescriber's guide: antidepressants: Stahl's essential psychopharmacology. Cambridge, UK: Cambridge University Press; 2014. 431 p.

Sun-Edelstein C, Tepper SJ, Shapiro RE. Drug-induced serotonin syndrome: a review. Expert Opin Drug Saf. 2008;7(5):587–96.

Sussman JC, Liu WM. Perceptions of two therapeutic approaches for palliative care patients experiencing death anxiety. Palliat Support Care. 2014;12(4): 251–60.

Teunissen SCCM, de Graeff A, Voest EE, de Haes JCJM. Are anxiety and depressed mood related to physical symptom burden? A study in hospitalized advanced cancer patients. Palliat Med. 2007;21(4):341–6.

Thekdi SM, Irarráazaval ME, Dunn LB. Psychopharmacological interventions. In: Clinical psycho-oncology. Wiley; 2012. p. 109–26.

Udo I, Gash A. Challenges in management of complex panic disorder in a palliative care setting. BMJ Case Rep [Internet]. 2012. https://doi.org/10.1136/bcr-2012-006800.

Valentine AD. Anxiety disorders. In Holland JC, Golant M, Greenberg DB, Hughes MK, Leverson JA, Loscalzo MJ, Pirl WF (eds) Psycho-oncology: a quick reference on the psychosocial dimensions of cancer symptom management. New York. Oxford University Press.

Watson M, Kissane D. Management of clinical depression and anxiety. New York: Oxford University Press; 2017. 96 p.

Widera EW, Block SD. Managing grief and depression at the end of life. Am Fam Physician. 2012;86(3):259–64.

Willmarth EK. Clinical hypnosis in pain therapy and palliative care: a handbook of techniques for improving the patient's physical and psychological well-being by Brugnoli, Maria Paola. Am J Clin Hypn. 2017; 59(3):318–20.

Wilson KG, Chochinov HM, Skirko MG, Allard P, Chary S, Gagnon PR, et al. Depression and anxiety disorders in palliative cancer care. J Pain Symptom Manag. 2007;33(2):118–29.

Wise MG, Rieck SO. Diagnostic considerations and treatment approaches to underlying anxiety in the medically ill. J Clin Psychiatry. 1993;54(Suppl):22–6. discussion 34–6

Zigmond AS, Snaith RP. The hospital anxiety and depression scale. Acta Psychiatr Scand. 1983;67(6):361–70.

Zweers D, de Graaf E, Teunissen SCCM. Non-pharmacological nurse-led interventions to manage anxiety in patients with advanced cancer: a systematic literature review. Int J Nurs Stud. 2016;56:102–13.

Part VIII

Ethics of Palliative Care and End-of-Life Decision-Making

End-of-Life Decisions

86

Kenneth Chambaere and Jan Bernheim

Contents

K. Chambaere (✉) · J. Bernheim
End-of-Life Care Research Group, Vrije Universiteit Brussel (VUB) and Ghent University, Brussels, Belgium
e-mail: kenneth.chambaere@vub.be; jan.bernheim@vub.be

R. D. MacLeod, L. Van den Block (eds.), *Textbook of Palliative Care*,
https://doi.org/10.1007/978-3-319-77740-5_91

Abstract

This chapter deals with the topic of medical decisions and decision-making that occur at the end of life and have the potential to allow the patient to die or hasten death. These decisions include: withholding and withdrawing treatment, intensified management of pain and other symptoms, active shortening of life without explicit patient request, euthanasia, physician-assisted suicide, and voluntary stopping eating and drinking. Evidently, such decisions are subject to considerable ethical deliberation and scrutiny, apart from their applicability in the legal framework of some jurisdictions. In this contribution, the main ethical principles – autonomy, beneficence, nonmaleficence and justice – are considered in the context of end-of-life decision-making. We go on with a discussion of intensely debated special topics such as: proportionality, the principle of double effect, (medical) futility, nonabandonment, and vulnerability. Next a glossary is provided of the most pertinent issues inherent in each type of end-of-life decision. Examples include: opioid phobia in pain management, the "slippery slope" argument in the assisted dying debate, and the relationship between palliative care and assisted dying. Finally, attention turns to a number of important topics related to communication in end-of-life decision-making: truth-telling, shared decision-making, advance care planning & advance directives, conflict, and cultural issues.

1 Introduction and Aims

Over the past decades, momentous progress has been made in the form of changes in living conditions and substantial and significant advances in science and technology, including in the realm of medicine. This has brought about important epidemiological, demographic, and social changes and hence also new challenges. Everywhere, but nowhere to the same extent as in the developed countries of the Americas, Australasia, central and western Europe, and the Asia-Pacific basin, life expectancy has risen sharply and consistently since the 1950s and will continue to increase (Kontis et al. 2017). Increased life expectancy, which might break the 90-year threshold in 2030, is accompanied by global population ageing. Both the increase of life expectancy and the growing proportion of people at old age – outnumbering younger generations – will globally challenge key aspects of health-care management.

Improved medicine and living conditions have changed not only the manner in which people live but also the way people die. Old age often brings frailty and failing health and illnesses with a heavy symptom burden. Death nowadays comes more often – generally in about two third of all cases – after a chronic, protracted illness trajectory with mostly noncommunicable conditions such as cancer, dementia, cardiovascular disease or lung disease, rather than suddenly due to communicable infectious disease or violence (accidental or conflictuous). Death is very often foreseeable and expected. This can be seen as the downside of medicine having provided us and continuing to provide us with the means to overcome health crises and prolong our lives. The corollary of many more life years for much of the population is that at a certain stage in a person's illness trajectory the "standard" or "straightforward" decision of providing life-saving, life-sustaining, or life-prolonging treatment can become disputable, undesirable, and/or unadvisable. Over the years, the extended period of declining health preceding death has incited people to become more involved in discussions and decisions on how they want to live in the final stages of life as well as how they want to die.

Historically, the dominant paradigm in medicine has been geared toward preservation of life at all costs, even in the very late stages of severe, incurable, and even terminal disease. Particularly when it comes to people with advanced chronic illness, this focus on "quantity of life" has recently become questioned and is being challenged by a movement – a societal movement, but also within medicine itself – advocating a shift in focus and perspective toward "quality of life" (Gawande 2016). This socio-cultural perspective shift is within medicine mainly represented by the palliative care movement, which has developed considerably in the past decades. As concerns treatment plans and decisions to be made in advanced illness and/or when death is approaching, considerations about quality of life and comfort care will increasingly come into play. The focus on life prolongation and therefore the relevance and appropriateness of burdensome and costly treatment for patients will increasingly be disputed. In this context, end-of-life decisions (i.e., decisions that allow the patient to die or that have the potential to hasten death) will be made primarily between the physician and the patient, and with the patient's family and other involved caregivers. These decisions will range anywhere on the spectrum between withdrawal of futile treatment and active life termination.

While there is a wide variety of clinical situations and ensuing therapeutic attitudes, and a great many variables need to be considered in each individual end-of-life decision, there are a number of tenets and ethical principles underlying each type of decision. The aim of this chapter is to provide an overview of the various types of end-of-life decisions and to discuss the ethical considerations and dilemmas (whether or not grounded in a specific legal framework) that come up in each of them. This will give the reader some insights into the complexities and pitfalls of end-of-life decision-making. Given that it remains a highly contested topic in academic, medical, and legal circles, this chapter will also highlight the fault lines of debates about acceptability and applicability of the conditions of certain types of end-of-life decisions.

2 Typology of End-Of-Life Decisions

Recognizing that medical practice at the end of life is extremely complex and does not always lend itself to clear-cut categorizations, classification is nonetheless necessary for an orderly discussion of the ethical and practical aspects. Though there is some occasional academic dissent, the typology of end-of-life decisions used in this chapter is widely accepted, largely uncontroversial, and empirically validated in research. The following types are discerned:

- *Withholding or withdrawing medical treatment*

  These are decisions forgo or discontinue (potentially) life-prolonging treatment. Examples of such decisions include forgoing radiation or chemotherapy, artificial respiration, resuscitation, antibiotics treatment, artificial administration of food and fluid, etc. Physicians can decide to withhold or withdraw treatment taking into account that the patient may die or explicitly intending to allow the patient to die.
- *Intensified management of pain or other symptoms*

  These decisions concern the administration of drugs for pain and/or symptom relief in doses that may also have a life-shortening effect. Life shortening can in these cases be taken into account as a foreseeable but unintended side-effect, or cointended.

  A special form of this type of end-of-life decision, in fact the most far-reaching form, is palliative or terminal sedation. If applied appropriately, i.e., according to professional and ethical guidelines, this practice will not influence the moment of death. However, when due care criteria are not followed or when applied in patients with special risk factors, a life-shortening effect cannot be precluded. The next chapter is focused solely on this practice (see ▶ Chap. 87, "Palliative Sedation: A Medical-Ethical Exploration").
- *Euthanasia*

  Euthanasia can be defined as the administration of drugs by someone else than the patient with the explicit intention of hastening the patient's death, at the patient's explicit request.

This definition excludes "passive" decisions such as withholding or withdrawing life-sustaining or life-prolonging treatment, which have often been termed "passive euthanasia." This is a misnomer. Similarly, "nonvoluntary euthanasia" or "involuntary euthanasia," oft-used terms for the act of administering lethal drugs without the patient's explicit request, constitute misnomers. Euthanasia is by definition active and voluntary.

- *Physician-assisted suicide*

  Physician-assisted suicide can be defined as the physician's act to supply or prescribe a lethal dose of drugs to be taken by the patient him/herself, with the explicit intention of hastening the patient's death, at the latter's explicit request.
- *Voluntary stopping eating and drinking*

  This is the conscious and voluntary decision of the patient to halt all food and fluids intake with patient's explicit aim of hastening his/her death.

The pervasive issues in each of these end-of-life decisions will be discussed extensively further in this chapter. Euthanasia and physician-assisted suicide are often subsumed together under the umbrella terms "assisted dying," "medical assistance in dying," or "physician-assisted dying." For the remainder of this chapter both practices will be discussed together.

Perhaps not unexpectedly – but nonetheless important to point out here – it appears that there is an inverse relationship between the ethical contestedness of an end-of-life decision and its actual incidence in end-of-life practice. Though euthanasia and assisted suicide are by far the most controversial of all end-of-life decisions, and illegal in most parts of the world, empirical studies show that even in jurisdictions where they can be legally practiced they make up only a small minority of all deaths. Hence, the vast majority of end-of-life decisions concern cases of withholding or withdrawing treatment and cases of intensified management of pain or other symptoms, regardless of jurisdiction or medical culture.

Empirical studies into end-of-life decision-making have also pointed to considerable overlap, grey zones, and even confusion among physicians and other clinicians regarding the various types of end-of-life decisions (Deyaert et al. 2014). Vignette studies on and studies into the labelling of end-of-life decisions, for instance, have revealed faulty interpretations and a potentially problematic lack of understanding of differences between types of end-of-life decisions (Smets et al. 2012). On the other hand, these studies also show that clear-cut classification of end-of-life decisions in clinical practice is wishful thinking. Readers should keep this in mind at all times in this chapter.

3 Legal Contexts

Before discussing the various ethical principles and rationales, it is important to note upfront that the legal and regulatory context in a jurisdiction or country form the stage for practical ethical reasoning and concrete medical decision-making in that jurisdiction or country. There is extreme variation across countries worldwide in the legal status of the various end-of-life decisions, not only with regard to what is legally permissible and what is not but also to what extent relevant aspects for end-of-life decision-making are explicitly regulated. This latter aspect signifies that there are a great number of countries where the legal status of end-of-life decisions is undetermined and therefore uncertain. This compounds the difficulty of making such decisions. An oft-cited example concerns the legal status of withdrawing life-sustaining treatment in a patient in persistent vegetative state. In some countries this may be explicitly illegal, in others the permissibility needs to be determined through court rulings, while elsewhere it might be legally permitted by means of laws on patient autonomy and self-determination (Schneiderman 2011). Generally speaking, (legal) permissibility of end-of-life decisions in more developed countries is higher than in less-developed countries.

Obviously, it is imperative for clinicians and other involved actors to be well-informed on the permissibility of various end-of-life decisions, as well as the specific legal criteria and interpretive intricacies. For instance, in countries that allow medical assistance in dying, the patient must fulfil a number of substantive criteria and the physician must follow mandatory procedural criteria for due care in decision-making. Also, in some jurisdictions withdrawing treatment will only be permitted under a number of specific circumstances. Awareness of specific legal frameworks is vital in order not to expose oneself to criminal charges and to avoid overly aggressive and/or unjustified treatment courses. Moreover, the legal context may conflict with the personal stance and individual ethical standards of one or more of the actors involved, e.g., when the patient or family request a hastened death, at which point the physician can explain that this is not a legal option. Legal developments generally tend to lag behind ethical and philosophical debate.

4 General Medical-Ethical Principles in Relation to End-of-Life Decisions

Medical decision-making is also ethical decision-making: there are always several ethical considerations to be reckoned with. As concerns medical end-of-life decision-making, this is particularly true given that these decisions are made literally about life and death. Though the main ethical principles are systematically taught in clinical education (Beauchamp and Childress 1979) and widely known by clinicians, it is worth repeating in short here the content and the context of the basic four ethical principles that permeate all end-of-life decisions and that should always be heeded when forming end-of-life decisions.

4.1 (Respect for) Autonomy

The most fundamental of medical-ethical principles is respect for autonomy. It is increasingly recognized that patients have the last word in judging and deciding on the often many available treatment options and their consequences that are submitted to their informed consent. Basically, this entails that the patient has sovereignty over their own body and what does and does not happen to it. In the end-of-life context, this translates into the right of the patient to determine which treatment that is medically indicated according to the physician may be given and which may not. The final decision for a clinical course thus ultimately lies in the hands of the patient who is to receive it. This presupposes that the patient should be always fully informed about diagnosis, prognosis, and the benefits and drawbacks of the treatment plan.

The right to autonomy has not always been as central as it is today. It has gained considerable momentum in the past decades, as part of a societal and cultural shift from medical paternalism to patient and physician shared decision-making, the focus on quality of life, self-determination, and individualism. For this movement, the wish for self-control is considered fundamental as individuals are seen as planning agents, not only of their life but also of their death (which is inherent in life itself). In this context, openness and acceptance of death as well as the concept of "good death" (i.e., with dignity and according to one's personal preferences, which mostly feature being free from pain, dying at home, being surrounded by loved ones, being conscious until the final moments, being at peace, etc.) have come to centre-stage. In the philosophy of palliative care – and in its various definitions – attention to the needs and respect for the wishes of the patient (i.e., person-centeredness) is paramount. Many countries have even set legal parameters for patient autonomy, like the Patient Self-Determination Act in the USA or the Law on Patient Rights in Belgium. Lastly, advance care planning, advance directives, and living wills are aimed at allowing patients to exercise their autonomy in case or in anticipation of becoming incompetent (see below).

The counterpart of autonomy is usually termed paternalism – whereby someone else than the subject decides about what is in the interest of the subject and what is to happen to him/her. A sometimes useful distinction is between "strong" paternalism, where decisions are taken against the wishes of the subject end "weak" paternalism, where the subject has not expressed wishes. With the ascent of autonomy as the overarching principle in medical ethics, paternalism has been increasingly imbued with pejorative connotations and has an aura of being undesirable and unethical. Particularly in the case of "vulnerable patient groups," i.e., groups that are less well able to stand-up for themselves and thus more prone to medical misconduct such as the elderly or the cognitively impaired (see below), the issue of paternalism is heavily discussed. Recent academic contributions have attempted to requalify this negative perspective, e.g., claiming that the perspectives of other involved moral agents – such as the physicians, care team, and the family – are also highly relevant in decision-making. They argue that the ethical pendulum may have swung too far in the direction of patients' autonomy (Wancata and Hinshaw 2016) and that patient autonomy should not supersede physician responsibility, which must not be dodged (Roeland et al. 2014; Levy 2014; Specker 2016). Middle-ground solutions such as shared decision-making are discussed further in this chapter.

4.2 Beneficence and Nonmaleficence

Beneficence signifies that the physician and involved care team are at all times concerned with "doing good" for the patient and acting in the patient's best interests. Nonmaleficence is closely related to beneficence and signifies that, above all, a physician should refrain from inflicting harm upon the patient. Beneficence and nonmaleficence can be served by active (doing well) versus passive (omission of doing harm) behavior. Both beneficence and nonmaleficence represent a fundamental tenet in the code of medical ethics. Especially in cases where the patient has not clearly communicated his/her preferences or wishes, the physician must adhere to these principles to ensure ethically sound end-of-life decision-making and the patient dying with dignity. These principles should for instance shield patients from the potential pitfalls of strong paternalistic decision-making.

In real-life clinical end-of-life situations, the application of the principles of beneficence and nonmaleficence is not always as straightforward as one would perhaps expect. The best course of action often hinges on a multitude of factors on various levels, rendering medical end-of-life decision-making highly complex. In such instances, they are essentially cost-benefit judgments. Dilemmas often arise e.g., when improving a patient's situation entails inflicting considerable harm upon the patient. Naturally, medical-ethical debate has focused on the central question concerning what constitutes a "harm" for the patient. In the context of end-of-life decisions, the question becomes whether death itself should be seen by definition as a harm (Clark et al. 2002). A corollary of this is that in some cases, some patients can see further irreversibly suffering life as a harm. Adherents of the recent cultural and societal paradigm shift toward quality of life over quantity of life may formulate permissive stances toward allowing patients to die, accepting potential life-shortening effects of medical actions, and in some cases even intentional ending of life. Diametrically opposed to this view and at the other extreme is the religiously inspired sanctity of life doctrine, rooted in the conviction that life is a gift from the Supreme Being, and therefore cannot be put at risk or given up but needs to be protected at any cost.

4.3 Justice

The principle of justice or fairness relates to the equal treatment of patients under equal conditions. It is more of a transversal principle that can be formulated and applied on two levels: the level of the individual and the societal level.

At the level of the individual, the tenet requires that patients are treated fairly and adequately. This applies particularly to the most vulnerable in society who are most at risk of not receiving the treatment they need, while others in similar situations would receive that treatment. In such cases, patients are denied access to adequate healthcare and services by virtue of a characteristic that should be irrelevant in the decision whether or not to treat. A prime example of this is ageism i. e., different treatment of older people based purely on their age. However, the line can be very fine. For instance, age can arguably be a contributing factor in end-of-life decisions, so long as it has demonstrable relevance in the clinical parameters underlying the decision. An illustration of this is the decision not to operate on a patient when their advanced age entails an unacceptable risk.

At the societal level, the principle of justice translates into a just distribution of (scarce) healthcare resources. It regulates fair and equal treatment of patients from a higher level by rationing interventions based on the costs of end-of-life care and the available resources. It is the duty of governments, clinical networks, and medical institutions and departments to continuously strive for adequate allocation of resources based on the needs of the population and/or on issues of equality.

4.4 Usefulness of General Principles in Clinical Practice

As mentioned above, the general medical-ethical principles are commonly known among healthcare practitioners. They are the backdrop of ethically sound decisions; much care must be taken to arrive at a defensible decision. However, to apply them adequately requires quite some rigor and experience. "Principlism" certainly also has its limitations in clinical practice. At best, it constitutes a practical heuristic on which to base the reasoning toward an end-of-life decision. The principles can be seen as fundamental though not absolute, as they can easily come into conflict with each other, and the hierarchical relative weights they are ascribed will likely lead to different end decisions and outcomes. In any case, the principles are represented in basic clinical criteria for treatment decision-making: every treatment must be directed toward alleviating a clear indication (= beneficence, achieving benefits), the treatment goal must be achievable (= nonmaleficence, avoiding unnecessary harm) and informed consent must be obtained from the patient or the proxy decision maker in case the patient is no longer capable (= autonomy). (Justice is more of a relational ethical principle and is presupposed in clinical treatment decision models.)

5 Special Considerations in End-of-Life Decision Making

To further the application of the general medical-ethical principles, there are a number of special considerations central to ethical, clinical, and academic debate on end-of-life decisions. These considerations are germane to the ethical intricacies inherent in medical treatment decisions at the end of life.

5.1 Proportionality

Proportionality denotes the idea that the choice whether or not to provide a treatment should be based on a harm-benefit judgment. It requires one to weigh the potential benefits of the treatment against its potential harms and burdens for the patient. In view of the general clinical situation of a patient, the prognosis, all available treatment options and their consequences in terms of achieved or foreseen benefits should outweigh the harms, i.e., be proportional to the harms. Only then can the treatment be suggested to and discussed with the patient. In the end-of-life context, harms will most often relate to disproportionally prolonging the dying process and consequently the suffering of patients, with an unacceptably low quality of life. As a basic rule, treatment that fulfils the proportionality principle may be chosen in agreement between both the physician and the patient, and disproportionate treatment should be forgone. Even if this results in hastened death, there is no obligation to provide disproportionate treatment (Ko and Blinderman 2013).

Naturally, identifying and weighing the harms and benefits of a given treatment will never be a straightforward task. It presupposes the ability of the physician and care team to estimate the outcomes of the treatment, including among others the likelihood of success, the severity of potential side effects, the impact on the intended treatment goal and knock-on effects for the patient's well-being. Also, the judgment of the patient plays a cardinal role in deciding on the relative values of the benefits and harms. For instance, to one patient nausea may be a totally intolerable side effect of palliative chemotherapy whereas another may feel it is an acceptable price to pay to live a while longer. These considerations make proportionality decisions at the end of life a highly complex process requiring accurate information and extensive discussions between healthcare professionals, preferably from various disciplines, between physicians and their patients and the patients' relatives.

The proportionality principle has largely replaced the concept of distinguishing between "extraordinary" and "ordinary" treatment as a means to make end-of-life decisions – with extraordinary treatment being more difficult to justify. The distinction proved not useful in clinical practice because it was unclear as to which criteria (usualness, complexity, artificiality, availability, cost) should be used to define "extraordinary" treatment.

5.2 Double Effect

The principle of double effect was first formulated by Thomas Aquinas (thirteenth century) to justify homicide in self-defence. An agent applies the principle of double effect when he/she wishes to do good but cannot do so without also causing harm. In its most stringent classic formulation, the principle of double effect can be licitly applied if all of four conditions are fulfilled: (1) the nature of the act must be morally good or neutral, (2) the harmful effect may be foreseen but should not be intended, (3) the good effect is not the product of the harm, and (4) the good effect must outweigh the harmful effect (cf. above: proportionality, the benefit must be proportional to the harm) (Mangan 1949).

The doctrine is applied mainly in the context of administration of opioids and/or sedatives, e.g., when mechanical ventilation is withdrawn or when pain and other symptoms become extremely discomforting for the dying patient, where the dosages are high and where causation of death due to e.g., respiratory depression, may be foreseen or expected by the physician (Thorns and Sykes 2000; Boyle 2004; López-Saca et al. 2013).

An authoritative study of intention in general has shown that it is a brittle criterium for acting morally (Anscombe 1958). There is an old utilitaristic tradition of criticism on the originally catholic doctrine of the double effect (Mill 1863). Though the concept has been often used in the justification of rapid dose increases in symptom treatment near the end of life, beyond philosophical considerations, its practical usefulness and appropriateness in clinical situations has been disputed (Quill et al. 1997). By involving the notions of redescription (alternative definitions) of acts and proportionality of consequences, a "weak" form of double effect principle has been proposed (Boyle 2004).

Whereas in criminal law intention is crucial, e.g., to distinguish manslaughter from murder, it is a disputed criterion for the ethical acceptability of end-of-life practices. First, is "absence of intention" a serious proposition when it contradicts or denies a high probability and a reasonable expectation, as when life support is forgone? When one relies on intention, one is dependent on self-reporting and risks self-delusion. People can fabricate an intention they at heart do not have or to obfuscate an intention they do have. The double-effect principle relies heavily on the individual clinical-ethical stance of the physician and supposes that physicians will always be conscious, honest, and clear about their ethical motives. This is problematic as it is extremely difficult or even impossible to cognitively separate intention to hasten death from expecting or foreseeing a hastened death. This applies to the person who makes the decision, and even more so to third parties such as the family. Secondly, the same action can be described in different ways, without there being an objective way to determine which description is correct. In many end-of-life situations, there are multiple layers of intention, and these layers, like a cascade, are related by a chain of causalities and consequences. For example, in euthanasia, the proximate intention is killing, the next is relief of suffering, and the next respect for patient autonomy. Similarly, for end-of-life sedation, the proximate intention is reducing consciousness, the next is relief of suffering, and the next respect for patient autonomy if it is done at the patient's request. If the patient has expressed no wish, the physician's beneficence is applied paternalistically. Which level of intention is privileged can thus be highly subjective. Acts almost always serve multiple intentions. Establishing a hierarchy between them is very difficult (Quill et al. 1997).

Thirdly, the rule obviously refers to the intention of the physician. This disregards that multiple actors are involved in palliative care, foremost the patient, but also nurses, other paramedics, informal caregivers, clergy, etc. and these different actors may well have different intentions. Focusing solely on the physician's intention is unduly paternalistic and ignores the concept of care as a *process* involving multiple parties (indeed a central tenet of palliative care). The intentions of the person who is dying cannot be ignored, and those requesting the withdrawal of life-sustaining treatment or continuous deep sedation may intend to hasten their death, even when their physician harbors no such intention.

As such, invoking the principle of double effect can be an obfuscation of the "elephant in the room" and a weak safeguard against abuse of the practice of intentionally hastening the death of the patient through administration of medication. Actually, the only effective and somewhat objectifiable aspect of the double-effect principle may be the proportionality criterion which could be a sufficient condition. The necessity of the principle of double effect comes into question for commentators who submit that it is sufficient to let care of the dying patient be guided by patients' informed consent, the degree of suffering and the absence of preferable alternatives.

5.3 Futility

Futility, simply put, can be understood as the opposite of utility, which is the result of beneficence, i.e., the state of meaningfulness or benefit. An act is futile when it generates no utility, or when its performance entails drawbacks that exceed its benefits. Deciding that something is futile requires a judgment. This judgment can be by the person performing the act, by the person undergoing its consequences or – ideally in clinical settings – jointly by both.

At the end of life, futility relates foremost to unwarranted initiation or continuation of disease-directed treatments, thereby forgoing or delaying palliative care. Secondarily, especially in jurisdictions (countries and states) having depenalized-assisted dying, some patients may (come to) declare (further) palliative care futile and request assisted dying.

We will successively deal with these two cases of futility at the end of life.

There comes a time when during the disease-directed therapeutic stage of a fatal disease the pursuit of, e.g., chemotherapy or of life support is judged futile. Qualitative research suggests that, e.g., oncologists are well aware of the minimal response rate at the cost of nonnegligible drawbacks of aggressive treatments in many cases of advanced cancer. However, they feel that they cannot deny patients even largely illusory hope. The motives to discourage or curb medical futility are at the same time clinical, ethical, and economical (Bagheri 2014). It has proven a difficult task because of poor acceptance of death: both public expectation of what medicine can achieve and professional perception of what ethics and law require drive an unhelpful alliance that often results in futile courses of medical action (Ashby 2011). As for fee-for-service remuneration of doctors and health-care facilities, we are not aware of data supporting the contention that it is associated with more medically futile interventions, but, logically, such remuneration might compound the problem.

The use of the concept of futility in clinical practice has its problems as there are many complications in attempting to define or operationalize it. Futility may lie in the total lack of a physiological benefit for the patient, e.g., treatments that would not *at all* alter the course of the disease, the time of the fatal outcome or the prevalence or intensity of symptoms and complaints. .Such a binary judgment is often based on objective and evidence-based criteria and is thus relatively feasible for well-trained doctors and well-informed patients. More frequently, futility is quantitative, a continuous variable. It can relate to an unacceptably low probability of success, or to so small a benefit that it is outweighed by the drawbacks of the course of action. This type of futility draws on proportionality and the balancing of benefits and drawbacks. Treatment can also be deemed futile if the financial cost is too great to justify the low probability and/or magnitude of the effect. The goal of this higher-level approach is cost control and justice in the allocation of resources (Baily 2011). The overarching principle for these considerations is the obligation to always do a cost-benefit analysis, where costs can be both economical and clinical (e.g., side effects and other adverse consequences of treatment), and benefits can be physiological, psychological, or social. Cost-benefit analysis can be considered as belonging to the obligatory means of clinical practice.

"Physiologically" futile treatment at the request of the patient or proxies poses a difficult problem of conflicting interests: the values of the requesting agent are then at odds with the physician's. Most cases ought to be resolved by complete information and full deliberation.

Uncertainty also abounds according to *who* decides whether a certain course of action is useful or futile. Ideally, after a process of shared decision-making all those involved concur, but when they differ, problems arise. A decision of forgoing a course of action that is medically futile, if taken unilaterally by the physician, can be closely related to paternalism: "strong" if against patient preferences or "weak" if without input from the patient. As long as the decision is based on clear physiological or clinical indicators, and the patient has declined involvement in decision-making, such reasoning may be perfectly justified. But, of course, it is always advisable to consult with the patient and others. A judgement of futility should not serve as a justification to forgo difficult but ultimately beneficial conversations to address unrealistic expectations and prepare for the end of life. Conversely, medical futility may be a judgment by the informed patient against the "physiologic" judgment of the physicians. This is what has been termed "normative futility" (Youngner and Arnold 2016) or "qualitative futility" where a treatment may be physiologically effective but not psychologically beneficial (ten Have and Janssens 2002).

The second issue on futility at the end of life is whether there is such a thing as "palliative futility" and, if so, whether in permissive jurisdictions this justifies a request of assisted dying. A debate is ongoing regarding the (non)sense of the concept of "palliative futility." It has been argued that "meaningfulness" is not absolute, but inseparable from the question "for whom?". Caregivers, for whom palliative care is always meaningful, will always offer it, but a patient not. According to this reasoning, one can take a hard look at any a priori subordination of the view of the patient to that of the caregiver. Such a hierarchy, it is argued, violates the central position and autonomy of the patient (Bernheim and Raus 2017). Especially in jurisdictions with legal assisted dying, some patients may consider the initiation or continuation of palliative care as futile, and request assisted dying (Bernheim et al. 2008; Bernheim and Raus 2017). In general, respect for patients' autonomy encompasses patients' fundamental right to refuse perceived futile treatment (Bagheri 2017). Logically, this also applies to palliative care. However, many dispute that palliative care can ever be futile (Jaspers et al. 2009; Materstvedt and Bosshard 2013). This is also the formal European Association of Palliative Care's (EAPC) normative stance: "Palliative care is provided up until the end of life and is by definition never futile" (Radbruch et al. 2016). A reconciliating consideration could be a distinction between palliative "treatment" which may for the odd patient be or become futile and palliative "care" which is always meaningful from a human solidarity perspective (ten Have and Janssens 2002). In Belgium, for instance, palliative caregivers may see euthanasia as a last exercise of care and refusing further palliative care does not disqualify a patient from assisted dying (Vanden Berghe et al. 2013).

In any case, the question is particularly pertinent in the assisted dying debate: if palliative care can always alleviate all suffering, then a standard condition for eligibility for assistance in dying, i. e., that suffering cannot be alleviated, is never fulfilled. Conversely, if palliative care is not always able to sufficiently alleviate suffering and if some patients consider (further) palliative care as futile, then at least some requests for assisted dying could be considered legitimate and legal in permissive jurisdictions. In the Benelux countries with depenalized euthanasia and/or assisted suicide options, some patients' well-considered perception of further palliative care being futile can be honored and acted upon (Bernheim et al. 2008, 2013; Bernheim and Raus 2017).

5.4 Nonabandonment

Another oft-cited ethical consideration related to end-of-life care and decision-making relates to the idea of nonabandonment, also referred to as fidelity, on the part of the physician and care team toward the patient. It entails a duty of responsibility and accountability of the physician and the care team toward continued care for their patient. This may seem evident, yet there exist a number of not infrequent situations in which this duty conflicts with other values or priorities.

One situation very often encountered in palliative and end-of-life care relates to patients feeling a sense of abandonment from their physician when a decision needs to be made to focus treatment on palliation – instead of cure or life prolongation – or the withdrawal of life-sustaining treatment. This is closely tied to the reluctance of physicians to bring such a message and "take away hope."Nevertheless, this communication is important and when it happens the patient needs to be reassured that any change in treatment goals and any withholding or withdrawal of treatment will be accompanied by an appropriate and effective care plan focusing on the patient's comfort. This also implies that a physician will not abandon the patient by failing to consult the necessary palliative care experts when they themselves do not possess this expertise. A special case of this is when the physician has to refuse a request of futile treatment.

A different type of situation concerns the case in which a palliative patient explicitly requests a certain course of action that goes against the morals or beliefs of the physician. This will concern assistance in dying in most but certainly not all cases; a patient's refusal of clinically beneficial treatment, for instance, may also be difficult for a physician to accept. If clear and explicit communication does not reconcile the conflicting views, the physician may decide to withdraw from the therapeutic relationship on grounds of conscientious objection. In the Benelux countries there is no legal obligation to transfer the patient into the care of another permissive physician, team or unit, thus assuring the patient continuity of care whilst preserving one's personal ethical principles. However, it has argued that failing to do this in order not to be an accessory of something one disapproves of, comes near to abandoning one's patient (Vanden Berghe et al. 2013). A final type of situation relates to the physician being faithful in following the choices and decisions of the patient and even defending them when the patient can no longer speak for himself or herself.

5.5 Vulnerability

Vulnerability constitutes an important reflection in palliative care and end-of- life decision-making, closely tied to the ethical principle of justice. Over and beyond the fact that severely ill and dying patients are by definition vulnerable, physicians need to pay special attention to the protection of people who are unable or not sufficiently able to defend their own interests. Categories often mentioned in this regard are: children; the elderly; the disabled; the mentally incapacitated; psychiatric patients, cultural, and ethnic minorities. Referring to the nonabandonment consideration discussed above, physicians can be expected to defend these interests in lieu of the patient. Particularly those with reduced competence or complete incompetence are most vulnerable to unethical and unjust treatment. Persons from a cultural or ethnic minority might lack the necessary health literacy or language skills to navigate their way to appropriate, tailored care. These persons also adhere to specific belief systems different from the cultural majority of a country and are therefore more at risk of receiving treatment that is inappropriate to their moral values.

6 Notes on Specific End-of-Life Decisions

In this section, a number of points particular to the specific types of end-of-life decisions are highlighted and discussed. These points are nonexhaustive but give the reader an understanding of the "lay of the land" with regard to modern academic, ethical, and clinical debate on each decision.

6.1 Withholding and Withdrawing Medical Treatment

Medical treatments that are commonly withheld or withdrawn at the end of life are: cardio-pulmonary resuscitation, intubation, mechanical ventilation, artificial nutrition and hydration, kidney dialysis, surgery, and antibiotics treatment. However, a nontreatment decision may also concern the decision not to run diagnostic tests or not to transfer the patient to hospital, as the finality of these conscious choices is to no longer pursue curative or disease-directed options for one or more given problems.

Many philosophers, ethicists and legal scholars have long studied the existence, necessity and/or usefulness of a moral distinction between withholding treatment and withdrawing treatment. This is referred to as the act-omission or commission-omission distinction. While the general debate does not look to be settled for some time, the consequentialism-inspired consensus view related to end-of-life treatment seems to be geared toward moral equivalence between withholding and withdrawing. Jurisprudence in most developed countries has ruled in favor of this view as well. This said, while there may not be a legal or ethical distinction, a considerable psychological and moral effect for the physician and others involved can be expected. It is arguably much more difficult and confronting to remove mechanical ventilation than it is to not initiate it. This psychological and moral impact should not be ignored in clinical practice.

The legal status of nontreatment decisions (withholding and withdrawing treatment) varies greatly from country to country. In most modern industrialized countries, they are largely unproblematic under the necessary conditions, though even recently some cases elicit heated debate and legal proceedings are necessary to clarify the possibility of treatment limitation. The most thought-provoking cases concern withdrawing life support or artificial nutrition and hydration in people in a persistent vegetative state, especially minors (cf. the Alfie Evans case in Britain, in which the parents of a terminally ill toddler in a semivegetative state lost their legal battles over the hospital's decision to withhold further prolonging life support as well as the option to transfer their son to a Vatican hospital in Rome for further treatment (Evans 2018)). In less developed and non-Western countries the law might severely restrict clinicians' possibilities to forgo life-saving, life-sustaining, or life-prolonging treatment. Clinicians are strongly advised to inform themselves about the legality in their country of forgoing various treatments at the end of life.

According to some, artificial administration of nutrition and hydration represents a special case in end-of-life treatment, as it can be regarded as standard and obligatory practice to provide food and water to the patient. It also has particular symbolic meaning; the argument states that while it does entail a technical intervention, it does not constitute a medical treatment but rather basic human care. While this is an understandable perspective on the issue, the consensus view disputes this, arguing that artificial nutrition and hydration, just as any other medical treatment, must adhere to all standard requirements: a clear indication, a reasonably achievable treatment goal and informed consent (Ko and Blinderman 2013). If not subject to these requirements, artificial nutrition and hydration, a notably invasive treatment, could be performed against the wishes of the patient. Moreover, studies have shown that providing it at the end of life does not procure much benefit and that in end-of-life settings starvation is extremely unlikely (Druml et al. 2016). As not providing nutrition and hydration may seem harsh and unacceptable, especially for the family, it is important to reassure them – as well as the patient – of these medical requirements and that adequate comfort care will be provided to prevent unwanted effects of dehydration.

6.2 Intensified Management of Pain or Other Symptoms

As mentioned above, intensified pain and symptom management at the end of life mostly concerns the administration of increasingly high doses of morphine and/or sedatives, as these drugs are thought to contribute to a hastened death in certain doses.

The literature describes the reportedly widespread phenomenon of "opioid phobia." This term refers to a fear or reluctance on the part of physicians to provide morphine or other opioids in high or even only moderate doses. Outside the end-of-life setting, this concern is also based on fears of causing addiction and dependency in patients, but in an end-of-life situation the concern lies mostly with patients developing tolerance leading to ever higher doses being needed, and with the possibility that high doses will cause respiratory depression in already very weak patients and lead to a premature, nonnatural death. While such fears are reasonable, cf. the sharp increase of unintended deaths due to prescribed opioids in the USA (López-Saca et al. 2013), according to experts, the effects of high-dose opioids in general are largely overstated, especially in patients where the dosage increase is gradual (in opioid-naïve patients, however, more caution is needed) (Thorns and Sykes 2000). Notwithstanding the complexity of calculating dose equivalences between the various opioid products, opioid rotation, i.e., switching regularly between opioids, is recommended as in order to avoid tolerance and the need for rapid dose increases. The importance of assuaging unsubstantiated fears in physicians to use opioids in adequate doses cannot be overestimated: opioid phobia could well lead to undertreatment and therefore ineffective relief of pain (and other symptoms) at the end of life (Macauley 2012).

Of course, there will be instances in which e.g., respiratory depression under treatment with opioids occurs. These and other situations are typical examples of where the proportionality principle, the rule of double effect and risk-benefit balancing are highly useful to justify high dosages of opioids. Respectively, the reasoning goes as follows: the administered dose is as high as necessary to alleviate the patient's pain (proportionality), the objective is achieving adequate pain relief, with respiratory depression and death as an unintended but acceptable consequence/effect (double effect) and the risk of hastened death is of less importance than the need to avoid protracted suffering. As discussed in the section above, it is may be important to communicate clearly with all involved – patient, family, and care team alike – about the explicit treatment goal and the possibility of unintended consequences.

At the end of life, high doses of sedatives (mostly benzodiazepines, or sometimes barbiturates) are increasingly used to achieve palliative or terminal sedation. Here, the same considerations of proportionality and double effect apply in order to avoid misuse as "slow euthanasia," as research has suggested. Therefore, guidelines for adequate performance have been issued, and in some countries there are initiatives to register the practice (e.g., Belgium) and it has even be legally regulated (i.e., France's *Loi Leonetti*). See ▶ Chap. 87, "Palliative Sedation: A Medical-Ethical Exploration" for a thorough discussion of palliative sedation.

6.3 Euthanasia and Assisted Suicide (Assisted Dying)

An increasing number of countries and jurisdictions are legalizing assisted dying. Euthanasia is, at the time of this writing, legal in six jurisdictions worldwide: the Netherlands (since 2002), Belgium (since 2002), Luxembourg (since 2009), Colombia (since 2015), Canada (since 2016), and Victoria in Australia (as of 2019). In the Netherlands, the legalization of euthanasia was preceded by a period between the mid-1980s and 2001 of legal tolerance of the practice, as long as certain requirements of careful practice, suggested by the Royal Dutch Medical Association, were complied with (Griffiths et al. 1998). The first jurisdiction to have legal euthanasia was actually the Northern Territories in Australia in 1995; however, the law only held 9 months and was overturned by the federal Parliament of Australia. The legalization in Canada was a result of a ruling of the Supreme Court in the Carter versus Canada case, which ordered the provinces to draft laws legalizing euthanasia by February 2016, later extended to June 2016. Medically assisted suicide, but not euthanasia, is legal in a number of states in the USA and in Switzerland.

Euthanasia and assisted suicide – for the remainder of the chapter together referred to as "assisted dying" – are arguably the most controversial topic in end-of-life debates today. Heated discussion continues to rage whether or not assisted dying can be morally acceptable at all. Obviously, for proponents of assisted dying (notably the "Right to Die" or "Pro Choice" movement) the autonomy and right to self-determination of the patient takes primacy over any other ethical principle. However, they also argue that assisted dying need not violate the principles of beneficence and nonmaleficence as death can be considered as the curtailing of unnecessary and pointless suffering – suffering that cannot otherwise be alleviated – and thus as beneficial and a good in itself. Moreover, similarly to other bioethical issues such as in the sexual or reproduction domains, assisted dying belongs to the personal province, and its legalization, as is argued, does not impinge on the rights and values of those who want no part in it.

Invoked pragmatic advantages of legally regulated assisted dying include: bringing into the open practices that were clandestine and solitary, allowing better peer and societal scrutiny and control; protection of caregivers against prosecution; boosting the development of palliative care insofar as universal access to palliative care is an ethical and political precondition for euthanasia, and; promoting reflection by members the public on what they want for their end of life.

Opponents (often called "Pro Life" thinkers) dismiss these views, arguing either that one ethical principle cannot dominate or dismiss another or that beneficence and nonmaleficence have primacy over autonomy (with regard to assisted dying) (Callahan 2008; Foster 2009). Proponents of the sanctity-of-life argument label the idea of death being beneficial or good as preposterous (when completely contrary to human nature). On a more general level, they argue that legal-assisted dying would denature medicine and corrupt society.

Apart from philosophical and theoretical-ethical arguments against the practice, international concerns of societal ratification of euthanasia focus on undesirable pragmatic developments, also referred to as the slippery slope. The various aspects of the slippery slope argument (or hypothesis as it is mostly composed of expectations and presuppositions) can be classified as follows:

1. *Effects for patients*, e.g., vulnerable patients such as the oldest old being pressured into requesting assisted dying (cf. "a duty to die?") (Lewis and Black 2013), patients not receiving adequate end-of-life or palliative care (Hudson et al. 2015), erosion of trust in their relationship with their physicians (Hall et al. 2005);
2. *Effects for physicians*, e.g., stress, burnout, and emotional problems or conversely desensitization from ending patients' lives (van Marwijk et al. 2007), confusion over deontological rules (Cohen-Almagor 2013), feeling pressured into granting assisted dying requests;
3. *Uncontrollable "runaway" practice*, e.g., nonadherence to legal requirements, hastening death without the patient's explicit request (Cohen-Almagor 2009; Pereira 2011), and expanding ("overstretching") interpretations of eligibility criteria (Shariff 2012).

4. *Effect for palliative care*, i.e., regulated euthanasia is also anticipated to undermine or overshadow the palliative care movement striving to improve quality of life for people with life-threatening conditions, particularly at the end of life (Materstvedt et al. 2003; Bernheim et al. 2008).

Many of these aspects have been subject to empirical research, mostly in the euthanasia-permissive Benelux countries and Oregon. Important to bear in mind here is that trends in time – as opposed to single-point-measurements – need to be studied in order to corroborate or assuage the concerns expressed in the slippery slope argument. To the extent that scientific research is able to examine this, the evidence shows that since legalization, overall, there have been no significant adverse "slippery-slope" effects (Battin et al. 2007; Chambaere et al. 2015; Chambaere and Bernheim 2015; van der Heide et al. 2017). However, given the fact that the practice is still fairly recent and evolving even in the Low Countries, developments need to be monitored closely.

All jurisdictions that have regulated assisted dying have installed safeguards, including both substantive and procedural requirements for assisted dying. While the safeguards slightly differ between the jurisdictions, there are commonalities (Emanuel et al. 2016). Substantive requirements include:

- A person's request must be voluntary, well-considered, and sustained/reiterated.
- That person must have a serious and incurable condition caused by either an illness or an accident (in Canada, Colombia, and Victoria [Australia] the person must also be expected to die soon).
- That person's suffering is unbearable and cannot be alleviated.
- There is no reasonable treatment alternative.
- That person must be informed about his/her health condition and prospects by the physician and both parties must together have come to the belief that no reasonable prospect of improvement can be expected.

Procedural requirements include:

- The treating physician must consult another independent physician before proceeding with the act of euthanasia.
- The physician must notify the case of euthanasia, a posteriori, for review by a multidisciplinary control and evaluation committee (with the exception of Colombia where this needs to happen a priori).

While the existing laws do not prescribe what substances should be used and, in principle, physicians can use several types of drugs to perform euthanasia, the recommended drugs in the jurisdictions where it is legal are usually a combination of benzodiazepine (optionally as a means to relax the patient), a high dose of a barbiturate such as thiobarbital (which usually suffices to cause the death) followed by a muscle relaxant, if required.

The concept of suffering lies at the heart of the assisted dying debate. The legal regulations and initiatives for legalization in various countries implicitly recognize that there can exist suffering that is both unbearable and irremediable. Opponents have attempted to point out flaws inherent in both aspects. First, unbearable suffering has been argued to be unobjectifiable and therefore precarious and untrustworthy when considering so grave and irreversible act as ending life. It is impossible to assess for a clinician in many cases, and best not left to the subjective judgment of the patient alone. Moreover, there might be underlying motives and fears (e.g., fear of abandonment, existential distress, solitude, perception of being a burden, socio-economic issues) that remain unsaid and unexplored. Second, opponents also argue that suffering is never irremediable, i.e., that there are always other ways to alleviate suffering than death, no matter how intolerable, with adequate palliative care and/or terminal sedation. This reasoning brings us back to the discussion of palliative futility (see above).

A final note relates to the relationship between palliative care and assisted dying: are these compatible practices or not? Arguments negating their compatibility point to the authoritative WHO definition of palliative care which excludes assisted dying in the phrase "...intends neither to postpone nor hasten death." (World Health Organisation 2018). In fact, the foundation of palliative care (by Dame Cicely Saunders in the UK) was explicitly predicated on preventing assisted dying requests. As such, allowing assisted dying into palliative care practice would alter the mission and deontological code of palliative care altogether; in some scenarios palliative care would be tainted to the extent that it would become completely synonymous with ending life (Bernheim and Raus 2017). Adherents of the compatibility view on the other hand argue that a dismissal of assisted dying in palliative care departs from the palliative care tenets of patient centeredness, by prioritizing caregivers' values over patients' values, and of pluralism, by rejecting divergent but respectable views on decision-making at the end of life. Also, the canonical adherence to the WHO definition of palliative care is found to be objectionable in a number of respects. Lastly, there would be practical consequences to a separation in clinical practice in euthanasia-permissive countries (Bernheim and Raus 2017). In Belgium, the Flemish Federation for Palliative Care has explicitly assumed the position of "euthanasia embedded in palliative care" (Vanden Berghe et al. 2013) and was therein followed by the Brussels and Wallonia federations, based on considerations of continuity of care and empirical evidence in Flanders showing that euthanasia already was often provided in the context of palliative care (Vanden Berghe et al. 2013).

6.4 Active Hastening of Death Without Explicit Patient Request

Related to the subject of assisted dying but very distinct from it, drugs may also be used at the end of life explicitly to hasten death without the consent of the patient. Needless to say, this constitutes an extremely problematic practice in ethical and legal terms. It is considered illegal worldwide. It also violates many ethical principles, first and foremost the autonomy principle, signals the "malfunction" of rules as proportionality and double effect, and is not in accordance with the deontological code. This practice does occur, though it is rare; it has been observed in empirical studies in every country where it has been studied, including in countries where assisted dying is not legalized (van der Heide and Rietjens 2012). An in-depth analysis of empirically reported cases revealed that a somewhat nuanced view may be advisable: the drugs (mostly opioids and benzodiazepines) were administered with a focus on symptom control; a hastened death was highly unlikely; and/or the act was in accordance with the patient's previously expressed wishes (Chambaere et al. 2014). Nonetheless, having an explicit intention to hasten death without explicit consent from the patient is very difficult to justify as good clinical practice. The kinship with intensified pain treatment, palliative sedation, and euthanasia looks to be close, perhaps pointing to a considerable empirical "grey zone" between these archetypes of end-of-life practices. Ethical principles and considerations draw clear lines between them, but clinical cases cannot always be sharply categorized.

A distinction can be made between nonvoluntary and involuntary shortening of life (Materstvedt and Bosshard 2013). Nonvoluntary shortening of life refers to instances in which the patient lacks the ability to make decisions, e.g., children, the demented and unconscious patients. Involuntary shortening of life points to cases in which patients explicitly reject life-shortening acts. Though both forms still constitute unacceptable medical practice it is clear that the latter form aggravates any moral evaluation.

6.5 Voluntary Stopping Eating and Drinking (Self-Starvation)

Voluntary stopping of eating and drinking is a relatively recently addressed phenomenon that is gaining scholarly attention. It is mostly considered by older people with (an array of) serious but not terminal afflictions (polypathology) who experience high symptom burden, in a context where assisted dying is illegal or not possible due to ineligibility of the patient or situational factors (Wax et al. 2018). As such, self-starvation is viewed as an alternative to assisted dying, and one that is ethically and legally less problematic given that there is no intervention from a physician to achieve death. Though strictly speaking it is not a "medical" end-of-life decision, it ideally does involve the supervision of an experienced clinician. To be sure, stopping the intake of nutrients entails an entirely new array of issues, not only physiological but also emotional and psychological in nature, which require the attention of medical professionals. It remains the clinician's task to keep the patient comfortable and address problems such as thirst, hunger, weakness, delirium, and restlessness. If a clinician does commit to medically accompanying the patient who decides to self-starve, and self-starvation amounts to suicide to some extent, then ethically speaking that medical accompaniment could be viewed by some to equate to assisted suicide (Jox et al. 2017). An ethical motivation in favor of assisting these patients, particularly used in countries where it is accepted practice, is taken from the nonabandonment principle. In any case, according to many observers, self-starvation is a less dignified way to die and therefore not a superior alternative to assisted dying.

7 Communication in the End-of-Life Decision-Making Process

To arrive at ethically sound end-of-life decisions, good information and communication are imperative. This section will briefly touch on a number of issues that deserve special attention in communication between the actors involved.

7.1 Truth-Telling

Correct, intelligible, and comprehensive information about diagnosis, prognosis, possible treatments and their pros and cons is a necessary condition for patients to be able to exercise their autonomy and to consent to or refuse treatment. This is what is signified in the "informed" in informed consent. Physicians should also provide ongoing accurate information about the patient's condition when appropriate (Emanuel and Johnson 2013). This may seem straightforward but research has found that information provided to patients is often lacking in clarity and comprehensiveness, and physicians are reluctant to disclose all information fully and timely to their dying patients for fear of taking away hope or eliciting requests of assisted dying and/or due to a lack of adequate communication skills (Sleeman 2013; Visser et al. 2014).

7.2 Shared Decision-Making

The principle of patient autonomy is often misunderstood as meaning that patients should make decisions on their own. Especially in end-of-life care, decision-making should rather be regarded as a process between partners, in which the actors each fulfil unique roles and have equally valuable perspectives in the face of the decisions that need to be made (Emanuel and Emanuel 1995; Makoul and Clayman 2006). Ideally, there is ongoing active and open dialogue between patient, family, physician(s), and care team, in order to come to a mutual understanding of the values and goals underlying treatment decisions. Clinicians can then provide recommendations and explain possible options based on their expertise, while the patient can use these recommendations as input to make an educated decision, taking into account the perspective of their family. This novel model of shared decision-making allows for the patient to exercise autonomy while at the same time retaining the positive aspects of paternalistic decision-making. Paternalism has been dismissed by research suggesting that physicians are bad at predicting their patients' wishes and tend to underestimate their quality of life (Uhlmann et al. 2004). It will only apply when the patient explicitly defers discussion and decision-making to the physicians, care team, and/or family. We suggest that such a patient chooses a filial position and mandates the doctor to be paternal (as distinct from paternalistic, where it is the doctor, rather than the patient, who decides on the type of relationship).

7.3 Advance Care Planning and Advance Directives

The patient does not always have the ability to be directly involved in decision-making. In many cases patients nearing the end of life lose their (full) competences and/or their capacity to communicate clearly, let alone to make an informed decision about a given treatment course. Decision-making capacity relates to five distinguishable cognitive abilities: understanding the factors relevant to making a decision, appreciating the nature and importance of the decision, understanding the risks as well as the benefits of the decision, ability to communicate about the decision, and deliberation based on personal values. When one or more of these capabilities is compromised, the care team has to liaise with the family, who represent the default surrogate decision makers, to make end-of-life decisions together. (Note that this burden of deciding may lead to considerable emotional distress for the family.) To counter this suboptimal situation, guidelines, tools, and interventions are increasingly being developed to achieve what is termed “extended autonomy,” encouraging patients to make advance decisions about their preferred care plan at the end of life, before they become incapacitated. This can be done via advance care planning initiatives, advance directives, and/or living wills.

Advance care plans and advance directives can designate the surrogate decision maker and/or set out the patient’s values, goals, and treatment preferences. The advantages are evident: they allow for clear values and goals to abide by when an end-of-life decision needs to be made; they create trust between patient and physician; they prevent or at least reduce the risk of uncertainty and confusion, and they offer peace of mind to the patient and their family (Detering et al. 2010). However, some pitfalls exist to their use in end-of-life practice: patients often find it extremely difficult to predict their future preferences; advance care plans can lead to conflicts between patients and family and they may be difficult to locate or access when urgently needed.

7.4 Conflicts

Conflict between patient, family, and/or caregivers may occasionally occur (Mehter et al. 2015). When faced with such disagreement or conflict, it is important to thoroughly analyze the problem and involve the appropriate parties to resolve the issue. First, what is the nature of the conflict: ethical dilemma, legal uncertainty, or clinical uncertainty? When the conflict cannot be handled/resolved by the protagonists, additional parties to be involved would be, respectively, an ethics committee, a legal counsellor, and a clinical expert. Second, between which parties has the conflict arisen? Many conflict resolution techniques are available for the clinical setting, but the problem in an end-of-life setting is that the situation is often dire and in urgent need of resolution as the condition of the patient could change rapidly.

7.5 Cultural Issues in End-of-Life Communication

In our increasingly pluralistic and multicultural societies, the odds of patients and caregivers not sharing the same ethnic background or religious beliefs increase. This in turn increases the risk of conflicting views and perspectives. In all cases, mutual understanding of and respect for one another’s views is of the utmost importance. Clinicians need to be sensitive to the intricacies of cultural and religious beliefs and how they influence attitudes toward end-of-life decision-making. Examples of this influence abound: patients may adhere to certain spiritual beliefs that disallow some avenues of treatment (e.g., blood transfusion for Jehovah’s Witnesses); the family is highly influential in medical decision-making in some cultures, and bad news is to be conveyed to the family instead of the patient ("familism"); in other cultures there rests a considerable stigma on the use of opioids, even in the very last stages of life; etc.

Yet, valuing diversity and being sensitive to these and other culturally determined issues does not automatically imply a necessity to comply with them; certain beliefs may clash with the legal, ethical, and deontological norms that predominantly prevail in the healthcare context. In certain cases, clinicians walk a fine line between respecting culturally specific norms and adhering to local laws and regulations. Thorough and clear communication constitutes the best way to avoid and defuse conflicts. In this regard, physicians may do well to communicate on the patient's level and in their language (by involving an interpreter) and offer additional assistance for adequate decision-making (Kogan et al. 2002).

8 Summary and Conclusion

Nowadays, increase in life expectancy is considered as one of the highest achievements of humankind. However, despite the rising standards of medicine and living conditions, the prevalence of health problems and disability is not decreasing. On the contrary, whereas in the past most people died at a younger age and more unexpectedly of acute infectious and parasitic diseases, this and future generations are confronted with a diversity of chronic degenerative diseases at an older age. This happens at a time of a paradigmatic shift in human endeavors away from survival and procreation to quality of life.

Over the past decades, the medical culture has moved from medical paternalism (characterized by phyisicians' sovereignty in medical decision-making) to shared medical decision-making, balancing physicians' expert knowledge and values with patients' autonomous choice that best aligns with their own individual values. As a consequence, focus has shifted from striving for longer survival to striving for optimal quality of life. In the end-of-life context, these fundamental changes incite more and more people to reflect on end-of-life decisions that may curtail their life but also their suffering. With informed consent at the core of shared decision-making, more patients are in charge to decide, express, and specify what forms of medical treatment they would like to receive or refuse, ranging from all available medical interventions prolonging their life to hastening their death.

Providing a high standard of end-of-life care requires physicians to be well-informed of the legal framework in which a range of end-of-life decisions (from withdrawing and withholding treatment over palliative sedation to euthanasia) can be legally justifiable. It also requires sufficient interiorization of the basic four ethical principles in an end-of-life context (the principle of autonomy, beneficence, nonmaleficence, and justice). However, each of these principles is in its essence fundamental though not absolutely inviolable, as these principles can (seem to) conflict. In the assisted dying context, for example, the principle of nonmaleficence may be perceived as in conflict with respecting a patient's autonomous request to hasten death. In attempts to solve such conflicts, the double effect doctrine is often invoked, though it only provides partial justification and hence furthers continuing, unresolved discussions between proponents and opponents. Over and beyond these potentially competing ethical principles, there is also broad dissent on more specific principles. For example, there is a lack of consensus on the mere existence of medical futility: the situation in which there is no reasonable prospect that the intended therapeutic goals can be achieved in a reasonable period of time nor the patient's medical condition and/or quality of life can be sufficiently improved. Even a more incontrovertible principle as nonabandonment seems not always to be adequately translated in clinical practice, as scientific evidence shows too many patients still experience some degree of abandonment in their end-of-life context.

In order to acknowledge and coordinate these tenets, sharpening physicians' basic communication skills (based on truthful, accurate, intelligible assessment of what patients need and want to know in order to be able to make informed consent decisions) is quintessential; not only to avoid or solve ethical dilemmas but also to strengthen the patient-physician relationship.

References

Anscombe E. Intention. Oxford: Basil Blackwell; 1958.

Ashby MA. The futility of futility: death causation is the "elephant in the room" in discussions about limitation of medical treatment. J Bioeth Inq. 2011;8(2):151–4.

Bagheri A. Medical futility. London: World Scientific and Imperial College Press; 2014.

Bagheri A. Futility. In: ten Have H, editor. Encyclopedia of global bioethics [Internet]. Cham: Springer; 2017. p. 1–10. https://doi.org/10.1007/978-3-319-05544-2_204-1

Baily MA. Futility, autonomy, and cost in end-of-life care. J Law, Med Ethics. 2011;39(2):172–82.

Battin MP, van der Heide A, Ganzini L, van der Wal G, Onwuteaka-Philipsen BD. Legal physician-assisted dying in Oregon and the Netherlands: evidence concerning the impact on patients in "vulnerable" groups. J Med Ethics. 2007;33(10):591–7.

Beauchamp TL, Childress JF. Principles of biomedical ethics. New York: Oxford University Press; 1979.

Bernheim JL, Raus K. Euthanasia embedded in palliative care. Responses to essentialistic criticisms of the Belgian model of integral end-of-life care. J Med Ethics. 2017;43(8):489–94.

Bernheim JL, Deschepper R, Distelmans W, Mullie A, Bilsen J, Deliens L. Development of palliative care and legalisation of euthanasia: antagonism or synergy? BMJ [Internet]. 2008;336(7649):864–7.

Bernheim JL, Vansweevelt T, Annemans L. Medical futility and end-of-life issues in Belgium. In: Bagheri A, editor. Medical futility: a cross-national study. London: World Scientific and Imperial College Press; 2013. p. 59–83.

Boyle J. Medical ethics and double effect: The case of terminal sedation. Theor Med Bioethics. 2004;25(1):51–60.

Callahan D. When self-determination runs amok. Hast Cent Rep. 2008;22(2):52–5.

Chambaere K, Bernheim JL. Does legal physician-assisted dying impede development of palliative care? The Belgian and Benelux experience. J Med Ethics. 2015;41(8):657–60.

Chambaere K, Bernheim JL, Downar J, Deliens L. Characteristics of Belgian "life-ending acts without explicit patient request": a large-scale death certificate survey revisited. CMAJ Open. 2014;2(4):E262–7.

Chambaere K, Vander Stichele R, Mortier F, Cohen J, Deliens L. Recent trends in euthanasia and other end-of-life practices in Belgium. N Engl J Med. 2015;372(12):1179–81.

Clark D, ten Have H, Janssens R. Conceptual tensions in European palliative care. In: ten Have H, Clark D, editors. The ethics of palliative care. Philadelphia: Open University Press; 2002.

Cohen-Almagor R. Euthanasia policy and practice in Belgium: critical observations and suggestions for improvement. Issues Law Med [Internet]. 2009;24(3):187–218.

Cohen-Almagor R. First do no harm: pressing concerns regarding euthanasia in Belgium. Int J Law Psychiatry [Internet]. 2013;36(5–6):515–21.

Detering KM, Hancock AD, Reade MC, Silvester W. The impact of advance care planning on end of life care in elderly patients: randomised controlled trial. BMJ [Internet]. 2010;340(mar23 1):c1345–c1345.

Deyaert J, Chambaere K, Cohen J, Roelands M, Deliens L. Labelling of end-of-life decisions by physicians. J Med Ethics. 2014;40(7):505–7.

Druml C, Ballmer PE, Druml W, Oehmichen F, Shenkin A, Singer P, Soeters P, Weimann A, Bischoff SC. ESPEN guideline on ethical aspects of artificial nutrition and hydration. Clin Nutr. 2016;35(3):545–56.

Emanuel EJ, Emanuel LL. Four models of the physician-patient relationship. JAMA. 1995;267(16):2221–6.

Emanuel LL, Johnson R. Truth telling and consent. In: Cherny N, Fallon M, Kaasa S, Portenoy RK, Currow DC, editors. Oxford textbook of palliative medicine. Oxford University Press New York; 2013.

Emanuel EJ, Onwuteaka-Philipsen BD, Urwin JW, Cohen J. Attitudes and practices of Euthanasia and physician-assisted suicide in the United States, Canada, and Europe. JAMA [Internet]. 2016;316(1):79.

Evans & Anor v Alder Hey Children's NHS Foundation Trust & Ors. EWCA Civ 805. British and Irish Legal Information Institute; 2018. 16 Apr 2018.

Foster C. Choosing life, choosing death [Internet]. In: The tyranny of autonomy in medical ethics and law. Oxford and Portland: Hart Publishing; 2009. 189 p.

Gawande A. Quantity and quality of life: Duties of care in life-limiting illness. JAMA. 2016;315(3):267–9.

Griffiths J, Bood A, Weyers H. Euthanasia and law in the Netherlands. Amsterdam: Amsterdam University Press; 1998.

Hall MA, Trachtenberg F, Dugan E. The impact on patient trust of legalising physician aid in dying. J Med Ethics. 2005;31(12):693–7.

Hudson P, Hudson R, Philip J, Boughey M, Kelly B, Hertogh C. Legalizing physician-assisted suicide and/or euthanasia: pragmatic implications. Palliat Support Care. 2015;13(5):1399–409.

Jaspers B, Müller-Busch HC, Nauck F. Integral palliative care: a contradiction in Terms? (in German). Z. Palliativmed. 2009; 10:162–6.

Jox RJ, Black I, Borasio GD, Anneser J. Voluntary stopping of eating and drinking: is medical support ethically justified? BMC Med. 2017;15(1):186.

Ko DN, Blinderman CD. Withholding and withdrawing life-sustaining treatment (including artificial nutrition and hydration). In: Cherny N, Fallon M, Kaasa S, Portenoy RK, Currow DC, editors. Oxford textbook of palliative medicine. New York: Oxford University Press; 2013.

Kogan S, Blanchette P, Masaki K. Talking to patients about death and dying: improving communication across cultures. In: Braun KL, Pietsch JHP, Blanchette PL, editors. Cultural issues in end-of-life decision making. Thousand Oaks: Sage Publishing; 2002. p. 305–26.

Kontis V, Bennett JE, Mathers CD, Li G, Foreman K, Ezzati M. Future life expectancy in 35 industrialised countries: projections with a Bayesian model ensemble. Lancet. 2017;389(10076):1323–35.

Levy N. Forced to be free? Increasing patient autonomy by constraining it. J Med Ethics. 2014;40(5):293–300.

Lewis P, Black I. Reporting and scrutiny of reported cases in four jurisdictions where assisted dying is lawful: a review of the evidence in the Netherlands, Belgium, Oregon and Switzerland. Med Law Int. 2013;13(4): 221–39.

López-Saca JM, Guzmán JL, Centeno C. A systematic review of the influence of opioids on advanced cancer patient survival. Curr Opin Support Palliat Care. 2013; 7(4):424–30.

Macauley R. The role of the principle of double effect in ethics education at US medical schools and its potential impact on pain management at the end of life. J Med Ethics. 2012;38(3):174–8.

Makoul G, Clayman ML. An integrative model of shared decision making in medical encounters. Patient Educ Couns. 2006;60(3):301–12.

Mangan J. An historical analysis of the principle of double effect. Theol Stud. 1949;10:41–61.

Materstvedt LJ, Bosshard G. Euthanasia and palliative care. In: Cherny N, Fallon M, Kaasa S, Portenoy RK, Currow DC, editors. Oxford textbook of palliative medicine. New York: Oxford University Press; 2013.

Materstvedt LJ, Clark D, Ellershaw J, Forde R, Gravgaard AM, Muller-Busch HC, et al. Euthanasia and physician-assisted suicide: a view from an EAPC Ethics Task Force. Palliat Med. 2003;17:97–101.

Mehter HM, Clark JA, Wiener RS. Physician approaches to provider-family conflict associated with end-of-life decision-making in the ICU: a qualitative study. Am J Respir Crit Care Med [Internet]. 2015;191.

Mill JS. Utilitarianism. London: Parker, Son and Bourn; 1863. p. 26.

Pereira J. Legalizing euthanasia or assisted suicide: the illusion of safeguards and controls. Curr Oncol. 2011;18(2):e38–45.

Quill TE, Dresser R, Brock D. The rule of double effect – a critique of its role in end-of-life decision making. New Eng J Med. 1997;337:1768.

Radbruch L, Leget C, Bahr P, Müller-Busch C, Ellershaw J, De Conno F, et al. Euthanasia and physician-assisted suicide: a white paper from the European Association for Palliative Care. Palliat Med. 2016;30:104–16.

Roeland E, Cain J, Onderdonk C, Kerr K, Mitchell W, Thornberry K. When open-ended questions don't work: the role of palliative paternalism in difficult medical decisions. J Palliat Med. 2014;17(4):415–20.

Schneiderman LJ. Defining medical futility and improving medical care. J Bioeth Inq. 2011;8(2):123–31.

Shariff MJ. Assisted death and the slippery slope – finding clarity amid advocacy, convergence, and complexity. Curr Oncol [Internet]. 2012;19(3):143–54.

Sleeman KE. End-of-life communication: let's talk about death. J Roy Coll Phys Edinburgh. 2013;43(3):197–9.

Smets T, Cohen J, Bilsen J, Van Wesemael Y, Rurup ML, Deliens L. The labelling and reporting of euthanasia by Belgian physicians: a study of hypothetical cases. Eur J Pub Health. 2012;22(1):19–26.

Specker SL. Medical maternalism: beyond paternalism and antipaternalism. J Med Ethics. 2016;42(7):439–44.

ten Have H, Janssens R. Futility, limits and palliative care. In: ten Have H, Clark D, editors. The ethics of palliative care. Philadelphia: Open University Press; 2002.

Thorns A, Sykes N. Opioid use in last week of life and implications for end-of-life decision-making. Lancet [Internet]. 2000;356(9227):398–9.

Uhlmann AT, Uhlmann DR, Workman S. Distress of clinicians with decisions to withhold or withdraw life-support measures (multiple letters). J Crit Care. 2004; 19:118–20.

van der Heide A, Rietjens J. End-of-life decisions. In: Cohen J, Deliens L, editors. A public health perspective on end of life care. New-York: Oxford University Press; 2012.

van der Heide A, van Delden JJM, Onwuteaka-Philipsen BD. End-of-life decisions in the Netherlands over 25 Years. N Engl J Med. 2017;377(5):492–4.

van Marwijk H, Haverkate I, van Royen P, The AM. Impact of euthanasia on primary care physicians in the Netherlands. Palliat Med. 2007;21(7):609–14.

Vanden Berghe P, Mullie A, Desmet M, Huysmans G. Assisted dying – the current situation in Flanders: euthanasia embedded in palliative care. Eur J Palliat Care. 2013:20(6).

Visser M, Deliens L, Houttekier D. Physician-related barriers to communication and patient- and family-centred decision-making towards the end of life in intensive care: a systematic review. Crit Care. 2014;18(6):604.

Wancata LM, Hinshaw DB. Rethinking autonomy: decision making between patient and surgeon in advanced illnesses. Ann Transl Med. 2016;4(4):77.

Wax JW, An AW, Kosier N, Quill TE. Voluntary stopping eating and drinking. J Am Geriatr Soc. 2018; 66(3):441–5.

World Health Organisation. WHO definition of palliative care [Internet]. World Health Organisation. 2018 [cited 2018 Apr 29]. Available from http://www.who.int/cancer/palliative/definition/en/

Youngner SJ, Arnold RM. The Oxford handbook of ethics at the end of life. [Internet]. 2016; Available from http://ovidsp.ovid.com/ovidweb.cgi?T=JS&PAGE=reference&D=psyc13&NEWS=N&AN=2016-26125-000

Palliative Sedation: A Medical-Ethical Exploration

87

Jeroen Hasselaar

Contents

Abstract

Palliative sedation involves the intentional lowering of consciousness in the last phase of life to relieve refractory symptoms. Most ethical controversies concern the application of continuous deep palliative sedation. After an introduction about prevalence and terminology, the concept of a refractory symptom is discussed from an ethical viewpoint in particular with regard to existential suffering. After this, several ethical approaches to the topic of artificial hydration in relation to life expectancy are considered. This is followed by a reflection on decision-making for palliative sedation, in particular the role of informed consent and the possible emotional burden for family and professional caregivers. After this, the rule of double effect is discussed. Finally, the debate about palliative sedation and (hidden) euthanasia is introduced. Continuous deep palliative sedation as a last resort option for patients at the end of life operates at an

J. Hasselaar (✉)
Department of Anesthesiology, Pain and Palliative Medicine, Radboud University Medical Center, Nijmegen, The Netherlands
e-mail: Jeroen.Hasselaar@radboudumc.nl

R. D. MacLeod, L. Van den Block (eds.), *Textbook of Palliative Care*,
https://doi.org/10.1007/978-3-319-77740-5_92

ethical fine line and should avoid both postponing and hastening of death. However, it is concluded that palliative sedation is rightly considered part of palliative care. Nevertheless ongoing concerns need further attention, for example, a need for up to date, ethically balanced, and well-implemented practice guidelines and a careful communication with patients and families.

1 Introduction

In the Western world, cancer and other chronic diseases have replaced infectious diseases as the major cause of death. Due to improved hygienic and medical interventions, people live longer than ever before. Medical interventions however allow people to live longer, but not always to live better lives. In the 1960s people Dame Cicely Saunders founded the hospice movement focusing on the care of the dying, initially in cancer. Since then, this movement has expanded to encompass a broader concept of palliative care, including symptom management for patients with advanced disease. One of the first studies that mentioned sedation in the context of palliative care is a prospective study from 1990 of Ventafridda et al. who investigated symptom prevalence in 120 terminal cancer patients and concluded that about half of them died with physical suffering that could only be relieved by palliative sedation (Ventafridda et al. 1990). During the past decade, surveys of physicians have shown that palliative sedation became a more common and accepted practice. However, ethical debate continues with concerns that palliative sedation contributes to the medicalization of death and dying.

1.1 Palliative Sedation: Not Only a Medical Debate

In 2013, Papavasiliou et al. showed that sedation has been discussed in many fields (for example, oncology, nursing, health sciences & services, neurology, ethics, and law). This shows that palliative sedation is not only a technical medical act but touches upon important ethical and societal values. When sedation for the dying was firstly debated, it was mostly referred to as terminal sedation. The word terminal refers to the terminal state of the patients who received sedation but it does not say much about what the procedure actually involves. Also, the adjective "terminal" was sometimes used to argue that sedation itself would imply the termination of life, because it has been considered, by some, as a slow euthanasia. Slow because during sedation, dosages of medication may be gradually increased to help the patient die sooner, quietly, and without suffering. Or slow because sedated patients are not able to take fluids anymore and may slowly die because of dehydration. These are important ethical considerations that will receive more attention in this chapter, but for now, it is important to see how much confusion the adjective "terminal" in "terminal sedation" has caused. And although still preferred by some, the majority of the scientific and medical community has departed from this term and turned to the term palliative sedation (Hasselaar et al. 2009a). Notwithstanding, there have been societal concerns that continuous deep palliative sedation may be used as a slow or hidden alternative for euthanasia. As an answer to these concerns, professional guidelines have been developed to define terms and frameworks for the appropriate application of palliative sedation.

The aim of this chapter is to give an overview of the ethical debate surrounding palliative sedation with a discussion of the most prominent dilemmas. This chapter, however, does not give a detailed overview of the medical aspects involved in palliative sedation, like drugs and dosages. The first part will consider the definition of palliative sedation and some practice characteristics. The second part will discuss ethical issues in the context of the clinical preconditions of palliative sedation. The third part will move into possible life shortening effects, the rule of double effect, and the debate surrounding palliative sedation and (hidden) euthanasia. Finally, the conclusion will discuss the role of the caring professions in relation to a need for societal trustworthiness.

2 Part I Terminology and Prevalence of Palliative Sedation

2.1 What Is Palliative Sedation?

Already in 2002, Morita et al. performed a literature review and formulated two core elements of palliative sedation, namely, (1) the presence of severe distress refractory to standard palliative treatment, and (2) the use of sedative medication with the primary aim of relieving distress by reduction of consciousness (Morita et al. 2002). However, they also noticed differences in the degree and duration of sedation, symptoms, and targeted patients which are currently still often found.

For palliative sedation, a distinction is often made between light or intermittent sedation and deep and/or continuous sedation. Light sedation means that a patient is still able to communicate, whereas during deep sedation this is no longer possible, at least not verbally. Intermittent sedation (also called respite sedation) can, for example, be applied during the night to provide a time-out. Continuous deep sedation involves sedation that is continued until the moment of death. Continuous deep sedation raised a lot of societal controversy because it was thought that it could be used to hasten the death of the patient. It has been proposed to distinguish several types of sedation: ordinary sedation, proportionate sedation, which is the minimum amount of sedation needed to relieve physical refractory symptoms, and sedation until unconsciousness with the intended endpoint of unconsciousness (Quill et al. 2009). Cellarius and Henry (2010), however, correctly noted that all sedations should be proportionate to the aim of relief of suffering. Sometimes this will involve intermittent or light sedation with lower dosages of sedatives; sometimes this may involve continuous and deep sedation with a higher and longer lasting administration of sedatives.

Currently, guidelines are available in several countries including Ireland, the USA, Belgium, Italy, Austria, Spain, Canada, the Netherlands, Norway, and Japan (Abarshi et al. 2017). The Dutch guideline for palliative sedation (2005, revised 2009) was one of the first clinical guidelines to define palliative sedation as *"the intentional lowering of consciousness in the last phase of life"* (KNMG 2009). In 2009, the EAPC recommended a framework for palliative sedation in which palliative sedation is considered as *"the monitored use of medications intended to induce a state of decreased or absent awareness in order to relieve the burden of otherwise intractable suffering, in a manner that is ethically acceptable to patient, family, and healthcare providers"* (Cherny et al. 2009). An overview of definitions can be found in a review of Schildmann and Schildmann (2014). Schildmann and Schildmann (2014) made an inventory of guidelines listing and comparing the topics that were addressed and noticed a considerable variation in recommendations with regard to artificial hydration and aspects of indication and decision-making. De Graef and Dean (2007) were among the first to list recommendations for palliative sedation. They concluded that most recommendations were based on expert opinion. Recently, Abarshi et al. (2017), in a review of sedation guidelines, concluded that most guidelines are conceptually similar, resembling the EAPC recommended framework, but that there are striking differences in the terminology used. Studies from the Netherlands (Hasselaar et al. 2009b; Swart et al. 2012) indicate practice improvements after the launch of a national guideline for palliative sedation, in particular with regard to the aims and goals of palliative sedation and the involvement of patients and their family in the decision-making process. However, in general, there is little known about the effect of guideline development and structured implementation is scarce.

The vast majority of literature and accompanying ethical discussions about palliative sedation concern continuous deep sedation until death, and the remaining part of this chapter about palliative sedation will be focused on this. However, from a clinical perspective, palliative sedation is often considered as a continuum from light to deep and from superficial to continuous sedation.

2.2 Prevalence and Cultural Acceptance of Palliative Sedation

The use of palliative sedation as a medical practice is considerable. In 2017, a Japanese survey among palliative care specialists showed that palliative sedation was used for symptom relief and decrease of consciousness level. About 4 out of 10 respondents aimed to preserve consciousness as much as possible, and 1 out of 10 also intended to shorten patient survival to some extent (Hamano et al. 2017). In a survey from the United States, 1 out of 10 physicians had applied palliative sedation the past 12 months with the aim to make the patient unconscious until death, while 8 out of 10 accepted unconsciousness as a side effect only (Putman et al. 2013). One study reported different perceptions between American and Dutch physicians regarding the use of sedation at the end of life and found more open and proactive discussion in the Netherlands (Rietjens et al. 2014). A vignette study with French speaking physicians in Quebec (Canada) and Switzerland showed that their attitudes towards palliative sedation were similar: not legal considerations but the perceived suffering and diagnosis of the patient were leading in decisions for sedation, although Canadian physicians seemed more open to take existential suffering into account (Dumont et al. 2015).

For Europe, a comparative death certificate study from Miccinesi et al. (2006) showed that the prevalence of continuous deep sedation until death as a percentage of the total number of deaths differed between Belgium (8.2%), Denmark (2.5%), Italy (8.5%), The Netherlands (5.7%), Sweden (3.2%), and Switzerland (4.8%). However, it is not unlikely that these figures need updating by now. Recent Dutch research showed significant increase in continuous deep sedation in the Netherlands from 8% of all deaths in 2005 to 18% of all deaths in 2015 (Van der Heide et al. 2017). Interestingly, the prevalence of continuous deep palliative sedation until death in Flanders decreased from 15% in 2007 to 12% in 2013 (Robijn et al. 2016). The prevalence of palliative sedation based on a physician survey was estimated at 19% in the UK in 2010 (Seale 2010). Looking at German speaking countries, a study among 2,414 patients from 23 Austrian palliative care units showed that 21% received sedation, which in 4 out of 5 concerned continuous deep sedation, with an average duration of 48 h (Schur et al. 2016). Research under 281 members of the German ethics academy with and without medical background showed 98% acceptance of palliative sedation for physical suffering in dying patients (Simon et al. 2007).

Fainsinger et al. (2003) starting from the observation that psycho-existential suffering has a much larger role in palliative sedation in Spain compared to Canada, studied differences in values of cognition and information disclosure between 100 Spanish and 100 Canadian patients and their families in hospital palliative care consultation settings. Canadian families put more emphasis on clear thinking towards the end of life and full disclosure compared to Spanish patients and families, who were also less agreeing with each other. Núñez Olarte and Guillen (2001) related the use of palliative sedation for psycho-existential suffering in Spain and Latin America to a so-called external locus of control influenced by a (Catholic) worldview, where life events and circumstances are highly regarded beyond one's own control. This is contrasted with Anglo-Saxon cultures including North-Western Europe with a so-called internal locus of control where life events and circumstances are highly considered as being influenced by one's own actions. Although relevant, this seems not the only demarcation line for the use of palliative sedation. Qualitative research from the Unbiased study in three Western European countries indicated that physicians in the United Kingdom use palliative sedation differently than physicians in Belgium and in The Netherlands. While in the UK this seems to involve titration of dosages with the aim to preserve consciousness as much as possible, in the Netherlands and Belgium continuous and deeper levels of sedation were more often considered and the start of palliative sedation was more often organized as a final farewell (Seale et al. 2015).

Although the abovementioned studies give an idea of the use of palliative sedation, one should be cautious to conclude that palliative sedation is more or less prevalent in one country compared to the other because the methodology of the studies, the definitions and interpretations of palliative sedation, and the investigated target groups are diverse (from epidemiological to more clinical studies). Moreover, it needs to be considered that the increased media attention for palliative sedation may have increased the popularity of the practice over time but may have also lead to a more precise understanding of what it actually involves. Finally, cultural differences exist in how palliative sedation is approached and used.

3 Part II Ethical Issues in a Clinical Context

Nowadays, there is broad consensus that palliative sedation has two important preconditions, namely, that palliative sedation is restricted to patients who are severely suffering from refractory symptoms and to patients who are in the last phase of life. This paragraph will first discuss the concept of refractory symptoms and the ethical questions that are related to this. After this, the ethical discussion about artificial hydration, in particular, in the context of deep palliative sedation until death, will be discussed.

3.1 First Precondition for Palliative Sedation: Refractory Symptoms

Sometimes, symptoms cannot be treated without unacceptable side effects given the clinical situation of the patient or symptom relief cannot be expected in due time. In these cases, a symptom can become refractory, which means that it cannot be relieved by conventional medication or in due time (De Graef and Dean 2007). In a review by Maltoni et al. (2012), the most prevalent (refractory) symptoms were: delirium (54%), dyspnea (30%), psychological distress (19%), pain (17%), and vomiting (5%). Delirium is a prevalent symptom at the end of life. Especially agitated delirium can cause a lot of stress for patient and families and can become refractory (Bush et al. 2014). In such circumstances, before (continuous deep) palliative sedation is considered, regular symptom treatment needs to be evaluated thoroughly. Figure 1 introduces a stepwise approach to determine the refractoriness of a symptom. In addition, the Dutch guideline mentions a non-linear combination of different dimensions of symptoms that can lead to unbearable suffering of the patient, like for example extreme dyspnea producing severe anxiety. The untreatable nature of symptoms must however be demonstrated beyond reasonable doubt (KNMG 2009).

Refractory suffering is not limited to somatic symptoms and therefore a multidimensional approach is needed in order for these to be fully assessed and managed. In this respect, especially the presence of existential suffering needs further attention.

It is challenging to define existential suffering. Most descriptions suggest a perceived loss of meaning, loss of perspective, or a perceived loss of dignity (Van Deijck et al. 2015). There are intercountry and cultural differences regarding the extent of existential suffering as an accepted

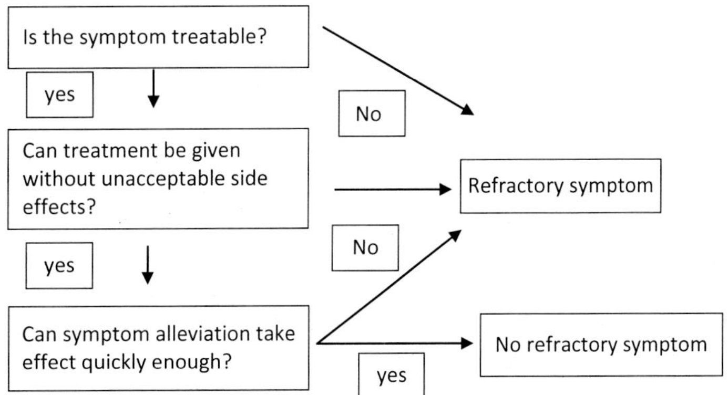

Fig. 1 Stepwise approach to identify refractory symptoms. (Dutch guideline for palliative sedation KNMG 2009)

reason for palliative sedation. Literature from Japan for example is hesitant at this point (Morita et al. 2005a). The majority of physicians from the United States also seems quite hesitant (Putnam et al. 2013), whereas Belgian and Dutch physicians seem to accept this to some extent as part of refractory suffering. When refractoriness is considered an aggregation of several symptoms, it can be imagined that some form of existential suffering will often be a part of this. Patients in the last phase of their lives can suffer when facing their own mortality. It can be considered a part of the normal dying phase that patients struggle or even wrestle with this. However, when existential suffering is the predominant reason to start palliative sedation, caution is needed because it can be questioned whether palliative sedation, in particular continuous deep sedation until death, is the right answer in this case. With continuous deep palliative sedation, patient awareness is suppressed, and, if applied for existential suffering only, important stages of loss and finishing life may be distorted. Hence, the first argument to be hesitant with palliative sedation in these cases comes from the perspective of providing good palliative care. A second argument is that patients who predominantly experience existential suffering are often not yet in the terminal stage of life, which would frustrate the second precondition for palliative sedation, namely the imminence of death.

Juth et al. (2010), in a critical reaction to the EAPC recommended framework for palliative sedation, argue that the concept of intolerable suffering needs more clarification. Suffering is a highly subjective experience and it can be difficult to distinguish existential or physical causes of suffering. Juth et al. point out that more clarification is needed about the perspective of patients and physicians in particular regarding concepts of intolerable distress and refractory symptoms, and how these relate in the context of identifying necessary and sufficient criteria for palliative sedation. This also echoes the viewpoint of Cassell and Rich (2010) who consider suffering to be a human and personal experience and warn that distinguishing causes of suffering may lead to an undesirable mind-body distinction. In a reply to this view, Jansen argued that philosophical mind-body distinctions are not needed to introduce a difference between neurocognitive and agent-narrative causes of suffering. She concludes that "Compared with neurocognitive suffering, it is exceedingly more difficult to establish that agent-narrative suffering is truly refractory" (Jansen 2010). A recent review of Rodrigues et al. (2018) identified several relevant concepts in the discussion surrounding existential suffering and palliative sedation, namely, mind-body dualism, existential suffering, refractoriness, terminal condition, and imminent death and concluded that more clarification in the ethical debate is needed at this point.

The last word has probably not been said about this issue. Therefore, in more complex cases of assessing refractory suffering, especially the application of deep and continuous sedation may call for multidisciplinary decision-making, which is also mentioned in the EAPC framework for palliative sedation.

3.2 Second Precondition for Palliative Sedation: A Limited Life Expectancy

During palliative sedation, a patient is not able to take fluids orally. The ethical concern has been that this could lead to a life shortening effect, in particular when deep sedation occurs over a prolonged period. In most guidelines therefore, it is stressed that continuous palliative sedation should be restricted to the last phase of life. Most guidelines also argue that the application of palliative sedation and the decision not to apply artificial hydration are two separate medical decisions that need separate evaluation. However, this "dual procedure" has raised critical remarks from an ethical viewpoint because both decisions are often implemented at the same time and especially in sedation trajectories with a longer duration, sedation without artificial hydration would prevent the patient from taking fluids which could result in life shortening due to dehydration (Den Hartogh 2016).

The work of Callahan (1992) assists in understanding this critique better. Callahan introduced a thought "test" to distinguish "allowing to die," from killing. A central notion in this "test" is that an act of allowing to die only causes death in a very ill patient and not in a healthy person. Applied to palliative sedation, it can be argued that during continuous deep palliative sedation every person, whether healthy or ill, will eventually die from dehydration if continuously kept under sedation without (artificial) hydration. On the one hand it has been argued that during deep and continuous sedation, "often the patient dies of dehydration from the withholding of fluids, not of the underlying disease" (Quill et al. 1997). On the other hand, as mentioned before, continuous deep sedation is mainly applied in dying patients and maintained for a limited period of time (about 48 h). In these cases, the risk of dehydration due to sedation may be limited in practice. However, when the prolonged administration of sedatives frustrates the oral intake of the patient and eventually causes a life shortening effect due to dehydration, this may be morally problematic.

To avoid this problem and to clearly distinguish palliative sedation from hastening of death, guidelines restrict continuous deep sedation until the last phase of life, more precisely the last 1 or 2 weeks of life. A closer view learns that this last phase can be interpreted as the recognition of the approaching death like being bedbound, having cachexia, severe weakness, being disoriented, and limited or absent oral intake (KNMG 2009). In addition, some guidelines have used a reference to medical futility, by stating that the possible harmful effects of artificial hydration during sedation may outweigh the possible benefits. The Dutch guideline for example is hesitant about artificial hydration during continuous deep sedation, pointing to the possible negative effects of supplying artificial hydration in a dying patient like edema. Also the Belgian guideline is more hesitant at this point and stresses that it is a separate decision next to the decision to start sedation (Broeckaert 2012). The EAPC framework (Cherny et al. 2009) admits that practices vary and considers this as a separate decision which is left with the care teams and patients in their specific situations: for some it is a humane continuation of life support, for other it is superfluous and can be withdrawn because it does not contribute to goals of comfort care. If adverse effects however appear, withdrawal should be considered. This reflects an approach that artificial hydration can be withdrawn if it can be considered futile care.

Futility is a layered and much debated concept and agreed definitions are largely lacking (Macfadyen and Mcconnell 2016). One influential approach comes from Schneiderman et al. (1990), who argue that futility involves both a quantitative aspect, referring to the probability of success (5% or 10% etc.), and a qualitative aspect, related to the goals of care. In a later publication, they note that a patient is not merely a collection of organs or an individual with desires but a person who seeks healing (Schneiderman 2011). They remark that on the one hand physicians cannot be expected to deliver medical care with low probability of success, but on the other hand they should move beyond "pull the plug" and "nothing to offer" discussions. Truog (2018) agrees that futility often refers to the limits of medicine in the context of mortality, but he emphasizes that physicians as medical professionals should be hesitant to make judgments about essential human values. For this reason he criticizes the statement that treatment which merely preserves permanent unconscious life is as such futile care. According to Rinehart (2013), the diversity of our cultural values can make it difficult to agree on the goals of care. Therefore Rinehart proposes to adopt shared decision-making with a thorough inventory of a patient's values and life goals. In those cases however where agreement with patient and family is not possible, it may be wise to adopt a (narrow) concept of physiologic futility together with a careful procedural approach that takes into account values of patient, family, and society at large (Truog 2018).

In most clinical practices, with a short expected duration of palliative sedation, the discussion about artificial hydration may be considered less relevant because dehydration is not expected to happen in such a short timeframe or because the patient already stopped drinking as part of an approaching death. However, it is important to be aware of the underlying ethical discussion. Although at first sight futility seems to refer to a rather technical decision aid, moral values are at stake. In the case of palliative sedation, a discussion about the medical futility of artificial hydration can involve the physiological effects of hydration, but it can also bring forth a discussion about whether it is ethically obliged to artificially prolong the life of otherwise dying patients. The well known WHO palliative care (WHO 2002) definition states that palliative care does not aim to prolong the dying process but also does not aim to shorten life. In decisions concerning palliative sedation, this can be a fine line, which requires medical and ethical sensitivity, preferably in a multidisciplinary deliberation, together with compassionate communication with patients and families.

3.3 Decision Making for Palliative Sedation and Emotional Distress

So far, the ethical issues in the context of the clinical preconditions of palliative sedation have been discussed. However, the EAPC framework for palliative sedation also mentions that palliative sedation needs to be ethically acceptable for patients, caregivers, and family members. This refers to the position and interaction of the several stakeholders involved in a palliative sedation process, to begin with the patient.

Informed consent is a procedure to obtain the written or oral consent of a patient for a medical treatment. It reflects respect for the patients' autonomy as a right to make his/her own decisions, including also the right to refuse medical treatment. Therefore, attaining informed consent of the patient for a medical treatment can be regarded as a general obligation for all caregivers, before the treatment starts. But this can become difficult when the patient has a reduced capacity for decision-making which is often the case for patients who are near to death. There are however several ways in which the application of medical treatment without the consent of the patient can be justified. If the patient is incompetent for decision-making, family members may act as proxies also called "surrogate decision-makers." A proxy should comply to the wishes, values, and perspectives of the patient as good as possible. To some extent, the physician might act as proxy, serving the best interests of the patient. In addition, advanced directives, whether oral or written, may be used, although these donot seem to play a major role in the context of palliative sedation. However, specific national laws may differ at this point.

Patient consent for palliative sedation has been addressed in several studies. A general concern has been that this consent is not always obtained, in particular with regard to continuous deep sedation. After the introduction of the Dutch guideline, patient involvement in decision-making increased from 72% to 82% (Hasselaar et al. 2009b). Interestingly, Morita et al. (2005b), in a Japanese prospective study, found that 67% of the patients expressed explicit wishes for sedation and families were involved in the other cases. This is an interesting outcome as research also showed that the general public is not always aware of terms related to palliative care and palliative sedation (Hirai et al. 2011; van der Kallen et al. 2013). Sometimes, patients can have different understandings about palliative sedation than their caregivers. It is an ethical duty of the physician to correctly inform patient and family about the available treatment options in a way that is understandable for him/her in order to make an informed decision. Often in palliative care, a shared decision-making process will be strived for.

In a survey about family experiences during palliative sedation (intermittent and continuous deep sedation) from Japan, 78% of 185 interviewees were satisfied with treatment but 25% expressed emotional distress (Morita et al. 2004a). In a review of Bruinsma et al. (2012), investigating 36 studies, family members appeared to be involved in the decision-making for continuous deep sedation in 69–100% of cases. Although in general, family members seem to be comfortable with palliative sedation, cases of distressed family members were also mentioned. Possible reasons for distress are that the patient still suffers, that the patient isn't able to communicate, feeling a burden of decision-making, concerns about a possibly hastened death, a long duration of sedation, and ideas about more appropriate alternatives.

The Unbiased study, based on interviews with 78 nurses, 82 physicians, and 32 family members of deceased patients, has provided more insight in the everyday moral reasoning about palliative sedation in three Western European countries: UK, Belgium, and the Netherlands. Raus et al. (2014) found that dimensions of "closeness" to the patient determine the distress that caregivers experience with continuous palliative sedation until death. Firstly, in particular nurses, involved in the daily care for the patient experienced emotional closeness, especially when the patient is younger. Secondly, physical closeness was felt when caring for a patient. Thirdly, decisional closeness occurs when the interviewee was closer involved in the decision-making. And finally causal closeness occurred when administering sedatives can cause a feeling of distress in case the patient dies shortly thereafter. Feelings of distress were often associated with continuous palliative sedation, but could also be balanced with the relief it brings to a severely suffering patient.

In a large survey among nurses in hospitals and palliative care units, Morita et al. (2004b) found that a significant percentage (12%) of nurses felt serious emotional burden related to continuous deep sedation, for example, the experience of unclear patient wishes, insufficient time, belief that a diagnosis of refractor symptoms is difficult, and a perceived lack of skills. Feelings of burden were related to shorter clinical experience and younger age. Rietjens and colleagues (2007) published an interview study with 16 nurses about their memorable cases of palliative sedation, reporting that for many nurses being involved in palliative sedation is more than "just carrying out a medical order." Although palliative sedation is generally considered a good death, it is also a process that brings forth reflections about its appropriateness and conditions of adequate practices.

In sum, in many cases of palliative sedation patients and family members are involved in decision-making in some way. Reports from studies with bereaved family members show that many are satisfied with the care that has been received during a palliative sedation trajectory, although concerns and emotional distress remain in a considerable number of cases. Studies under nurses show that the application of palliative sedation is not considered a routine task and can be a burden. Data concerning medical doctors, however, was less easy to find. Care for the carer, in particular for younger professionals with less clinical experience, is needed. Care for the bereaved family members, in particular when unclarities remain, seems also important.

4 Part III Two Moral Dilemmas Surrounding Palliative Sedation

In the next paragraphs, two ethical problems surrounding palliative sedation will be discussed more in-depth. One has been around in the literature for a longer time, namely, the rule of double effect. And the other is an important but sometimes neglected topic, namely, the ethical value of consciousness.

4.1 The Rule of Double Effect

The past decade, the possible occurrence of life shortening effects during palliative sedation has been an important concern. The so-called rule of double effect has often been used for an ethical evaluation of palliative sedation, in particular continuous deep sedation.

The doctrine of double effect describes an act as having two effects, one positive and one negative. The good effect in palliative sedation can be defined as the relief of suffering. The negative effect is the possible shortening of life which may be foreseen but should not be intended. The rule is subdivided in four parts and reads as follows (Sulmasy and Pellegrino 1999):

1. The act is not in itself immoral.
2. The act is undertaken with the intention to achieve the good effect and without intention

to achieve the bad effect, even though the latter might be foreseen.

3. The act does not bring about the good effect by means of the bad effect (since that would imply that the bad effect is intended, too).
4. The act is undertaken for a grave and proportional reason.

In the literature, attempts have been made to apply this rule to palliative sedation in order to distinguish it from active euthanasia. The first criterion reads that the act should not be immoral in itself. The act, namely, the use of sedatives for the relief of suffering, is not immoral in itself. Relief of suffering is one of the basic tasks of medicine. Secondly life shortening effects, if present, may be foreseen but not intended. Therefore, according to this second criterion, the act of prescribing medication should be intended or titrated towards the effect of symptom relief, and not to the effect of shortening life. Drugs and dosages that are used for palliative sedation should reflect this intention by being proportional to the goal of symptom relief. The third criterion holds that the act of symptom relief is not achieved by means of life shortening. According to the rule of double effect, palliative sedation is cumbersome if it serves as a means to hasten death. In that case, the sedation is used to shorten life. According to the fourth criterion, proportionality and a grave indication for palliative sedation are needed to justify an act of palliative sedation. Proportionality means that there are no less harmful alternatives available to attain the good effect of symptom relief. This refers to the idea that palliative sedation is a last resort option, only to be applied in case of refractory symptoms when more conventional treatment is not (longer) available. Also it reflects the idea that intermittent or light sedation, if possible, is preferred above continuous palliative sedation.

Some authors have doubted the suitability of the rule of double effect for palliative sedation. Sykes and Thorns (2003), for example, argued that there are no life shortening effects reported for palliative sedation, and that, in fact, there is no life-shortening effect that needs to be morally justified. The actual occurrence of life shortening effects during continuous palliative sedation has been a topic of heavy debate. Maltoni et al. (2012) in a review about palliative sedation described 11 studies of which one reached statistical significance. This study, from Mercadante et al. (2009), reported that nonsedated patients had a shorter survival compared to sedated patients, measured in days from the moment of admission, with a mean sedation time of 22 h. One study of Kohara et al. (2005) reported a mean sedation duration of 3.4 days, with a statistically non-significant shorter survival after admission for sedated patients (28.9 vs. 39.5 days). However, they included mild to deep sedations which make their figures less comparable to studies that are limited to continuous deep sedation. One of the most robust studies so far about life shortening during palliative sedation involved a secondary analysis of a prospective research in 58 palliative care centers in Japan. In the sample of 1827 patients, 15% of the patients received continuous palliative sedation (Maeda et al. 2016). They did not evidence an increased risk of life shortening due to continuous deep palliative sedation. Based on this article, Caraceni (2016) called for more empirical data in this debate and less opinions.

The rule of double effect has been criticized because it relies heavily upon the distinction between intended and foreseen consequences. Surveys under caregivers from – among others – Belgium and Japan reported that palliative sedation is sometimes applied with a more or less explicit intention to hasten death (Hamano et al. 2017; Rys et al. 2014). According to the rule of double effect, this will be problematic in particular regarding the second criterion. However, intentions can be ambiguous. When confronted with a terminally ill patient, is it wrong to hope that suffering will soon be over and death will come soon? In addition, the methodological validity of asking after life shortening effects via surveys is not beyond doubt. Statements from general surveys should be interpreted with caution. On the one hand, intentions are important to consider in an ethical evaluation, but it does make a difference whether shortening of life is a matter of fact (or not). On the other hand, literature reporting that palliative sedation is used with the implicit or explicit intention to shorten life, even when compassionate care is the main motive, cannot be neglected and deserves further ethical exploration.

Notwithstanding, the rule of double effect may be relevant to take into account in individual patients care. In terminal patients, symptom relief may require a delicate balance between the type of drugs, monitoring, dosage, and titration schedule chosen. In particular because the effects of medication in a terminal patient can vary due to, for example, renal problems and loss of weight. Hence, the precise effects may be difficult to estimate or predict beforehand. In 2005, Morita et al. reported a prospective research where serious complications occurred in 20% of sedated patients, with a respiratory or cardiac arrest in 4% of patients (Morita et al. 2005c). In such cases, if palliative sedation is applied as a proportional last resort of symptom relief, according to best possible standards of care, life shortening effects due to fatal complications may be accepted as an unintentional side effect of symptom relief.

4.2 The Ethical Value of Consciousness

The capacity to express oneself and to make one's own decision is considered important for human beings and a basic ethical value. At first sight it is clear that consciousness, also in the last phase of life, is important. For example, to say goodbye to loved ones, to make final arrangements, or simply to be consciously reacting to caregivers and family members. In principle, awareness is a basic requirement to express oneself in many ways. Although many patients who approach death suffer from a gradual decline of consciousness due to the natural course of terminal disease, to actively decline or suppress awareness until death by using medication is a serious intervention that calls for a convincing ethical justification. Considering that many persons experience periods of unawareness, for example, during anesthesia in a hospital, intermittent sedation for symptom control seems to be ethically justifiable at prima facie. When sedation occurs as a side effect of symptom treatment, symptom treatment will be the primary goal and sedation will be the foreseen but unintended side effect. But if sedation is the direct aim or intention, in particular in the case of continuous deep sedation until death, it is less obvious how the rule of double effect can be applied. Concerning the first criterion, for example, continuous suppression of consciousness may not be morally desirable as a general ethical value. However, it may be acceptable in some cases like patients near to death who suffer unbearably. It is not totally clear how the rule of double effect can fully account for such context related elements. In any case, the continuous suppression of consciousness needs a thorough medical and ethical justification.

In particular for deep and continuous sedation, fundamental ethical values are at stake. It is therefore important that continuous deep palliative sedation is used as a last resort only, to be justified only by grave reasons like refractory symptoms and excruciating suffering, and to be considered in a continuum of palliative care at the end of life.

5 Part IV the Debate About (Hidden) Euthanasia

The relation between euthanasia and continuous deep palliative sedation (then called "terminal" sedation) was firstly questioned during the discussion about the US Supreme court cases Vacco v. Quill and Washington v. Glucksberg. Here, the Supreme Court rejected a constitutional right to physician assisted suicide and insisted on the distinction between – accepted – withdrawal of life sustaining treatment and – prohibited – assisted suicide or euthanasia. Representatives of the medical profession wrote to the court that even the most intolerable pain can eventually be resolved by so-called terminal sedation. Orentlicher (1997), in an article heading that the court rejects assisted suicide but embraces euthanasia, argued that with terminal sedation, the unconscious state of the patient is initiated deliberately by the physician and as a consequence a process of dehydration is initiated by the same intentional decision for sedation of the physician (see our discussion of this topic earlier). Moreover, as terminal sedation may also be applied without the explicit permission of the patient, its application may be more vulnerable to abuse than euthanasia (see also Quill et al. 1997 for similar concerns).

Raus et al. (2011), analyzed these court decisions and concluded that continuous sedation is not to be considered a morally preferable alternative to assisted suicide. Their article raised many reactions, of which we highlight only one. Broeckaert (2011), in a critical reply, outlined the differences between palliative sedation and euthanasia in (a) their intent, (b) their procedure, and (c) their consequence. For palliative sedation, physicians in general do not aim to kill the patient, the drugs and dosages differ, and the result of palliative sedation is that the patient dies as a result of the illness and not because of lethal medication. However, to accept palliative sedation in principle as a part of palliative care does not imply that possible concerns about the practice should be neglected. For example , in November 2017, the Belgian minister of healthcare has raised concerns about palliative sedation being applied as a hidden euthanasia and pleaded for a legal procedure (newspaper de Standaard 2017). In the recent third evaluation report of the Dutch law on termination of life, concerns were raised about a possible grey area between euthanasia and intensified symptom treatment, with a call for more research into the practice of continuous deep palliative sedation (Onwuteaka-Philipsen et al. 2017).

How to continue with ongoing concerns surrounding palliative sedation? Perhaps we should look at the trustworthiness of medical practice as a whole. It can be argued that autonomy is often exercised in a relational context with family members and professional caregivers. Therefore, the first and most important safeguard regarding palliative sedation should be grounded in the patient-physician relationship. This is not primarily to be considered a contractual relationship between two contract partners, but an ethical relationship based upon mutual respect, sharing values, and shared decision-making (see also Emanuel and Emanuel 1992). Virtues like integrity and courage are needed in combination with excellent skills for communication and symptom management in a context of advance care planning to early detect preferences and possibilities in the palliative phase. In addition, the caring professions have a role here. When palliative sedation is principally regarded a part of palliative care, the medical and nursing professions have the primary responsibility to establish and support adequate practices, together with other multidisciplinary professions. They should address societal concerns about palliative sedation by ensuring well-established practice standards, with an adequate implementation, monitoring of current practices, and where needed medical disciplinary law. Its policies and practices should be directed at improving quality and trustworthiness for patients, families, and society at large.

6 Conclusion

David Clark (2002) argued that palliative care may have contributed to a certain medicalization of death and dying in their efforts to provide better symptom relief. In line with this observation, he does not recommend to totally avoid medical interventions at the end of life but to "reconcile high expectations of technical expertise with calls for a humanistic and ethical orientation." The ongoing debate about palliative sedation emphasizes the importance of such a reconciliation. In principle, palliative sedation including deep and continuous sedation can be considered part of palliative care. Probably the often debated problem of artificial hydration is not the most pertinent problem currently, given that sedations at the end of life last about 48 hours on average and current guidelines restrict continuous deep sedation to the last days of life. In the context of longer during sedations, for example, in case of existential suffering, caution is needed and this remains controversial in the literature. More research is needed to investigate palliative sedation to further answer medical and ethical questions, for example, about how to establish refractory symptoms and what this exactly involves.

Considering palliative sedation as a palliative care intervention, the question as to whether more safeguards are needed needs to be primarily answered within the palliative care and medical community. Regular updating and further implementation of ethically and medically balanced clinical guidelines are recommended together with ongoing education of care professionals and patients to avoid confusion about terms and conditions in daily practice. When it comes about concerns for hidden euthanasia however, societal values at large also come into play.

The task to provide humane care till the end is an important "raison d'etre" for palliative care. For patients with refractory symptoms, palliative sedation can bring comfort as a last resort. To exclude palliative sedation as a palliative care intervention would be highly problematic for the comfort care of many terminally ill patients. From an ethical viewpoint, palliative sedation can be acceptable in principle, but it remains important to (a) avoid both undertreatment leading to discomfort and overtreatment leading to unnecessary medicalization of death and dying, and (b) avoid both postponing and hastening of death. In finding the right middle, practical wisdom, the right skills and expertise, and a careful interaction with patient and family are pivotal.

References

Abarshi E, Rietjens J, Robijn L, Caraceni A, Payne S, Deliens L, Van den Block L, EURO IMPACT. International variations in clinical practice guidelines for palliative sedation: a systematic review. BMJ Support Palliat Care. 2017;7(3):223–9.

Broeckaert B. Palliative sedation, physician-assisted suicide, and euthanasia: "same, same but different". Am J Bioeth. 2011;11(6):62–4.

Broeckaert B. Palliatieve sedatie. Federatie Palliatieve Zorg Vlaanderen. 2012. http://www.pallialine.be/template.asp?f=rl_palliatieve_sedatie.htm. Last accessed March 2018.

Bruinsma SM, Rietjens JA, Seymour JE, Anquinet L, van der Heide A. The experiences of relatives with the practice of palliative sedation: a systematic review. J Pain Symptom Manag. 2012;44(3):431–45.

Bush SH, Leonard MM, Agar M, Spiller JA, Hosie A, Wright DK, Meagher DJ, Currow DC, Bruera E, Lawlor PG. End-of-life delirium: issues regarding recognition, optimal management, and the role of sedation in the dying phase. J Pain Symptom Manag. 2014;48(2):215–30.

Callahan D. When self-determination runs amok. Hast Cent Rep. 1992;22(2):52–5.

Caraceni A. Palliative sedation: more data and fewer opinions. Lancet Oncol. 2016;17(1):15–7.

Cassell EJ, Rich BA. Intractable end-of-life suffering and the ethics of palliative sedation. Pain Med. 2010;11(3):435–8.

Cellarius V, Henry B. Justifying different levels of palliative sedation. Ann Intern Med. 2010;152(5):332.

Cherny NI, Radbruch L, Board of the European Association for Palliative Care. European Association for Palliative Care (EAPC) recommended framework for the use of sedation in palliative care. Palliat Med. 2009;23(7):581–93.

Clark D. Between hope and acceptance: the medicalisation of dying. BMJ. 2002;324(7342):905–7.

de Graeff A, Dean M. Palliative sedation therapy in the last weeks of life: a literature review and recommendations for standards. J Palliat Med. 2007;10(1):67–85.

'De Standaard', November 2017. http://www.standaard.be/cnt/dmf20171126_03208014.

Den Hartogh GD. Continuous deep sedation and homicide: an unsolved problem in law and professional morality. Med Health Care Philos. 2016;19:285–97.

Dumont S, Blondeau D, Turcotte V, Borasio GD, Currat T, Foley RA, Beauverd M. The use of palliative sedation: a comparison of attitudes of French-speaking physicians from Quebec and Switzerland. Palliat Support Care. 2015;13(4):839–47.

Emanuel EJ, Emanuel LL. Four models of the physician-patient relationship. JAMA. 1992;267(16):2221–6.

Fainsinger RL, Núñez-Olarte JM, Demoissac DM. The cultural differences in perceived value of disclosure and cognition: Spain and Canada. J Palliat Care. 2003;19(1):43–8.

Hamano J, Morita T, Ikenaga M, Abo H, Kizawa Y, Tunetou S. A nationwide survey about palliative sedation involving Japanese palliative care specialists: intentions and key factors used to determine sedation as proportionally appropriate. J Pain Symptom Manag 2017.

Hasselaar JG, Verhagen SC, Vissers KC. When cancer symptoms cannot be controlled: the role of palliative sedation. Curr Opin Support Palliat Care. 2009a;3(1):14–23.

Hasselaar JG, Verhagen SC, Wolff AP, Engels Y, Crul BJ, Vissers KC. Changed patterns in Dutch palliative sedation practices after the introduction of a national guideline. Arch Intern Med. 2009b;169(5):430–7.

Hirai K, Kudo T, Akiyama M, Matoba M, Shiozaki M, Yamaki T, Yamagishi A, Miyashita M, Morita T, Eguchi KJ. Public awareness, knowledge of availability, and readiness for cancer palliative care services: a population-based survey across four regions in Japan. Palliat Med. 2011;14(8):918–22.

Jansen LA. Intractable end-of-life suffering and the ethics of palliative sedation: a commentary on Cassell and Rich. Pain Med. 2010;11(3):440–1. discussion 442

Juth N, Lindblad A, Lynöe N, Sjöstrand M, Helgesson G. European Association for Palliative Care (EAPC) framework for palliative sedation: an ethical discussion. BMC Palliat Care. 2010;9:20.

KNMG Committee on the National Guideline for Palliative Sedation. Guideline for palliative sedation. Utrecht. 2009. Available via https://www.knmg.nl/advies-richtlijnen/dossiers/palliatieve-sedatie.htm. Accessed 2 Feb 2018.

Kohara H, Ueoka H, Takeyama H, Murakami T, Morita T. Sedation for terminally ill patients with cancer with uncontrollable physical distress. J Palliat Med. 2005;8 (1):20–5.

Macfadyen R, Mcconnell P. Ethics in practice: is it futile to talk about 'futility'? Eur J Anaesthesiol. 2016;33: 473–4.

Maeda I, Morita T, Yamaguchi T, Inoue S, Ikenaga M, Matsumoto Y, Sekine R, Yamaguchi T, Hirohashi T, Tajima T, Tatara R, Watanabe H, Otani H, Takigawa C, Matsuda Y, Nagaoka H, Mori M, Tei Y, Kikuchi A, Baba M, Kinoshita H. Effect of continuous deep sedation on survival in patients with advanced cancer (J-Proval): a propensity score-weighted analysis of a prospective cohort study. Lancet Oncol. 2016;17(1): 115–22.

Maltoni M, Scarpi E, Rosati M, Derni S, Fabbri L, Martini F, Amadori D, Nanni O. Palliative sedation in end-of-life care and survival: a systematic review. J Clin Oncol. 2012;30(12):1378–83.

Mercadante S, Intravaia G, Villari P, Ferrera P, David F, Casuccio A. Controlled sedation for refractory symptoms in dying patients. J Pain Symptom Manag. 2009;37(5):771–9. https://doi.org/10.1016/j.jpainsymman.2008.04.020. Epub 2008 Nov 28

Miccinesi G, Rietjens JA, Deliens L, Paci E, Bosshard G, Nilstun T, Norup M, van der Wal G, EURELD Consortium. Continuous deep sedation: physicians' experiences in six European countries. J Pain Symptom Manag. 2006;31(2):122–9.

Morita T, Tsuneto S, Shima Y. Definition of sedation for symptom relief: a systematic literature review and a proposal of operational criteria. J Pain Symptom Manag. 2002;24(4):447–53.

Morita T, Ikenaga M, Adachi I, Narabayashi I, Kizawa Y, Honke Y, Kohara H, Mukaiyama T, Akechi T, Uchitomi Y, Japan Pain, Rehabilitation, Palliative Medicine, and Psycho-Oncology Study Group. Family experience with palliative sedation therapy for terminally ill cancer patients. J Pain Symptom Manag. 2004a; 28(6):557–65.

Morita T, Miyashita M, Kimura R, Adachi I, Shima Y. Emotional burden of nurses in palliative sedation therapy. Palliat Med. 2004b;18(6):550–7.

Morita T, Bito S, Kurihara Y, Uchitomi Y. Development of a clinical guideline for palliative sedation therapy using the Delphi method. J Palliat Med. 2005a;8(4):716–29.

Morita T, Chinone Y, Ikenaga M, Miyoshi M, Nakaho T, Nishitateno K, Sakonji M, Shima Y, Suenaga K, Takigawa C, Kohara H, Tani K, Kawamura Y, Matsubara T, Watanabe A, Yagi Y, Sasaki T, Higuchi A, Kimura H, Abo H, Ozawa T, Kizawa Y, Uchitomi Y, Japan Pain, Palliative Medicine, Rehabilitation, and Psycho-Oncology Study Group. Ethical validity of palliative sedation therapy: a multicenter, prospective, observational study conducted on specialized palliative care units in Japan. J Pain Symptom Manag. 2005b;30 (4):308–19.

Morita T, Chinone Y, Ikenaga M, Miyoshi M, Nakaho T, Nishitateno K, Sakonji M, Shima Y, Suenaga K, Takigawa C, Kohara H, Tani K, Kawamura Y, Matsubara T, Watanabe A, Yagi Y, Sasaki T, Higuchi A, Kimura H, Abo H, Ozawa T, Kizawa Y, Uchitomi Y, Japan Pain, Palliative Medicine, Rehabilitation, and Psycho-Oncology Study Group. Efficacy and safety of palliative sedation therapy: a multicenter, prospective, observational study conducted on specialized palliative care units in Japan. J Pain Symptom Manag. 2005c;30(4):320–8.

Núñez Olarte JM, Guillen DG. Cultural issues and ethical dilemmas in palliative and end-of-life care in Spain. Cancer Control. 2001;8(1):46–54.

Onwuteaka-Philipsen B, Legemaate J, van der Heide A, van Delden H, Evenblij K, Hammoud I, Pasman R, Ploem C, Pronk R, van de Vathorst S, Willems D. Derde evaluatie: wet toetsing levensbeeindiging op verzoeken hulp bij zelfdoding. Den Haag: ZonMw; 2017.

Orentlicher D. The Supreme Court and physician-assisted suicide – rejecting assisted suicide but embracing euthanasia. N Engl J Med. 1997;337:1236–9.

Papavasiliou E, Payne S, Brearley S, Brown J, Seymour J. Continuous sedation (CS) until death: mapping the literature by bibliometric analysis. J Pain Symptom Manag. 2013;45(6):1073–82.

Putman MS, Yoon JD, Rasinski KA, Curlin FA. Intentional sedation to unconsciousness at the end of life: findings from a national physician survey. J Pain Symptom Manag. 2013;46(3):326–34.

Quill TE, Lo B, Brock DW. Palliative options of last resort: a comparison of voluntarily stopping eating and drinking, terminal sedation, physician-assisted suicide, and voluntary active euthanasia. JAMA. 1997;278(23): 2099–104.

Quill TE, Lo B, Brock DW, Meisel A. Last-resort options for palliative sedation. Ann Intern Med. 2009;151(6): 421–4.

Raus K, Sterckx S, Mortier F. Is continuous sedation at the end of life an ethically preferable alternative to physician-assisted suicide? Am J Bioeth. 2011;11(6): 32–40.

Raus K, Brown J, Seale C, Rietjens JA, Janssens R, Bruinsma S, Mortier F, Payne S, Sterckx S. Continuous sedation until death: the everyday moral reasoning of physicians, nurses and family caregivers in the UK, The Netherlands and Belgium. BMC Med Ethics. 2014;15:14.

Rietjens JA, Hauser J, van der Heide A, Emanuel L. Having a difficult time leaving: experiences and attitudes of nurses with palliative sedation. Palliat Med. 2007;21 (7):643–9.

Rietjens JA, Voorhees JR, van der Heide A, Drickamer MA. Approaches to suffering at the end of life: the use of sedation in the USA and Netherlands. J Med Ethics. 2014;40(4):235–40.

Rinehart A. Beyond the futility argument: the fair process approach and time-limited trials for managing dialysis conflict. Clin J Am Soc Nephrol. 2013;8(11):2000–6.

Robijn L, Cohen J, Rietjens J, Deliens L, Chambaere K. Trends in continuous deep sedation until death between 2007 and 2013: a repeated nationwide survey. PLoS One. 2016;11(6):e0158188.

Rodrigues P, Crokaert J, Gastmans C. Palliative sedation for existential suffering: a systematic review of argument-based ethics literature. J Pain Symptom Manag. 2018;55(6):1577–90.

Rys S, Deschepper R, Mortier F, Deliens L, Bilsen J. Continuous sedation until death with or without the intention to hasten death – a nationwide study in nursing homes in Flanders, Belgium. J Am Med Dir Assoc. 2014;15(8):570–5.

Schildmann E, Schildmann J. Palliative sedation therapy: a systematic literature review and critical appraisal of available guidance on indication and decision making. J Palliat Med. 2014;17(5):601–11.

Schneiderman LJ. Defining medical futility and improving medical care. J Bioeth Inq. 2011;8(2):123–31. Epub 2011 Mar 20

Schneiderman LJ, Jecker NS, Jonsen AR. Medical futility: its meaning and ethical implications. Ann Intern Med. 1990;112(12):949–54. Review

Schur S, Weixler D, Gabl C, Kreye G, Likar R, Masel EK, Mayrhofer M, Reiner F, Schmidmayr B, Kirchheiner K, Watzke HH, AUPACS (Austrian Palliative Care Study) Group. Sedation at the end of life – a nation-wide study in palliative care units in Austria. BMC Palliat Care. 2016;15:50.

Seale C. Continuous deep sedation in medical practice: a descriptive study. J Pain Symptom Manag. 2010; 39(1):44–53.

Seale C, Raus K, Bruinsma S, van der Heide A, Sterckx S, Mortier F, Payne S, Mathers N, Rietjens J, UNBIASED consortium. The language of sedation in end-of-life care: the ethical reasoning of care providers in three countries. Health (London). 2015;19(4):339–54.

Simon A, Kar M, Hinz J, Beck D. Attitudes towards terminal sedation: an empirical survey among experts in the field of medical ethics. BMC Palliat Care. 2007; 6:4.

Sulmasy DP, Pellegrino ED. The rule of double effect: clearing up the double talk. Arch Intern Med. 1999;159(6):545–50. Review

Swart SJ, van der Heide A, Brinkkemper T, van Zuylen L, Perez R, Rietjens J. Continuous palliative sedation until death: practice after introduction of the Dutch national guideline. BMJ Support Palliat Care. 2012;2(3): 256–63.

Sykes N, Thorns A. Sedative use in the last week of life and the implications for end-of-life decision making. Arch Intern Med. 2003;163(3):341–4.

Truog RD. The concept of futility: recognizing the importance of context. Perspect Biol Med. 2018;60(3):428–32.

Van Deijck RH, Hasselaar JG, Krijnsen PJ, Gloudemans AJ, Verhagen SC, Vissers KC, Koopmans RT. The practice of continuous palliative sedation in long-term care for frail patients with existential suffering. J Palliat Care. 2015;31(3):141–9.

Van der Heide A, van Delden JJM, Onwuteaka-Philipsen BD. End-of-life decisions in the Netherlands over 25 years. N Engl J Med. 2017;377(5): 492–4.

Van der Kallen HT, Raijmakers NJ, Rietjens JA, van der Male AA, Bueving HJ, van Delden JJ, van der Heide A. Opinions of the Dutch public on palliative sedation: a mixed-methods approach. Br J Gen Pract. 2013;63 (615):e676–82.

Ventafridda V, Ripamonti C, De Conno F, Tamburini M, Cassileth BR. Symptom prevalence and control during cancer patients' last days of life. J Palliat Care. 1990; 6(3):7–11.

World Health Organization. WHO definition of palliative care. WHO. 2002. http://www.who.int/cancer/palliative/definition/en/. Last accessed March 2018.

Nutrition and Hydration in Palliative Care and Their Diverse Meanings

88

Jean B. Clark and Lesley S. Batten

Contents

J. B. Clark (✉)
Hospital Palliative Care Service Palmerston North Hospital, MidCentral Health, Palmerston North, New Zealand

School of Nursing, Massey University, Palmerston North, New Zealand
e-mail: J.Clark@xtra.co.nz

L. S. Batten
College of Health, Massey University, Palmerston North, New Zealand
e-mail: L.Batten@massey.ac.nz

Abstract

Essential for life, food and fluids are regarded as basic care, professionally, ethically, and legally. This chapter seeks to contextualize and explore the significance and meaning of compromised nutrition and hydration in contemporary adult palliative care. The internationalization of Western medicine, Western bioethics, and palliative care generates new perspectives and can challenge established practices. It is important that evidence of the relevance, efficacy, and appropriateness of

R. D. MacLeod, L. Van den Block (eds.), *Textbook of Palliative Care*,
https://doi.org/10.1007/978-3-319-77740-5_117

artificially intervening in the natural course of terminal illnesses is developed; however, that knowledge will not necessarily resolve the issues associated with the reality that food and fluids mean different things to those involved.

Universally, food and fluid, its preparation, use, symbolism, and value are inherently meaningful. Discussions, opinions and decisions vary regarding supporting oral intake, and clinically assisted nutrition and hydration, particularly towards the end of life. Inevitably, the perspectives of the ill person, their companions, and informal and professional caregivers are not necessarily consistent or static.

Endeavors to address declining oral intake must be individualized, congruent with care goals, and cognizant of cultural values, religious, and personal beliefs. It is an aspect of care (and dying) that should not be taken for granted nor considered problematic. Rather, it is inevitable for many people and no lasting resolution should be anticipated or desired. Professional knowledge and curiosity towards the multiple meanings surrounding eating, food, nutrition, and hydration, and their meaning is the proposed aspiration.

1 Key Points

- Declining oral intake is meaningful for patients, family members and clinicians.
- Perceptions that food and fluid intakes influence lifetime are essentially well founded.
- Refractory cachexia in people with a progressive life-limiting illness is not ameliorated by clinically assisted nutrition and hydration.
- There is a paucity of evidence to provide unequivocal guidance for clinicians regarding artificial nutrition and hydration, although facts alone are unlikely to change clinical practice and patients' and families' expectations.
- Clinicians hold diverse views regarding forgoing, providing, and withdrawing clinically assisted nutrition and hydration.
- The goals of care regarding nutrition and hydration require on-going review with informed and meaningful dialogue between patients, family members, and clinicians.

2 Introduction

Vignette one: A close family member of a person recently diagnosed with a terminal illness and with probably months to live focuses on the "not eating": "He doesn't seem to want to eat, if I make it for him he does, but I don't think he is bothering to eat anything except pudding if I am not there. Should I get him some [supplement] or something? But then, does it matter? I know it is illogical to worry about that at this time, but I do."

As is identified in this vignette, food and fluids, eating and not eating are everyday challenges and also key flags of actual or impending change for the person, their family and friends when someone has a life-limiting condition. This chapter explores this complex issue, reviews the goals of care in palliative and end of life care, and contextualizes the meaning of food and fluid and **clinically assisted nutrition and hydration (CANH)** in life-limiting illness. Basic care includes food and fluids, while CANH is regarded as a medical intervention (Druml et al. 2016). The ethical principles drawn on in palliative and end-of-life care, including autonomy, beneficence, nonmaleficence, and justice are applicable to the provision of food and fluids and decisions to forgo, utilize, or withdraw CANH (Druml et al. 2016). Exploring and contextualizing the diverse meanings of oral food and fluids and CANH in the adult palliative care population in relation to bioethics requires consideration of many interconnected elements (Fig. 1).

In this chapter, small vignettes have been developed from the authors' combined clinical practice and research experience to illustrate and explore the most pertinent issues. There are consistent elements:

- A person's life is ending.
- Food and fluids are meaningful and essential for life.

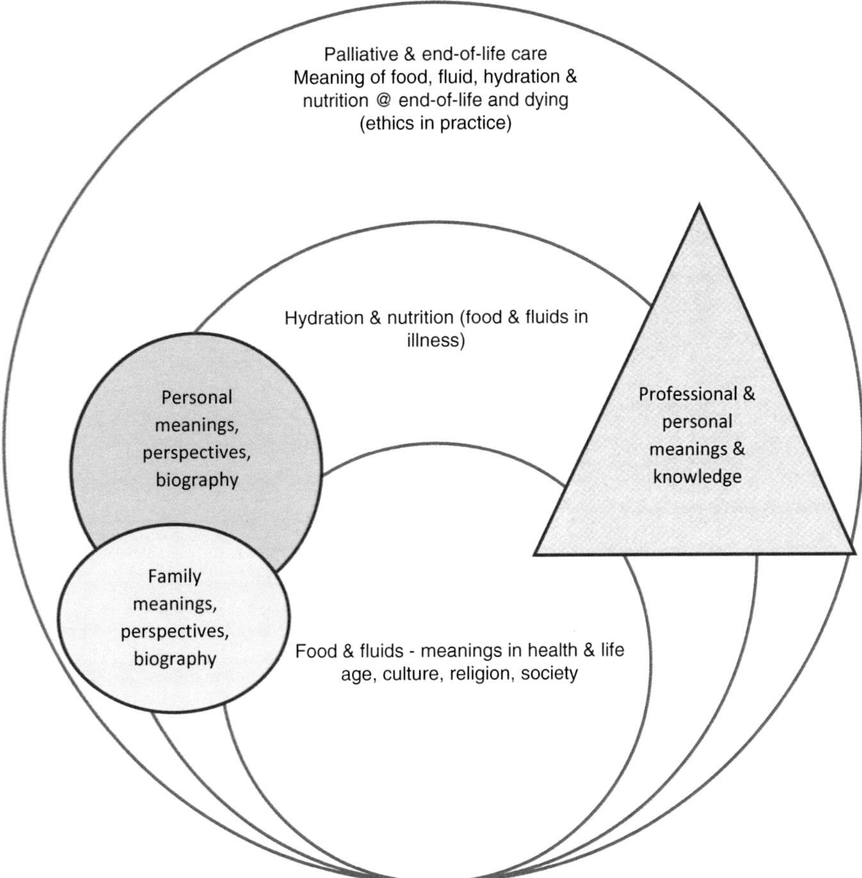

Fig. 1 The multiple contexts of food and fluids in palliative care

- The dying process results in the loss of oral intake.
- CANH is available but does not reverse the dying process.
- Suffering should be mitigated.

Ethical discussions regarding dilemmas associated with food and fluids and CANH are inevitable in palliative and end-of-life care, because nutrition and hydration are requisites for life. Factual clinical data related to this topic, while important, is unlikely to significantly ameliorate this challenging and complex aspect of clinical practice because all parties experience hydration and nutrition as meaningful. The intention of this chapter is to inform, support dialogue, and encourage professional reflection and acceptance of the inevitable ambiguity and complexity for patients, families, and their companions, so providers of palliative care are enabled to meet their dynamic needs ethically.

3 Oral Food, Fluids and Clinically Assisted Nutrition and Hydration in Palliative Care

Addressing the unmet needs of people dying from malignant conditions in acute care was the main catalyst for the modern hospice movement, established in London in 1967 (Fallon and Smyth 2008). Subsequently extensive efforts to promote and mainstream palliative care have occurred. This has influenced where palliative care is delivered (acute hospital settings, home, aged care facilities), expanded the population focus to include people with progressive nonmalignant illnesses (e.g., congestive heart failure, chronic obstructive pulmonary disease, or neurological conditions), and the integration of palliative care earlier in the disease trajectory (Fallon and Smyth 2008; World Health Organization 2002). Additionally, previously well people who experience acute life-threatening events may require and benefit from palliative care. In this latter cohort interventions like CANH may be in place while the person is fully assessed and the likely outcome determined. Sudden changes in physical condition, devoid of anticipated and witnessed deterioration can make decisions regarding CANH more fraught for all parties.

The majority of people with progressive disease from malignant and nonmalignant causes experience declining oral intake and will eventually struggle to take food and fluid safely (Royal College of Physicians and British Society of Gastroenterology 2010; Watson et al. 2009). These changes are often associated with weight loss, altered physical appearance, declining function, and increasing fatigue (Watson et al. 2009). The person, family members, companions, and clinicians all bear witness to these changes. All parties may have differing perceptions of the need, purpose, and benefits of food and fluids and CANH (del Rio et al. 2011). Additionally, perceptions of the benefits and burdens of oral food and fluids and CANH may not be congruent amongst clinicians and the recipients of care. Indeed the differences in the utilization of CANH identified in literature reviews indicates that clinical practice (del Rio et al. 2011; Raijmakers et al. 2011; Torres-Vigil et al. 2012), as well as family members' and patients' perceptions of food and fluid and CAHN are influenced by multiple factors, not just knowledge (del Rio et al. 2011).

In diverse societies globally, food and fluid are meaningful in life, health, culture, religion, and society. They have roles and functions other than the avoidance of dehydration and starvation. Food and fluids are often central to social interactions, be this within daily family life, among friends, for celebrations and as gifts (Raijmakers et al. 2013; Rozin 2005; Wallin et al. 2015). The importance of food and fluid is not confined to the factual, calorific, and measurable because in most, if not all societies, food and fluids have meanings that extend beyond nutritional values (Rozin 2005). Therefore, it is understandable that questions will arise regarding what is adequate and appropriate, and how food and fluids will, could, or should be obtained or provided in palliative care.

In their simplest and most poignant, the issues that underpin the complexity of food and fluids and CANH in palliative and end-of-life care can be seen as a battle between an illness ending a life and perceptions of being deprived of the essentials for life. Mal Morgan (1999), an Australian poet living and dying with terminal lung cancer, captured this dichotomy in the following extract from one of his poems (p. 56).

> . . . I look at the stick-man
> In my bathroom mirror
> every morning.
> There he is.
> Cancer can do this.
> Ethnic cleansing
> can do this. . . .

Morgan's (1999) poem illustrates cancer cachexia and inflicted starvation as highly visible threats to a person's embodied existence.

The perception that lack of food and fluids leads to death is well founded. When nutrition is withheld in a previously well person, death may take weeks (up to 10); however, in the absence of fluids, it is estimated to be between 3 and 14 days and is more rapid in the unwell (Royal College of Physicians and British Society of Gastroenterology 2010). "If water is given in the absence of food, survival is long enough for death from nutritional deprivation to occur. Whilst giving hydration seems a humane act, it may prolong dying" (Royal College of Physicians and British Society of Gastroenterology 2010, p. 16). The latter point is important in the context of progressive life-threatening illness and in acute catastrophic events where recovery is not expected. Usually the ethical doctrine of double effect, whereby an action is justified if the intention is good, is related to the use of opioid analgesics in palliative care. The action itself should not be the direct cause of death. If a person's death is not foreseen, withholding CANH may be a direct cause of death. In those people close to death, the doctrine of double effect can however be applied to the use of CANH, as "...withholding feeding may foreseeably end the life of the patient. This effect is not aimed at death but is aimed at avoiding the suffering or burdens associated with (artificial) feeding therapies, relative to their possible benefits" (Royal College of Physicians and British Society of Gastroenterology 2010, p. 42).

Changes in the patient population, diagnoses, place of care, and the point in the illness trajectory when palliative care may be appropriate have not altered the central tenets of palliative care. Alleviating suffering, the relief of symptoms, quality of life, neither hastening nor postponing death, the unit of care (patient and family), and a holistic approach (World Health Organization 2002) remain and are pertinent in relation to CANH.

Proponents for and against CANH in the context of palliative and end-of-life care are committed to negating suffering and harm. Nevertheless, perceptions differ regarding what is more likely to be harmful. Families, in particular, perceive the person as suffering in the absence of fluids (Bear et al. 2017). Conversely, advocates of palliative care often accept changes in oral intake as part of the natural dying process and focus on ameliorating symptoms such as a dry mouth (Watson et al. 2009). The continuation or initiation of CANH when it is apparent a person is dying is usually regarded as clinically futile, harmful rather than beneficial, prolonging dying, and diverging from focusing on quality of life. Questions related to CANH can occur along the palliative care continuum and across all diagnoses; however, it often arises when oral intake declines, becomes more arduous, and when the oral route is no longer possible. The intended palliative care goals to neither hasten nor postpone death (World Health Organization 2002) is not a neatly delineated dichotomy. Decisions regarding forgoing, administering, or withdrawing of CANH may contribute to hastening or postponing death. Intervening when oral feeding difficulties arise has a long history, and new developments bring complex challenges about their appropriate utilization.

4 Ancient and New: Interventions That Have Been, Are, and Could Be Utilized

People have been attempting to redress or overcome difficulties and deficiencies related to oral food and fluids for millennia. The history of enteral nutrition "... dates back as far as 3500 bc to the ancient Egyptians, Indians, and Chinese. Their medical practices were the first reports of enteral feeding therapy, provided via the rectum with enemas of wine, milk whey, wheat and barley" (Vassilyadi et al. 2013, p. 209). Relatively, more recent experimentation related to the parenteral route occurred in the twelfth century (Vassilyadi et al. 2013), and in the twentieth century, substantial advances were made with improvements in equipment, techniques, nutritional knowledge, and developments in formula to meet specific nutritional requirements (Royal College of Physicians and British Society of Gastroenterology 2010; Vassilyadi et al. 2013).

The goals of enteral feeding have become increasingly complex, moving towards aiding recovery, healing, improving immunity, the treatment of illness and injury, and the ability to provide a person's full nutritional requirements (Royal College of Physicians and British Society of Gastroenterology 2010; Vassilyadi et al. 2013). Hence many therapeutic options are available to clinicians when declining oral intake occurs; however, the challenge is not solely related to the capacity to intervene. In this vein, Barrocas refers to the troubling trichotomy – the "... conflicts between can (technology), should (ethics) and must (law) as they apply to nutrition support" (2016, p. 295). The challenge is often not the therapies themselves, rather that there are other underlying considerations like an unresolvable illness that continues to progress (Royal College of Physicians and British Society of Gastroenterology 2010; Truog 2014). Indeed, the intentions of CANH, to maintain a person's nutritional and hydration status by securing alternative routes to meet their ongoing metabolic needs, may be at odds with a palliative care approach, particularly at the end of life (Orrevall 2015; Royal College of

Physicians and British Society of Gastroenterology 2010).

The European Society for Parenteral and Enteral Nutrition's (ESPEN) definition of artificial nutrition includes oral nutritional supplements, which are not usually controversial, as well as enteral (nasogastric and nasogastrojejunal percutaneous tubes and endoscopic gastrostomy) and parenteral nutrition (peripheral intravenous, central venous line) (Druml et al. 2016). Artificial hydration includes fluid for hydration delivered by means other than the oral route (Druml et al. 2016). Contemporary developments regarding the ability to provide CANH gives rise to questions about whether CANH should (ethically) be provided and if indeed CANH must (legally) be provided (Barrocas 2016).

The ethical principles of beneficence, nonmaleficence, and the provision of care that reflects the principles of justice inform health care generally and are applicable in relation CANH in palliative and end-of-life care (Barrocas 2016; Bear et al. 2017; Druml et al. 2016; Royal College of Physicians and British Society of Gastroenterology 2010; Watson et al. 2009). Alongside obligations to treat, cure (when possible), and relieve symptoms, is the relief of suffering and the provision of comfort (Royal College of Physicians and British Society of Gastroenterology 2010). Clinicians have a duty of care to meet people's needs and to act in their best interests. However, there is a paucity of unequivocal evidence regarding CANH to guide clinicians providing palliative and end-of-life care (del Rio et al. 2011; Ganzini 2006; Good et al. 2014; Kozeniecki et al. 2017; Royal College of Physicians and British Society of Gastroenterology 2010). This includes the care of cancer patients in the last week of life (Raijmakers et al. 2011). No clear benefit of one route of CANH administration over another has been identified among cancer patients, although there was a greater risk of infection with parenteral nutrition over enteral nutrition and neither improved survival (Chow et al. 2016). Parenteral nutrition was also noted to be twice as expensive (Chow et al. 2016), providing a resource argument to support the preferred use of enteral nutrition along with the benefits to gastrointestinal health and function. Route may also influence the place of care, leading to resource implications alongside social and cultural considerations.

A recent review of the literature (Bear et al. 2017) identified a number of arguments for and against the provision of clinically assisted hydration (CAH) at the end of life with both potentially enhancing comfort. Arguments in support included that the provision of fluid is a basic human need, preventing complications of other treatments and relieving thirst (Bear et al. 2017). Arguments against CAH at the end of life include its provision impeding the acceptance of the terminal situation, prolonging a person's suffering and dying, and contributing to uncomfortable symptoms like edema and ascites. These authors also cite the argument that the accumulation of metabolic by-products in dehydration may reduce pain perception and improve comfort (Bear et al. 2017). The potential benefits and burdens of different methods of CANH (enteral and parenteral) have also been tabulated (Kozeniecki et al. 2017). While all may provide a sense of relief for patients and families, all have significant risks and no clear outcomes to guide clinicians have been identified (Bear et al. 2017; Good et al. 2014; Kozeniecki et al. 2017; Raijmakers et al. 2011). Importantly, significant limitations in the evidence available was noted, with authors suggesting there may be a subset of this population who may derive some benefit (Kozeniecki et al. 2017). Research to obtain evidence is challenging when the population may be significantly debilitated, cognitively impaired or actively dying. Alongside these challenges are the risk of injustices occurring, specifically among vulnerable population groups, when evidence is lacking resulting in inequitable care (Bear et al. 2017). The absence unequivocal evidence makes ethical decision-making more challenging.

Justice is one of the ethical principles relevant to the provision of appropriate care which does no harm and is beneficial for the recipient. Fairness, treating people equally and the equitable distribution of resources, is also inherent in the ethical principle of justice (Bear et al. 2017; Royal College of Physicians and British Society of Gastroenterology 2010; Watson et al. 2009).

ESPEN offers guidance for clinicians regarding ethical aspects of CANH, proposing the following three prerequisites be considered, with the key priorities to do no harm, to do good and respect autonomy (Druml et al. 2016, p. 546).

1. An indication for a medical treatment
2. The definition of a therapeutic goal to be achieved
3. The will of the patient and his or her informed consent

Indications for CANH (or not) will vary significantly over the course of a life-limiting illness and in acute events, as will the goals, preferences, and perceptions of its purpose. Utilizing CANH may be indicated and uncontroversial early in an illness to ameliorate the side effects of therapies, to treat concurrent or incidental illness, improve a person's health status, and to enable therapeutic treatment to be given. The difficulties encountered require consideration of reversible causes and the natural progression of an illness alongside the goals of care.

5 Natural Progression Versus Reversible Causes

Screening for malnourishment, identifying those underweight, and enquiring about unintended weight loss so reversible causes may be redressed is common in health care (O'Hara 2017). Prior to the more imminently terminal phase, the goal is to enable and support oral intake by assisting with feeding, providing appropriate food and fluid, oral care, and a providing a conducive environment. The primary goal regarding "nutrition in palliative care is to maximise food enjoyment and minimise food discomfort" (O'Hara 2017, p. 24). To facilitate this, identifying and addressing symptoms, reversing reversible causes, and accessing and providing appropriate nutritional advice or support is central to maximizing quality of life and is basic care. Oral intake can be adversely impacted by candida infections of the mouth and upper gastrointestinal tract, the side effects of medications or treatments, dry mouth, taste changes, nausea, indigestion, malodourous wounds, dyspnea, fatigue, early satiety, and bowel obstruction (Royal College of Physicians and British Society of Gastroenterology 2010; Watson et al. 2009). Unfortunately, the effects of an illness and the changes wrought are not always reversible.

Cachexia is the consequence of a number of progressive life-limiting illnesses and general cachexia, unrelated to malignancy, has been defined as (Evans et al. 2008, p. 794):

> . . . a complex metabolic syndrome associated with underlying illness and characterized by loss of muscle with or without loss of fat mass. The prominent clinical feature of cachexia is weight loss in adults (corrected for fluid retention) or growth failure in children (excluding endocrine disorders). Anorexia, inflammation, insulin resistance and increased muscle protein breakdown are frequently associated with cachexia. Cachexia is distinct from starvation, age-related loss of muscle mass, primary depression, malabsorption and hyperthyroidism and is associated with increased morbidity.

Subsequently, an international consensus defined cancer cachexia as (Fearon et al. 2011, p. 499):

> . . . a multifactorial syndrome characterised by an on-going loss of skeletal muscle mass (with or without loss of fat mass) that cannot be fully reversed by conventional nutritional support and leads to progressive functional impairment. The pathophysiology is characterised by a negative protein and energy balance driven by a variable combination of reduced food intake and abnormal metabolism.

The important distinguishing characteristic of cachexia (all causes) is that unlike malnutrition, which may be concurrent, or starvation, it cannot be adequately redressed by nutrition (Evans et al. 2008; Fearon et al. 2011; Royal College of Physicians and British Society of Gastroenterology 2010; Watson et al. 2009). Commonalities are evident between the general and cancer cachexia definitions, with both acknowledging metabolic changes, changes to the body composition, and the impact on the person. In defining cancer cachexia, guidance is offered for staging, covering a spectrum which includes precachexia, cachexia and refractory cachexia (Fearon et al. 2011). Malignancies differ in terms of their cachexic impact and an individual's progress across the spectrum to refractory cachexia before death is uncertain. Cancer cachexia, which remains poorly understood, affects approximately 80% of this population and is usually accompanied by other symptoms (Fearon et al. 2011; Watson et al. 2009). These changes, acknowledged in the staging of cancer cachexia, include anorexia, loss of appetite, weight loss, metabolic changes, inflammatory changes, changes in performance status, and expected survival (Fearon et al. 2011). For both cancer and non-cancer related cachexia, clinicians are reliant on the clinical context, a history of unplanned weight loss, body mass index, anorexia, declining oral intake, performance status, inflammatory, and other biomarkers (Evans et al. 2008; Fearon et al. 2011). Confronted by difficulties in eating and drinking in advanced illness, patients, families, and some clinicians may consider CANH.

The metabolic changes occurring with cachexia can inform clinical decisions to forgo or utilize CANH. Orrevall (2015, p. 615) suggests trying to "estimate if the cancer spread allows the patient a survival longer than 3 months. No benefit can theoretically be expected by an active nutritional support if a starving patient is going to die of tumour progression within that time interval." Starving is an emotive word that is frequently used, especially by family members. However, patients' and family members' perceptions of and attention to mitigating starvation may obscure the real issue; the person is not dying because of nutrient deprivation (Kozeniecki et al. 2017).

Importantly CANH is unable to reverse refractory cachexia in advanced illness and it is not a source of pleasure (Cohen et al. 2012; Orrevall et al. 2005). Indeed CANH may become a source of discomfort and can be contrary to the nutritional goals of palliative and end of life care (O'Hara 2017; Orrevall 2015). Unfortunately, the pleasure of oral intake is often lost, adversely affected by taste changes, difficulty eating and drinking, and associated with anxiety, worry, and physical discomfort (Watson et al. 2009). Refusing oral intake to hasten death is an alternative to navigating the uncertainty of disease progression.

6 Choosing to Stop Eating and Drinking

Voluntarily choosing to stop eating and drinking (VSED) is the action of a competent and capable person to deliberately forgo oral intake. The "primary intention [is] to hasten death because unacceptable suffering persists" (Ivanović et al. 2014, p. 1). They exchange what is unacceptable suffering for them for the suffering often perceived by families and companions when the oral route is lost in advanced illness. VSED leads to death within days to two weeks, depending on the person's preceding health status (Ivanović et al. 2014; Wax et al. 2018). Reasons for choosing to VSED include being ready to die, believing continuing to live is futile, perceiving their quality of life as poor, and a desire to control the circumstances and method of their death (Ganzini et al. 2003; Ivanović et al. 2014). VSED is considered a more accessible and less bureaucratic option than seeking euthanasia or physician-assisted suicide, and it can occur in the absence of a terminal diagnosis and without requiring medical input (Wax et al. 2018). Ethically and legally, given certain requirements, VSED is defendable (Ivanović et al. 2014; Wax et al. 2018). The following criteria are proposed for physician-supported VSED (Wax et al. 2018). Firstly, there is a "terminal or serious debilitating illness with intolerable suffering which remains after access to high-quality palliative care evaluation and support" (Wax et al. 2018, p. 443). Additionally, it is necessary to establish that the person has capacity, is informed of the risks, benefits, and possible alternatives. It also requires ascertaining that the choice is voluntary and verifying that mental illness or cognitive impairment are not factors. Support by the person's main caregivers is considered important, as is confirming VSED is consistent with the values of the person (Wax et al. 2018).

Understanding the often multidimensional suffering associated with choosing VSED to hasten death and responding appropriately is crucial (Ivanović et al. 2014; Wax et al. 2018). Included is the impeccable management of symptoms and psychosocial and existential support (Ivanović et al. 2014; Wax et al. 2018). All competent people can change their mind regarding the plan of care. However, carers and clinicians may be morally and ethically challenged when a person's cognitive state is impaired in the dying process and they express a wish for fluids or food which may prolong their dying, contrary to their previously expressed wishes (Wax et al. 2018).

Choosing VSED results in end of life symptoms that are described as similar to those experienced by the withdrawal of CANH. Thirst, dry mouth, hunger, dysuria, weakness, delirium, and somnolence are anticipated and require management (Wax et al. 2018). Hospice nurses in Oregon, who responded to a survey (72%), perceived patients choosing VSED "... as suffering less and being more at peace in the last two weeks of life" than those who chose physician assisted suicide (Ganzini et al. 2003, p. 362). They noted that 85% of deaths occurred within 15 days, the stand-down period required for physician-assisted suicide in Oregon (Ganzini et al. 2003). VSED appeared to be accepted by the nurses and not a source of moral distress or ethical concern for them, although this is not explicitly explored. The perceived lack of suffering may be comforting for the nurses and reflects European findings that decisions to withdraw or forgo CANH did not lead to suffering based on the comparative use of end-of-life medications for symptom management (Buiting et al. 2007).

Authors (Ivanović et al. 2014) argue that VSED has received marginal attention within palliative care. Although commentary is emerging, there is a paucity of systematic approaches to assess people choosing to VSED and to provide guidance to clinicians (Wax et al. 2018).

7 Oral Intake: Focusing on Eating and Not Eating

The introduction to this chapter began with a vignette illustrating the relatively common challenge of declining appetite and oral intake and the endeavors of those who care for them to prepare and offer tempting and nutritional food and fluids. As a clinical and ethical issue, it may be overlooked by clinicians and overshadowed by debates regarding the appropriateness or otherwise of CANH when illness is advanced and the end of life near. In addressing oral feeding difficulties and dilemmas, it is proposed that three questions are considered (Royal College of Physicians and British Society of Gastroenterology 2010, p. 9–10):

1. What is the underlying diagnosis?
2. What is the mechanism of the oral feeding problem?
3. Can the person eat and drink and if so, at what risk?

These are critical questions in relation to oral intake in palliative care and can inform thoughtful consideration and appropriate responses. Knowledge of the underlying diagnosis is important as is the extent of the disease and prognosis. As discussed earlier, clinicians have a responsibility to identify and address potentially reversible causes for declining or poor oral intake (Royal College of Physicians and British Society of Gastroenterology 2010; Watson et al. 2009). Eating and drinking when there is a risk of aspiration, coughing, and the potential for choking may or may not be acceptable to the person and ultimately, they should be able to exercise their autonomy whenever possible. Indeed, the pleasure of eating may override difficulties, including the unpleasantness of vomiting (Orrevall et al. 2005).

Declining oral intake in the presence of life threatening illness is full of meaning for patients (Wallin et al. 2015) and family members (Amano et al. 2016; Hopkinson 2016; Raijmakers et al. 2013; Reid et al. 2009a, b; Reid et al. 2010). For patients, changes in oral intake have been described as "... existentially loaded markers of impending death" (Wallin et al. 2015, p. 123). Declining oral intake and appetite is also meaningful for clinicians in terms of prognosis (Royal College of Physicians and British Society of Gastroenterology 2010; Watson et al. 2009) and is one of the ten phenomena identified by palliative care experts as indicating approaching death (Benedetti et al. 2013).

For relatives, food can symbolize love, concern, and compassion and result in significant efforts to tempt and provide favorite foods (Raijmakers et al. 2013; Reid et al. 2009b). Food and fluid also represent nourishment, preserving life, enjoyment, special memories, social activities, providing a routine to daily life, a way to care, express love, and meet the ill person's wishes (Raijmakers et al. 2013). Relatives' responses to declining oral intake include laboring to prepare special food, tempting them to eat and drink, and endeavoring to maintain routines and ordinariness in their daily lives (Raijmakers et al. 2013; Wallin et al. 2013). Awareness of the life-threatening context informs relatives' responses and they often expend significant thought and effort. Internationally researchers have noted tensions between family members and the ill person regarding declining oral intake (Amano et al. 2016; Raijmakers et al. 2013; Reid et al. 2009b, 2010; Wallin et al. 2015).

Tensions can arise when a person who is debilitated, fatigued, and experiencing loss of appetite endeavors to eat to please, is no longer able to eat as expected, or at all (Raijmakers et al. 2013; Reid et al. 2009b). Conflict as a result of declining oral intake can result in patients feeling "... like they were constantly in an environment focused on food from which they could not escape"(Reid et al. 2009b, p. 441). Relatives could become embroiled in what they described as a "vicious circle" (Raijmakers et al. 2013, p. 670) whereby they and their ill relative were trying to please each other to avoid worry and conflict, which was recalled vividly when it had occurred. Some relatives accepted changes as part of the process of dying, while others perceived this change, in part, as the person's choice (Raijmakers et al. 2013).

These experiences and their complex meanings are not exclusive to European societies. Amano et al. (2016) found Japanese relatives also pressured ill family members to eat in the belief that this would be beneficial and they went to significant effort to entice and encourage oral intake. Conflict could occur. Their findings inferred there was a higher risk of bereavement depression for relatives who felt they had forced oral intake and who believed they had inadequate information about weight loss, cachexia, and nutrition (Amano et al. 2016).

The desires of patients and relatives for more information and greater understanding is well documented (Amano et al. 2016; Raijmakers et al. 2013; Reid et al. 2009b, 2010; Wallin et al. 2015, 2013). Openly discussing the changes occurring (when this is what the patient and relatives want) may appear obvious yet it may not occur. Communication regarding food and fluids, hydration and nutrition is acknowledged as difficult even for palliative care clinicians (Clark et al. 2017; Millar et al. 2013). Interestingly, bereaved relatives recalled little information being conveyed to them by health professionals regarding declining oral intake (Raijmakers et al. 2013), yet health professionals in the same service richly described how they respond, inform, and guide relatives, although they tended to wait for cues and opportunities. A mismatch in experience and perceptions was revealed (Clark et al. 2017).

The lack of open acknowledgement of weight loss by health professionals, even when apparent, concerned relatives and patients alike (Reid et al. 2010). They wanted their weight loss acknowledged, information and a response regarding appropriate interventions; however, health professionals' lack of engagement damaged patients' and families' confidence in them (Reid et al. 2010). Awareness of the significance of cachexia and tacit acceptance of its inevitability have been identified as potential contributors to clinicians' avoidance (Millar et al. 2013). The authors (Millar et al. 2013) believed palliative care staff avoided the issue less than nonpalliative care staff and were more holistic in their approach. The relative silence regarding weight loss and cachexia encountered by patients and family members from health professionals may be related to the paucity of therapeutically effective interventions (Reid et al. 2010). Inaccurate knowledge can result in nurses and doctors relying on a nutritional response, even when they knew it would not be effective (Millar et al. 2013). In addition to knowledge, dialogue needs to be effective and the active integration of patients, families, and nurses into clinical decision-making is recommendation (del Rio et al. 2011).

Issues associated with declining oral intake are likely to arise over a longer timeframe than dilemmas associated with CANH. A degree of burden and potential harm for both the ill person and their family members is evident in relation to declining oral intake, as are the challenges of exercising autonomy when unwell. The concept of autonomy, that a person has the right to accept, refuse or decline care and treatments is widely accepted in Western bioethics (Bear et al. 2017; Royal College of Physicians and British Society of Gastroenterology 2010; Watson et al. 2009). Nevertheless, few people act or make choices about health care completely independently of other influences. Included may be the wishes of others, hopes, prior knowledge or experience, cultural influences, and religious beliefs. Having the capacity to act autonomously does not necessarily translate into one's personal choice being fulfilled.

Failing to meet the needs of both relatives and patients reveals a significant burden, a potential source of harm, and the possibility of undermining autonomy. All have implications for justice in care delivery. The ethical principle of justice also relates to how health professionals engage with those they care for and includes honesty in terms of not imposing one's own wishes, values, and preferences (Truog et al. 2015). Clinicians should be cognizant of this when they are enveloped in and perhaps invested in not only the philosophy of palliative care but also what is routine and standard practice. Acceptance of the status quo or professional comfort may adversely impact on care. In the presence of declining or compromised oral intake, patients, families, and clinicians may consider the use of CANH.

8 Clinically Assisted Nutrition and Hydration: Forgoing, Providing, and Withdrawing

Vignette two: Nasogastric feeding commenced amidst rapid deterioration from an undiagnosed illness. In the family meeting, the irreversible cause could finally be explained to the patient's family, with death anticipated very soon. The partner requested feeding continue. A sibling recalled the person's preceding loss of appetite and interest in food, another noted how unsightly the feeding tube was on their now severely debilitated and barely responding brother. Tearfully the partner responded, "I can't bear the thought of him starving to death. I don't want him to think we have given up and I have abandoned him."

Family members are not alone in perceiving the forgoing or withdrawal of CANH as harmful and a sign of care being abandoned. Ethically, the focus in palliative care is often on CANH, its appropriate and timely provision and decisions to withdrawal or forgo it (Royal College of Physicians and British Society of Gastroenterology 2010; Truog 2014).

Clinicians often feel more comfortable withholding (acts of omission) rather than withdrawing (acts of commission) therapies such as CANH, although the two are often regarded as ethically the same (Royal College of Physicians and British Society of Gastroenterology 2010; Truog 2014). Withdrawing CANH is a decision to stop a therapy after commencement, while withholding or forgoing CANH is the decision not to start. All decisions around CAHN require careful consideration, including if it is appropriate in the last weeks to days of life (Royal College of Physicians and British Society of Gastroenterology 2010). Differing views are held by individual practitioners and professional groups, including physicians (Chambaere et al. 2014; Morita et al. 2002; Torres-Vigil et al. 2012) and nurses (Stiles 2013) regardless of professional and ethical frameworks. Those most affected by these decisions are patients and family members.

9 Patients and Families

Many people receiving palliative care experience declining oral intake over the course of their illness. In the terminally ill, causes of declining oral intake are often multifactorial and include swallowing difficulties, loss of appetite, nausea and vomiting, and physical obstruction (Raijmakers et al. 2011). In the presence of weight loss, and difficulties with oral feeding, it is common for standard care concerning food and fluid to be questioned, leading to discussions on how best to redress perceived needs for nutrition and hydration. Although there is an obligation to use ordinary means to support food and fluids, there is no firm obligation to use extraordinary measures, which require consideration of both the benefit and burdens of medical therapies, CANH included (Druml et al. 2016; Royal College of Physicians and British Society of Gastroenterology 2010). Despite this clear description of CANH as a medical therapy rather than ordinary care, it is more complex in practice. Artificial hydration and nutrition can be a controversial topic in specialist palliative care yet it is often, but not always, perceived positively by patients and families. Table 1 illustrates some of the meanings and perceptions of patients and family members.

The attentiveness, loss of shared mealtimes, and social isolation experienced when supporting a person receiving CANH are similar to challenges described by family members in relation to declining oral intake (Raijmakers et al. 2013; Wallin et al. 2013). Significantly, CANH does not redress these aspects of daily life. The perceived benefits and burdens of CANH should not obscure the necessity to engage in efforts to consider the less tangible elements which influence the experiences of care giving and receiving, like ethics, culture, and emotions (del Rio et al. 2011).

Potential benefits, clinical risks, and burdens can be and are tabulated (del Rio et al. 2011; Kozeniecki et al. 2017; Royal College of Physicians and British Society of Gastroenterology 2010). However, there is a paucity of clinical evidence to guide and inform (Good et al. 2014; Royal College of Physicians and British Society of Gastroenterology 2010). A review of the literature regarding the emotional impact, perceptions, and decision-making among patients, families, and clinicians associated with CANH identified that insufficient information and misunderstandings prevailed (del Rio et al. 2011).

Patients and family members have expressed similar preferences in relation to CANH at the end of life and patients were usually very clear about their preferences (Bükki et al. 2014). However, relatives tended to be more conservative when deciding for others rather than themselves. Older age was associated with deciding to decline CANH by relatives and patients, with relatives more concerned about the physical impact of withdrawing CANH than patients. Importantly, more than one third of the participants (patients and relatives) would forgo CANH and the authors (Bükki et al. 2014) noted this differed from other qualitative studies.

Vignette two illustrates complex yet familiar challenges in palliative care. Routine intravenous fluids had commenced when the severity of the patient's illness was unclear and the patient could exercise autonomy. He consented to the nasogastric tube (NGT) when swallowing became difficult but his wishes if the prognosis was poor were not explored. Opportunities for advanced care planning were missed, compromising his autonomy. When the prognosis became clear, the patient's verbal and written communication abilities had been lost. The siblings, alarmed at the partner's determination to maintain CANH, recalled his anorexia. They did not perceive him as hungry nor the feeding as beneficial and believed he would not want his life prolonged in this context. The partner acknowledged their concerns but could not reconcile feeding withdrawal with her sense of abandoning him. A compromise was reached; the IV fluids would be reduced and stopped when the line occluded. Feeding would be reduced and the NGT removed when he became unconscious.

Continuing CANH could be conceived as poor resource use, and contrary to the principle of justice. Endeavors were made to minimize staff time and optimize resources with reduced IV fluids and feeding volumes. Negotiating a compromise minimized risks of unnecessary current and future suffering for the patient, partner, and siblings. The clinicians endeavored to care for the patient and family unit and to do so holistically. The ethical challenges resulted from an initially unknown prognosis, the absence of clear communication, and recording of the patient's wishes combined with differing family perspectives, and the lack of robust scientific evidence regarding the benefits and burdens of CANH at the end of life. Although utilization of CANH as a resource could not be justified due to the poor prognosis (Orrevall 2015; Royal College of Physicians and British Society of Gastroenterology 2010), it could be argued that it was in their psychological best

Table 1 The meaning of CANH for patients and families

Population	Key points	Authors
Positive perspectives for patients and families		
The meaning of CAH for hospice patients and family carers (USA)	Hope Of prolonging life Supporting dignity Improved quality of life through reducing symptoms Provided comfort By reducing pain Enhancing the efficacy of analgesics Nourishing holistically	Cohen et al. (2012)
Patients' and relatives' perceptions of CAH (Italy)	IV fluids perceived as highly effective Nourishing Positive psychologically (>90%) IV fluids were perceived as more effective and not burdensome IV fluids were preferred over SC fluids even at home	Mercadante et al. (2005)
Patients' and relatives' perceptions of home parenteral nutrition (Sweden)	Relief and security that nutritional needs were being met Positive effect on QOL, weight, energy, strength and activity Relieved the pressure to eat Shared burden with the home visiting clinicians (distinguished between enteral and parenteral routes),	Orrevall et al. (2005)
Family members experiences of caring for patients receiving tube feeding (Canada)	Negotiating a new "normal" Supported their priority to provide adequate hydration and nutrition Reduced family tension over intake	Penner et al. (2012)
Limitations or burdens for patients and families		
The meaning of CAH for hospice patients and family carers of (USA)	They knew it wouldn't cure, nor replace eating	Cohen et al. (2012)
Patients' and relatives' perceptions CAH (Italy)	SC route not as effective nor less troublesome	Mercadante et al. (2005)
Patients' and relatives' perceptions of home parenteral nutrition (Sweden)	Restricted family and social life Checking on overnight administration – "free" and not free evenings Only partially solves issues by delivering nutrition (social aspects of eating not redressed)	Orrevall et al. (2005)
Family members' experiences of caring for patients receiving tube feeding (Canada)	Negotiating a new "normal" Changed roles Little choice and redefined from spouse to caregiver Challenge of multiple roles (old and new) responsibility of new skills, providing feeds, responding to symptoms Physical toll, disturbed sleep, and psychological burden Altered lifestyle Lack of freedom, less personal time, fitting life in between feeding, being tied down in their caregiving role and diminished social contact Changes to their oral intake (guilt and to reduce food odors)	Penner et al. (2012)

interests (Royal College of Physicians and British Society of Gastroenterology 2010). In clinical discussions, the issue of prolonging dying by providing fluids in the absence of nutrition should be addressed (Royal College of Physicians and British Society of Gastroenterology 2010).

10 Clinicians

Vignette three: Lucy, diagnosed with metastatic bowel cancer, presented to the hospital emergency department overnight with intractable vomiting. An abdominal x-ray revealed a high bowel obstruction. Treatment commenced with an NGT and IV fluids, and a scan planned for the morning. Lucy declined the scan and surgical review and requested hospice transfer for terminal care. This was arranged on the understanding that IV fluids would stop. At the morning clinical meeting, hospice staff discussed Lucy's impending transfer and plan of care. Lucy's goals and wishes had previously been documented by a hospice community nurse. Included were her intention to decline further surgery if a bowel obstruction occurred and her wish to die in the hospice. A doctor questioned Lucy's decision because she was not significantly cachexic when seen the previous week and chose to explore Lucy's decision. Lucy described her previous complicated postoperative journey, becoming increasingly distressed and eventually angry that her decisions were revisited. Her husband remained beside her, tense and silent. The doctor looked to the husband who eventually spoke. He did not want Lucy to die but he could not stop it happening. He explained he would never ask her to experience again what she had already endured. Silence followed. Eventually, the nurse asked Lucy what her wishes and priorities were now. She wanted to be comfortable, supported to live, if possible, until her daughter and grandchildren arrived. Then she wanted the clinical team to stop anything that might prolong her life. A plan was agreed, including a NGT on free drainage, oral intake as desired, trialling medical management of the obstruction, medications subcutaneously, and subcutaneous fluids overnight until the family arrived.

Endeavors to ensure ethical principles and professional obligations are appropriately met can result in tensions between the triad of patients, family members and clinicians, and within families and among clinicians. Peoples' hopes and expectations, including those of clinicians, are often not uniform and static. Palliative care nurses hold heterogeneous attitudes towards CANH, including whether it was a medical treatment or a minimum standard of care (Stiles 2013). Their views varied in recognition of the complex interaction of multiple influences including legal, ethical, social, clinical, and professional elements. Others, including patients, family members, doctors, and nursing colleagues influenced them. Although significant variation across the six research studies reviewed (Byron et al. 2008; L. Ke et al. 2008a; L. S. Ke et al. 2008b; Konishi et al. 2002; Miyashita et al. 2008; van der Riet et al. 2008) was identified and the influence of culture noted, nurses perceived the patient's autonomy as most important. In four studies from Asia, family rather than individual decision-making was identified as predominant although in all publications CANH was a significant issue and nurses experienced moral distress when family wishes prevailed over patient autonomy (Stiles 2013).

Physicians, like nurses, have differing attitudes regarding whether CANH is a medical treatment or a minimum standard of care (Morita et al. 2002), including those in specialist palliative care (Torres-Vigil et al. 2012). Internationally, practices regarding physicians' decisions to forgo or withdraw CANH for patients at the end of life differ (Buiting et al. 2007; Morita et al. 2002; Raijmakers et al. 2011; Torres-Vigil et al. 2012). In the care of patients with cancer in the last week of life, the utilization of CANH can vary widely with CAN administration varying from 3% to 53% while the utilization of CAH ranged from 12% to 88%. (Raijmakers et al. 2011). Mixed results were identified from this literature review, with some studies reporting positive effects and others negative and no studies focused solely on CAN. Utilization of CANH was less common in specialist palliative settings where death may be more likely to be predicted. While focused on the last week of life, reviewers noted the paucity of evidence regarding CANH's efficacy, and the positive perception of it by family members and patients (Raijmakers et al. 2011). The prevalence of studies from Asia, particularly in relation to CAH was noted and ongoing enquiry concerning CANH from the Asia Pacific region has continued (Bükki et al. 2014).

Decisions regarding withdrawing or forgoing life-prolonging treatments also differed across six Western European countries (Belgium [Flanders], Denmark, Italy, The Netherlands, Sweden, and Switzerland) (Buiting et al. 2007). Forgoing CAH occurred least in Italy (2.6%) and most frequently in the Netherlands (10.9%). Withholding CANH was more common than withdrawing and occurred more often for older people

(≥80 yrs), females, a malignant diagnosis and diseases of the nervous system. It was least common in hospitals, except for Sweden (Buiting et al. 2007). A more recent survey of physicians in Flanders, Belgium, found "... a decision to forego ANH occurred in 6.6% of all deaths (4.2% withheld, 3.0% withdrawn)" (Chambaere et al. 2014, p. 501). Patient characteristics were similar to the earlier study (Buiting et al. 2007). Variation in prescribing practices also occurs outside Europe and among palliative care physicians.

Prescribing practices of palliative care physicians (n = 238) in a Latin American study were not congruent with usual palliative care practices where CANH is more likely to be forgone at the end of life (Torres-Vigil et al. 2012). Over half (60%) prescribed CAH for their patients in the last week of life and beliefs that it was beneficial clinically and psychologically were the main reasons. The physicians were more likely to disagree with the premise that withholding CAH was beneficial for symptom management. They believed CAH met minimum standards of care and the SC route was preferred. Hospital in-patients were more likely to receive parenteral hydration (57%) and receive it IV (59%) than patients at home (45%) who were more likely to receive fluids SC (68%). Practical issues inhibited in-home CAH.

Physicians do believe CANH impacts on life time, with European physicians reporting decisions related to CANH and other measures as foreshortening life, most often by less than a week, although it could be longer (Buiting et al. 2007). Interestingly, with the exception of Belgium, when CANH was forgone fewer medications were given for symptom management than for other patients, leading the authors to conclude this did not add to symptom burden and suffering (Buiting et al. 2007). Physicians in Belgium (Chambaere et al. 2014) estimated that in 77% of cases the decision had some influence in foreshortening life. "An explicit intention of hastening death was present in a quarter of cases where ANH was withheld and in half where it was withdrawn" (Chambaere et al. 2014, p. 502). This needs to be considered in the legislative context of patients' rights, euthanasia, and palliative care in Belgium. Including patients in discussions may not have been possible because of their cognitive status, and in Belgium, physicians can autonomously withdraw futile treatment (Chambaere et al. 2014).

Clinician experience is one of many influences on clinical practice. A 2002 study of Japanese physicians (n = 584, a response rate of 53%) identified that comfort and experience with end-of-life care influenced their perceptions of the appropriateness of IV hydration in terminally ill cancer patients (Morita et al. 2002). Those less involved in end of life gave greater volumes of fluid and believed there were greater benefits than harm. While 96% agreed with patients' right to decline CAH, declining oral intake in the terminal stage was not seen as part of the natural dying process for 53% of respondents. Nearly one-third (32%) agreed that it was not ethically permissible to allow patients to die dehydrated, while 40% believed IV fluid was the minimum standard of care rather than a medical treatment. Once again a tension is revealed between the professional position that CANH is a medical treatment, established palliative care practice, acceptance of the dying process as natural and individual physician's practices. Diverse perceptions and decision-making regarding the influence of CANH in postponing or hastening death adds to the complexity of the palliative care goals to do neither.

The need for early discussions with patients to identify their preferences has been noted, as was the need for clinicians to be well informed due to their significant influence on decision-making regarding CANH (Mercadante et al. 2005). Knowledge is crucial to dispel myths and engage confidently with patients and families (Bükki et al. 2014). Nevertheless, education alone may not be sufficient. An education program in Taiwan focusing on CANH did not override the influences of the food and family culture to change clinical behavior (L. Ke et al. 2008a).

Returning to vignette three, the clinical staff had a responsibility to ensure Lucy was making an informed decision and understood possible benefits and burdens. Justice was evident in offering a surgical review and an acceptable level of care negotiated. Importantly, with death anticipated, clinical staff rechecked if Lucy's wishes had changed. Unfortunately, this was distressing for her. The appropriate utilization of resources, with the offer to explore surgical options, could be questioned (Royal College of Physicians and British Society of Gastroenterology 2010). However, as it transpired, the resources to support her wishes were modest and met the psychosocial needs of the patient and family and were congruent with palliative care goals of care (World Health Organization 2002). This vignette illustrates the complexity of autonomy, the uncertainty of what may be a benefit or a burden and the importance of having courage in difficult conversations. It also reinforces the importance of knowledge, quality communication, advanced care planning, and appreciating the diverse meanings of food and fluids and CAHN for all parties.

11 Summary and Conclusion

Clinicians draw on clinical evidence, ethical frameworks, protocols, guidelines, and established practice, but these do not eliminate emotional responses, anxiety, cultural and religious influences, and misunderstandings. They are embedded in their own life biographies, a milieu of spiritual, societal, and cultural influences including ethnic, workplace, and professional cultures. Equally, the people they care for are also embedded in their life experience and influenced by their spiritual belief system, society, culture, family culture, and relationships. These factors in the context of living and dying, food and fluids, experiences with and the meaning of food and fluid creates a complex dynamic. With such diversity, freely exercising autonomy and perceptions of benefit and burden and fairness are unlikely to be congruent. Disparity and the need for early, repeated, collaborative, and ethical dialogue is inevitable and should be anticipated and accepted.

Clinician communication is a recurring theme in relation to the meaning of food and fluids, CANH and the perceptions of patients, families. The potential to moderate the focus on food and fluids which can be constraining and oppressive is an important clinical and ethical issue. The changes that occur in advanced illness and dying require open acknowledgement and early engagement whenever possible. These discussions should include the goals of care in relation to the use of CANH, its benefits, burdens, role in symptom management, the patient's and family's wishes, their values, beliefs, and cultural practices. Communication is clearly important although it alone is unlikely to assuage all concerns.

The development and refinement of CANH continues to be discussed, questioned, and researched regarding its place in the context and provision of palliative care. Perceptions of basic care and medical treatment in relation to CANH is not homogenous within professions. Additionally, the established palliative care approach of accepting declining in oral intake and dehydration as natural at the end of life is not universally accepted. The diversity identified and challenges faced, including those by palliative care clinicians, raises issues not addressed here regarding how to best support the mainstreaming of palliative care practices, and the growing international specialty in managing these ethical issues.

The commonality is a desire to alleviate suffering. However, the lack of certainty regarding the type and amount of suffering underpins the need to keep knowledge current and personalize care. Clinicians will have encountered conversations where the desire to give food and fluids prevails in the absence of a patient narrative that indicates they desire it or feel they are suffering in its absence.

Clear evidence of the acceptable benefits of CANH would probably be more readily accepted and acceptable than clear evidence of unacceptable burdens. Importantly, not all benefits related to CAHN are nutritional. A definitive answer appropriate for people with malignant and nonmalignant conditions with advanced progressive illness at the end of life is unlikely. Therefore, in the absence of certainty, current knowledge, effective appropriate dialogue, clinical case-by-case consideration and negotiated compromise are appropriate. Individualized care for patients and their companions that is respectful of their biographies, varied rather than homogenous, and founded on curiosity rather than a prescribed dialogue is indicated. Food and fluids and CANH are likely to remain enduring ethical challenges in palliative and end-of-life care; however, when these issues arise and decisions are made in partnership, there are important opportunities to improve care at the end of life.

References

Amano K, Maeda I, Morita T, Okajima Y, Hama T, Aoyama M, et al. Eating-related distress and need for nutritional support of families of advanced cancer patients: a nationwide survey of bereaved family members. J Cachexia Sarcopenia Muscle. 2016;7:527–34.

Barrocas A. The troubling trichotomy 10 years later: where are we now. Nutr Clin Pract. 2016;31(3):295–304.

Bear AJ, Bukowy EA, Patel JJ. Artificial hydration at the end of life. Nutr Clin Pract. 2017;32(5):628–32.

Benedetti FD, Ostgathe C, Clark J, Costantini M, Daud ML, Grossenbacher-Gschwend B, et al. International palliative care experts' view on phenomena indicating the last hours and days of life. Support Care Cancer. 2013;21(6):1509–17. https://doi.org/10.1007/s00520-012-1677-3.

Buiting HM, van Delden JJM, Rietjens JAC, Onwuteaka-Philipsen BD, Bilsen J, Fischer S, et al. Forgoing artificial nutrition or hydration in patients nearing death in six European countries. J Pain Symptom Manag. 2007;34(3):305–14.

Bükki J, Unterpaul T, Nübling G, Jox RJ, Lorenzl S. Decision making at the end of life – cancer patients' and their caregivers' views on artificial nutrition and hydration. Support Care Cancer. 2014;22:3287–99.

Byron E, de Casterie BD, Gastman C. Nurses' attitudes towards artificial food or fluid administration in patients with dementia and in terminally ill patients: a review of the literature. J Med Ethics. 2008;34(6):431–6.

Chambaere K, Loodts I, Deliens L, Cohen J. Forgoing artificial nutrition or hydration at the end of life: a large cross-sectional survey in Belgium. J Med Ethics. 2014;40:501–4.

Chow R, Bruera E, Chiu L, Chow S, Chiu N, Lam H, et al. Enteral and parenteral nutrition in cancer patients: a systematic review and meta-analysis. Ann Palliat Med. 2016;5(1):30–41.

Clark J, Raijmakers N, Allan S, van Zuylen L, van der Heide A. Declining oral intake towards the end of life: how to talk about it? A qualitative study. Int J Palliat Nurs. 2017;23(2):74–62.

Cohen M, Torres-Vigil I, Burbach BE, de la Posa A, Bruerea E. The meaning of parenteral hydration to family caregivers and patients with advanced cancer receiving hospice care. J Pain Symptom Manag. 2012;43(5):855–65.

del Rio MI, Shand B, Bonati P, Palma A, Maldonado A, Taboada P, Nervi F. Hydration and nutrition at the end of life: a systematic review of emotional impact, perceptions and decision-making amongst patients, families and health care staff. Psycho-Oncology. 2011; 21(9):913–21.

Druml C, Ballmer PE, Druml W, Oehmichen F, Shenkin A, Singer P, et al. EPSN guideline on ethical aspects of artificial nutrition and hydration. Clin Nutr. 2016;35: 545–56.

Evans WJ, Morley JE, Argile's J, Bales C, Baracos V, Guttridge D, et al. Cachexia: a new definition. Clin Nutr. 2008;27:793–9.

Fallon M, Smyth J. Terminology: the historical perspective, evolution and current usage – room for confusion? Eur J Cancer. 2008;44:1069–71.

Fearon K, Strasser F, Anker SD, Bosaeus I, Bruera E, Fasinger RL, et al. Definition and classification of cancer cachexia: an international concensus. Lancet Oncol. 2011;12:489–95.

Ganzini L. Artificial nutrition and hydration at the end of life: ethics and evidence. Palliat Support Care. 2006; 4:135–43.

Ganzini L, Goy ER, Miller LL, Harvath TA, Jackson A, Delorit MA. Nurses' experiences with hospice patients who refuse food and fluids to hasten death. N Engl J Med. 2003;349:359–65.

Good P, Richard R, Syrmis W, Jenkins-Marsh S, Stephens J. Medically assisted hydration for adult palliative care patients (publication no. 10.1002/14651858.CD006273). The Cochrane Database of Systematic Reviews from Wiley. 2014.

Hopkinson JB. Food connections: a qualitative exploratory study of weight-and eating-related distress in families affected by advanced cancer. Eur J Oncol Nurs. 2016; 20:87–96.

Ivanović N, Büche D, Fringer A. Voluntary stopping of eating and drinking at the end of life – a 'systematic search and review' giving insight into an option of hastening death in capacitated adults at the end of life. Br Med J Palliat Care. 2014;*13*(1):1–8. http://www.biomedcentral.com/1472-684X/13/1. https://doi.org/10.1186/1472-684X-13-1.

Ke L, Chiu T, Hu W, Lo S. Effects of educational intervention on nurses' knowledge, attitudes, and behavioral intentions toward supplying artificial nutrition and hydration to terminal cancer patients. Support Care Cancer. 2008a;16:1265–72. https://doi.org/10.1007/s00520-008-0426-0 .

Ke LS, Chiu TY, Lo SS, Hu WY. Knowledge attitudes and behavioral intentions of nurses toward providing artifical nutrition and hydration for terminal cancer patients in Taiwan. Cancer Nurs. 2008b;31(1):67–76.

Konishi E, Davis AJ, Aiba T. The ethics of withdrawing artificial food and fluid from terminally ill patients: an end of life dilemma for Japanese nurses and families. Nurs Ethics. 2002;9(1):7–19.

Kozeniecki M, Ewy M, Patel JJ. Nutrition at the end of life: It's not what you say, it's how you say it. Curr Nutr Rep. 2017;6(3):261–5.

Mercadante S, Ferrera P, Girello D, Casuccio A. Patients' and relatives' perceptions about subcutaneous hydration. J Pain Symptom Manag. 2005;30(4):354–8.

Millar C, Reid J, Porter S. Health care professionals' response to cachexia in advanced cancer: a qualitative study. Oncol Nurs Forum. 2013;40(6):393–402.

Miyashita M, Morita T, Shima Y, Kimura R, Takahashi M, Adachi I. Nurses' views of the adequacy of decision making and nurses' distress regarding artificial hydration for terminally ill cancer patients: a nationwide survey. Am J Hosp Palliat Care. 2008.

Morgan M. Beautiful veins. Wollongong: Five Islands Press; 1999.

Morita T, Shima Y, Adaci I. Attitudes of Japanese physicians towards terminal dehydration: a nationwide survey. J Clin Oncol. 2002;20(24):4699–704.

O'Hara P. The management of nutrition for palliative care patients. Links Health Soc Care. 2017;2(1):21–38.

Orrevall Y. Nutritional support at the end of life. Nutrition. 2015;31:615–6.

Orrevall Y, Tishelman C, Permert J. Home parenteral nutrition: a qualitative interview study of the experiences of advanced cancer patients and their families. Clin Nutr. 2005;24:941–70.

Penner JL, McClement S, Lobchuck M, Daeninck P. Family members' experiences caring for patients with advanced head and neck cancer recieving tube feeding: a descriptive phenomological study. J Pain Symptom Manag. 2012;44(4):563–51.

Raijmakers NJH, van Zuylen L, Costantini M, Caraceni A, Clark J, Lundquist G, et al. Artificial hydration and nutrition in the last week of life in cancer patients. A systematic review of practices and effects. Ann Oncol. 2011;22(7):1477–86.

Raijmakers NJH, Clark JB, van Zuylen L, Allan S, van der Heide A. Bereaved family members' perspectives of the patient's oral intake towards the end of life. Palliat Med. 2013;27(7):665–72.

Reid J, McKenna H, Fitzsimons D, McCance T. The experience of cancer cachexia: a qualitative study of advanced cancer patients and their family members. Int J Nurs Stud. 2009a;46:606–16.

Reid J, McKenna H, Fitzsimons D, McCance T. Fighting over food: patient and family understanding of cancer cachexia. Oncol Nurs Forum. 2009b;36(4):439–45.

Reid J, McKenna HP, Fitzsimons D, McCance TV. An explorations of the experience of cancer cachexia: what patients and their families want from health professionals. Eur J Cancer Care. 2010;19(682–689): 682–9.

Royal College of Physicians and British Society of Gastroenterology. Oral feeding difficulties and dilemmas: a guide to practical care, particularly towards the end of life. London: Royal College of Physicians; 2010.

Rozin P. The meaning of food in our lives: a cross-cultural perspective on eating and well-being. J Nutr Educ Behav. 2005;37(2):107–12.

Stiles E. Providing artificial nutrition and hydration in palliative care. Nurs Stand. 2013;27(20):35–42.

Torres-Vigil I, Mendoza TR, Alonso-Babarro A, DeLima L, Cardenas-Turanzas M, Hernandez M, et al. Practice patterns and perceptions about parenteral hydration in the last weeks of life: a survey of palliative care physicians in Latin America. J Pain Symptom Manag. 2012;43(1):47–58.

Truog RD. Withholding and withdrawing life sustaining treatments. In: Quill ET, Miller FG, editors. *Palliative care and ethics*. Oxford: Oxford University Press; 2014. p. 187–98.

Truog RD, Brown SD, Browning D, Hundert EM, Rider EA, Bell SK, Myer EC. Microethics: the ethics of everyday clinical practice. Hast Cent. 2015;45(1):11–7. https://doi.org/10.1002/hast.413.

van der Riet P, Good P, Higgins I, Sneesby L. Palliative care professionals' perceptions of nutrition at the end of life. Int J Palliat Nurs. 2008;14(3):145–51.

Vassilyadi F, Panteliadou A, Panteliadis C. Hallmarks in the history of enteral and parenteral nutrition: from antiquity to the 20th century. Nurtr Clin Pract. 2013;28(2):209–17.

Wallin V, Carlander I, Sandman PO, Ternestedt BM, Hakanson C. Maintaining ordinariness around food: partners' experiences of everyday life with a dying person. J Clin Nurs. 2013;23:2748–56.

Wallin V, Carlander I, Sandman PO, Hakanson C. Meanings of eating deficiencies for people admitted to palliative home care. Palliat Support Care. 2015;13:1231–9.

Watson M, Lucas C, Hoy A, Wells J. Oxford handbook of palliative care. 2nd ed. Oxford: Oxford University Press; 2009.

Wax JW, An AW, Kosier N, Quill TE. Voluntary stopping eating and drinking. J Am Geriatr Soc. 2018;66:441–5. https://doi.org/10.1111/jgs.15200.

World Health Organization. National cancer control programmes: policies and managerial guidelines. Geneva: World Health Organization; 2002.

Attending to the Suffering Other: A Case Study of Teleconsultation in Palliative Care at Home

89

Jelle van Gurp, Jeroen Hasselaar, Evert van Leeuwen, Martine van Selm, and Kris Vissers

Contents

J. van Gurp (✉)
IQ healthcare/Ethics of healthcare, Radboud University Medical Center, Nijmegen, The Netherlands
e-mail: Jelle.vanGurp@radboudumc.nl

J. Hasselaar · K. Vissers
Department of Anesthesiology, Pain and Palliative Medicine, Radboud University Medical Center, Nijmegen, The Netherlands

E. van Leeuwen
Professor Emeritus of IQ healthcare/Ethics of healthcare, Radboud University Medical Center, Nijmegen, The Netherlands

M. van Selm
Amsterdam School of Communication Research, University of Amsterdam, Amsterdam, The Netherlands

R. D. MacLeod, L. Van den Block (eds.), *Textbook of Palliative Care*,
https://doi.org/10.1007/978-3-319-77740-5_119

Abstract

Although this chapter has its origins in the Dutch practice of palliative care at home, its message is relevant to all countries in which a considerable percentage of the population prefers to die at home. These people usually depend to a great extent on general practitioners to realize such a death at home. Although there are exceptions, many generalists lack experience with and/or knowledge of palliative care. These limitations show themselves most in complex cases and often result in the patient being hospitalized. This chapter provides a perspective on a potential (part of the) solution to integrate generalist and specialist palliative care at the patient's home: teleconsultation. It describes how to empirically and ethically study such a complex, technological intervention within a particular care practice, with a focus on the fit of the technology. Teleconsultation technology should be considered non-neutral. It mediates the relationships between patients and their accompanying professionals, while also coshaping experiences of virtual proximity and real-time autonomy. It can also be a constant reminder of an approaching death. Teleconsultation appears to provide opportunities for professionals to experience responsibility for a patient's suffering and to address it adequately, although its scripts do not fill the need for meaningful moments of silence. In the end, this chapter claims that teleconsultation can be of value to the practice of palliative homecare, if special consideration has been given to its careful use by professionals. Teleconsultation requires an open and humble attitude toward both patients and colleagues, as well as sensitivity for privacy issues.

1 Introduction

Ms. K., in her mid-60s, suffers from recurrent bladder cancer. During her last visit at the hospital, it appeared that the disease was already in an advanced stage and metastasized into the liver, the lungs, and the bones. Her oncologist recently told her that recovery was very unlikely and that she would advise her to opt for a palliative care approach. Such an approach would focus on preserving her quality of life as long as possible by trying to prevent and relieve pain, other physical discomfort, as well as psychosocial and spiritual problems. She agreed with her oncologist and discussed her future care and treatment plan with the hospital-based palliative care specialists. During this discussion the question arose where Ms. K. would like to spend the last phase of her life. She immediately responded that home is where her heart is. Her husband is there, as well as her little dog. Moreover, her home contains 30 years of personal history. She hopes she can stay at home until she dies, but she fears that dying at home might be impossible due to all the complex problems that will probably come with her physical decline. How can treatment and care be organized in such a way that Ms. K. is able to pass away peacefully in her own home?

Each year, a lot of people like Ms. K. are in need of palliative care. The continuously increasing aging of Western populations will induce an increase of chronic diseases, such as cancer, heart failure, and dementia, leading to a steep rise of non-sudden deaths in the nearby future Statistics Netherlands (2017). This chapter focuses on a potentially important shift in healthcare policy, namely, to provide adequate care for most of these chronically ill people in *their own homes*. This includes providing adequate palliative and end-of-life care at home. One of the challenges is to make expert palliative care available for those home-based palliative care patients who develop complex problems and needs and for whom the general palliative care delivered by primary care physicians is no longer sufficient. Such expert palliative care is supposed to prevent burdensome transitions to specialist palliative care facilities and/or hospitals in the last phase of life. Communication technologies supplying synchronous audiovisual contact are considered potential solutions for the transfer of expert palliative care, but the fit of these technologies in existing palliative care practices is only limitedly explained (e.g., Pols 2012). This chapter aims to show and explain the fit of teleconsultation in the practice of palliative care at home, with particular attention to the ethical dimensions of palliative telecare.

2 Ethics: Will Palliative Telecare Contribute to Attending to a Patient's Suffering?

Literature of patient narratives demonstrates that suffering quite often is an alienating experience for (palliative care) patients (Cassell 1991; Frank 2001). When patients are suffering, their wounded body or mind preoccupies them, hindering subjectivity, intentionality, and involvement in everyday life (Charmaz 1983; Van Hooft 2003). Healthcare professionals only have limited practical tools to heal these wounds and are often confronted with patients who continue to be socially and aesthetically out of sync with healthy others around them, as well as with their own previous lives (Frank 2001). Those who suffer as a result of life-threatening illnesses often no longer have the "enchantment of a future," (Cassell 1991) and they have often also lost what "they valued and enjoyed in the past" (Charmaz 1983).

2.1 Introducing the Perspective of Levinas

Healthcare professionals get acquainted with a patient's suffering through what Levinas refers to as the *Face* (Box 1).

Box 1

Why the ideas of Emmanuel Levinas (France, 1906–1995) are relevant to current medical practice?

- Levinas' life's work concerned hospitality, intersubjectivity, and lived immediacy.
- Levinas has written on what precedes (medical) ethics, about the responsibility to our patients before we even begin to think about it.
- Levinas offers a unique phenomenological description of the intersubjective relation between, for example, a patient and a healthcare professional before they start trying to categorize one another in work and words.
- Levinas challenges us to become aware that every conversation, every type of communication always demands a response: a responding to another. The patient who is in the immediacy of healthcare professionals already summons these professionals, even before a de facto command is uttered.
- Levinas' work about the face-to-face encounter, which is essential in patient-professional communication, forms a solid base to think over the mediation of patient-professional communication by modern communication technologies.

Levinas' Face can be understood as all those elements of a suffering being that express a pre-reflexive, ethical, demanding appeal: crying, bodily gestures, becoming rigid, the skin, et cetera (Burggraeve 1986). The capital "F" emphasizes the pureness of the suffering – its nakedness as a consequence of an extreme vulnerability – that appeals to other human beings through its uncoveredness and finitude. A patient's Face is disruptive; it commands humility while not representing something else but itself (Peperzak 1991; Levinas 1996, 2005).

The Face communicates suffering as an intangible and untranslatable part of the human being. It defines the patient as an Other, as one who is appealing beyond the reach of common comprehension and rational analysis (Pinchevsky 2005). Healthcare professionals may experience standing face-to-face with their suffering patients: a patient's suffering urges healthcare professionals to surpass their professional ability to appropriate and objectify the patient and his/her suffering in words (medical diagnosis) and work (treatment) (Levinas 2011). The Face commands caregivers to openly and unconditionally engage *with* the patient, to greet and "welcome" the patient as a fellow human being before anything else can be communicated or done.

2.2 "Welcoming" a Patient: Proximity in Technology-Mediated Communication

A patient's suffering forces healthcare professionals to maintain the wondrous orientation, the welcoming, that precedes all (communicative) action. It offers the opportunity to open up to the patient without knowing for sure how he/she will be able to be involved in actual communication and further action (Levinas 2011). Such a humble communicative stance precedes any procedural frameworks of physician competences and activities. It implies an awareness of the "communicating of communication," wherein previous images and concepts are still irrelevant and patients are unconditionally welcomed. For the patient, such an original and silent invitation of the healthcare professional creates a way out of the isolation into which the suffering has forced him. A humble attitude enables proximity and, figuratively, an engaged wandering in patients' stories that will redefine the healthcare professional's personal, medical role. This being said, how could this idea about welcoming a suffering human being be related to teleconsultation technologies? These Internet-based communication technologies, at least, call into question (a) the appearance of suffering (the Face) within these communication technologies, (b) the pre-communicative orientation toward a suffering patient, and (c) proximity.

2.3 The Need for Empirical-Ethical Research

The innovative application of teleconsultation to the practice of palliative homecare should be considered "a complex practice still under construction" (Pols 2012). A long-term, naturalistic approach is considered essential to study such complex practices still under construction in which patients, informal caregivers, and healthcare professionals continuously try to reshape and refine teleconsultation in palliative care at home. A qualitative, naturalistic approach helps to uncover the interactional patterns, participants' continuous adaptations to teleconsultation, as well as unanticipated results. The knowledge resulting from a long-term and naturalistic investigation could determine how teleconsultation changed the existing palliative homecare, if at all (Corbin and Strauss 2008; Pols 2012). Teleconsultations can be considered crossings where various perspectives and actions meet, bringing about new perspectives and actions in the home of patients, in the primary care practice, and in the hospital (Ihde 1990). Such an approach implies the use of several qualitative methods, such as observations, interviews, and group interviews, to follow participants over time to learn about their experiences, stories, and practical knowledge (Pols 2012). Analyses should then lead to a conceptual understanding of the practice of teleconsultation in palliative homecare based on participant perspectives and experiences, which would enable discussions and negotiations between different professionals (Charmaz 2009).

Don Ihde's *postphenomenology* functions as a conceptual base for empirical research on teleconsultation in palliative care. The post-phenomenological approach indicates, in line with pragmatism, that people continuously interact with their physical and social environment (Ihde 2009). By adding teleconsultation to the environments of patients, family caregivers, and healthcare professionals, participants' interactions with both these environments and the persons being engaged in them are likely to change. How teleconsultation technology is presented to its participants is highly dependent on how the technology "fits" into daily practice: will the technology magnify its users' worlds without being too noticeable? Will physicians, for example, be able to assess a patient's physical status without being too restrained by the use of real-time, audiovisual communication technologies? The question of fit is not solely restricted to these particular embodiment relations, but extends itself to the question of the "fit" of the teleconsultation technology within existing and historically emerged care practices. Ihde and others propose a "concrete empirical study of technologies in the plural," just like this study of teleconsultation technologies (Ihde 2009; Pols 2012). How does teleconsultation technology, in the course of a palliative care process, appear in and impact relationships between home-based palliative care patients and healthcare professional(s), between different professionals embedded in different care cultures, and between all participants and their personal and/or professional environments?

Central to both postphenomenology and the applied ethics of technology is Ihde's notion that technology is "non-neutral." Technology changes our perceptions of the surrounding world, thereby forcing people, however subtle, to think and act differently. Technologies mediate human (inter)actions (Ihde 1990; Swierstra and Waelbers 2012). Teleconsultation technologies redefine the original situation (e.g., all of a sudden, a hospital-based healthcare professional is virtually present in the living room of a seriously ill patient) and mediate the practical options (e.g., a distance diagnosis is made easier due to the addition of vision, but a private room to make these diagnoses is no longer available). Such a magnification/reduction scheme that is inherent to a technology calls for ethical reflection: if one knows how technology mediates the situation and the practical options, what then "ought to be done"? This question gains relevance when it is translated to questions on stakeholders, on consequences, and on considerations of the good life.

Research projects on telehealth solutions in palliative care practices should be designed to explore and describe the normative issues that arise with telehealth in the practice of palliative care, to reflect on them with "common moral vocabularies," and to study how these issues are resolved in practice. The normative issues and their practical solutions need to be critically evaluated in order to control the normative power of the factual. This chapter will further focus on what teleconsultation in palliative care means to the caring relationships between a suffering patient and healthcare professionals, which are considered to be at the heart of palliative care. In addition, a description and analysis of normative issues as a consequence of teleconsultation-induced changes in interprofessional relationships will be given.

3 Context to the Research Project on Teleconsultation

A cross-national study on preferred place of death in Europe shows that "at least two thirds of people prefer a home death in all but one country studied [Portugal]" when confronted with advanced cancer (Gomes et al. 2012). Deaths occurring at home, however, are not common practice in Europe (Cohen et al. 2010) and vary largely based on country-specific cultural, social, and healthcare factors. One can thus conclude that a considerable amount of patients with advanced cancer do not and/or cannot realize their wish to die at home. Moreover, the chances of dying at home steadily decrease for chronically ill patients from the age of 70 years and beyond (Van der Velden et al. 2009).

Let us start with the presumption that access to expert palliative care supports home-based patients in receiving high-quality palliative care and also, therefore, in dying at home. In the Dutch case, primary care physicians, the professionals responsible for palliative care at home, report having mainly general knowledge of treatment options but limited knowledge and competencies (through lack of education and experience) with respect to applying specific medical-technical treatments required for complex palliative care (Groot et al. 2007). Such data imply that primary care in general would benefit from some form of specialized support and/or education to provide adequate palliative care to patients suffering from complex problems. Therefore specific collaborations between primary care and expert palliative care, in which treatment and care are continuously attuned to the individual patient's problems and needs, have to be explored.

3.1 Early Steps in the Generalist and Specialist Palliative Care Integration Process

Home-based palliative care patients are ideally adequately cared for by their primary care physicians. However, patients who suffer from complex problems require more integrated generalist and expert palliative care at home (Quill and Abernethy 2013; Den Herder-van der Eerden et al. 2017). The integration of different professional palliative care services in Europe is still in an incipient stage (Wright et al. 2014; Den Herder-van der Eerden et al. 2018).

Still being an inceptive form of interprofessional integration, "primary care physicians-expert palliative care" consultations already showed some essential barriers to a far-reaching integration of services. Primary care physicians, for example, mostly consult expert palliative care services at their patients' (very) end of life, thereby strongly focusing on medical-technical aspects (Desmedt and Michel 2002; Abarshi et al. 2011). Interprofessional consultations do not automatically evoke an early integration of multidimensional palliative care at home. Despite this narrow use of interprofessional consultation, different collaboration initiatives positively impacted patient outcomes such as dyspnea and sleep, anxiety, and spiritual problems and needs (Marshall et al. 2008; Rabow et al. 2004), while also improving advance care planning and reducing urgent care visits. The collaborations examined, however, were less favorable to extensive information sharing, joint decision-making, and interdisciplinary teamwork in a homecare culture. Apart from some promising results, current consultations (usually by phone) demonstrate shortcomings. Therefore, new services and technologies are needed that support continuous care and sharing responsibilities (professional integration), while at the same time guaranteeing a patient and informal caregiver focused perspective (clinical integration) (Valentijn et al. 2013).

3.2 Patient and Informal Caregiver Participation in Integrated Palliative Care?

Palliative (home)care asks caregivers to be open to various contexts and care practices and to different patient values and experiences in order to guarantee a patient-centered, flexible palliative care process. This care is about being attentive to the individual patient and to give room to the patient as a person and as an agent (Randall and Downie 2006). Most patients would like to have a relationship with their doctors and nurses that provides them with the opportunity to decide on treatment and care in line with personal goals and values. Integration in palliative (home)care, from a patient perspective, means being able to work flexibly with a "pool of professionals" (Randall and Downie 1999) who are all well-informed, mutually attuned, and focused on common aims but have different ways and expertise to solve a variety of problems.

3.3 Innovative Use of Synchronous, Audiovisual Teleconsultation to Align Home-Based Patients' Interests with Generalist and Expert Palliative Care

As shown by the paragraphs above, the integration of generalist and expert palliative care to serve home-based patients is mainly based on communication. Inspired, among others, by the Michigan telehospice project (Whitten et al. 2004) and Canadian research on telehomecare supporting hospital-home transitions of severely ill children (Young et al. 2006), the Radboud

University Medical Center developed and researched an innovative integrated palliative care service, centered around synchronous audio-visual teleconsultations between home-based palliative care patients, primary care physicians, and a hospital-based specialist palliative care team. Those earlier projects showed that patients appreciated the direct contact with the hospice or healthcare organization, especially when they were living in rural areas. Telehospice proved to reassure patients and family caregivers, to enable physical and pain assessment, and to provide information and support (Whitten et al. 2004). The study of Gagnon et al. (2006) showed that, as a consequence of telehomecare, intensified relationships between patients and homecare nurses came about. Continuity and closer follow-up care were believed to contribute to a better quality of care, with healthcare professionals experiencing an improved trust in relationships with colleagues. Patients did not consider the lack of physical presence to be a major issue. However, part of the healthcare professionals did experience a loss of the "personal touch and hands-on care tailored for each individual" (Whitten et al. 2005). This loss of physical presence combined with a diminished flexibility of the working agenda and doubts about the perceived convenience for vulnerable patients led providers to reject telehospice more often, compared to patients.

3.4 The Nijmegen Palliative Care Teleconsultation Service and Its Devices

The Dutch Radboud UMC is a university medical center serving a big area in which approximately two million people reside. In contrast with the Northern American projects, the aim of the teleconsultation service central to the Radboud University Medical Center research project was to include both interprofessional communication ("telemedicine") and patient-professional communication ("telecare") (Pols 2012) in order to create a high-quality, interdisciplinary palliative care service that would include patients. This teleconsultation service aimed to digitally connect home-based patients, their primary care physicians, and a hospital-based specialist palliative care team (Fig. 1). During the research period, the teleconsultation technology was employed for (bi-)weekly videoconferencing interactions between a hospital-based specialist palliative care team and palliative care patients living at home. Primary care physicians were invited to attend the teleconsultations at the patient's home so as to construct the triangular consultation between patient, primary care physician, and specialist palliative care team. Easy to use software that adequately supported *digital* triangular consultations at reasonable costs was unfortunately not available at the start of the study. In the Netherlands, approximately 95% of the households have access to the Internet, making it a fruitful environment for telecare and interprofessional teleconsultation. At the start of this project's implementation process in 2010, just under 60% of the Dutch people aged between 65 and 75 used the Internet, compared to 75% in 2012. In 2012, the generation that will most often require palliative care in the foreseeable future, those between the ages of 50 and 65, used the Internet. Due to technological progress during our research project, two teleconsultation devices were subsequently utilized in this study: (1) a simplified desktop computer called a "Bidibox" and (2) an iPad2. Encryption of the digital teleconsultations guaranteed the privacy of health information.

4 How Teleconsultation Fits Palliative Care at Home: The Relationship Between Patient and Professional

The following paragraphs will show teleconsultation technologies' "multistability" (Ihde 1990): the technologies present themselves in different forms and functions in the palliative care practice, and they mediate different relationships. In these paragraphs the focus is on the relationship (a) between patient and professional and (b) between research participants – patients, informal carers, and healthcare professionals – and their

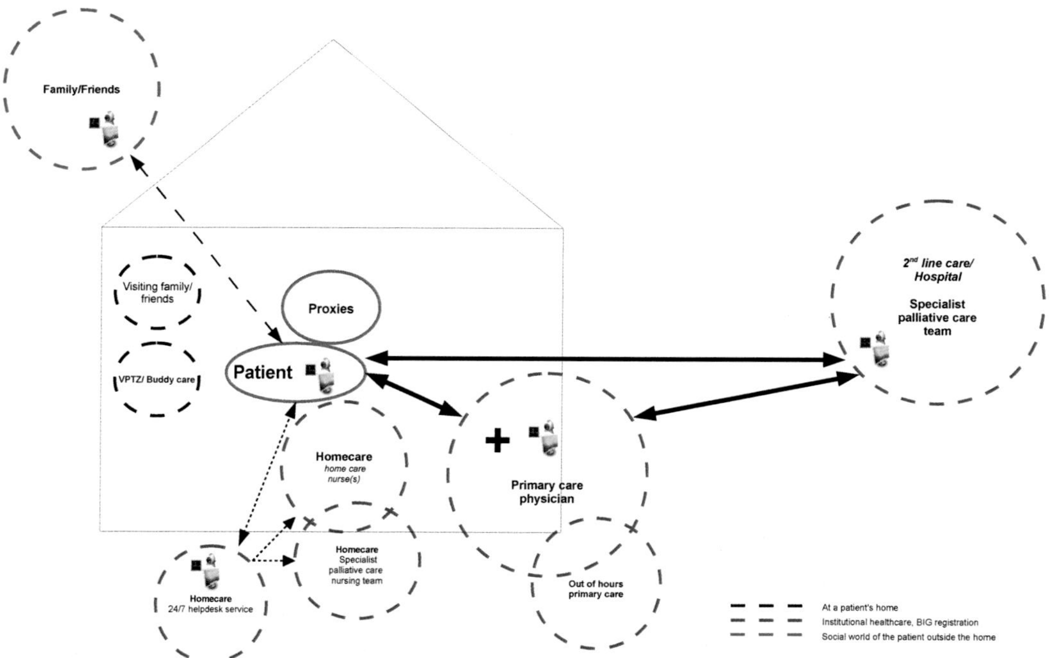

Fig. 1 **A Dutch home-based palliative care patient** is usually supported by her proxies, her primary care physician, and various homecare nurses. Teleconsultation offers possibilities to digitally connect the patient with a specialist palliative care team, primary care physician, the homecare help desk, and relatives living further away. A triangular connection also seems possible

practical environments, i.e., home and hospital. The full results of the empirical-ethical study with 18 home-based palliative care patients (16 suffering from cancer, 2 from COPD; age range 24–85 years old), their family/friends, 12 hospital-based specialist palliative care team clinicians, and 17 primary care physicians are published elsewhere (Van Gurp et al. 2015, 2016). Central to this study were serial observations of teleconsultations in home and hospital contexts, as well as serial interviews with everyone involved (patients, family members, palliative care specialists, and primary care physicians).

4.1 Physical Proximity and Diagnosis

Palliative care professionals, and healthcare professionals in general, consider face-to-face communication and physical proximity with their vulnerable and dying patients prerequisites for good clinical practice. These clinical contacts usually lead to an adequate clinical touch and solid clinical knowledge. In this study, the palliative care specialists' need for clinical contact resulted in a strong demand to see the patient in the hospital at least once before teleconsultation could start. In practice, however, these first, physical visits did not always take place, a fact that turned out not to hinder the development of long-term and meaningful digital relationships with patients and their primary care physicians. Without wanting to disregard the value of clinical contacts with patients, the research shows on more occasions that physical proximity between healthcare professionals and patients is not always necessary, and sometimes even undesirable, to address many forms of patients' suffering.

> Specialist palliative care team nurse 1: "[right after a teleconsultation] sigh… that was intense [and cries]. You just notice that you're far away [...]. This man will deteriorate rapidly from now on [...]. I would really prefer to sit next to him now. A bit more personal. However, that's how it is."

Patient 1: "I cried during the conversation. [I: Yes, and afterwards. . .] I'm calm again. Relieved too [. . .] You just have the opportunity to pour your heart out."

With respect to monitoring a patient's physical state, the professionals' need for physical proximity appears justified most of the time. Teleconsultation technologies (a combination of hardware, software, and the Internet) not only exclude sensory information such as smell and touch, but the technologies' information encoding-decoding schemes are so opaque that palliative care professionals cannot be certain of the accuracy of the translation of a patient's color and physical details into an image. Instead, professionals can only rely on the general information that these images provide, such as physical progression or regression and the most prominent nonverbal cues. During teleconsultations, this less detailed information can still be used in an extensive clinical reasoning process wherein the visual is but one source of information for clinical reasoning. An extensive clinical reasoning process also includes stories of patients, observations, and accounts of informal caregivers and primary care physicians. To gather these pieces of information from other (non-)professionals, to qualify them, and to relate them to other stories requires palliative care expertise and advanced interviewing skills. Palliative care specialists need to learn how to incorporate teleconsultation's images in their clinical reasoning in order to draw reliable conclusions.

Specialist palliative care team clinician 4: "And the image, it's additional and supportive. You see someone's status [. . .], which makes the picture complete."

4.2 Patient-Centered Care by Means of Teleconsultation

The lack of physical proximity caused by teleconsultation did not hamper patient-centered care and knowing the patient as a person per se (in contrast to Demiris et al. 2006). For patients, a teleconsultation meant that they did not have to make a sometimes burdensome journey to their palliative care specialists. In addition, being at home and not in a hospital also left patients feeling less of an ill and/or dying person, as well as feeling more in control of treatment, care, and conversation. The physical distance caused by teleconsultation technology can contribute to patients experiencing more autonomy, as they are less hindered by the physical presence of a hospital and/or healthcare professionals. To allow patients to remain at home as long as possible, palliative care specialists can use teleconsultation to build trusting relationships with the patient and his/her social system, as well as with their primary care physician. Teleconsultation offers palliative care specialists an opportunity to build and commit to long-term relationships with patients who reside at home. With continuous digital care and/or contact, professionals can prevent patients from experiencing abandonment in the last phase of life.

Informal caregiver: ". . . at that moment, she was no longer capable of going to the hospital. And contact with the specialist palliative care team, through the video screen, came in handy then. Because if she had to go to the hospital every time, she would have been just too tired for that."

4.3 Virtual Proximity Counterbalances Rationalization

A common response to the use of technologies in the medical domain (such as Internet-based communication technologies) is that of a fear for "cold care" (Bauer 2001; Pols 2012). Especially in palliative care, intensive use of technology is often associated with dehumanization and rationalization, turning the suffering patient into an object and medicalizing the intimate sphere of dying (Randall and Downie 2006). Research, however, shows that although Internet-based communication technologies sometimes dehumanize or rationalize parts of palliative care, they can also enable empathic care and intimate relationships at a distance. Teleconsultation technologies supply intimate views of patients' daily lives, offer room for personal stories, and provide contact with important informal caregivers.

Teleconsultation technologies proved to center their users' attention, thereby fostering a hyper-focus on the conversation partner's face. In addition to Pols' observations of "topologically reversed telepresence," where participants experience visiting one another in the physical space of the other (e.g., the experience of "sharing a cup of coffee" at the patient's home/in the hospital), this study recorded moments of actual telepresence, the shared experience of meeting one another in a virtual space, during discussions of intimate topics related to illness and dying (Savenstedt and Knudsen in Pols 2011). This actual telepresence is characterized by a physical orientation toward the other (e.g., bending over to the screen; "serious" facial expressions) as well as becoming totally absorbed in the virtual encounter. Virtual proximity is simply about two faces and two minds directed toward each other via the screen.

4.4 Teleconsultation Penetrating into the Daily Lives of Patients

The value of the different devices utilized for this study in the daily life of patients is best illustrated with two observations: (1) the large and immobile desktop device that was first used in this study was too visually dominant. It was usually installed in the living room. The devices were often placed close to the patients' beds or places of comfort due to the limited mobility of both patients and devices. The device remained constantly in sight, reminding the patient and informal caregivers of their inability to get rid of the device when desired, their precarious situations, as well as the approaching death of the patient. Some could not stand the sight of the devices anymore and handed them back. This observation came closest to the presumption that "medical" technology intrudes into and disrupts the home as a peaceful place (Sandman 2005).

> Patient: "[a teleconsultation device] is not something you have at home when you're in full glory... It reminds you of going toward an ending."

(2) The tablet computers were better suited to the patients. Tablet computers could be easily taken up and put away when needed. They functioned as handheld portals to a different world where patients could find medical expertise, attention, and comfort. One patient even called his tablet computer affectionately "his little painting," a strong reference to the characteristic of a two-dimensional painting that evokes different and distant worlds. Tablet computers fitted well into the daily, often impaired, lives of the patients. Interestingly however, the use of tablet computers in the hospital practice paved the way for privacy infringement, as these mobile devices were more often used in public rooms and in between other activities.

5 How Teleconsultation Fits Palliative Care at Home: The Mediation of Professional Relationships

During our research, two teleconsultation models emerged. In the first model of teleconsultation-induced team care, which occurred most frequently during our study, palliative care specialists and primary care physicians decided to work as a multidisciplinary team. This means that both primary care physicians and specialists engage in private conversations with the patient. The latter engages with the patient by means of teleconsultation technology, and the former usually by physically visiting the patient. In addition, the palliative care specialists and the primary care physicians use interprofessional backstage conversations to share their insights about the patient and attune treatment and care.

This form of collaboration strongly requires standardization of backstage communication in order to prevent the occurrence of ambiguous and/or parallel care and medical treatment (Gardiner et al. 2012). This backstage communication relies on the commitment and discipline of all professionals involved to promptly and accurately inform one another when the patient's situation changes. Furthermore, multidisciplinary teams require prudence from all members in order to appear to the patient as a complementary team with an attuned perspective and treatment plan. In multidisciplinary team care, there is less room for primary care physicians to work solo. Specialist palliative care teams also have to exercise restraint in their teleconsultation approach to the patient in order to sustain a central coordinating position of the primary care physician in homecare. One of the most striking examples of such a competence is primary care physicians providing hands-on end-of-life care for patients at home. A pitfall of multidisciplinary team care, with and without teleconsultation, is for professionals to communicate with one another via the patient. In the research, this occasionally resulted in patients feeling insecure, being confronted with opposing care perspectives.

If team members can maintain a prudent attitude, teleconsultation can lead to a long-term "personal liaison" between the healthcare professionals involved. Such liaisons will result in a sharing of the burden of the palliative care provision at home, mutual understanding of each others' professional practices, profound and patient-centered decision-making and advance care planning, and finally mutual trust.

In the second teleconsultation model, a real-time tripartite, and therefore interdisciplinary consultation, is organized. This collaboration model occurred in our research in only one instance. As the teleconsultation technology used only allowed for high-quality *bilateral* videoconferencing by connecting no more than two locations, one healthcare provider had to be prepared to travel to join the patient (or the other professionals) in order to set up interdisciplinary treatment and care conversations. Most primary care physicians mentioned that difficulties in attuning the different professional agendas were the main reason for not being able to engage in this type of interdisciplinary care (Gardiner et al. 2012).

In *tripartite* teleconsultations the negotiation of responsibilities between professionals became more obvious due to the instant reciprocity between patient, primary care physician, and specialist palliative care team clinician(s). This reciprocity demands a modest and open attitude from professionals: they need to have the ability to deal with criticisms and comments in front of the patient as well as an open mind to new perspectives (Esterle and Mathieu-Fritz 2013). Tripartite teleconsultation requires relinquishing personal control over communication, planning, treatment, and care. Interdisciplinary dialogues make medical-technical jargon inappropriate, as not every conversation partner will be able to understand it. Instead, professionals need to find a common language with an appropriate level of complexity in tripartite teleconsultations.

5.1 Teleconsultation in Palliative Care at Home Requires Careful Use of Technology

Instead of dehumanizing and rationalizing the intimate sphere of suffering and dying, as is suggested by the literature (Seymour 1999; Randall and Downie 2006), recurring teleconsultations by means of synchronous audiovisual contact showed the potential to install a valuable patient-professional ritual in which the mutually focused gaze and mutual chatter can form the prelude to a proximity in which the suffering patient appears as a Face: an original, provoking Other that demands responsiveness. In their response, healthcare professionals have to surpass the usual, medical-technical imperative ordering: the wondrous orientation on the suffering human being can only be revived when the healthcare professional is prepared to offer a digital welcome to home-based patients. Thus, palliative care specialists do not have to fear losing their ability to "touch upon a patient's personality" in teleconsultation. They rather have to fear their own inability to adopt a humble attitude that facilitates an open space in which the patient can appear (DasGupta 2008). Palliative care specialists' reluctance to discuss sensitive topics in teleconsultation due to an experienced lack of control about what happens on the other side easily closes the door to virtual proximity.

During the teleconversation, the tablet computer used for the teleconsultations is held at arm's length, thereby shaping and showing a rather detailed portrait of the other person. The tablet computer magnifies (the importance of) the human face and, as a consequence, can stimulate an intense hyper-focus toward this face. This technology-led orientation allows the suffering patient to emerge as someone who asks his/her healthcare professionals to leave the realm of medical discourse, in which the patient is easily transformed into a "distinctive manifestation." However, the occurrence of such an open and welcoming orientation is not obvious, as the technology's ambivalent nature equally enables the reduction of another's face into a smaller, two-dimensional *object* that can be placed next to other objects in the physical viewing environment (Pols 2012). Professionals therefore have to make a conscious effort to avoid the objectification of the patient.

Easing the suffering of a patient does not require physical proximity per se: the distance created by technology can also support an openness with new dimensions. The original thinking of Levinas that proximity is independent from space seems to be reflected in some of the results from our qualitative study. The virtual proximity observed in this teleconsultation study, however, implies two problematic situations.

First, moments of virtual proximity usually ended in moments of silence, but teleconsultation technologies' scripts continuously invite participants to verbally interact with one another (Akrich 1992; Verbeek 2006). In other words, the hyper-focus demanded by audiovisual communication technologies requires participants to speak as soon as the image of one's conversation partner appears. Underlying the technology-instilled chatter, however, remains what Levinas calls Saying (Levinas 2011): an inclination toward a mutual, open orientation between interactants in which one may suddenly touch upon the ineffable presence of suffering. In our empirical study, we captured the story of an apparently superficial teleconversation starting with a healthcare professional asking a simple opening question "How are you doing today?" The ensuing talk gradually transformed into a conversation about the existential topic of an approaching death. The early conversation already seemed to contain an implicit, joint wandering (the Saying) that slowly but surely laid the foundation for a proximity wherein the patient eventually felt free enough to approach the healthcare professional with his deepest thoughts about not having much time left and the intense sorrow that accompanied these thoughts. Technology supports patients in creating their stories as a bricolage (Ihde 1990; Radley 2004): patients can use their facial and some of their bodily expressions, their physical positions, and their words to communicate a composed personal aesthetic (Chouliaraki 2006). Patients use these technologized aesthetics mostly for downplaying their suffering. They put on a brave face and avoid giving free reign to their inner feelings. However, the Saying within such aesthetic chatter can create moments in which the aesthetic façade is taken off and the patient shows her-/himself at her/his most vulnerable. However, such intense communicative moments are accompanied by the conversation partners falling silent, as there is nothing left to say. Interestingly, these silences did *not* fit with the technology's continuous invitation for hyper-focus and chatter. The silence feels awkward and out of place, whereas sitting with someone in silence is considered essential in the approach of suffering human beings (Randall and Downie 1999). In this study, participants did not yet find appropriate ways to insert moments of silence in teleconsultations. Instead, long silences led to conversation partners ending the teleconsultations.

Second, the digital hyper-focus and virtual proximity are vulnerable to disturbing elements from the home or the hospital that pierce their fragile exclusiveness. Intrusions of unannounced others – nurses, colleague physicians, or informal caregivers – bring about immediate disruptions of exclusive conversations. As a consequence of these disruptions, conversation partners feel caught, their intimacy betrayed, and their privacy infringed. The intimate connectedness that is needed to converse truthfully about a patient's situation, hope, and/or suffering does not allow for the presence of unknown others.

The empirical study also exposed healthcare professionals' (natural) inclination to act upon patient suffering. Observations showed that *after* teleconsultations, notwithstanding the discussion of private and/or emotional topics, patients usually expressed a feeling of relief and/or gratitude and a desire to continue with their daily lives. In contrast, the observed healthcare professionals were regularly left with a strong desire to be physically close to their suffering and vulnerable patients after such consultations. This desire for physical closeness does not only stem from a need to reinforce proximity through a comforting touch or a caress but also from a need to regain valuable senses such as smell and touch with which healthcare professionals attempt to master their patients' suffering. This strong desire to work on the patient's suffering, however, is hampered by technology. In this way, the technology seems to be able to guard the privacy of the home against the inclination of healthcare professionals to physically control patients and their contexts. By possibly making the physical presence of healthcare professionals superfluous, teleconsultation technology breaks open the traditional, asymmetric relationship between professional and patient. Interestingly, proximity, which Levinas already thought of as being independent from space, is now maintained by the distance created by the technology: palliative care teleconsultations show that physical presence and face-to-face communication are not prerequisites per se for proximity and meaningful communication.

6 Conclusion

Through Internet-based communication technologies that provide synchronous audiovisual contact, healthcare professionals can offer their patients short moments of reconnection with a social albeit medical world that, if professionals display open and attentive communication, can be receptive to their patients' suffering. However, this chapter also shows that teleconsultation technology is in itself non-neutral and has to be used carefully by professionals in order to contain the rationalizing and dehumanizing scripts that are also present in these technologies. What follows are some concluding statements accompanied by suggestions for careful use:

1. Communication technologies supporting synchronous audiovisual communication tempt healthcare professionals to make the visual element dominant in teleconsultations. During teleconsultations, however, the visual should always be compared with the medical history and stories/information provided by proxies and primary care physicians in an extensive clinical reasoning process, so as to triangulate information and come to reliable conclusions. In this way, technology's limited transparency and opaque encoding-decoding schemes can be overcome.
   1a. Palliative care specialists should learn about how the teleconsultation technology encodes and decodes visual information. In other words, they have to learn about the quality of the images as well as about the appropriate probing questions for checking the images. Expert palliative care teleconsultations thus require (a) excellent interviewing skills with which they can, via *teleconsultation, elicit truthful stories from patients and proxies, (b) professionals capable of interacting with people on different levels and different topics (patients, proxies, physicians), and (c) professionals capable of "connecting the dots" between all these information to gain credible clinical knowledge.*
2. Teleconsultation technology enables continuous and long-term commitment to a patient, regardless of physical distance. Teleconsultation thereby neutralizes a patient's fear of abandonment. Patients experience a sense of relief and safety, knowing that expert palliative care is available at home and believing that this will prevent distressing hospital visits to occur due to the combination of generalist and specialist palliative care.
   2a. Palliative care patients can find comfort and relief in staying at home, where they feel less of a dying person and more in control with respect to their own care. With this in mind, teleconsultation should be offered to (a) patients who require a gradual transfer from high-technological care settings to the home and who will suffer from feelings of

abandonment as a result of these transfers, (b) patients who desire to maintain their personal autonomy and control, and (c) patients at home who are in need of specialist palliative care treatment and support.

3. Patients do not necessarily experience a sense of medicalization of the home with teleconsultation. In fact, they may experience more comfort and autonomy in their homes, which will help them to better express themselves and to feel more in control with respect to decisions on treatment and care. The physical distance created by teleconsultation can contribute to the experience of autonomy as it complicates physical apprehension by healthcare professionals and/or healthcare settings.
   3a. In order to prevent patients from being constantly reminded of a medical system that monitors their last phase of life, the devices used for teleconsultation in palliative care settings should be as "transparent" as possible. They have to be mobile (WiFi) and light. Moreover, they have to blend in with the households in order not to become a continuous reminder of an approaching death.
4. If well applied, teleconsultation can foster a hyper-focus on the conversation partner that induces the acknowledgment of the patient as an original human being and true contact.
5. Teleconsultation technology invites conversation partners to involve in chatter, which can serve as a breeding ground for creating *virtual* proximity with the patient as a person.
6. Both the hyper-focus and the small talk bear implicit elements of being oriented toward the patient as an Other person and as such are preludes to moments of intimate yet technology-mediated contact in which truthful dialogues can come about.
7. Such intimate, humane contact through teleconsultation gives room for the suffering of a patient to appear, but appropriate endings for these intimate contacts on suffering have not yet been found: it appears difficult to sit with a patient in silence as the teleconsultation technologies continuously invite participants to verbally interact.
   7a. As patients (and proxies) experience feelings of intimacy and relief as a consequence of virtual proximity, palliative care specialists should adapt a humble and open attitude so as to establish the virtual proximity in which the patient can fully appear as another person. Through an open orientation and closely listening to the patient, palliative care specialists "welcome" the patients and their stories. The innocent small talk has to be cherished as, especially in teleconsultation, one reaches virtual proximity only through sharing of and building on stories.
   The disruption of the fragile virtual proximity by the intrusion of unannounced others led to patients experiencing being looked at, betrayed, and deprived of their privacy. To prevent such experiences from occurring, private teleconsultation rooms should be used.
8. Patients desire to be able to flexibly work with a "pool of professionals" (Randall and Downie 1999) who nevertheless appear as a cohesive team with a shared perspective on treatment and support. Interprofessional collaborations as a consequence of teleconsultation are, therefore, best supported by a modest and prudent attitude of the practitioners. Professionals should explore each other's strengths and weaknesses and deploy this knowledge for the provision of maximum complimentary team care.
   8a. Long-term engagement of palliative care specialists by means of teleconsultation results in solid knowledge of the patient's situation and an interprofessional trust based on thorough knowledge of palliative care specialists' and primary care physicians' medical practices.
9. Professionals should make a deliberate choice between working from a multidisciplinary and interdisciplinary team care perspective. With multidisciplinary team care, professionals should commit to and invest in intensive backstage communication to make this kind of team care work. With interdisciplinary team care, professionals and patients should work on a form of communication

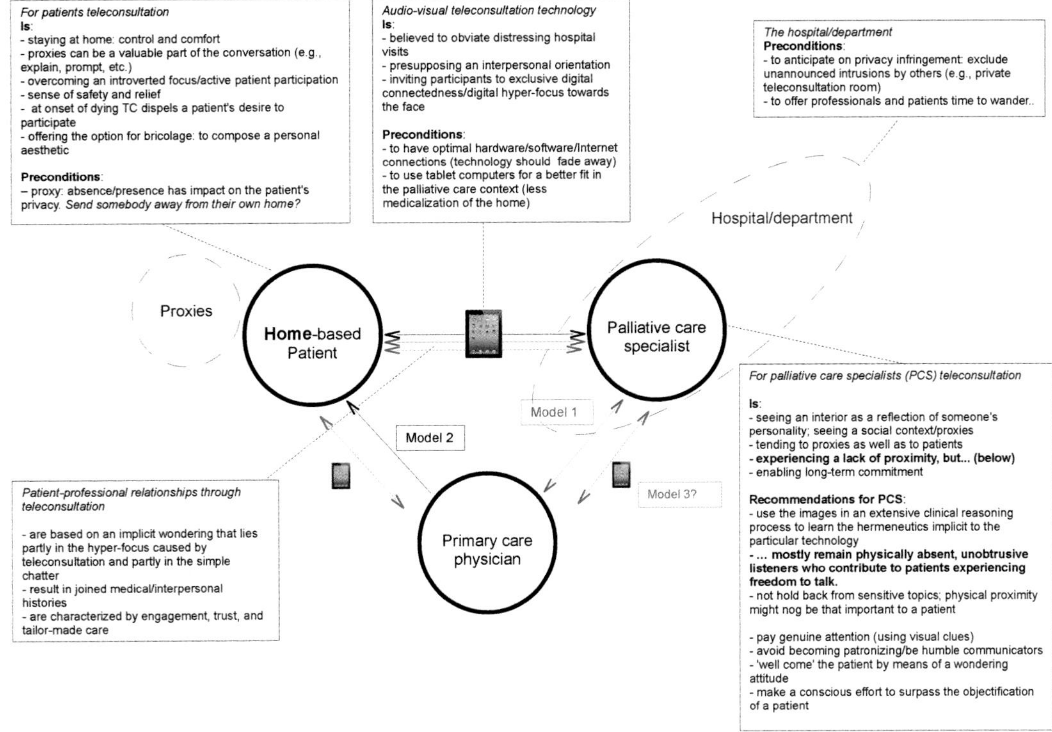

Fig. 2 Transmural palliative care by means of teleconsultation

in which all participants, but especially the patient, feel free to express their thoughts.

9a. Teleconsultation in a palliative homecare setting requires an active and continuous tuning and division of responsibilities. In multidisciplinary team collaborations, professional freedom seems more guaranteed. In contrast, in tripartite, interdisciplinary team collaborations, the direct digital contact between patient, primary care physician, and palliative care specialists results in a more concentrated responsiveness and mutual control.

10. Multidisciplinary and interdisciplinary team care both require backstage work. For that reason, standardization of and technological support (e.g., sharing patient files, opportunities for e-mail) for this backstage work are required. Solid backstage work is a high priority as it prevents patients from getting caught between two or more different perspectives on their treatment and care.
11. Especially interdisciplinary care requires strict agenda management to bring professionals, proxies, and the patient together at the same time.

In Fig. 2 this study's most important findings have been translated into an informative map.

Disclaimer This chapter is an adaptation of three unpublished chapters from the PhD dissertation "Teleconsultation: enhancing personalized palliative care at home. An empirical-ethical analysis." A PDF of this PhD dissertation is hosted at the Radboud Repository of the Radboud University Nijmegen.

References

Abarshi E, Echteld MA, Van den Block L, Donker G, Bossuyt N, Meussen K, et al. Use of palliative care services and general practitioner visits at the end of life in the Netherlands and Belgium. J Pain Symptom Manage. 2011;41:436–48.

Akrich M. The de-scription of technical objects. In: Bijker WE, Law J, editors. Shaping technology/building society: studies in sociotechnical change. Cambridge, MA: MIT Press; 1992. p. 205–24.

Bauer KA. Home-based telemedicine: a survey of ethical issues. Camb Q Healthc Ethics. 2001;10(2):137–46.

Burggraeve R. Man and fellow man, responsibility and God: the metaphysical ethics of Emmanuel Levinas [Dutch: Mens en medemens, verantwoordelijkheid en God: de metafysische ethiek van Emmanuel Levinas]. 1st ed. Leuven/Amersfoort: Acco; 1986.

Cassell EJ. The nature of suffering: and the goals of medicine. New York: Oxford University Press; 1991.

Charmaz K. Loss of self: a fundamental form of suffering in the chronically ill. Sociol Health Illn. 1983;5: $32#168–95.

Charmaz K. Constructing grounded theory. A practical guide through qualitative analysis. London: Sage; 2009.

Chouliaraki L. The spectatorship of suffering. London/Thousand Oaks: Sage; 2006.

Cohen J, Houttekier D, Onwuteaka-Philipsen B, Miccinesi G, Addington-Hall J, Kaasa S, et al. Which patients with cancer die at home? A study of six European countries using death certificate data. J Clin Oncol. 2010;28(13):2267–73.

Corbin JM, Strauss AL. Basics of qualitative research. Techniques and procedures for developing grounded theory. 3rd ed. Thousand Oaks: Sage; 2008.

DasGupta S. Narrative humility. Lancet. 2008; $32#371(9617):980–1.

Demiris G, Oliver DP, Courtney KL. Ethical considerations for the utilization of tele-health technologies in home and hospice care by the nursing profession. Nurs Adm Q. 2006;30(1):56–66.

Den Herder-van der Eerden M, et al. Towards accessible integrated palliative care: perspectives of leaders from seven European countries on facilitators, barriers and recommendations for improvement. J Integr Care. 2017;25(3):222–32.

Den Herder-van der Eerden M, et al. How continuity of care is experienced within the context of integrated palliative care: a qualitative study with patients and family caregivers in five European countries. Palliat Med. 2018;31(10):946–955. https://doi.org/10.1177/0269216317697898 (forthcoming).

Desmedt M, Michel H. Palliative home care: improving co-operation between the specialist team and the family doctor. Support Care Cancer. 2002;10(4):343–8.

Esterle L, Mathieu-Fritz A. Teleconsultation in geriatrics: impact on professional practice. Int J Med Inform. 2013;82(8):684–95.

Frank AW. Can we research suffering? Qual Health Res. 2001;11(3):353.

Gagnon MP, Lamothe L, Hebert M, Chanliau J, Fortin JP. Telehomecare for vulnerable populations: the evaluation of new models of care. Telemed J E Health. 2006; 12:324–31.

Gardiner C, Gott M, Ingleton C. Factors supporting good partnership working between generalist and specialist palliative care services: a systematic review. Br J Gen Pract. 2012;62:e353–62.

Gomes B, Higginson IJ, Calanzani N, et al. Preferences for place of death if faced with advanced cancer: a population survey in England, Flanders, Germany, Italy, the Netherlands, Portugal and Spain. Ann Oncol. 2012;$32#23(8):2006–15.

Groot MM, Vernooij-Dassen MJ, Verhagen SC, Crul BJ, Grol RP. Obstacles to the delivery of primary palliative care as perceived by GPs. Palliat Med. 2007;$32#21(8): 697–703.

Ihde D. Technology and the lifeworld. From garden to earth. Bloomington: Indiana University Press; 1990.

Ihde D. Postphenomenology and technoscience. The Peking University lectures. Albany: SUNY Press; 2009.

Levinas E. Proper names. Stanford: Stanford University Press; 1996.

Levinas E. The human face. Essays [Dutch: Het menselijk gelaat. Essays]. 9th ed. Amsterdam: Ambo; 2005.

Levinas E. Otherwise than being. Or beyond essence. 11th ed. Pittsburgh: Duquesne University Press; 2011.

Marshall D, Howell D, Brazil K, Howard M, Taniguchi A. Enhancing family physician capacity to deliver quality palliative home care: an end-of-life, shared-care model. Can Fam Physician. 2008;54(12):$32#1703–1703.e7.

Peperzak A. The one for the other – the philosophy of Emmanuel Levinas. Man World. 1991;24:427–59.

Pinchevsky A. The ethics of interruption: toward a Levinasian philosophy of communication. Soc Semiot. 2005;15:211–34.

Pols J. Wonderful webcams: about active gazes and invisible technologies. Sci Technol Hum Values. 2011;36:451–73.

Pols J. Care at a distance. On the closeness of technology. Amsterdam: Amsterdam University Press; 2012.

Quill TE, Abernethy AP. Generalist plus specialist palliative care – creating a more sustainable model. New Engl J Med. 2013;368(13):1173–5.

Rabow MW, Dibble SL, Pantilat SZ, McPhee SJ. The comprehensive care team: a controlled trial of outpatient palliative medicine consultation. Arch Intern Med. 2004;164(1):83–91.

Radley A. Pity, modernity and the spectacle of suffering. Paper for symposium Human dignity, narrative integrity, and ethical decision-making at the end of life; 2004.

Randall F, Downie RS. Palliative care ethics: a companion for all specialties. 2nd ed. Oxford: Oxford University Press; 1999.

Randall F, Downie RS. The philosophy of palliative care: critique and reconstruction. Oxford: Oxford University Press; 2006.

Sandman L. A good death: on the value of death and dying. Maidenhead: Open University Press; 2005.

Seymour JE. Revisiting medicalisation and 'natural' death. Soc Sci Med. 1999;49(5):691–704.

Statistics Netherlands [Internet]. The Hague/Heerlen: CBS. December 2017. Deaths; underlying cause of death (short list), sex, age; [cited 2018 Feb 4]. Available from: http://statline.cbs.nl/Statweb/publication/?DM=SLNL&PA=7052_95&D1=a&D2=0&D3=0&D4=0,10,20,30,40,50,60,(l-1)-l&VW=T

Swierstra T, Waelbers K. Designing a good life: a matrix for the technological mediation of morality. Sci Eng Ethics. 2012;18:157–72.

Valentijn PP, Schepman SM, Opheij W, Bruijnzeels MA. Understanding integrated care: a comprehensive conceptual framework based on the integrative functions of primary care. Int J Integr Care. 2013;13:e010.

Van der Velden LF, Francke AL, Hingstman L, Willems DL. Dying from cancer or other chronic diseases in the Netherlands: ten-year trends derived from death certificate data. BMC Palliat Care. 2009;8:4.

Van Gurp J, Van Selm M, Vissers K, et al. How outpatient palliative care teleconsultation facilitates empathic patient-professional relationships: a qualitative study. PLoS One. 2015;10:e0124387.

Van Gurp J, Van Selm M, Van Leeuwen E, Vissers K, Hasselaar J. Teleconsultation for integrated palliative care at home: a qualitative study. Palliat Med. 2016;$32#30(3):257–69.

van Hooft S. Pain and communication. Med Health Care Philos. 2003;6(3):255–62.

Verbeek PP. Materializing morality: design ethics and technological mediation. Sci Technol Hum Values. 2006;31:361–80.

Whitten P, Doolittle G, Mackert M. Telehospice in Michigan: use and patient acceptance. Am J Hosp Palliat Care. 2004;21(3):191–5.

Whitten P, Doolittle G, Mackert M. Providers' acceptance of telehospice. J Palliat Med. 2005;8(4):730–5.

Wright et al. in WHO. Global Atlas of Palliative Care at the End of Life. http://www.who.int/nmh/Global_Atlas_of_Palliative_Care.pdf?ua=1. Published January 2014. Accessed February 4, 2018.

Young NL, Bennie J, Barden W, Dick PT. An examination of quality of life of children and parents during their Tele-Homecare experience. Telemed J E Health. 2006;12(6):663–71.

Request for Assisted Suicide

90

Rachel E. Diamond, Puneeta Khurana, and Timothy E. Quill

Contents

Abstract

Physician-assisted dying (PAD) is receiving increasing media and academic attention, and legalization is expanding internationally. The potential legitimization of this practice is laden with medical, legal, and ethical considerations. Regardless of legality or willingness to participate, clinicians must be able to respond to enquiries about this topic, whether the patient's aim is information gathering or a formal request to end his or her life.

R. E. Diamond · P. Khurana · T. E. Quill (✉)
Palliative Care Division, Department of Medicine, University of Rochester Medical Center, Rochester, NY, USA
e-mail: Rachel_Diamond@urmc.rochester.edu; Puneeta_Khurana@urmc.rochester.edu; Timothy_Quill@urmc.rochester.edu

R. D. MacLeod, L. Van den Block (eds.), *Textbook of Palliative Care*,
https://doi.org/10.1007/978-3-319-77740-5_90

1 Introduction

The goal of this chapter is to use a real clinical case to outline the process by which clinicians might counsel a patient requesting help to end his or her life. This includes the process by which to assess the clinical context of the request, as well as the associated legal and ethical considerations.

Case Presentation: Over the past year, you have been in conversation with a patient with a brain tumor about what options he might have if he develops severe intractable headaches or if he begins to lose capacity to make his own decisions. He was particularly afraid of being "out of his mind" at the very end, a condition he felt would be "worse than death." He had read about Brittany Maynard and wondered if this option might be open to him in New York and was disappointed that it was not. He wanted to hear about the possibilities for a controlled death that might be available either legally or illegally. He was not ready to act now, but potential situations in the future that appeared far worse than death loomed large in his imagination.

Over the last few decades, the concept of PAD has made its way into both the medical and public worldview through various academic and media outlets. Some of these stories have captured the public's imagination in compelling ways, like Brittany Maynard, and others have been more problematic and polarizing like some of Jack Kevorkian's actions (It's over, Debbie 1988; Quill 1991). All these cases seem to strike a chord in our society and raise serious discussions about possibilities and practices in our communities. At the heart of the issue lies the boundaries and options for how clinicians and society should respond to genuine human suffering and/or to the fear of future suffering, associated with a debilitating illness.

Given the increased public exposure PAD is receiving, as well as an increasing trend toward legalization in the developed world, it is important that clinicians are well versed in these issues. Although physicians are directly involved in PAD, all healthcare professionals should understand the medicolegal and ethical arguments involved. Responses should be considered in advance of receiving a request for PAD, keeping in mind whether it is legal or not in the states or countries in which the clinician practices. It is also important to know what other tools are available to practitioners, when treating seemingly intractable physical and psychological suffering in patients with a life-limiting condition.

2 Defining Terminology and Practice

2.1 Physician-Assisted Dying

PAD is defined as the process through which a physician provides the means (a lethal drug potentially taken orally by the patient him or herself) to a competent patient fitting certain criteria, at the patient's request, to end his or her life voluntarily and independently (Fins and Bacchetta 1995). This practice has been referred to as "physician-assisted suicide" mainly by opponents of the practice, but, given negative connotations of the word "suicide," "physician-assisted dying" or "physician aid-in-dying" is often preferred when discussing the issue with patients. The criteria that a patient has to meet to be considered for PAD are different around the world. In parts of the USA where the practice is legal, a patient must be terminally ill and fully capable of decision-making and of self-administration. In the USA, after the patient meets agreed criteria, which usually includes a 2-week waiting period, a physician writes a prescription for a specific drug. Most often a barbiturate is prescribed, which the patient will then obtain at a pharmacy and take at the time he or she decides is most appropriate (Quill and Battin 2017a).

2.2 Voluntary Active Euthanasia

Voluntary active euthanasia (VAE) is a practice in which a clinician both provides and then administers the means to directly cause death for a patient, who has voluntarily requested to die and otherwise meets agreed criteria (Fins and Bacchetta 1995). This is typically done with lethal drugs delivered intravenously by the patient's physician. In Belgium, the Netherlands, and Colombia, this is the preferred practice because it is more reliably effective and because it does not depend on the ability of a very sick patient to self-administer. In these countries, there is also more emphasis on the presence of intolerable suffering that is refractory to treatment, deemed unacceptable by the patient without the patient necessarily being imminently terminal (Quill and Battin 2017a).

3 Additional Alternatives to PAD

When a patient requests PAD or VAE as an option, either in the present or future, it is critically important for him or her to know alternatives that could also help alleviate suffering. A palliative care consultation should always be pursued if possible and should ideally include access to an interdisciplinary team, including but not limited to a physician, nurse and/or nurse practitioner, social worker, pharmacist, chaplain, and massage and music therapists. In addition to providing expertise on managing challenging symptoms, the palliative care consultation can provide holistic care and counseling around end of life. The goal is to understand the basis of the request for PAD or VAE and address underlying suffering as effectively as possible. Hospice services (specifically referring to the U.S. model of an insurance benefit supporting comfort-oriented care at the end of life), potentially in the setting of an acute inpatient setting if symptoms are severe, should be instituted to maximize expert symptom management and also enhance social supports. Not only might the seemingly intolerable symptoms be addressed in these circumstances, but such consultations can also be a source of support for the patient and his or her family, potentially extending into the bereavement period after the patient dies. A systematic approach to this process is outlined in Fig. 1 below and will be discussed in the following sections.

Patients should have access to more formalized psychological/psychiatric services, especially if there is a concern that the request is associated with or stemming from an underlying mental health illness such as depression. Such a step may also be built in to criteria or steps required for a formal PAD request in places where it is offered as a legal option.

3.1 Intensification of Symptom Management

The first step in addressing requests for PAD is to ensure that the request is not a direct result of inadequate symptom control. If symptoms are being inadequately addressed, it is appropriate to proportionally escalate palliative treatments. Sometimes the doctrine of double effect will come into play in the process of intensification of symptom management (Quill et al. 1997a). According to this ethical principle, effects that would normally be seen as unethical if performed intentionally are permissible as long as they are foreseen but unintended. In this situation, administering larger doses of medications to proportionately relieve intractable suffering in a terminal illness may have the unintended, but

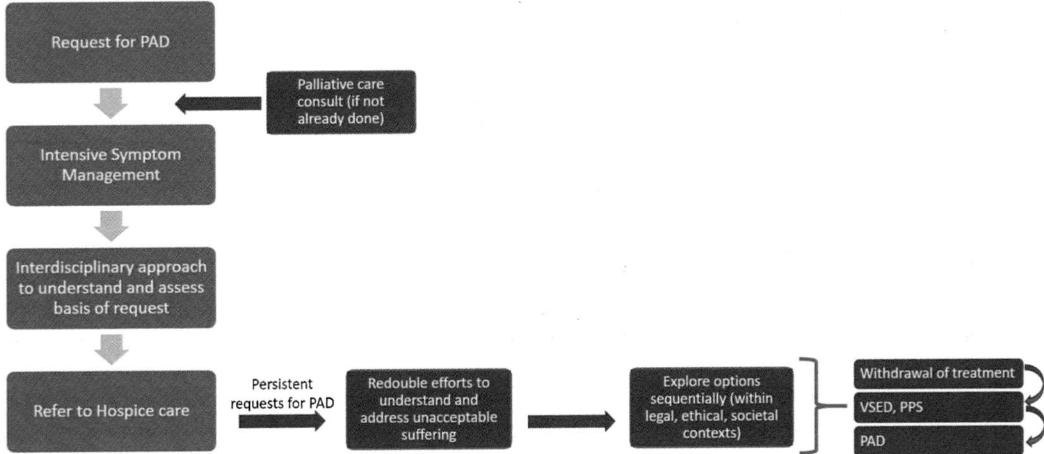

Fig. 1 Practical approach to requests for PAD

potentially foreseen effect of sedating the patient and even hastening/causing death. Because the appropriate medications are dosed strictly in *proportion* to, and with the intent to relieve the patient's *physical* suffering and not to cause death, the act is ethically permissible under this rule or principle. In the vast majority of cases, expert symptom management does not shorten life (and may sometimes even lengthen it) and certainly enhances the quality of the patient's life.

3.2 Withdrawing Life-Sustaining Therapy

In keeping with the ethical concept of personal autonomy, patients are given authority over their own bodily integrity (i.e., the patient must give informed consent to receive any medical treatment). Similarly, it is widely accepted that a patient can chose to refuse (i.e., either withhold or withdraw) any medical therapy even if the patient's intent is to die more quickly. This may include more invasive therapies such as a ventilator or dialysis or less invasive therapies such as oral diuretics, insulin for type 1 diabetes, or steroids for brain cancer. Despite the generalized legality, the motives for why a patient is choosing to make a treatment withdrawal decision at a particular point in time must still be thoroughly explored and understood.

3.3 Palliative Sedation and Voluntary Stopping Eating and Drinking

Both palliative sedation (PS) and voluntary stopping eating and drinking (VSED) are considered interventions of "last resort," meaning that they are available to patients experiencing extreme suffering at the end of life who do not respond to standard palliative treatment (Quill et al. 1997b).

Palliative sedation (PS) is defined as deliberately decreasing a patient's level of consciousness, to relieve severe and refractory symptoms that cannot be otherwise addressed despite other intensive palliative efforts (KNMG Guideline for Palliative Sedation 2009). This is generally achieved by giving medications specifically designed to reduce consciousness as a means of escaping suffering, but can also occur as an unintended side effect of symptom-targeted therapy (Quill et al. 1997b).

PS is generally considered when death is imminent from the patient's underlying disease and is administered continuously from initiation until the time of death. Proportionate palliative sedation (PPS) means that the lowest amount of sedation is used that can adequately relieve the patients suffering. If a relatively small dose of the sedating medication can relieve the adverse symptoms and still preserve some level of awareness, the dose would be held at that level. Sometimes sedation must be taken all the way to unconsciousness in progressive steps (e.g., severe agitated delirium), but this is done relatively gradually and would stop at the least level of sedation that would achieve the desired goal. On rare occasions, a patient may also be sedated all the way to unconsciousness in one step ("palliative sedation to unconsciousness" or PSU), usually for more severe, acute, catastrophic medical events (e.g., bleeding out from a carotid artery perforation from cancer) (Schildmann et al. 2015). One of the prerequisites for PSU is that the patient's death is expected to occur within a few weeks at most. While it has been suggested that PPS or PSU hastens the dying process directly or indirectly, the clinician's primary intention of this treatment is not to shorten life, but rather to relieve otherwise intractable symptoms and decrease suffering.

PS is most commonly used for refractory symptoms such as pain, dyspnea, and delirium or a combination of symptoms. The working definition of "refractory" is that existing palliative interventions cannot provide relief in an acceptable period of time. The clearest indication for PS would be to treat otherwise refractory, predominantly physical suffering, but the specifics may vary for each patient and family depending on their concepts of suffering, dignity, and symptom relief.

Another option that can be considered in cases of unacceptable suffering at end of life is voluntary stopping eating and drinking (VSED). VSED is an action of a legally competent person, who is still physically able to eat and drink, but who voluntarily decides to completely stop eating and drinking with the primary intention to hasten death to escape unacceptable suffering (Quill and Byock 2000).

The main ethical argument in favor of supporting VSED is based on the principle of autonomy. A competent patient with a terminal illness has the legal right to decline life-sustaining measures, including forms of artificial nutrition, even if his desire is to achieve an earlier death. Choosing to stop eating and drinking can similarly be considered a waiver of life-sustaining measures to not further prolong suffering, but it differs from forgoing medical treatment (such as *artificial* hydration and nutrition) in that it involves a conscious choice to stop taking ordinary food and liquids, despite being physically able to partake (Quill et al. 1997b).

4 Putting the Request into Context

4.1 Clinical Context

In exploring the demographic data from Oregon and the Netherlands where PAD is legal, it is possible to gain some understanding of the characteristics of patients that request PAD. They are mostly of higher socioeconomic class, married, insured, and almost all Caucasian. Male to female ratio is about equal, and most are in their sixties and seventies. The most common diagnoses are cancer and ALS (Battin et al. 2007).

Regardless of legality, many patients wish to explore PAD as an option in response to real-time or fear of future physical and/or emotional suffering, as well as real or threatened loss of autonomy and dignity. If the request is to gain information and reassurance from the clinician about what options the patient might have in the future, the clinician should be honest about which "last resort" options he can, and which he cannot, support if it comes to that in the future. If the request is for consideration of PAD *right now*, the clinician has to explore what is happening with the patient at this point in time to trigger such a request. The first step should be a detailed assessment of current symptom management, including anxiety and depression, and redoubling of efforts to adequately address those symptoms. This can be done through a primary care physician or subspecialist (often oncologist) but should also include an expert in palliative care medicine if possible. If a patient is nearing the end of life, it would be appropriate to discuss the benefits of hospice care in supporting the patient and family as well as aiding in symptom management.

The most common inquiry about PAD is not reactive to immediate suffering, rather it is from the proactive planning standpoint (Quill et al. 2016). Often the motives driving the enquiry are fears of losing control of the circumstances surrounding death and perhaps wanting to die at home rather than a facility of some kind. Most patients who make such enquiries fear loss of dignity, independence, quality of life, and self-care ability (Ganzini et al. 2007). Whether living in an area where PAD is legal or not, the request deserves exploration by and understanding from the clinicians involved. In addition, regardless of the clinician's stance on directly assisting with PAD, they should reassure the patient that he or she will not be abandoned in a time of need. Physicians should discuss with patients what options are legally available in their place of residence and also which of those options the clinicians can personally support. In addition to exploring the full range of "last resort" options outlined above, this discussion should also include reviewing advance care directives and filling out a MOLST (medical order for life-sustaining treatment) or equivalent form. It is important to understand the patient's views and values via these documents and also rationalize and adjust their medications based on their current situation and goals.

Another important aspect to explore with patients is whether they might like to know what the very terminal stages of their disease may look like. This discussion would ideally begin with the patient describing the kinds of deaths they have witnessed among their own families or friends.

Knowing how such deaths might be approached by the clinician or hospice team might be very reassuring depending on the patient's main concerns (i.e., if someone that the patient knew died in severe pain, because the doctor was afraid to prescribe opioids in proper doses, the doctor can reassure them that they would be very aggressive if needed with future pain management). Sometimes this exploration may alleviate some of the patient's fears about the future; however it may also exacerbate anxieties, depending on the patient's experiences, views, and values.

As with any patient interaction, these discussions should be focused on responsiveness to the particulars of the patient and her values, as well as respect for her autonomy. Reviewing the legal status of PAD in the patient's particular jurisdiction, in conjunction with the interdisciplinary team's approach and commitment to the patient, develops a crucial, ongoing, and committed partnership to address her suffering. Both patient and physician will need to establish and voice their own goals and limits, amidst the legal milieu in which they live.

4.2 Legal Context

The legal status of PAD across the USA is varied and rapidly changing. As of April 2017, there are six states in the USA that have legalized PAD (Oregon, Vermont, Washington State, California, Colorado, and the District of Columbia) (Quill and Battin 2017b).

State	Law
Oregon	Oregon Death with Dignity Act Passed by simple majority of voters in November 1994 Law enacted in October 1997 Upheld by the U.S. Supreme Court in January 2006
Washington	Washington Death with Dignity Act Passed by Washington State voters in 2008 Came into effect March 2009
Vermont	Patient Choice and Control at End of Life Act Signed by Vermont Governor in May 2013
California	End of Life Option Act Signed in October 2015 Came into effect June 2016
Colorado	End of Life Options Act Passed by Colorado voters in November 2016 Came into effect December 2016
District of Columbia	Death with Dignity Act Signed in January 2017 Came into effect February 2017

In the state of Montana, the Supreme Court ruled that state law currently does not prohibit a physician from participating in PAD, but there is no legislation or regulatory framework guiding the process, so it is in a legal "gray zone."

Outside of the USA, there are a number of countries that have legalized PAD and/or voluntary active euthanasia (VAE): the Netherlands, Belgium, Luxembourg, Colombia, and Switzerland (Quill and Battin 2017b).

In February 2015, the Supreme Court of Canada ruled in Carter v. Canada that certain sections of the Criminal Code are unconstitutional in that they prohibit competent adults who are not terminally ill from having access to PAD and VAE (Government of Canada 2017). The ruling mandated that assisted dying should be available to all adults with a "grievous and irremediable medical condition that causes enduring suffering that is intolerable to the individual in the circumstances of his or her condition (Quill and Battin 2017b)." In June of 2016, the Canadian Parliament passed a bill to legalize and regulate assisted dying in Canada, although there has been continuing debate about the degree to which the bill limits the Supreme Court's directive. To avoid "suicide tourism," only individuals eligible for health services funded by the Canadian government can be eligible for assisted dying in Canada (Government of Canada website 2017).

The Australian state of Victoria passed a bill in November 2017 making it the first state to pass PAD legislation, since the Northern Territory's "Rights of the Terminally Ill Act (1995)" was overturned in 1997. There are certain criteria that will be put into place, such as residency in the state of Victoria for at least 12 months before a request can be made. The bill is planned to be implemented into law in June 2019 (Victoria 2018).

As in the USA, laws around PAD and VAE are changing in the developed world, so it is important that clinicians are aware of the laws in the regions in which they are practicing.

4.3 Moral/Ethical Context

There are a number of arguments that have been made for and against the practices of PAD and VAE.

Part of the debate centers around patient autonomy. Autonomy in medicine means that a competent patient is able to make decisions for him or herself, based on adequate information and free from controlling interference from others (Varelius 2006). Proponents argue that patient autonomy dictates that they have the right to determine what kind of life is worth living, and this includes being able to choose when and how to die. Critics of this argument say that patient autonomy cannot include the ending of one's own life, because such an act would mean ending the possibility of further exercising autonomy (Fromme and Smith 2017). There are also societal factors to consider. Every individual who is living as a part of a civilized society accepts that there are limitations placed on their autonomy in order to properly function in that society. Hence in considering PAD, the autonomy of the individual should be considered alongside the effects upon the rest of the society, according to the ethical principle of justice for all.

The principles of beneficence and nonmaleficence also apply in context of PAD and VAE. If a patient is experiencing physical or psychological suffering that is not alleviated by palliative care, an assisted death may be perceived to be the only way to adequately relieve that suffering. Critics argue that eliminating the suffering by eliminating the sufferer cannot possibly be beneficial and that the number of patients that continue to experience pain and suffering, after providing adequate palliative care, is too small to justify permitting the use of PAD or VAE. They argue further that medicine cannot relieve all suffering and that society should focus in improving access to quality palliative care for a much broader group of patients who might otherwise "choose" this path.

Proponents also argue that PAD or VAE can be considered an extension of withdrawal of life-sustaining treatment, which is generally agreed to be ethically acceptable. They argue that in both cases, patients consent and accept death, the physician participates in the action that results in patient's death, and the final result of the intervention is death for the patient. Critics argue that intention plays an important role here. In withdrawal of life-sustaining treatment, the physician's intent is not to cause death, but rather to remove or avoid treatments that are futile or adversely impact quality of life. They argue that in PAD or VAE, the intent is to specifically end the patient's life, and this potentially sets it apart and cannot be ethically justified in the way withdrawal of life-sustaining treatment can. The end result of the patient dying is also not consistent between the two scenarios. There have been numerous cases, such as that of Karen Ann Quinlan, where the patient lived for an extended period of time after withdrawal of treatment. Finally, the need for life supports to sustain life restricts the practice by definition to seriously ill patients, whereas PAD and VAE could potentially achieve death for patients with no discernable illness (Fromme and Smith 2017).

5 Clinician Limitations

In situations where patients and/or families are considering PAD or VAE, there may still be barriers that exist beyond the legal context. Clinicians may have personal values that prohibit them from participating in PAD or VAE even where it is legal, and these values should be honored regardless of other circumstances. The interdisciplinary team involved with these patients should meet at the onset of care and periodically thereafter to explore such limits, debrief, and make sure everyone is "on the same page." Professional caregivers should be encouraged to be clear about their own limitations, avoiding ambiguous or false promises about their ability to participate. Referral to another clinician who would be prepared to take over this aspect of the patient's care should be considered as early as possible, should the patient desire such a change. Before that occurs, the clinician should be honest about what kinds of assistance he or she can, or cannot, provide, always looking for some kind of common ground to satisfactorily meet the patient's needs.

It is important for the clinician to take time to evaluate possible psychosocial consequences for him or herself in participating in PAD, or any other last resort options, even in environments where the practice is legal. It can be helpful to confer with another clinician who has palliative care experience and who could provide clinical consultation as well as support. In the USA, one such service is Doc2Doc, hosted by the advocacy organization Compassion & Choices, which provides information for clinicians about numerous end-of-life practices including PAD (Fromme and Smith 2017). In the final analysis, after an assiduous attempt to find a mutually acceptable way to respond to the patient's situation, clinicians must be able to live with their decisions and personal principles. Consultation and conversation with trusted colleagues is essential.

6 Approach to the Patient Who Refuses Palliative Care Involvement

There may be patients along the way who express interest in PAS or VAE however refuse any alternatives, including a palliative care consultation. While every patient has the right to refuse treatment, it is imperative to unpack the reasoning behind the patient's refusal. It may be a misunderstanding of the role of palliative care or a previous personal experience that has affected his or her opinion. Some patients may feel uncomfortable voicing their requests to additional practitioners – they may even feel betrayed that a trusted primary care provider or specialist is suggesting the involvement of another party into such a deeply personal conversation. Reassuring the patient that their current trusted care team remains actively involved and that palliative care is involved to make sure they have considered all options to potentially improve his or her quality of life before making such a final decision.

Identifying a main medical provider that the patient trusts and has a trusted relationship with the patient in such situations is crucial. This may be a PCP, an oncologist, or others. If it seems like roadblocks are being encountered in exploring and evaluating a patient's request for PAD, involving such a provider may help move the conversation forward.

Involvement of social work can also sometimes be very helpful. They can help assess for psychosocial, financial, and other stressors, potentially putting services and supports in place.

Pastoral care may also be beneficial depending on the patient's underlying views and values. Components of a patient's underlying suffering may be spiritual or religious in nature. Having the opportunity to meet with a chaplain or other spiritual guide and voice this suffering may bring some peace and understanding of the full nature of their suffering.

Patients clearly have a right to refuse palliative care consultation or consultation of any kind. Yet physicians have the right not to participate in PAD even where it is legal, especially if they do not feel all alternatives have been thoroughly explored (or if they don't feel they can live with the consequences of participation). As always, every effort should be made to find common ground without violating fundamental values on all sides.

Case Resolution: In discussing future options, the patient was informed that PAD was illegal in New York State and that while his doctor was not personally opposed to the practice, he did not feel comfortable prescribing the medication under this circumstance. He was told his symptoms related to headache, seizures, or confusion would be aggressively managed with standard hospice care. If his symptoms in those domains were severe, he would get proportionate doses of sedating medication, even if it required heavily sedating him to escape the unacceptable suffering. He was also told that he could stop his steroids at a time of his choosing if his desire was to die more quickly and that any associated headache and confusion would be aggressively managed. He could also stop eating and drinking if he chose to do so, though this would probably not be necessary if he were to stop his steroids. He was made aware that there are groups such as Compassion & Choices who advise patients who want additional options which may be illegal such as PAD in the state of New York.

The patient and doctor agreed that at some point in the future stopping the steroids along with aggressive symptom management would probably be the best of the available options. About a month later, the patient began to develop more severe pain that was harder to treat with opioids along with higher dose steroids. He and his doctor began a conversation about whether it was time to initiate the plan to stop his steroids and aggressively palliate when the patient developed headache, confusion, and/or a seizure. Before he made any potentially death hastening decision, the patient had a grand mal seizure, and when he awoke in the hospital on the palliative care floor, he was quite frightened, but was very clear that he felt the time to withdraw treatment and begin more aggressive symptom management was now. The primary doctor, the palliative care specialist, the patient, and family all agreed, and a plan was made to stop his steroids and provide proportionate sedation with benzodiazepines and analgesia with a continuous opioid infusion. The benzodiazepine and opioid required considerable upward adjustment over the first 24 h until the patient appeared peacefully sedated after which it was maintained at that level. He died 48 h later in the presence of family. While all agreed he would have preferred PAD had it been legal and available to him, they were appreciative that the clinical team found a way to allow him an escape his suffering.

References

Battin MP, van der Heide A, Ganzini L, van der Wal G, Onwuteaka-Philipsen BD. Legal physician-assisted dying in Oregon and the Netherlands: evidence concerning the impact on patients in “vulnerable” groups. J Med Ethics. 2007;33(10):591–7.

Fins JJ, Bacchetta MD. Framing the physician-assisted suicide and voluntary active euthanasia debate: the role of deontology, consequentialism, and clinical pragmatism. J Am Geriatr Soc. 1995;43(5):563–8.

Fromme EK, Smith MD. Ethical issues in palliative care. UpToDate. Accessed 14 May 2017.

Ganzini L, Goy ER, Dobscha SK. Why Oregon patients request assisted death: family members’ views. J Gen Intern Med. 2007;23(2):154–7.

Government of Canada website: Medical Assistance in Dying. https://www.canada.ca/en/health-canada/services/medical-assistance-dying.html#a2. Accessed 12 May 2017.

Quill TE. Death and dignity. A case of individualized decision making. N Engl J Med. 1991;324:691–4.

Quill TE, Battin M. Responding to requests for physician-assisted death. UpToDate. Accessed 14 May 2017.

Quill TE, Byock IR. Responding to intractable terminal suffering: the role of terminal sedation and voluntary refusal of food and fluids. ACP-ASIM end-of-life care consensus panel. American College of Physicians-American Society of internal medicine. Ann Intern Med. 2000;132:408–14.

Quill TE, Dresser R, Brock DW. The rule of double effect – a critique of its role in end-of-life decision making. N Engl J Med. 1997a;337:1768–71.

Quill TE, Lo B, Brock DW. Palliative options of last resort: a comparison of voluntarily stopping eating and drinking, terminal sedation, physician-assisted suicide, and voluntary active euthanasia. JAMA. 1997b;278:2099–104.

Quill TE, Back AL, Block SD. Responding to patients requesting physician-assisted death. JAMA. 2016;315(3):245–6.

Royal Dutch Medical Association (KNMG). Guideline for Palliative Sedation [Internet]. 2009. Available from: https://www.knmg.nl/contact/about-knmg.htm.

Schildmann EK, Schildman J, Kiesewetter I. Medication and monitoring in palliative sedation therapy: a systematic review and quality assessment of published guidelines. J Pain Symptom Manag. 2015;49(4):734–46.

Varelius J. The value of autonomy in medical ethics. Med Health Care Philos. 2006;9(3):377–88.

Victoria becomes first state to legalise assisted dying as parliament passes bill. https://www.theguardian.com/society/2017/nov/29/victoria-becomes-first-state-to-legalise-assisted-dying-as-parliament-passes-bill. Accessed 28 Jan 2018.

William D, Fiorini MD. It’s over, Debbie. JAMA. 1988;259:272.

Part IX

Research in Palliative Care

Public Health and Epidemiological Research in Palliative Care

91

Lara Pivodic and Joachim Cohen

Contents

Abstract

Palliative care has been declared an important topic for public health. In turn, concepts of public health such as health promotion are highly relevant for populations in need of palliative care. In recent decades, public health and epidemiological research methods have been applied to study the circumstances of dying, including palliative care provision, in large communities or populations. This chapter starts by outlining several characteristics that distinguish public health from clinical research in palliative care. It subsequently gives an illustrative, rather than exhaustive, overview of several different methodological approaches that have been used in public health research in palliative care, as well as their advantages and limitations. The focus is on quantitative, epidemiological methods, which reflects the current dominant approach in public health research. These include population-based survey research and specifically the mortality follow-back design, the use of death certificate data to study place of death, studies of routinely collected administrative data on the population-level, and the use of existing epidemiological monitoring tools. Finally, the chapter describes the importance and contributions of qualitative and mixed methods public health research in palliative care. It does so by describing examples of community-centered

L. Pivodic (✉) · J. Cohen
End-of-Life Care Research Group, Vrije Universiteit Brussel (VUB) and Ghent University, Brussels, Belgium
e-mail: lara.pivodic@vub.be; joachim.cohen@vub.be

R. D. MacLeod, L. Van den Block (eds.), *Textbook of Palliative Care*,
https://doi.org/10.1007/978-3-319-77740-5_106

palliative care initiatives and research in less visible populations. Acknowledging that no single of these methods can answer all relevant questions about a topic, this chapter argues that it is the combination of a diverse set of research methodologies that will lead to the best possible view on and understanding of the circumstances of dying and provision of palliative care in populations.

1 Palliative Care as Public Health

Public health has been defined as the combination of sciences, skills, and beliefs directed toward the protection, promotion, and restoration of people's health through organized collective or social actions (Sallnow et al. 2016a). "Protection, promotion, and restoration" of health does not imply an exclusively curative approach to illness. It is to be interpreted in the context of the commonly accepted definition of health that has been put forward by the founders of the World Health Organization (WHO). According to this, "health is a state of complete physical, mental and social well-being and not merely the absence of disease or infirmity"(World Health Organization 2018). This definition detaches health from categories of disease or mortality and places it in a broader context of human well-being and includes mental and social, next to physical, well-being. Consequently, health promotion, as a crucial component of public health practice, encompasses, next to curative and restorative approaches, attention to well-being in a broader sense, including personal and social resources and physical capacities (Sallnow et al. 2016a).

This conceptualization of public health and health promotion makes apparent that both are highly relevant for people affected by life-threatening illness, dying, death, and bereavement. Indeed, the central ideas of public health and health promotion – attention to mental, social, and physical well-being – are reflected in the WHO definition of palliative care, which includes attention to physical, psychosocial, and spiritual problems (WHO 2002). Public health approaches to palliative care focus on maintaining and improving well-being of dying people and those affected by dying, death, and bereavement (Sallnow et al. 2016a). The reference to "collective or social actions" in the definition of public health suggests that it is a collective counterpart to individual patient care in a patient-professional relationship. As a result, public health practice and research in palliative care look at total populations – local, regional, national, or global – rather than limiting its focus to the health of individual patients and families or persons at risk or those receiving certain health services (Cohen and Deliens 2011).

Not only are the aims of palliative care and public health compatible, palliative care has in fact the typical characteristics of a public health priority: the need for palliative care places great burden on societies given the large number of people who die from diseases for which it is indicated (Murtagh et al. 2013); it has a major impact with respect to health consequences for populations and costs for individuals as well as the public; and it harbors potential for prevention and harm reduction (Glasgow et al. 1999). Addressing the challenge of providing high-quality palliative care in populations therefore requires applying public health methods to palliative care research.

While there are some paradigmatic differences between "classical" and "new" public health approaches, both approaches to public health research in palliative care have several important characteristics that distinguish them from clinical and health services research:

1. Focus on communities rather than on individuals who are at risk of developing a specific health problem or who are receiving a particular health service or treatment
2. Inclusion of social science alongside medical research methods
3. Recognition of the importance of non-professional actors (e.g., family, friends, wider networks) in palliative care alongside professional services
4. Attention to social and economic determinants of health as opposed to a focus solely on the immediate health services or interventions under study

5. Recognition of community involvement and empowerment as essential to maintaining and improving well-being toward the end of life
6. Evaluation of the impact of policy changes and societal debate on palliative care on a larger scale and less strong focus on impact of isolated interventions

Public health research in palliative care uses a variation of research methods, ranging from experimental and quasi-experimental studies, through classic epidemiological research methods, to methods from qualitative and action research. It would vastly exceed the scope and possibilities of this chapter to provide an exhaustive overview of possible methods to use in public health research on palliative care. The aim of this chapter is rather to highlight the potential of public health research in this field by giving an illustrative overview of several different methodological approaches that have been used, as well as their advantages and limitations. We describe population-based survey research and specifically the mortality follow-back design, the use of death certificate data to study place of death, studies of routinely collected administrative data on the population level, the use of existing epidemiological monitoring tools, and studies using qualitative and mixed methods in less visible populations.

The selection of research methods included in this chapter was guided by the aim to present different methods that can be applied to study palliative care either in full populations or in population-based samples. In the tradition of classic public health research methods, all of these methods are quantitative. Additionally, we included a section explaining the importance and advantages of including qualitative public health research alongside quantitative population-based methods. The specific studies that are used to illustrate the different methods were chosen based on the research that the authors of this chapter are experienced in. In our selection of studies presented, and where possible, we paid particular attention to include cross-national comparative studies. In doing so, we aimed to highlight the particular advantage that public health research offers in studying the same phenomena in different countries using standardized and comparable research methods. This approach was shown to be very useful for generating hypotheses regarding the impact of public policy on palliative and end-of-life care.

2 Population-Based Survey Research and the Mortality Follow-Back Design

Population-based surveys are conducted in representative samples of populations or communities. Most surveys have in common that they ask people questions and then analyze these responses quantitatively, using statistics (Addington-Hall 2007). The quantitative data are collected (i.e., the questions are being asked) in a standardized way in order to obtain comparable results across the sample. Once the results are summarized and analyzed, inferences are drawn from the sample to the entire population about which one aims to make conclusions. Surveys may be used to describe attributes, attitudes, opinions, knowledge or beliefs, as well as intended and/or actual behavior regarding a population at a given time point.

As the central purpose of a population-based survey is to draw reliable, valid, and unbiased inferences about the population, and not just about the sample, it is crucial to ensure that the sample is representative of the population. Therefore, particular attention needs to be paid to the sampling frame. The sampling frame is a list of all the units in the population of interest who are eligible to be sampled. It is important to ensure that the sampling frame is well chosen, because a sample can only be representative of the sampling frame. An incomplete sampling frame is therefore a threat to the representativeness and generalizability of a survey (Addington-Hall 2007).

A core feature of population-based surveys in palliative and end-of-life care is their aim to provide information that is generalizable to whole (national) populations or communities. They offer important insights about the health problems of entire populations of dying individuals and other people affected (e.g., family carers). The sampling frames of population-based studies in palliative and end-of-life care have included, for instance, all registered deaths in a country (as identified on death certificates) or all deaths among patients of representative samples of general practitioners (see studies in Boxes 1 and 4). Drawing population-based samples prevents bias that would be introduced by other sampling methods that systematically, explicitly or implicitly, exclude certain subpopulations. For instance, a sample of older cancer patients attended by a palliative care service excludes those dying without receiving this service. Hence, based on this sample, no general conclusions can be made about the full population of older people who are dying from cancer.

A very frequently applied design in population-based surveys in palliative and end-of-life care is the mortality follow-back design. It allows for the identification of individual deaths and thus creates a clear population-based sampling frame that is relevant to studying the end of life. Researchers conducting surveys in palliative care that use a mortality follow-back design typically select a random population-based sample of deaths and subsequently ask relevant respondents to retrospectively describe or evaluate the care the deceased person received shortly before death (i. e., the final hours, days, or weeks of life). The sampling frame for these studies is often death certificates, although other methods, such as deaths identified by GPs belonging to epidemiological surveillance networks, have also been applied (see Box 4). The respondents typically are groups who have relevant knowledge on the deceased person's end of life such as bereaved relatives (see VOICES study in Box 1), the treating physician (see ELD study in Box 1), or care home nurses (see PACE study in Box 1).

The frequent use of retrospective designs in population-based studies is largely due to difficulties in prospectively obtaining information from representative samples of dying people. This would entail following large numbers of persons for extended periods of time, in numerous care settings, and thus would be hardly feasible (Chambaere et al. 2008; Earle and Ayanian 2006). Furthermore, those who are most ill would have a high risk of being underrepresented due to their likely non-response, attrition, or decisions by researchers, healthcare staff or family not to overburden them. Additionally, it is difficult to prospectively identify who is dying. Research has indicated that clinicians perform poorly at predicting expected survival and usually overestimate it (Tavares et al. 2018). Retrospective studies offer a realistic possibility to researchers to study population-based samples of people nearing the end of life rather than nonrandomly selected subsets of patients defined by a disease characteristic (e.g., diagnosis of metastatic cancer), care setting (e.g., enrolled in a palliative care service), or specific event that identifies them as dying (e.g., assignment of a formal "palliative status" linked to reimbursement of healthcare costs) and thus provides a more inclusive approach (Earle and Ayanian 2006). They provide a clear denominator or sampling frame for the population under study (e.g., all non-sudden deaths in the ELD study and Euro-Sentimelc study; see Boxes 1 and 4) and allow limiting the analyses to a clearly defined time period, such as the last 3 months of a person's life. This is particularly important when examining aspects of care that are a function of time, such as the time of initiation of palliative care prior to death or frequency of palliative care service use.

Mortality follow-back studies also carry several challenges. Firstly, selecting the most adequate respondent to report on the care received by a deceased person requires careful consideration. The treating physician, nurses, and relatives are suitable respondents for different kinds of research questions. For instance, a physician or nurse may better report on medications administered and their dosages than a family carer. However, both the physician and the family carer can report on symptoms experienced by the patient (Klinkenberg et al. 2003). Secondly, there is a risk of recall bias because periods before death need to be cognitively reconstructed by the respondent. Therefore, the period on which respondents are asked to report is usually limited (e.g., the last 3 days or the last 3 months of life), and respondents are not asked to report on deaths that occurred more than a few months ago (Pivodic et al. 2016a). This also means that this method is particularly useful for studying the circumstances of the imminent dying phase rather than the longer course of disease until death. Thirdly, an important challenge is obtaining good response rates in mortality follow-back surveys. While there are studies where this is less of a problem (e.g., registrations by epidemiological surveillance networks; Pivodic et al. 2016b), it has been particularly difficult to get high response rates from bereaved relatives (Pivodic et al. 2016a).

Box 1 describes three examples of mortality follow-back studies: VOICES, the End-of-Life Decisions study, and the epidemiological study of the PACE project. They were chosen to represent different topics surveyed, populations, sampling frames, and respondents.

Box 1 Three Examples of Mortality Follow-Back Studies

National Survey of Bereaved People (VOICES)

The first large-scale population-based mortality follow-back survey was the National Survey of Bereaved People (VOICES), in England. The first VOICES study examined the quality of care in the last year of life given to patients aged 15 years or over who died from a range of conditions (e.g., cancer, stroke, chronic obstructive pulmonary disease) and in different locations. The authors conducted structured interviews with bereaved relatives and asked about their perceptions of the care given to recently deceased persons (Addington-Hall and McCarthy 1995). The Office for National Statistics (ONS) identified from death registrations deaths eligible for inclusion in the study and, for each death, the person who had notified authorities of the death. This was usually a relative or friend of the deceased. In later editions of the VOICES study, instead of conducting interviews, structured questionnaires were mailed to respondents by the ONS (Burt et al. 2010). The respondents then mailed the completed questionnaires

Box 1 (continued)

directly to the research team. Furthermore, the period before death studied changed from 1 year to 3 months. The VOICES questionnaire covers the following topics: details about the deceased (sociodemographic and clinical characteristics including cause of death, care settings where she/he had received care), perceptions of the quality of care delivered in each setting (e.g., home, hospital, hospice), coordination of care, quality of care in the last 2 days of life, decision-making toward the end of life, preferences for place of death, respondents' views on the ultimate place of death, and support provided to family/friends in the last 3 months of life and after the death. Numerous research articles have resulted from this study, including analyses of these topics for specific groups according to cause of death, place of death, or age (Burt et al. 2010; Young et al. 2009; Hunt et al. 2014).

Following the publication of the End-of-Life Care Strategy in the United Kingdom, the Department of Health commissioned a modified VOICES study to monitor key aspects of the quality of care identified in the strategy. The National Survey of Bereaved People was conducted by the Office for National Statistics on behalf of NHS England for the first time in 2011 and has been repeated annually thereafter. For this purpose, the original VOICES questionnaire was redesigned to meet the requirements of the End-of-Life Care Strategy (Hunt et al. 2017). This government-funded monitoring program of the quality of end-of-life care has continued until today and is regularly collecting survey data and publishing findings through government reports.

End-of-Life Decisions (ELD) study

The End-of-Life Decisions (ELD) study is a mortality follow-back survey carried

(*continued*)

Box 1 (continued)

out in Belgium (Flanders), the Netherlands, Switzerland, Italy, Denmark, and Sweden (van der Heide et al. 2003). Its aim was to obtain reliable and valid incidence estimates of ELDs and their characteristics as well as data on the decision-making process prior to ELDs and the treatments and care provided to people at the end of life. The ELD study design is based on a method first developed in the Netherlands in 1990 (Van Der Maas et al. 1991).

The sampling frame consisted of individual deaths. A sample of death certificates was taken, corresponding to almost 25% of deaths in a 6-month period. The sample was stratified proportionally for month of death (and, where applicable, province) and disproportionately for cause of death, as ELDs are known to vary by these factors (Chambaere et al. 2008). Both minors and adult deaths were included, using separate questionnaires for both groups, and they were analyzed separately. From the sampled death certificates, the research team identified the physician who certified the death and who was the information unit for the study. Physicians received the study questionnaire by regular mail. If the certifying physician was not the patient's treating physician, they were advised to forward the questionnaire to the treating physician (or to discard the questionnaire, if the treating physician's identity was unknown) and to inform the research team of this. The respondents returned the completed questionnaires to a trusted third party (TTP; e.g., a lawyer in Belgium) whose task it was to safeguard anonymity by removing any possible identifying information from the questionnaires. The TTP also linked the returned questionnaires to anonymized sociodemographic and morbidity information they received from national death certificate processing agencies for each identified deceased person. The TTP then

Box 1 (continued)

transmitted the anonymized and linked data to the research team.

The physician was asked at the beginning of the questionnaire to indicate whether the death was sudden and completely unexpected. Only if this was not the case, i.e., if the death was non-sudden and expected, were they instructed to complete the further sections. This was done to ensure that only those deceased people were included for whom ELDs had been a realistic option. The questionnaire concerned the last weeks of life of the deceased person and included sections on the types of ELDs made and decision-making process, characteristics of care and involvement of palliative care services, as well as several questions on palliative sedation. Next to providing important insights into end-of-life decisions and the decision-making process in several European countries (Chambaere et al. 2015a; Cohen et al. 2007a), the ELD study has been an important monitoring tool of the incidence of euthanasia which has been legalized in Belgium in May 2002 (Dierickx et al. 2018; Chambaere et al. 2015b).

Palliative Care for Older People (PACE) study: mortality follow-back study in nursing homes

The international Palliative Care for Older People (PACE) study included a cross-sectional epidemiological study of deceased residents in nursing homes in Belgium, Italy, Finland, the Netherlands, Poland, and England (Van den Block et al. 2016). It is an example of a mortality follow-back survey in a specific care setting (i.e., nursing homes). Its overall aim is to generate international data regarding the quality and costs of palliative care in several types of nursing homes in different countries across Europe. The specific aims of the PACE study are situated on two levels, that

(*continued*)

Box 1 (continued)
of the resident and that of care staff (i.e., nurses and care assistants). The study aim on the resident level is to examine the quality of dying as well as costs of end-of-life care in nursing homes. The study aim on the staff level is to examine palliative care knowledge and attitudes among care staff. The PACE study uses the term "nursing home" to refer to "collective institutional settings where care, on-site provision of personal assistance in daily living, and on-site or off-site provision of nursing and medical care, is provided for older people who live there, 24 h a day, 7 days a week, for an undefined period of time" (Van den Block et al. 2016).

In each country, a sample of nursing homes was drawn through proportionally stratified random sampling to obtain representative samples in terms of region within country, facility type, and bed capacity. Sampling was done based on national lists of nursing homes in all countries, except Italy, where no national lists exist and a previously created cluster of nursing homes with interest in research participation was used. The English research team additionally recruited through ENRICH, a network of nursing homes with interest in research participation, to improve the participation rate. The sampling frame consisted of all deaths of the previous 3 months among residents of the sampled nursing homes. Questionnaires were distributed to four different respondents linked to each death: (1) the nurse most involved in the care of the deceased resident or a care assistant in case a nurse could not be identified, (2) the nursing home administrator/manager/head nurse, (3) the resident's treating physician (GP or elderly care physician), and (4) a closely involved relative (family or friend). Questionnaires for care staff were distributed to all care staff on duty on the day the

Box 1 (continued)
researchers visited the nursing home for data collection.

The resident-level questionnaires assessed residents' quality of dying, health-related quality of life of residents and relatives, quality and processes of palliative and end-of-life care (including psychosocial and spiritual care, advance care planning, medication use, life-prolonging treatments, treatments discontinued or not initiated, palliative sedation), and costs and resource use. The staff-level questionnaires assessed staff knowledge and attitudes regarding palliative care, self-efficacy in providing palliative care, interdisciplinary communication and ethics in the work environment, and communication with residents and family. The PACE study has provided evidence from six countries regarding the quality of dying and quality of end- of-life care of nursing home residents (Pivodic et al. 2018), as well as palliative care knowledge of nursing home care staff (Smets et al. 2018).

3 Death Certificate Data to Study Place of Death

Most countries worldwide register deaths in a systematic and standardized manner using death certificates that are handled by a government agency. These records primarily serve administrative purposes, but they are also being used in public health research. The analysis of information from death certificates is a classic method applied in epidemiology. All major descriptions and projections of mortality, including causes of death and life expectancy, such as those regularly published by the WHO, rely on death certificate data. Death certificates typically contain information on the deceased's identity; birth details; gender; date, cause, and location of death; date on which the death was registered; informant details; name of coroner (in case the death was referred to one); details of the registrar handling the registration; and the date on which the death certificate was produced. These are limited data, but they are highly standardized across most countries worldwide which makes them particularly useful for cross-national comparisons.

The research potential of death certificates has also been recognized in palliative care (Cohen et al. 2007b). Death certificate data on place of death have become one of the most frequently used tools in public health research in palliative care (Pivodic et al. 2016c; Gao et al. 2013; Sleeman et al. 2014). Studies using place of death data have shown to be useful for identifying the care settings that have an important role in the delivery of end-of-life care in different countries (Cohen et al. 2007b). This has made them a cornerstone in the planning, implementation, and evaluation of policies aimed at enabling people to die in their place of choice. Data on where people die can also provide a scientific evidence base for the allocation of financial, material, and human resources for palliative care (Pivodic et al. 2016c).

The major advantage of death certificate data is that they allow phenomena to be studied in full populations (e.g., all deaths of one country during 1 year) rather than samples and thus do not carry the risk of sampling bias. This fact, together with the high level of standardization of death certificate data, facilitates cross-national comparisons of place of death (Pivodic et al. 2016c; Cohen et al. 2015). Several cross-national studies of the place of death have been conducted to date and revealed countries with higher or lower proportions of deaths in certain locations (Houttekier et al. 2010; Cohen et al. 2008; Pivodic et al. 2015; Cohen et al. 2015). Next to cross-national standardization, there is also standardization of place of death data over time *within* countries. This has made death certificates the tool of choice for monitoring trends over time in place of death in different populations (Sleeman et al. 2014; Houttekier et al. 2011; Gao et al. 2013). These analyses can be used, for instance, to study the potential impact of changes in healthcare policy (e.g., additional funding for home palliative care) or societal changes (e.g., decrease in availability of family care).

The unique identifiers on death certificates, which unambiguously link them to a particular individual, usually enable linkages across population-level databases administered by government agencies. This has been important for obtaining relevant predictor variables in analyses of place of death that are not recorded on death certificates, such as certain sociodemographic data, economic indicators, or regional indicators of healthcare resources (e.g., hospital bed capacity) (Pivodic et al. 2016c). In principle, there lies even greater potential in linking individual death certificate data to other population-level data, such as health claims data. These possibilities are discussed in the next section. A further advantage of death certificate data lies in the large sample size one can obtain with them. This provides sufficient statistical power for studying subpopulations (e.g., people who died from lung cancer, people living in regions with low socioeconomic indicators) and for conducting tests of association with a large number of independent variables (Cohen et al. 2007b).

Studies of place of death using death certificate data carry several challenges. Firstly, the primary use of these data is administration and not research. As a result, important information for research purposes (e.g., sociodemographic information, individual socioeconomic status rather than regional aggregates) is often not included in them. Death certificates do not contain some information that is important for predicting a person's place of death, such as information on the course of disease, treatments received toward the end of life, or the persons' preferred place of death (Cohen et al. 2007b). Although it is possible to study the place of death in a population that could potentially benefit from palliative care as judged by the cause of death (Pivodic et al. 2016c), we cannot know from death certificates whether palliative care was a realistic option for a specific individual. Secondly, despite the high level of cross-national standardization of death certificates, place of death is not uniformly coded across countries. Some countries register it only in a limited way, for instance, by distinguishing merely "home" versus "other" (Pivodic et al. 2016c). This calls for a more complete registration and better standardization of place of death records across countries (Pivodic et al. 2013). Finally, studies using death certificates may be affected by issues of validity regarding the cause of death (Burger et al. 2012). This seems less of a problem when aggregated categories of causes of death are used (e.g., cancer versus non-cancer disease), but it appears particularly problematic when dementia is concerned. A study using linked administrative data showed that only around half of people who die with dementia have it listed as their cause of death on the death certificate (Perera et al. 2016). The likelihood of having dementia recorded was higher if the person died in a nursing home rather than at home. These findings should warn researchers to be cautious in their conclusions from studies that investigate associations between cause and place of death.

Box 2 describes the International Place of Death study as an example of a population-level investigation of place of death. This study has been conducted in multiple countries, allowing for cross-national comparisons, as well as multiple times within the same country (Belgium) with the aim to study trends in place of death.

Box 2 Example of a Study Using Death Certificate Data

International Place of Death (IPoD) study

The International Place of Death (IPoD) study investigated the place of death in the total population of deaths of 1 year in 14 countries worldwide (Cohen et al. 2007b). The study collected complete death certificate data in countries that are situated across different levels of palliative care integration into mainstream healthcare. Next to place of death, the death certificates provided limited clinical (i.e., cause of death) and sociodemographic data. In some countries, sociodemographic and environment-related variables are not recorded on death certificates and were obtained by linking death certificates with other databases (e.g., census data). Additionally, healthcare resource statistics per capita (e.g., number of hospital beds/1000 inhabitants) and data on the degree of urbanization were linked with the deceased's municipality/local authority of residence.

These data were used for large-scale studies of the place of death in different populations (e.g., people in potential need of palliative care (Pivodic et al. 2016c), people who died from cancer (Cohen et al. 2015)) as well as for trend analyses (Houttekier et al. 2011). Among other findings, these analyses revealed that people who die from cancer were more likely to die at home rather than in hospital in many countries, but not all. This led to the hypothesis that the relatively predictable course of disease of cancer might facilitate a home death only in those countries where cancer care is not centered in hospitals (Pivodic et al. 2016c). IPoD data also revealed important similarities across countries, such as the finding that people who died from hematological cancer were more likely to die in hospital than people who died from a solid tumor in 14 countries across four continents. This raises the possibility that there might be clinical characteristics that make a certain place of death more likely, independent from healthcare organization (Cohen et al. 2015).

4 Routinely Collected Population-Level Administrative Data

A growing body of public health research in palliative care makes use of routinely collected health data. These data are generated by and serve administrative and clinical processes, as opposed to data generated solely for research purposes, such as survey data. Routinely collected data in palliative care research include, for instance, death registry data; activity data from primary, secondary, and tertiary care settings; health claims data; and cancer registries (Davies et al. 2016; Maetens et al. 2016).

Routine health data can be collected at three different levels, and this has an influence on their possibilities for research use: (1) the personal level, which includes disaggregated information about individual people including clinical records of care received; (2) the service level, which includes summary information about a healthcare service, e.g., number of patients seen in a year; and (3) the area level, which includes summary information about an area, e.g., proportion of home deaths or number of hospitals (Davies et al. 2016). The second and third levels allow comparisons to be made between areas and services. The first level, the person level, contains the richest information about a patient's clinical and sociodemographic characteristics and treatments. It is this level on which the most meaningful data on quality of care can be collected. Hence this section focuses on the use of person-level routine data in palliative care research.

Earle and colleagues were among the first to explore the potential of using systems of routinely collected data in palliative care research, specifically to assess and implement quality indicators for end-of-life cancer care (Earle 2003). Since then, increasing digitalization has further facilitated the process of generating, storing, and exchanging large amounts of individual patient data that can be used for public health research in palliative care (Murdoch and Detsky 2013). Routinely collected health data are a source of comprehensive information concerning service and medication use and associated costs, as these are well-recorded for billing purposes in many countries (Maetens et al. 2016).

The use of routinely collected administrative data has several important advantages for public health research in palliative care. Just like death certificates, they are population-level data and hence not prone to sampling bias. They allow different subpopulations, including difficult-to-reach subgroups to be studied (Billings 2003). Individual person-level routine data can be aggregated on multiple levels (e.g., by diagnosis, treatment, service provider, geographical region), which gives them an important advantage over routinely collected data on the service level that do not offer the possibility to identify unique cases. Given that most administrative data are collected at regular intervals, they permit time trend analyses and longitudinal studies. Lastly, obtaining administrative data is relatively inexpensive compared to original large-scale data collection (Maetens et al. 2016).

Using routine administrative data in research also carries limitations (Maetens et al. 2016). Obtaining comprehensive routine data for research purposes often requires linking data from different sources. This process brings about potential challenges for researchers, including identifying relevant data, completeness of data, obtaining access to data from different organizations, technical difficulties when linking data, creating useful variables for research purposes, and maintaining strict ethics and privacy procedures (Davies et al. 2016; Maetens et al. 2016). Health services not covered by insurers are usually not included in these databases, and it may be region- and country-specific which services are and are not covered. This places additional demands on researchers to identify the regulations applicable to the region or country they intend to study. Furthermore, the use of certain services cannot be identified because there is no individual reimbursement per patient (e.g., mobile hospital palliative care teams in Belgium) or because reimbursements are not regulated or generalized (e.g., consultations of a psychologist in Belgium) (Maetens et al. 2016). An additional limitation is linked to the fact that administrative databases are not primarily research instruments. This means that they do not contain more in-depth data on quality of care (e.g., patient reported outcome measures), quality of dying, and details of the course of disease and symptoms experienced.

Box 3 describes a study that used linked administrative data to study palliative and end-of-life care in Belgium.

Box 3 Example of a Study Using Routinely Collected Administrative Data

Belgian study using linked data from eight administrative databases (Inter-Mutualistic Agency [IMA] study) (Maetens et al. 2016)

(*continued*)

Box 3 (continued)

The Inter-Mutualistic Agency (IMA) study was conducted in Belgium and linked eight administrative databases from three different administrators with the aim of studying the use, quality, and costs of end-of-life care on the population level and their association with various clinical, socio-demographic, socioeconomic, and environmental factors.

The data sources included:

1. Sociodemographic database of all individuals with health insurance (legally mandatory in Belgium)
2. Medical claims database containing health and medical care use characteristics of all reimbursed healthcare services of home, nursing home, and hospital care, except medication dispensed in public pharmacies
3. Pharmaceutical database containing medication supply characteristics of medications dispensed in public pharmacies
4. Belgian Cancer Registry database with diagnostic information on all new cases of cancer including type of cancer and date of diagnosis
5. Death certificate database containing causes of all reported deaths
6. Population registry database including household composition
7. Census database including housing characteristics and educational level
8. Fiscal database including net taxable income

The combination of these databases can provide information for the full population of deceased persons on formal healthcare use and related costs, medication prescription, causes of death, main diagnoses, and various sociodemographic and socioeconomic information. However, the data will likely be an underestimation of costs for end-of-life care given that services not covered by insurers are not included and neither are out-of-pocket costs.

A published research article describes the procedures for accessing and linking these databases, the information they contain, and which data handling procedures were necessary to prepare the data for analysis (Maetens et al. 2016). This can help researchers in navigating possibilities for using routine data in Belgium. It also provides a thorough description of the possibilities and limitations, as well as procedures and considerations to make, when using routinely collected administrative data for palliative care research internationally.

Research that has resulted from this method includes an investigation of resource use in the last 6 months of life of people who died with versus from Alzheimer's Disease (Faes et al. 2018), as well as a study of quality indicators for end-of-life care in the population who died from cancer (De Schreye et al. 2017).

5 Existing Epidemiological Monitoring Tools

A further research method derived from public health research to examine large population-based samples of people at the end of life includes the monitoring of care through epidemiological surveillance networks, such as sentinel networks of general practitioners (GPs) (Van den Block et al. 2013). Sentinel networks are networks of practices or community-based physicians who conduct epidemiological surveillance of one or more specific health problems on a regular basis (Fleming et al. 2003; Deckers and Schellavis 2004; Vega et al. 2006). The networks are typically set up and managed by national public health institutes to monitor various health problems such as the incidence of flu, diabetes, stroke, or suicide

(Fleming et al. 2003; Devroey et al. 2003; Lobet et al. 1987). In doing so, they monitor the health of the entire population in a country or wider region (Fleming et al. 2003; Deckers and Schellavis 2004). The general objectives of sentinel networks are (1) to evaluate public health problems and their importance within the general population; (2) to observe the change in certain health problems over time to evaluate, for instance, the impact of prevention campaigns; and (3) to study the management and follow-up of health problems in general practice (Van den Block et al. 2013).

Epidemiological surveillance through sentinel networks of GPs has a long tradition in scientific research. In countries in which close to everyone has a GP these networks capture representative samples of the population and thereby constitute a good research tool for studying population health (Van den Block et al. 2013). General practice is highly accessible in Europe; in the countries included in the Euro-Sentimelc study (see Box 4), almost all of the population have a GP whom they consult regularly (Schäfer et al. 2010; García-Armesto et al. 2010; Gerkens and Merkur 2010; Ferré et al. 2014). The yearly turnover of GPs in the sentinel networks is low which contributes to the scientific quality of the data collected. In contrast to death certificates and other routinely collected data, data generated by sentinel networks have primarily a research rather than an administrative purpose. This means that they are more comprehensive and include important sociodemographic and health- and healthcare-related information that is not captured in administrative databases and often not even in patients' medical files (e.g., whether GPs were aware of a patient's preferred place of death). Furthermore, researchers can rely on the routine quality assurance procedures employed by the public health institutes that manage the networks. This includes checks of data for inconsistencies and completeness, measures to reduce non-response, and instructions to physicians to use patient records and information coming from hospitals when registering information. Sentinel networks have regular and frequent registration intervals (e.g., weekly registration of deaths in the study described in Box 4), which makes recall bias less likely than in retrospective surveys with non-continuous registration where the interval between a person's death and data collection is typically longer (see Box 1).

Studies using sentinel networks of GPs also carry challenges. Obtaining in-depth data of care aspects is usually not possible as registration forms have to be kept short and simple so as not to overburden GPs. GPs are also asked to report on care that patients received outside of general practice (e.g., in hospital) of which they may not be fully informed. Hence there may be an underestimation of certain treatments provided or decisions taken by hospital physicians. It was also shown that GPs underreport deaths that occurred in hospital (Van den Block et al. 2013). Lastly, some countries' healthcare organization poses specific challenges to this research method. For instance, Belgium does not have patient lists per practice which means that the population denominator cannot be precisely defined. In the Netherlands, sentinel networks of GPs do not capture deaths in nursing homes as the treating physicians in these facilities are specialized nursing home physicians.

Box 4 describes one, and so far the only, study that used population-based data from sentinel networks of GPs to study end-of-life care.

Box 4 Example of a Population-Based Study Using an Existing Epidemiological Surveillance Network to Study Palliative Care

European Sentinel Network Monitoring End-of-Life Care (Euro-Sentimelc) study

The European Sentinel Network Monitoring End-of-Life Care (Euro-Sentimelc) study is a continuous cross-national mortality follow-back study with the aim to examine end-of-life care in the population of four European countries (Van den Block et al. 2013). It is called continuous because, unlike in the VOICES or ELD studies (Box 1), deaths were not identified at one point in time but continuously over a 3-year period. The sampling frame was individual

(*continued*)

Box 4 (continued)

adult deaths that were registered by general practitioners (GPs) belonging to sentinel networks of Belgium, the Netherlands, Italy, and two autonomous communities in Spain, i.e., the Valencian Community and Castile and Leon.

The GPs belonging to the sentinel networks completed a standardized registration form for every deceased patient of their practice and answered questions regarding several aspects of their end-of-life care. GPs registered deaths on a weekly basis to keep response bias at a minimum. The information collected by the registration forms is anonymous, and the topics surveyed include places of care and place of death, transitions between care settings, communication between physician and patient/family, advance care planning, palliative care provision, symptoms in the last week of life, and costs and burden of end-of-life care for patients and family carers. A particular characteristic of this study is that GPs were asked to indicate whether the death they were reporting on was "sudden and totally unexpected." The authors excluded sudden deaths from the analyses in order to focus on patients for whom care in the terminal phase of life, including palliative care, was a realistic option (Van den Block et al. 2013).

An analysis of deaths registered by the sentinel networks showed that they were representative for all deaths in the participating countries in terms of age, gender, and place of death (Van den Block et al. 2013). Deaths in nursing homes in the Netherlands were an important exception to this, as nursing home residents are treated by specialized elderly care physicians as opposed to GPs. Furthermore, GPs underreported a small number of sudden hospital deaths in all countries as well as non-sudden hospital deaths and deaths of people under 65 years in Belgium (Van den Block et al. 2013).

Box 4 (continued)

Over several years of data collection, the Euro-Sentimelc study (and its predecessor studies in Belgium and the Netherlands Meeussen et al. 2011) provided monitoring data on several aspects of end-of-life care in the last 3 months of life in four European countries.

These include, but are not limited to, transitions between care settings (Van den Block et al. 2007, 2015), hospital admissions at the end of life (Pivodic et al. 2016b), trends over time in specialist palliative care involvement in Belgium (Penders et al. 2018), preferred and actual place of death (Ko et al. 2013), and patient-GP communication about end-of-life topics (Evans et al. 2014).

6 Qualitative Methods in Public Health Research in Palliative Care

Public health research is dominated by quantitative research methods, and public health research in palliative care is no exception to this. As a result, there are many *descriptions* of end-of-life care processes and outcomes in populations but few studies that aim to provide *understanding* or *meaning* to these phenomena (Sallnow et al. 2016a). The spread of traditional, quantitative, methods in public health research across a growing number of health topics has led to calls for more reflection on the appropriateness of the questions asked in public health research, the ways in which they are addressed, and the conclusions drawn from research into health practice and policies (Faltermaier and Faltermaier 1997). Authors have argued that the complexity inherent to public health initiatives in palliative care is insufficiently captured by the dominant quantitative methods outlined in the previous sections (Sallnow et al. 2016a). They do not provide sufficient information to answer questions such as when and where people with a life-threatening illness seek professional help, how they perceive and interpret their illness, how they view the care provided to them, their preferences for care, and how this is shaped by societal factors. Understanding these phenomena, all of which influence the circumstances in which people die, can aid in the development of appropriate and effective public health interventions. However, studying them places new demands on study designs.

Qualitative methods provide a possibility to study the complexity inherent to public health approaches in palliative care. Qualitative research has been particularly used and promoted within "new public health" approaches to palliative care (Sallnow et al. 2016b). It is seen as the method of choice for studying social, personal, and environmental resources for health, next to curative and restorative approaches that have guided "classic" conceptions of public health. According to this view, qualitative methods are essential for research that represents patients not as mere objects of compliance to expert-based interventions but as active and conscious individuals capable of making informed decisions, seeking professional help only under certain circumstances, with special needs and expectations (Faltermaier and Faltermaier 1997). Box 5 presents two studies as examples of the research questions asked, methods applied, and insights gained from qualitative approaches to public health research in palliative care.

Box 5 Examples of Qualitative Public Health Research in Palliative Care

The impact of a community volunteer program in Uganda

This study explored the impact of a Community Volunteer Program (CVP) run by Hospice Africa Uganda that provides practical, emotional, physical, and spiritual support to people with cancer and HIV/AIDS in their own home (Jack et al. 2011). It engages members from the local community (i.e., community volunteers) to augment the work of a local hospice team by identifying patients, who often live in rural

Box 5 (continued)

communities and who would normally not be seen by the hospice team, or even know of it. Community volunteers are acting as a link between patients in the community and healthcare professionals. The research was conducted with a sample of key stakeholders involved with the service, i.e., 21 patients (who had been attended by the CVP team for at least 3 months), 11 hospice clinical staff, and 32 community volunteer workers (CVWs). Data from patients and CVWs was collected through group interviews using a semi-structured schedule. Hospice clinical staff participated either in focus groups or individual semi-structured interviews. Data collection focused on the participants' experience of the CVW program. Data were analyzed using thematic analysis. The authors found that the CVP was having a positive impact on patients and families by being a "bridge" to the hospice and enabling palliative care to reach out into the rural community. Identified challenges included distances that volunteers are required to travel on poor transport (bicycles in bad condition) and expected reductions in funding.

Usefulness of digital stories as research method for palliative care in Māori communities

Digital stories are short first-person videos comprised of images, video clips, voice-overs, text, and music that tell a story of great significance to the creator. They have been described as a useful emergent method for public health research and specifically community-based participatory research (Williams et al. 2017). This study explored how this method might be applied in palliative care and specifically for studying Māori(Indigenous people of New Zealand) experiences of caring for their older relatives at the end of life. This method is based on the position that

(*continued*)

Box 5 (continued)
community-centered palliative care approaches call for community-centered research methods, especially ones that can be adapted to the particularities of a certain locality. Previous research using digital storytelling (DST) with indigenous communities suggested that it might fulfill the imperative for culturally appropriate methods.

This study adopted an exploratory qualitative research design using a constructivist conceptual framework. Constructivism acknowledges the presence of multiple realities; the understanding of phenomena is derived through participants' subjective views that have been shaped by social interaction with others and from their own personal histories (Williams et al. 2017). The research approach involved making Māori concerns and priorities the focal point of the research, which was centered within Māori culture and practice. Participants, who had to be involved in the care of an older relative, were recruited through snowball sampling based on a group of Māori who had participated in previous research. The digital stories were created in a workshop facilitated by the researchers. Additionally, participants were asked to complete an anonymous, written questionnaire consisting of open-ended questions on their views of the workshop and digital story. Thematic analysis was used to analyze the questionnaires.

The authors identified several facilitating factors for this method as well as hindering factors with regard to recruitment, use of technology, and integration of the pōwhiri process (Māori formal welcome of visitors) into the research. Overall, they concluded that DST is a useful method to study Māori end-of-life caregiving. Differences between cultures among countries worldwide mean that people face different palliative and end-of-life care scenarios. This diversity necessitates a diversity in research

Box 5 (continued)
methods to better understand ways in which care can be most effectively delivered in different communities. DST may be a useful method for studying palliative care in a participatory research environment built on community involvement and specifically with indigenous groups.

7 Conclusion

Public health research is an essential element of palliative care research. It allows us to study circumstances of dying, patients' and families' needs, and the provision and quality of care toward the end of life, including palliative care, in populations. This chapter provides an illustrative overview of quantitative and qualitative methods that have been used in public health research in palliative care. All methods described here, both quantitative and qualitative, are well-established in public health research. This chapter explains how they can be applied in the specific field of palliative care and which knowledge can be gained through them. We distinguished several quantitative approaches according to their sampling frame, the data source and the primary purpose of the data (administrative versus research), and types of respondents (in the case of surveys). Next to the dominant quantitative methods, this chapter also pays attention to qualitative public health research methods, which are increasingly being employed, particularly in the context of community-centered approaches to dying and palliative care. This chapter aimed to highlight their importance and the potential they offer for a better understanding of public health phenomena in palliative care that are insufficiently or not at all captured by quantitative data.

Next to showing the possibilities that public health research offers to palliative care, this chapter also makes apparent that no single method can answer all relevant questions. In this regard, public health research is no different from other domains, including clinical research. Recognizing this, this chapter describes the advantages and limitations of each method presented and gives examples of research questions they are particularly suited to address.

We acknowledge that our illustrative overview of research methods and studies likely overlooks several other public health research designs that have led to important insights in palliative care. Likewise, there are many examples of studies using the methods we presented that we did not mention. However, we do hope that the examples presented in this chapter convey to interested readers the diversity and possibilities of public health research in palliative care, help them identify similar studies in the literature, appraise their possibilities and limitations, and guide future research endeavors.

Ultimately, we argue that the best possible view on and understanding of the circumstances of dying and provision of palliative care in populations can be achieved only by applying a diversity of public health research methods, each of which is suited to answer specific sets of questions.

References

Addington-Hall J. In: Addington-Hall J, Bruera E, Higginson IJ, Payne S, editors. Research methods in palliative care. Oxford: Oxford University Press; 2007.

Addington-Hall J, McCarthy M. Regional study of care for the dying: methods and sample characteristics. Palliat Med. 1995;9:27–35.

Billings J. Using administrative data to monitor access, identify disparities, and assess performance of the safety net. Agency for Healthcare Research and Quality; U.S. Department of Health and Human Services. 2003. Available at: https://archive.ahrq.gov/data/safetynet/billings.htm. Accessed 7 Mar 2018.

Burger EH, et al. Validation study of cause of death statistics in Cape Town, South Africa, found poor agreement. J Clin Epidemiol. 2012;65:309–16.

Burt J, Shipman C, Richardson A, Ream E, Addington-Hall J. The experiences of older adults in the community dying from cancer and non-cancer causes: a national survey of bereaved relatives. Age Ageing. 2010;39:86–91.

Chambaere K, et al. A post-mortem survey on end-of-life decisions using a representative sample of death certificates in Flanders, Belgium: research protocol. BMC Public Health. 2008;8:299.

Chambaere K, Cohen J, Robijn L, Bailey SK, Deliens L. End-of-life decisions in individuals dying with dementia in Belgium. J Am Geriatr Soc. 2015a;63:290–6.

Chambaere K, Vander Stichele R, Mortier F, Cohen J, Deliens L. Recent trends in euthanasia and other end-of-life practices in Belgium. N Engl J Med. 2015b;372:1179–81.

Cohen J, Deliens L. In: Cohen J, Deliens L, editors. A public health perspective on end of life care. Oxford: Oxford University Press; 2011. p. 3–18.

Cohen J, et al. End-of-life decision-making in Belgium, Denmark, Sweden and Switzerland: does place of death make a difference. J Epidemiol Commun Health. 2007a;61:1062–8.

Cohen J, et al. Using death certificate data to study place of death in 9 European countries: opportunities and weaknesses. BMC Public Health. 2007b;7:283.

Cohen J, et al. Population-based study of dying in hospital in six European countries. Palliat Med. 2008;22:702–10.

Cohen J, et al. International study of the place of death of people with cancer: a population-level comparison of 14 countries across 4 continents using death certificate data. Br J Cancer. 2015;113:1397–404.

Davies JM, et al. Using routine data to improve palliative and end of life care. BMJ Support Palliat Care. 2016;6:257–62.

De Schreye R, et al. Applying quality indicators for administrative databases to evaluate end-of-life care for cancer patients in Belgium. Health Aff. 2017;36:1234–43.

Deckers J, Schellavis F. Health information from primary care: final report December 1, 2001 – March 31, 2004. 2004.

Devroey D, Van Casteren V, Buntinx F. Registration of stroke through the Belgian sentinel network and factors influencing stroke mortality. Cerebrovasc Dis. 2003;16:272–9.

Dierickx S, Deliens L, Cohen J, Chambaere K. Involvement of palliative care in euthanasia practice in a context of legalized euthanasia: a population-based mortality follow-back study. Palliat Med. 2018;32:114–22.

Earle CC. Identifying potential indicators of the quality of end-of-life cancer care from administrative data. J Clin Oncol. 2003;21:1133–8.

Earle CC, Ayanian JZ. Looking back from death: the value of retrospective studies of end-of-life care. J Clin Oncol. 2006;24:838–40.

Evans N, et al. End-of-life communication: a retrospective survey of representative general practitioner networks in four countries. J Pain Symptom Manag. 2014;47:604–19.

Faes K, Cohen J, Annemans L. Resource use during the last 6 months of life of individuals dying with and of Alzheimer's disease. J Am Geriatr Soc. 2018. https://doi.org/10.1111/jgs.15287.

Faltermaier T, Faltermaier T. Why public health research needs qualitative approaches. Eur J Pub Health. 1997;7:357–63.

Ferré F, et al. Italy: health system review. Health Syst Transit. 2014;16:1–168.

Fleming DM, Schellevis FG, Paget WJ. Health monitoring in sentinel practice networks. Eur J Pub Health. 2003;13:80–4.

Gao W, Ho YK, Verne J, Glickman M, Higginson IJ. Changing patterns in place of cancer death in England: a population-based study. PLoS Med. 2013;10: e1001410.

García-Armesto S, Abadía-Taira MB, Durán A, Hernández-Quevedo C, Bernal-Delgado E. Spain: health system review. Health Syst Transit. 2010;12: 1–295.

Gerkens S, Merkur S. Belgium: health system review. Health Syst Transit. 2010;12:1–266.

Glasgow RE, et al. If diabetes is a public health problem, why not treat it as one? A population-based approach to chronic illness. Ann Behav Med. 1999;21:159–70.

Houttekier D, et al. Place of death of older persons with dementia. A study in five European countries. J Am Geriatr Soc. 2010;58:751–6.

Houttekier D, Cohen J, Surkyn J, Deliens L. Study of recent and future trends in place of death in Belgium using death certificate data: a shift from hospitals to care homes. BMC Public Health. 2011;11:228.

Hunt KJ, Shlomo N, Addington-Hall J. End-of-life care and preferences for place of death among the oldest old: results of a population-based survey using VOICES-Short Form. J Palliat Med. 2014;17:176–82.

Hunt KJ, Richardson A, Darlington A-SE, Addington-Hall JM. Developing the methods and questionnaire (VOICES-SF) for a national retrospective mortality follow-back survey of palliative and end-of-life care in England. BMJ Support Palliat Care . bmjspcare-2016-001288. 2017. https://doi.org/10.1136/bmjspcare-2016-001288.

Jack BA, Kirton J, Birakurataki J, Merriman A. 'A bridge to the hospice': the impact of a community volunteer programme in Uganda. Palliat Med. 2011;25:706–15.

Klinkenberg M, et al. Proxy reporting in after-death interviews: the use of proxy respondents in retrospective assessment of chronic diseases and symptom burden in the terminal phase of life. Palliat Med. 2003;17: 191–201.

Ko W, et al. Awareness of general practitioners concerning cancer patients' preferences for place of death: evidence from four European countries. Eur J Cancer. 2013;49:1967–74.

Lobet MP, et al. Tool for validation of the network of sentinel general practitioners in the Belgian health care system. Int J Epidemiol. 1987;16:612–8.

Maetens A, et al. Using linked administrative and disease-specific databases to study end-of-life care on a population level. BMC Palliat Care. 2016;15:1–10.

Meeussen K, et al. End-of-life care and circumstances of death in patients dying as a result of cancer in Belgium and the Netherlands: a retrospective comparative study. J Clin Oncol. 2011;29:4327–34.

Murdoch TB, Detsky AS. The inevitable application of big data to health care. JAMA. 2013;309:1351.

Murtagh FE, et al. How many people need palliative care? A study developing and comparing methods for population-based estimates. Palliat Med. 2013. https://doi.org/10.1177/0269216313489367.

Penders YW, Gilissen J, Moreels S, Deliens L, Van den Block L. Palliative care service use by older people: time trends from a mortality follow-back study between 2005 and 2014. Palliat Med. 2018;32:466–75.

Perera G, Stewart R, Higginson IJ, Sleeman KE. Reporting of clinically diagnosed dementia on death certificates: retrospective cohort study. Age Ageing. 2016;45:667–72.

Pivodic L, Higginson IJ, Sarmento VP, Gomes B. Health metrics: standardize records of place of death. Nature. 2013;495:449.

Pivodic L, et al. Place of death in the population dying from diseases indicative of palliative care need: a cross-national population-level study in 14 countries. J Epidemiol Community Health. 2015;70:17–24.

Pivodic L, et al. Home care by general practitioners for cancer patients in the last 3 months of life: an epidemiological study of quality and associated factors. Palliat Med. 2016a;30:64.

Pivodic L, et al. Hospitalisations at the end of life in four European countries: a population-based study via epidemiological surveillance networks. J Epidemiol Community Health. 2016b;70:430–6.

Pivodic L, et al. Place of death in the population dying from diseases indicative of palliative care need: a cross-national population-level study in 14 countries. J Epidemiol Community Health. 2016c;70:17–24.

Pivodic L et al. Quality of dying and quality of end-of-life care of nursing home residents in six countries: an epidemiological study. Palliat Med. In press. 2018.

Sallnow L, Tishelman C, Lindqvist O, Richardson H, Cohen J. Research in public health and end-of-life care – building on the past and developing the new. Prog Palliat Care. 2016a;24:25–30.

Sallnow L, Richardson H, Murray SA, Kellehear A. The impact of a new public health approach to end-of-life care: a systematic review. Palliat Med. 2016b;30:200–11.

Schäfer W, et al. The Netherlands: health system review. Health Syst Transit. 2010;12:1–229.

Sleeman KE, et al. Reversal of English trend towards hospital death in dementia: a population-based study of place of death and associated individual and regional factors, 2001–2010. BMC Neurol. 2014;14:59.

Smets T et al. The palliative care knowledge of nursing home staff: The EU FP7 PACE cross-sectional survey in 322 nursing homes in six European countries. Palliat Med. In press. 2018.

Tavares T, et al. Predicting prognosis in patients with advanced cancer: a prospective study. Palliat Med. 2018;32:413–6.

Teno JM, et al. Change in end-of-life care for Medicare beneficiaries: site of death, place of care, and health care transitions in 2000, 2005, and 2009. JAMA. 2013;309:470–7.

Van den Block L, Deschepper R, Bilsen J, Van Casteren V, Deliens L. Transitions between care settings at the end of life in Belgium. JAMA. 2007;298:1638–9.

Van den Block L, et al. Nationwide continuous monitoring of end-of-life care via representative networks of general practitioners in Europe. BMC Fam Pract. 2013;14:73.

Van den Block L, et al. Transitions between health care settings in the final three months of life in four EU countries. Eur J Pub Health. 2015. https://doi.org/10.1093/eurpub/ckv039.

Van den Block L, et al. Comparing palliative care in care homes across Europe (PACE): protocol of a cross-sectional study of deceased residents in 6 EU countries. J Am Med Dir Assoc. 2016;17:566.e1–7.

van der Heide A, et al. End-of-life decision-making in six European countries: descriptive study. Lancet. 2003; 362:345–50.

Van Der Maas PJ, Van Delden JJ, Pijnenborg L, Looman CW. Euthanasia and other medical decisions concerning the end of life. Lancet. 1991;338:669–74.

Vega T, et al. Guide to the principles and methods of health sentinel networks in Spain. Gac Sanit. 2006;20:52–60.

WHO. WHO Definition of palliative care. 2002.

Williams L, et al. Can digital stories go where palliative care research has never gone before? A descriptive qualitative study exploring the application of an emerging public health research method in an indigenous palliative care context. BMC Palliat Care. 2017;16:1–9.

World Health Organization. Constitution of WHO: principles. 2018. Available at: http://www.who.int/about/mission/en/. Accessed 4th Apr 2018.

Young AJ, Rogers A, Dent L, Addington-Hall JM. Experiences of hospital care reported by bereaved relatives of patients after a stroke: a retrospective survey using the VOICES questionnaire. J Adv Nurs. 2009;65:2161–274.

Development and Evaluation of Complex Interventions in Palliative Care

92

Nilay Hepgul, Wei Gao, Matthew Maddocks, and Irene J. Higginson

Contents

Abstract

Evaluations of complex interventions are of utmost importance to identify and deliver clinically and cost-effective palliative and end-of-life care for future populations. They are however challenging and resource intensive. The Medical Research Council (MRC) framework together with the Methods Of Researching End of Life Care (MORECare) collaboration provides clear standards on best research practice in evaluating services and treatments. These guidelines emphasize the need to consider implementation at all phases of evaluation, rather than only at the end. Furthermore, they highlight the need for flexible and pragmatic approaches to develop, examine, and evaluate complex interventions in palliative and end-of-life care. In this chapter we outline what a complex intervention is, discuss the challenges of developing and evaluating complex interventions in palliative and end-of-life care, and provide examples of complex interventions which have reached the evaluation phase.

1 Introduction

Conducting research in palliative and end-of-life care can be demanding, especially when evaluating the effectiveness of complex palliative care interventions. There are multiple challenges associated with involving people with advanced illness in research, for example, people have

N. Hepgul (✉) · W. Gao · M. Maddocks · I. J. Higginson
Cicely Saunders Institute of Palliative Care, Policy and Rehabilitation, King's College London, London, UK
e-mail: nilay.hepgul@kcl.ac.uk; wei.gao@kcl.ac.uk; matthew.maddocks@kcl.ac.uk; irene.higginson@kcl.ac.uk; ea_irenehigginson@kcl.ac.uk

R. D. MacLeod, L. Van den Block (eds.), *Textbook of Palliative Care*,
https://doi.org/10.1007/978-3-319-77740-5_108

progressive and unpredictable illness trajectories, and high attrition from studies is common (Lorenz et al. 2008). The "gold standard" randomized controlled trial (RCT) is particularly challenging to conduct, as it demands a position of equipoise and a readiness to allocate to trial arms, by chance, people living with troublesome symptoms and a high level of need. A flexible and pragmatic approach is therefore needed to identify, examine, and evaluate palliative care interventions.

In 2000, the Medical Research Council (MRC) published its landmark framework for developing and evaluating complex interventions (Craig et al. 2008; Medical Research Council 2000). This provided an internationally agreed definition of what is meant by a "complex" intervention and a robust framework for the design of evaluative trials in this area. Complex interventions in health care were said to comprise a number of separate elements that seem essential to the proper functioning of the intervention, although the "active ingredient(s)" of the intervention are difficult to specify (Medical Research Council 2000). In their guidance the MRC advocates for the use of distinct iterative phases of intervention development, feasibility/piloting, evaluation, and implementation. Subsequent to this, the MRC jointly with the UK National Institute for Health Research (NIHR) established the Methods Of Researching End of Life Care (MORECare) collaboration. The aim was to identify, appraise, and synthesize best practice methods for research evaluating palliative and end-of-life care. In particular, it focused on the evaluation of complex interventions around service delivery and reconfiguration. In this chapter we outline what a complex intervention is, discuss the challenges of developing and evaluating complex interventions in palliative and end-of-life care, and provide examples of complex interventions which have reached the evaluation phase.

2 What Is a Complex Intervention?

There are several definitions of complex interventions. Most highlight the presence of multiple, interacting components and emphasize variability in the content, context, and mode of delivery, as well as the unpredictability of the overall effect (Lewin et al. 2017; Petticrew 2011; Wells et al. 2012). According to the MRC definition, a complex intervention (e.g., treatment, service) is one with several interacting components which may act both independently and interdependently. The components usually include behaviors, parameters of behaviors (e.g., frequency, timing), and methods of organizing and delivering those behaviors (e.g., type(s) of practitioner, setting, and location) (Medical Research Council 2000). As such, it can be difficult to know which are the "active ingredients." Complex interventions may be delivered at the individual, organizational, or population level and be targeted toward patients either directly or indirectly via health professionals and/or health systems. Taking these defining attributes into account, palliative and end-of-life services are clearly complex interventions, which comprise multiple interacting components and dimensions (Campbell et al. 2007).

Box 1 What Makes an Intervention Complex?

- The number of and interactions between components within the experimental and control interventions.
- Number and difficulty of behaviors required by those delivering or receiving the intervention.
- Number of groups or organizational levels targeted by the intervention.
- Number and variability of outcomes.
- Degree of flexibility or tailoring of the intervention.

Taken from Craig et al. (2008)

3 Evaluation

There is a growing interest in understanding the effectiveness of complex interventions in order to accurately describe and replicate them. Evaluation of a complex intervention is key to help identify and examine the "active ingredients" and how they tend toward an effect. Through this understanding, it becomes possible to know how an intervention can be transferred to other contexts, how generalizable an intervention might be, and how it can be most effectively implemented in clinical practice. A challenging aspect of evaluating a complex intervention is defining the intervention itself, to standardize its content and delivery by determining the critical components of the intervention and how they relate to and impact on each other (Medical Research Council 2000). Evaluations of complex interventions can be problematic simply because the researchers have not fully defined and developed the intervention prior to undertaking a trial. Added to this, the evaluation of palliative and end-of-life care interventions can be particularly difficult due to patients having complex and often multiple needs (physical, psychological, social, and spiritual) making standardization of the intervention more difficult. There are also often many people involved, not just patients but their families and those who support and care for them. Finally, there are issues around recruitment and retention of patients into studies and defining and measuring outcomes on a background of rapidly changing clinical situations and limited survival times.

4 MRC Framework/Guidance

In 2000 the MRC presented a stepwise approach to the evaluation of complex interventions. These steps can be compared with the sequential phases of drug development from the initial preclinical experiments through to post-marketing surveillance studies (Campbell et al. 2000). The sequential framework is useful as it sets out the objectives to be met at each stage prior to moving forward. However, it fits more readily with typical routes for drug development, and therefore for complex interventions, not all stages will be relevant for all research questions. Nonetheless, as a definitive effectiveness trial can be highly costly, it is important to systematically develop, test, and refine an intervention and the research methods before one takes place. The guidance was intended to help researchers choose and implement rigorous methods to develop and evaluate complex interventions, leading to theory-driven interventions with well-understood components.

Preclinical or theoretical phase – The first step is to establish the theoretical basis and identify evidence that suggests the intervention might lead to the expected effect. Reviewing the theoretical basis for an intervention may lead to changes in the hypothesis and improved specification of potentially active ingredients (Campbell et al. 2000). Some interventions may already be widely practiced or have evidence from previous studies from different contexts, and therefore a theoretical phase may not be essential. Consulting available evidence may help to eliminate implausible interventions or highlight any facilitating factors or barriers in developing a specific intervention.

Phase I or modelling – This phase involves identifying the components of the intervention as well as their underlying mechanisms and interrelationships. Paper modelling (diagrams or flowcharts) or simulations may be used. It is essential to clarify important components in order to devise clear and reasoned protocols for subsequent trial design. This phase may also involve qualitative testing, for example, through focus groups, preliminary surveys, case studies, or small observational studies. Qualitative testing during this early phase can also be helpful to understand how the intervention might work and to identify potential barriers to it being delivered.

Phase II or exploratory trial – In this phase, all the evidence gathered so far is put to the test to develop the optimal intervention and trial design. This can involve testing the feasibility of delivering the intervention as well as its acceptability to patients and providers. It may be appropriate to experiment with the intervention by adjusting different components to see what effect each change has on the intervention as a whole and to understand which variations seem to be the most appropriate for a full-scale effectiveness trial. Evidence can be obtained to support the theoretically expected treatment effect and to identify an appropriate control group, outcome measures, and recruitment estimates for a main trial.

Phase III or main trial – The central step in the evaluation of a complex intervention is the main randomized controlled trial. This requires addressing the issues usually posed by RCTs such as adequate sample size, eligibility criteria, adequate randomization and blinding (where feasible), appropriate outcome measures, and informed consent of participants. Complex interventions can pose challenges in these areas. Individual randomization may not always be feasible, for example, if the intervention requires training and upskilling staff who will interact with all trial participants. Allocation concealment or blinding is often not possible given that treatments involve face-to-face contact.

Phase IV or long-term implementation – The purpose of the final phase is to examine the implementation of the intervention into practice and establish the long-term, real-life clinical effectiveness. This can help inform about the stability of the intervention, the broader applicability, and the safety profile, including adverse effects that might not become apparent until large groups of people experience the intervention.

In 2008, the MRC framework was updated to provide a more cyclical model that placed greater emphasis on early phase piloting and evaluation work and recognized that complex interventions work best when tailored to local contexts rather than being completely standardized (Fig. 1) (Craig et al. 2008). The framework superseded the 2000 guidance, and this updated version presented a more iterative process of development, feasibility/piloting, evaluation, and implementation. As an example, the theoretical basis and components of an intervention may be reexamined following the results of an exploratory trial. The 2008 guidance has a broader scope than the 2000 version, covering observational and experimental methods as well as implementation of interventions (Anderson 2008).

Development – Before any substantial evaluation occurs, the intervention must be developed to the point where it can reasonably be expected to lead to an effect (Craig et al. 2008). This requires the identification of an evidence base, which may be achieved through a systematic review of the existing literature. Based on the available evidence, a theory or model of how the proposed intervention is going to work can be developed. Often it can be useful to draw on disciplines outside of palliative care and end-of-life care and even beyond health sciences.

Feasibility/piloting – Piloting is crucial to assess and test intervention procedures and their acceptability. An important step is to estimate likely recruitment and retention rates in order to inform sample size calculations (that take attrition into account) and avoid smaller than expected effect sizes (Eldridge et al. 2004). Similarly, missing data is to be expected; therefore piloting can help determine the expected level of missing data in advance. Pilot studies do not need to be a scale model of the planned evaluation but function to

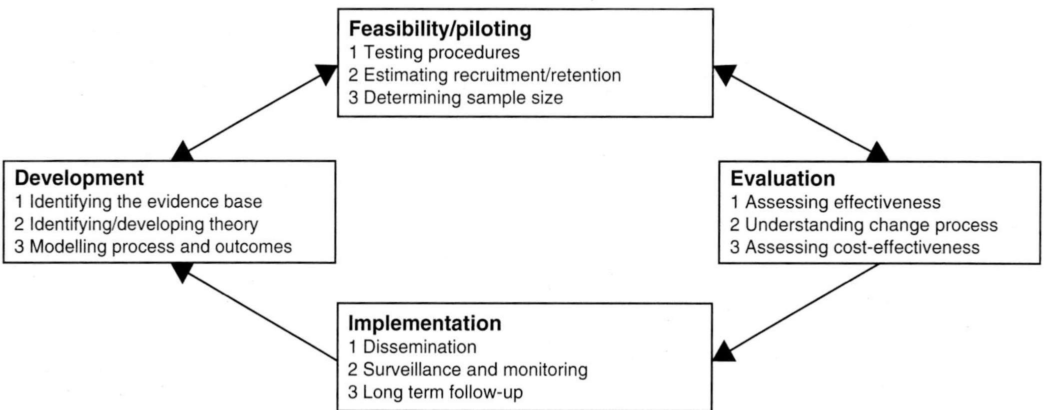

Fig. 1 Key elements of the development and evaluation process. (Taken from Craig et al. 2008)

examine the key uncertainties that have been identified during the development (Craig et al. 2008).

Evaluation – The choice of study design and how the intervention will be evaluated need careful consideration. Randomization should always be considered where possible in order to avoid selection bias. It is critical to think about the outcome measures, most importantly the primary outcome but then also secondary outcomes. The chosen timing of data collection is also important, and long-term follow-up may be required to establish whether any immediate effects of an intervention persist. Understanding the processes involved in the implementation and delivery of an intervention can provide valuable insights into why an intervention works or fails and how it can be optimized in clinical practice. An embedded process evaluation can be helpful to assess implementation fidelity and understand the contextual factors associated with variations in outcomes (Oakley et al. 2006).

Implementation – Reports of evaluations should include detailed description of the intervention to enable replication, evidence synthesis, and wider implementation (Craig et al. 2008). It is critical to utilize the findings from an evaluation of a complex intervention either for clinical practice or to inform policy.

5 MORECare

A major barrier to progress the science of palliative and end-of-life care is the lack of high-quality research (Higginson 2004). While the number of clinical trials in palliative and end-of-life care is on the increase (Tieman et al. 2008), questions remain about the quality of research being undertaken, particularly with regard to rigorous designs. Reviews have concluded that palliative care studies are largely descriptive, with wide variations in sample size, demographic and clinical aspects, and a lack of recognized standardized measures (Aoun and Nekolaichuk 2014; Bakitas et al. 2006; Hui et al. 2011). A recent review of evidence-based practice in palliative care highlights common problems including underpowered studies, recruitment difficulties and high attrition, inadequate follow-up periods, difficulty defining outcomes, and performance bias (Visser et al. 2015). In response to this need, the UK Medical Research Council (MRC) and National Institute for Health Research (NIHR) established the Methods Of Researching End of Life Care (MORECare) collaboration. The aim of the collaboration was to identify, appraise, and synthesize "best practice" methods for research evaluating palliative and end-of-life care. In particular, it focused on complex service delivery reconfiguration interventions (Higginson et al. 2013).

Building on the MRC guidance, MORECare involved systematic literature reviews, transparent expert consultations (involving consensus methods of nominal group and online voting), and stakeholder workshops to identify challenges and best practice in palliative and end-of-life research (Higginson et al. 2013). The transparent expert consultations identified three shortcomings for the MRC guidance:

- Moving from feasibility and piloting to implementation without robust evaluation;
- Failing to develop the feasibility of the evaluation methods alongside the feasibility of the intervention;
- Lack of a theoretical framework underpinning interventions.

There is a need to build simultaneously the intervention and research methods and consider implementation at all phases of evaluation rather than only at the end (Higginson et al. 2013). The findings were synthesized to develop a guidance statement (the MORECare statement) on the best methods to research end-of-life care. The statement provides a first step in setting common, much-needed standards for evaluative research in palliative and end-of-life care. It is designed to be used alongside existing reporting statements, e.g., CONSORT and STROBE. The MORECare statement is relevant to all research stakeholders, researchers, funders, ethical committees, and editors, and presents 36 best practice solutions to improve study quality and set the standard for future research. In addition it includes 13 recommendations to improve the national/international environment for complex intervention research in palliative and end-of-life care (Higginson et al. 2013). The recommendations focus in particular on five key areas of uncertainty, as identified by the literature reviews, of: ethics (Gysels et al. 2013); outcome measurement (Evans et al. 2013a); statistics (managing missing data and attrition) (Preston et al. 2013); mixed methods research (Farquhar et al. 2013); and health economics (Preston et al. 2012). We discuss ethics, outcome measurement, and statistics in more detail below.

Participation and Ethics – Whether patients who are at the end of their lives should be invited to participate in research has been debated (Casarett and Karlawish 2000; Gysels et al. 2012, 2013). It can be difficult to obtain informed consent in circumstances where time is restricted, and patients may have fluctuating/declining mental capacity (Vig et al. 2010). In such situations the likely influence of family members on research participation must be considered, and their concerns must be addressed. These ethical issues must be taken into account when designing and evaluating complex interventions in palliative and end-of-life care. The MORECare transparent expert consultation reasoned that it can be unethical to assume that patients should not be offered research opportunities purely because they have advanced disease (Higginson et al. 2013). In fact there is evidence suggesting patients and families are willing to engage in research near the end of life and find it a positive, rewarding experience (Gysels et al. 2012). Steps should be taken during the study design stage to ensure studies are flexible and researchers are equipped with methods that can enable patients and carers to participate (Gysels et al. 2012).

Box 2 MORECare Considerations for Participation and Ethics

- Work within legal frameworks on mental capacity and consent to ensure that those who may benefit from interventions are offered the opportunity to participate.
- Collaborate with patients and caregivers in the design of the study, vocabulary used in explaining the study, consent procedures, and any ethical aspects.
- Attend the ethics committee meeting with a caregiver or patient to help the committee better understand the patient perspective.
- Ensure proportionality in patient and caregiver information sheets, appropriate to the study design and level of risk, as excessive information in itself can be tiring/distressing for very ill individuals.
- Adjust eligibility criteria to recruit those patients who may benefit most from the intervention, ensuring equipoise.

Taken from Higginson et al. (2013)

Outcome measurement – Outcomes in palliative and end-of-life care can be equally as complex as interventions. There is a need to capture change in needs across a variety of functional domains (physical, emotional, social, and spiritual) at a time when participants may be deteriorating rapidly or approaching death. In both research and clinical practice, multiple measures exist including many which have often not been validated in palliative care populations (Harding et al. 2011). The use of outcome measures which have not been developed or validated in palliative care populations, compromises the evaluation of intervention/service effectiveness (Harding et al. 2010; Tang and McCorkle 2002; Zimmermann et al. 2008). The nature of palliative and end-of-life care requires outcome measures with properties that accommodate multiple domains of care, change over time and increasing levels of debility, the use of proxies, and the timing to detect change (Evans et al. 2013a). The MORECare transparent expert consultation identified three main areas which are of critical importance for the evaluation of palliative care interventions: priority measurement properties, incorporating proxy data, and identifying time points. These aspects each require careful consideration during the development and feasibility/piloting phases.

Box 3 MORECare Considerations for Outcome Measures

- Choose outcome measures which:
  - Have established validity and reliability in the relevant population;
  - Are responsive to change over time;
  - Capture clinically important data;
  - Are easy to administer and interpret;
  - Are applicable across care settings (e.g., patients' home, hospital, hospice);
  - Are able to be integrated into clinical care;
  - Minimize problems of response shift.
- Consider including patients' experience of care.
- Select time points of outcome measurement to balance the value of early recording, to reduce attrition, but to allow enough time for the intervention to have had an effect.
- Consider the potential effect of response shift (that is, a change in a person's internal conceptualization of the aspects measured). Questionnaires that include anchor points or descriptions of each response category may be less problematic.

Taken from Higginson et al. (2013)

Missing data – Attrition and missing data are inevitable in palliative and end-of-life care research. A recent systematic review of missing data in published RCTs of palliative care interventions found 23% of data was missing for the primary endpoint of included studies (Hussain et al. 2016). This level of missing data can make statistical analysis problematic, especially when evaluating complex interventions as it results in the loss of statistical power and the introduction of bias. When designing studies in palliative and end-of-life care, it is recommended that high rates of attrition should not be seen as indicative of poor design (Preston et al. 2013). The causes of "missingness" should be clearly recorded, and an analysis plan should consider how to account for missing data and attrition based on cause. In keeping with the considerations for the choice of outcome measurement, data from proxies may be used to account for missing data as appropriate. The feasibility/piloting phase can provide valuable estimates of attrition which may occur in a full-scale evaluation, and these should be used to test and model the impact of different forms of imputation.

Box 4 MORECare Considerations for Missing Data and Attrition

- Estimate in advance levels of, and reasons for, attrition and missing data, integrating these into sample size estimates and planned collection of data from proxies.
- Monitor and report all levels of, and reasons for, attrition and other missing data.
- Assume missing quantitative data not to be at random unless proven otherwise.
- Test results from different methods of imputation – noting that "using only complete cases" is a form of imputation.
- Use the MORECare classifications of attrition: attrition due to death (ADD), attrition due to illness (ADI), and attrition at random (AaR).
- Consider reasons for missing data which are not due to attrition, and consider these in the analysis and the potential imputations.

Taken from Higginson et al. (2013)

6 Real Case Examples

The examples below demonstrate the successful use of an iterative and phased approach to developing complex interventions in palliative care. The knowledge in each stage of development helps build and improve the design, execution, and generalizability of these large-scale effectiveness trials.

The OPTCARE Neuro Trial – This is a multicenter, mixed methods Phase III trial investigating the clinical and cost-effectiveness of short-term integrated palliative care (SIPC) for patients with long-term neurological conditions. The SIPC being trialed is a complex intervention in that it:

- Contains several components (assessment, symptom management, future care planning, follow-up visits);
- Aims to change behaviors by those staff delivering the intervention, those providing usual care to this patient group, and some changes on the part of patients and families;
- Targets patients, families, and staff in primary, hospital, and voluntary care, thus including different groups and organizational levels;
- Has several complex outcomes, including change in symptom management and hospital admissions;
- Is tailored to individual patient need and circumstances by those delivering the SIPC;
- Operates in a context where there may be some variability between patient groups and settings in the usual care provided to patients with long-term neurological conditions.

The SIPC was developed following the MRC guidance and modelled on previous work. This included a literature review (Gruenewald et al. 2004) and qualitative studies (Edmonds et al. 2007a, b) to determine need and to develop the theoretical underpinning of the intervention, appraisal of trial methods (Higginson et al. 2006a, b), service modelling, and a successful phase II trial randomizing 52 patients (Edmonds et al. 2010; Higginson et al. 2008, 2009). The main trial will randomize 356 patients with a range of long-term neurological conditions, a sample size which accounts for 20% attrition in keeping with recent evidence and the MORECare considerations.

Following MORECare recommendations, the trial has involved a patient and public involvement group at all stages with a particular emphasis on the vocabulary used in explaining and promoting the trial. In the early stages of the trial, further development work included a mapping exercise (van Vliet et al. 2016) and an online survey of professionals (Hepgul et al. 2017) in order to explore the current levels of integrated working between palliative care and neurology services. The complexity of delivering and evaluating a palliative care intervention requires the accumulation of knowledge from multiple sources and will depend on interprofessional behaviors (Craig et al. 2008; Evans et al. 2013b). Furthermore, the effects of an intervention may be dependent on the existing clinical context and provider factors (Lewin et al. 2017). It is therefore valuable to explore clinicians' views and opinions when implementing and evaluating emerging services and informing future requirements. The recruitment of participants into the trial as well as the delivery of the intervention has relied heavily on "buy-in" from clinicians, and so this early work exploring their views has contributed greatly to building good working relationships. As this is a multicenter trial, a key aspect of evaluating the intervention will be implementation fidelity. The SIPC requires individualized care and may become ineffective if any of its vital interacting components are left out. Therefore, understanding how to maintain and improve implementation fidelity in palliative care is especially important in order to avoid errors of poor implementation of complex interventions (Ang et al. 2017).

The Breathlessness Intervention Service (BIS) – This program of work aimed to establish the effectiveness and cost-effectiveness of a Breathlessness Intervention Service (BIS) as compared to standard care, for patients with advanced cancer or non-cancer conditions. The program followed the MRC framework for the development and evaluation of complex interventions. The preclinical phase included a literature review followed by a qualitative study which explored the experience of breathlessness for patients and carers living with cancer or COPD. This provided the evidence around the need for the intervention, its role, and the way it should work, for example, it should be community based and address carer, as well as patient need (Booth et al. 2003). This was followed by a Phase I qualitative evaluation of the first model of the BIS (Booth et al. 2006), the results of which led directly to the refinement of the complex intervention to be tested in a Phase II exploratory trial (Farquhar et al. 2009, 2010). In addition, the Phase I data informed the choice of primary outcome for the Phase II RCT: patient distress due to breathlessness.

The Phase II used a mixed methodology which integrated qualitative interviews with quantitative outcome measures for patients and carers as well as qualitative interviews with referrers to, and providers of, the intervention. The development and evaluations of complex interventions in palliative care benefit from the application of mixed methodology as this can provide evidence from a variety of sources, enabling better understanding of how an intervention does or does not work and inform the design of subsequent studies (Farquhar et al. 2011). Indeed, this mixed methods approach allowed for further refinement of the BIS, for example, it provided evidence that the length of intervention should be reduced – an important finding for a palliative care intervention. The BIS subsequently underwent a Phase III RCT with two sub-protocols: one for advanced cancer and one for advanced nonmalignant disease (due to differing service models) (Farquhar et al. 2014, 2016).

7 Conclusion and Summary

Developing and evaluating complex interventions in palliative and end-of-life care involves overcoming many challenges. The complexity involved requires the accumulation of knowledge to fully understand the processes and mechanisms of palliative care interventions. Evaluations provide important information irrespective of trial outcome. If a trial is negative, it can be unclear if that was due to the intervention being truly ineffective or whether the intervention was poorly applied or used in an inappropriate context. If a trial demonstrates a positive effect, it can be hard to judge how the results of the trial might be applied to a different context if the active ingredients and mechanisms are not well understood (Campbell et al. 2007). The use of an iterative and phased approach where knowledge can build should improve the design, execution, and generalizability of large-scale effectiveness trials. Mixed methods can be employed at all phases of development and evaluation. The MORECare statement sets clear standards on best research practice in evaluating services and treatments in palliative and end-of-life care. It emphasizes the need for considerations about implementation to be integrated into all phases of evaluation rather than only at the end. This approach ensures that when the intervention is ready to be implemented more widely, it is feasible, and the context and processes of implementation are understood, planned for, and resourced (Higginson et al. 2013).

References

Anderson R. New MRC guidance on evaluating complex interventions. BMJ. 2008;337:a1937.

Ang K, Hepgul N, Gao W, Higginson IJ. Strategies used in improving and assessing the level of reporting of implementation fidelity in randomised controlled trials of palliative care complex interventions: a systematic review. Palliat Med. 2017. https://doi.org/10.1177/0269216317717369.

Aoun SM, Nekolaichuk C. Improving the evidence base in palliative care to inform practice and policy: thinking outside the box. J Pain Symptom Manag. 2014; 48:1222–35.

Bakitas MA, Lyons KD, Dixon J, Ahles TA. Palliative care program effectiveness research: developing rigor in sampling design, conduct, and reporting. J Pain Symptom Manag. 2006;31:270–84.

Booth S, Silvester S, Todd C. Breathlessness in cancer and chronic obstructive pulmonary disease: using a qualitative approach to describe the experience of patients and carers. Palliat Support Care. 2003;1:337–44.

Booth S, Farquhar M, Gysels M, Bausewein C, Higginson IJ. The impact of a breathlessness intervention service (BIS) on the lives of patients with intractable dyspnea: a qualitative phase 1 study. Palliat Support Care. 2006;4:287–93.

Campbell M, Fitzpatrick R, Haines A, Kinmonth AL, Sandercock P, Spiegelhalter D, Tyrer P. Framework for design and evaluation of complex interventions to improve health. BMJ. 2000;321:694–6.

Campbell NC, Murray E, Darbyshire J, Emery J, Farmer A, Griffiths F, Guthrie B, Lester H, Wilson P, Kinmonth AL. Designing and evaluating complex interventions to improve health care. BMJ. 2007; 334:455–9.

Casarett DJ, Karlawish JH. Are special ethical guidelines needed for palliative care research? J Pain Symptom Manag. 2000;20:130–9.

Craig P, Dieppe P, Macintyre S, Michie S, Nazareth I, Petticrew M, Medical Research Council Guidance. Developing and evaluating complex interventions: the new Medical Research Council guidance. BMJ. 2008;337:a1655.

Edmonds P, Vivat B, Burman R, Silber E, Higginson IJ. 'Fighting for everything': service experiences of people severely affected by multiple sclerosis. Mult Scler. 2007a;13:660–7.

Edmonds P, Vivat B, Burman R, Silber E, Higginson IJ. Loss and change: experiences of people severely affected by multiple sclerosis. Palliat Med. 2007b; 21:101–7.

Edmonds P, Hart S, Wei G, Vivat B, Burman R, Silber E, Higginson IJ. Palliative care for people severely affected by multiple sclerosis: evaluation of a novel palliative care service. Mult Scler. 2010;16:627–36.

Eldridge SM, Ashby D, Feder GS, Rudnicka AR, Ukoumunne OC. Lessons for cluster randomized trials in the twenty-first century: a systematic review of trials in primary care. Clin Trials. 2004;1:80–90.

Evans CJ, Benalia H, Preston NJ, Grande G, Gysels M, Short V, Daveson BA, Bausewein C, Todd C, Higginson IJ, Morecare. The selection and use of outcome measures in palliative and end-of-life care research: the MORECare International Consensus Workshop. J Pain Symptom Manag. 2013a;46:925–37.

Evans CJ, Harding R, Higginson IJ, Morecare. 'Best practice' in developing and evaluating palliative and end-of-life care services: a meta-synthesis of research methods for the MORECare project. Palliat Med. 2013b;27:885–98.

Farquhar MC, Higginson IJ, Fagan P, Booth S. The feasibility of a single-blinded fast-track pragmatic randomised controlled trial of a complex intervention for breathlessness in advanced disease. BMC Palliat Care. 2009;8:9.

Farquhar M, Higginson IJ, Fagan P, Booth S. Results of a pilot investigation into a complex intervention for breathlessness in advanced chronic obstructive pulmonary disease (COPD): brief report. Palliat Support Care. 2010;8:143–9.

Farquhar MC, Ewing G, Booth S. Using mixed methods to develop and evaluate complex interventions in palliative care research. Palliat Med. 2011;25:748–57.

Farquhar M, Preston N, Evans CJ, Grande G, Short V, Benalia H, Higginson IJ, Todd C, Morecare. Mixed methods research in the development and evaluation of complex interventions in palliative and end-of-life care: report on the MORECare consensus exercise. J Palliat Med. 2013;16:1550–60.

Farquhar MC, Prevost AT, Mccrone P, Brafman-Price B, Bentley A, Higginson IJ, Todd C, Booth S. Is a specialist breathlessness service more effective and cost-effective for patients with advanced cancer and their carers than standard care? Findings of a mixed-method randomised controlled trial. BMC Med. 2014;12:194.

Farquhar MC, Prevost AT, Mccrone P, Brafman-Price B, Bentley A, Higginson IJ, Todd CJ, Booth S. The clinical and cost effectiveness of a Breathlessness Intervention Service for patients with advanced non-malignant disease and their informal carers: mixed findings of a mixed method randomised controlled trial. Trials. 2016;17:185.

Gruenewald DA, Higginson IJ, Vivat B, Edmonds P, Burman RE. Quality of life measures for the palliative care of people severely affected by multiple sclerosis: a systematic review. Mult Scler. 2004;10:690–704.

Gysels MH, Evans C, Higginson IJ. Patient, caregiver, health professional and researcher views and experiences of participating in research at the end of life: a critical interpretive synthesis of the literature. BMC Med Res Methodol. 2012;12:123.

Gysels M, Evans CJ, Lewis P, Speck P, Benalia H, Preston NJ, Grande GE, Short V, Owen-Jones E, Todd CJ, Higginson IJ. MORECare research methods guidance development: recommendations for ethical issues in palliative and end-of-life care research. Palliat Med. 2013;27:908–17.

Harding R, Higginson IJ, Prisma. PRISMA: a pan-European co-ordinating action to advance the science in end-of-life cancer care. Eur J Cancer. 2010;46:1493–501.

Harding R, Simon ST, Benalia H, Downing J, Daveson BA, Higginson IJ, Bausewein C, Prisma. The PRISMA Symposium 1: outcome tool use. Disharmony in European outcomes research for palliative and advanced disease care: too many tools in practice. J Pain Symptom Manag. 2011;42:493–500.

Hepgul N, Gao W, Evans CJ, Jackson D, Van Vliet LM, Byrne A, Crosby V, Groves KE, Lindsay F, Higginson IJ, Neuro O. Integrating palliative care into neurology services: what do the professionals say? BMJ Support Palliat Care. 2017. https://doi.org/10.1136/bmjspcare-2017-001354.

Higginson IJ. It would be NICE to have more evidence? Palliat Med. 2004;18:85–6.

Higginson IJ, Hart S, Silber E, Burman R, Edmonds P. Symptom prevalence and severity in people severely affected by multiple sclerosis. J Palliat Care. 2006a; 22:158–65.

Higginson IJ, Vivat B, Silber E, Saleem T, Burman R, Hart S, Edmonds P. Study protocol: delayed intervention randomised controlled trial within the Medical Research Council (MRC) Framework to assess the effectiveness of a new palliative care service. BMC Palliat Care. 2006b;5:7.

Higginson IJ, Hart S, Burman R, Silber E, Saleem T, Edmonds P. Randomised controlled trial of a new palliative care service: compliance, recruitment and completeness of follow-up. BMC Palliat Care. 2008;7:7.

Higginson IJ, Mccrone P, Hart SR, Burman R, Silber E, Edmonds PM. Is short-term palliative care cost-effective in multiple sclerosis? A randomized phase II trial. J Pain Symptom Manag. 2009;38:816–26.

Higginson IJ, Evans CJ, Grande G, Preston N, Morgan M, Mccrone P, Lewis P, Fayers P, Harding R, Hotopf M, Murray SA, Benalia H, Gysels M, Farquhar M, Todd C,

Morecare. Evaluating complex interventions in end of life care: the MORECare statement on good practice generated by a synthesis of transparent expert consultations and systematic reviews. BMC Med. 2013;11:111.

Hui D, Parsons HA, Damani S, Fulton S, Liu J, Evans A, De La Cruz M, Bruera E. Quantity, design, and scope of the palliative oncology literature. Oncologist. 2011; 16:694–703.

Hussain JA, White IR, Langan D, Johnson MJ, Currow DC, Torgerson DJ, Bland M. Missing data in randomized controlled trials testing palliative interventions pose a significant risk of bias and loss of power: a systematic review and meta-analyses. J Clin Epidemiol. 2016;74:57–65.

Lewin S, Hendry M, Chandler J, Oxman AD, Michie S, Shepperd S, Reeves BC, Tugwell P, Hannes K, Rehfuess EA, Welch V, Mckenzie JE, Burford B, Petkovic J, Anderson LM, Harris J, Noyes J. Assessing the complexity of interventions within systematic reviews: development, content and use of a new tool (iCAT_SR). BMC Med Res Methodol. 2017;17:76.

Lorenz KA, Lynn J, Dy SM, Shugarman LR, Wilkinson A, Mularski RA, Morton SC, Hughes RG, Hilton LK, Maglione M, Rhodes SL, Rolon C, Sun VC, Shekelle PG. Evidence for improving palliative care at the end of life: a systematic review. Ann Intern Med. 2008;148:147–59.

Medical Research Council. A framework for development and evaluation of RCTs for complex interventions to improve health. London: Medical Research Council; 2000.

Oakley A, Strange V, Bonell C, Allen E, Stephenson J, RIPPLE Study Team. Process evaluation in randomised controlled trials of complex interventions. BMJ. 2006;332:413–6.

Petticrew M. When are complex interventions 'complex'? When are simple interventions 'simple'? Eur J Pub Health. 2011;21:397–8.

Preston N, Short V, Hollingworth W, Mccrone P, Grande G, Evans C, Anscombe E, Benalia A, Higginson IJ, Todd C. MORECare research methods guidance development: recommendations for health economic evaluation in palliative and end of life care research [abstract]. Palliat Med. 2012;26:419.

Preston NJ, Fayers P, Walters SJ, Pilling M, Grande GE, Short V, Owen-Jones E, Evans CJ, Benalia H, Higginson IJ, Todd CJ, Morecare. Recommendations for managing missing data, attrition and response shift in palliative and end-of-life care research: part of the MORECare research method guidance on statistical issues. Palliat Med. 2013;27:899–907.

Tang ST, Mccorkle R. Appropriate time frames for data collection in quality of life research among cancer patients at the end of life. Qual Life Res. 2002;11:145–55.

Tieman J, Sladek R, Currow D. Changes in the quantity and level of evidence of palliative and hospice care literature: the last century. J Clin Oncol. 2008;26: 5679–83.

Van Vliet LM, Gao W, Difrancesco D, Crosby V, Wilcock A, Byrne A, Al-Chalabi A, Chaudhuri KR, Evans C, Silber E, Young C, Malik F, Quibell R, Higginson IJ, Neuro O. How integrated are neurology and palliative care services? Results of a multicentre mapping exercise. BMC Neurol. 2016;16:63.

Vig E, Irwin S, Casarett D. Can my patient make that decision? Assessing capacity to make decisions about clinical care and research participation (516). J Pain Symptom Manag. 2010;39:413.

Visser C, Hadley G, Wee B. Reality of evidence-based practice in palliative care. Cancer Biol Med. 2015; 12:193–200.

Wells M, Williams B, Treweek S, Coyle J, Taylor J. Intervention description is not enough: evidence from an in-depth multiple case study on the untold role and impact of context in randomised controlled trials of seven complex interventions. Trials. 2012;13:95.

Zimmermann C, Riechelmann R, Krzyzanowska M, Rodin G, Tannock I. Effectiveness of specialized palliative care: a systematic review. JAMA. 2008; 299:1698–709.

Mixed Method Research in Palliative Care

93

Catherine Walshe

Contents

Abstract

This chapter focuses on the use of mixed methods research designs in palliative care. Mixing methods is increasing in popularity as a research approach, but study quality can be poor. This chapter highlights key issues and resources for those interested in mixed methods research, to encourage researchers to focus on important principles and debates to inform study planning. First, the defining features of mixed methods research are explored and definitions presented. Second, the paradigm challenges of mixed methods research are discussed, with a focus on current epistemological thinking in the area. Third, the issues of design are presented. This includes consideration of the purpose of mixed methods studies, a continuum of study characteristics, and a typology of core mixed methods designs. Approaches to mixing data are given particular consideration. Barriers to high-quality mixed methods studies are presented and recommendations on mixed methods research in palliative care discussed. Throughout, contemporary examples from palliative care mixed methods research are used to illustrate key points.

C. Walshe (✉)
International Observatory on End of Life Care,
Lancaster University, Lancaster, UK
e-mail: c.walshe@lancaster.ac.uk

R. D. MacLeod, L. Van den Block (eds.), *Textbook of Palliative Care*,
https://doi.org/10.1007/978-3-319-77740-5_109

1 Introduction

Humans, it is argued, are intuitively mixed methods researchers. When we make decisions in our day-to-day lives, we frequently draw from a range of data sources. For example, when making a decision on which household appliance to purchase, we may turn to quantitative data such as energy efficiency ratings, price, or customer review ratings. We are also likely to be influenced by qualitative data such as feedback from friends and colleagues about their experiences and decisions. Our final choice will probably involve weighing up these different strands of information. Mixed methods research can tap into that instinctive approach to understanding the world around us and is gaining popularity with funders and researchers, although it still represents less than 3% of published health services research (O'Cathain et al. 2007; Coyle et al. 2016; Wisdom et al. 2012). Mixed methods research is, essentially, shorthand for research that uses qualitative and quantitative research approaches within a single project, where there are likely a combination of methods and where the data are mutually illuminating, and inferences are drawn using both (or multiple) approaches (Bryman 2012; Tashakkori and Cresswell 2007). This integration is frequently seen as vital, as without it the contribution to knowledge is the same as that from a qualitative and quantitative study undertaken independently, rather than the whole being the sum of the parts (O'Cathain et al. 2010).

The focus of this chapter is to explore the issues associated with mixed methods research, highlight important debates, present essential information, and illustrate with examples from palliative care research. The focus is on why, when, and how mixed methods research can be appropriately used in palliative care, to facilitate apt research choices and enable high-quality, impactful work. While much of the focus of this chapter is on research involving empirical data collection, mixed method systematically constructed research reviews are also possible, and similar considerations apply (Pearson et al. 2015; Sandelowski et al. 2012).

2 Defining Mixed Methods Research

Mixed methods research is often characterized as a "third" methodological movement or paradigm, following the examinations and developments of quantitative and qualitative research (Tashakkori and Teddlie 2010; Johnson and Onwuegbuzie 2004). There is clear evidence of an evolving trajectory of thinking about what mixed methods research is and how it is characterized. The focus of definitions has shifted and developed from those focusing on methods to methodology, philosophy, purpose, and characteristics (Creswell and Plano Clark 2018). An analysis of 19 definitions of mixed methods research identified a number of important themes within existing definitions, which are explored in Box 1 (Johnson et al. 2007).

Box 1 Analysis of Definitions of Mixed Methods Research

What is mixed: Qualitative and quantitative research but may also include within paradigm mixing (e.g., two forms of qualitative research).

The mixing stage: May occur at data collection, analysis, or throughout the research phases. Some considerations that there are perspectives on the same research question.

Breadth: Definitions can encapsulate mixing of data, mixing at all stages, and mixing of worldviews and paradigms.

Why mixing occurs: Definitions include a number of purposes for mixing including breadth, corroboration, understanding, validation, and social justice.

Orientation: Some definitions are "bottom-up," where the research question drives the approach, others are "top-down" where the philosophy or paradigm of the researcher drives the approach.

Johnson et al. (2007, pp. 118–123)

Johnson et al. (2007) conclude by offering a general definition:

> Mixed methods research is the type of research in which a researcher or team of researchers combines elements of qualitative and quantitative research approaches (e.g., use of qualitative and quantitative viewpoints, data collection, analysis, inference techniques) for the broad purposes of breadth and depth of understanding and corroboration.
>
> This definition refers to mixed methods research as a type of research:
>
> A mixed methods study would involve mixing within a single study; a mixed method program would involve mixing within a program of research and the mixing might occur across a closely related set of studies. (Johnson et al. 2007, p. 123)

What this definition does not address, however, is an understanding of the social world, and worldview, of the researcher nor an acknowledgment of the importance of paradigmatic, epistemological, or ontological issues in this field. These issues are explored in the writings of Jennifer Greene (2006, 2007, 2008). She argues that a methodology for social inquiry engages four domains of issues and assumptions: philosophical assumptions and stances, inquiry logics, guidelines for practice, and sociopolitical commitments in science (Greene 2006). These issues are debated later in this chapter, but the argument that mixed methods offer different ways of framing an understanding of the world is important to acknowledge in definitions. Mixed methods research draws on the strengths and perspectives of different methods, recognizing the existence and importance of the physical, natural world as well as the importance of reality and influence of human experience (Johnson and Onwuegbuzie 2004).

Creswell and Plano Clark (2018) and Creswell et al. (2011) offer a number of evolving definitions which incorporate these core characteristics, including a highly cited definition provided as part of commissioned guidance for the National Institutes of Health and which is used in this chapter:

Mixed methods research will be defined as a research approach or methodology:

> focusing on research questions that call for real-life contextual understandings, multi-level perspectives, and cultural influences; employing rigorous quantitative research assessing magnitude and frequency of constructs and rigorous qualitative research exploring the meaning and understanding of constructs; utilizing multiple methods (e.g., intervention trials and in-depth interviews); intentionally integrating or combining these methods to draw on the strengths of each; and framing the investigation within philosophical and theoretical positions. Creswell et al. (2011 p. 4)

3 Foundations of Mixed Methods Research: History and Philosophy

A good overview of the evolution of mixed methods is provided by Creswell and Plano Clark (2018), who identify five overlapping stages. They characterize these stages as formative (arguing for the use of mixed methods), the paradigm debate (discussing stances, reconciliation), procedural development (rationales, design, typologies), expansion (positioning as a distinctive approach), and reflection and refinement (mapping onto frameworks, critique, presenting new paradigms). Despite these stages, the existence of mixed methods studies is not new but has not always been explicitly labelled as such (Pelto 2015). Suffice to say here that palliative care researchers interested in adopting mixed methods may wish to consider these developments, so that their work is grounded in contemporary understandings of mixed methods approaches. As with most areas of health service research, there has been an expansion in the use of mixed methods approaches in palliative care, but not necessarily with an explicit description of how developments in the ways that mixed methods are conceptualized have informed designs (Farquhar et al. 2011a). A more important focus for this chapter is the exploration of philosophical and theoretical debates in mixed methods research and a consideration of how this can and should shape palliative care research in the field.

A framework for how to consider different domains of thinking associated with issues of ontology, epistemology, methodology, design, and purpose is offered by Jennifer Greene (2008) and outlined in Table 1, together with key questions for consideration.

Table 1 A framework for social science methodology

Domain	Descriptor	Issues for mixed methods research
Philosophical assumptions and stances	Philosophical and theoretical stance. Anchored in philosophy of science and includes assumptions about *ontology* (nature of social world) and *epistemology* (social knowledge)	Is it possible to hold competing or contrasting assumptions?
		What influences the decisions made by researchers in the field?
		Is mixed methods an alternative paradigm itself?
Inquiry logics	Justificatory logic. The *methodology* considerations, such as purpose, question, and design which are internally congruent and coherent	How best can methods follow purpose and question?
		How can research designs be developed and better focus on integration?
		How do we judge the quality of mixed methods research?
Guidelines for practice	Practical advice. The "*how to*" of research, with guidance on specifics such as sampling, data collection, etc.	How best to mix different approaches?
		How to choose best methods in an inquiry context?
Sociopolitical commitments	Location of the design in society The *interests* and *purpose* of the research in *context*	Is mixed methods a distinctive methodology?

Derived from Greene (2008)

The arguments against mixed methods research primarily fall into the epistemological domain. Some consider that because qualitative and quantitative research are believed to be separate paradigms, encapsulating different ways that the world can be understood and interpreted, it is not possible, or desirable, to mix them (Bryman 2012). While there are technical arguments associated with this debate, with discussions of the practical aspects of data collection and analysis, understanding arguments associated with a paradigmatic debate is an important conceptual first step for a researcher. A number of different positions have been articulated (Greene 2008; Creswell et al. 2011):

PURIST STANCE: The assumptions of qualitative and quantitative research are incompatible, and so it is not possible to combine them in research. The paradigms are coherent wholes that must be respected (Lincoln and Guba 1985; Sale et al. 2002).

COMPLEMENTARY STRENGTHS STANCE: Rather than seen as incompatible, paradigms have valuable differences that should be maintained. Methods are kept separate from one another, but within a single study (Brewer and Hunter 1989; Morse 2003).

DIALECTIC STANCE: Paradigmatic assumptions are different and valuable, but the paradigms are historical and social constructions and are not immune to change. Engagement can bring new, transformative, insight, but must be made explicit (Greene 2007, 1997; Maxwell and Loomis 2003; Greene and Hall 2010). *Dialectical pluralism suggests that different world views should be carefully considered, stakeholder values should guide projects, and collaborations conducted with attention to fairness, justice and equality* (Burke Johnson and Stefurak 2013; Stefurak et al. 2015).

*ALTERNATIVE PARADIGM: Emergent paradigms (*e.g. *pragmatism, realism, transformative) actively promote mixing of methods* (Johnson and Onwuegbuzie 2004). *This thinking has been expanded to a consideration of a 'best' worldview for mixed methods* (Creswell and Plano Clark 2018). *Some authors privilege pragmatism as an approach that prioritises the question over the paradigm, focusing on 'what works', and recommend abandoning* *a dichotomy between approaches* (Morgan 2007; Florczak 2014). *Others suggest transformative paradigms* (Mertens 2003)*, or critical realism* (Maxwell and Mittapalli 2010) *as perspectives which support aspects of combining qualitative and quantitative approaches.*

A-PARADIGMATIC STANCE: Assumptions of paradigms are logically independent, and hence can be mixed. Priority given to demands of the research problem (Patton 2002). *Worldviews may relate to different designs, related to different project phases, but need to be explicit* (Creswell and Plano Clark 2018). *These views may be tied to a common perspective from the community of scholars relevant to the research, who form a shared identity, with common problems* (Morgan 2007; Denscombe 2008).

SUBSTANTIVE THEORY STANCE: Paradigmatic assumptions embedded with or intertwined with substantive theories relevant to conduct of study. They enable thinking, but do not guide practice.

Contemporary thinking on mixed methods tends toward adopting dialectic, pragmatic, realistic, or transformative approaches. Examples of mixed methods studies guided by the realist, pragmatic, and transformative perspectives are summarized in Tables 2, 3, and 4.

4 Mixed Method Research Designs

Mixed methods study designs should take account of standard considerations when planning any robust research study, and each study is likely to have unique features. However, there are concepts that are particular to, or emphasized within, mixed methods research studies that require attention. First, the purpose of the mixed methods study needs to be considered. Second, operationalising a continuum of study characteristics. Third, selecting a core design from a typology of studies. These are now considered in turn.

4.1 Purpose of Mixed Methods Research

Five primary purposes of mixed methods research have been determined, based on a conceptual framework developed from theoretical literature and refined through the analysis of 57 empirical mixed method evaluations:

Table 2 Example palliative care study using a REALIST perspective

Question/aim	To find if how and under what circumstances palliative care registrations are made for patients with nonmalignant diseases in primary care
Design	GP practice data were analyzed statistically, and qualitative data was collected from healthcare professionals and members of relevant organizations
Perspective	Realism
Findings	The Integrated Care Pathway began to enable the reduction of inequalities in care by identifying, registering, and managing an increasing number of palliative patients with nonmalignant diseases. Consensual and inclusive definitions of palliative care were developed in order to legitimize the registration of such patients
Contribution of mixed methods	Mixed methods uncovered not only whether palliative care registrations are increasing but also for whom, by what means, and in which circumstances
Key references	Dalkin SM, Jones D, Lhussier M, et al. Understanding integrated care pathways in palliative care using realist evaluation: a mixed methods study protocol BMJ Open 2012;2:e001533. https://doi.org/10.1136/bmjopen-2012-001533
	Dalkin SM, Lhussier M, Philipson P. et al. Reducing inequalities in care for patients with non-malignant diseases: Insights from a realist evaluation of an integrated palliative care pathway. Palliat Med 2016;30(7):690–697
	(Dalkin et al. 2012, 2016)

Table 3 Example palliative care study using a PRAGMATIC perspective

Question/aim	To examine the use of specialist palliative care in relation to age, after controlling for need
Design	Mixed methods: focused ethnography of specialist palliative care services, systematic literature review, cross-sectional survey
Perspective	Pragmatic philosophy, drawing upon a health capability account of equitable healthcare
Findings	The findings suggest equitable use of specialist palliative care. However, a comprehensive account of equity must consider both use and quality of care. There were some suggestions that, within a resource-limited context, the quality of care may vary
Contribution of mixed methods	Mixed methods enabled broader research questions and deeper inferences. Ideas about need were interwoven with need measurement. Pragmatic grounding enabled use of best-fit methods to answer questions
Key references	Burt JA. Equity, need and access in health care: a mixed methods investigation of specialist palliative care use in relation to age. Doctoral thesis, UCL (University College London). 2010 http://discovery.ucl.ac.uk/19633/1/19633.pdf [accessed 12.10. 17]
	Burt JA, Plant H, Omar R, Raine R. Equity of use of specialist palliative care by age: cross-sectional study of lung cancer patients. Palliat Med. 2010; 24(6):641–50 https://doi.org/10.1177/0269216310364199
	Burt J, Raine R. The effect of age on referral to and use of specialist palliative care services in adult cancer patients: a systematic review, Age Ageing. 2006; 35(5):469–76, https://doi.org/10.1093/ageing/afl001
	(Burt 2010; Burt et al. 2010; Burt and Raine 2006)

Table 4 Example palliative care study using a TRANSFORMATIVE perspective

Question/aim	To report the meta-synthesis of a research project investigating delirium epidemiology, systems of care, and nursing practice in palliative care units
Design	A two-phase sequential transformative mixed methods design with knowledge translation as the theoretical framework. The project answered five different research questions about delirium epidemiology, systems of care, and nursing practice in palliative care units. Data integration and meta-synthesis occurred at project conclusion
Perspective	Transformative
Findings	There was a moderate to high rate of delirium occurrence in palliative care unit populations; and palliative care nurses had unmet delirium knowledge needs and worked within systems and team processes that were inadequate for delirium recognition and assessment. The meta-inference of the DePAC project was that a widely held but paradoxical view that palliative care and dying patients are different from the wider hospital population has separated them from the overall generation of delirium evidence and contributed to the extent of practice deficiencies in palliative care units
Contribution of mixed methods	The meta-inference was that a widely held but paradoxical view that palliative care and dying patients are different from the wider hospital population has separated them from the overall generation of delirium evidence and contributed to the extent of practice deficiencies in palliative care units
Key references	Hosie A, Agar M, Lobb E, Davidson PM, Phillips J. Online First. Improving delirium recognition and assessment for people receiving inpatient palliative care: a mixed methods meta-synthesis. Int J Nurs Stud. https://doi.org/10.1016/j.ijnurstu.2017.07.007
	Hosie et al. (2017) https://www.journalofnursingstudies.com/article/S0020-7489(17)30157-8/fulltext

triangulation, complementarity, development, initiation, and expansion (Greene et al. 1989).

1. ***Triangulation:*** *This implies convergence, corroboration, correspondence of results from different methods. The emphasis can be on seeking corroboration between qualitative and quantitative data.*
2. ***Complementarity:*** *This implies elaboration, enhancement, illustration or clarification of*

Table 5 Example palliative care study for a DEVELOPMENT purpose

Question/aim	To refine and evaluate a practical, clinical tool (SPICT) to help multidisciplinary teams in the UK and internationally, to identify patients at risk of deteriorating and dying in all care settings
Design	Participatory research with ongoing peer review process via an open-access web page, followed by prospective case-finding study in an acute hospital
Perspective	Instrument development
Findings	The SPICT was refined and updated to consist of readily identifiable, general indicators relevant to patients with any advanced illness and disease-specific indicators for common advanced conditions
Contribution of mixed methods	Enabled second phase of case finding to be informed by international development work
Key references	Highet G, Crawford D, Murray SA et al. Development and evaluation of the supportive and Palliative Care Indicators Tool (SPICT): a mixed-methods study BMJ Support Palliat Care 2014;4:285–290. (Highet et al. 2014)

findings from one method with the results from another. Methods can be used to explore different aspects of phenomena to yield an elaborated understanding or explanation. This may include off-setting weaknesses of some approaches (Bryman 2006). *Complementarity differs from triangulation, as convergence requires that methods assess the same phenomenon.*

3. ***Development:*** *This implies sequential use of results from one method to help develop or inform the other method. This may include instrument development, or development of sampling approaches* (Bryman 2006).
4. ***Initiation:*** *This implies discovery of paradox and contradiction, such that results from one method can inform changes in the other. These may emerge rather than be a planned intent, or be intentionally analysed for fresh insights.*
5. ***Expansion:*** *This seeks to extend breadth and range by using different methods for different or multiple components. For example, qualitative methods can be used to assess processes and quantitative methods to assess outcomes, or qualitative data to generate hypotheses, and quantitative data to test them* (Greene et al. 1989).

When this categorization was used to explore health services research, the main purposes were complementarity, expansion, and development (O'Cathain et al. 2007), while triangulation and expansion were common in social sciences (Bryman 2006). Inherent in this categorization of purpose is that some imply fixed designs, planned in advance, and others a more flexible or emergent approach where the use of mixed methods develops or commences during the research (Creswell and Plano Clark 2018). Researchers should be clear and explicit about the purpose of their study and why a mixed methods design is appropriate to meet this purpose. A critique of this categorization is that it focuses too much on analysis (Collins et al. 2006). Example palliative care studies, categorized by the purpose of the study, are summarized in Tables 5 and 6.

4.2 The Characteristics of Mixed Methods Research

Once the overarching purpose of the research is determined, attention can be paid to specific design characteristics of the study. These are often typified on a sliding scale, continuum, or dichotomy depending on the specific characteristic and the choices available within that characteristic. Greene et al. (1989) identified seven characteristics in their study: methods, phenomena, paradigms, status, independence, timing, and study. These are displayed in Table 7, interspersed with three exemplars from palliative care research. These are a study of a breathlessness intervention (Farquhar et al. 2009, 2011b, 2014, 2016), a study of spiritual well-being (Selman et al. 2013),

Table 6 Example palliative care study for a CONVERGENT, TRIANGULATION purpose

Question/aim	To investigate the interactions between organization and culture as conditions for integrated palliative care in hospital and to suggest workable solutions for the provision of generalist palliative care
Design	A convergent parallel mixed methods design. Two independent studies: a quantitative study, in which three independent datasets were triangulated to study the organization and evaluation of generalist palliative care, and a qualitative, ethnographic study exploring the culture of generalist palliative nursing care in medical department
Perspective	Theories of integrated care, convergent design
Findings	Two overall themes emerged: (1) "generalist palliative care as a priority at the hospital," suggesting contrasting issues regarding prioritization of palliative care at different organizational levels, and (2) "knowledge and use of generalist palliative care clinical guideline," suggesting that the guideline had not reached all levels of the organization
Contribution of mixed methods	Valuable in addressing the complexity of palliative care provision in hospital culture and organization
Key references	Bergenholtz H, Jarlbaek L, Hølge-Hazelton B. Generalist palliative care in hospital – Cultural and organisational interactions. Results of a mixed-methods study. Palliat Med. 2016;30(6):558–66 (Bergenholtz et al. 2016)

Table 7 The characteristics of mixed methods research

<table>
<tr><td rowspan="2">SIMILAR</td><td>Methods</td><td rowspan="2">DIFFERENT</td></tr>
<tr><td>Degree to which methods selected are similar to or different from each other in form, assumptions, strengths, or limitations (Greene et al. 1989). Most health service studies prioritized quantitative methods or gave equal weighting to methods. Rare that qualitative methods given priority (O'Cathain et al. 2007)</td></tr>
<tr><td colspan="3">DIFFERENT: Farquhar et al., used a wait-list randomized controlled trial and qualitative interviews</td></tr>
<tr><td colspan="3">SIMILAR: Selman et al. used cognitive interviews and outcome scales</td></tr>
<tr><td colspan="3">DIFFERENT: Morita et al. used a pre-post survey study and qualitative interviews and focus groups</td></tr>
<tr><td rowspan="2">SAME</td><td>Phenomena</td><td rowspan="2">DIFFERENT</td></tr>
<tr><td>Degree of intention to assess different, similar, or the same phenomena. This can be caused by a response to different research questions. Mixed methods tend to be used with broad and complex questions, with multiple facets (Tariq and Woodman 2013)</td></tr>
<tr><td colspan="3">SIMILAR: Farquhar et al. investigated the phenomena of both response to treatment (same) and the experience of treatment (different)</td></tr>
<tr><td colspan="3">SIMILAR: Selman et al. investigate constructs of peace and well-being through two different means</td></tr>
<tr><td colspan="3">DIFFERENT: Morita et al. examine a complex range of outcome and process phenomena</td></tr>
<tr><td rowspan="2">SAME</td><td>Paradigms</td><td rowspan="2">DIFFERENT</td></tr>
<tr><td>Degree to which different method types implemented within same or different paradigms. This is a dichotomous choice</td></tr>
<tr><td colspan="3">DIFFERENT: Farquhar et al. used a trial and qualitative interviews from different paradigms</td></tr>
<tr><td colspan="3">SIMILAR: Selman et al.'s cognitive interviewing and outcomes both examined different aspects of validity</td></tr>
<tr><td colspan="3">DIFFERENT: Morita et al. used a pre-post survey and qualitative data collection from different paradigms</td></tr>
<tr><td rowspan="2">EQUAL</td><td>Status</td><td rowspan="2">UNEQUAL</td></tr>
<tr><td>Degree to which methods have equally important or central roles to meet the study objectives</td></tr>
<tr><td colspan="3">UNEQUAL: Farquhar et al. give prominence to trial results in reporting</td></tr>
<tr><td colspan="3">EQUAL: Selman et al. give equal weight to both methods in reporting</td></tr>
<tr><td colspan="3">UNEQUAL: Morita et al. give prominence to survey data in reporting</td></tr>
</table>

(*continued*)

Table 7 (continued)

INTERACTIVE	***Independence***	INDEPENDENT
	Continuum of how qualitative and quantitative methods are conceptualized, designed, and implemented interactively or independently	
INTERACTIVE: Farquhar et al. appear to have designed and implemented the methods interactively		
INTERACTIVE: Selman et al. appear to have designed and implemented the methods interactively		
INDEPENDENT: Morita et al. appear to have conducted the methods in independent phases		
SEQUENTIAL	***Timing***	SIMULTANEOUS
	Methods typically implemented concurrently or sequentially but can be interspersed. Decisions important on sequencing and timing (Morgan 1998)	
SIMULTANEOUS: Farquhar et al. conduct data collection using multiple methods simultaneously		
SIMULTANEOUS: Selman et al. conduct data collection using multiple methods simultaneously		
SEQUENTIAL: Morita et al. conduct data collection sequentially, but with qualitative and quantitative methods interspersed		
MULTIPLE	***Study***	ONE
	Categorical choice between one or multiple studies. Typically one study	
ONE STUDY: Farquhar et al.'s study is a single study		
ONE STUDY: Selman et al.'s study is a single study		
SINGLE STUDY: Morita et al.'s study appears to be a single study, although the protocol recognizes design changes over time		

Greene et al. (1989), Farquhar et al. (2009, 2011, 2014, 2016), Selman et al. (2013), Morita et al. (2012, 2013), and Morgan (1998)

and the study of a program of interventions on palliative care for people with cancer (Morita et al. 2012, 2013).

4.3 Typology of Mixed Methods Research

Many authors have created typologies of mixed methods designs, including those who have changed and refined their typology over time (Creswell and Plano Clark 2018). Creswell and Plano Clark (2018) tabulate 15 typologies, and their own four iterations, refined over time. Their current typology has three core designs: explanatory sequential, exploratory sequential, and convergent designs. These are summarized in Table 8. They consider these parsimonious and practical, positing that one or more of these three core designs are at the heart of a mixed methods study. The labels reflect the *primary intent* of the researcher for using and integrating data – intent being the outcome that the researcher hopes to attain by mixing data. Intent is implied with the first label (e.g., explanatory, exploratory, and convergent). The sequencing of data is reflected in the second label (e.g., sequential). They consider that these changes shift the conceptualization from timing and sequence to purpose and intent (Creswell and Plano Clark 2018).

A review of mixed methods studies in healthcare published between 1999 and 2009 identified 168 papers, primarily from the USA, the UK, and Canada, categorized using an earlier typology of Creswell and Plano Clark (Östlund et al. 2011). Most common ($n = 98$) were approaches using parallel analysis, but with little articulation of purpose, method status, or expected outcomes. Other studies used sequential approaches ($n = 46$) both explanatory and exploratory, but concurrent approaches were rarer. Their critique of the papers highlights the lack of explicit theoretical assumptions and poor clarity on whether the conclusions primarily stemmed from qualitative or quantitative findings (Östlund et al. 2011).

The use of each of these core designs is now discussed with a worked example in palliative care.

4.3.1 Convergent Design

This design is illustrated with a study developing and evaluating the Dignity Talk framework for

Table 8 Outline of three core mixed methods research designs

Design	Features
Convergent design (previously called concurrent or parallel design)	To bring together results of quantitative and qualitative data analysis. Comparison may bring more complete understanding, validate one set of findings with another, etc.
	Example: conducting survey and focus group on same topic with similar group(s) of people. Separately analyzed, but datasets compared to see similarity and difference
	Also called simultaneous triangulation, parallel study, convergence model, concurrent triangulation
Explanatory sequential design (or explanatory design)	Occurs in two distinctive interactive phases. Starts with collection and analysis of quantitative data, followed by collection and analysis of qualitative data to explain or expand on first phase results
	Example: collect survey data on one topic, but find surprising association in data. Conduct focus group targeted at those who experience particular phenomenon to attempt to explain unexpected result
	Also called sequential model, sequential triangulation, qualitative follow-up, iteration design
Exploratory sequential design (or exploratory design)	Occurs in two phases but begins with and typically prioritizes the qualitative data in first phase. Quantitative feature is built on the exploratory results from the qualitative phase and typically incorporates a development phase (e.g., instrument development) followed by quantitative testing
	Example: collects interview data about a phenomenon, used to create a survey instrument, which is used to assess prevalence of activities
	Also called instrument development design

Extracted from Creswell and Plano Clark (2018)

people receiving palliative care (Guo et al. 2018) (Table 9).

4.3.2 Explanatory Sequential Design

This design is illustrated with a study designed to provide insight into what nurses know, do, and need to provide support to anxious patients in hospice care (Zweers et al. 2017) (Table 10).

4.3.3 Exploratory Sequential Design

This design is illustrated with a study to examine the effect of using the interRAI PC on the quality of palliative care in nursing homes (De Almeida Mello et al. 2015; Hermans et al. 2014, 2016, 2018) (Table 11).

4.4 Approaches to Mixing Data

The mixing of data is considered to be the most conceptually challenging and practically difficult areas of mixed methods research (Collins and O'Cathain 2009). The approach taken has to be grounded in the purpose and design of the research and occurs at different times, depending in this, as can be seen from the earlier discussions of core designs. With this in mind however, it is worth examining mixing and integrating data in more depth. Typical approaches include merging data, connecting data, building data, and embedding data (Creswell et al. 2011; Fetters et al. 2013).

Merging data is commonly used in convergent designs and implies combining both qualitative data (e.g., text) and quantitative data (e.g., numeric information). Some of the exemplar studies presented in this chapter achieve this through reporting quantitative results, followed by qualitative data that explore, support, or expand upon the quantitative data. Diagrams are also possible, for example, (Selman et al. 2013) display merged data figuratively. Different forms of data matrices or displays can also be used (Miles and Huberman 1984). Merging may also be possible through

Table 9 Palliative care example of a convergent mixed methods design

Feature	Discussion	Example
Guo Q, Chochinov HM, McClement S, Thompson G, Hack T. et al. Development and evaluation of the dignity talk question framework for palliative patients and their families: a mixed-methods study. Palliative Med. 2018 (First published 13 Nov 2017. https://doi.org/10.1177/0269216317734696)		
Intent	To obtain different but complementary data on the same topic, bringing together strengths and weaknesses of quantitative and qualitative methods (Patton 2002). Also corroboration, validation	To develop a novel means of facilitating meaningful conversations for palliative patients and family members, coined Dignity Talk, explore anticipated benefits and challenges of using Dignity Talk, and solicit suggestions for protocol improvement
Reasons for choice	Facilitates collection of both data types at once, when both sorts of data needed from participants, researchers, or team have both sorts of skills	Not explicitly stated
Assumptions	Pragmatic paradigm can be appropriate, as this worldview holds with merging qualitative and quantitative data	No paradigm explicitly stated
	If multiple philosophical frameworks, should be reported	
Procedures	(a) Collect both qualitative and quantitative data on the topic. Usually concurrent but separate, often equally important	Described as a convergent parallel mixed methods design
	(b) Separate and independent data analysis	The Dignity Talk guidelines and questions were evaluated using both quantitative and qualitative data. Data were collected simultaneously and priority was given to both forms of data
	(c) Merging results through comparison or transformation, e.g., joint data display table, graphical display, transforming qualitative data into counts	Descriptive statistics were used to describe demographic data. Feedback obtained from patients and family members regarding clarity, sensitivity, relevance, and importance of Dignity Talk questions was analyzed quantitatively (endorsement rate). Chi-square analysis was employed to compare the overall endorsement rate by patients and family members. Qualitative data were analyzed line by line using the constant comparative techniques to identify recurrent themes by the first two authors. Quantitative and qualitative results were finally merged and interpreted, based on which the Dignity Talk question framework was revised
	(d) Interpretation of convergence or divergence, relationships	
Advantages and disadvantages	Efficient, can be conducted by a team, gives a voice to participants	The research team included members from psychiatry, psychology, and nursing, as well as research personnel
	Consequences of different sample sizes and merging datasets of different sizes, how to explain divergence	Strengths of the study include Dignity Talk being developed and modified based on both qualitative and quantitative data. It is one of very few psychosocial interventions targeting patient/family dyads and is meant to be self-administered by patients and families. Limitations include a relatively small sample size, although rich qualitative data were collected

Creswell and Plano Clark (2018) and Guo et al. (2018)

transforming data to the same form, mostly commonly through counting within qualitative data (Sandelowski et al. 2009). Matrices can facilitate focusing attention on cases rather than variables or themes and allow patterns to be sought (O'Cathain et al. 2010).

Table 10 Palliative care example of an explanatory sequential mixed methods design

Feature	Discussion	Example
Zweers D, de Graaf E, Teunissen S. Suitable support for anxious hospice patients: what do nurses 'know', 'do' and 'need'? An explanatory mixed method study. BMJ Supportive & Palliative Care. 2017. (Published Online First: 30 June 2017. https://doi.org/10.1136/bmjspcare-2016-001187)		
Intent	To use a qualitative strand to explain initial quantitative results, to form groups based on quantitative results, sampling	The primary aim of this mixed methods study was to gain insight into what nurses know, do, and need to support patients in hospice care suffering from anxiety. The secondary aim was to explore which additional factors influence knowledge about anxiety, performed interventions, and the needs of hospice care nurses
Reasons for choice	Teams are more quantitatively oriented, important variables are known, ability to return to participants, time for two phases, only resource to collect one type of data at a time	Not explicitly stated
Assumptions	Often greater focus on quantitative aspects, leading to positivist assumptions, but which can shift to constructivism, be dialectic	No paradigm explicitly stated
Procedures	(a) Design and implement qualitative strand, analyze	A prospective explanatory and triangulated component design was conducted using quantitative and qualitative methods
	(b) Use quantitative results to determine which results will be explained, refine qualitative questions, sampling, etc.	
	(c) Design and implement qualitative strand, analyze	An online survey was conducted to establish a broad understanding of the current practice regarding anxiety management. Data were analyzed with descriptive and inferential statistics
	(d) Interpret connected results	
		The focus groups (FGs) provided a deeper and multifaceted insight with a subset of nurses who had completed the survey. Data were analyzed using thematic analysis
		Results presented in a connected manner.
Advantages and disadvantages	Appeals to quantitative researchers, straightforward and manageable design, and reporting requirements, second phase can be emergent	The combined quantitative and qualitative approach allowed the researchers to acquire an in-depth insight into the current practices of anxiety management
	Can take time for two phases, second phase not known in advance	They report nonrandom non-response to the online survey, with a risk of socially desirable answers. However the focus groups mitigated this risk as clear from the exchange of experiences that is perceived as safe environment to share practice

Creswell and Plano Clark (2018) and Zweers et al. (2017)

Building and connecting data share some characteristics and are more common in sequential designs. Connecting involves data links through the sampling frame and building through informing data collection approaches (Fetters et al. 2013). Two techniques which may be helpful both in connecting data and merging data are the use of a triangulation protocol and following a thread (O'Cathain et al. 2010). Triangulation protocols in mixed methods research usually take place at the interpretation stages of studies, examining data for convergence, complementarity, or contradiction. Again coding matrices are recommended to display data to consider where there is agreement, partial agreement, silence, or disagreement (O'Cathain et al. 2010). Following a thread means taking a question or theme from

Table 11 Palliative care example of an exploratory sequential mixed methods design

Feature	Discussion	Example
Hermans K, Spruytte N, Cohen J, Van Audenhove C, Declercq A. Informed palliative care in nursing homes through the interRAI Palliative Care instrument: a study protocol based on the Medical Research Council framework. BMC Geriatr. 2014; 14, 132		
Hermans K, Spruytte N, Cohen J, Van Audenhove C, Declercq A. Usefulness, feasibility and face validity of the interRAI Palliative Care instrument according to care professionals in nursing homes: A qualitative study. Int J Nurs Stud. 2016; 62, 90–99		
Hermans K, De Almeida Mello J, Spruytte N, Cohen J, Van Audenhove C, Declercq A. Does using the interRAI Palliative Care instrument reduce the needs and symptoms of nursing home residents receiving palliative care? Palliat Support Care. 2018; 1–9		
Intent	Results of first, qualitative method can help develop the quantitative method that follows, e. g., to develop a new tool or intervention based on experience/culture, etc.	Main research aims:
		(a) To evaluate the effect of the interRAI PC on the quality of palliative care in nursing homes
		(b) To evaluate the feasibility of using the interRAI PC in nursing homes
		(c) To evaluate the face validity of the instrument
Reasons for choice	Used when instruments not available, variables not known, no guiding framework, need for cultural adaption of measure/tool	Not explicitly stated
	Teams are qualitatively oriented, time is available for phased study, interested in transferability of new measure/tool/intervention	
Assumptions	Can start from constructivist stance and move to post-positivist stance	No paradigm explicitly stated, but individual papers reported in a way congruent with paradigms of individual phases
Procedures	(a) Collect and analyze qualitative data to explore phenomenon	The study has a longitudinal, quasi-experimental pretest-posttest design
	(b) Identify results on which quantitative feature will be built	Care professionals evaluated the needs and preferences of all nursing home residents receiving palliative care by means of the interRAI Palliative Care instrument. Data on the usefulness, feasibility, and face validity of the interRAI Palliative Care instrument were derived from notes, semi-structured interviews, and focus groups with participating care professionals and were thematically analyzed and synthesized
	(c) Development phase (instrument, measure, intervention)	
	(d) Implement quantitative strand to examine salient variables/test with new set of participants	
		Care professionals made a series of recommendations in order to optimize the usefulness of the instrument
		A quasi-experimental pretest-posttest study was conducted to compare the needs and symptoms of residents nearing the end of their lives. Care professionals at the intervention nursing homes filled out the interRAI PC over the course of a year for all residents aged 65 years and older who were nearing the end of their lives
Advantages and disadvantages	Sequential nature straightforward, qualitative aspect acceptable to some audiences as associated with quantitative component, clear product from research	Part of a large, funded, long-term study which facilitated the use of different study phases. This also means the study is reported across different papers, which makes the mixed-method element challenging to report comprehensively
	Time-consuming, can be difficult to specify in advance, may require multiple samples, need to determine which qualitative results to use, requires skilled team	

Creswell and Plano Clark (2018) and Hermans et al. (2014, 2016, 2018)

one component and following it through across methods, and potentially phases, of a study.

A particular form of integration is seen when one of the datasets has lesser priority and is embedded within a larger design. The classic example of this is an embedded qualitative process evaluation within a trial or other evaluation designs (Grant et al. 2013; Linnan and Steckler 2002; Oakley et al. 2006). Qualitative data collection embedded within a trial is increasingly common, although still only seen in a minority of published studies, especially in palliative care, and not always well conducted or described (Lewin et al. 2009; Flemming et al. 2008). Such embedded work can occur before the trial (e.g., to generate hypotheses, refine the intervention, or develop outcome measures), during the trial (e.g., to assess fidelity, change processes, or responses to the intervention), or after a trial (e.g., to explore reasons for the findings, generate further hypotheses) (Lewin et al. 2009).

5 Barriers to High-Quality Mixed Methods

Both Bryman (2007) and O'Cathain et al. (2009) studied barriers to mixed methods and the integration of data within studies. They identify eight issues:

Audience*: Mixed methods research is frequently written for publication as separate studies, with different parts of the research written for different audiences. An example is the research examining palliative care in nursing homes used as an exemplar earlier, reported across separate, multiple, publications* (Hermans et al. 2014, 2016, 2018). *Priority can be given to the reporting of quantitative data, particularly those from randomised controlled trials that are considered a 'gold standard' in health services research. An example here is some of my own research which mixed both randomised controlled trial and qualitative case study data, but where the trial report contained no qualitative data, as requested by reviewers* (Dodd et al. 2018; Walshe et al. 2016a, b, c).

Methodological preferences: *Researchers can report having particular skills in, predilection towards or a greater faith in a particular approach as a component of a mixed method study.*

Research structure: *Sometimes insufficient planning or conceptualisation of design mitigates against good data integration. Time issues in planning and conducting research can exacerbate these issues, as can funding which can limit the length of studies.*

Timelines: *A barrier can be that results from different parts of a study are available at different times, and sometimes to different parts of the research team(s).*

Research skills and specialisms: *Apposite skills need to be present within an individual or team. An issue to note is that the skill mix within a team may impede integration by compartmentalising roles, or privileging a particular form of data. There remain few opportunities to train in mixed methods research, and examples in the literature are scant due to the publication issues alluded to already.*

Nature of the data: *One set of data may be more intrinsically interesting or novel.*

Ontological divides: *Most mixed methods researchers are pragmatists, but the divide can lead to issues within teams and more widely*

Publication issues: *The requirements of journals, funders or institutions can shape the conduct of studies, with perceived preference assumed to be quantitative studies. Guidelines to publishing mixed methods studies exist, and should be consulted* (Leech et al. 2011). *However there are few examples of mixed methods research to draw from as exemplars as less than 3% of studies in health services research are mixed methods studies* (Wisdom et al. 2012).

The challenge of reporting mixed methods research and demonstrating that it has been conducted appropriately and rigorously is important and worth separate consideration. Methodological reviews point to deficiencies of reporting of mixed methods research, especially with regard to issues associated with rigor (Brown et al. 2015). Readers are pointed toward two resources: first the Good Reporting of a Mixed Methods Study (GRAMMS) reporting guidelines which should be used when reporting mixed methods studies (O'Cathain et al. 2008) and, second, a scoring system for mixed studies' reviews (Pluye et al. 2009).

Perhaps more complex are the debates surrounding how to ensure high quality in and subsequently judge mixed methods research. Disputes and inconsistencies are evident in understanding whether the qualitative and quantitative components of a study should be assessed separately and how to assess the "mixing" of methods and its appropriateness (Tashakkori and Teddlie 2010). One approach to rigor is legitimation, a term proposed to avoid the connotations associated with terms more usually used with purely qualitative or quantitative designs (Onwuegbuzie and Johnson 2006; Onwuegbuzie and Leech 2007). Legitimation in mixed research, rather than being viewed as a procedure that occurs at a specific step of the mixed research process, is better conceptualized as a continuous iterative, interactive, and dynamic process (Onwuegbuzie et al. 2011; Collins et al. 2012). In addition to the quality criteria inherent in GRAMMS (O'Cathain et al. 2008), quality criteria based on literature review and meta-summary are also proposed by (Fàbregues and Molina-Azorín 2017). Readers are encouraged to consider the recommendations of these writers and also directed to the textbook of Creswell and Plano Clark (2018).

5.1 Recommendations on Mixed Methods Research in Palliative Care

The MORECare study into methodological issues in palliative care research examined the use of mixed methods in this field using a transparent expert consultation design (Farquhar et al. 2013). They made nine recommendations, which they categorized as fully endorsed, partially endorsed, or refined draft recommendations (Table 12).

While the authors recognize that many of these recommendations are also apt to research outside palliative care, they also argue that mixed methods research may address some of the key challenges of palliative care research. In particular they highlight that mixed methods research approaches may mitigate some of the known issues of recruitment, attrition, respondent burden, and outcome measurement known to affect palliative care research (Higginson et al. 2014; Preston et al. 2013). They argue that this is because mixed methods could provide valuable data that could inform recruitment and sample-retention strategies, address issues of gatekeeping, and ensure that outcome measures are fit for purpose (Preston et al. 2016; White and Hardy 2008; Bausewein et al. 2016). Palliative care research often explores issues which are complex and context dependent, where interventions are complex, and with challenging ethical issues. Such complexity is likely to require research designs that are themselves more complex and mixed methods designs part of that picture.

6 Conclusions

Mixed methods research designs have much to offer the field of palliative care. Research in palliative care brings particular challenges, and the use of mixed methods can assist in ameliorating some of these. Caution must be exercised, as mixing methods requires particular considerations associated with understanding of paradigm and attention to design choices and the order and function of data collection and analysis. Hopefully there are pointers to these considerations in this chapter which will facilitate researchers in accessing resources to guide excellent mixed methods design choices. This should further the field of palliative care research and hopefully enhance the quality of palliative care in the future.

Table 12 The MORECare recommendations on mixed methods research in palliative care

Endorsement	Recommendation
Fully endorsed	Mixed methods (integrating quantitative and qualitative methods) research is a particularly useful approach for palliative and end-of-life care research: the exact choice of method will depend on the research question, and each method needs to be justified
	The degree of respondent burden needs careful consideration in palliative and end-of-life care research, and researchers should consider prioritization of key outcome measures and qualitative questions, whether splitting data collection sessions may be necessary, and the place and mode of data collection. Piloting and user involvement inform respondent burden concerns, but decisions about respondent burden should be taken with participants and not for them
Partially endorsed	Where justified, qualitative exploration of experiences of participation in randomized controlled trials and other "well-designed studies" should be carried out and should include all participant groups, e.g., patients, carers, and clinicians; this is in addition to qualitative exploration of experiences of the intervention
	Trial registers need to include fields for registration of qualitative components of the study or parallel qualitative studies, and similar non-trial registers should be established
	Depending on the research question, palliative and end-of-life care research may benefit from a multidisciplinary team-working approach; thus in most cases, teams will need to consist of requisite disciplines (clinical and academic) to answer the research question proposed
	Greater emphasis is required on implementation studies in palliative and end-of-life care research than is presently the case: this may develop naturally as the specialty establishes, but researchers should be encouraged to move from phase III RCTs to phase IV implementation studies and consider the contribution a mixed methods approach could make to them
	Researchers working on mixed methods studies need both quantitative and qualitative skills (and training) that should come from separate relevant professionals at the design stage and potentially also at the data collection stage, but given the sensitivity of research in palliative and end-of-life care, researchers conducting interviews need additional empathy and communication skills. Researchers from differing paradigms need an openness to, and understanding of, other paradigms within the team. Support and debriefing of all team members is important
Refined draft recommendations	Given the current state of (under-)development of palliative and end-of-life care research, the explicit use of theoretical perspective is encouraged from the outset, and investigators should be open to developing new theoretical frameworks for the field
	Given the nature of the sensitivities involved in palliative and end-of-life care research, there are potentially particular problems of therapeutic effects of research interviews that can be confounding: this should be considered when designing studies and interpreting findings. The lack of evidence of the nature and duration of therapeutic effects requires further research

Farquhar et al. (2013, pp. 1157–1158)

References

Bausewein C, Daveson BA, Currow DC, Downing J, Deliens L, Radbruch L, et al. EAPC white paper on outcome measurement in palliative care: improving practice, attaining outcomes and delivering quality services – recommendations from the European Association for Palliative Care (EAPC) task force on outcome measurement. Palliat Med. 2016;30(1):6–22.

Bergenholtz H, Jarlbaek L, Hølge-Hazelton B. Generalist palliative care in hospital – cultural and organisational interactions. Results of a mixed-methods study. Palliat Med. 2016;30(6):558–66.

Brewer J, Hunter A. Multimethod research: a synthesis of styles. Thousand Oaks: Sage; 1989.

Brown KM, Elliott SJ, Leatherdale ST, Robertson-Wilson J. Searching for rigour in the reporting of mixed methods population health research: a methodological review. Health Educ Res. 2015;30(6):811–39.

Bryman A. Integrating quantitative and qualitative research: how is it done? Qual Res. 2006;6(1):97–113.

Bryman A. Barriers to integrating quantitative and qualitative research. J Mixed Methods Res. 2007;1(1):8–22.

Bryman A. Social research methods. 4th ed. Oxford: Oxford University Press; 2012.

Burke Johnson R, Stefurak T. Considering the evidence-and-credibility discussion in evaluation through the Lens of dialectical pluralism. N Dir Eval. 2013;2013 (138):37–48.

Burt J, Raine R. The effect of age on referral to and use of specialist palliative care services in adult cancer patients: a systematic review. Age Ageing. 2006;35(5):469–76.

Burt J, Plant H, Omar R, Raine R. Equity of use of specialist palliative care by age: cross-sectional study of lung cancer patients. Palliat Med. 2010;24(6):641–50.

Collins KM, O'Cathain A. Introduction: ten points about mixed methods research to be considered by the novice researcher. Int J Mult Res Approach. 2009;3(1):2–7.

Collins KM, Onwuegbuzie AJ, Sutton IL. A model incorporating the rationale and purpose for conducting mixed methods research in special education and beyond. Learn Disabil: Contemp J. 2006;4(1):67–100.

Collins KM, Onwuegbuzie AJ, Johnson RB. Securing a place at the table: a review and extension of legitimation criteria for the conduct of mixed research. Am Behav Sci. 2012;56(6):849–65.

Coyle CE, Schulman-Green D, Feder S, Toraman S, Prust ML, Plano Clark VL, et al. Federal funding for mixed methods research in the health sciences in the United States: recent trends. J Mixed Methods Res. 2016. https://doi.org/10.1177/1558689816662578.

Creswell JW, Plano Clark V. Designing and conducting mixed methods research. 3rd ed. Sage: Los Angeles; 2018.

Creswell J, Klassen A, Plano Clark V, Smith K, Research OoBaSS. Best practices for mixed methods research in the health science. Bethesda: National Institutes of Health; 2011.

Dalkin SM, Jones D, Lhussier M, et al. Understanding integrated care pathways in palliative care using realist evaluation: a mixed methods study protocol BMJ Open 2012;2:e001533. https://doi.org/10.1136/bmjopen-2012-001533.

Dalkin SM, Lhussier M, Philipson P, Jones D, Cunningham W. Reducing inequalities in care for patients with non-malignant diseases: insights from a realist evaluation of an integrated palliative care pathway. Palliat Med. 2016;30(7):690–7.

De Almeida Mello J, Hermans K, Van Audenhove C, Macq J, Declercq A. Evaluations of home care interventions for frail older persons using the interRAI home care instrument: a systematic review of the literature. J Am Med Dir Assoc. 2015;16(2):173.e1–10.

Denscombe M. Communities of practice: a research paradigm for the mixed methods approach. J Mixed Methods Res. 2008;2(3):270–83.

Dodd S, Hill M, Ockenden N, Algorta GP, Preston N, Payne S, Walshe C. 'Being with' or 'doing for'? How the role of an end-of-life volunteer befriender can impact patient wellbeing: interviews from a multiple qualitative case study (ELSA). Support Care Cancer 2018. https://doi.org/10.1007/s00520-018-4169-2

Fàbregues S, Molina-Azorín JF. Addressing quality in mixed methods research: a review and recommendations for a future agenda. Qual Quant. 2017;51(6):2847–63.

Farquhar M, Higginson I, Fagan P, Booth S. The feasibility of a single-blinded fast-track pragmatic randomised controlled trial of a complex intervention for breathlessness in advanced disease. BMC Palliat Care. 2009;8(1):9.

Farquhar MC, Ewing G, Booth S. Using mixed methods to develop and evaluate complex interventions in palliative care research. Palliat Med. 2011a;25(8):748–57.

Farquhar M, Prevost AT, McCrone P, Higginson I, Gray J, Brafman-Kennedy B, et al. Study protocol: phase III single-blinded fast-track pragmatic randomised controlled trial of a complex intervention for breathlessness in advanced disease. Trials. 2011b;12(1):130.

Farquhar M, Preston N, Evans CJ, Grande G, Short V, Benalia H, et al. Mixed methods research in the development and evaluation of complex interventions in palliative and end-of-life care: report on the MORECare consensus exercise. J Palliat Med. 2013; 16(12):1550–60.

Farquhar MC, Prevost AT, McCrone P, Brafman-Price B, Bentley A, Higginson IJ, et al. Is a specialist breathlessness service more effective and cost-effective for patients with advanced cancer and their carers than standard care? Findings of a mixed-method randomised controlled trial. BMC Med. 2014;12:194.

Farquhar MC, Prevost AT, McCrone P, Brafman-Price B, Bentley A, Higginson IJ, et al. The clinical and cost effectiveness of a breathlessness intervention service for patients with advanced non-malignant disease and their informal carers: mixed findings of a mixed method randomised controlled trial. Trials. 2016;17(1):1–16.

Fetters MD, Curry LA, Creswell JW. Achieving integration in mixed methods designs-principles and practices. Health Serv Res. 2013;48(6 Pt 2):2134–56.

Flemming K, Adamson J, Atkin K. Improving the effectiveness of interventions in palliative care: the potential role of qualitative research in enhancing evidence from randomized controlled trials. Palliat Med. 2008; 22(2):123–31.

Florczak KL. Purists need not apply: the case for pragmatism in mixed methods research. Nurs Sci Q. 2014; 27(4):278–82.

Grant A, Treweek S, Dreischulte T, Foy R, Guthrie B. Process evaluations for cluster-randomised trials of complex interventions: a proposed framework for design and reporting. Trials. 2013;14:15.

Greene JC. Advances in mixed-method evaluation: the challenges and benefits of integrating diverse paradigms. San Francisco: Jossey-Bass; 1997.

Greene JC. Toward a methodology of mixed methods social inquiry. Res School. 2006;13(1):93–8.

Greene JC. Mixed methods in social inquiry. San Francisco: Wiley; 2007.

Greene JC. Is mixed methods social inquiry a distinctive methodology? J Mixed Methods Res. 2008;2 (1):7–22.

Greene JC, Hall JN. Dialectics and pragmatism: being of consequence. In: Sage handbook of mixed methods in social & behavioral research. Los Angeles: Sage; 2010. p. 119–43.

Greene JC, Caracelli VJ, Graham WF. Toward a conceptual framework for mixed-method evaluation designs. Educ Eval Policy Anal. 1989;11(3):255–74.

Guo Q, Chochinov HM, McClement S, Thompson G, Hack T. Development and evaluation of the dignity talk question framework for palliative patients and their families: a mixed-methods study. Palliat Med. 2018;32(1):195–205. https://doi.org/10.1177/0269216317734696.

Hermans K, Spruytte N, Cohen J, Van Audenhove C, Declercq A. Informed palliative care in nursing homes through the interRAI palliative care instrument: a study protocol based on the Medical Research Council framework. BMC Geriatr. 2014;14:132.

Hermans K, Spruytte N, Cohen J, Van Audenhove C, Declercq A. Usefulness, feasibility and face validity of the interRAI palliative care instrument according to care professionals in nursing homes: a qualitative study. Int J Nurs Stud. 2016;62:90–9.

Hermans K, De Almeida Mello J, Spruytte N, Cohen J, Van Audenhove C, Declercq A. Does using the interRAI palliative care instrument reduce the needs and symptoms of nursing home residents receiving palliative care? Palliat Support Care. 2018;16(1):32–40. https://doi.org/10.1017/S1478951517000153.

Higginson I, Evans C, Grande G, Preston N, Morgan M, McCrone P, et al. Evaluating complex interventions in end of life care: the MORECare statement on good practice generated by a synthesis of transparent expert consultations and systematic reviews. BMC Med. 2014;11(111). https://doi.org/10.1186/741-7015-11-111.

Highet G, Crawford D, Murray SA, Boyd K. Development and evaluation of the supportive and palliative care indicators tool (SPICT): a mixed-methods study. BMJ Support Palliat Care. 2014;4(3):285–90.

Hosie A, Agar M, Lobb E, Davidson PM, Phillips J. Improving delirium recognition and assessment for people receiving inpatient palliative care: a mixed methods meta-synthesis. Int J Nurs Stud. 2017; 75:123–9.

Johnson RB, Onwuegbuzie AJ. Mixed methods research: a research paradigm whose time has come. Educ Res. 2004;33(7):14–26.

Johnson RB, Onwuegbuzie AJ, Turner LA. Toward a definition of mixed methods research. J Mixed Methods Res. 2007;1(2):112–33.

Leech NL, Onwuegbuzie AJ, Combs JP. Writing publishable mixed research articles: guidelines for emerging scholars in the health sciences and beyond. Int J Mult Res Approaches. 2011;5(1):7–24.

Lewin S, Glenton C, Oxman AD. Use of qualitative methods alongside randomised controlled trials of complex healthcare interventions: methodological study BMJ 2009; 339 :b3496

Lincoln YS, Guba EG. Naturalistic inquiry, vol. 1985. Beverley Hills: Sage; 1985.

Linnan L, Steckler A. Process evaluation for public health interventions and research. San Francisco: Jossey-Bass; 2002.

Maxwell JA, Loomis DM. Mixed methods design: an alternative approach. In: Handbook of mixed methods in social and behavioral research, vol. 1. Thousand Oaks: Sage; 2003. p. 241–72.

Maxwell JA, Mittapalli K. Realism as a stance for mixed methods research. In: Handbook of mixed methods in social & behavioral research. Thousand Oaks: Sage; 2010. p. 145–68.

Mertens DM. Mixed methods and the politics of human research: the transformative-emancipatory perspective. In: Tashakkori A, Teddlie C, editors. Handbook of mixed methods in social and behavioral research. Thousand Oaks: Sage; 2003. p. 135–64.

Miles M, Huberman A. Qualitative data analysis. London: Sage; 1984.

Morgan DL. Practical strategies for combining qualitative and quantitative methods: applications to health research. Qual Health Res. 1998;8(3):362–76.

Morgan DL. Paradigms lost and pragmatism regained: methodological implications of combining qualitative and quantitative methods. J Mixed Methods Res. 2007;1(1):48–76.

Morita T, Miyashita M, Yamagishi A, Akizuki N, Kizawa Y, Shirahige Y, et al. A region-based palliative care intervention trial using the mixed-method approach: Japan OPTIM study. BMC Palliat Care. 2012;11(1):2.

Morita T, Miyashita M, Yamagishi A, Akiyama M, Akizuki N, Hirai K, et al. Effects of a programme of interventions on regional comprehensive palliative care for patients with cancer: a mixed-methods study. Lancet Oncol. 2013;14(7):638–46.

Morse JM. Principles of mixed methods and multimethod research design. In: Tashakkori A, Teddlie C, editors. Handbook of mixed methods in social and behavioral research. 1. Thousand Oaks: Sage; 2003. p. 189–208.

O'Cathain A, Murphy E, Nicholl J. Why, and how, mixed methods research is undertaken in health services research in England: a mixed methods study. BMC Health Serv Res. 2007;7(1):85.

O'Cathain A, Murphy E, Nicholl J. The quality of mixed methods studies in health services research. J Health Serv Res Policy. 2008;13(2):92–8.

O'Cathain A, Nicholl J, Murphy E. Structural issues affecting mixed methods studies in health research: a qualitative study. BMC Med Res Methodol. 2009;9(1):82.

O'Cathain A, Murphy E, Nicholl J. Three techniques for integrating data in mixed methods studies. BMJ. 2010;341:c4587.

Oakley A, Strange V, Bonell C, Allen E, Stephenson J. Process evaluation in randomised controlled trials of complex interventions. BMJ. 2006;332(7538):413–6.

Onwuegbuzie AJ, Johnson RB. The validity issue in mixed research. Res Schools. 2006;13(1):48–63.

Onwuegbuzie AJ, Leech NL. Validity and qualitative research: an oxymoron? Qual Quant. 2007;41(2): 233–49.

Onwuegbuzie AJ, Johnson RB, Collins KM. Assessing legitimation in mixed research: a new framework. Qual Quant. 2011;45(6):1253–71.

Östlund U, Kidd L, Wengström Y, Rowa-Dewar N. Combining qualitative and quantitative research within mixed method research designs: a methodological review. Int J Nurs Stud. 2011;48(3):369–83.

Patton M. Qualitative research and evaluation methods. 3rd ed. Thousand Oaks: Sage; 2002.

Pearson A, White H, Bath-Hextall F, Salmond S, Apostolo J, Kirkpatrick P. A mixed-methods approach to systematic reviews. Int J Evid Based Healthc. 2015;13(3): 121–31.

Pelto PJ. What is so new about mixed methods? Qual Health Res. 2015;25(6):734–45.

Pluye P, Gagnon MP, Griffiths F, Johnson-Lafleur J. A scoring system for appraising mixed methods research, and concomitantly appraising qualitative, quantitative and mixed methods primary studies in mixed studies reviews. Int J Nurs Stud. 2009;46(4): 529–46.

Preston NJ, Fayers P, Walters SJ, Pilling M, Grande GE, Short V, et al. Recommendations for managing missing data, attrition and response shift in palliative and end-of-life care research: part of the MORECare research method guidance on statistical issues. Palliat Med. 2013;27(10):899–907.

Preston NJ, Farquhar MC, Walshe CE, Stevinson C, Ewing G, Calman LA, et al. Strategies designed to help healthcare professionals to recruit participants to research studies. Cochrane Database Syst Rev 2016(2).

Sale JE, Lohfeld LH, Brazil K. Revisiting the quantitative-qualitative debate: implications for mixed-methods research. Qual Quant. 2002;36(1):43–53.

Sandelowski M, Voils CI, Knafl G. On quantitizing. Journal of mixed methods research. 2009;3(3): 208–22.

Sandelowski M, Voils CI, Leeman J, Crandell JL. Mapping the mixed methods-mixed research synthesis terrain. J Mixed Methods Res. 2012;6(4):317–31.

Selman L, Speck P, Gysels M, Agupio G, Dinat N, Downing J, et al. 'Peace' and 'life worthwhile' as measures of spiritual well-being in African palliative care: a mixed-methods study. Health Qual Life Outcomes. 2013; 11(1):94.

Stefurak T, Burke Johnson R, Shatto E. Mixed methods and dialectical pluralism. In: Handbook of methodological approaches to community-based research: qualitative, quantitative, and mixed methods. New York: Oxford University Press; 2015. p. 345.

Tariq S, Woodman J. Using mixed methods in health research. JRSM Short Rep. 2013;4(6). https://doi.org/10.1177/2042533313479197.

Tashakkori A, Cresswell JW. The new era of mixed methods. J Mixed Methods Res. 2007;1(1):5.

Tashakkori A, Teddlie C. Sage handbook of mixed methods in social & behavioral research. Thousand Oaks: Sage; 2010.

Walshe C, Algorta GP, Dodd S, Hill M, Ockenden N, Payne S. Protocol for the end-of-life social action study (ELSA): a randomised wait-list controlled trial and embedded qualitative case study evaluation assessing the causal impact of social action befriending services on end of life experience. BMC Palliat Care. 2016a; 15:60. https://doi.org/10.1186/s12904-016-0134-3.

Walshe CD, Dodd S, Hill M, Ockenden N, Payne S, Perez Algorta G, Preston N. What is the impact of social action befriending services at the end-of-life? Evaluation of the end of life social action fund. Lancaster: Lancaster University; 2016b.

Walshe C, Dodd S, Hill M, Ockenden N, Payne S, Preston N, et al. How effective are volunteers at supporting people in their last year of life? A pragmatic randomised wait-list trial in palliative care (ELSA). BMC Med. 2016c;14(1):203.

White C, Hardy J. Gatekeeping from palliative care research trials. Prog Palliat Care. 2008;16(4):167–71.

Wisdom JP, Cavaleri MA, Onwuegbuzie AJ, Green CA. Methodological reporting in qualitative, quantitative, and mixed methods health services research articles. Health Serv Res. 2012;47(2):721–45.

Zweers D, de Graaf E, Teunissen S. Suitable support for anxious hospice patients: what do nurses 'know', 'do' and 'need'? An explanatory mixed method study. BMJ Supportive & Palliative CarePublished Online First: 30 June 2017. https://doi.org/10.1136/bmjspcare-2016-001187.

Ethics in Palliative Care Research

94

Kasper Raus and Sigrid Sterckx

Contents

Abstract

Today, there is near universal consensus on evidence-based medicine (EBM) as the preferred approach to medical practice. In palliative care, however, a strong evidence base is lacking in many respects, which could result in less than optimal care being provided to patients. Establishing a solid evidence base requires much research to be conducted in palliative care. Such research in palliative care faces both empirical and ethical challenges. In this chapter, we focus on several ethical issues and challenges that are relevant to palliative care research. Many legal and ethical

K. Raus (✉)
Ghent University Hospital, Ghent, Belgium
e-mail: Kasper.Raus@UGent.be

S. Sterckx
Department of Philosophy and Moral Sciences, Ghent University, Ghent, Belgium
e-mail: Sigrid.Sterckx@UGent.be

R. D. MacLeod, L. Van den Block (eds.), *Textbook of Palliative Care*,
https://doi.org/10.1007/978-3-319-77740-5_110

frameworks exist for dealing with research on ethical issues, but this chapter examines how these general frameworks apply more specifically to the domain of palliative care research. We will discuss the key issue of vulnerability in palliative care research. Other issues that will be touched upon are: (1) respect for research participants; (2) the need for independent review; (3) the requirement of social and/or scientific value; (4) issues related to informed consent; (5) challenges regarding scientific validity; (6) favorable risk-benefit ratio; and (7) fair participant selection. In touching upon these issues, most ethical challenges for palliative care research are examined. The chapter aims to show that although many ethical challenges may exist when conducting palliative care research, these challenges should in no way be deemed insurmountable. Research in palliative care is both needed and possible, provided sufficient attention is given to possible ethical sensibilities.

1 Introduction

Within medicine, there has been a clear paradigm shift toward the use of empirical evidence in both clinical practice and policy making. Today, there is near universal consensus on evidence-based medicine (EBM) as the preferred approach to medical practice (Sackett 1997). However, in this respect, palliative care has been argued to lag behind. The evidence base supporting palliative care is there, but is not as good as it could be (Higginson 1999). Other research suggests that there is an increasing amount of research in palliative care and that the level of evidence is rising (Tieman et al. 2008).

There are many reasons for this gap in research and evidence base. Part of it concerns the funding of palliative care research (Higginson 2016), but other factors include the challenges to conducting palliative care research that is both maximally scientifically valid and ethically justified. In this chapter, we will deal with the second of those challenges, namely, the research ethics challenges that arise when conducting palliative care research.

The need for palliative care research hardly requires justification. It is clear that more evidence is needed, as only good and solid evidence provides the best guarantee for good and ethical practices. An example is the well-known Liverpool Care Pathway for the Dying Patient which was developed in the UK as a care pathway to explore and implement good end of life care for all patients. It was widely used but sparked considerable controversy because it was seen by many as a mere tick box exercise. In 2013 an independent review found that there was no evidence on the potentially adverse events of the LCP and that "[n]o research has yet produced evidence by robustly comparing these pathways with other forms of care" (Neuberger et al. 2013). Subsequently, it was recommended that the LCP should be phased out and abandoned. This case provides a striking example of how the lack of research and evidence in palliative care might potentially lead to improper care being provided. This is but one example of the fact that there are strong ethical reasons, in addition to scientific ones, for conducting research in palliative care and thereby improving the evidence base.

Nevertheless, although necessary, palliative care research is also particularly challenging from an ethical perspective. In this chapter, we will look at some of the ethical issues that are particular to research in palliative care. Two remarks are in order. First, this chapter does not pretend to provide an exhaustive overview of all research ethics issues. Our goal is to discuss some of the most pertinent issues with regard to palliative care research. Second, this chapter does not pretend to address any of the issues at length. Each of the issues discussed in this chapter is themselves subject to considerable debate. We examine each issue in some detail and provide essential literature references for those interested in more in-depth discussions of that particular issue.

For sake of clarity, in the next two sections, we explain the focus of this chapter and the ethical framework that is used. Subsequently, we will discuss the key issue of vulnerability in palliative care research. Other issues that will be commented upon are (1) respect for research participants, (2) the need for independent review, (3) the requirement of social and/or scientific value, (4) issues related to informed consent, (5) challenges regarding scientific validity, (6) favorable risk-benefit ratio, and (7) fair participant selection.

2 The Focus of This Chapter

To avoid conceptual confusion, we believe it is important to be clear that we will focus on palliative care research, a category which should be distinguished from other types of research that will not be our focus.

Palliative care research ought to be distinguished from the more broad category of research involving terminally ill or dying patients. Although there may be significant overlap (since much of palliative care research involves terminally ill or dying patients), distinguishing them is essential. First, not all research involving terminally ill or dying patients constitutes palliative care research. For example, terminally ill or dying patients might be enrolled in clinical trials to test potential new *curative* drugs. No doubt the involvement of terminally ill or dying patients in such research raises specific and highly relevant ethical issues, yet these are not the focus of this chapter.

Second, not all palliative care research involves terminally ill or dying patients. Research can take many forms (survey, interview, focus group, clinical trial, etc.) and involve many different types of participants (nurses, relatives, caregivers, physicians). With regard to the ethical evaluation, this diversity in research types and research populations is particularly relevant. Although roughly the same ethical principles apply to all types of research, in the application of these principles, the research type and participant population recruited play an important role. For example, the ethical requirement for a favorable risk-benefit ratio applies to all research, but interventional research with terminally ill or dying patients evidently involves a different risk-benefit calculation compared to epidemiological research involving palliative care physicians. Nevertheless, both will be considered to be examples of palliative care research. Whenever relevant, we will explicitly distinguish between research types and participant population throughout the chapter.

In short, what characterizes palliative care research is not the population of participants it involves. Rather, palliative care research, as we use the concept, should be seen as *research of any type, regardless of participant population, that is intended to further the evidence or knowledge base of palliative care.*

3 Ethical Frameworks

When considering the ethical aspects of research ethics, a wide variety of possible ethical framework exists. There is currently no framework that enjoys universal consensus, although there is considerable overlap and near universal consensus on several items.

A first important source for clinical research ethics can be found in various authoritative international guidelines. An argument could be made that serious thinking about research ethics started only after WWII (Rothman 1987) and in the wake of particular scandals (e.g., the WWII research atrocities and the Tuskegee syphilis research scandal). Following these revelations, several international guidelines were drafted. Well known are the Nuremberg Code, the Declaration of Helsinki, and the CIOMS guidelines. Although not legally binding, many of these guidelines form the basis for national legislation in various countries.

However, these guidelines do not always provide definite answers to research ethical dilemmas in palliative care research. First, considerable differences exist between these guidelines. A recent study by Bernabe and colleagues, looking at the well-known international guidelines, found that:

> There is no consensus on the majority of the imperatives and that in only 8.2 % of the imperatives were [sic] there at least moderate consensus (i.e., consensus of at least 3 of the 5 ethics guidelines). (Bernabe et al. 2016: 1)

Second, these guidelines have a wide scope and thus rarely specifically address issues that are directly relevant to palliative care research. Therefore, merely consulting internationally recognized guidelines will not suffice to find definite research ethical recommendations for palliative care research.

Another often cited and highly influential framework is that of Emanuel and colleagues (Emanuel et al. 2000). This is an attempt to construct a coherent ethical framework based on the international guidelines cited above. More specifically, the framework consists of seven key ethical requirements that should all be met in order for any clinical research to be considered ethical. Ethical clinical research must (1) be valuable (enhance health or knowledge), (2) be scientifically valid, (3) select participants fairly, (4) have a favorable risk-benefit ratio, (5) be subject to independent ethical review, (6) have informed consent from participants, and (7) show respect for enrolled participants.

Although many other frameworks might be possible, for the present chapter we will make use of this framework. We believe the seven requirements provide a good overview of the key ethical issues in clinical research. As our chapter is focused on palliative care research, we will examine how these requirements relate to palliative care research.

4 Vulnerability of Terminally Ill Patients

Before dealing with the seven ethical requirements, we first want to highlight one of the most common concepts in research ethics: "vulnerability" (for a recent and extensive exploration of the concept, see Bracken-Roche et al. 2017). Some groups or individuals are considered to be vulnerable, meaning they are at increased likelihood of being harmed or wronged (The difference between harming and wronging is the topic of considerable debate. In general harming seems to involve some form of damaging (e.g., physical or psychological harm). Wronging is a more broad concept that refers to acts that are contrary to moral principles such as fairness, justice, and beneficence or acts which involve unjustified breaches of moral rights (e.g., the right not to be harmed or the right to privacy). Understood in this way, wronging does not necessarily coincide with harming. Although it is possible to wrong someone through the infliction of unjustifiable harm, one can also wrong someone without harming them (e.g., breaching someone's privacy without them ever knowing) or harm someone without wronging them (e.g., harm inflicted in a medically and ethically justified amputation).) *in research contexts*. All guidelines acknowledge the issue of vulnerability and maintain that when vulnerable individuals are recruited for health-related research, additional or special protective measures should be taken or considered. Classic examples are pregnant women, prisoners, and children.

It is important to emphasize two particular points. First, there are many different kinds of vulnerability, and the concept of vulnerability discussed here relates to the research context. The *Oxford English Dictionary*, for example, defines "vulnerable" as "susceptible of receiving wounds or physical injury" (*Oxford English Dictionary*). In this sense every human being is vulnerable by virtue of being human, but this broad interpretation of vulnerability is not helpful when considering protection for particular groups or individuals participating in palliative care research. Therefore, labelling potential research participants as either vulnerable or not vulnerable implies nothing with regard to these participants' vulnerability in other contexts. Second, it should be stressed that vulnerability is best interpreted as a comparative concept (Wendler 2017). When a particular group or individual is labelled as vulnerable, this should be taken to mean that this group or individual is *more likely* to be harmed or wronged in research and that therefore *additional* protective measures are in order. Considering a particular group or individual to be non-vulnerable hence does not necessarily mean that they cannot be harmed or wronged through their participation in research. Adequate protective measures should be taken for *all* research participants, but *additional* measures should be considered for vulnerable participants.

Vulnerability is an established concept in research ethics, but the relevant question for this chapter is whether participants in palliative care research should be considered vulnerable and, thus, be awarded additional or special protection. As argued above, palliative care research can include a variety of different participants (e.g., terminally ill patients, relatives, nurses, physicians, etc.). Within that group of possible research participants, the most likely candidates to be labelled as vulnerable are terminally or seriously ill patients. These potential participants have indeed been argued to be vulnerable. The influential CIOMS guideline argues that the category of potentially vulnerable participants includes "people with incurable or stigmatized conditions or diseases" (CIOMS 2016: 58). This position has also been taken in academic literature (Nickel 2006).

However, the usefulness of vulnerability as a concept has also been questioned to some degree (e.g., Levine et al. 2004). There seem to be several arguments against using vulnerability as a broad label, especially for terminally ill patients.

First, applying the concept in a way that automatically covers entire groups or populations might incorrectly consider these groups as more homogeneous than they really are. Those with terminal or serious illnesses form a highly heterogeneous group that cuts across age, gender, socioeconomic background, etc. Again, this is not to say that particular patients with serious terminal illnesses might not be considered vulnerable but rather that there seems to be no reason to *automatically* consider them to be vulnerable. Indeed, vulnerability could be argued to be a context-dependent rather than a category-wide concept. For example, a socioeconomically disadvantaged patient might be vulnerable to coercive financial offers to participate, but need not be vulnerable with regard to other ethically relevant risks. Many guidelines, for example, the CIOMS guideline, explicitly address this issue and seek "to avoid considering members of entire classes of individuals as vulnerable" (CIOMS 2016: 57).

Second, and related, there are no agreed upon criteria to determine vulnerability. The Declaration of Helsinki, for example, argues that some groups or individuals are potentially vulnerable, but provides no examples or criteria to help determine what constitutes such vulnerability. The CIOMS guideline and the WHO, on the other hand, use a very broad concept that may cover or include a large majority of patients, including seriously ill ones. However, if the concept of vulnerability is used in such a way that it covers nearly all potential research subjects, its usefulness in practice is limited (Levine et al. 2004).

Third, vulnerability as a broad concept has led to problematic practices. Many of the populations that have been labelled vulnerable have, as a result, been systematically excluded from research as this was sometimes seen as the only way to guarantee protection for vulnerable patients. However, this could lead to injustice and an unfair participant selection (for instance, if they are automatically withheld the benefits from participating in research). This could, paradoxically, actually lead to increased vulnerability for these patients. This might be relevant to the context of palliative care since, as mentioned earlier, palliative care lags behind in its evidence base. As we will explain below, there may be a significant extent of so-called gatekeeping in palliative care research whereby institutions, researchers, families, or health-care providers prevent access to research recruitment (see Sect. 10).

This has led to calls for a pragmatic conception of vulnerability. The question then is not so much "is this patient vulnerable or part of a vulnerable population" but rather "which steps should be taken to maximally protect the participants recruited within a particular study" (Wendler 2017). It would seem to be a fundamental ethical requirement that every participant in a research study should be granted the best possible protection, regardless of whether they should be deemed vulnerable or non-vulnerable. Therefore, in the remainder of this chapter, we will not focus on the question as to whether participants in palliative care research should be labelled vulnerable, but rather on particular potential ethical risks within palliative care research and ways of handling those risks.

As mentioned above, we will be using the well-known framework developed by Emanuel and colleagues which focuses on seven ethical requirements. Some of these requirements are more relevant than others in the context of palliative care research, but in the interest of completeness, we will discuss all of them.

5 Independent Review

There is widespread consensus that, for any study involving human participants to be ethical, a research protocol has to be in place which needs to be independently reviewed. Many jurisdictions around the world legally require ethics committees or Institutional Review Boards (IRBs) to be established. The drafting of a protocol is required to guarantee valid informed consent (see Sect. 7), since without it patients cannot know what they are consenting to, making their consent invalid. Such a protocol is also essential for guaranteeing scientific validity (see Sect. 8) since ad hoc changes to the research while underway are unlikely to positively benefit the ethical nature and scientific validity of the research.

It has been suggested that getting approval from an ethics committee or IRB may be particularly challenging for palliative care research involving terminally ill patients or their loved ones (Casarett and Karlawish 2000; Lee and Kristjanson 2003). Abernethy et al. (2014) suggest that many ethics committees or IRBs may not be familiar with the particularities of palliative care research or may be hesitant to approve research that involves terminally ill patients or their loved ones. In turn, this may shun researchers away from palliative care research which is seen as overly ethically contentious and not likely to obtain approval from an IRB.

There is no reason to assume, however, that palliative care research involving terminally ill patients or relatives cannot be done in an ethical manner. A strategy for getting approval that has repeatedly shown to be effective, is early communication with the ethics committee or IRB (e.g., Hickman et al. 2012; Abernethy et al. 2014). This allows researchers to more quickly respond to possible concerns from the ethical committee and to collaboratively create a palliative care research protocol that is scientifically valid and ethically justified.

6 Social or Scientific Value

Another general ethical requirement for research involving human participants is that the research that is being considered is expected to have social or scientific value. This is crucial since research puts patients at risk (however slight), and this should only be considered when social value can reasonably be expected. Additionally, social or scientific value is essential from the perspective of making responsible use of finite funds for research. It is therefore highly recommended for researchers to reflect in advance on the potential beneficial contributions of their research to science or society. Within the research community, there is a growing emphasis on translational research which focuses on translating research findings into everyday practice in order to improve health care for patients (Westfall et al. 2007; Woolf 2008).

When applied to palliative care research, this ethical requirement clearly strengthens the case for conducting palliative care research. In view of the gap in evidence base and the existing reservations toward palliative care, there is a huge potential for societal and/or scientific value of research in this area.

7 Informed Consent

Informed consent is the best known and often seen as the main requirement for research involving human participants. Hence we will devote a bit more attention to this requirement. Many of the well-known research scandals, such as the Nazi experiments or the Tuskegee study, raised (among other things) significant concern due to the lack of informed consent or even the lack of *any* consent whatsoever (Vollman and Winau 1996). Today, there is near universal consensus that informed consent is a conditio sine qua non for ethical research. Of course, ethical issues pertaining to research should not be limited to issues of consent. As famously argued by Emmanuel and colleagues, research can be unethical even when there is informed consent (Emanuel et al. 2000). As such, consent is a necessary condition, but it should not be considered a sufficient one.

Generally, a person is deemed to be able to provide informed consent if (1) she has the cognitive capacities to understand information about the study and the effects of participation and (2) she is not subject to coercion, manipulation, or undue influence. Those who cannot meet these conditions are deemed unable to provide consent.

Note that for this chapter we will use the formulation "unable to provide informed consent" rather than "incompetent," which has sometimes been used in the past. Competence is clearly task-specific, and labelling patients as incompetent might create the wrong impression that they have lost all capacity to consent. Persons unable to provide informed consent in a research context might still be able to provide informed consent in a variety of other contexts.

In palliative care research, the issue of informed consent is clearly pertinent, particularly with research involving dying patients or their relatives. We will deal with each of these two categories in turn.

7.1 Dying Patients

Dying patients may face an increased risk of failing to meet the two essential conditions of informed consent: the cognitive capacity to understand information and the absence of undue influence.

7.1.1 Reduced Cognitive Capacity

With regard to the capacity to understand information, dying patients may face an increased risk of having a reduced capacity to understand and assess information due to their life-threatening illness or general physical condition. This is the case for patients who suffer from conditions such as dementia or brain tumors, but also for imminently dying patients whose consciousness is frequently reduced. Hence, three possible scenarios might unfold. Terminally ill patients might be incapable of providing informed consent if they are not conscious, if they have reduced cognitive capacities that give reason to question their ability to provide informed consent, or if they lose their ability to provide consent while participating in the research study. We will briefly discuss each of these situations.

Scenario 1: Terminally Ill Patients Who Clearly Lack the Ability to Provide Consent
The Nuremberg Code drafted in response to the WWII atrocities includes the requirement that research may only be conducted following "the voluntary, well-informed, understanding consent of the human subject in a full legal capacity" (paragraph 1) (The full text of the Nuremberg Code can be found online at https://archive.hhs.gov/ohrp/references/nurcode.htm.). This clearly makes it impossible to conduct research with, for example, children and persons who are unable to consent. Since then the realization has grown that, if particular conditions are met, research involving persons who lack the ability to consent can be ethical. In fact the CIOMS guidelines provide that including patients who are unable to consent should be the default and that it is their exclusion which must be justified.

> Adults who are not capable of giving informed consent must be included in health-related research unless a good scientific reason justifies their exclusion. (CIOMS 2016, guideline 16)

Of course, all clinical research ethics guidelines agree that when research is done involving persons who are unable to provide informed consent, particular conditions must be met. **First** of all, research involving persons unable to consent should only be considered if the research cannot be conducted with patients able to provide consent. **Second**, even though patients may be unable to provide informed consent, they should always be informed and *refusal* to participate should always be respected. **Third**, informed consent has to be obtained from a legally recognized representative of the patients. **Fourth**, according to the Declaration of Helsinki, persons unable to provide consent should not be included in research that is unlikely to benefit them, unless "it is intended to promote the health of the group represented by the potential subject" (World Medical Association 2013, section 28). **Fifth**, research involving participants unable to provide informed consent must present no more than minimal risk.

For palliative care research, the fourth condition seems to be particularly relevant. It has been observed that one of the challenges of palliative care research with terminally ill patients is that it is less likely to be directly beneficial to these patients. However, according to the Declaration of Helsinki, this does not automatically invalidate the study but requires the study to be intended to promote the health of palliative care patients. It is clear that in this respect "health" should be interpreted broadly, as in the well-known WHO definition which states that health is: "a state of complete physical, mental and social well-being and not merely the absence of disease or infirmity" (WHO).

Scenario 2: Terminally Ill Patients Who Have Reduced Cognitive Capacities

Although sensitive, this scenario does not seem to pose an insurmountable ethical challenge. Patients are normally believed to be able to provide consent unless there is reason to believe otherwise, and capacity assessment tools exist to determine the presence or absence of capacity (Karlawish 2008). Dying patients should thus be assessed for this purpose. In cases where these patients are found to lack the ability to provide informed consent, scenario 2 effectively collapses into scenario 1 in which case special provisions apply.

Scenario 3: The Situation Changes While the Study Is Ongoing

A less often discussed scenario concerning palliative care research with dying patients is the scenario where a patient has given informed consent beforehand, but *becomes* unable to provide informed consent during the study period. This raises problems because the requirement of informed consent should be seen as more than merely required before the study is initiated. It revolves around respect for the patient as a person and also covers the patient's right to withdraw consent (and thus participation) at any given time. If participants become unable to provide informed consent during the study, they might thereby lose the ability to protect their own interests. How should such participants be protected? Note that for research protocols that require participants' full cognitive capacities throughout the study, this is less of an issue. Participants who are likely to become unable to provide informed consent will then fail to meet the inclusion criteria and hence will be excluded. However, studies that do not require participants' full cognitive capacities throughout the study are faced with an ethical challenge.

A far-reaching protective measure would be to automatically exclude from *any* study patients who are likely less able or unable to provide informed consent during the study. The effect of such an automatic exclusion, however, would be that those in physically poor condition (and therefore more likely to become less able to provide consent) would be systematically excluded from research. This could result in an evidence gap for those patients, which in turn might lead to a higher likelihood of improper palliative or end of life care. Less far-reaching protective measures therefore seem to be preferable.

As mentioned earlier, all international guidelines allow health research to be conducted on participants incapable of providing informed consent, provided that various additional conditions are met. It would thus seem obvious that when participants *become* unable to provide informed consent during the study, the same additional conditions apply. For example, there is widespread agreement that research on participants incapable of consenting can only take place either if an advance directive for participation is available or if the participant's legal representative approves. For participants who *become* incapable of providing consent, continued participation in the study must, in our view, also be justified by an advance directive and/or a proxy consent. For studies including participants who are likely to become less able or unable to provide consent, this scenario needs to be addressed beforehand.

Another crucial requirement for research involving participants unable to provide informed consent is that the research can reasonably be expected to benefit the participant directly or to serve the health needs of the group of which the participant is a member. As argued above, a significant need exists for valuable research on end of life care, and the concept of health is a broad concept, so this condition can arguably be met by palliative care research. However, this should never automatically be assumed.

In short, we would argue that even when participants becoming unable to provide informed consent have provided informed consent beforehand, this does not automatically justify their continued participation in the study. Continued participation must be justified by an advance directive or a proxy consent, and in this context the abovementioned additional ethical requirements apply. For studies involving terminally ill patients who are more likely to become less able or unable to provide informed consent, these situations should be addressed beforehand.

7.1.2 Undue Influence

Another particular concern that is relevant to dying patients is the risk that the presence of a terminal illness might unduly influence them in their decision to participate in palliative care research (Agrawal et al. 2006).

In this regard, we should first and foremost mention the risk of therapeutic misconception (Appelbaum and Roth 1982) which has become a standard concept in research ethics. Therapeutic misconception has been defined in many different ways (Henderson et al. 2007). It can be argued to occur when participants in a study:

> Do not understand that the defining purpose of clinical research is to produce generalizable knowledge, regardless of whether the subjects enrolled in the trial may potentially benefit from the intervention under study or from other aspects of the clinical trial. (Henderson et al. 2007: 1736)

Some studies indicate that dying patients might be willing to undergo significant risks in the expectation of a mere glimmer of therapeutic hope (e.g., Agrawal et al. 2006). In doing so, they might overestimate the benefits of participating in a particular research. If they are willing to try anything, dying patients might find it impossible to refuse an offer to participate in a study. This would invalidate their informed consent.

Although the issue of therapeutic misconception is most pertinent in research pertaining to therapeutic interventions, it is also a source of concern in palliative care research. For informed consent to be valid, it is essential that potential participants have a realistic understanding of the risks and benefits of participation. Therefore, when a study includes dying patients, who are well known for being at risk of therapeutic misconception, particular attention should be paid to this issue. This is true even for palliative care research where no possibility of therapeutic effect is present.

Another matter of concern is the relationship between the dying patients and their treating physician. There is no doubt that terminally ill or dying patients may depend to a considerable extent on their treating physician or health-care institution. If the physician then asks for their participation in a research study, they may well feel unable to refuse. This may be due to gratitude or alternatively to a fear that refusal will negatively affect their relationship with their physician or even the quality of their care. As regards the fear that refusal will adversely affect care, it is an established ethical principle that refusal to participate in a study or a decision to withdraw from a study should never adversely affect the patient-physician relationship. However, this in no way excludes the possibility that dying patients may perceive this to be the case and, as a result, *experience* an inability to refuse, however unfounded this may be. Particular care must therefore be taken in such cases to avoid this perception.

In general, there seems to be a potential risk when dying patients are asked to participate in a research study by the health-care professional responsible for their care. The Helsinki Declaration specifically discusses this issue and recommends the following:

> When seeking informed consent for participation in a research study the physician must be particularly cautious if the potential subject is in a dependent relationship with the physician or may consent under duress. In such situations the informed consent must be sought by an appropriately qualified individual who is completely independent of this relationship. (WMA 2013, paragraph 27)

The CIOMS guideline provides a similar recommendation in the case of a dependent relationship. We would argue that, in cases of palliative or terminally ill patients, there is definitely a relationship of strong dependency. Due to their physical condition the patients may not be easily transferable, and due to their limited life expectancy, there may be no opportunity to establish a relationship with a new physician.

7.2 Relatives or Loved Ones

It is important not to limit issues regarding informed consent in palliative care research to research involving dying patients. Indeed, relatives or loved ones might also be involved in palliative care research, either directly as research participants or as proxy for involvement of a participant who is unable to provide consent.

As with dying patients, relatives or loved ones may be influenced by considerations of gratitude toward physicians involved in treating their relative or loved one. Moreover, the risk of therapeutic misconception may also exist for relatives or loved ones who operate as a proxy for a participant unable to provide consent. They are expected to protect the interests of their relative or loved one, and they are only fully able to do so when they have an adequate and correct understanding of the risks and benefits.

8 Scientific Rigor or Validity

Any research study must be as scientifically rigorous as possible. As was made clear by Emmanuel and colleagues in their classic ethical framework for clinical research, scientific validity is a key ethical requirement. Having patients participate in a study that is not conducted in a way that it can reasonably be expected to generate valid results is simply unethical as it amounts to (potentially) harming patients for no reason.

For palliative care research this might result in somewhat of a catch-22. The "gold standard" of clinical research is still the randomized controlled trial (RCT). However, in some palliative care research, for example, studies involving terminally ill patients, randomization might be particularly challenging (Grande and Todd 2000) or even ethically unjustified (de Raeve 1994). Hence research would only be ethical when maximally scientifically rigorous, but cannot be made maximally scientifically rigorous due to other ethical considerations. By way of example, let us consider the question of whether continuous deep sedation at the end of life (often referred to as palliative sedation) shortens life. The scientifically most valid way of testing this assumption is by performing an RCT with dying patients, half of whom would receive continuous deep sedation and half of whom would not. Obviously this would not be possible for ethical reasons (Beller et al. 2015). The question of whether continuous deep sedation shortens life therefore remains a topic of considerable debate (Sterckx et al. 2013).

Unsurprisingly, in view of the above, research indicates that RCTs are rare in palliative care research and often methodologically flawed. Rinck and colleagues have conducted a systematic review of all RCTs investigating the effectiveness of palliative care services (Rink et al. 1997). They examined 11 trials and found that all had methodological shortcomings. A more recent study from 2008, reviewing 25 Cochrane systematic reviews, found that RCTs in palliative care remain small scale and methodologically problematic (Wee et al. 2008). This conclusion was reaffirmed in a 2017 systematic review (Bouça-Machado et al. 2017). In a framework that judges the gold standard of evidence to be evidence gathered through RCTs, palliative care may be at an inherent disadvantage. This might in turn affect the ethical acceptability of palliative care research.

As a proposed way out of this, catch-22 calls have been made to rethink the framework of evidence for palliative care research (Aoun and Kristjanson 2005) and to move away from RCTs as the only "gold standard." Many commentators indeed emphasize the need to further the evidence base of palliative care using other research methodologies than RCTs, for example, qualitative research, mixed method methodologies, etc. (e.g., Aoun and Nekolaichuk 2014; Visser et al.

2015). Such a shift does not necessarily imply a loss of scientific validity, since, as argued in a highly influential article on trial design, large-scale observational trials can be scientifically equivalent to RCTs (Concato et al. 2000). Numerous other commentators likewise challenge the RCT as being the one and only gold standard (e.g., Grossman and Mackenzie 2005; Bothwell et al. 2016). Of course, RCTs are not necessarily impossible in palliative care research and are often used to good effect. However, if an RCT can only be performed in an ethical way with far-reaching concessions on scientific validity, different research designs need to be considered.

We would submit that it is possible for researchers in palliative care research to fulfill their ethical obligation or scientific validity even where RCTs are not possible. In fact, there is reason to believe that finding valid alternatives for RCTs in palliative care may in some case actually be the ethically correct way of moving forward. Researchers in palliative care research thus have a continuous ethical obligation to critically select the research methodology that best meets both ethical and scientific requirements.

9 Favorable Risk-Benefit Ratio

Another fundamental ethical requirement on which near universal consensus exists is that every study should have a favorable risk-benefit ratio. This is notoriously difficult since, as emphasized in international guidelines and in the academic literature, there is no clear mathematical formula for determining risks and benefits or for determining what constitutes an acceptable or favorable ratio.

In order to determine risk, researchers need to consider (1) the magnitude of possible physical, psychological, social, or other harms and (2) the likelihood of that harm occurring. A low likelihood of substantial harm can in this way be compared to a high risk of minor harm. For palliative care research, especially research involving seriously or terminally ill patients, careful harm assessment needs to be undertaken in advance. What represents minor harm for a healthy participant might be a more substantial harm for a vulnerable patient. Interviews or surveys, for example, might take a limited amount of time, but for patients with a terminal illness, this may represent a serious investment of time they would rather spend otherwise. For relatives, on the other hand, there exists the risk that they become distressed.

As regards the benefits, there are two kinds of benefits to consider. First, the direct benefits for the research participants, and, second, there are potential benefits for the group of which the research participant is a member. Both kinds of benefits can be considered in a risk-benefit analysis. As regards palliative care research with terminally ill patients, it has been suggested that there is little chance of real benefit for the participants themselves as they have a limited life expectancy (De Raeve 1994). Nevertheless, this has been argued to potentially underestimate the variety of potential benefits. A systematic review of research into the attitudes of terminally ill patients and their relatives toward participation in palliative care research suggests that these groups are often interested in participation in research and may even experience some form of benefit (White and Hardy 2010). Participation in palliative care research has, for example, been found to provide some palliative and/or dying patients with an increased sense of meaning because of the opportunity "to give something back." According to other studies, participation in palliative care research "assisted [palliative care patients] in coping in their situation and reduced their feelings of isolation" (White and Hardy 2010).

Finally, there must be an acceptable or favorable balance between the risks and the benefits of a study. What counts as acceptable or favorable is a matter of debate, but seems to depend on two things. First, and most obviously, a risk-benefit ratio is acceptable or favorable when the risks are offset by the study's benefits. The higher the risk (more likely or more substantial harm), the higher the potential benefits should be in order for the study to be justified.

A related and equally important condition is not only that the risks and benefits should weigh up but also that they should be divided fairly. If a particular group bears all the risks while another group enjoys the potential benefits, this is arguably unfair and even exploitative (for a good and extensive overview of exploitation in clinical research, see Wertheimer 2008). It is thus not sufficient for researchers in palliative care to list the potential risks and benefits; they should also reflect on the allocation of those risks.

10 Fair Participant Selection and Gatekeeping

A final important requirement for a research study to be ethical is that participants be selected fairly. This involves the formulation of clear and justified inclusion and exclusion criteria. The inclusion of a certain participant population must not be based on mere convenience, but must be both ethically and scientifically justified. Care must also be taken that no individuals or groups are unjustifiably excluded from research.

For palliative care research, a particular challenge arises concerning fair participant selection. A well-known issue in research is gatekeeping, which has been defined as "the ad hoc denial of access to individual patients or systematic denial for particular groups of patients for reasons outside the framework of the trial eligibility criteria" (Sharkey et al. 2010: 363). Such gatekeeping has repeatedly been reported in palliative care research contexts (Hudson et al. 2005; Kars et al. 2016). The reasons for gatekeeping are often paternalistic concerns for the well-being of the research participant (White et al. 2008). Although no doubt often well-intended, the result of such gatekeeping is that recruitment in palliative care research becomes ad hoc and dependent on the willingness of physicians to recruit patients or relatives. This might not only threaten the scientific validity of a study; it might also be ethically unfair if potential participants are not even given the opportunity to consider participation in a research study. It has been reported that for palliative care trials a high percentage of patients are willing to participate (Ling et al. 2000), strengthening the argument that paternalistic gatekeeping might be unjustified.

Therefore, care must be taken to minimize gatekeeping. Strategies that have been suggested include anticipating possible misconceptions, continuously checking the inclusion for potential biases, and involving clinicians. Of course, there may still be ethical grounds for excluding particular vulnerable individuals, but that exclusion should be based on clear and study-wide criteria rather than on ad hoc grounds for exclusion.

11 Respect for Potential and Enrolled Subjects

Although respect for enrolled subjects is no doubt essential, it might be somewhat unclear how this requirement should be translated into the practice of doing research. What does it mean to show respect for potential and enrolled subjects?

In philosophy, perhaps one of the most famous elaborations of the concept of respect for persons is that of Immanuel Kant (2012 (1785)). The precise interpretation of Kant's idea of "respect" is a matter of extensive philosophical debate. However, key to the Kantian interpretation is that persons, by virtue of being rational human beings, should never be treated solely as a means, but always also as an end in themselves. One fails to respect human beings when one treats them as mere passive instruments, means, or objects in the achievement of a certain goal, however good that goal might be. This is particularly relevant for a research context, since in research involving human participants, human beings *are* used as a means to gather data and/or generate knowledge.

However, although human beings are used as a means in this context, investigators can still make sure they are shown respect and are not *solely* or *merely* used as a means. For example, when persons freely and autonomously consent to participation, they can be said to subscribe to the goal of the research study, thereby making it their own. In this scenario the participant is not a passive object, but an active participant. In essence, the principle of respect revolves around the researchers' attitudes and the acknowledgment that every single participant in a research study is a human being with dignity, dreams, desires, beliefs, and interests that need to be protected. As the Declaration of Helsinki states:

> While the primary purpose of medical research is to generate new knowledge, this goal can never take precedence over the rights and interests of individual research subjects. (WMA 2013)

Fulfilling the requirements of clinical research is in the *interest of the participants* and should not be seen as a mere safety measure for the (legal) protection of researchers.

Although the requirement of respect for research participants is not limited to palliative care research, it is too important to leave out. When applied to palliative care research, it requires researchers to be aware of and concerned for the situations that are specific to the participants in their study. In research including terminally ill patients and/or their loved ones, care must be taken to always take a respectful attitude toward these participants and to do this *throughout* the entire research study. The requirement to show respect does not stop when, for example, the informed consent form is signed nor when the active involvement of the participant is finished. Data gathered from patients should equally be treated with sufficient respect when stored, analyzed, and put into publishable form. Participants have a continued interest in what happens to their data, and this interest may even continue to apply when they pass away (a situation that is more likely to occur in palliative care research involving seriously ill patients). No matter how scientifically relevant or valuable one might deem the research to be, the dignity, integrity, and general interests of participants should always come first.

12 Concluding Remarks

In this chapter we have sought to provide an overview of some of the relevant ethical issues pertaining to palliative care research. In general it is hard to make broad and general statements on this topic, for palliative care research can involve a great variety of research methodologies and a wide diversity of participant populations.

What is clear, however, is that palliative care research can be ethically justified, and we arguably even have a moral obligation to engage and invest in palliative care research in order to create a much more solid evidence base. It is also clear that particular ethical requirements give rise to particular challenges in the field of palliative care research. For example, for research involving terminally ill patients, scientific validity and informed consent may be particularly problematic. However, none of these challenges are impossible to overcome.

References

Abernethy AP, Capell WH, Aziz NM, Ritchie C, Prince-Paul M, Bennet RE, et al. Ethical conduct of palliative care research: enhancing communication between investigators and institutional review boards. J Pain Symptom Manag. 2014;48(6):1211–21.

Agrawal M, Grady C, Fairclough DL, Meropol NJ, Maynard K, Emanuel EJ. Patients' decision-making process regarding participation in phase I oncology research. J Clin Oncol. 2006;24(27):4479–84.

Aoun SM, Kristjanson LJ. Challenging the framework for evidence in palliative care research. Palliat Med. 2005;19(6):461–5.

Aoun SM, Nekolaichuk C. Improving the evidence base in palliative care to inform practice and policy: thinking outside the box. J Pain Symptom Manag. 2014;48(6):1222–35.

Appelbaum PS, Roth LH. The therapeutic misconception: informed consent in psychiatric research. Int J Law Psychiatry. 1982;5:319–29.

Beller EM, van Driel ML, McGregor L, Truong S, Mitchell G. Palliative pharmacological sedation for terminally ill adults (Review). Cochrane Database Syst Rev. 2015;1:1–40.

Bernabe RDLC, van Thiel GJMW, van Delden JJM. What do international ethics guidelines say in terms of the scope of medical research ethics? BMC Med Ethics. 2016;17(23):1–18.

Bothwell LE, Greene JA, Podolsky SH, Jones DS. Assessing the gold standard – lessons from the history of RCTs. N Engl J Med. 2016;374(22):2175–81.

Bouça-Machado R, Rosário M, Alarcão J, Correia-Guedes L, Abreu D, Ferreira JJ. Clinical trials in palliative care: a systematic review of their methodological characteristics and of the quality of their reporting. BMC Palliat Care. 2017;16(10):1–12.

Bracken-Roche D, Bell E, Macdonald ME, Racine E. The concept of "vulnerability" in research ethics: an in-depth analysis of policies and guidelines. Health Res Policy Syst. 2017;15(8):1–18.

Casarett DJ, Karlawish JHT. Are special ethical guidelines needed for palliative care research? J Pain Symptom Manag. 2000;20(2):130–9.

Concato J, Shah N, Horwitz RI. Randomized, controlled trials, observational studies, and the hierarchy of research designs. N Engl J Med. 2000;342(25): 1887–92.

Council for International Organizations of Medical Sciences (CIOMS). International ethical guidelines for health-related research involving humans. 4th ed. Geneva; 2016. Available at https://cioms.ch/wp-content/uploads/2017/01/WEB-CIOMS-EthicalGuidelines.pdf.

de Raeve L. Ethical issues in palliative care research. Palliat Med. 1994;8(4):298–305.

Emanuel EJ, Wendler D, Grady C. What makes clinical research ethical? J Am Med Assoc. 2000;283(20): 2701–11.

Grady C. Payment of clinical research subjects. The Journal of Clinical Investigation. 2005;115(7):1681–7.

Grande GE, Todd CJ. Why are trials in palliative care so difficult? Palliat Med. 2000;14:69–74.

Grossman J, Mackenzie FJ. The randomized controlled trial: gold standard, or merely standard? Perspect Biol Med. 2005;48(4):516–34.

Henderson GE, Churchill LR, Davis AM, Easter MM, Grady C, Joffe S, et al. Clinical trials and medical care: defining the therapeutic misconception. PLoS Med. 2007;4(11):1735–8.

Hickman SE, Cartwright JC, Nelson CA, Knafl K. Compassion and vigilance: investigators' strategies to manage ethical concerns in palliative and end-of-life research. J Palliat Med. 2012;15(8):880–9.

Higginson IJ. Evidence based palliative care: there is some evidence – and there needs to be more. Br Med J. 1999;319:462–3.

Higginson IJ. Research challenges in palliative and end of life care. BMJ Support Palliat Care. 2016;6(1):2–4.

Hudson P, Aranda S, Kristjanson LJ, Quinn K. Minimising gate-keeping in palliative care research. Eur J Palliat Care. 2005;12(4):165–9.

Kant I. Groundwork of the metaphysics of morals. Cambridge: Cambridge University Press; 2012 (1785).

Karlawish JHT. Measuring decision-making capacity in cognitively impaired individuals. Neurosignals. 2008; 16(1):91–8.

Kars MC, van Thiel GJMW, van der Graaf R, Moors M, de Graeff A, van Delden JJM. A systematic review of reasons for gatekeeping in palliative care research. Palliat Med. 2016;30(6):533–48.

Kelley AS, McGarry K, Fahle S, Marshall SM, Du Q, Skinner JS. Out-of-Pocket Spending in the Last Five Years of Life. National Bureau of Economic Research Bulletin on Aging and Health. 2010;2:3–4.

Lee S, Kristjanson LJ. Human research ethics committees: issues in palliative care research. Int J Palliat Nurs. 2003;9(1):13–8.

Levine C, Faden RR, Grady C, Hammerschmidt D, Eckenwiler L, Sugarman J. The limitations of "Vulnerability" as a protection for human research participants. Am J Bioeth. 2004;4(3):44–9.

Ling J, Rees E, Hardy J. What influences participation in clinical trials in palliative care in a cancer centre? Eur J Cancer. 2000;36:621–6.

Macklin R. On paying money to research subjects: "due" and "undue" inducements. IRB. 1981;3(5):1–6.

Miller FG, Joffe S. Benefit in phase 1 oncology trials: therapeutic misconception or reasonable treatment option? Clinical Trials: Journal of the Society for Clinical Trials. 2008;5(6):617–23.

Nickel PJ. Vulnerable populations in research: the case of the seriously ill. Theor Med Bioeth. 2006;27(3): 245–64.

Nueberger J, Guthrie C, Aaronovitch D, Hameed K, Bonser T, Pentregarth H, et al. More care, less pathway: a review of the liverpool care pathway. 2013. https://www.gov.uk/government/uploads/system/uploads/attachment_data/file/212450/Liverpool_Care_Pathway.pdf.

Rink GC, van den Bos GA, Kleijnen J, de Haes HJ, Schadé E, Veenhof CH. Methodologic issues in effectiveness research on palliative cancer care: a systematic review. J Clin Oncol. 1997;15(4):1697–707.

Rothman DJ. Ethics and human experimentation. N Engl J Med. 1987;317:1195–9.

Sackett DL. Evidence based medicine. Semin Perinatol. 1997;21(1):3–5.

Sharkey K, Savulescu J, Aranda S, Schofield P. Clinician gate-keeping in clinical research is not ethically defensible: an analysis. J Med Ethics. 2010; 36:363–6.

Sterckx S, Raus K, Mortier F. Continuous sedation at the end of life: ethical, clinical and legal perspectives. Cambridge: Cambridge University Press; 2013. (Bioethics and Law).

Tieman J, Sladek R, Currow D. Changes in the quantity and level of evidence of palliative and hospice care literature: the last century. J Clin Oncol. 2008;26(35): 5679–83.

Visser C, Hadley G, Wee B. Reality of evidence-based practice in palliative care. Cancer Biol Med. 2015;12(3):193–200.

Vollman J, Winau R. Informed consent in human experimentation before the Nuremberg code. Br Med J. 1996;313:1445–7.

Wee B, Hadley G, Derry S. How useful are systematic reviews for informing palliative care practice? Survey of 25 Cochrane systematic reviews. BMC Palliat Care. 2008;7:13.

Wendler D. A pragmatic analysis of vulnerability. Bioethics. 2017;31(7):515–25.

Wertheimer A. Exploitation in Clinical Research. In: Emanuel EJ, editor. The Oxford Textbook of Clinical Research Ethics. Oxford: Oxford University Press; 2008. p. 201–10.

Westfall JM, Mold J, Fagnan L. Practice-based research – "Blue Highways" on the NIH roadmap. J Am Med Assoc. 2007;297(4):403–6.

White C, Hardy J. What do palliative care patients and their relatives think about research in palliative care? – A systematic review. Support Care Cancer. 2010;18:905–11.

White C, Gilshenan K, Hardy J. A survey of the views of palliative care healthcare professionals towards referring cancer patients to participate in randomized controlled trials in palliative care. Support Care Cancer. 2008;16:1397–405.

Williams EP, Walter JK. When Does the Amount We Pay Research Participants Become "Undue Influence"? J Am Med Assoc. 2015;17(12):1116–21.

Woolf SH. The meaning of translational research and why it matters. J Am Med Assoc. 2008;299(2):211–3.

World Medical Association. World medical association declaration of Helsinki: ethical principles for medical research involving human subjects. J Am Med Assoc. 2013;310(20):2191–4.

Evidence-Based Practice in Palliative Care

95

Lieve Van den Block and Jan Vandevoorde

Contents

Abstract

Many of the chapters in this Textbook provide state of the art, that is, evidence-based recommendations for the practice of palliative care and palliative medicine. This chapter on "Evidence-based practice in palliative care" will focus on the principles, advantages, and limitations of evidence-based medicine (EBM) and evidence-based practice (EBP) in general and specifically within the field of palliative care. We will discuss the concepts of EBM/EBP from a historical perspective, their role within the field of palliative care, the way EBM/EBP is practiced by a clinician in a stepwise approach, and critically reflect on how these concepts have developed over the past decade. The development of EBM/EPB has had an enormous impact on the way medicine is practiced today. It should not however be considered cookbook medicine. Its future lies

L. Van den Block (✉)
VUB-UGhent End-of-Life Care Research Group, Department of Family Medicine and Chronic Care and Department of Clinical Sciences, Vrije Universiteit Brussel (VUB), Brussels, Belgium
e-mail: lvdblock@vub.be

J. Vandevoorde
Department of Family Medicine and Chronic Care, Vrije Universiteit Brussel (VUB), Brussels, Belgium
e-mail: Jan.Vandevoorde@vub.be

R. D. MacLeod, L. Van den Block (eds.), *Textbook of Palliative Care*,
https://doi.org/10.1007/978-3-319-77740-5_111

in generating useable evidence that can be combined with context, professional expertise, and patient preferences to provide optimal treatment and care to individual patients.

1 What Is Evidence-Based Medicine (EBM) and Evidence-Based Practice (EBP)?

For over a century (between the eighteenth and nineteenth century), physicians have debated the role of statistics, mathematics, and probabilistic knowledge in the practice of medicine, particularly in Europe and the USA. Only by the start of the twentieth century, medicine had moved from the empirical observation of cases to the scientific application of basic sciences to determine best therapies or diagnoses (Mayer 2010). After 1950, the randomized clinical trial became the standard for excellent research, following the work of British men such as Sir Ronald Fisher, Austin Bradford Hill, and particularly Archie Cochrane. The latter was the first to publish a quality-rated systematic review of the literature on a particular topic in medicine (Mayer 2010). This was the beginning of a true paradigm shift in thinking and reasoning in medicine. The Cochrane Collaboration Network, founded in 1993, grew out of this work.

In 1996, Sackett published his ground-breaking publication in the *British Medical Journal*, defining **evidence-based medicine (EBM)** as "the conscientious, explicit, and judicious use of the best evidence in making decisions about the care of individual patients" (Sackett et al. 1996). More simply stated, EBM concerned the application of the best possible evidence from medical literature to the individual patient's problem, resulting in the best possible care for each patient (Mayer 2010). The movement of EBM that grew out of this work has led to a profound innovation in medical teaching and medical research. It resulted in the development of professional guidelines and standards of care to support professionals in making decisions in individual patient care (Dutch Council for Public Health and Society 2017).

Evidence-based practice (EPB) – sometimes referred to as evidence-based clinical practice (EBCP) – is a term that was introduced later. While both terms EPB and EBM considerably overlap, the term "EBP" is considered "broader" than EBM, and it implies the use of evidence-based knowledge by multiple professional disciplines in health care. Historically, EBM primarily involved physicians and concentrated on the treatment aspect of medicine. EBP is considered to be more multidisciplinary, targeting nurses, clinicians, nurse practitioners, physical and occupational therapists, hospital administrations, etc. (Adriaenssens et al. 2018). For reasons of readability and because of the broader concept of EBP, we will use this term throughout the chapter.

Initially, EBP focused primarily on the use of evidence in clinical decision-making, while at the same time de-emphasizing other important determinants of clinical decisions such as the individual clinical experiences. In later definitions, it was emphasized more that research evidence alone is not sufficient to guide clinical decisions. Clinicians should apply their expertise to assess the patient's problem and incorporate the evidence together with patient preferences and values. Evidence-based decision-making was then defined as the integration of best research evidence with clinical expertise and patient values. This model is depicted in Fig. 1.

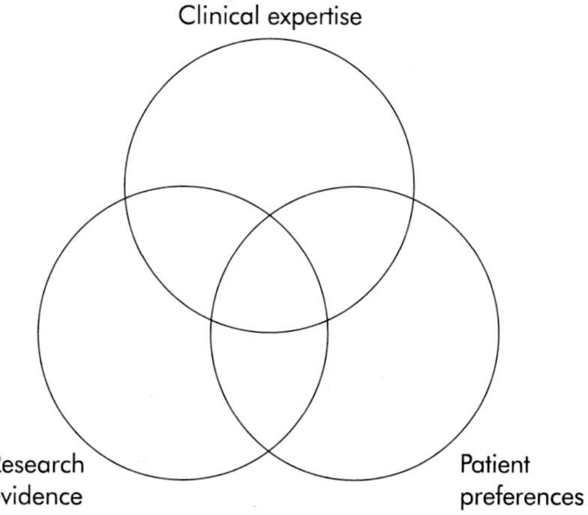

Fig. 1 Early model of the key elements for evidence-based clinical decisions. (Reproduced from Haynes et al. 2002, with permission from BMJ Publishing Group Ltd)

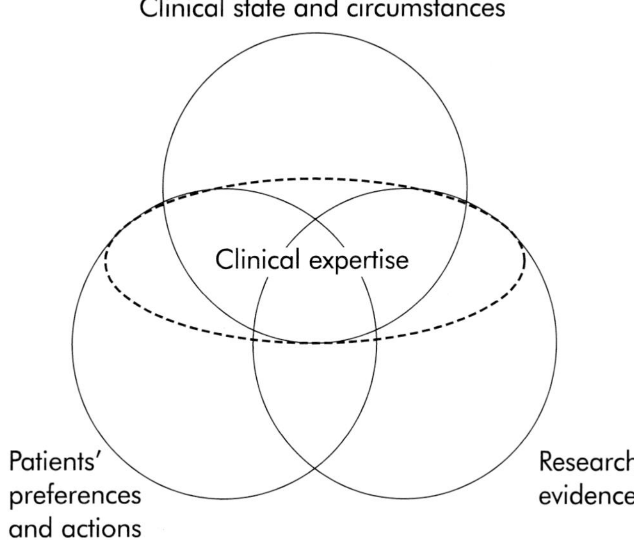

Fig. 2 An updated model for evidence-based clinical decisions. (Reproduced from Haynes et al. 2002, with permission from BMJ Publishing Group Ltd)

In a more advanced and recent model, as shown in Fig. 2, **evidence-based health care combines the best available evidence, clinical situation of the patient, patient preferences and actions, all bound together by clinical experience** (Mayer 2010; Adriaenssens et al. 2018; Haynes et al. 2002). At the top of Fig. 2 are the patient's clinical state, the clinical setting, and clinical circumstances she/he is in, which are dominant factors in clinical decisions. Regarding preferences, patients might have varying views on treatment options (or they might have no clear preference) depending on several factors such as previous experiences, personal values or traits, or the values of their families. Such preferences should be explored and taken into account. In particular for end-of-life and palliative care, with its important focus on patient values and preferences in decision-making, this component in the updated EPB model is highly relevant. The factor "patient actions" was mainly added due to the inconsistencies that might occur between patient preferences or physician's advice and actual patient behavior, for example, patients who prefer to stop smoking but still smoke. A third obvious factor is the research evidence available, which includes all sorts of observational and interventional studies in basic and applied health research. However, a lot of research evidence will not easily or automatically apply to the individual patient at hand. Hence, personalizing the evidence to fit a patient's specific circumstances is a key part of evidence-based decision-making. Finally, the role of clinical expertise is very central and important in evidence-based decision-making. This includes the general basic skills of clinical practice as well as the experience of the individual practitioner. It is the clinical expertise that integrates and balances the other elements in the model and often involves sorting through trade-offs (Haynes et al. 2002).

The EBP community has grown rapidly over the past 20 years to become an "energetic intellectual community committed to making clinical practice more scientific and empirically grounded and thereby achieving safer, more consistent, and more cost-effective care" (cited from Pope 2003; in Greenhalgh et al. 2014). The EBP community has achieved to set up the Cochrane Collaboration to summarize evidence from clinical trials; it has set methodological and publication standards for research, built national and international infrastructures for developing and updating clinical practice guidelines, and developed resources and courses for teaching critical appraisal and building the knowledge base for implementation and knowledge translation (Greenhalgh et al. 2014). Regarding the latter, a whole body of literature has developed regarding EBP development, dissemination, and implementation. It addresses the importance of three distinct stages as part of the evidence-based process: knowledge creation and distillation; diffusion and dissemination; and adoption, implementation, and institutionalization (Nieva et al. 2005; Adriaenssens et al. 2018). Additionally, EPB has also gained a lot of attention within health-care policy work. EBP can provide important means to improve efficacy, efficiency, and quality of care, and sometimes it might help in keeping health-care expenses under control (Adriaenssens et al. 2018). Developing methods to produce evidence-based policies in health care has become an important research field of its own.

Although these developments are highly relevant in the field of EBP, this chapter will focus mainly on the viewpoint of the individual clinician and how he/she uses EBP in real practice. We will first highlight the need for more evidence in palliative care and on how EBP can/should be practiced or what skills are needed by clinicians to perform EBP adequately. Because the model of EPB outlined here is not without critics, we will also discuss these further on in the chapter.

2 Evidence-Based Practice in Palliative Care: The Need for High-Quality Evidence

EBP has grown rapidly over the past 20 years across the field of medicine and has resulted in much improvement in clinical practice for patients. Every year, an enormous amount of trials and reviews are produced in the medical research community (Visser et al. 2015). It has been argued that palliative care has been lagging behind compared to other medical disciplines and that the evidence-base is still too limited in terms of high-quality trials to ensure high-quality practice (Aoun and Nekolaichuk 2014; Higginson et al. 2013; Dy et al. 2012).

The number of researchers in the field of palliative care has grown substantially over the past decades. Multiple disciplines – medicine, public health, social health, sociology, psychology, anthropology, etc. – are studying this highly complex and multidisciplinary field using different methodological approaches. The number of clinical trials in palliative care has also grown accordingly. For example, a 2017 Cochrane review on the effects of early palliative care in cancer patients summarized the work of 7 published trials, but also reported 20 additional trials that are currently ongoing (Haun et al. 2017). A systematic review of published clinical trials assessing therapeutic interventions in palliative care (up to 2015) retrieved 107 trials in Medline (Bauça-Machado et al. 2017).

However, a number of reviews (Bauça-Machado et al. 2017; Dy et al. 2012; Hui et al. 2012; Kaasa and Radbruch 2008; Visser et al. 2015, Wee et al. 2008b) evaluating the strength of the evidence in palliative care have highlighted some important problems with current evidence:

- RCTs are proportionately limited in number, for example, while the proportion of original studies have increased between 2004 and 2009, the proportion of interventions studies remained stable over time (Hui et al. 2012).
- Many clinical trials are methodologically flawed. Existing study designs show important quality deficiencies including poor recruitment, high attrition, small sample sizes leading to a lack of study power, and lack of thoroughly executed pilot studies to carefully select outcome measures or understand possible biases or confounders, the absence of an explicit defined primary outcome, etc. (Aoun and Nekolaichuk 2014; Dy et al. 2012; Luckett et al. 2014; Smith et al. 2014).
- Even trials that are judged to be of high quality are often underpowered (Wee et al. 2008b).
- The overall quality of the reporting of key trial methodology is too poor (e.g., lack of reporting of random sequence generation, allocation concealment, blinding (Bauça-Machado et al. 2017, Hui et al. 2012)).
- Due to a lack of well-designed and well-executed studies, reviews "fail to provide good evidence to guide clinical practice because the primary studies are few in number, small, clinically heterogeneous, and of poor quality and validity" (cited from Wee et al. 2008b).

Hence, effectiveness research in palliative care has been described as lacking the quality to contribute to evidence-based medicine or to inform practice and policy-making well enough. This lack of high-quality research and evidence is considered to be a major barrier to improving quality of care provided in the final phases of life (Higginson et al. 2013).

Recently, important work was done to improve the design and conduct of intervention research in palliative care, which resulted in the MORECare statements for palliative care research (Higginson et al. 2013). It starts from the idea that all palliative care interventions are inherently complex interventions. The development and evaluation of such interventions can follow the UK Medical Research Council's guidance on developing and evaluating complex interventions, but because of the complexities and specificities in palliative and end of life care research, the MORECare work leads researchers through all phases of intervention development and provides advises on how to optimize research methods. In this Textbook, a whole chapter ("Development and Evaluation of Complex Interventions in Palliative Care") is devoted to this important work and the reader is referred to that chapter for further information.

With these efforts, researchers in palliative care have attempted to increase the quality of their research with the aim of providing better evidence to improve EBP decision-making. Nevertheless, a number of authors have also argued that some of the fundamental assumptions underlying EBP are incompatible with palliative care, and the methodologies used in randomized controlled trials are often not feasible in the palliative care context. A review outlining the challenges of conducting high-quality research in palliative care and the limitations attached to the traditional EBP approach in the field of palliative care was published in 2015 by Visser et al. We will address these criticisms more in detail at the end of this chapter, after describing in detail how EBP should be practiced.

3 How to Practice Evidence-Based Practice: A Stepwise Approach

Three skills are identified as important for practitioners practicing evidence-based medicine: (1) information mastery, (2) critical appraisal, and (3) knowledge translation (Mayer 2010). These skills are used throughout the different steps involved in the process of EBP. While different authors have identified slightly different versions of this stepwise approach, they all involve the same processes. From a learner's perspective, it would be best to start learning EBP by learning and practicing the different steps, taking a specific patient scenario as a starting point. For details, we refer the reader to other Textbooks on EBM and EBP, of which there have been written many, for many different disciplines and professions. Here, we will summarize the different steps involved in the complete process of EBP.

3.1 Step 1: From Clinical Problem to Clinical Question

A first step is the translation of a clinical problem of a patient to an adequately formulated clinical question. Clinical questions are usually formulated in the form of a PICO, that is, what is the problem of the patient (P), what is the intervention of interest (I), what is the control-intervention (C) that is used for comparison, and what is the outcome of interest (O)? This is a very important step since the answer to your clinical question will co-determine how you deal with the patient's problem.

In Table 1, a PICO is defined using an example. The clinical question could be for example: "Is medically assisted hydration more effective than no medically assisted hydration for maintaining quality of life in a patient who is considered in the last days of life and unable to maintain sufficient oral fluid intake?" In some cases, time is also added to PICO. This relates to the period over which the intervention is studied (i.e., whether the study was carried out for a sufficient amount of time).

3.2 Step 2: Searching for Evidence

There is an enormous amount of literature to be found in medicine. There are several types of research studies (e.g., case-control, cross-sectional, cohort, randomized controlled trials), many different peer-reviewed and non-peer-

Table 1 PICO is used to identify the clinical question (Mayer 2010)

Structure of the clinical question (PICO)	Explanation	Example from palliative care
The Patient	Population group to which your patient belongs	Adults who are considered to be in the last days of life and are unable to maintain sufficient oral fluid intake
The Intervention	The therapy, etiology, or diagnostic test you are interested in applying to your patient	Effect of medically assisted hydration
The Comparison	A comparison group (that is commonly encountered in clinical practice) to against which the intervention is measured	Compared to no medically assisted hydration
The Outcome of interest	The endpoint of interest to you or your patient. The most important outcomes are those that matter to the patient, often death, disability or full recovery	Quality of life

reviewed journals, focused on specific disciplines or a more general medicine audience. In step 2, the clinician needs to have good searching skills and use medical informatics, to search the literature for those studies that are most likely to give the best evidence to answer the identified question. This requires that one develops an effective, hence systematic search strategy for a clinical question. To ensure that all relevant information can be retrieved when searching the literature, it will be important to access several databases. One of the most widely known database is Medline. Medline was developed by the National Library of Medicine at the National Institutes of Health in the USA, and it is the world's largest general biomedical database. In psychological science, other databases are more relevant such as PsycINFO, or in the field of nursing and allied health studies, CINAHL. It is beyond the scope of this chapter to provide the reader with a full overview of databases available or specific instructions on how search strategies can be made in the different databases.

In this chapter, we will focus on the different sources available to clinicians when seeking the answer to a clinical question for a particular patient. When a clinician is looking for an answer to his question at the point of care, when the patient is "in his office," she/he will not perform comprehensive Medline searches, but instead will look for pre-appraised sources and high-quality meta-analyses such as those published by the Cochrane Collaboration, or search for clinical guidelines or decision supports available on the topic.

3.2.1 Knowledge Acquisition Pyramid

To help clinicians search for evidence among the large amount of publications and tools available to them, the Haynes **knowledge acquisition pyramid** (Haynes 2006, in Mayer 2010) was developed, sometimes also referred to as the "**waterfall or cascade" approach.** Following this approach would mean that clinicians should search the literature in a number of consecutive steps, as shown in Fig. 3.

Clinicians start by looking at the highest level of systems, standards, and guidelines to help with decision-making. Computerized decision support systems are newly developing approaches to providing clinicians with online support at the point of care via linking with patient file data. The IT system links directly to high-quality information needed "on the spot." There are a few of these systems being developed to support the implementation of guidelines; some are local or national linked to specific institutions (further details are provided later in this chapter). Second, clinicians should search for summaries and synopses which provide critical overviews of reviews and studies. These can be evidence-based textbooks or critical overviews of reviews and studies such as *BMJ* best practice or ACP Journal Club

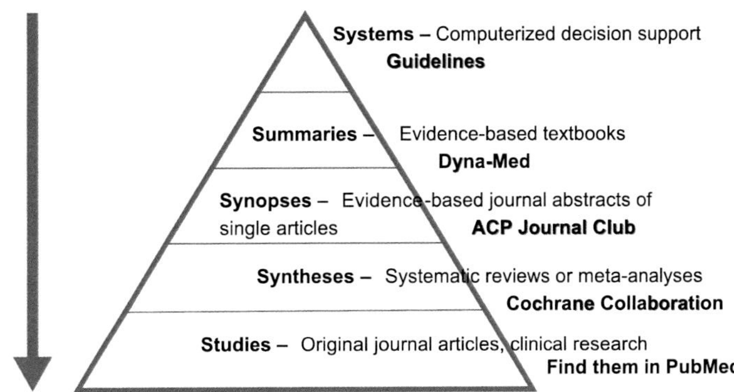

Fig. 3 The knowledge acquisition pyramid of Haynes. (Reproduced from Mayer 2010, by permission of Oxford University Press)

(these sources can also have different names in different countries). A third source of evidence concerns the systematic reviews and meta-analyses of which Cochrane reviews is one of the most important. Lastly, when all other sources do not provide clinical guidance, clinicians are bound to evaluate primary sources of evidence and look for original studies in different databases such as Medline or Cinahl.

Clinicians go "down the pyramid" and stop when they have (or estimate that they have) sufficient high-quality information to answer their clinical question. For all these steps, it will be crucial to also understand the quality of the evidence or the strength of recommendations that are made by these different sources. Hence, step 3 of EBP is a crucial element of decision-making.

3.3 Step 3: Critical Appraisal of Available Evidence

Once the evidence has been found, a third step in EBP is to perform a critical appraisal of the evidence found. When appraising individual studies, clinicians should search in this step for sources of bias within those studies. More specifically, they should systematically evaluate whether a study addresses a clearly focused question, whether valid methods were used to address that question, and whether the valid results of the study are important. When appraising clinical practice guidelines or other aggregate sources of evidence, they should evaluate the development process of these sources, and several important tools have been developed to help clinicians in this task. This section addresses the most important elements to consider when appraising the available evidence for the different types of sources identified in the knowledge acquisition pyramid, starting with individual studies up to guidelines and decision-support systems.

3.3.1 The Appraisal Pyramid: From Animal Research to Meta-analyses

Clinicians usually are taught to appraise literature following an **appraisal pyramid**. Such pyramids exist in multiple formats with slightly different terminologies used. Important is the distinction between literature that is already critically and systematically appraised by others and individual studies of various designs. An example of such a pyramid can be found in Fig. 4. The higher on the appraisal pyramid, the easier the source is to use, and the least amount of critical appraisal is needed by the user, of course considering the quality of the methods used in the different studies or analyses.

In recent literature, there have been some alternative proposals for this evidence pyramid. Murrad et al. (2016) have proposed to chop off the meta-analyses and systematic reviews from the pyramid top. Instead, reviews should be a lens through which evidence is viewed and applied. Also, in their new pyramid, the lines separating the study designs have become wavy instead of fixed, referring to the fact that studies might differ substantially in the quality with which they are performed. The wave going up and down reflects the GRADE approach of rating up and down based on the various domains of the

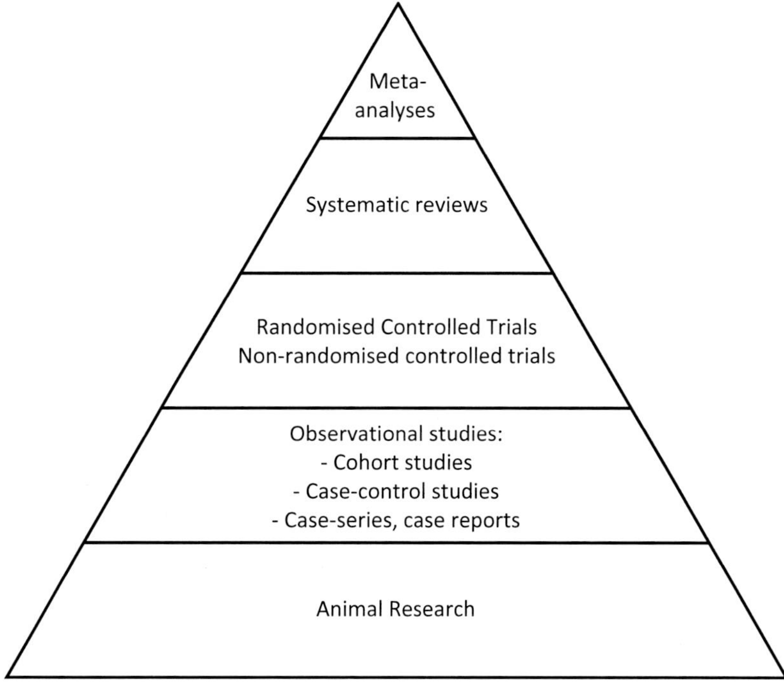

Fig. 4 The pyramid of appraisal of the literature (Mayer 2010)

quality of evidence (see further). The quality of studies, and not only the study design, determines how high or low they should be rated. For example, even though RCTs are considered high on the pyramid, there are also several biases that might lead an RCT to have a lower quality of evidence, and this should be taken into account by clinicians when evaluating the literature (Murrad et al. 2016).

In the following section of this chapter, we have highlighted what is most important for clinicians when appraising the literature and information available to them. First, meta-analyses and reviews are discussed. Secondly, the most important issues related to individual studies (RCT and other) are addressed. Finally, the strengths and weaknesses of summaries and guidelines available to clinicians are described.

3.3.2 Meta-analyses and Systematic Reviews

Meta-analyses or systematic reviews are techniques that aim to provide a comprehensive and objective analysis of all clinical studies on a specific topic. In many cases, statistical techniques are applied to quantify the combined effect of selected studies (Mayer 2010). (An important organization occupied with producing meta-analyses on a variety of topics in health care is the Cochrane Collaboration http://www.cochrane.org/). Cochrane is an international nonprofit organization that aims to "gather and summarize the best evidence from research to help you make informed choices about treatment." It is a global independent network of researchers, professionals, patients, carers, and people interested in health. Worldwide, there are more than 37,000 Cochrane contributors from 130 countries. It is organized via different Cochrane groups such as review groups, thematic networks, groups concerned with methodology of systematic reviews, and regional centers (with a regional focus for Cochrane activities within a defined geographical or linguistic area).

The Cochrane Library (http://www.cochranelibrary.com/) is a collection of databases that contain different types of high-quality, independent evidence:

- Cochrane database of systematic reviews (CDSR): preparing peer-reviewed systematic reviews following the *Cochrane Handbook*

for Systematic Reviews of Interventions and the *Cochrane Handbook for Diagnostic Test Accuracy Reviews* (Higgins and Green 2011)
- The Cochrane Central Register of Controlled Trials (CENTRAL), a highly concentrated source of reports (usually the abstract with bibliographical details) of randomized and quasi-randomized controlled trials
- Cochrane Clinical Answers (CCA) providing a digestible clinically focused entry point to rigorous research from Cochrane Systematic Reviews, aiming to inform point-of-care decision-making

In the field of palliative care, the work of the PaPaS Cochrane Pain, Palliative Care and Supportive Care Collaborative Review Group is an important resource (http://papas.cochrane.org/). PaPaS is based in Oxford, UK, founded in 1998, and funded by the National Institute of Health Research (NIHR) as part of the Research and Development program. They are one of the Cochrane review groups that specialize in different areas of health based in different countries around the world. Their scope is defined as studies of interventions for:

- Acute pain arising accidentally or through deliberate injury
- Chronic pain (lasting 3 months or longer)
- Headache and migraine
- Palliative care for those with life-limiting disease or illness
- Supportive care of patients and significant others living with serious illness, defined as "the multi-disciplinary holistic care of patients with malignant and non-malignant chronic diseases and serious illness, and those that matter to them, to ensure the best possible quality of life. It extends as a right and necessity for all patients, is available throughout the course of the condition, concurrent to condition management and is given equal priority alongside diagnosis and treatment. It should be individualised, taking into account the patient's past life experiences, their current situation and personal goals" (Cramp and Bennett 2012).

Cochrane reviews are performed following a very strict methodology described in the *Cochrane Handbook for Systematic Reviews of Interventions* (Higgins and Green 2011). While Cochrane Reviews are considered of very high quality, not all systematic reviews follow the methodologies used by Cochrane. The quality of reviews might vary considerably; hence, it is important for clinicians to critically appraise them. To help with this process, checklists have been developed to assess the methodological quality of systematic reviews. Next to Cochrane (Higgins and Green 2011), there are several organizations who have produced such checklists among others the AMSTAR checklist (Shea et al. 2017), the CASP Systematic review checklist developed by the Critical Appraisal Skills Programme (https://casp-uk.net/), the Centre for Evidence-Based Medicine in Oxford (UK) (https://www.cebm.net/2014/06/critical-appraisal/), the Joanna Briggs Institute (http://joannabriggs.org/research/critical-appraisal-tools.html), and the toolkits provided by BMJ Best Practice, to name a few. Finally, important aspects for a clinician to take into account when appraising a review are the seven domains identified by Shea et al. (2017) that can critically affect the validity of a review and its conclusions: (1) Is the protocol registered before commencement of the review? (2) Is the literature search performed adequately? (3) Is the exclusion of individual studies justified well? (4) Does the review include an evaluation of risk of bias from individual studies; (5) Are the meta-analytical methods appropriate? (6) Is the risk of bias when interpreting the results of the review considered? and (7) Is there an assessment of presence and likely impact of publication bias?

3.3.3 Critical Appraisal of Individual Studies

While the evidence pyramid in Fig. 4 provides guidance on which study design is considered of better quality, it will also be important to evaluate the quality of the methods used for each of these studies. To determine the validity of individual study results, it will be important to understand the characteristics, strengths, and weaknesses of different study designs used in science and the different sources of bias of each design. There are several manuals available describing validated checklists for critical appraisal of different types of study designs. Several organizations or centers specializing in EBP have critical appraisal checklists available online such as the Critical Appraisal Skills Programme (https://casp-uk.net/), the Centre for Evidence-Based Medicine in Oxford (UK) (https://www.cebm.net/2014/06/critical-appraisal/), the Joanna Briggs Institute (http://joannabriggs.org/research/critical-appraisal-tools.html), and the toolkits provided by BMJ Best Practice. Because the methodological assessment of the study design of reviews and individual studies is key in determining the validity of the results and conclusion drawn, clinicians in most countries have extensive courses on research methods, designs, statistics, and critical appraisal of them.

Since one of the most important skills when appraising the evidence is understanding and recognizing different sources of bias, we will elaborate on this issue here. In Table 2, different sources of bias that can occur in clinical studies are summarized (Mayer 2010). As defined by the Cochrane Collaboration, bias is a systematic error or deviation from the truth, in results or in inferences (Higgins and Green 2011). Bias can lead to over- as well as underestimation of an intervention effect. Some biases are small, but others might be substantial and limit the validity of the results found in a study. Cochrane has produced a Risk of Bias Tool to be used by authors performing systematic reviews. It explains the most important sources of bias in clinical trials. Clinicians should be aware of these types or sources of bias when critically appraising the literature.

The most likely limitations that have been identified in randomized controlled trials that result in biased results (Schünemann et al. 2013) are the following:

– Lack of allocation concealment
– Lack of blinding

Table 2 An overview of different sources of bias in clinical studies (Mayer 2010; The Cochrane Risk of Bias Tool in Higgins and Green (2011))

Sources of bias	When does this occur?
Selection or sampling bias	When patients are selected in a manner that will systematically influence the outcome of the study, for example, inadequate randomization or inadequate concealment of allocation
Referral bias	When patients are selected after being referred for a specific type of care. This is a special form of selection bias that particularly limits the external validity thus generalizability of the study
Performance bias	When participants and personnel are not blinded hence are knowledgably of the allocated interventions during the study
Detection bias	When patients are preferentially included if they have been exposed to a particular risk factor. This is also a form of selection bias where exposure causes a sign or symptom that precipitates a search for the disease and then is blamed for causing the disease
Attrition bias	Patient attrition occurs when patients drop out of a study or are lost to follow-up, leading to a loss of valuable information. Patients who drop out may do so because a treatment or placebo is ineffective or there are too many unwanted side effects
Recall bias	Occurs most often in a retrospective study, either a case control or nonconcurrent cohort study. When asked about certain exposures, subjects with the outcome in the study are more likely than controls to recall the factors to which they were exposed
Reporting bias	When there is selective outcome reporting
Observer bias	When there is conscious or unconscious distorting in perception of reporting the measurement by an observer
Nonrespondent bias	Is a bias in the results of a study because of patients who do not respond to a survey or who drop out of a study; it occurs because those people who do not respond to a survey may be different in some fundamental way from those who do respond
Confounding	The presence of several variables that can explain the apparent connection between the cause and effect, for example, when there is no adequate statistical adjustment for possible confounders
Contamination	When the control group receives the same therapy as the experimental group

- Incomplete accounting of patients and outcome events
- Selective outcome reporting
- And other such as stopping a trial early for benefit, use of unvalidated outcome measures, carry-over effects in crossover trials, and recruitment bias in cluster RCTs

Key study limitations identified in observational studies that can introduce bias are (Schünemann et al. 2013):

- Failure to develop and apply appropriate eligibility criteria (inclusion of control population)
- Flawed measurement of both exposure and outcome
- Failure to adequately control confounding
- Incomplete or inadequately short follow-up, especially within prospective cohort studies

These sources of bias are determining factors to what is called "**internal validity**" of a study. Internal validity exists when precision and accuracy are not distorted by bias in the study. A study that is judged to be internally valid, measures precisely and accurately what is intended. Another important type of validity to consider, in particular for clinical studies and trials, is "**external validity**." External validity means that the results of the study can be generalized or extrapolated beyond the study population to other clinical situation or populations. When a population of a study is too narrow or the actual intervention delivered cannot be implemented in real practice, external validity is threatened (Mayer 2010).

Finally, an important network involved with improving quality in health research is the **EQUATOR network**. The EQUATOR network "Enhancing the QUAlity and Transparency Of health Research" is an international initiative that seeks to improve the reliability and value of published health research literature by promoting transparent and accurate **reporting** and wider use of robust **reporting guidelines**. The EQUATOR website (http://www.equator-network.org/) provides an overview of all types of reporting guidelines available for different study design:

- CONSORT for RCTs (with several extensions for cluster trials, pilot trials, etc.) and SPIRIT for trial protocols
- STROBE for observational studies
- PRISMA for systematic reviews
- SRQR and COREQ for qualitative research
- AGREE for clinical practice guidelines
- SQUIRE for quality improvement studies
- CARE for case reports
- STARD and TRIPOD for diagnostic and prognostic studies
- CHEERS for economic evaluations

We refer the reader to http://www.equator-network.org/ for up-to-date information on all reporting guidelines for main study types and their recent extensions. The reporting guidelines are intended for authors and researchers to help them in adequately reporting as well as designing their studies. They can also be an important tool to teach clinicians to evaluate and appraise the quality of studies performed within the broad domain of health care.

3.3.4 Synopses and Summaries

Summaries and synopses aim to provide critical overviews of reviews and studies to be available and usable by clinicians at the point-of care. These can be evidence-based textbooks or critical overviews of reviews and studies. They aim to provide high-quality, frequently updated, and easily digestible evidence-based recommendations for clinical practice, in particular those that are available online. Examples are UpToDate, DynaMed, and BMJ Best Practice. They are usually logically grouped around common medical scenarios and translated into alternative options related to diagnosis, treatment, and management (Banzi et al. 2010, 2011). They are also advocated and advertised as products with regular updating systems.

It is however very important to consider that recent analyses have criticized these textbooks and point-of-care summaries. The authors (Banzi et al. 2010; Jeffery et al. 2012; Kwag et al. 2016) compared different sources and showed that they include evidence relevant to practice at different speeds, that the proportion of topics with potentially outdated treatment recommendations varies substantially and that topic coverage varies substantially. Generally, a high proportion of the 200 common topics had potentially out-of-date conclusions, missing information from one or more recently published studies (Banzi et al. 2010; Jeffery et al. 2012; Kwag et al. 2016). Jeffery et al. (2012) concluded that "although there is variation in the rate at which the leading textbooks are updated, all of them can benefit from more frequent processing of high quality, clinically relevant, recently published studies."

3.3.5 Clinical Practice Guidelines and Decision Support Systems

Systematic reviews of the effects of certain health-care interventions are essential to perform; however, they often do not provide sufficient information for making well-informed decisions. Clinical guidelines are systematically developed statements to assist practitioner and patient decisions about appropriate health care for specific clinical circumstances (Legido-Quigley et al. 2013). Clinicians should be aware that not all clinical practice guidelines available to clinicians are evidence-based. Quite a few guidelines, also in palliative care, are based on expert opinions and lack the necessary studies to substantiate the guidance provided. Some guidelines also combine statements that are evidence-based with consensus-based statements when there is no evidence concerning one of the clinical questions. It will be important for readers to consider how statements are developed and preferably guidelines make this explicit (e.g., via the GRADE approach).

Regarding palliative care guidelines, several institutions and organizations exist that produce guidelines for palliative or end-of-life care. While some organizations (e.g., NICE, ESMO) produce palliative care guidelines next to a wide range of other health-care topics, there are also several national palliative care organizations who have specific units working to develop guidelines for palliative care, and there are international organizations developing international guidelines, including the European Association of Palliative Care.

High-quality guidelines should be based on high-quality evidence or in the absence of such evidence, on high-quality consensus procedures. Preferably of course, high-quality evidence is available to guide decision-making. The AGREE criteria to evaluate guidelines can help professionals to evaluate the development process of a guidelines. The AGREE working group has developed six domains for the evaluation of the quality of the process of making a practice guideline: scope/purpose, stakeholder involvement, rigor of development, clarity of presentation, applicability, and editorial independence. However, these criteria only indirectly assess quality of the content of the guideline by focusing on the way it was developed. To evaluate the extent to which a recommendation is based on evidence (and the level of that evidence), GRADE quality assessment criteria have been developed.

GRADE Approach

The **GRADE (Grading of recommendations assessment, development, and evaluation)** working group was founded in 2000. Because guidelines varied in how they rated the quality of evidence and how they graded the strength of recommendations, this group of researchers developed a new approach to grading quality (or certainty) of evidence and strength of recommendations, which is now considered the standard in guideline development internationally. A systematic and explicit grading approach can help prevent errors, facilitate critical appraisal, and help to improve communication of the information.

Table 3 displays an overview of the GRADE approach to quality of the evidence. Although quality of evidence is a continuum, four grades are distinguished and specific instructions for guidelines panels and authors of systematic reviews are described in detail in the Grade Handbook as it was updated in 2013 (Schünemann et al. 2013). We refer the reader to the http://www.gradeworkinggroup.org/ for up-to-date information on the grading approach.

In the GRADE approach, the quality of evidence is determined by several factors. The rating begins with the study design (trials or observational studies) and then addresses several factors that can reduce the quality of evidence and factors that can increase the quality rating. These are

Table 3 Quality of evidence grades. (Reproduced from Schünemann et al. 2013, with permission from the editors)

Grade	Definition
High	We are very confident that the true effect lies close to that of the estimate of the effect
Moderate	We are moderately confident in the effect estimate: The true effect is likely to be close to the estimate of the effect, but there is a possibility that it is substantially different
Low	Our confidence in the effect estimate is limited: The true effect may be substantially different from the estimate of the effect
Very low	We have very little confidence in the effect estimate: The true effect is likely to be substantially different from the estimate of effect

Table 4 Factors determining the quality of evidence in the GRADE approach. (Reproduced from Schünemann et al. 2013, with permission from the editors)

Factors than can reduce the quality of the evidence	Consequence for the evidence level assigned
Limitations in study design or execution (risk of bias)	Decrease 1 or 2 levels
Inconsistency of results	Decrease 1 or 2 levels
Indirectness of evidence	Decrease 1 or 2 levels
Imprecision	Decrease 1 or 2 levels
Publication bias	Decrease 1 or 2 levels
Factors than can increase the quality of the evidence	Consequence for the evidence level assigned
Large magnitude of effect	Increase 1 or 2 levels
All plausible confounding would reduce the demonstrated effect or increase the effect if no effect was observed	Increase 1 level
Dose-response gradient	Increase 1 level

summarized in Table 4. The GRADE Handbook explains all these elements in further detail (Schünemann et al. 2013).

GRADE also makes explicit how to go from evidence to recommendation. The strength of a recommendation reflects the extent to which a guideline panel is confident that desirable effects of an intervention outweigh undesirable effects or vice versa, across a range of patients for whom the recommendation is intended (Schünemann et al. 2013). A strong recommendation signifies that the guideline panel judges the desirable effects of an intervention outweigh its undesirable effects (strong recommendation for an intervention) or that the undesirable effects of an intervention outweigh its desirable effects (strong recommendation against an intervention).

GRADE has also identified implications for different users of guidelines (i.e., patients, clinicians, as well as policy makers) of strong and weak recommendations, to aid with the interpretation. These are shown in Table 5.

Finally, GRADE has suggested how quality of evidence and strength of recommendations should be visually or symbolically represented. Table 6 summarizes the different symbols and letters that are used in guidelines to summarize these evaluations.

Implementation of Guidelines and Clinical Decision Support Systems

It has become clear over the past decades that guidelines do not implement themselves. While there has been a lot of literature related to the development and identification of evidence-based practices and programs, it has become clear that the mere existence of this knowledge does not change practice (Eyssen and Sikken 2018). Real impact in practice can only be achieved if effective intervention practices are combined with effective implementation practices. Consequently, several models have been developed to explain and visualize the implementation process of EBP (Nilsen 2015; Benahmed et al. 2017), such as the PARiHS framework (Kitson et al. 2008), the "research-to-practice-pipeline" model (Glasziou and Haynes 2005), and the GUIDE-M model (Brouwers et al. 2014). It is beyond the scope of this chapter to describe these models in detail. A meta-analysis of Fretheim et al. (2015) concluded that strategies that will increase adherence to clinical practice guidelines with moderate certainty include: clinical decision-support systems (including reminders), educational outreach visits (including practice facilitation), audit and feedback, local opinion leaders, tailored interventions, and educational meetings. In particular the clinical decision-support systems (CDS), also called computerized decision support systems, are important EPB initiatives currently under development.

Table 5 Implications of strong and weak recommendations for different users of guidelines. (Reproduced from Schünemann et al. 2013, with permission from the editors)

	Strong recommendation	Weak recommendation
For patients	Most individuals in this situation would want the recommended course of action and only a small proportion would not	The majority of individuals in this situation would want the suggested course of action, but many would not
For clinicians	Most individuals should receive the recommended course of action. Adherence to this recommendation according to the guideline could be used as a quality criterion or performance indicator. Formal decision aids are not likely to be needed to help individuals make decisions consistent with their values and preferences	Recognize that different choices will be appropriate for different patients and that you must help each patient arrive at a management decision consistent with her or his values and preferences. Decision aids may well be useful helping individuals making decisions consistent with their values and preferences. Clinicians should expect to spend more time with patients when working toward a decision
For policy makers	The recommendation can be adapted as policy in most situations including for the use as performance indicators	Policy making will require substantial debates and involvement of many stakeholders. Policies are also more likely to vary between regions. Performance indicators would have to focus on the fact that adequate deliberation about the management options has taken place

Table 6 Suggested GRADE representations of quality of evidence and strength of recommendations. (Reproduced from Schünemann et al. 2013, with permission from the editors)

Quality of evidence	Symbol	Letter (varies)
High	⊕⊕⊕⊕	A
Moderate	⊕⊕⊕○	B
Low	⊕⊕○○	C
Very low	⊕○○○	D
Strength of recommendation	**Symbol**	**Letter (varies)**
Strong for an intervention	↑↑	1
Weak for an intervention	↑?	2
Weak against an intervention	↓?	2
Strong against an intervention	↓↓	1

CDS is a technology that provides patient-specific medical knowledge at the point of need, that is, during medical or other consultations, via linking with patient file data. An EU-funded project GUIDES (Guideline Implementation with Decision Support) aims to develop a checklist and tools to improve the use of CDS. Organizations such as Duodecim Medical Publications have, for example, developed EBMeDS (Evidence-Based Medicine electronic Decision Support), a platform-independent service which can be integrated into electronic health records containing structured patient data. The EBMeDS system brings evidence into practice by means of context-sensitive guidance at the point of care. It receives structured patient data from electronic health records (EHRs) and returns reminders, therapeutic suggestions, and diagnosis-specific links to guidelines. Such systems will become an important tool for clinicians in the future to help at the point of care.

3.4 Step 4: Apply Evidence to the Individual Patient

In the application of evidence, step 3 is of course crucial. The quality of the studies found and/or the strength of recommendations in guidelines should be carefully considered. However, a number of other factors are crucial for translating this evidence to the individual patient at hand. The last EBP step is the process of knowledge transition (Haynes 2010) and concerns the application or interpretation of the evidence found in clinical studies to an individual or specific patient. Instead of generalizing evidence, EBP focuses on individualizing evidence to a specific problem or patient. This process is often the most difficult for a clinician.

A first important element to consider is the **clinical significance or importance** of a result of a study. Often in research, odds ratios and relative risks are reported to describe whether an intervention works compared to a control group. They are limited in providing information about how well the intervention works, that is, the size of the effect. Effect size reporting is one method of estimating the amount of benefit. A useful help in interpreting effect sizes is offered by Cohen, indicating that an effect size or standardized mean difference of around 0.2 is considered a small effect, 0.5 a moderate effect, and 0.8 or higher a large effect (Schünemann et al. 2013). An effect size quantifies the difference between two groups. For example, in the case of a comparison between an intervention and a control group in an intervention study, an effect size of 0.8 means that the score of the average person in the intervention group is 0.8 standard deviations above the average person in the control group and hence exceeds the scores of 79% of the control group.

Another highly relevant method for determining clinical significance is the **NNT or number-needed-to-treat** to get benefit and the **NNH or number-needed-to-harm** or number needed to treat to get harm. The NNT is the number of patients that must be treated with the therapy or intervention for a duration equal to the study period, in order to have one additional person experience a beneficial outcome. Ideally, NNT would be small as this means that the new intervention is a lot better than the standard or control (a "perfect" NNT would be 1). NNH is the number of patients that are needed to be exposed to a risk factor before an additional patient is harmed by side effects of the treatment or intervention. Hence, NNT and NNH are meant to help clinicians balance the benefit and risks of a therapy or intervention for an individual patient (Mayer 2010).

Next to these important elements for clinicians to consider when using evidence, Figure 2 also clearly indicated that clinical decisions are a result of four factors, that is, available evidence, the clinical situation, the patients' preferences, and clinical experience. Most evidence produced by research studies is not straightforward. Research designs all have strengths and weaknesses. Also, studies often have a specific target population that might not correspond to the individual patient of a clinician. That individual patient might have different characteristics in terms of gender, age, socio-economics, pathophysiology, compliance, comorbidity, risk of adverse events or other. Hence, clinicians often need to make decisions with relative uncertain or not easily transferable evidence. EBP has been advocated as an approach in which an experienced clinician decides whether and how external evidence applies to a particular patient (Wiebe 2000). It is not cookbook medicine.

If the application of evidence were a simple process, there would not be so much variability in actual practice as there is now. Research studies from various domains have shown there are large variations in diagnostic and therapeutic approaches between physicians from the same and other disciplines. Additionally, sometimes research studies clearly show the benefits of certain treatment or lack thereof, while clinicians do not act upon that evidence. One example is the observation that palliative care physicians all over the world use anticholinergic medications for the treatment of a "death rattle" at the end of life, while several studies including a systematic Cochrane review showed that there is no evidence of benefit of this medication (Wee and Hillier 2008). Qualitative research in this area showed that other factors were at play (e.g., feeling pressured, relatives that were distressed by the sound) that could explain clinician behavior (Wee et al. 2008a; Hirsch et al. 2013; Visser et al. 2015).

There are multiple factors contributing to or influencing actions and decisions of physicians. The complexity of the clinical problems, the uncertainty of outcomes of certain decisions, the lack of high-quality evidence, the feeling of physicians that they "need to act" and do something for their patients, patient expectations, examples of peers, or changes in reimbursement schemes, are only a few factors causing variability in practice. Medical decision-making can be very complex. Hence, clinical expertise does have a major role to play in the EBP process.

To increase the likelihood that physicians will make the best possible decisions, we must perform the best possible clinical research and improve the quality of the evidence, and at the same time train physicians in all parts of the EBP process, from evaluating to applying evidence.

Finally, the factor "patient preferences" in the decision-making process cannot be underestimated. As most clinical decisions might have both advantages and disadvantages for patients, patients and clinicians must discuss the different treatment options together to make joint and well-informed decisions (Adriaenssens et al. 2018). The process is called "shared decision-making." Optimal patient care results out of the optimal interaction between evidence-based medicine and patient-centered communication skills, that is, shared decision-making (Hoffmann et al. 2014). Without shared decision-making, authentic EBP cannot occur (Greenhalgh et al. 2014; Hoffmann et al. 2014). Over recent decades, this process of shared decision-making has gained considerable attention and research has shown how difficult it is to put into practice. Health-care professionals do not always have the necessary skills and competences and there is a lack of good tools to support this process in practice, also in palliative care.

3.5 Step 5: Evaluate Own Performance as Clinician

Clinicians should evaluate the results of applying the evidence to their patient or patient population. Evaluating one's own performance as a clinician was already recommended by Sackett early 1990s and remains very necessary today (Sackett et al. 1991). Questioning yourself and regularly monitoring whether you are asking answerable questions, how efficiently you search the literature using current technologies, whether you can efficiently and critically appraise the literature, and what are determinants in applying evidence, can help in remaining an active and lifelong learner. Today, a whole body of literature has evolved around quality monitoring and quality management, aimed at monitoring performance of clinicians or practices or services using quality indicators, quality circles, or other methods for continuous quality improvement.

4 A Critical Reflection on EBP

The evidence-based movement has made important contributions to improving the quality of medical care. Scientific evidence has received a much more central and explicit role in medicine, reducing uncertainty, subjectivity, and bias. Ineffective or even harmful care or treatment can be identified better and prevented. It also helps to identify domains that lack sufficient evidence and can prevent new technologies from being advocated before sufficiently proven. EBP has also led to a critical reflection about the care we offer patients and has made the generating and dissemination of knowledge considerably easier. Consequently, research methodologies and statistical methods are improving consistently (Dutch Council for Public Health and Society 2017).

Nevertheless, EBP has not been left without criticism. One of the critiques on EBP in general is that the EBP model has become too focused on a "top-down" approach which emphasized "populations, statistics, risk and spurious certainty." Consequently, there might be too little flexibility needed to provide real person-centered care, focusing on the individual needs of patients (Greenhalgh et al. 2014).

An important essay published in the *BMJ* in 2014 by Greenhalgh et al. argues that, although EBP has had many benefits, it has also had some negative unintended consequences. Some of the problems highlighted today concern: the influence of industry (drug and medical devises companies) on setting the research agenda (Adriaenssens et al. 2018); the volume of evidence (in particular clinical guidelines) which has become unmanageable (Aoun and Nekolaichuk 2014); statistically significant benefits which may be marginal in clinical practice (Banzi et al. 2010); a danger of care being management-driven (e.g., computerized decision-support systems, point of care prompts, or structured templates) instead of patient-centered (Banzi et al. 2011); and EBP guidelines that often map poorly to complex multi-morbidity (Bauça-Machado et al. 2017).

These authors suggest refocusing on providing useable evidence that can be combined with context and professional expertise so that individual patients get optimal treatment. They advocate to return to "real EBM," that is, to the movement's founding principles, instead of rejecting EBM as a failed model: "to individualise evidence and share decisions through meaningful conversations in the context of a humanistic and professional clinician-patient relationship." Fig. 6 further explains "real EBM" as defined by these authors.

The importance of context in EBP has received progressively more attention by different organizations. The Dutch Council for Health and Society in the Netherlands has published a report in 2017 entitled "Without context, no proof: concerning the illusion of evidence-based practice in health care" (in Dutch). The Belgian Health Care Knowledge Centre has also highlighted the importance of context by adding a fourth dimension to the definition of the concept of EPB. "A fourth dimension, contextual factors (such as costs and availability of resources) is added as this is an element that affects the strength of a recommendation and can hamper implementation of a guideline." This is depicted in Fig. 5. The Centre states that "solely using scientific evidence in health care decision making without taking into account professional expertise, context and patient' preferences (called 'cookbook medicine') does not result in high quality healthcare provision" (Adriaenssens et al. 2018).

Greenhalgh et al. (2014), the Dutch Council for Health and Society, and the Belgian Health Care Knowledge Centre do not advise to fully abandon EBM, EBP, or the search for evidence. As stated

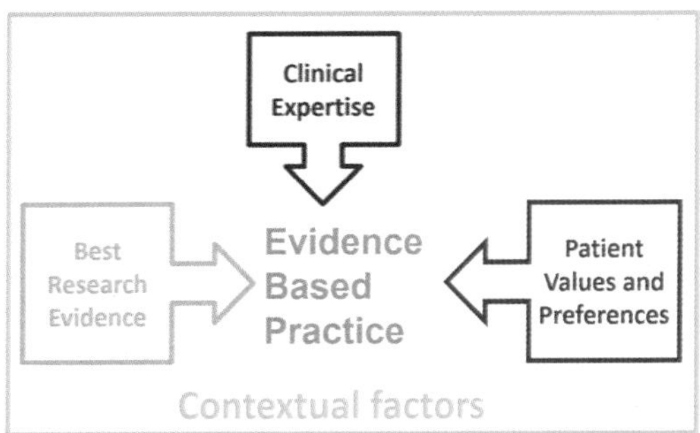

Fig. 5 Visualization of the concept of EBP including the importance of context. (From Adriaenssens et al. 2018, with permission (CC-BY-NC-ND license); no changes made)

by the Dutch Council for Health and Society, what is needed, is evidence in multiple forms. If daily reality of health and social care can be seen from multiple angles, the search for conclusive evidence is an illusion and would lead to over-simplification of good care. "The" evidence as a basis for good care is an illusion. To deliver good patient-centered care, external knowledge or evidence as such is not enough. Clinical expertise, local knowledge, knowledge from patients, and knowledge of the context – the circumstances of living, patient preferences, the care setting, are also of utmost importance. Care professionals should embrace uncertainty in evidence and take the context in which their patients live into account. Researchers should acknowledge that scientific evidence is always incomplete. Healthcare insurance companies, the government, and inspectors should also allow a more experimental approach in health care and value the ability of care professionals and care organizations to learn and improve via such experiments. The Council pleads for a context-based practice instead of pure evidence-based practice.

5 A Critical Reflection on EPB in Palliative Care

In principle, the same issues addressed in EBP apply to palliative care, as this is one branch of medicine, although a highly complex one. Decisions concerning patients and families should be evidence-based or evidence-informed, depending on the evidence at hand. However, several authors in the field of palliative care have also criticized the EBM and EBP approach where RCTs are considered the gold standard. They indicate that while well-executed RCTs can minimize the different sources of bias via the use of universal and objective methodological criteria (e.g., via CONSORT guidelines, Moher 1998), conducting such high-quality research studies is very challenging in the context of palliative care – both ethically and methodologically. The population at hand as well as the complexity of the interventions in palliative care are both reasons that complicate doing high-quality RCTs. Visser et al. (2015)

Box 2: What is real evidence based medicine and how do we achieve it?

Real evidence based medicine:

- Makes the ethical care of the patient its top priority
- Demands individualised evidence in a format that clinicians and patients can understand
- Is characterised by expert judgment rather than mechanical rule following
- Shares decisions with patients through meaningful conversations
- Builds on a strong clinician-patient relationship and the human aspects of care
- Applies these principles at community level for evidence based public health

Actions to deliver real evidence based medicine

- Patients must demand better evidence, better presented, better explained, and applied in a more personalised way
- Clinical training must go beyond searching and critical appraisal to hone expert judgment and shared decision making skills
- Producers of evidence summaries, clinical guidelines, and decision support tools must take account of who will use them, for what purposes, and under what constraints
- Publishers must demand that studies meet usability standards as well as methodological ones
- Policy makers must resist the instrumental generation and use of "evidence" by vested interests
- Independent funders must increasingly shape the production, synthesis, and dissemination of high quality clinical and public health evidence
- The research agenda must become broader and more interdisciplinary, embracing the experience of illness, the psychology of evidence interpretation, the negotiation and sharing of evidence by clinicians and patients, and how to prevent harm from overdiagnosis

Fig. 6 Box 1 Real EBM. (Reproduced from Greenhalgh et al. 2014, with permission from BMJ Publishing Group Ltd)

highlight, for example, that recruitment is inherently difficult in palliative care because of the gatekeeping role of relatives or clinical staff which prevents studies from achieving adequate sample sizes. They also show that the high attrition rates are probably often caused by symptomatic deterioration of patients which is problematic for intention-to-treat analyses in RCTs that rely on completeness of data sets. Furthermore, in palliative care trials, interventions are often multi-componential targeting multiple problems and symptoms of patients and/or their families (physical, psychological, social, and/or spiritual) which makes it very difficult to identify one primary outcome and link outcomes clearly to the intervention components.

Visser et al. (2015) have highlighted the need for improving palliative care research not only by improving the quality of RCTs where possible but also to devote more attention to alternative research methodologies, including high-quality observational studies. Some important work outside of the field of palliative care (Benson and Hartz 2000; Concato et al. 2000) has shown that high-quality methodologically valid observational prospective studies with adequately large sample sizes can yield equivalent results to RCTs, challenging the hierarchy of evidence traditionally put forward in EBP. Based on an evaluation of the current literature, Visser et al. (2015) highlight that – although promising – currently the quality of observational studies is not sufficient enough to rival RCTs. Hence, both improving methodologies of trials as well as other study design will be of utmost importance in palliative care to ensure that clinical practice is informed by adequate levels of evidence. They also conclude that "the EBM model is likely to grow more flexible as the traditional unimodal top-down approach is replaced by the use of multiple diverse methodologies as a research tool kit. Such a mixed-method approach will be viewed not as a means by which to dodge the challenge of conducting methodologically rigorous work in palliative care. Instead, a multi-faceted approach can be regarded as a more valuable scheme with which to address the complex and subtle questions that define the objective of the palliative care research agenda" (cited from Visser et al. 2015).

6 Conclusion

EBP has enormously transformed clinicians' approach to practicing their profession. It was responsible for a true paradigm shift in medicine and improving the standards of treatment and care for all people. To ensure patients in palliative care receive the best possible care, decisions should be taken in conjunction with them, based on their preferences and wishes and the best available evidence on treatments and care. The research community in palliative care must strive to provide high-quality research, high-quality reviews, and high-quality guidelines of that research and ensure that clinicians can easily access and use the best available evidence at the point of care. To produce this evidence and considering the complexity and large diversity of the palliative care population at hand combined with the multi-component nature of palliative care, there is a need for research groups and trial centers to work together across multiple disciplines – medical and social science disciplines, quantitative and qualitative research methods. The future of EBP lies in generating useable evidence that can be combined with context and professional expertise to provide individual patients optimal treatment and care.

References

Adriaenssens J, Benahmed N, Eyssen M, Paulus D, Mertens R. Towards an integrated evidence-based practice plan in Belgium – Part 1: literature, Belgian situation and end-user needs. Brussels: Belgian Health Care Knowledge Centre (KCE); 2018. Health Services Research (HSR), KCE Reports 291. D/2018/10.273/12.

Aoun SM, Nekolaichuk C. Improving the evidence base in palliative care to inform practice and policy: thinking outside the box. J Pain Symptom Manag. 2014;48:1222–35.

Banzi R, Liberati A, Moschetti I, Tagliabue L, Moja L. A review of online evidence-based practice point-of-care information summary providers. J Med Internet Res. 2010;12:e26.

Banzi R, Cinquini M, Liveratir A, Mschetti I, Pecoraro V, Tagliabue L, Moja L. Speed of updating online evidence based point of care summaries: prospective cohort analyses. BMJ, 2011; 23;343:d5856.

Bauça-Machado R, Rosária M, Alarcao J, Correia-Guedes L, Abreu D, Ferreira JJ. Clinical trials in palliative care: a systematic review of their methodological characteristics and of the quality of their reporting. BMC Palliat Care. 2017;16(10)

Benahmed N, Adriaenssens J, Christiaens W, Paulus D. Towards tailoring of KCE guidelines to users' needs. Method. Brussels: Belgian Health Care Knowledge Centre (KCE); 2017. KCE reports 284.

Benson K, Hartz AJ. A comparison of observational studies and randomized, controlled trials. N Engl J Med. 2000;342:1878–86.

Brouwers M, Bhattacharyya O, Team TG-MR. Guideline implementability for decision Excellence Model GUIDE-M [Web page]. 2014. Available from http://www.agreetrust.org/agree- research-projects/guide-m/.

Concato J, Shah N, Horwitz RI. Randomized, controlled trials, observational studies, and the hierarchy of research designs. N Engl J Med. 2000;342:1887–92.

Cramp F, Bennett MI. Development of a generic working definition of "supportive care". BMJ Support Palliat Care. Published online first 02 Aug 2012. https://doi.org/10.1136/bmjspcare-2012-000222.

Dutch Council for Public Health and Society (Raad voor Volksgezondheid en Samenleving) of the Netherlands. No proof without context: concerning the illusion of evidence-based practice in care (in Dutch: Zonder context geen bewijs: over de illusive van evidence-based practice in de zorg), The Hague; 2017.

Dy SM, Aslakson R, Wilson RF, et al. Closing the quality gap: revisiting the state of thze science (Vol 8: Improving health care and palliative care for advanced and serious illness). Evidence Report No. 208. Baltimore: Johns Hopkins University evidence-based practice center; 2012. (Prepared by Johns Hopkins university evidence-based practice center under contract No. 290–2007-10061-I.)

Eyssen M, Sikken BJ. Towards an integrated evidence-based practice plan in Belgium: part 4 – EBP implemenationa in primary healthcare in Belgium. Brussels: Belgian Health Care Knowledge Centre (KCE); 2018. Health Services Research (HSR), KCE reports 291. D/2018/10.273/15

Fretheim A, Flottorp S, Oxman A. NIPH systematic reviews: executive summaries. In: Effect of interventions for implementing clinical practice guidelines. Oslo: Knowledge Centre for the Health Services at The Norwegian Institute of Public Health (NIPH); 2015.

Glasziou P, Haynes B. The paths from research to improved health outcomes. Evid Based Nurs. 2005;8 (2):36–8.

Greenhalgh T, Howick J, Maskreay N. Evidence based medicine: a movement in crisis? BMJ. 2014;348: g3725.

Haun MW, Estel S, Rücker G, Friederich H, Villalobos M, Thomas M, Hartmann M. Early palliative care for adults with advanced cancer. Cochrane Database Syst Rev, June, 2017.

Haynes RB. Of studies, syntheses, synopses, summaries and systems: the '5S' evolution of information services for evidence-based health care decisions. ACP J Club. 2006;145:A8–9.

Haynes RB, Devereaux PJ, Guyatt GH. Clinical expertise in the era of evidence-based medicine and patient choice. BMJ, EBM Notebook. 2002;7:36–8.

Higgins JPT, Green S, editors. Cochrane handbook for systematic reviews of interventions. London: The Cochrane Collaboration; 2011.

Higginson IJ, Evans CJ, Grande G, et al. Evaluating complex interventions in end of life care: the MORECare statement on good practice generated by a synthesis of transparent expert consultations and systematic reviews. BMC Med. 2013;11:111.

Hirsch CA, Marrio JF, Faull CM. Influences on the decision to prescribe or administer anticholinergic drugs to treat death rattle: a focus group study. Palliat Med. 2013;27:732–8.

Hoffmann TC, Montori VM, Del Mar C. The connection between evidence-based medicine and shared decision-making. JAMA. 2014;312(13):1295–6.

Hui D, Arthur J, Dalal S, Bruera E. Quality of the supportive and palliative oncology literature: a focused analysis on randomized controlled trials. Support Care Cancer. 2012;20:1779–85.

Jeffery R, Navarro T, Lokker C, Haynes RB, Wilczynski NL, Farjou G. How current are leading evidence-based medical textbooks? An analytic survey if hour online textbooks. J Med Internet Res. 2012;14(6):e175.

Kaasa S, Radbruch L. Palliative care research – priorities and the way forward. Eur J Cancer. 2008;44:1175–9.

Kitson AL, Rycroft-Malone J, Harvey G, McCormack B, Seers K, Titchen A. Evaluating the successful implementation of evidence into practice using the PARiHS framework: theoretical and practical challenges. Implement Sci. 2008;3(1).

Kwag KH, Gonzalez-Lorenzo M, Banzi R, Bonovas S, Moja L. Providing doctors with high-quality information: an updated evaluation of web-based point-of-care information summaries. J Med Internet Res. 2016;18(1):e15.

Legido-Quigley H, Panteli D, Car J, McKee M, Busse R. Clinical guidelines for chronic conditions in the European Union. Copenhagen: The European Observatory on Health Systems and Policies, World Health Organization; 2013.

Luckett T, Phillips J, Agar M, Virdun C, Green A, Davidson PM. Elements of effective palliative care models: a rapid review. BMC Health Serv Res. 2014;14:136.

Mayer D, editor. Essential evidence-based medicine. 2nd ed. Cambridge, UK: Cambridge University Press; 2010.

Moher D. CONSORT: an evolving tool to help improve the quality of reports of randomized controlled trials. Consolidated standards of reporting trials. JAMA. 1998;279:1489–91.

Moher D, Liberati A, Tetzlaff J, Altman DG, The PRISMA Group. Preferred reporting items for systematic reviews and meta-analyses: The PRISMA statement. PLoS Med. 2009;6(7):e1000097. https://doi.org/10.1371/journal.pmed1000097.

Murrad MH, Assi N, Alsawas M, Alahdab F. New evidence pyramid. Evid Based Med. 2016;21(4).

Nieva V, Murphy R, Ridley N, Donaldson N, Combes J, Mitchell P, et al. Advances in patient safety: from research to implementation. Rockville: Agency for Healthcare Research and Quality (AHRQ); 2005. (From science to service: a framework for the transfer of patient safety research into practice).

Nilsen P. Making sense of implementation theories, models and frameworks. Implement Sci. 2015;10:53.

Pope C. Resisting evidence: the study of evidence-based medicine as a contemporary social movement. Health. 2003;7:267–82.

Sackett DL, Haynes RB, Guyatt GH, Tugwell P. Introduction: how to review your own performance. In: Sackett DL, Haynes RB, Guyatt GH, Tugwell P, editors. Clinical epidemiology: a basic science for clinical medicine. Boston: Little, Brown; 1991. p. 305–33.

Sackett DL, Rosenberg WM, Gray JA, Haynes RB, Richardson WS. Evidence based medicine: what it is and what it isn't. BMJ. 1996;312:71–2.

Schünemann H, Brożek J, Guyatt G, Oxman A, editors. Handbook for grading the quality of evidence and the strength of recommendations using the GRADE approach. Updated October 2013. http://gdt.guidelinedevelopment.org/app/handbook/handbook.html

Shea BJ, Reeves BC, Wells G, Thuku M, Hamel C, Moran J, Moher D, Tugwell P, Welch V, Kristjansson E, Henry DA. AMSTAR 2: a critical appraisal tool for systematic reviews that include randomised or non-randomised studies of healthcare interventions, or both. BMJ. 2017;358:j4008.

Smith S, Brick A, O'Hara S, Normand C. Evidence on the cost and cost-effectiveness of palliative care: a literature review. Palliat Med. 2014;28(2):130–50.

Visser C, Hadley G, Wee B. Reality of evidence-based practice in palliative care. Cancer Biol Med. 2015;12:193–200.

Wee B, Hillier R. Interventions for noisy breathing in patients near to death. Cochrane Database Syst Rev. 2008:CD005177.

Wee B, Coleman P, Hillize R, Holgate S. Death ratlle: its impact on staff and volunteers in palliative care. Palliat Med. 2008a;22:173–6.

Wee B, Hadley G, Derry S. How useful are systematic reviews for informing palliative care practice? Survey of 25 Cochrane systematic reviews. BMC Palliat Care. 2008b;7:13.

Wiebe S. The principles of evidence-based medicine. Cephalalgia. 2000;20(Suppl 2):10–3.

Part X

Public Health Approach in Palliative and End-of-Life Care

New Public Health Approaches to End-of-Life Care

96

Libby Sallnow and Sally Paul

Contents

Abstract

The palliative and end-of-life care movement worldwide has been a success story in many respects. Palliative care services exist in many countries throughout the world and are increasingly integrated into mainstream health services. Despite these achievements, the movement continues to face challenges from demographic trends, changing patterns of illness, and social contexts of care, which suggest an increasing need for services. Questions have been raised regarding the appropriateness of building further services, as compared with new perspectives on care, which see communities and professionals working in partnership. These perspectives are collectively known as the new public health perspective and this chapter details the emergence of new public health perspectives in end-of-life care.

L. Sallnow (✉)
Palliative Care Physician, University College London Hospital and Central and North West London NHS Trust, London, UK
e-mail: libby.sallnow@nhs.net

S. Paul
School of Social Work and Social Policy, University of Strathclyde, Glasgow, UK
e-mail: sally.paul@strath.ac.uk

R. D. MacLeod, L. Van den Block (eds.), *Textbook of Palliative Care*,
https://doi.org/10.1007/978-3-319-77740-5_97

1 End-of-Life Care in Need of New Public Health Approaches

The end-of-life care movement worldwide has been a success story in many respects. Palliative care services exist in many countries throughout the world and are increasingly integrated into mainstream health services. The experiences of those dying in pain have been highlighted as a human rights issue at both national and global levels (Knaul et al. 2017), and the impact of early palliative care is increasingly recognized in certain disease groups (Temel et al. 2010).

Despite these achievements, the movement continues to face challenges from demographic trends, changing patterns of illness, and social contexts of care which suggest increasing need for services. Further to this, the movement is increasingly facing criticisms that the original vision of holistic care is being interpreted in a more restrictive manner, focusing on physical or psychological symptoms at the expense of social concerns. The proliferation of professionals in the discipline has led some to reflect that communities no longer feel confident or able to respond to end-of-life issues, depending increasingly on professional responses which both disempower people and place further demands on services.

One response to these concerns has been to redefine how end-of-life care is understood. Rather than holding it as a medical issue, under the remit of health and social care professionals, it should be reframed as a social experience. This then allows individuals, families, and communities to take an active role in the issues affecting them, working with professional services to meet the needs of the dying. This approach of working in partnership with communities is named the new public health approach to end-of-life care.

This chapter will begin by detailing the emergence of the new public health movement and the key documents that have shaped its development. It will go on to discuss the relevance of a new public health approach to end-of-life care, identifying key theoretical models that seek to develop and conceptualize this area of practice. It finishes by highlighting examples of new public health approaches to end-of-life care to illustrate the different ways in which this approach is being used in practice.

2 An Introduction to New Public Health

The new public health movement emerged in the later part of the twentieth century. While it emerged from and was built on the traditional or classical public health movement of centuries before, the movement was "new" in that it challenged and redefined certain components of the approach. New public health continued to endorse many aspects such as the role of policy in improving health and the importance of prevention of disease or ill-health, but it also represented a departure from classical public health, through its radical reframing of health as everyone's responsibility. This included identifying the importance of the social determinants of health alongside biomedical factors and the positioning of patients, carers, communities, and citizens as experts in their own health. New public health approaches have equity as their core focus and seek to bring healthy lives within everyone's reach. As a result they take a much broader view of the causes and solutions for health and well-being, going beyond medicine, biomedical approaches, and professional responses.

Fran Baum, in her book *The New Public Health* (2015), describes five innovative features of a new public health approach (see Box 1).

Box 1: Features of a new public health approach

1. Puts the pursuit of equity at the center of public health endeavors
2. Is based on the assumption that social and environmental factors are responsible for much ill-health
3. Argues for health-promoting health services that are based on a strong system of primary health care

(continued)

Box 1: (continued)
4. Stresses the role of all sectors in impacting on health and the importance of health in all policies
5. Stresses the importance of participation and involvement in all new public health endeavors

As the new public health approach was formalized, it galvanized a range of different approaches from preexisting global movements such as community development, behavioral, health education, and environmental approaches and indigenous and lay medicine. This has led to a diverse and inclusive field.

2.1 Key Documents that Have Shaped the New Public Health

A series of documents and declarations have helped define the field of new public health.

1) The so-called *Lalonde Report,* after the then ruling Canadian Health Minister, was published in 1974 (formally titled "A New Perspective on the Health of Canadians") and provided an important articulation of the broad range of factors, beyond the biomedical health-care system, understood to influence and determine health. It recognized the role of environmental, political, and lifestyle factors and health-care services, through the health field concept (Lalonde 1974).

2) The *Alma-Ata Declaration*, published by the World Health Organization (WHO) in 1978, positioned primary health care as participatory health care, in which people have both a right and a duty to participate. It provided a new model for affordable, sustainable, and universal primary health care (see Box 2).

3) The *Ottawa Charter for Health Promotion* (World Health Organisation 1986) (see Box 3) defined the new practice of health promotion as the process of enabling people to increase control over, and to improve, their health. While it has provided a framework for a new public health approach globally, there have been some criticisms voiced over the extent to which it incorporates the diversity of perspectives globally, focusing on individual rather than collective approaches to health (McPhail-Bell et al. 2013).

Box 2: An excerpt from the Alma-Ata Declaration (WHO 1978)
Primary health care is essential health care based on practical, scientifically sound and socially acceptable methods and technology made universally accessible to individuals and families in the community through their full participation and at a cost that the community and country can afford to maintain at every stage of their development in the spirit of self-reliance and self-determination.

Box 3: The Ottawa Charter for Health Promotion (WHO 1986): the five pillars
1. Building healthy public policy
2. Creating supportive environments
3. Strengthening community action
4. Developing personal skills
5. Reorienting health-care services toward prevention of illness and promotion of health

Subsequent documents from the WHO have further embedded this approach, including the *Millennium Development Goals* and the subsequent *Sustainable Development Goals* (Sachs 2012), but new public health approaches go beyond the WHO principles. Much grassroots community action can be considered under the umbrella term of new public health approaches. The balance of power between such local and informal initiatives and those supported by health-care organizations and institutions continues to inform, challenge, and redefine the field.

3 New Public Health Approaches and End-of-Life Care

The hospice and palliative care movement has made great strides in challenging the conditions in which the dying and their close family are cared for and supported. It is argued, however, that these movements have become predominantly a professional or service-based response, and this has led to over-professionalization of care and a disempowerment of communities in relation to these issues (Kellehear 2005). Further concerns have been raised regarding the inequity of care provided at the end of life (Dixon et al. 2015) or the international variation (Economist Intelligence Unit 2015). The predicted demographic changes, relating to rising numbers of older people and the prevalence of chronic illness, will place further stress on the system (Etkind et al. 2017).

For these reasons, alternative approaches to supporting death, dying, loss, and care can offer more holistic, empowering, and sustainable models of support. The new public health approach to end-of-life care integrates principles of health promotion, equity, social and environmental responses to ill-health, and professional/lay power sharing and partnerships. The broad natures of both new public health and end-of-life care have meant that a range of examples is in existence today. The two common terms used to describe these approaches are health-promoting palliative care and compassionate communities.

Health-promoting palliative care describes the application of the five pillars of health promotion to end-of-life care (Kellehear 1999). It aims to change the practice of end-of-life care and provides a structure for services to develop health-promoting practices. This model focuses heavily on the role of professional services, and the subsequent movement of compassionate communities moves beyond end-of-life care services to look at the role lay communities, schools, businesses, or councils play in end-of-life care.

One of the key principles of new public health is working with communities as partners, often termed community engagement and defined by the authors as:

> An umbrella terms for a process which enables communities to work together to understand, build capacity and address issues to improve their experience of end-of-life and bereavement and related wellbeing. It exists on a spectrum of engagement that extends from informing through to empowering, depending on a range of factors such as the degree of participation from the local community and the intention of the work. Community engagement activities in end-of-life care services go beyond working in the community to working with the community to improve the experiences of end-of-life care. (Sallnow and Paul 2015)

4 Current Practices in End-of-Life Care

Examples of new public health approaches to end-of-life care are developing around the world and represent a diverse set of approaches, shaped both in response to local need and the differing approaches contained within the new public health field. Such work includes, but is not limited to, mobilizing existing or facilitated community networks and/or resources; working with community organizations to influence perceptions of and responses to death and bereavement; awareness raising, education, and/or training activities around specific end-of-life issues; and policy reform (Sallnow et al. 2016). The significance of these activities for meaningful end-of-life care, and the challenge of applying a new way of thinking to this area of practice, has resulted in a number of frameworks that attempt to define and develop how new public health approaches to end-of-life care are conceptualized and how they are different to service delivery approaches.

4.1 The Theory: What Defines a New Public Health Project?

Allan Kellehear's (2005 p.156) "Big Seven Checklist" offers a guide to understanding "genuine" health-promoting palliative care activities (see Box 4). It highlights the significance of community ownership, collaboration, and participation in employing a health-promoting approach to end-of-life care. The checklist also identifies the importance of developing activities that are based on early intervention and harm reduction that involves normalizing death, dying, and bereavement: proactively preparing individuals and communities for related experiences.

Box 4: The Big Seven Checklist

1. In what way does the project help prevent social difficulties around death, dying, loss, or care?
2. In what way do they harm-minimize difficulties we may not be able to prevent around death, dying, loss, or care?
3. In what ways can these activities be understood as early interventions along the journey of death, dying, loss, or care?
4. In what ways do these activities alter/change a setting or environment for the better in terms of our present or future responses to death, dying, loss, or care?
5. In what way are the proposed activities participatory – borne, partnered, and nurtured by community member?
6. How sustainable will the activities or programs be without your future input?
7. How can we evaluate their success of usefulness so that we can justify their presence, their funding, and their ongoing support?

The Spectrum for Community Engagement in End-of-Life Care (Sallnow and Paul 2015) offers a framework for end-of-life care service providers to both understand and develop new public health approaches (see Box 5). It employs a hierarchical model that represents five types of work along a continuum involving different levels of power sharing and participation. This extends from informing the people or communities that they work with to consulting with them, co-producing, collaborating, and finally empowering them. The spectrum thus distinguishes a new public health approach from more traditional forms of service provision by placing emphasis on the development of community capacity and resilience.

4.2 Practice: Examples of Existing New Public Health Approaches in End-of-Life Care

This section discusses four existing practice examples that are illustrative of new public health approaches to end-of-life care. It follows the earlier theoretical sections by exploring what these approaches look like in practice and how they have been understood and evaluated.

Box 5: The Spectrum for Community Engagement in End-of-Life Care: developing community capacity [EoLC – End-of-life care]. Reproduced with permission from Sallnow and Paul (2015)

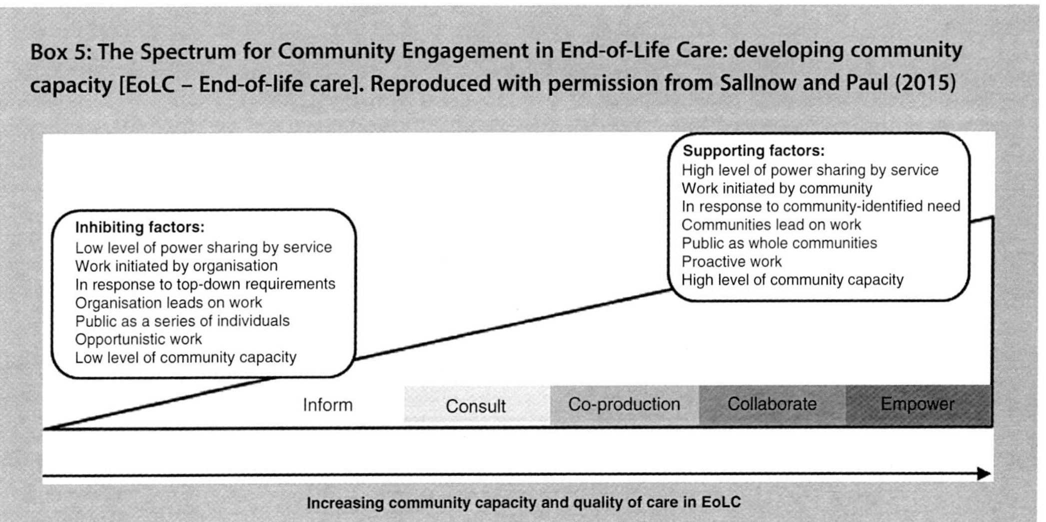

4.2.1 Example 1: Compassionate Neighbours, London

The Compassionate Neighbours project recruits and trains local people to become Compassionate Neighbours. Compassionate Neighbours are local people who support those nearing the end of their lives in their own homes. The project focuses on supporting people to be good neighbors rather than training them in a new role. The aim is to support those at the end of life and their families through companionship, practical support, connecting people to their communities, or helping people to access services they need.

Recruitment is through a series of open days that culminate in a selection day, where participants select whether they would like to participate in the project and the project managers determine if there are any reasons they may not participate. Once enrolled in the project, participants complete a training course. This is either over 4 full days or over 2 weekends. Approximately 15 participants take part in each training program. At the end of the training program, a DBS (Disclosure and Barring Service) check is carried out. The project managers and Compassionate Neighbour then jointly consider the roles most appropriate for them. For some, they are matched with people in the community immediately, but for others, a different role within the project is selected. Not everyone begins with being matched to someone in the community; some participate in other aspects of the project, and some are never matched yet remain with the project. The focus is less on matching set numbers of people but instead on developing the capacity of members of the community to make their own contribution.

The project holds supportive and reflective monthly meetings for all Compassionate Neighbours. In these meetings, participants can reflect on their relationship with the person they are visiting but are also encouraged to reflect on themselves and their own personal development. These are based on a model of personal and group learning and are termed practice development meetings (PDM). In addition to these more formal modes of support, the project hosts a weekly coffee morning in a public space in the hospice open to all participants and the general public. These meetings allow people to come and learn about the project and for the Compassionate Neighbours to meet with each other and develop the network of peer support. Internal and external speakers come and speak about topics related to the project such as how to support someone with dementia or that can be of general relevance, such as managing fuel poverty.

The project has developed to have over 200 trained Compassionate Neighbours matched with over 90 people in the community at the time of writing and has won many prestigious national awards. It has two full-time members of staff coordinating the project and, although initially set up outside the traditional volunteer department, is working increasingly closely with it today.

The project has been the subject of a mixed methods evaluation (Sallnow et al. 2017). The study showed how participating in the project improved participants sense of well-being, connection, and feelings of loneliness. Interestingly, although those being visited at the end of life described these changes, the most significant changes were observed for the Compassionate Neighbours. Their membership of a large network, the time taken to develop new skills and make new friends, and the development of a sense of meaning and purpose were seen to have the most significant impact. These outcomes illustrate how this functioned as a new public health project, acting to prevent and reduce social isolation and disconnection in people before they reached the end of life. The outcomes for those training were seen as important as those receiving the care, illustrating how this sits distinctly from a service-based approach focusing only on outcomes for the recipient.

4.2.2 Example 2: Work with Schools, Central Scotland

Strathcarron Hospice, in Stirlingshire, Scotland, undertook an action research study to identify how hospice staff could work with schools in their catchment area. This was because the hospice catchment area covered 160 schools and received numerous ad hoc requests from schools for pre- and post-bereavement support for pupils, education sessions relating to end-of-life care, and presentations on the role of the hospice due to local fundraising initiatives. The study therefore aimed to explore how the hospice could work with these schools in a more structured and meaningful way that involved advancing education and support around end-of-life and bereavement care. Through a process that involved working in partnership with staff, parents, and children aged 9 to 12, several practice developments were identified that were found to be useful for the school curriculum and the relationship between hospices and school communities (Paul et al. 2016). Four activities were subsequently co-created, piloted, and then delivered as part of normal service delivery at both the hospice and participating schools. These innovations include:

- The Resilience Project – an education program for all 9–12-year-olds that aims to introduce death as a normal part of the life cycle, develop an understanding of what happens to the body at death, nurture the skills and capacity of children to cope when someone dies, and support an awareness of other people's needs when someone dies and how to respond appropriately. The program is delivered over five core lessons but is adapted according to the needs, and questions, of each group of children.
- Bereavement training to school staff – a 2-hour free training session that is offered to all schools in the hospice catchment area. It seeks to assist staff to develop confidence and skills in engaging and supporting children experiencing bereavement while also dispel myths associated with hospice care and ensure that any referrals for specialist bereavement support are appropriate.
- Hospice information leaflets – children and hospice staff co-designed a leaflet that explains the role of the hospice in the community. This leaflet is included in all hospice fundraising materials that are sent to/used with schools so that school staff are able to communicate to children what the hospice does in an age-appropriate way.
- A Schools Bereavement Policy – a document sent to all schools that provides a framework for school staff on what to do if a child and/or staff member is bereaved. The policy seeks to support staff to feel more confident when dealing with bereavement experiences and where to access appropriate support and resources if needed.

Box 6: Role of the hospice in working with schools: a model for integrated practice. Reproduced with permission from Paul et al. (2016)

Role of hospice	Goal	Practice innovation(s)
Awareness raising	Dispel myths associated with hospice care, end-of-life care, and bereavement	Develop existing fundraising campaigns that focus on raising awareness of hospice care
Education and training	Increase awareness of childhood bereavement Develop capacity of school staff to manage childhood bereavement within the school setting and at home	Plan and deliver bereavement training for school staff
Leadership in death education and bereavement	Influence policy makers and/or management teams to establish death, dying, and bereavement affirming activities, policies, and procedures	Engage with school communities to raise awareness of palliative care issues Work with school staff to develop a death and life-affirming curriculum Work with school staff to develop bereavement policies and procedures

These practice innovations sit apart from the hospices previous work with schools as they do not involve the hospice delivering specific services but mobilizing those involved in caring for children to be actively involved in providing support and education around hospice, end-of-life, and bereavement care. The learning about what these activities means for hospices in working with school communities is outlined in Box 6.

4.2.3 Example 3: Compassionate City Charter

The Compassionate City Charter focuses on sectors of society outside traditional palliative care or even health and social care services. The reason for this is the potential hit-and-miss nature of services developed by discrete community interests or services, where some communities may be involved, while others are unaware of the projects. The Compassionate City Charter takes a civic approach by developing a program of work through local governments, mayor's offices, or other municipal agencies and engaging broadly with all the cultural, religious, commercial, or leisure organizations in a locality, both to engage with a broader part of the local community and also to explicitly situate issues around death and dying as outside the remit of health and social care. It then becomes everybody's business.

Kellehear (2016) has outlined the steps a local government should take to develop their local area as a Compassionate City (see Box 7).

Box 7: The Compassionate City Charter (Kellehear 2016)

Compassionate Cities are communities that recognize that all natural cycles of sickness and health, birth and death, and love and loss occur every day within the orbits of its institutions and regular activities. A Compassionate City is a community that recognizes that care for one another at times of crisis and loss is not simply a task solely for health and social services but is everyone's responsibility.

Compassionate Cities are communities that publicly encourage, facilitate, support, and celebrate care for one another during life's most testing moments and experiences, especially those pertaining to life-threatening and life-limiting illness, chronic disability, frail, ageing and dementia, death in childhood, grief and bereavement, and the trials and burdens of long-term care. Though local government strives to maintain and strengthen quality services for the most fragile and vulnerable in our midst, those persons are not the limits of our experience of fragility and vulnerability. Serious personal crises of illness, dying, death, and loss may visit any of us, at any time during the normal course of our lives. A Compassionate City is a community that squarely recognizes and addresses this social fact.

Through the auspices of the Mayor's office or equivalent body, a Compassionate City will – by public marketing and advertising, by the use of the city's network and influences, and by virtue of collaboration and cooperation, in partnership with social media and its own offices – develop and support the following *13 social changes* to the cities key institutions and activities:

1. Our schools will have annually reviewed policies or guidance documents for dying, death, loss, and care.
2. Our workplaces will have annually reviewed policies or guidance documents for dying, death, loss, and care.
3. Our trade unions will have annually reviewed policies or guidance documents for dying, death, loss, and care.
4. Our places of worship will have at least one dedicated group for end-of-life care support.
5. Our city's hospices and nursing homes will have a community development program involving local area citizens in end-of-life care activities and programs.
6. Our city's major museums and art galleries will hold annual exhibitions on the experiences of ageing, dying, death, loss, or care.
7. Our city will host an annual peacetime memorial parade representing the major sectors of human loss outside military campaigns –

cancer, motor neuron disease, AIDS, child loss, suicide survivors, animal companion loss, widowhood, industrial and vehicle accidents, the loss of emergency workers and all end-of-life care personnel, etc.

8. Our city will create an incentive scheme to celebrate and highlight the most creative compassionate organization, event, and individual/s. The scheme will take the form of an annual award administered by a committee drawn from the end-of-life care sector. A "Mayor's Prize" will recognize individual/s for that year who most exemplify the city's values of compassionate care.
9. Our city will publicly showcase, in print and in social media, our local government policies, services, funding opportunities, partnerships, and public events that address "our compassionate concerns" with living with ageing, life-threatening and life-limiting illness, loss and bereavement, and long-term caring. All end-of-life care-related services within the city limits will be encouraged to distribute this material or these web links including veterinarians and funeral organizations.
10. Our city will work with local social or print media to encourage an annual citywide short story or art competition that helps raise awareness of ageing, dying, death, loss, or caring.
11. All our compassionate policies and services, and in the policies and practices of our official compassionate partners and alliances, will demonstrate an understanding of how diversity shapes the experience of ageing, dying, death, loss, and care – through ethnic, religious, gendered, and sexual identity and through the social experiences of poverty, inequality, and disenfranchisement.
12. We will seek to encourage and to invite evidence that institutions for the homeless and the imprisoned have support plans in place for end-of-life care and loss and bereavement.
13. Our city will establish and review these targets and goals in the first 2 years and thereafter will add one more sector annually to our action plans for a Compassionate City – e.g., hospitals, further and higher education, charities, community and voluntary organizations, police and emergency services, and so on.

4.2.4 Example 4: To Absent Friends Festival, Scotland

To Absent Friends, a People's Festival of Storytelling and Remembrance is a Scotland-wide event that is held on the 1st–7th of November each year. The festival was initiated by the Scottish Partnership for Palliative Care, through the Good Life, Good Death, Good Grief Alliance, and aims to empower Scottish society to reassert control of death in their own lives by making it acceptable to share memories and stories of people who have died. The festival has a number of supporters but is not owned by one particular group, instead it seeks to provide an opportunity for individuals and groups to remember people who have died in whatever way is meaningful for them and their communities, in public or private.

Since the first festival in 2014, the range and breadth of activities have expanded and now occur across Scotland. Patterson et al. (2017) detail some of these activities that include:

- Public events that are open to all, such as concerts, storytelling, and poetry events
- Community events that are run by organizations for their own members and invitees, such as activities ran by local hospices, nursing homes, and charitable organizations that encourage the sharing of memories
- Private events that are held by individuals, families, and groups of friends, such as making memory boxes, lighting remembrance candles, and visiting cemeteries
- Online activities, such as using the festival website to dedicate music videos or leave messages on the wall of remembrance

The festival has been subject to an evaluation that identified its potential to engage people from a variety of social and economic communities (Scottish Partnership for Palliative Care 2015). This evaluation also identified that the success of the festival was related to local ownership of the events. The time, knowledge, and skills of the Scottish Partnership for Palliative Care in growing the festival were also highlighted yet this time were viewed as necessary in supporting the promotion of activities that would, in turn, generate wider participation.

5 Summary

This chapter has explored the emergence of new public approaches to end-of-life care and their establishment as an integral component of end-of-life care for the future. The range of approaches that have evolved recognize the diversity of need that exists for individuals, families, communities, and society when faced with issues relating to death, dying, loss, and care: a new public health approach represents a broad inclusive model for meeting these needs collectively. Four practice examples have been provided that identify the breadth of the approach but by no means define the scope, as projects must be locally relevant and tailored. Such activities sit apart from traditional, clinical-based, service delivery approaches by working *with* communities as equal partners to identify and respond to their own end-of-life and bereavement needs.

References

Baum F. The new public health. 4th ed. Melbourne: Oxford University Press; 2015.

Dixon J, King D, Matosevic T, Clark M, Knapp M. Equity in the provision of palliative care in the UK: review of evidence. London: London School of Economics and Political Science; 2015.

Economist Intelligence Unit. The 2015 quality of death index, London; 2015.

Etkind SN, Bone AE, Gomes B, Lovell N, Evans CJ, Higginson IJ, Murtagh FEM. (2017) How many people will need palliative care in 2040? Past trends, future projections and implications for services. BMC Medicine 15 (1).

Kellehear A. Health promoting palliative care. Melbourne: Oxford University Press; 1999.

Kellehear A. Compassionate cities. London: Routledge; 2005.

Kellehear A. The compassionate city charter: inviting the cultural and social sectors into end of life care. In: Compassionate communities: case studies from Britain and Europe. Oxon: Routledge; 2016. p. 76–87.

Knaul FM, Farmer PE, Krakauer EL, De Lima L, Bhadelia A, Kwete XJ, et al. Alleviating the access abyss in palliative care and pain relief – an imperative of universal health coverage: the Lancet commission report. Lancet. 2017;391(10128):1391–454. https://doi.org/10.1016/S0140-6736(17)32513-8.

Lalonde, M.. A new perspective on the health of Canadians. Ottawa, ON: Minister of Supply and Services Canada. Retrieved from Public Health Agency of Canada website. 1974. http://www.phac-aspc.gc.ca/ph-sp/pdf/perspect-eng.pdf.

McPhail-Bell K, Fredericks B, Brough M. Beyond the accolades: a postcolonial critique of the foundations of the Ottawa Charter. Glob Health Promot. 2013; 20(2):22–9.

Sachs JE. From millennium development goals to sustainable development goals. Lancet. 2012;379:2206–11.

Sallnow L, Richardson H, Murray SA, Kellehear A. The impact of a new public health approach to end-of-life care: a systematic review. Palliat Med. 2016; 30(3):200–11.

Sallnow L, Richardson H, Murray SA, Kellehear A. Understanding the impact of a new public health approach to end-of-life care: a qualitative study of a community led intervention. Lancet. 2017;389(s88)

Sallnow L, Paul S. Understanding community engagement in end-of-life care: developing conceptual clarity. Crit Public Health. 2015;25(2):231–8.

Scottish Partnership for Palliative Care. To Absent Friends, a people's festival of storytelling and remembrance: activity and evaluation report. Edinburgh: SPPC; 2015.

Patterson R, Peacock R, Hazelwood M. To Absent Friends, a people's festival of storytelling and remembrance. Bereavement Care. 2017;36(3):119–26.

Paul S, Cree V, Murray SA. Integrating palliative care into the community: the role of hospices and schools. BMJ Support Palliat Care. 2016; https://doi.org/10.1136/bmjspcare-2015-001092.

Temel JS, Greer JA, Muzikansky A, Gallagher ER, Admane S, Jackson VA, et al. Early palliative care for patients with early non-small cell lung cancer. NEJM. 2010;363:733–42.

WHO-UNICEF. Primary health care. A joint report by the Director General of the World Health Organization and the Executive Director of the United Nations Children's Fund. New York: WHO; 1978.

World Health Organisation. The Ottawa Charter for Health Promotion. Ottawa: WHO/Canadian Public Health Association/Health Canada; 1986.

A Public Health Approach to Integrate Palliative Care into a Country's Health-Care System: Guidance as Provided by the WHO

97

Arno Maetens, Joachim Cohen, and Richard Harding

Contents

The following chapter is largely based by on the following publication by the WHO:

World Health Organization. Planning and Implementing Palliative Care Services: A Guide for Programme Managers. World Health Organization. 2016.

The full report can be downloaded for free at: apps.who.int/iris/bitstream/10665/250584/1/9789241565417-eng.pdf

A. Maetens · J. Cohen (✉)
End-of-Life Care Research Group, Vrije Universiteit Brussel (VUB) and Ghent University, Brussels, Belgium
e-mail: Arno.Maetens@vub.be; joachim.cohen@vub.be; jcohen@vub.ac.be; joachim.cohen2@gmail.com

R. Harding
Cicely Saunders Institute, Department of Palliative Care Policy and Rehabilitation, Florence Nightingale Faculty of Nursing, Midwifery and Palliative care, King's College London, London, UK
e-mail: richard.harding@kcl.ac.uk

R. D. MacLeod, L. Van den Block (eds.), *Textbook of Palliative Care*,
https://doi.org/10.1007/978-3-319-77740-5_122

Abstract

Many people across the globe are in need of quality palliative care (PC), of which a majority live in low- and middle-income countries. However, many still see their needs unmet. It is estimated that only 14% of people in need of PC actually receive it. To improve access to PC as a core component of health systems, the WHO developed evidence-based tools on how to integrate PC into national health systems, across disease groups and levels of care. The current chapter provides an overview of this WHO Public Health Approach to Palliative Care, and discusses the seven components that were set out as a practical guidance for policy makers and program managers at national or subnational level to plan and implement PC services integrated into existing healthcare services. The components discussed are: (1) the development of appropriate PC policies, (2) the scaling up and integration of PC into the healthcare system, (3) the improvement of pain relief medicines access, (4) the strengthening of human resources for PC, (5) the establishment of palliative care services, (6) the setting of standards for evaluating PC services, and (7) the costing of PC services.

1 The Need for Palliative Care Globally

Every year, an estimated 20 million people globally are in need of palliative care in the last year of their life, with even more requiring palliative care in their preceding years (Connor and Bermedo 2014). Of these people in need, 78% live in low- and middle-income countries. For children, 98% of those needing palliative care live in low- and middle-income countries, with almost half of them living in Africa. For these children, the evidence of models and outcomes of care is very scarce (Harding et al. 2014a). In 2014, it was estimated that only 14% of people needing palliative care at the end of life actually receive it. An analysis of global palliative care provision found that 33% of countries had no known activity (Connor and Bermedo 2014). In recent years the field of global health has begun to address the underdeveloped field of palliative care, with growing evidence of need, models, and outcomes that are appropriate for local health systems (Harding and Higginson 2014).

With other organizations, the WHO sees access to palliative care as a fundamental right. In 2014, the first ever global resolution on palliative care, WHA 67.19, called upon WHO and member states to improve access to palliative care as a core component of health systems, with an emphasis on primary health care and community-/home-based care. Member states have requested WHO to develop evidence-based tools on integrating palliative care into national health systems, across disease groups and levels of care. This has been further strengthened by the WHO universal health coverage (UHC) policy which “means that all people have access to the health services they need (prevention, promotion, treatment, rehabilitation and palliative care) without the risk of financial hardship when paying for them” (World Health Organization 2018a). The current chapter provides an overview of the approach and practical guidance suggested by the WHO for policy-makers or program managers at national or subnational level to plan and implement palliative care services, integrated into existing health-care services. It is a condensed version of the WHO document “Planning and Implementing Palliative Care Services: A Guide for Programme Managers” (World Health Organization 2016). In proposing the approaches, the WHO has paid specific attention to feasibility for low- and middle-income settings.

2 Definitions

The World Health Organization has defined palliative care as an approach that improves the quality of life of patients (adults and children) and their families who are facing problems associated with life-threatening illness (World Health Organization 2018b). It prevents and relieves suffering through the early identification, correct assessment, and treatment of pain and other problems. Palliative care is the prevention and relief of suffering of any kind – physical, psychological, social, or spiritual – experienced by adults and children living with life-limiting health problems. It promotes dignity, quality of life, and adjustment to progressive illnesses, using best available evidence.

Palliative care for children represents a special field in relation to adult palliative care. Palliative care for children is the active total care of the child's body, mind, and spirit and also involves giving support to the family. It begins when illness is diagnosed and continues regardless of whether or not a child receives treatment directed at the disease.

Primary palliative care refers to the core elements of palliative care (e.g., aligning treatment with a patient's preferences, basic symptom management) that are provided by all physicians and health-care workers caring for chronically or terminally ill patients.

Specialist or specialized palliative care refers to palliative care provided by health-care professionals or teams that mostly care for chronically or terminally ill patients, are specialized in addressing more complex palliative care needs (e.g., negotiating a difficult family meeting, addressing hidden existential distress, and managing refractory symptoms), and have received specific training for these skills (Quill and Abernethy 2013).

The published strategy builds on the WHO Public Health Strategy pioneered in the 1990s (Stjernswärd et al. 2007). The strategy assumes a responsibility for national health systems to include palliative care in the continuum of care for people with serious chronic, life-limiting health problems, linking it to prevention, early detection, and treatment programs. A good palliative care system is one that is integrated into primary health care, community- and home-based care, but also into informal care, such as care provided by family and community volunteers. Integrated palliative care implies that specialist palliative care is just one component of palliative care service delivery. All health-care providers are to be trained in pain management and the needs of patients with life-threatening illness.

A comprehensive approach to strengthening palliative care requires addressing **seven essential components:**

1. The development of appropriate (national) palliative care *policies*
2. *Scaling up and integration* of palliative care into the health-care system
3. Improving access to *medicines* for pain relief (especially oral morphine) and to palliative care
4. Strengthening *human resources* for palliative care (i.e., education of policy-makers, health-care workers, and the public)
5. Establishing palliative care *services* in accordance with the principles of universal health coverage
6. Setting standards and *evaluating* palliative care services
7. *Costing* palliative care services

3 Core Aspects of the WHO Public Health Approach for Palliative Care

What constitutes a comprehensive public health strategy?

All these components of the comprehensive approach are addressed below, with a more detailed elaboration on how to develop policies, establish services, and integrate palliative care into the health-care system.

3.1 Component 1: Developing a Palliative Care Policy (Including Assessment of the Current Situation)

A first essential element of a comprehensive approach is to develop appropriate palliative care policies. A palliative care policy can take many forms. Whether it is a stand-alone policy, part of a national health plan, or an element of a national NCD, HIV/AIDS, or cancer control strategy, the principles remain the same.

A national palliative care policy should seek to address the following elements:

- Service delivery through a continuum of care (through primary health care, community- and home-based care, and specialist palliative care services)
- Strategies to provide palliative care to all patients in need (e.g., noncommunicable diseases, HIV/AIDs, tuberculosis, older adults, children) and with attention to reaching vulnerable groups (e.g., poor, ethnic minorities, people living in institutions)
- Defining the government–civil society interface in establishment and delivery of palliative care
- Universal coverage of palliative care, through financing and insurance mechanisms
- Ensuring support for carers and families (social protection)
- Identification and allocation of resources for palliative care
- Development of national standards and mechanisms to improve quality of palliative care (see also component 6)
- Setting up a monitoring of palliative care need, access, and quality (e.g., by identifying indicators), at national and subnational levels (see also component 6)

When planning the policy, it is important to involve partners who can provide helpful input, assistance, and maybe funding:

- The Ministry of Health, but other ministries may also become involved.
- Health workers and their professional bodies.
- Social workers (or their organizations).
- NGOs.
- Academic institutions.
- National ethics committees.
- Funding bodies (including potentially private-sector groups).
- International partners should also be considered (especially the WHO country office, but also representatives of other United Nations agencies, international NGOs working on palliative care, and international technical experts).

Development of a palliative care policy takes a step-by-step approach, in order to make sure that all concerns are taken into account and that there is sufficient support and a firm legal basis. Figure 1 provides an example of what this stepwise process is likely to involve.

Ideally, developing a palliative care policy should begin with an assessment of the current situation and a description of the population in need for palliative care. A needs assessment survey can be adapted to the different levels of existing information in countries. It is important to consider factors such as the following:

- *The policy situation related to palliative care:* Has palliative care been included in any major health policy documents (e.g., national health strategies, national cancer control plans, HIV plans, healthy aging strategies)?
- *Availability and coverage of existing palliative care services:* Where are palliative care services currently delivered (e.g., types of patients, in which geographical areas, at what cost)? What dimensions of care are provided? How many patients currently receive care?
- *Current availability of palliative medicines:* Are all essential palliative care medications for adults (World Health Organization 2015a) and children (World Health Organization 2015b) available in the country, including oral morphine and liquid formulations? What is the availability and affordability of opioids

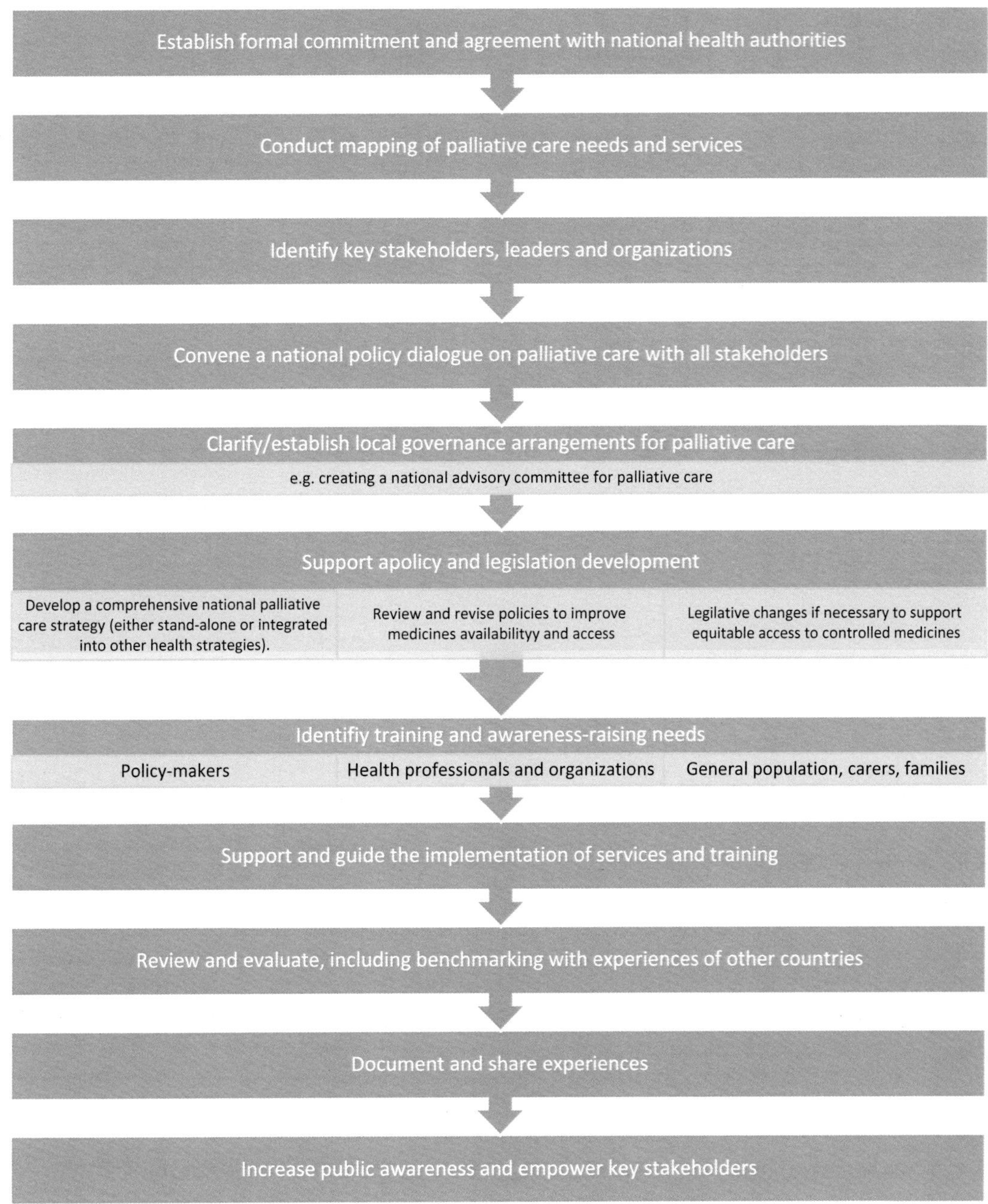

Fig. 1 Example of a stepwise process for developing palliative care strategies and programs

for pain relief and what restrictions are in place? However, evaluation of innovative programs to roll out opioids such as the Ugandan program (Merriman and Harding 2010) found that following enactment of policies to enable opioid availability, supply problems persisted due to unwillingness to prescribe (Logie and Harding 2005).

- *Quantitative estimate of the need for palliative care:* Several approaches to determining the number of persons needing palliative care can be used (see Box 1 below). The health workforce and the number of inpatient beds/services needed to meet the need also need to be estimated.

- *Qualitative assessment*, e.g., interviews with patients and their families to identify any unmet needs for care as well as strengths, weaknesses, and barriers of the current system. This allows evaluating the capacity of key services (e.g., primary care, hospitals) for providing palliative care and identifying settings that can help in implementing actions decided upon.

Box 1 Useful Methods for Calculating Population Need for Palliative Care

There are a number of ways to estimate the numbers of people in a population who are likely to need palliative care at any one time, and several approaches have been proposed (Higginson et al. 2007; Murtagh et al. 2014):

– *Estimates based on disease prevalence*: The WHO has used a method (based on prevalence of pain) for estimating the proportion of people with various diseases who require palliative care in the last year of their lives (Connor and Bermedo 2014). This method can be used for adults and children. The need for palliative care at the end of life should be doubled to account for patients needing palliative care prior to the last year of life.
– *Estimates based on mortality*: Death registration data, where there is reliable reporting, can give good estimates of the population-based need for palliative care without the need for symptom or hospital activity data. Methods used in 14 middle- to high-income countries estimate that 38–74% of those who die need palliative care (Morin et al. 2017).

3.2 Component 2: Developing a Strategy to Gradually Scale Up and Integrate Palliative Care into the Health-Care System

Based on the needs assessment, a plan will be developed for scaling up coverage of palliative care services in the population. The WHO advises to plot a timeline that projects the growth in what percentage of need is being met every year. The plan clearly identifies where the need is greatest geographically and where resources already exist.

Again, there is not one single approach to expanding coverage: expanding from population centers to rural areas, from regional centers to other centers, from private to public providers, and from states or districts to national strategies are all possible scaling up strategies.

In the absence of any system of palliative care, a stepwise approach to introducing a palliative care program is advised covering policy actions, health-care financing, service delivery, workforce development, access to medicines, and information and research.

These strategies must take into account the WHO building blocks of health systems, which in palliative care take into account finance (to ensure services are part of the mainstream health system), workforce (training in palliative care), governance (to ensure that opioid restrictions are well adhered to), information systems (to understand outcomes of care), and access to essential medicines (which is a common problem at all stages of the WHO pain ladder) (Harding et al. 2014b).

3.3 Component 3: Improving Access to Medicines for Pain Relief and Palliative Care

The national medicine policy needs to use the concept of essential medicines. This will help to set priorities for the health-care system, promote equity and sustainability in the pharmaceutical sector, and provide a framework for identifying national goals and commitments.

Table 1 WHO model list of essential medicines for palliative care (extract from the detailed list, limited to only the drug types; for details see the published WHO strategy document World Health Organization 2015b)

		General	Children
Non-opioids and non-steroidal anti-inflammatory medicines (NSAIMs)	Acetylsalicylic acid	X	
	Ibuprofen	X	X
	Paracetamol	X	X
Opioid analgesics	Codeine	X	
	Morphine (alternatives limited to hydromorphone and oxycodone)	X	X
Medicines for other common symptoms in palliative care	Amitriptyline	X	X
	Cyclizine	X	X
	Dexamethasone	X	X
	Diazepam	X	X
	Docusate sodium	X	X
	Fluoxetine	X	X
	Haloperidol	X	
	Hyoscine butylbromide	X	
	Hyoscine hydrobromide	X	X
	Lactulose	X	X
	Loperamide	X	
	Metoclopramide	X	
	Midazolam	X	X
	Ondansetron	X	X
	Senna	X	X

Source: Adapted from World Health Organization 2015b

To determine what are the essential medicines, the WHO has published model lists of essential medicines for palliative care in adults and in children (see Table 1). They include medicines for pain relief and for the most common symptoms in palliative care. From these model lists, countries, regions, or districts can propose a list of essential medicines that is in line with their own needs (cfr. component 1) and resources. When an essential medicine list is finalized, it should be made widely available. The intended use, legitimacy, and authority of the list should be clear to all.

A next step is access to the medicines for those in need. The vast majority of patients with palliative care needs do not have access to essential medicines. Countries should, therefore, implement strategic plans to ensure access to many medications, including internationally controlled medications. The WHO has published guidelines to help countries to develop and implement a policy to make these medicines available to all those who need it (World Health Organization 2015a).

Continuing barriers to opioid availability for medical use in, for instance, sub-Saharan Africa include overly restrictive controlled medicines' laws; use of stigmatizing language in key documents; inaccurate actual opioid consumption estimation practices; knowledge gaps in the distribution, storage, and prescription of opioids; critical shortage of prescribers; and high out-of-pocket financial expenditures for patients against a backdrop of high levels of poverty (Namisango et al. 2017).

3.4 Component 4: Strengthening Human Resources for Palliative Care

The fourth component of the comprehensive strategy is concerned with training and education. Increasing the skills and awareness of palliative care among the health workforce is critical to improving access to and quality of palliative care. While specialist training in palliative care is important, a basic training in palliative care principles and good pain management should also be implemented for all health professionals by integrating it into their training. Because most practicing health professionals have received limited or no training in palliative care in their preservice training, strategies should also include in-service training.

Because much of the care for dying persons and those with advanced chronic conditions with palliative care needs will occur in the community and in various health-care settings (see Fig. 2) and will include health professionals who are generalists and not specialist practitioners, palliative care training in primary care and community care is essential. This training should include a focus on increasing the ability for primary care professionals to identify people potentially in need of palliative care.

The WHO strategies to strengthen human resources for palliative care assume that different health workers are able to perform palliative care tasks safely and effectively (see Table 2). The level of skills, and hence the level of training required for different types of health providers as suggested by the WHO, can be as follows:

- *Expert palliative care skills* for specialist palliative care professionals who will work in specialized palliative care units and will help to train others
- *Advanced palliative care skills* for health-care professionals seeing a large number of patients with advanced illnesses – e.g., cancer, HIV/AIDS, dementia
- *Core palliative care skills* for all health-care professionals – e.g., doctors, nurses, pharmacists, social workers, psychologists (including trainees and practicing professionals)

Ensuring that core tasks and skills are built requires training to various health-care professionals and to informal carers:

- *All palliative care providers* have a responsibility for communication and smooth information transfer and need training in management of both physical and emotional problems, as well as in communication.
- *Community health workers and other community workers dedicated to palliative care* have a range of tasks related to assisting other members of the palliative care team as well as giving guidance and support to the patient and family members, e.g., including developing an individualized home-based care plan for each patient, routinely conducting comprehensive assessments of palliative care needs, answering questions and providing information, providing treatments and instructing the family in this task, training the patient and family in care and comfort-giving

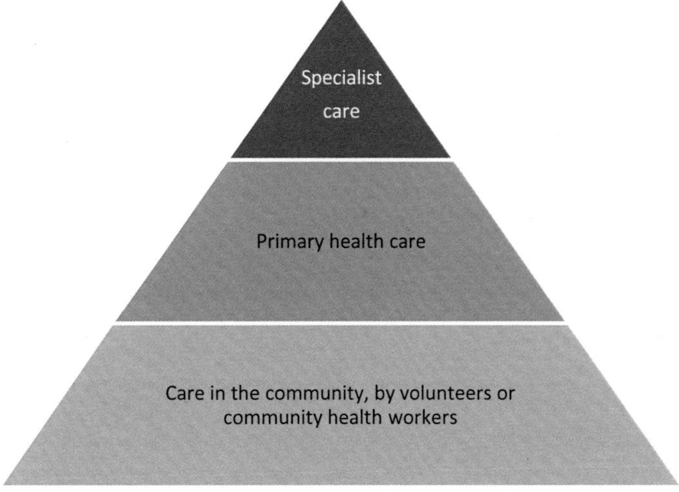

Fig. 2 Where palliative care is provided. (Source: adapted from Kumar and Numpeli 2005 and Government of India 2014)

Table 2 Trained health workers are able to perform palliative care tasks safely and effectively

	Medical doctor	Non-physician clinician	Nurse	Community health worker
Pain management				
Conduct pain assessment(s)	x	x	x	x
Treat mild, moderate, and severe pain using chronic pain management guidelines, including oral morphine	x	x	x	
Teach the patient and caregiver how to give pain medicine, including oral morphine	x	x	x	x
Prevent, recognize, and treat the side effects of pain medications	x	x	x	
Advise on non-pharmacological methods of controlling pain	x	x	x	x
Treat extreme, nonresponsive pain appropriately, including through the use of steroids where indicated	x	x		
Symptom management				
Manage other common symptoms (weight loss, nausea, fever, diarrhea, trouble sleeping, anxiety, etc.)	x	x	x	
Psychosocial support and end-of-life care				
Counseling, psychosocial and spiritual support	x	x	x	x
Support for the patient at end of life	x	x	x	x
Support for caregivers, family members, and children	x	x	x	x
Supervision				
Supervise non-physician clinicians, nurses, and community health workers in above activities	x			
Supervise nurses and community health workers in above activities	x	x		
Supervise community health workers in above activities	x	x	x	

Source: WHO guidelines on task shifting (Task shifting: rational redistribution of tasks among health workforce teams 2008)

procedures, and checking that they are being carried out.

- *Staff nurses at primary, secondary, and tertiary care facilities* have a range of supervisory, coordination, and teaching roles, provide specialist nursing procedures such as care of lymphedema and stoma, and ensure documentation of home care.
- *Physicians and authorized prescribers at primary and secondary care facilities* are able to provide management of severe symptoms, prescribe medicines, and train and advise staff, patients, and families.
- *Providers at tertiary care level (including the hospital)* are skilled to provide inpatient care for patients with intractable pain and other symptoms, including, e.g., radiotherapy and other treatments available only at this level. They are able to maintain patients pain-free.
- *Family* has to understand the nature and prognosis of the disease and recommended treatment. It is the health worker's role to ensure this, to involve the family in joint decision-making, and to guide the family in best practices of palliative care. Both family and other informal carers can be taught to provide home-based care.

Finally, an effort should also be made in educating the public and policy-makers to make sure that they understand what it is, who can use it, and how to benefit from it. This will increase the chance that people who need palliative care will ask for it and access it. One strategy includes involvement of the media to disseminate information of educational value while avoiding sensationalism.

3.5 Component 5: Establishing Palliative Care Services

Establishing and implementing palliative care services is a next core component of the comprehensive strategy. Before establishing palliative care services, it is good to determine the minimum tasks of palliative care services.

3.5.1 Minimum Tasks of Services

Palliative care services can be provided in any health-care setting and also in patients' homes and should at a minimum:

- Identify patients who could benefit from palliative care.
- Assess and reassess patients for physical, emotional, social, and spiritual distress, and (re) assess family members for emotional, social, or spiritual distress.
- Relieve pain and other distressing physical symptoms.
- Address spiritual, psychological, and social needs.
- Care for families and caregivers.
- Clarify the patient's values and determine culturally appropriate goals of care.

The essential practices for palliative care include physical care, psychological/emotional/spiritual care, care planning and coordination, and communication.

(i) *Identifying who could benefit from palliative care and assessing and reassessing needs*

First, a system of timely identification of palliative care needs to become a feature of all health-care settings. Pain that disrupts daily life activities, breathlessness at rest, or functional decline can, for instance, be clinical indicators that result in further palliative care assessment. A multidimensional assessment of physical, emotional, social, spiritual, and cultural needs, values, and preferences of both patients and families is then needed. This can be done with validated short screening instruments such as the Edmonton Symptom Assessment Scale (ESAS) and the Palliative Outcome Score (POS) as adapted by the African Palliative Care Association (African POS). As needs can change, assessments should be repeated regularly throughout the course of the disease.

(ii) *Relieving pain and other symptoms*

Palliative care services need to treat pain and other symptoms experienced by adults and children and should aim to maintain or improve the quality of life and optimize physical and cognitive function throughout the course of illness. This requires (1) treatment of the underlying causes of symptoms (respecting a balance between expected benefit and burden from the intervention), pharmacological (see list of essential medicines above) and/or non-pharmacological (e.g., mouth or skin care, lymphatic drainage, physiotherapy) treatment of any symptom, and attention to each patient's values and needs. The patient and/or family caregivers, as appropriate, should be involved in decision-making about the treatment plan. A key task for low- and middle-income countries is to ensure that the relief of pain and symptoms is evidenced – it is not enough to develop and deliver services; their outcomes must be proven at the individual and facility level. This has been successfully achieved in sub-Saharan Africa (Defilippi and Downing 2013).

(iii) *Addressing spiritual, psychological, and social needs*

Palliative care services pay attention to the psychological, emotional, social, and financial well-being of patients and family members. Bereavement support is also a core component of palliative care. In low- and middle-income countries, spiritual concerns may be the greatest contributing factor to quality of life in advanced illness (Selman et al. 2011), and caring for a family member can push poor families into greater poverty (Streid et al. 2014).

Another core task for palliative care services is to support family caregivers. This includes assessing their needs as they too often have unmet needs and problems including, for instance, physical and psychological morbidity and social isolation.

3.5.2 Setting Up Services

Palliative care services can be established in a number of different ways. There is no single best starting point, and the approaches suggested by the WHO need to be seen as complementary and depending on capacity and context and taking into account the country's social and health system context. However, in all cases, it is important to assess which services are already providing palliative care, including in the nongovernmental sector, and to build on these existing resources.

Depending on the local situation, a country may, for instance, decide to begin by:

1. Setting up a palliative home-care service or integrating palliative home care into existing home-care services
2. Establishing palliative care in a community setting
3. Integrating palliative care services into a district or general hospital
4. Establishing a palliative care service for children, including neonates
5. Setting up a stand-alone palliative care center or hospice
6. Taking an integrated approach in a district

Table 3 provides an overview of different categories of palliative care services. The WHO manual provides a guideline for establishing each of these services.

Setting Up a Palliative Home-Care Service or Integrating Palliative Home Care into Existing Home-Care Services

Home-based palliative care provides care to people with chronic, life-limiting health problems such as cancer; advanced cardiac, renal, and respiratory diseases; HIV/AIDS; and chronic neurological disorders, in the home in which the patient lives. It is best delivered by a multidisciplinary team trained in palliative care, including doctors, nurses, community health workers, and volunteers. A basic home-based palliative care service can be set up quite simple. The minimum essential requirements for a home-care service are listed in Table 4.

Establishing Palliative Care in a Community Setting

Community-based palliative care services are those offered at a community health center or that are run with community participation. Community-based palliative care services can be a way to achieve significant coverage of services for patients with chronic, life-limiting health problems. Wherever possible, this should be initiated in collaboration with the local health authorities and should follow the planning processes used in the health system. Typically these services are provided by both health-care professionals and community health workers/volunteers (Table 5).

Table 3 Categories of palliative care services

		Palliative care		
	Palliative care approach	Specialist support for general palliative care		Specialist palliative care
Acute care	Hospital	Volunteer hospice service	Hospital palliative care support team	Palliative care unit
Long-term care	Nursing home, residential home		Home palliative care teams	Inpatient hospice
Home care	General practitioners, community nursing teams			Home palliative care teams, day-care center

Source: EAPC (Radbruch et al. 2009) adapted from (Nemeth and Rottenhofer 2004)

Table 4 Minimum requirements for a home-based palliative care service

Basic infrastructure	Central meeting point
	Storage facilities (including for controlled drugs)
	Transport for team and home-care kit
	Method of communication (e.g., mobile telephone)
Personnel	Doctor
	Nurse
	Volunteers or community health workers
Home-care kit	Medications (including morphine)
	Equipment
	Documentation
Finance	Salaries for team members
	Transportation/vehicle hire
	Rental for room/storage facility
	Communication and printing
	Medication and equipment costs

Table 5 Key human resources required for a community-based palliative care service

	Tasks	Suggested minimum training
Community volunteers/health workers		
Untrained sensitized volunteers	Provide support to the palliative care service (e.g., transport, food for patients, fund-raising)	Sensitization course (approx. 2 h) covering basics of palliative care, home care, communication
Trained volunteers	Contribute to patient home care, offering:	Basic palliative care course for volunteers (approx. 16 h theory plus 4 home visit days) covering communication skills, emotional support, patient assessment, nursing care, home care, basics of symptom management, reporting to higher level
	Emotional support	
	Basic nursing tasks	
	Help with mobility	
	Reporting of uncontrolled distress to higher level	
Community health workers	Contribute to patient home care, offering:	Basic palliative care course for community health workers (approx. 3–6 h) covering communication skills, emotional support, patient assessment, reporting to higher level
	Emotional support	
	Basic nursing chores	
	Help with mobility	
	Reporting of uncontrolled distress to higher level	
Health-care professionals		
Nurses	Key professionals in the team, providing nurse-led home care and/or care at CHCs	Staff nurses with mid-level training in palliative care supported by nurses or auxiliary nurses with basic foundation training in palliative care (3 months/400 h)
Doctors	Provide medical support and supervision for nurses and CHCs, home visits, and outpatient and inpatient care	Physicians with training in palliative care

Source: Adapted from (Guidelines for developing palliative care services 2009)

Integrating Palliative Care Services into a Regional or General Hospital

In sub-Saharan Africa, 38–46% of patients at a national referral hospital were found to have life-limiting illness (Lewington et al. 2012; Jacinto et al. 2015). All hospitals involved in the treatment of patients with cancer should have a palliative care service, and this can enable improvements in costs and outcomes for patients and families in low- and middle-income countries (Desrosiers et al. 2014). Any hospital that caters for people with other chronic diseases – such as

Table 6 Minimum staffing required for a hospital-based palliative care service

	Role	Capacity/skills required	Position	Availability
Doctor (required)	Team manager/ member	Training in palliative care and communication skills. As a minimum, a course with a theoretical component and at least 10 days practical. Ideally a specialist qualification in palliative care	Regular staff	Full-time or part-time, depending on workload
Nurses (required)	Team member	Training in palliative care and communication skills. As a minimum, a course with a theoretical component and at least 10 days practical. Ideally a more specialized qualification in palliative care	Regular staff	Full-time
Psychologists or counselors (recommended)	Team member	Trained counselor with orientation to special needs in palliative care	Regular/ visiting	Full-time
Auxiliary nurses/ palliative nursing aides	Team member	Assisting staff nurses in clinical work	Regular staff	Full-time
Pharmacist	Team member		Regular staff	Part-time
Social workers (recommended)	Team member	Trained social worker with orientation to special needs in palliative care	Regular/ visiting	Full-time/part-time
Volunteers (recommended)	Additional support to the team	Specific to their role	Visiting	Part-time

Source: Adapted from (Guidelines for developing palliative care services 2009)

HIV/AIDS, chronic respiratory diseases, heart failure, and chronic renal diseases – should also consider a palliative care service. The on-site availability of various specialities and diagnostic procedures makes the care more comprehensive and makes it easier to control symptoms. Hospital-based palliative care also facilitates the discussion of the patient's values, diagnosis, prognosis, and agreement about the goals of care (Table 6).

Establishing a Palliative Care Service for Children, Including Neonates

Palliative care for children includes physical, emotional, spiritual, and social care; it also takes into account the developmental needs from neonate to young adult. The family (including siblings and the extended family) is seen as the unit of care. Although palliative care for persons of any age has many similarities, palliative care for children represents a special area of care. It involves active total care of the child's body, mind, and spirit and also involves giving support to the family. It begins when illness is diagnosed and continues regardless of whether or not the child receives treatment directed at the disease. The role of the health providers is to both evaluate and alleviate a child's physical, psychological, and social distress (Table 7).

Setting Up a Stand-Alone Palliative Care Center or Hospice

A stand-alone palliative care center or hospice may have several roles and functions. When planning to set up such a center, it is important to be clear which function it will have and, if more than one function is envisaged, in what order they should be established. The basic elements of palliative care should be present – medical, nursing, psychological, social, and spiritual support – but the level of care depends on local resources, the availability and capabilities of staff, and their training. Depending on the target group of patients, the care provided may need to include financial support and basic necessities – such as food, utilities, mobile telephone and travel subsidy, and the lending of equipment (Table 8).

Taking an Integrated Approach in a Region

There is no one-size-fits-all public health approach to integrating palliative care into

Table 7 Ideal health workforce for a pediatric palliative care service

	Role	Competencies	Position	Availability
Doctor with pediatric knowledge or pediatrician	Team member and as consultant/attending physician	Palliative care for children; 10-day course includes theory and practical experience	Regular staff	Part-time, as required
		Communication skills with children and families		
		Understanding of childhood development and children's rights		
Registered nurses – preferably with pediatric experience and knowledge	Team members/ coordinator	Palliative care for children; 10-day course includes theory and practical experience	Regular staff	Full-time
		Communication skills with children and families		
		Understanding of childhood development and children's rights		
Staff and auxiliary nurses	Team members	Palliative care for children; 10-day course includes theory and practical experience	Regular staff	Full-time
		Communication skills with children and families		
		Understanding of childhood development and		
		Children's rights		
		Nutrition		
Social worker	Team member for psychosocial care, with access to social security/grants where available	Palliative care for children; 10-day course includes theory and practical experience	Regular staff – not all countries have access to social workers and may use a trained counselor or child psychologist	Full- or part-time
		Communication skills with children and families		
		Understanding of childhood development and children's rights		
Teacher	Team member	Palliative care for children; 10-day course includes theory and practical experience	Regular staff	Full- or part-time
		Communication skills with children and families		
		Understanding of childhood development and children's rights		

(*continued*)

Table 7 (continued)

	Role	Competencies	Position	Availability
Chaplain/spiritual care worker	Team member	Palliative care for children; 10-day course includes theory and practical experience	Ideally regular staff; often a volunteer	Part-time
		Communication skills with children and families		
		Understanding of childhood development and children's rights		
Care workers/ community caregivers for home care and day care	Team members	30-day course on all aspects of palliative care, pediatric care, childhood development and play, and children's rights	Regular staff	Full-time
Occupational therapist/ physiotherapist/ nutritional therapist/speech, play, music therapists	Team members	Introduction to pediatric palliative care; 5-day course	Ad hoc consultants or volunteers	Part-time
Child psychologist	Team member	Introduction to pediatric palliative care; 5-day course	Ad hoc consultant	Part-time
Neonatologist	Consultant or team member depending on the focus of the program and number of neonates cared for	Palliative care for children; 10-day course includes theory and practical experience	Consultant/advisor	Part-time
		Communication skills with children and families		
		Understanding of childhood development and children's rights		

Source: WHO Planning and implementing palliative care services (World Health Organization 2016)

different levels of care or types of services as much depends on services already existing. Nevertheless, there are a number of general principles for success:

- The approach must acknowledge the resources and structures that a health system in an area has at its disposal and respect its values.
- The approach must be dynamic and responsive to the needs of the area.
- It should be based on co-production and co-development of services set in a context of shared knowledge about palliative care.
- Palliative care is not to be seen as a medical approach that belongs only to health providers; it is an approach everyone needs to embrace for effective working in a health-care area.

Palliative care integration requires different steps: invitation, initiation, innovation, and implementation.

Step 1: Invitation
This step requires:

Table 8 Different roles and functions of a stand-alone palliative care center or hospice

Role or function	Advantages	Disadvantages
Hospice home-care service	Can be a very cost-effective service, serving the most patients with the least resources	Less convenient for teaching and training except on a one-to-one basis
	Needs little space – only office space with workstations and storage space for medications and equipment	Difficult for donors to see the service and how their donations make a difference
	Most patients prefer to stay in their own homes; many may not be fit to travel to seek health care	Volunteers do not have a center to meet, as they are scattered, working with patients at their homes
		May be difficult for staff to travel to visit patients in challenging localities or at night
Inpatient hospice service	The environment can be controlled and adjusted to provide hospitable, respectful, and individualized care	Highly skilled medical and nursing care, if provided, is the most expensive form of palliative care, costing as much or possibly more than hospital care
	Patients and families can be given intensive care and support at a level not possible in a hospital, whether it is physical care of the patient or psychosocial care of both patient and family	Patients may prefer to be cared for or to die in their own homes and may not wish to be at a hospice
	With both patients and staff present in the same place, training and education is facilitated	Because of distance, cost, or convenience, it may not be practical for families to visit often
	Donors have a clear view of the effect of their donations	If many deaths occur at a hospice, patients may become unsettled. The hospice may be labeled as a death house
	Volunteers may congregate and have a better sense of belonging	
	It is easier to do community outreach as there is a place where people can meet	
Hospice day-care service	Patients can stay at their own homes and still receive specialized care at a hospice	Transportation often has to be provided unless the family can bring the patient
		Specialized transport (e.g., ambulances with wheelchair facilities or stair crawls) may be needed
	The hospice day care may provide custodial care for the patient during the day when family members are at work, thus enabling the patient to stay at home, at least until such time as the patient is unable to travel	Travel is constrained by travel time as much as by distance
	A good place to deploy volunteers and engage the community	Patients may be exhausted by the time they reach the day-care center
		Group activities may not suit all patients
Education center	Patients are concentrated in one location, providing enough clinical material for teaching	The patient's and family's privacy must be safeguarded
	Groups of trainees may be accommodated if proper facilities are available	Requirement for clinical staff to do teaching necessitates a reduction in their workload
	Requirement for clinical staff to do teaching will drive their own learning and raise standards	Having positions for trained teaching staff involves more costs
Research center	An academic culture is good for attracting staff of high caliber	Research requires considerable investment in time and money. Most clinicians are not trained in research and need to be trained. Time must be reserved for research, and trained staff must be dedicated to doing it

Source: WHO Planning and implementing palliative care services (World Health Organization 2016)

1. Engaging political leadership. Regional health-care bodies are in most cases government entities, structured as part of local and national government. Therefore engaging with the political leadership of a region is an important process.
2. Advocating about palliative care: sustained advocacy about palliative care that is open and explicit, non-threatening and positive.
3. Providing information about need: evidence of need will be required, i.e., informed data that illustrate the local burden of disease, end-of-life care requirements, and inpatient, outpatient, discharge, and follow-up processes. Political leadership needs to understand the current and foreseeable problems if need is not addressed. Those who can best inform leaders of the need are the staff of hospitals, health centers and clinics, persons living with non-curable illnesses, their caregivers, local faith communities, educators, and local businesses – all of whom interact directly or indirectly with individuals who need care. Data are often available through health information systems, hospital and clinic records, records from community health workers and volunteers, NGOs, and private services. However, such data are often neither standardized nor accessible to those who can use it most effectively.

   There are a number of ways to estimate the numbers of people in a population who are likely to need palliative care at any one time (see ▶ Chap. 5, "Development of Palliative Care: Past, Present, and Future").

Step 2: Initiation

Once an invitation (however broad or wide) to develop an integrated approach has been established, initiation of the approach can begin. This requires:

1. Wide stakeholder engagement, including with isolated centers of care. Bypassing existing institutions which have delivered specific care in isolation from the rest of the health service rarely contributes to effective integration. Recognizing the strengths of these individual centers and the challenges they face allows them to become stakeholders in the larger conversation.
2. Making a business case for developing an integrated approach to palliative care by showing how the integrated approach will demonstrate effectiveness and efficiency. Gaps and barriers in services must also be identified (e.g., beliefs about death, views on dying, geographical distance).

Step 3: Innovation

Having created the awareness and the openness to begin developing changes in services, opportunities need to be found to develop and trial new ways of delivering care. Some districts have engaged local businesses to run competitions in schools and companies to elicit innovative ideas on new ways of developing and delivering services and ways of engaging all community members in understanding palliative care.

Step 4: Implementation

Key success factors are likely to be:

- Senior management agrees that palliative care is part of the role of all health workers, rather than seeing palliative care as a speciality that requires separate health workers.
- Palliative care is embedded in the health-care continuum, making it an essential component of primary care. It is seen as a normal health-care activity rather than a specialist one.
- Opportunities in the national palliative care context (e.g., training, financing, legislation, regulation of drugs) are used to build ownership of them at regional level.
- The infrastructure for delivery is in place. This usually does not mean setting up new services but rather uniting separate services and systems to become part of the whole. The system enables services to be in the right place at the right time, supported by people with the right skills and the right resources to care.

3.6 Component 6: Setting Standards and Evaluating Palliative Care Services

All providers of palliative care should be committed to continuous improvement of the quality of their services. Data collected from quality indicators are a primary source of information for improving services. When possible, palliative care services should be able to compare their quality indicator results with other similar services. Services can be compared with similar initiatives in other locations, which will provide the technical basis for political decisions about the development of the service, including the provision of further funding and support. Both the African Palliative Care Association and the Hospice Palliative Care Association of South Africa have developed standards that have been widely taken up and offer useful templates (African Palliative Care Association 2018).

Evaluation of national/regional programs allows monitoring to progress toward the predefined program goals and the targets of different phases, enables comparisons between different population groups, and provides an opportunity for continuous quality improvement interventions in critical areas. Populations with disproportionately high risk factors can be given specific attention.

3.7 Component 7: Costing Palliative Care Services

To cost palliative care services, both direct costs and indirect costs can be determined. The total annual budget, cost per day, cost per patient per month, cost per inpatient day, cost per inpatient episode of care, or cost per home or clinic visit needs to be presented. The highest costs are related to personnel costs, unlike in other health-care services in which the costs of treatments are higher.

The total costs can be compared with the expected sources of funding. Additionally it may be worthwhile comparing the costs to the possible reduction in health-care costs by the establishment of palliative care services. By reducing avoidable hospitalization, emergency department presentations, and unnecessary treatments, palliative care can save health-care resources and costs while providing a better quality of life (Smith et al. 2014).

4 Conclusion

The WHO has developed a comprehensive public health approach to integrate palliative care into a national health-care system that provides policy-makers or program managers at national or subnational level with practical guidance. The seven components of this approach need to be addressed: (1) developing a palliative care policy, (2) scaling up and integrating palliative care into the health-care system, (3) improving access to medicines for pain relief and palliative care, (4) training and education those who hold a stake in palliative care, (5) establishing and implementing palliative care services, (6) setting quality standards for palliative care services and evaluating these, and (7) costing the palliative care services.

The WHO insists that there is no one-size-fits-all approach. A country's specific context needs to be acknowledged and respected. Countries may, for instance, differ in needs, prevailing views and values, availability of resources, basic health-care characteristics, and services already existing. Low- and middle-income countries have an even greater need to deliver cost-effective services that are developed to meet prevailing health conditions, fit within cultural preferences and practices, and are feasible within existing health systems. Therefore, the WHO palliative care public health strategy requires local evidence to inform development of services (Harding et al. 2013).

References

African Palliative Care Association. Standards for quality improvement [Internet]. Quality palliative care integrated into health systems using APCA standards. 2018. Available at https://www.africanpalliativecare.org/integration/standards-for-quality-improvement/

Connor S, Bermedo M. Global atlas of palliative care at the end of life. 2014. Available at http://www.who.int/cancer/publications/palliative-care-atlas/en/.

Defilippi K, Downing J. Feedback from African palliative care practitioners on the use of the APCA POS. Int J Palliat Nurs. 2013;19(12):577–8, 580–1.

Desrosiers T, Cupido C, Pitout E, van Niekerk L, Badri M, Gwyther L, et al. A hospital-based palliative care service for patients with advanced organ failure in sub-Saharan Africa reduces admissions and increases home death rates. J Pain Symptom Manag. 2014;47(4): 786–92.

Government of India. Narcotic drugs and psychotropic substances amendment act 2014. Gazette of India, 2014. Available at http://www.indiacode.nic.in/acts$32#2014/16%20of%202014.pdf.

Guidelines for developing palliative care services. Hyderabad: MNJ Institute of Oncology & Regional Cancer Centre; 2009.

Harding R, Higginson IJ. Inclusion of end-of-life care in the global health agenda. Lancet Glob Health. 2014;2(7):e375–6.

Harding R, Selman L, Powell RA, Namisango E, Downing J, Merriman A, et al. Research into palliative care in sub-Saharan Africa. Lancet Oncol. 2013;14(4):e183–8.

Harding R, Albertyn R, Sherr L, Gwyther L. Pediatric palliative care in sub-Saharan Africa: a systematic review of the evidence for care models, interventions, and outcomes. J Pain Symptom Manag. 2014a;47(3): 642–51.

Harding R, Simms V, Penfold S, Downing J, Powell RA, Mwangi-Powell F, et al. Availability of essential drugs for managing HIV-related pain and symptoms within 120 PEPFAR-funded health facilities in East Africa: a cross-sectional survey with onsite verification. Palliat Med. 2014b;28(4):293–301.

Higginson IJ, Hart S, Koffman J, Selman L, Harding R. Needs assessments in palliative care: an appraisal of definitions and approaches used. J Pain Symptom Manag. 2007;33(5):500–5.

Jacinto A, Masembe V, Tumwesigye NM, Harding R. The prevalence of life-limiting illness at a Ugandan National Referral Hospital: a 1-day census of all admitted patients. BMJ Support Palliat Care. 2015;5(2): 196–9.

Kumar S, Numpeli M. Neighborhood network in palliative care. Indian J Palliat Care. 2005;11(1):6.

Lewington J, Namukwaya E, Limoges J, Leng M, Harding R. Provision of palliative care for life-limiting disease in a low income country national hospital setting: how much is needed? BMJ Support Palliat Care. 2012;2(2):140–4.

Logie DE, Harding R. An evaluation of a morphine public health programme for cancer and AIDS pain relief in sub-Saharan Africa. BMC Public Health. 2005;5:82.

Merriman A, Harding R. Pain control in the African context: the Ugandan introduction of affordable morphine to relieve suffering at the end of life. Philos Ethics Humanit Med PEHM. 2010;5:10.

Morin L, Aubry R, Frova L, MacLeod R, Wilson DM, Loucka M, et al. Estimating the need for palliative care at the population level: a cross-national study in 12 countries. Palliat Med. 2017;31(6):526–36.

Murtagh FEM, Bausewein C, Verne J, Groeneveld EI, Kaloki YE, Higginson IJ. How many people need palliative care? A study developing and comparing methods for population-based estimates. Palliat Med. 2014;28(1):49–58.

Namisango E, Allsop MJ, Powell RA, Friedrichsdorf SJ, Luyirika EBK, Kiyange F, et al. Investigation of the practices, legislation, supply chain, and regulation of opioids for clinical pain management in southern Africa: a multi-sectoral, cross-national, mixed methods study. J Pain Symptom Manag. 2017;55:851–63.

Nemeth C, Rottenhofer I. Abgestufte Hospiz- und Palliativversorgung in Österreich. Vienna: Österreichisches Bundesinstitut für Gesundheitswesen; 2004. Available at http://www.hospiz.at/pdf_dl/oebig_studie.pdf.

Quill TE, Abernethy AP. Generalist plus specialist palliative care – creating a more sustainable model. N Engl J Med. 2013;368(13):1173–5.

Radbruch L, Payne S, the Board of Directors of the European Association for Palliative Care. White paper on standards and norms for hospice and palliative care in Europe. Part 1. Recommendations from the European Association for Palliative Care. Eur J Palliat Care. 2009;16(6):278–89.

Selman LE, Higginson IJ, Agupio G, Dinat N, Downing J, Gwyther L, et al. Quality of life among patients receiving palliative care in South Africa and Uganda: a multi-centred study. Health Qual Life Outcomes. 2011;9:21.

Smith S, Brick A, O'Hara S, Normand C. Evidence on the cost and cost-effectiveness of palliative care: a literature review. Palliat Med. 2014;28(2):130–50.

Stjernswärd J, Foley KM, Ferris FD. The public health strategy for palliative care. J Pain Symptom Manag. 2007;33(5):486–93.

Streid J, Harding R, Agupio G, Dinat N, Downing J, Gwyther L, et al. Stressors and resources of caregivers of patients with incurable progressive illness in sub-Saharan Africa. Qual Health Res. 2014;24(3):317–28.

Task shifting: rational redistribution of tasks among health workforce teams. Global recommendations and guidelines. Geneva: World Health Organization; 2008. Available at http://www.who.int/healthsystems/TTR-Task-Shifting.pdf.

World Health Organization. WHO model list of essential medicines, 19th list. [internet]. Geneva: World Health Organization; 2015a. Available at http://www.who.int/selection_medicines/committees/expert/20/EML_2015_FINAL_amended_JUN2015.pdf?ua=1.

World Health Organization. WHO model list of essential medicines for children, 5th list [Internet]. Geneva: World Health Organization; 2015b. Available at http://www.who.int/selection_medicines/committees/expert/20/EMLc_2015_FINAL_amended_JUN2015.pdf?ua=1.

World Health Organization. Planning and implementing palliative care services: a guide for programme managers [Internet]. 2016. Available at http://www.who.int/ncds/management/palliative-care/palliative_care_services/en/.

World Health Organization. Questions and answers on universal health coverage [Internet]. WHO. 2018a. Available at http://www.who.int/healthsystems/topics/financing/uhc_qa/en/.

World Health Organization. WHO definition of palliative care [Internet]. Geneva: World Health Organization. 2018b. Available at http://www.who.int/cancer/palliative/definition/en/.

Part XI

Financial Aspects and Cost-Effectiveness in Palliative Care

Measuring Cost-Effectiveness in Palliative Care

98

Charles Normand and Peter May

Contents

Abstract

Resources for health care will always be scarce and choices have to be made within palliative care as well as between palliative care and other services. Good choices are based on good evidence on value for money. In principle, we can compare the benefits of all health care interventions using the quality-adjusted life year (QALY) measure. However, there are multiple reasons to question the fitness for purpose of QALY analyses in evaluating palliative and end-of-life care. Tools are needed that measure and value services against the objectives of care, that take account of the wider group of beneficiaries and that value good processes as well as outcomes. Measuring costs and cost-effects in this field faces additional obstacles. Studies estimating the effect of palliative care on costs have identified substantive variation by intervention timing and comorbidity count. A critical challenge is posed by the complexity and heterogeneity of the interventions and populations under assessment.

C. Normand (✉)
Centre for Health Policy and Management, Trinity College Dublin, Dublin, Ireland

Cicely Saunders Institute Of Palliative Care, Policy and Rehabilitation, King's College London, London, UK
e-mail: normandc@tcd.ie

P. May
Centre for Health Policy and Management, Trinity College Dublin, Dublin, Ireland

The Irish Longitudinal study on Ageing (TILDA), Trinity College Dublin, Dublin, Ireland
e-mail: mayp2@tcd.ie

R. D. MacLeod, L. Van den Block (eds.), *Textbook of Palliative Care*,
https://doi.org/10.1007/978-3-319-77740-5_101

1 Introduction: What Is the Purpose of Cost-Effectiveness Analysis?

There is a simple logic to cost-effectiveness analysis. We cannot individually or collectively provide all possible health and social care services (just as few of us are able to buy all housing and holidays we would like), so the best strategy is to provide those services that yield the best value for the resources used. This involves assessing the costs and benefits of all potentially useful services. In our normal lives, we choose to use our resources on goods and services that provide us with the greatest benefits. Similarly, collectively in principle, we should give priority to those services that give the best return. Priorities should be set in order of the ratio of benefits to costs (since this rule provides the highest gains for any level of spending). In principle, it does not matter who the payer is – we should not choose to buy ourselves any services that are not worth the cost, insurance should not cover services that are poor value for money, governments should only fund services where benefits exceed the costs, and for any given budget, any decision-maker should prioritize those choices that provide the greatest value.

To make this a reality, we need evidence on the cost-effectiveness of different services. However, since not all individuals will benefit equally from health-care interventions, it does not always make sense in general to describe a service as being cost-effective or not cost-effective. What we really need evidence on is the cost-effectiveness of each intervention for each type of person and each circumstance. The capacity to benefit from treatment may depend on factors such as the presence or absence of disability and comorbidity and the availability of family support, lifestyle choices and habits, goals, or objectives of the individual. Clearly this heterogeneity in the wants and needs of patients (and their families) poses significant challenges for the application of cost-effectiveness analysis to services for older people and for people with complex needs. These contextual issues are compounded by some of the measurement issues discussed in this chapter.

The use of cost-effectiveness analysis needs evidence, but it also needs mechanisms by which this evidence can be fairly and efficiently used. Even discussing rationing in health care can be controversial, but the reality is that care is rationed in all countries. It may be rationed by ability to pay out of pocket, by insurance status, or by the local availability of services, but one way or another there are some limits to what is provided to at least some people in the population. Since in most cases at least some of the cost of care is paid by third parties (e.g., government agencies or insurance companies), much of the care provided is free or subsidized *at the point of use*. If something is provided free, then naturally people will want it even if it is poor value for money – economists call this problem "moral hazard." From the point of view of the service users, the question is whether the value to them of the service is higher than the cost to them. There are very good reasons for removing financial barriers to accessing some health care – indeed evidence shows that high user fees deter people from using high value as well as low value care, but an inevitable consequence of providing care without charges is that people will choose to use services that are poor value for money in their case.

We see this in the case of some new drugs, which have only a small extra effect on health but a very high cost. Those with insurance and who therefore may pay nothing will naturally want it – for them there is a gain and no apparent cost. Since every dollar spent for little gain cannot be spent on services that provide more benefit, in principle it is desirable to limit use of services that are poor value. Insurance companies limit the coverage of services or in some cases require patients to make a co-payment to limit use. Rationing by government (or government agencies) is sometimes done on the basis of specifying coverage limits, sometimes also by the use of co-payments, and sometimes simply by unavailability of services and long waiting times. Ideally the decision on what should be available for whom should be made on the basis of evidence on cost-effectiveness.

In some services, particularly those aimed at treating a single health problem, the measurement of costs and benefits can be relatively straight forward – we have the trials that have shown improved survival or better health, and this can be compared to the cost. Cataract surgery usually cures vision problems for many years. Emergency cardiology services can prevent deaths and extend life. Hip replacements can restore mobility and reduce pain.

Since the 1970s, a consensus has developed around two dimensions of effectiveness – longer life and better "health-related quality of life" (HRQoL). Using data from various sources and surveys, these two dimensions have been combined into a single measure – the quality-adjusted life year (QALY) (Weinstein et al. 2009). Effectiveness of an intervention is measured by the difference between QALYs for those treated (the number of years of life, adjusted to account for HRQoL) and the number of QALYs for those who did not receive the treatment.

It has been argued that this approach has the advantage that the same measures can be applied regardless of the type of treatment and the health problem being treated (Williams 1991). *In principle*, the benefits of a new cancer drug can be compared to those of cataract surgery, and hip replacements can be compared to coronary angioplasty. Life-extending treatments can be compared with ones that reduce disability. In this sense, the approach compares benefits on a "level playing field." There are many new drugs (and many existing drugs), and we can compare the evidence on costs and effectiveness, typically in terms of cost per QALY. While the evidence on effectiveness is not always perfect (e.g., drug trials do not always include older patients so there may be some uncertainty about effects), there is often a reasonable basis for judging if a new product is good enough to justify the cost. The results of cost-effectiveness studies are widely used in setting health-care priorities and for decisions to reimburse new treatments.

It is hard to argue against this approach where the health problems being addressed are simple, the treatments make a difference that can readily be measured, and the effectiveness is easily characterized in terms of extra years of life and improvements in HRQoL with a predictable duration. While there are vigorous intellectual debates about how quality of life is best measured, and how to take account of the timing of costs and benefits, in the context of simple problems and treatments with well-calibrated effects, there is much to recommend the use of these metrics. Equally, it is obvious that where the needs of patients are complex, where evidence on effects of treatment is often lacking or of poor quality, and where the context of patient and carer needs is very varied, it is more difficult to apply this approach (Normand 2009).

2 What Are the Goals in Palliative Care and How Can We Assess Cost-Effectiveness?

What makes cost-effectiveness studies in palliative care difficult is first, that the objectives of treatment tend to be complicated, focusing on both the patient and the wider family and friends and covering domains that are outside what is conventionally considered to be HRQoL; second, the degree to which objectives are met is not easily measured using simple metrics; third, it is hard to characterize the timing of benefits of palliative care since they occur not only at time of delivery but also in anticipation and in the memory of this period in someone's life; fourth, palliative care is often delivered alongside a range of other interventions so it can be difficult to identify the unique costs or unique contribution of palliative care. As will be discussed below, these problems generate significant challenges in the measurement of costs and benefits and can make it difficult to compare the cost-effectiveness of palliative care and other health and social care.

It is now recognized that palliative care is not end-of-life care (although may be of particular importance near the end of life) and is not necessarily an alternative to services with a disease-modifying or curative intent. In many ways, this is a false dichotomy, since good control of symptoms may require disease-modifying treatments and good control of symptoms may be life-extending. Palliative care is concerned with optimal management of symptoms and the best achievable quality of life, and this inevitably bring a focus both on disease and its effects and on wider psychological, social, and spiritual needs of patients and their carers.

There is often a trade-off between the different goals – some people may choose to live with more pain if that allows them to be more alert, and sometimes people will prefer pathways of care that reduce stress on family and informal carers. There may be a choice between different probabilistic outcomes, for example, a very small chance of much longer life, and a statistically longer life expectancy but one where the longest possible survival is quite short. There remains a popular belief that this is commonly the choice, but evidence in general suggests that good symptom management does not shorten life and in some instances may offer survival advantages. The more important point is that there are legitimate choices to be made between different care pathways, and it is quite legitimate to choose different balances of disease-modifying and more direct symptom management interventions.

There are particular problems in people wanting optimal experiences of care – it is not only the services that are used that are valued but also their availability, the linkages, and the processes that people encounter. In many cases, the experience of the processes is as important as the content of care – patients do not expect palliative care professionals to have all the answers but do value evidence of availability, caring, and engagement. In studies of patient and family preferences, a common theme is being able to navigate the access to appropriate care and being free of the frequent system failures that make it difficult to get necessary support (Douglas et al. 2005). People value the services they use, but also value availability of services that do not in fact use, but which are likely to play a crucial role in achieving the optimal pathway should the need arise. Put simply, it is a big enough challenge to have multiple health problems and to be approaching the end of life, and people simply do not want the additional challenge of confronting a complex and apparently hostile care environment.

The implication is that we need to understand the goals of patients and their carers and assess effectiveness against these (possibly complex) goals. Since the objectives are not simply to live longer or to have better (narrowly defined) HRQoL, there is a need to include a wider range of benefits and to include benefits to a wider range of people. In addition, two particular issues have become apparent in assessing effectiveness (Johnston 2017). First, it is not only what is delivered but also how it is delivered that can matter. Second, to a significant extent, people are interested in the whole experience of care when faced with life-limiting disease.

3 Measuring Effectiveness and Benefits in Palliative Care

Studies that have attempted to apply the QALY framework in palliative care have typically found that the measured benefits are small, but when asked, people put a high value on the effects of the services. This is not surprising. Palliative care does not normally contribute long periods of additional survival, and QALYs tend to be driven by achievement of longer life. It is also unsurprising given that QALYs measure only some of the intended quality of life and quality of experience benefits – those that conform to the domains typically included in HRQoL. QALYs typically use quality of life tools that focus on ability to perform activities of daily living and pain. While pain is clearly relevant to palliative care objectives, interventions may not focus strongly on improving mobility and self-care skills. QALYs also ignore benefits to families, friends, and other carers. Similar problems have been found when these measures have been attempted in other areas of complex care, such as in mental health – simple quality of life measurement tools do not measure some relevant dimensions and do not measure others very well (Chisholm D et al. 1997).

There are ongoing debates about how to deal with this problem (Williams 1996; Hughes 2005; Round 2012; NICE 2013; Normand 2012). One suggested approach has been to give extra weighting to benefits that are measured near the end of life – in essence to say that a day or a year is intrinsically more valuable if it is near the end.

This has the effect of making it more likely that palliative care interventions will be deemed to be cost-effective, and as a result more resources might become available. However, it does little to tackle the underlying measurement issues. In particular, it is not likely that this approach will be very helpful in looking at the *relative* cost-effectiveness of different palliative care services, since the tools used remain insensitive to important objectives of care, so inherently they will fail to identify more or less useful care.

Other approaches have used different types of measure that aim to include dimensions of benefits that go beyond those captured in QALYs and include benefits to families and carers as well as patients. This is more promising in that it specifically addresses the underlying measurement issue. A number of scales relating specifically to palliative care have been developed (such as the POS and IPOS), and these help to give a focus on the declared objectives in palliative care, although they were not specifically designed for use in economic evaluation (Dzingina et al. 2017). Other measures, such as ICECAP, aim to be more generic and can in principle be applied in a range of disease and treatment contexts and have versions of the measure that are aimed at carers (Huynh et al. 2017). In principle, the advantages of these developments are that benefits in palliative care can be compared to those of other services, especially other services that aim to tackle complex needs.

A further approach has been to look at the preferences of those using the services (e.g., using discrete choice experiments Malhotra et al. 2015) and to assess the extent to which services delivered achieve these objectives. Some interesting findings have come from this (relatively underdeveloped) body of work. One is that the quality of the process can be very important. People want to know that they can get access when needed *even if they do not in fact use the service*. Difficulty in accessing and navigating the care system is strongly disliked even when the services are in other ways appropriate and effective. At what is often a very stressful time for patients and carers, the additional stress of complex and poorly coordinated care delivery, financial obstacles, and unintended barriers to access increase the stress and reduce the benefits.

There is also some evidence that people can only cope with a certain amount of information and choices and will tend to deal initially only with the most important issues. Economists call this having lexicographic preferences. For example, while there may be high value given to recreational activities and support to improve appearance, these are only valued when people are assured access to good symptom management and support for basic needs. In effect people like to ensure that their more basic needs are being met well before they engage with the issues of their other wants.

There are particular issues with regard to the role of informal carers. Patients are keen to avoid excessive burdens (both financial and caring) on carers and may choose a trajectory of care that suits them less well but suits the carers better. In addition, there is now some evidence that links better care experiences with better bereavement experiences for families and carers, so that some benefits of good palliative care should be measured after the death occurs (Addington-Hall and O'Callaghan 2009; Gelfman et al. 2008). In terms of achieving the best possible bereavement trajectory, good quality experiences of end-of-life care has a key role.

One reason for low QALY scores in palliative care, and some judgments that it is not cost-effective, is that the time over which benefits can be enjoyed is often short. The logic is simple. While cataract surgery or angioplasty may affect health and quality of life for many years, palliative care may affect outcomes only for days or weeks. When asked to value palliative care, patients and families tend to emphasize its importance and substantial benefits, but the short time limits any QALY gain. Even a very large increase in quality of life from 40% to 90% will only generate 0.125 QALYs over 3 months. Even if QALYs are weighted at the end of life (as discussed above), it is unlikely that the measured effectiveness will be large over a short period. One possible argument is that in fact the benefits are enjoyed not only at the time but also before and after the end-of-life period – the knowledge of good care at the end of life may provide reassurance in preceding years, and good care may reduce stress and sadness in bereaved relatives. A more radical approach is to question if in fact units of time can simply be added up. Evidence from economic psychology suggests that they cannot. The work of Daniel Kahneman suggests that people value whole experiences, and a longer experience is not necessarily valued more highly than a shorter one with some better features (Kahneman 2011). There is, as yet, no definitive evidence in the context of palliative care, but this understanding does suggest that new approaches to measuring cost-effectiveness of palliative care near the end of life should try to value the whole experience and not to assume that we can add up the value of packages of time that have specified quality and value.

In summary, while debates continue about the best ways to measure effectiveness in palliative care, and the different innovations are continuing to develop new approaches, it is clear that the nature of the objectives in palliative care, the context in which care is provided, and the wide range of potential beneficiaries make conventional economic evaluation metrics inadequate, and a broader range of tools is needed. This inevitably leads to problems of comparability with cost-effectiveness studies in some other fields of health care. Since all services are in some sense competing for the limited pool of resources, it brings some disadvantages to palliative care if it is not feasible to measure effectiveness in the same ways as those for other elements of care.

4 Measuring Palliative Care Activities and Costs

While there are important conceptual and practical difficulties in measuring palliative care activities and costs, the body of high-quality evidence is growing, and some important results have emerged. The key issues in measurement have been the fact that palliative care is often delivered by a range of specialist and generalist professionals, that palliative care is not always distinct from care with some disease-modifying intent, and that interventions in one setting can affect services and costs in other settings (or importantly to families and informal carers).

Palliative care professional skills are scarce, and in many cases, the best strategy is to use these to encourage other care professionals to adopt a palliative care approach. Time is spent on training and education activities as well as direct advice to care staff, and this can be difficult to record and very difficult to link to specific care of individual patients or families. In general, this important role of palliative care does not get fully recorded, and overall the activity and costs are therefore underestimated.

Palliative care is often provided by teams, and in many cases, team include people with skills across other aspects of medicine and care. From the perspective of estimating volumes of activity and costs of care, it is not always clear where the boundary lies between palliative care costs and other costs. This problem is compounded by the fact that there is no simple boundary between what is and what is not best classified as palliative care.

A more serious difficulty in assessing costs in palliative care comes from the fact that palliative care services in one setting may significantly affect activity and costs in another. When specialist palliative care teams provide consultation in hospital, this affects the pattern of services during that hospital stay but may also affect the care provided and costs after discharge from hospital and may affect the likelihood and the services provided in future hospital admissions. If an intervention is successful in reducing hospital stays and admissions, this reduces hospital costs but may increase costs of community health services and may increase costs to families. Economists call this "cost shifting," since what is happening decreases cost to one payer but may increase them to another. In principle the only way to avoid this problem is to estimate the patterns of services and costs in all settings (including costs to families), ideally till the end of life. The cost of an intervention is therefore the amount spent on it plus any increase in costs elsewhere as a consequence, minus any savings in costs elsewhere.

5 Assembling Evidence on Cost-Effectiveness of Palliative Care

There are good reasons to focus on costs of palliative care in hospital settings, and the effects of interventions on hospital costs, since typically this is the setting in which costs of care are highest. Palliative care interventions can lead to decisions not to receive treatments that, given the overall circumstances, are not likely to be useful. There is good and growing evidence that timely palliative care consultations for patients admitted to hospital with life-limiting disease generally lead to fall in the cost of the stay by reducing expensive surgical and pharmacological treatments (and resulting intensive and high dependency care) (May et al. 2014a). This is (unsurprisingly) particularly the case where the patient has several comorbidities and is therefore unlikely to benefit from intensively treating one disease (May et al. 2016a) (see Example 2). For some groups of patients, it has also been shown that future costs in total are lower following a hospital consultation and that this change in treatment usually improves the experience of patients and families (Bausewein et al. 2011) and can be associated with longer survival (Temel et al. 2010).

The obvious conclusion from this evidence is that palliative care consultations can be effectively free or even have a negative cost, since the total cost (including the cost of the consultation) is lower. Any service with zero or negative costs is inevitably cost-effective if it does some good or at least does no harm. While the objective of this type of intervention is not limited to lowering cost, where it does reduce cost, it can actually release rather than use health-care resources and should have the highest priority. Ongoing studies are seeking to understand where palliative care consultations are most likely to bring gains at no cost, but the current evidence suggests that this is where patients are most frail and have many chronic conditions (May et al. 2018).

While cost-saving services (which at least do no harm) are always cost-effective, there is some evidence that people who receive more palliative care will often have higher overall cost, and better outcomes, and then the question is whether the additional gains outweigh the additional costs. Better outcomes include a lower risk of dying in an acute hospital, improved patient quality of life and symptom management, and better experiences of family and carers. Differences in reported costs are usually small, so the better experiences and outcomes are likely to be considered good value.

6 Conclusion: The Importance of Measuring Cost-Effectiveness in Palliative Care

This chapter has outlined the serious difficulties in measuring benefits and costs in palliative care. The problems in cost estimation are largely technical, and the evidence base on costs of palliative care and effects of other costs is developing well. The problems in measuring effectiveness and benefits are less tractable. On one hand, there is a strong case for trying to present evidence on the cost-effectiveness of palliative care that is compatible and comparable to that presented for other types of treatment. On the other hand, this may be largely pointless, since palliative care outcomes will almost certainly look weak even when there is evidence that they are highly valued by service users. If the measurement tools are not fit for purpose, then they will not provide a robust basis for choices.

But as has been argued at the start of the chapter, resources for health care will always be scarce, and choices have to be made within palliative care as well as between palliative care and other services, and good choices are based on good evidence on value for money. To some extent, the measures used in the standard cost-effectiveness analysis of many other services are not fit for purpose. They have been shown to be insensitive in areas such as mental health and may often be inappropriate when applied to a wider range of services used by people with complex needs. Since more than half of all health-care encounters are for people with two or more chronic conditions, it is likely that the issues that are clearly seen in palliative care cost-effectiveness studies apply more widely. Increasingly the needs are complex, the choices may differ between seemingly similar individuals, and the goals of care can be varied and personal. Tools are needed that will measure and value services against the objectives of care, that take account of the wider group of beneficiaries, and that value good processes as well as (simply measured) good outcomes.

Example 1 Importance of Cost-Effectiveness Evidence: The Case of Ireland

Adapted from: May et al. (2014b).

In 2001, Ireland became one of the first countries in the world to publish a dedicated national policy on palliative care (National Advisory Committee on Palliative Care 2001). The policy recommended comprehensive national provision of specialist-led care, free at the point of use, nationwide. There was broad support for the policy among political leaders and society: palliative care in certain regions of Ireland dates back to the nineteenth century, and the Irish Hospice Foundation, founded in 1986, is active and high profile in promoting high-quality end-of-life care.

Even in this supportive environment, the policy document was extremely ambitious. The estimated annual cost of comprehensive national provision in 2001 was €144 million, requiring more than a three-fold increase in the existing budget of €44 million. Additional to this was the one-off construction costs of new inpatient hospices and other capital facilities in regions that had not enjoyed historical political and volunteer support, and so had limited capacity in palliative care.

Moreover, there was no ring-fenced budget to fund the policy. Rather, funding was to be secured from the general health budget. The 2001 policy coincided with unusually large increases in that budget. Competition for these new resources was fierce after two decades of recessionary spending cuts. The international literature on the economics of palliative care was small and of variable quality, and in the face of competing demands, policymakers in the Irish health service found the relevant evidence on cost-effectiveness to be wanting (May et al. 2014b; Murray 2009).

Significant increases in palliative care spending were observed following publication of the policy, reaching €76 million in 2007 before the start of the Great Recession. But these increases were consistent with funding increases across the Irish health system at the time (Fig. 1).

(*continued*)

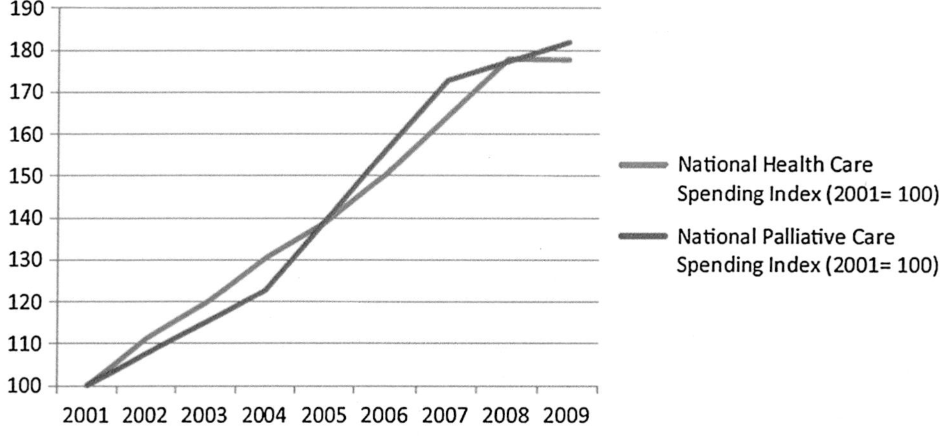

Fig. 1 Health care and palliative care budgets in Ireland (2001–2009)

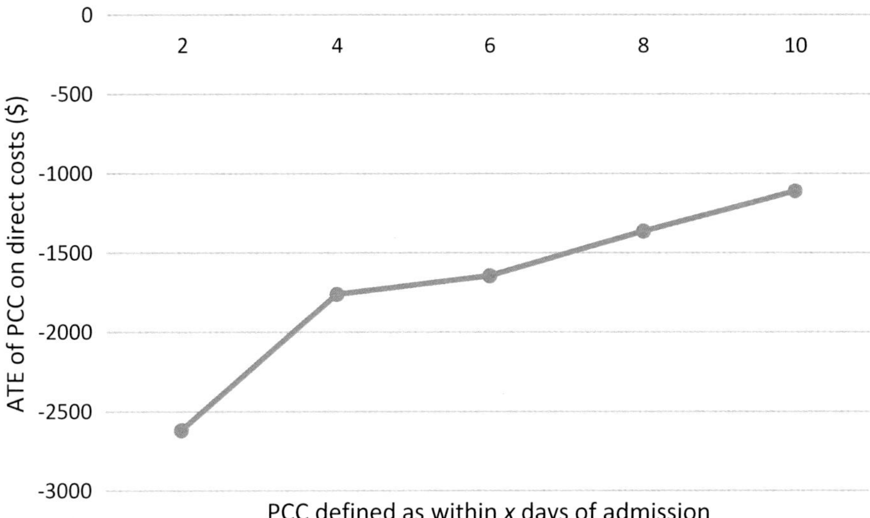

Fig. 2 Estimated impact of PCC on direct costs ($), by time from admission to PCC consult. ATE: Estimated average treatment effect for PCC compared to UC only. For detailed methods and results see (May et al. 2015) or contact authors. Results are robust to myriad sensitivity analyses, details from authors

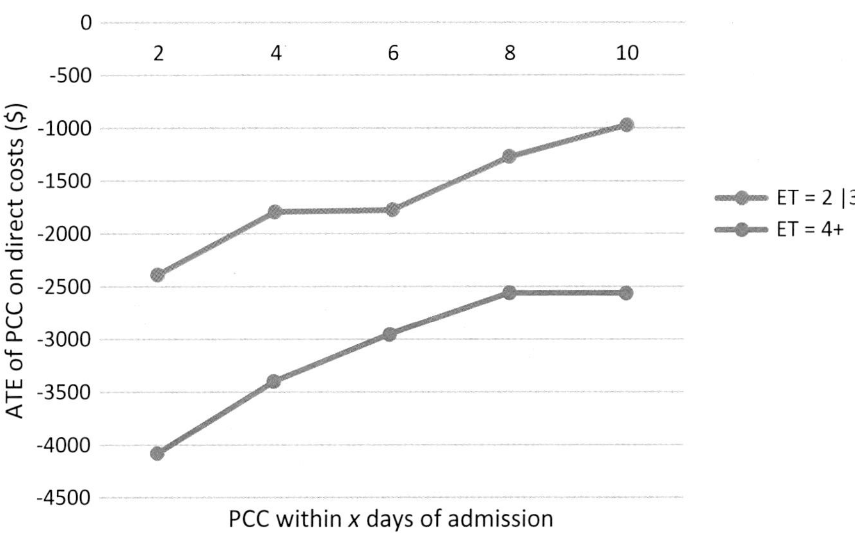

Fig. 3 Estimated impact of PCC on direct costs ($), by time from admission to PCC consult & comorbidity count. ATE: Estimated average treatment effect for PCC compared to UC only. ET: Elixhauser total of comorbidities (Elixhauser et al. 1998). Results are robust to myriad sensitivity analyses, details from authors. Copyrighted and published by Project HOPE/Health Affairs as (May et al. 2016a). The published article is archived and available online at www.healthaffairs.org/. See (May et al. 2016a) or contact authors for details. Results are robust to myriad sensitivity analyses, details from authors

A high-profile, widely embraced palliative care policy at a time of budgetary increase was insufficient to secure palliative care priority status or to realize the ambition of universal provision. Cost-effectiveness evidence was also essential to convince policymakers that new resources would yield most value in palliative care, and this evidence did not exist.

Other factors included a lack of readiness of underserved areas to avail of available funding. There was competition not only between palliative care and other areas of the health service but also within palliative care between different regions of the country. Historically well-served areas were most likely to have representation at the table when policies were being developed and decisions made about funding allocation. Underserved areas did not have the structures and processes, established and well-positioned advocates, and communication networks to seek and implement programs of funding.

Subsequently during years of austerity, the emphasis of policy debate shifted away from "ethics" (i.e., a case for universal palliative care provision to manage pain and symptom burden, and to ensure a good death for all) and towards "economics" (i.e., a case based on the cost-effectiveness of services) (Murray 2011). However, to an economist there is no such distinction. In both times of austerity and surplus, available healthcare budgets must be allocated to those services that provide the greatest value.

Despite enormous strides in the last 10 years (May et al. 2017a; Smith et al. 2014), palliative care requires further evidence to meet this standard and so ensure the widest possible access to appropriate care for the seriously ill.

Example 2 Complexity: Key to Cost-Effectiveness in Palliative Care

In Example 1, we highlighted the importance of economic evidence on palliative care in order to secure funding in competition with other healthcare services. Another important dimension is the allocation of available resources *within* palliative care.

Palliative care is widely recognized as an inherently multifaceted concept – accessed in a wide range of settings, provided by a wide range of professionals, and benefitting a wide range of patients with different diagnoses, prognoses, symptoms, and needs. As such, it stands to reason that different models of care will have different impacts for different populations in different circumstances. Understanding these dynamics is particularly important in the context of staff shortages (Spetz et al. 2016): Palliative care staff are a scarce resource and must be used where they have the greatest impact. Recent evidence from a study of hospital-based palliative care consultation (PCC) teams for adult inpatients has provided new and provoking insights into *when* and *for whom* palliative care is most impactful (May et al. 2015, 2016a, b, 2017b, c).

The results of the timing enquiry are presented in Fig. 2 (May et al. 2015). When the treatment group is restricted to those who received palliative care within two days of admission, there is an estimated $2619 cost-saving associated with PCC. Moving rightwards along the x-axis eases the definition of treatment to include later consults and the estimated cost-saving effect lessens in magnitude and statistical significance. The authors' conclusion, that early palliative care consultation is associated with larger cost-saving effect all things being equal, has been confirmed in follow-up studies (May et al. 2017c; May and Normand 2016).

The results of the multimorbidity enquiry are presented in Fig. 3 (May et al.

(*continued*)

2016a). For a subsample of patients with 2–3 comorbidities, PCC within 2 days is estimated to save $2392 in direct hospital costs. For a subsample with four or more comorbidities, the equivalent estimate is significantly larger: $4081. This disparity remains for other definitions of the intervention along the x-axis: as later consults are included in the treatment group, the estimated cost-saving effect diminishes in each subsample; the estimated effect for the 4+ comorbidities group is always larger than the 2–3 comorbidities group.

From these results the authors infer that, contingent on some basic assumptions about how outcomes for patients and their families are impacted by the intervention, palliative care is more cost-effective for patients with a higher illness burden. More research is required to pick apart the associations and causal relationships, but it is hypothesized that palliative care is more effective for people with more serious conditions because palliative care fundamentally reflects complex decision-making and is an approach more appropriate in more complex cases than a single-disease-focused alternative.

As the field of palliative care looks to grapple with the challenges of cost-effectiveness in the field, a critical factor is going to be complexity and heterogeneity of everything: differences among complex patient groups; differences between interventions in terms of timing, settings, and skill mix; and differences in how those interventions effect those populations.

References

Addington-Hall JM, O'Callaghan AC. A comparison of the quality of care provided to cancer patients in the UK in the last three months of life in in-patient hospices compared with hospitals, from the perspective of bereaved relatives: results from a survey using the VOICES questionnaire. Palliat Med. 2009;23(3):190–197. https://doi.org/10.1177/0269216309102525.

Bausewein C, Daveson BA, Benalia H, Simon ST, Higginson IJ. Outcome measurement in palliative care: the essentials. London: King's College London; 2011.

Chisholm D, Healey A, Knapp M. QALYs and mental health care. Soc Psychiatry Psychiatr Epidemiol. 1997;32(2):68–75.

Douglas HR, Normand CE, Higginson IJ, Goodwin DM. A new approach to eliciting patients' preferences for palliative day care: the choice experiment method. J Pain Symptom Manag. 2005;29(5):435–45.

Dzingina M, Higginson IJ, McCrone P, Murtagh FEM. Development of a Patient-Reported Palliative Care-Specific Health Classification System: The POS-E. Patient. 2017;10(3):353-365. https://doi.org/10.1007/s40271-017-0224-1.

Elixhauser A, Steiner C, Harris DR, Coffey RM. Comorbidity measures for use with administrative data. Med Care. 1998;36(1):8–27. Epub 07 Feb 1998. PubMed PMID: 9431328.

Gelfman LP, Meier DE, Morrison RS. Does palliative care improve quality? A survey of bereaved family members. J Pain Symptom Manage. 2008;36(1):22–28. https://doi.org/10.1016/j.jpainsymman.2007.09.008.

Hughes J. Palliative care and the QALY problem. Health Care Anal. 2005;13(4):289–301.

Huynh E, Coast J, Rose J, Kinghorn P, Flynn T. Values for the ICECAP-Supportive Care Measure (ICECAP-SCM) for use in economic evaluation at end of life. Soc Sci Med. 2017;189:114–128. https://doi.org/10.1016/j.socscimed.2017.07.012.

Johnston BM. PhD thesis. Centre for Health Policy and Management, University of Dublin; 2017.

Kahneman D. Thinking, fast and slow. New York: Farrar, Straus and Giroux; 2011.

Malhotra C, Farooqui MA, Kanesvaran R, Bilger M, Finkelstein E. Comparison of preferences for end-of-life care among patients with advanced cancer and their caregivers: a discrete choice experiment. Palliat Med. 2015;29(9):842–50.

May P, Normand C. Analyzing the impact of palliative care interventions on cost of hospitalization: practical guidance for choice of dependent variable. J Pain Symptom Manag. 2016;52(1):100–6. https://doi.org/10.1016/j.jpainsymman.2016.01.009. PubMed PMID: 27208867.

May P, Normand C, Morrison RS. Economic impact of hospital inpatient palliative care consultation: review of current evidence and directions for future research. J Palliat Med. 2014a;17(9):1054–63.

May P, Hynes G, McCallion P, Payne S, Larkin P, McCarron M. Policy analysis: palliative care in Ireland. Health Policy. 2014b;115(1):68–74. https://doi.org/10.1016/j.healthpol.2013.07.016. Epub 13 Aug 2013. PubMed PMID: 23932413.

May P, Garrido MM, Cassel JB, Kelley AS, Meier DE, Normand C, Smith TJ, Stefanis L, Morrison RS. Prospective cohort study of hospital palliative care teams for inpatients with advanced cancer: earlier consultation is associated with larger cost-saving effect. J Clin Oncol. 2015;33(25):2745–52. Epub 08 June 2015.

May P, Garrido MM, Cassel JB, et al. Palliative care teams' cost-saving effect is larger for cancer patients with higher numbers of comorbidities. Health Aff (Millwood). 2016a;35(1):44–53.

May P, Garrido MM, Cassel JB, Morrison RS, Normand C. Using length of stay to control for unobserved heterogeneity when estimating treatment effect on hospital costs with observational data: issues of reliability, robustness and usefulness. Health Serv Res. 2016b;51(5):2020–43. https://doi.org/10.1111/1475-6773. Epub 21 Feb 2016. PMCID: 26898638.

May P, Morrison RS, Murtagh FE. Current state of the economics of palliative and end-of-life care: a clinical view. Palliat Med. 2017a;31(4):293–5. https://doi.org/10.1177/0269216317695680. PubMed PMID: 28281405.

May P, Garrido MM, Aldridge MD, Cassel JB, Kelley AS, Meier DE, Normand C, Penrod JD, Smith TJ, Morrison RS. Prospective cohort study of hospitalized adults with advanced cancer: associations between complications, comorbidity, and utilization. J Hosp Med. 2017b;12(6):407–13. https://doi.org/10.12788/jhm.2745. PubMed PMID: 28574529.

May P, Garrido MM, Cassel JB, Kelley AS, Meier DE, Normand C, Smith TJ, Morrison RS. Cost analysis of a prospective multi-site cohort study of palliative care consultation teams for adults with advanced cancer: where do cost-savings come from? Palliat Med. 2017c;31(4):378–86. https://doi.org/10.1177/0269216317690098. PubMed PMID: 28156192.

May P, Normand C, Cassel JB, Del Fabbro E, Fine RL, Menz R, Morrison CA, Penrod JD, Robinson C, Morrison RS. Economics of Palliative Care for Hospitalized Adults With Serious Illness: A Meta-analysis. JAMA Intern Med. 2018;178(6):820–829. https://doi.org/10.1001/jamainternmed.2018.0750.

Murray E. How advocates use health economic data and projections: the Irish experience. J Pain Symptom Manag. 2009;38(1):97–104. https://doi.org/10.1016/j.jpainsymman.2009.04.017. PubMed PMID: 19615633.

Murray E. Maximizing palliative care provision in economic downturns. Int J Palliat Nurs. 2011;17(1):4, 6. Epub 01 Feb 2011. PubMed PMID: 21278667.

National Advisory Committee on Palliative Care. The report of the National Advisory Committee on palliative care. Dublin: Department of Health and Children; 2001.

NICE. Measuring effectiveness and cost effectiveness: the QALY. 2013. Accessed 21 Feb 2013.

Normand C. Measuring outcomes in palliative care: limitations of QALYs and the road to PalYs. J Pain Symptom Manag. 2009;38(1):27–31.

Normand C. Setting priorities in and for end-of-life care: challenges in the application of economic evaluation. Health Econ Policy Law. 2012;7(4):431–9.

Round J. Is a QALY still a QALY at the end of life? J Health Econ. 2012;31(3):521–7.

Smith S, Brick A, O'Hara S, Normand C. Evidence on the cost and cost-effectiveness of palliative care: a literature review. Palliat Med. 2014;28(2):130–50. https://doi.org/10.1177/0269216313493466. Epub 11 July 2013. PubMed PMID: 23838378.

Spetz J, Dudley N, Trupin L, Rogers M, Meier DE, Dumanovsky T. Few hospital palliative care programs meet national staffing recommendations. Health Aff (Millwood). 2016;35(9):1690–7. https://doi.org/10.1377/hlthaff.2016.0113. Epub 09 Sept 2016. PubMed PMID: 27605652.

Temel JS, Greer JA, Muzikansky A, et al. Early palliative care for patients with metastatic non-small-cell lung cancer. N Engl J Med. 2010;363(8):733–42.

Weinstein MC, Torrance G, McGuire A. QALYs: the basics. Value Health. 2009;12(1):S5–9.

Williams A. Is the QALY a technical solution to a political problem? Of course not! Int J Health Serv. 1991;21(2): 365–9; discussion 371-362.

Williams A. QALYS and ethics: a health economist's perspective. Soc Sci Med. 1996;43(12):1795–804.

Financial Aspects of Inpatient Palliative Care

99

Peter May and R. Sean Morrison

Contents

Abstract

The economics of hospital inpatient palliative care is a subject of significant policy interest internationally. Older people, and particularly those with multiple serious chronic conditions, account disproportionately for hospital admissions (McCusker et al. 2003), and up to half of recorded deaths worldwide occur in hospital (Bekelman et al. 2016; Broad et al. 2013). Hospitalization costs represent the main component of end-of-life costs across healthcare settings (Simoens et al. 2010a). Economic studies of palliative care for adult hospital inpatients suggest that persons who receive palliative care have lower costs and earlier discharge than matched patients who receive usual care only, as well as improved outcomes. Additionally, palliative care's effect is larger when provided earlier (raising questions of when palliative care should be introduced in the trajectory of illness for people both inside and outside the hospital) and is also larger for adults with higher numbers of comorbidities (suggesting that complex interdisciplinary interventions are more effective for complex clinical cases, an insight with major potential policy relevance worldwide).

Further economic evaluations of palliative care beyond the hospital silo to evaluate

P. May
Centre for Health Policy and Management, Trinity College Dublin, Dublin, Ireland

The Irish Longitudinal study on Ageing (TILDA), Trinity College Dublin, Dublin, Ireland
e-mail: mayp2@tcd.ie

R. S. Morrison (✉)
Brookdale Department of Geriatrics and Palliative Medicine, Icahn School of Medicine at Mount Sinai, New York, NY, USA
e-mail: sean.morrison@mssm.edu

R. D. MacLeod, L. Van den Block (eds.), *Textbook of Palliative Care*,
https://doi.org/10.1007/978-3-319-77740-5_102

impacts across whole trajectories of care are needed. Only then will policymakers have the full story on the costs and benefits of complex care for those with complex illness.

1 Introduction

The economics of hospital inpatient palliative care is a subject of significant policy interest internationally. Older people, and particularly those with multiple serious chronic conditions, account disproportionately for hospital admissions (McCusker et al. 2003), and up to half of recorded deaths worldwide occur in hospital (Bekelman et al. 2016; Broad et al. 2013). Hospitalization costs represent the main component of end-of-life costs across healthcare settings (Simoens et al. 2010a).

Thus, hospital care for people with palliative care needs raises major resource allocation concerns. In the United Kingdom's National Health Service, an estimated fifth of hospital bed days are accounted for by end-of-life care (Hatziandreu et al. 2008). In the United States, the 49% of Medicare beneficiaries with persistently high utilization in the last year of life are more likely to visit hospital and receive high-intensity treatments during these stays (Davis et al. 2016). Also in the United States, where spiraling cost of cancer care is a particular threat to the long-term viability of the healthcare system (Smith and Hillner 2011), a third of direct medical cancer costs are incurred in hospital (American Cancer Society 2015). In some cases, high hospital costs reflect appropriate treatment choices, but in many cases these represent avoidable admissions, overtreatment, and delayed discharge (Teno et al. 2013). Palliative care is one mechanism by which inappropriate high hospital costs may be mitigated with improved decision-making by clinicians and their families.

In turn, this poses questions of funding and organizing hospital palliative care provision itself. Multiple models termed "palliative care" are observable internationally. The most common is the interdisciplinary consultation (PCC) team, led by a specialist physician with nurse, social worker, and allied health supports (Morrison 2013; Davies and Higginson 2004). Dedicated units (PCU) where palliative care clinicians lead treatment rather than consulting in are also observable, particularly at large hospitals in the United States (Smith et al. 2012), and there is growing interest in evaluating the impact of palliative care expertise among generalist staff given that not all people with serious and life-limiting illness can or should receive specialist care (Radbruch and Payne 2010). While it is common for palliative care proponents to argue for improved use of budgets within overall healthcare systems, it is also essential resources within palliative care are allocated appropriately, including optimal allocation of hospital palliative care staff.

2 Early Evidence from the United States

The first economic studies of hospital inpatient palliative care were reported in the early 2000s in the United States, where cost-savings were reported from both the PCC (Penrod et al. 2006; Ciemins et al. 2007; Bendaly et al. 2008; Hanson et al. 2008; Morrison et al. 2008) and PCU (Smith et al. 2003) models of care. These early studies played a critical role in the development of palliative care in that country due to an artifact of the system: American hospitals are reimbursed a fixed sum according to diagnosis-related group (DRG), meaning that where an intervention lowers cost of admission, it in turn increases a hospital's profit margin on that admission. It has been estimated that an average hospital in the United States saves $3 million a year through having a palliative care program (Morrison et al. 2011), a significant factor in the prodigious growth of such programs over the last 20 years: 67% of hospitals with 50 beds or more had palliative care programs in 2015, compared to 15% in 1998 (Dumanovsky et al. 2015). There is now almost universal access in large (300+ bed) US hospitals, although access remains associated with geographical region (Dumanovsky et al. 2015).

In 2014, a review of the economic evidence on PCC found a total of ten studies, all from the United States (May et al. 2014). These ten were substantively consistent, reporting similar findings (a pattern of cost-saving in the 5–25%

Table 1 Summary of strategies that control for LOS in analysis of treatment effect on hospital utilization outcomes using observational data

Use of LOS	Definition – potential justifications	Potential problems	Examples from PC cost literature
I. Covariate	LOS employed as an independent variable/ predictor in regression analysis	Use of LOS as a covariate risks introducing endogeneity into analysis, since LOS is not an independent predictor of resource consumption or cost. Rather, it is associated with both treatment (long hospital stay suggests clinical complexity) and outcome (LOS and other utilization data are typically closely correlated), thus undermining estimation of the causal relationship of interest (Amporfu 2010; Garrido et al. 2012)	Whitford et al. (2014)
	Covariate intended to control for:		
	Unobserved heterogeneity, including hard-to-capture clinical complexity. LOS may be a useful proxy for complexity		
	Uneven accumulation of costs, higher costs being accrued early in hospitalization		
II. Sample parameter	Short- and/or long-stay outliers trimmed from sample	Defining a sample ex ante by a factor that is associated with both treatment and outcome risks biasing results and obscuring true treatment effect (Garrido 2014; Imbens 2004). Where propensity score matching is used[a], ex ante trimming is antithetical to the research framework, which aims to estimate a counterfactual using baseline data (Rubin 2007). LOS is not known at admission so evidence of treatment efficacy for a patient group defined by LOS is of limited practical use	McCarthy et al. (2015)
			Morrison et al. (2008)
	Sample parameter(s) intended to control for:		Starks et al. (2013)
	Unobserved heterogeneity, including clinical complexity. LOS outliers may be unrepresentative of the study sample in ways that are hard to capture – removing LOS outliers attempts to make the sample more homogenous		
	Outliers skewing distribution of utilization data such as LOS and cost, distorting and disguising treatment effects		
III. Outcome denominator	Average daily cost (the ratio of total cost to LOS) employed as primary outcome of interest	Estimated effect on average daily costs is of limited practical value because this is a ratio and not overall resource use: a treatment that reduces daily cost by 10% but increases LOS by 50% (thus increasing total cost) is not necessarily delivering desirable clinical or financial outcomes (Weinstein et al. 1996). Per diem ratios change systematically with LOS and must be interpreted carefully (Ishak et al. 2012). If LOS differs between treatment and comparison groups then daily cost (total cost/LOS) is a fundamentally different outcome to total cost	Ciemins et al. (2007)
	Outcome denominator intended to:		Penrod et al. (2010)
	Indirectly limit impact of unobserved heterogeneity for which LOS is a proxy by accounting for long LOS		
	Reduce skew and leptokurtosis common to healthcare utilization data distributions		
	Address specific stakeholders, e.g., a hospital reimbursed a fixed daily rate, who may prioritize average daily cost over total cost		

First published in May et al. (2016) in Health Services Research (May et al. 2016) and reprinted with thanks

[a]All examples cited in this table also used propensity scores to account for observed confounders, with the exception of Ciemins, who used DRG matching to account for observed differences

range, no significant impact on length of stay (LOS), cost-savings accruing through reduced intensity of stay) and limitations (nine of the ten were retrospective cohort studies with no original data collection, outcome measurement, or follow-up past discharge). Important methodological advances were observable across this literature. In particular, later studies had widely used advanced techniques to managing confounding (propensity scoring (Garrido 2014) or instrumental variable (Penrod et al. 2009)) where earlier studies had used simple matching approaches raising concerns about bias (Starks et al. 2009). Later studies had also used nonlinear modeling (e.g., generalized linear models (Manning et al. 2005)) to manage the distinct distributional properties of healthcare utilization data, where earlier studies had not adequately addressed important statistical issues such as the retransformation problem (Jones 2010; Manning 1998).

At the same time, an important limitation was also identified in the most robust of these studies. Common practice had been to control for LOS in analyses either as a covariate in regression, by removing LOS outliers ex ante or by estimating effect on daily cost instead of cost of admission. A summary of these strategies is provided in Table 1. The key thinking behind LOS controls was that in a field where observational designs (and those relying on routine data collection specifically) dominate, unobserved heterogeneity is a substantial concern. In particular, multiple investigators cite the risk that those receiving palliative care are significantly sicker in ways that matching techniques cannot control for, and since sicker people stay longer in hospital, controlling for LOS may indirectly control for illness burden.

However, these approaches also had a number of important weaknesses (also detailed in Table 1) (May et al. 2016). First, defining the analytic sample by LOS has an endogeneity problem: LOS is not a baseline factor but an outcome that itself may be impacted by the intervention under evaluation. Second, such results are not useful for policy or practice because LOS is not known at hospital admission. Third, since policymakers are most interested in the high-cost multimorbid minority who drive healthcare utilization, analyses that exclude complex long-stay outliers are excluding the priority population.

Nevertheless, multiple investigators had found that controlling for LOS markedly improved the performance and accuracy of their treatment effect estimates. This raised the question of which baseline factors are systematically associated with hospital length of stay. Using such factors to characterize and balance treatment groups, and more accurately define the intervention, would improve economic evidence for policy and practice as well as informing future methods in the field.

3 The Importance of Timing

Following identification of the problems summarized in Table 1, investigators on a new prospective study estimated the effect of PCC on costs for the whole sample and when LOS outliers were removed. They found results consistent with prior studies: PCC was associated with lower cost of hospital admission when the 5% of patients who stayed longer than 20 days were removed from the analysis, but when outliers were retained, no association was observable within the whole sample (Table 2). In Table 2, palliative care does not appear effective for a sample of adults with advanced cancer; it does appear effective for those who are discharged within 20 days. However, as summarized in the previous section, these findings are neither reliable nor useful – this cannot inform policy or practice.

They therefore devised two potential hypotheses for *baseline* factors systematically associated with hospital length of stay:

H1: Timing of first consultation. Longer-stay patients by definition have scope to accrue more days and costs in hospital prior to receiving the intervention, utilization that is included in the outcome of interest but that the exposure (receipt of palliative care) cannot impact. Therefore earlier interventions may be more cost-effective than later ones, *ceteris paribus*.

H2: Illness burden of patients. Longer-stay patients have on average more comorbidities and other health problems, potentially creating

Table 2 Estimated effect of PCC on cost of hospital admission, for the whole sample and the 95% of shortest stayers

Sample definition	UC (*n*=)	PCC (*n*=)	All (*n*=)	Estimated incremental effect (95% CI)	*P* value	Implied saving
LOS<=20 days	705	263	968	**−1165 (−2321 to −8)**	**0.04**	**13%**
All	734	286	1020	−117 (−1780 to +1546)	0.89	1%

UC usual care only. Estimates derived using propensity scores and generalized linear model with a gamma distribution and a log link, see May et al. (2016) or contact authors for details. Implied saving is calculated as estimated incremental effect/mean cost for UC patients. Results are robust to myriad sensitivity analyses, details from authors

Table 3 Estimated effect of PCC on cost of hospital admission, where definition of treatment is defined by timing after admission

Treatment defined as within _____ days of hospital admission	UC (*n*=)	PCC (*n*=)	All (*n*=)	Estimated incremental effect (95% CI)	*P* value	Implied saving
Any time	734	286	1020	−117 (−1780 to +1546)	0.89	1%
20	742	278	1020	−902 (−2201 to +397)	0.17	10%
10	750	270	1020	−1062 (−2339 to +214)	0.10	12%
6	767	253	1020	**−1664 (−2939 to −389)**	**0.01**	**19%**
2	811	209	1020	**−2719 (−3917 to −1521)**	**<0.01**	**30%**

UC usual care only. Estimates derived using propensity scores and generalized linear model with a gamma distribution and a log link. For full details see May et al. (2015) or contact authors. Results are robust to myriad sensitivity analyses, details from authors

a situation where a complex class incur intractably high costs that cannot be meaningfully altered by different decision-making via the PCC team (and this complexity cannot be controlled for using baseline data, only by also controlling for LOS).

Using data from a prospective multi-site cohort study of PCC for adults with advanced cancer in the United States, investigators examined H1 by altering the definition of "receiving palliative care" according to time to first consult after admission. Where prior studies had put in the treatment group all patients who received palliative care at any time during their index admission, the treatment group was instead variously defined as receiving PCC within 2, 6, 10, and 20 days of admission. The results revealed a systematic association (Table 3).

The top row of Table 3 is the same as in Table 2: There is no association between PCC at any time during the admission and cost of care. As we move down the table, later consults are excluded from the treatment group, and the estimated cost-saving effect grows. Palliative care within 2 days of admission is associated with a large and statistically significant cost-saving effect.

Follow-up work has since confirmed H1: Long-stay patients by definition have greater scope to accrue more costs prior to receiving the intervention, costs included in the outcome of interest but that the treatment cannot impact. Interventions are more cost-effective than later ones, *ceteris paribus* (May and Normand 2016). Controlling for intervention timing, instead of patient LOS, delivers results that are more robust and useful.

Palliative care for hospital inpatients therefore appears to be what economists call a dominant strategy: Patients who receive palliative care have lower costs and earlier discharge than matched patients who receive usual care only, and noneconomic literature suggests they also experience improved outcomes (Higginson et al. 2003).

4 New Insights from "Early" Palliative Care Economics

The development of timing-sensitive methods in economic analysis of hospital palliative care has led to a series of new insights for the field.

First, and most obviously, the importance of identifying patients with palliative care needs promptly following admission and ensuring early engagement. The association between timing and cost-effect is not linear: costs are accrued disproportionately in the early phase of a hospital admission (Ishak et al. 2012) and treatment decisions in that phase will likely result in some level of pathway dependency (Mierendorf and Gidvani 2014). Clearly this is a concern of the hospital palliative care field more widely – numerous checklists are available to identify new admissions with relevant needs, and much thought is given to improving engagement with primary physicians and their teams – but it is worth remembering that this kind of early engagement is also critical to realizing economic benefits. For the same reasons, palliative care late in an admission does not significantly reduce total cost of admission (although it appears to reduce costs from the point that it is administered) (May et al. 2017a). Palliative care any time in a hospital admission is not a strategy with notable economic benefits, even if it may have clinical ones. Precisely how "early" a consultation has to be following admission to reduce costs is methodologically complex and is yet to be definitively examined.

Second, contrary to Hypothesis 2 (above), patients with a higher illness burden were not associated with a lower cost-saving effect. Rather, the reverse turns out to be true. Follow-up analysis with the same data revealed that the estimated cost-effect of PCC was larger for patients with higher numbers of comorbidities (see also "Example 2" in ▶ Chap. 98, "Measuring Cost-Effectiveness in Palliative Care") (Maynard and Lynn 2016). A subsequent analysis showed that comorbidities and complications are the key drivers of hospital utilization in this sample, and so the increased effect of PCC for those sicker patients represents a key dynamic to improving cost-effectiveness of services to this high-priority population (May et al. 2017b). These are potentially influential discoveries – if complex interdisciplinary decision-making such as palliative care is more cost-effective for the most costly and complex patients, perhaps because management of symptoms and prescribing is more important for patients with multiple diseases, then palliative care ought to be targeted to that high-need population for whom the difference is greatest.

Third, where early studies found no consistent association between palliative care and hospital length of stay, evaluations incorporating intervention timing have found that early palliative care following admission does have a significant effect (May et al. 2017a). Researchers estimated that approximately two thirds of observed cost-savings from receiving a palliative care consult within 2 days of admission accrued through earlier discharge and only one third through reduced intensity of that stay. This finding is important not only in deepening our understanding of how palliative care "works" in reducing hospital costs but also in raising new research questions – notably, what happens to seriously ill people after they are discharged from hospital? Are these cost-savings in fact shifted onto patients and their families?

5 Future Research: Beyond the Hospital Silo and Beyond the United States

The significant contribution of studies to date notwithstanding the balance of evidence remains overwhelmingly in the United States, although exceptions are observable (Simoens et al. 2010b; Hwang et al. 2013). Both inside and outside that country, there remains a large and important research agenda in economics of hospital palliative care in the coming years:

- **Different models of patient care:** evidence to date has heavily emphasized PCC teams, but cost studies of PCUs, where specialist palliative care staff are the primary physicians with responsibility for directing care, have also reported cost-savings (Smith et al. 2003; Eti et al. 2014). Recently a comparison of the PCC and PCU models found that the latter are consistently more cost-saving than the former (Fig. 1) (May et al. 2017c). This difference is hypothesized to arise because consultations are

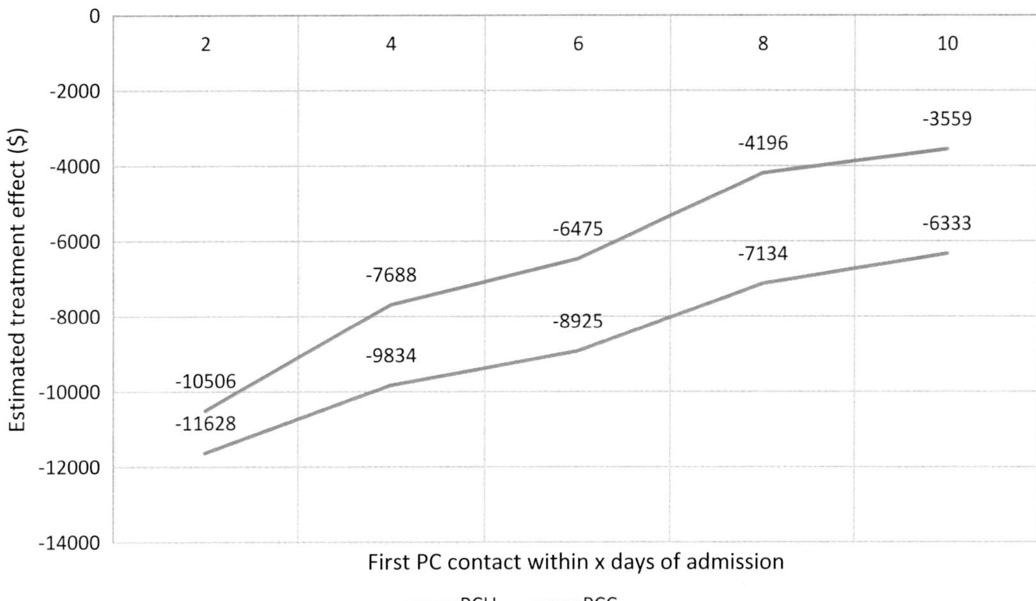

Fig. 1 Estimated treatment effect of PCC and PCU on direct hospital costs compared to UC only, by intervention timing. Each data point represents the ATE of the intervention compared to UC only where first PC interaction was within x days and x is given on the x axis. All ATEs in Fig. 2 are statistically significant ($p < 0.005$). First published as May et al. (2017c) in Journal of Pain and Symptom Management and reprinted with thanks

independent assessments, whereas PCU staff have more complete control over care, including medications and their dosages. This distinction deserves further examination. For example, should hospitals consider placing palliative care teams in direct charge of patient care from the moment of admission as happens with other specialisms in life-limiting illness? One possible location where palliative care staff could take a more prominent role earlier is the emergency department (ED): Many admissions of people with life-limiting illness occur through the ED (Mierendorf and Gidvani 2014; Latham and Ackroyd-Stolarz 2014), yet palliative care integration with the ED is often poor (Kistler et al. 2015; Quest et al. 2011; Elsayem et al. 2016; Grudzen et al. 2012).

- **Planning and education.** Staffing for hospital palliative care teams is found internationally to be underresourced (Spetz et al. 2016; Centeno et al. 2013). And the long-term projected growth of palliative care need is well-known (Etkind et al. 2017). Economic studies that demonstrate improved outcomes at lower costs (or modest increases) for these priority populations can contribute to the long-term planning of training for specialist palliative care staff. Additionally it is worth noting that studies to date exclusively focus on models of care that are led by specialist physicians. But it is surely also plausible that improving palliative care skills and capacity among non-palliative care staff could also yield economic benefits and studies of upskilling and education could be very informative to this set of questions.
- **Interdisciplinarity and complexity.** The recent discovery that palliative care is not ineffective but rather most cost-effective for people with more comorbidities (conditional on some basic assumptions about outcomes) invites further inquiry. This knowledge, which has demonstrable policy and practice relevance, is most plausibly explained by palliative care having its greatest impact in complex situations where disease-specific treatments are ill-equipped to address patient needs. For example, in the setting of multiple chronic conditions or serious illness, the application of

medications to adequately treat each condition may result in polypharmacy and enhancement of side-effects rather than appropriate treatment. Who, then, benefits most from palliative care? There are seven life-limiting illnesses typically observed in the literature: cancer; cardiovascular disease; respiratory, kidney, or liver failure; AIDS/HIV; and selected neurodegenerative conditions including dementia. Is palliative care more effective for some conditions than others? For different combinations of these? For specific primary diagnoses and other comorbidities such as complicated diabetes? At what point in the different disease trajectories are these benefits most realized? The inherent complexities of the population and the decision-making imply an almost infinite combination of important dynamics to be examined.

- **Beyond the hospital silo.** Hospitalizations for seriously ill people are a popular source of policy interest for the reasons cited at the start of this chapter: hospitals are the highest cost environment in which to receive care, many hospital admissions are avoidable or unnecessarily long, and many people die in hospital around the world. Nevertheless hospital admissions represent singular episodes – high-intensity care typically in response to adverse events. As populations age and people live longer with multiple serious conditions, hospital inpatient admissions will become less and less representative of the illness trajectory. Economic studies must broaden their scope to include but not be limited to hospital inpatient admissions, so as to establish when interventions are beneficial across the trajectory, when hospital-based care is optimal and when it is better substituted with care outside of institutions, and how the relationship between reported cost-savings and reported improvements in outcomes is best understood.

6 Conclusion

Economic studies of palliative care for adult hospital inpatients appear as a dominant strategy: persons who receive palliative care have lower costs and earlier discharge than matched patients who receive usual care only, as well as improved outcomes. Significant methodological progress has also been made, which future investigations can benefit from.

The findings from this literature have learnings for the field of palliative care more widely. In particular, palliative care's effect is larger when provided earlier (raising questions of when palliative care should be introduced in the trajectory of illness for people both inside and outside the hospital) and is also larger for adults with higher numbers of comorbidities (suggesting that complex interdisciplinary interventions are more effective for complex clinical cases, an insight with major potential policy relevance worldwide).

At the same time, significant limitations to this evidence remain. In particular investigators must look to take evaluations beyond the hospital silo to evaluate impacts across whole trajectories of care. Only then will policymakers have the full story on the costs and benefits of complex care for those with complex illness.

References

American Cancer Society. Cancer facts and figures 2015. Atlanta: American Cancer Society; 2015.

Amporfu E. Estimating the effect of early discharge policy on readmission rate. An instrumental variable approach. Health. 2010;2:504–10.

Bekelman JE, Halpern SD, Blankart CR, et al. Comparison of site of death, health care utilization, and hospital expenditures for patients dying with cancer in 7 developed countries. JAMA. 2016;315(3):272–83.

Bendaly EA, Groves J, Juliar B, Gramelspacher GP. Financial impact of palliative care consultation in a public hospital. J Palliat Med. 2008;11(10):1304–8.

Broad JB, Gott M, Kim H, Boyd M, Chen H, Connolly MJ. Where do people die? An international comparison of the percentage of deaths occurring in hospital and residential aged care settings in 45 populations, using published and available statistics. Int J Public Health. 2013;58(2):257–67.

Centeno C, Lynch T, Donea O, Rocafort J, Clark D. EAPC Atlas of palliative care in Europe. Milan: EAPC Press; 2013.

Ciemins EL, Blum L, Nunley M, Lasher A, Newman JM. The economic and clinical impact of an inpatient palliative care consultation service: a multifaceted approach. J Palliat Med. 2007;10(6):1347–55.

Davies E, Higginson IJ. The solid facts: palliative care. Copenhagen: World Health Organization, Regional Office for Europe; 2004. 9789289010917.

Davis MA, Nallamothu BK, Banerjee M, Bynum JP. Identification of four unique spending patterns among older adults in the last year of life challenges standard assumptions. Health Aff (Millwood). 2016;35(7):1316–23.

Dumanovsky T, Augustin R, Rogers M, Lettang K, Meier DE, Morrison RS. The growth of palliative care in U.S. hospitals: a status report. J Palliat Med. 2015;19:8.

Elsayem AF, Elzubeir HE, Brock PA, Todd KH. Integrating palliative care in oncologic emergency departments: challenges and opportunities. World J Clin Oncol. 2016;7(2):227–33.

Eti S, O'Mahony S, McHugh M, Guilbe R, Blank A, Selwyn P. Outcomes of the acute palliative care unit in an academic medical center. Am J Hosp Palliat Care. 2014;31(4):380–4.

Etkind SN, Bone AE, Gomes B, et al. How many people will need palliative care in 2040? Past trends, future projections and implications for services. BMC Med. 2017;15(1):102.

Garrido MM. Propensity scores: a practical method for assessing treatment effects in pain and symptom management research. J Pain Symptom Manag. 2014;48(4):711–8.

Garrido MM, Deb P, Burgess JF Jr, Penrod JD. Choosing models for health care cost analyses: issues of nonlinearity and endogeneity. Health Serv Res. 2012;47(6):2377–97.

Grudzen CR, Hwang U, Cohen JA, Fischman M, Morrison RS. Characteristics of emergency department patients who receive a palliative care consultation. J Palliat Med. 2012;15(4):396–9.

Hanson LC, Usher B, Spragens L, Bernard S. Clinical and economic impact of palliative care consultation. J Pain Symptom Manag. 2008;35(4):340–6.

Hatziandreu E, Archontakis F, Daly A. The potential cost savings of greater use of home-and hospice-based end of life care in England. Santa Monica: RAND CORP; 2008.

Higginson IJ, Finlay IG, Goodwin DM, et al. Is there evidence that palliative care teams alter end-of-life experiences of patients and their caregivers? J Pain Symptom Manag. 2003;25(2):150–68.

Hwang SJ, Chang HT, Hwang IH, Wu CY, Yang WH, Li CP. Hospice offers more palliative care but costs less than usual care for terminal geriatric hepatocellular carcinoma patients: a nationwide study. J Palliat Med. 2013;16(7):780–5.

Imbens GW. Nonparametric estimation of average treatment effects under exogeneity: a review. Rev Econ Stat. 2004;86(1):4–29.

Ishak KJ, Stolar M, Hu MY, et al. Accounting for the relationship between per diem cost and LOS when estimating hospitalization costs. BMC Health Serv Res. 2012;12:439.

Jones AM. Models for health care. York: Health Economics and Data Group, University of York; 2010.

Kistler EA, Sean Morrison R, Richardson LD, Ortiz JM, Grudzen CR. Emergency department-triggered palliative care in advanced cancer: proof of concept. Acad Emerg Med. 2015;22(2):237–9.

Latham LP, Ackroyd-Stolarz S. Emergency department utilization by older adults: a descriptive study. Can Geriatr J. 2014;17(4):118–25.

Manning WG. The logged dependent variable, heteroscedasticity, and the retransformation problem. J Health Econ. 1998;17(3):283–95.

Manning WG, Basu A, Mullahy J. Generalized modeling approaches to risk adjustment of skewed outcomes data. J Health Econ. 2005;24(3):465–88.

May P, Normand C. Analyzing the impact of palliative care interventions on cost of hospitalization: practical guidance for choice of dependent variable. J Pain Symptom Manag. 2016;52(1):100–6.

May P, Normand C, Morrison RS. Economic impact of hospital inpatient palliative care consultation: review of current evidence and directions for future research. J Palliat Med. 2014;17(9):1054–63.

May P, Garrido MM, Cassel JB, et al. Prospective cohort study of hospital palliative care teams for inpatients with advanced cancer: earlier consultation is associated with larger cost-saving effect. J Clin Oncol. 2015;33(25):2745–52.

May P, Garrido MM, Cassel JB, Morrison RS, Normand C. Using length of stay to control for unobserved heterogeneity when estimating treatment effect on hospital costs with observational data: issues of reliability, robustness and usefulness. Health Serv Res. 2016;51(5):2020–43.

May P, Garrido MM, Cassel JB, et al. Cost analysis of a prospective multi-site cohort study of palliative care consultation teams for adults with advanced cancer: where do cost-savings come from? Palliat Med. 2017a;31(4):378–86.

May P, Garrido MM, Aldridge MD, et al. Prospective cohort study of hospitalized adults with advanced cancer: associations between complications, comorbidity, and utilization. J Hosp Med. 2017b;12(6):407–13.

May P, Garrido MM, Del Fabbro E, et al. Does modality matter? Palliative care units associated with more cost-avoidance than consultations. J Pain Symptom Manag. 2017c;55:766. (epub ahead of print 2017/08/27).

Maynard L, Lynn D. Development of a logic model to support a network approach in delivering 24/7 children's palliative care: part one. Int J Palliat Nurs. 2016;22(4):176–84.

McCarthy IM, Robinson C, Huq S, Philastre M, Fine RL. Cost savings from palliative care teams and guidance for a financially viable palliative care program. Health Serv Res. 2015;50(1):217–36.

McCusker J, Karp I, Cardin S, Durand P, Morin J. Determinants of emergency department visits by older adults: a systematic review. Acad Emerg Med. 2003;10(12):1362–70.

Mierendorf SM, Gidvani V. Palliative care in the emergency department. Perm J. 2014;18(2):77–85.
Morrison RS. Models of palliative care delivery in the United States. Curr Opin Support Palliat Care. 2013;7(2):201–6.
Morrison RS, Penrod JD, Cassel JB, et al. Cost savings associated with US hospital palliative care consultation programs. Arch Intern Med. 2008;168(16):1783–90.
Morrison RS, Meier D, Carlson M. The healthcare imperative: lowering costs and improving outcomes. Washington, DC: Institute of Medicine; 2011.
Penrod JD, Deb P, Luhrs C, et al. Cost and utilization outcomes of patients receiving hospital-based palliative care consultation. J Palliat Med. 2006;9(4): 855–60.
Penrod JD, Goldstein NE, Deb P. When and how to use instrumental variables in palliative care research. J Palliat Med. 2009;12(5):471–4.
Penrod JD, Deb P, Dellenbaugh C, et al. Hospital-based palliative care consultation: effects on hospital cost. J Palliat Med. 2010;13(8):973–9.
Quest TE, Asplin BR, Cairns CB, Hwang U, Pines JM. Research priorities for palliative and end-of-life care in the emergency setting. Acad Emerg Med. 2011;18 (6):e70–6.
Radbruch L, Payne S. White paper on standards and norms for hospice and palliative care in Europe: part 2. Eur J Palliat Care. 2010;17(1):22–33.
Rubin DB. The design versus the analysis of observational studies for causal effects: parallels with the design of randomized trials. Stat Med. 2007;26(1):20–36.
Simoens S, Kutten B, Keirse E, et al. The costs of treating terminal patients. J Pain Symptom Manag. 2010a;40(3):436–48.
Simoens S, Kutten B, Keirse E, et al. Costs of terminal patients who receive palliative care or usual care in different hospital wards. J Palliat Med. 2010b;13(11):1365–9.
Smith TJ, Hillner BE. Bending the cost curve in cancer care. N Engl J Med. 2011;364(21):2060–5.
Smith TJ, Coyne P, Cassel B, Penberthy L, Hopson A, Hager MA. A high-volume specialist palliative care unit and team may reduce in-hospital end-of-life care costs. J Palliat Med. 2003;6(5):699–705.
Smith TJ, Coyne PJ, Cassel JB. Practical guidelines for developing new palliative care services: resource management. Ann Oncol. 2012;23(Suppl 3):70–5.
Spetz J, Dudley N, Trupin L, Rogers M, Meier DE, Dumanovsky T. Few hospital palliative care programs meet national staffing recommendations. Health Aff (Millwood). 2016;35(9):1690–7.
Starks H, Diehr P, Curtis JR. The challenge of selection bias and confounding in palliative care research. J Palliat Med. 2009;12(2):181–7.
Starks H, Wang S, Farber S, Owens DA, Curtis JR. Cost savings vary by length of stay for inpatients receiving palliative care consultation services. J Palliat Med. 2013;16(10):1215–20.
Teno JM, Gozalo PL, Bynum JP, et al. Change in end-of-life care for Medicare beneficiaries: site of death, place of care, and health care transitions in 2000, 2005, and 2009. JAMA. 2013;309(5):470–7.
Weinstein MC, Siegel JE, Gold MR, Kamlet MS, Russell LB. Recommendations of the panel on cost-effectiveness in health and medicine. JAMA. 1996;276(15):1253–8.
Whitford K, Shah ND, Moriarty J, Branda M, Thorsteinsdottir B. Impact of a palliative care consult service. Am J Hosp Palliat Care. 2014;31(2):175–82.

Financial Aspects of Outpatient Palliative Care

100

Sarina R. Isenberg, Rab Razzak, Mike Rabow, and Thomas J. Smith

Contents

S. R. Isenberg
Department of Health, Behavior and Society, Johns Hopkins Bloomberg School of Public Health, Baltimore, MD, USA

Temmy Latner Centre for Palliative Care and Lunenfeld-Tanenbaum Research Institute, Sinai Health System, Toronto, ON, Canada

Department of Family and Community Medicine, University of Toronto, Toronto, ON, Canada
e-mail: sisenbe2@jhu.edu

R. Razzak
Outpatient Palliative Medicine, Johns Hopkins Medicine, Johns Hopkins School of Medicine, Baltimore, USA
e-mail: rrazzak@jhmi.edu

M. Rabow
General Internal Medicine, University of San Francisco, San Francisco, CA, USA
e-mail: Mike.Rabow@ucsf.edu

T. J. Smith (✉)
JHMI, The Johns Hopkins Hospital, Baltimore, MD, USA
e-mail: tsmit136@jhmi.edu

R. D. MacLeod, L. Van den Block (eds.), *Textbook of Palliative Care*,
https://doi.org/10.1007/978-3-319-77740-5_103

Abstract

Community-based palliative care has become the focus of palliative care's growth and opportunity. Twelve of the largest randomized control trials on palliative care are community-based and result in equal or greater survival, positive satisfaction from patients and caregivers, and equal or less cost. Surprisingly, sometimes the business case is the easiest to make (Cassel et al. 2015). With health care financing that embraces value-based programs, such as serious-illness care models, shared savings, bundled payments, and global budget revenues, community-based palliative care shows great promise and may be part of the solution to provide better care for patients at an affordable cost. Some key obstacles include a shortage of practitioners and the necessity to perform as a public health system instead of a revenue-generating center. We provide examples of some successful programs that are reproducible.

1 Introduction

Studies from the United States, United Kingdom, and Canada suggest that most people prefer to both be cared for and die at home (Gomes et al. 2013a; Bell et al. 2009; Higginson and Sen-Gupta 2000). However, only a minority of deaths occur at home (Cohen et al. 2010). In the US in 2007, 24% of deaths occurred at home among those aged 65 years and older (Teno et al. 2013; Statistics 2010). In the UK in 2010, 21% of deaths occurred at home (Gomes et al. 2012). In Canada, from 1994 to 2004, 30% of deaths occurred at home (Wilson et al. 2009). In addition, the rapid rise of concurrent palliative care alongside disease-directed therapies for diseases like cancer and multiple sclerosis – where people may live a long time and not die – has made many programs retool for chronic ongoing care.

Varied initiatives in outpatient palliative care have focused on aligning care with people's preferences, improving clinical outcomes during and after treatment and increasing the proportion of people dying at home by decreasing hospital admissions near the end of life. In light of these trends and using a system-level international perspective, this chapter aims to explore what goes into the business planning for outpatient palliative care services.

This chapter describes research surrounding both "outpatient" (that is, clinic-based) and "home-based" palliative care. Clinic-based services may be associated with large health care systems. Home-based palliative care involves caring for seriously ill patients where they live, including private homes, nursing homes, and assisted living facilities. Both types of care may utilize telemedicine. Outpatient clinic-based and home-based palliative cares are sometimes referred to as Community-Based Palliative Care (CBPC).

CBPC developed differently in different countries. While it is outside the purview of this chapter to detail the development in each country, we will briefly list a few key points. In the USA, CBPC developed on a site-by-site basis, which largely reflects the health care system in that country. End-of -life care was and continues to be predominantly funded by the Medicare Hospice Benefit, which promotes community-based hospice models that rely on home care (Bull et al. 2012). In Canada, CBPC had a more organic development, and while palliative care services and availability vary widely across the country, various provincial initiatives (e.g., the Ontario Palliative Care Network) are working to standardize palliative care and improve access. In the UK, palliative care services were developed similar to the USA, in a haphazard manner, site by site, often as a feature of charities. Since the NHS Cancer Plan 2000 (https://www.thh.nhs.uk/documents/_Departments/Cancer/NHSCancerPlan.pdf) along with end of life (EOL) strategy in 2008, there has been a more systematic attempt to figure out the regional needs, led by the National Council for Palliative Care. The Royal College of Physicians has set target numbers of consultant palliative care physicians to per capita population. This will help identify under-resourced and recognize where there is a greater need for physicians.

In this chapter, we first present a literature review of the research in the finances of CBPC. Second, we provide case studies of organizations that have been successful in their implementation of outpatient and/or home-based palliative care. Third, we provide suggestions and a blueprint for steps to take to create a sustainable and replicable outpatient and/or home-based palliative care program.

2 Literature Review

When reviewing the literature, it is important to note that it is challenging to compare across programs and jurisdictions. As acknowledged by Gomes et al. in their 2014 systematic review of the effectiveness of home-based palliative care, what constitutes "home palliative care" varies – be it physician- or nurse practitioner-provided; daily, weekly, or monthly visits; the extent of care that can be provided in the home. Also, importantly, the comparator of "usual care" varies across setting. In the above systematic review, usual care included community care, that is, primary or specialist care at home, outpatient clinics or in nursing homes, and in some instances hospice care (Gomes et al. 2013b).

Others have noted that the existing cost effectiveness and costs savings research on CBPC have certain limitations, including ambiguous currency and cost information, and limited statistical information (e.g., t-test results, confidence intervals, ranges, and disaggregated data) (https://www.thh.nhs.uk/documents/_Departments/Cancer/NHSCancerPlan.pdf). In addition to the above-noted challenges, Davis et al.'s systematic review of trials featuring early integration of outpatient and home-based palliative care found that studies typically had high attrition rates, lack of mention regarding whether participants were blinded, infrequent power calculations, and minimal use of intention-to-treat analysis (Davis et al. 2015). Both reviews noted that many studies in this field do not incorporate family nonmedical factors, including productivity impacts (e.g., patients/caregivers taking time off work as a result of illness or caregiving), use of life savings to cover medical expenditures, and food and transportation. Similarly, a systematic review on the financial impact of caring for family members of patients receiving palliative care found that there is limited research on the financial burden of caregivers; however, the few available studies suggest the financial costs are substantial and result in caregiver burden (Gardiner et al. 2014).

3 Symptom Management in Home-Based Palliative Care

Gomes et al.'s recent Cochrane Systematic Review on home-based palliative care demonstrated that, compared to usual care, home-based palliative care increased the odds of dying at home (from their meta-analysis: odds ratio (OR) 2.21, 95%CI 1.31 to 3.71; $Z = 2.98$, P value $= 0.003$), and small but statistically significant benefits of reducing symptom burden for patients (https://www.thh.nhs.uk/documents/_Departments/Cancer/NHSCancerPlan.pdf). Davis et al.'s systematic review of trials featuring early integration of outpatient and home-based palliative found that most studies demonstrated improvement in depression and quality of life, decreased caregiver burden, and better maintenance of caregiver quality of life; however, they also noted that some trials demonstrate symptoms and quality of life did not improve (Gomes et al. 2013b). Sarmento et al. conducted a meta-ethnography to attempt to identify what components of home-based palliative care leads to these positive outcomes. The two overarching themes that emerged were that the 24/7 availability of home-based palliative care helped patients and families feel they had sufficient access to services, and that effective communication and symptom control made patients and their caregivers feel secure (Sarmento et al. 2017).

To our knowledge, only one trial has shown worse symptoms. Hoek et al. (2017) randomized 74 Dutch patients to weekly palliative care telemedicine sessions or "care as usual" without mandated palliative care consultations. In the intervention group, the Total Distress Score and anxiety scores (but not depression) were significantly worse at week 12. Their explanation was that the telemedicine allowed the patients to give excess attention to symptoms and suffering, and that the usual care had good palliative care as standard. But for the most part, these programs seemed to, according to the qualitative literature, allow patients and family caregivers to focus on living life and preparing for death at home, rather than dedicating time to the medical components of care (Gardiner et al. 2014).

There are specific examples of how concurrent palliative care improves symptoms. The UCSF outpatient team did an observational study of the outpatient cancer program that saw 266 patients at least twice. The only symptom that did not improve was nausea, but pain, depression, anxiety, quality of life, and spiritual wellbeing all improved clinically and statistically ($p < 0.002$ for all) (Bischoff et al. 2013). With US Oncology, Muir and colleagues embedded a palliative care advance practice or doctor or both (but not a social worker or chaplain) in oncology offices (Muir et al. 2010). The symptom burden was reduced by 21%, with ESAS scores falling from 49.3 to 39 (a meaningful difference). Oncology providers ranked satisfaction with the new PC service at 9/10, and consultation requests increased 87%, a doubling per oncology provider. The PC service saved the practice over 4 weeks of time, or 170 min per referral, used time-based billing by the PC group to calculate; this would allow the practice to see 121 new patients. Hospice length of stay, a marker of quality care, increased from 15 days to 24 days with palliative care consultation ($p < 0.001$) (Scheffey et al. 2014). In addition, opioid prescribing practices improved when palliative care saw the patient, with extended release analgesic prescriptions rising from 45% to 73% and pain scores dropping by 2/10 (Muir et al. 2013). The billing revenues from the palliative care providers paid their salaries, but the average half day session for a doctor and advance practice nurse included four new and six to eight follow-up visits in a half-day session, productivity which can be hard to sustain as a fulltime practice (Alesi et al. 2011).

3.1 Cost Effectiveness of Home-Based Palliative Care (United States)

While there is good penetration of inpatient palliative care programs in US hospitals, there are fewer outpatient palliative care programs. The total number of outpatient palliative care programs is not known but likely the current capacity in CBPC is inadequate to meet the current need (Bull et al. 2012; Kerr et al. 2015). To date, there have been some studies on the costs/benefits of home-based palliative care, but there is discordance in their findings. Overall, the aforementioned *Cochrane Review* of home palliative care services for adults with advanced illness and their caregivers deemed the evidence inconclusive regarding the cost effectiveness of this intervention as compared to hospital-based palliative care (6 studies). Similarly, Davis et al.'s systematic review of early integration of outpatient and home-based palliative care found that there is mixed evidence on whether these services reduce hospital length of stay and number of hospitalizations, as well as reduce costs. They suggest that the inconclusive nature of these results may stem from large variability in studies; standard deviations are often larger than the means suggesting lack of precision, skewed economic data, and heavy influence of outliers. Further, patient populations are often comprised of those with diverse primary diagnoses. Rabow et al.'s systematic review of outpatient palliative care interventions found that the evidence suggestions these programs reduce health care utilization. They suggest that while the delivery of outpatient palliative care is communication-rich, and staffing intensive, the program's ability to reduce overall health care utilization balances out the costs of delivery, especially in integrated health systems (e.g., accountable care organizations) (Rabow et al. 2013).

There are a few notable studies that examined the cost effectiveness of particular home-based and outpatient palliative care programs. One of the most cited cost-effectiveness studies is Brumley et al.'s work from Kaiser-Permanente in 2007 that entailed a randomized control trial in Hawaii and Colorado comparing home-based palliative care to usual care (Brumley et al. 2007). This study found that overall costs of care for those enrolled in the home-based palliative care program were 33% less than those receiving standard care ($P = 0.03$). Further, the average cost per day incurred by palliative care recipients (USD$95.30) was significantly lower than that of usual care group members (USD$212.80) ($P = 0.02$). This study and a similar one for inpatients convinced Kaiser-Permanente to adopt the palliative care interdisciplinary team in all their major markets.

Bookbinder et al. found a home-based palliative care model involving a nurse practitioner and social worker connected to a palliative care home team did not generate enough annual revenue from patient billings to offset the nurse practitioner's salary costs; however, a model of a nurse practitioner linked to a hospice program led to an increase in hospital referrals thereby generating sufficient revenue to support the nurse practitioner (Bookbinder et al. 2011). Indeed, an early study of outpatient palliative care practices suggested that billing revenue covers less than half of program budgets (Rabow et al. 2010).

Cassel et al. examined the cost impact of a concurrent care home-based program designed for individuals with advanced chronic illness found that, compared to a propensity-matched usual care control group, patients in the intervention group had less hospital use (mean hospital days per month of 0.69 (SD 1.84) vs. 2.62 (SD 3.44), p 0.001) and lower hospital costs (mean per month costs of $984 (SD $2,776) vs. $5,195 (SD $7,353), $p < 0.02$). In addition, overall, the cost of care in the last 6 months of life remained relatively the same in the intervention group ($1,550 4 months before death, $3,711 in the final month), compared to a significant increase in the control group ($2,631 4 months before death, $17,006 in the final month). The numbers included were for patients with a primary diagnosis of cancer. This home-based palliative program included in-home medical consultation, ongoing evidence-based prognostication of further survival, caregiver support, and advance health care planning (Brian Cassel et al. 2016).

Kerr et al. compared the costs of a community-based outpatient palliative care program featuring a hospice-private payer partnership to propensity-score matched control group, and found that outpatients costs were significantly lower for the intervention group at 2 weeks, 1 month, and 3 months, no difference at 6 months, and significantly higher at 1 year and 2 years (Kerr et al. 2014). Lustbader et al., examined the effect of a home-based palliative care program within an Accountable Care Organization, compared to usual care. The study found that the cost per patient during the final 3 months of life was $12,000 lower in the intervention compared to control group ($20,420 vs. $32,420; $p = 0.0002$). This decrease resulted from a 35% reduction in Medicare Part A ($16,892 vs. $26,171; $p = 0.0037$), and a 37% reduction in Medicare Part B ($3,114 vs. $4,913; $p = 0.0008$). The intervention group also resulted in a 34% reduction in hospital admissions, a 35%

increase in hospice enrollment, and a 240% increase in median hospice length of stay, compared to usual care (Lustbader et al. 2017).

Pouliot found that, in a pre-post study evaluating the impact of a home-based palliative care program, patients experienced decreased emergency department visits and inpatient hospital admissions (Pouliot et al. 2017).

In the study of concurrent palliative care embedded in oncologists offices described above, the practice was self-sustaining but may be difficult to sustain (Alesi et al. 2011). In our own practice (RR and TJS), billing revenues will cover at least half the salary (our arrangement with the institution) if the provider sees four patients; a busy practitioner see two new patients and four to six return visit patients in a half-day session and comes close to covering full salary.

It is important to recognize the importance of early versus late referral at their cancer in changing end of life practice patterns. At the UCSF Cancer Center, only 32% of decedents were referred to palliative care, with 68% referred less than 90 days before death (Scibetta et al. 2016). If the patients were referred 3 months before death, the health system saved $5198 due to fewer end of life hospital days with lower inpatient care costs ($19,067 vs. $25,754, $p < 0.01$), while outpatient costs were no different.

Besides the timing of referrals, the number of outpatient visits plays a role in reducing aggressive care at the end of life and resultant expenses. As shown in Fig. 1, as the number of visits increased, less aggressive care near the end of life was provided (less chemotherapy in the last month of life; fewer emergency visits, admissions, and Intensive Care Unit admissions) (Jang et al. 2015).

3.2 Cost Effectiveness of Home-Based Palliative Care (Canada)

Most figures from Canadian studies are 5–10 years old; therefore, there is a need for an updated cost-effectiveness analysis comparing home-based palliative care to hospital-based palliative care. Of note, while all hospital-based services are covered under public health insurance in Canada; home care and community care are only partially covered, depending on the province. For example, patients and families in Ontario cover 25–50% of the total costs (Dumont et al. 2009).

While models of palliative care exist across Canada, there are disparities and gaps in access across regions. One study compared costs of 6 months in a palliative care program in an urban versus rural setting and found that the total cost per patient was $26,652 in urban areas (with families covering 20.8% of the costs), while $31,018 in rural areas (with families covering 21.9% of the costs) (Dumont et al. 2015). Notably, these figures reflect inpatient, outpatient, and home-based palliative care, aggregated. Urban families tended to cover more costs related to formal home care, while rural families tended to cover more costs related to prescription medication,

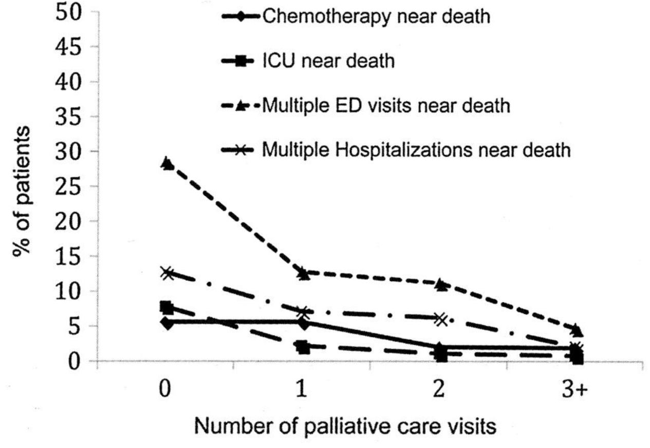

Fig. 1 Relationship between number of palliative care visits and end of life aggressive care

out-of-pocket costs, and transportation (Jang et al. 2015). There have also been province-based studies accessing disparities. In Quebec, where home-based palliative care services are provided by the Public Local Community-Based Health Care Service providers (Locaux de Services Communautaires [CLSC]), one study found large variation in delivery of these services to patients with cancer (Gagnon et al. 2015). Of the 53,316 cancer patients included in the study (representing patients with cancer who died in Quebec between 2003–2006), 52.1% received home visits during the 90 days before death, and of those, 72.5% received three visits or more.

The models of home-based palliative care programs have shifted over time. One study documented changing trends in services models from 2005 to 2015 in Ontario and found that the propensity and intensity to use home-based physician visits and personal support workers increased, while propensity and intensity of nurse visits deceased (Sun et al. 2017).

Regarding the cost effectiveness of these services, several studies have captured the impact of certain models of care on system costs. Klinger et al. tested a model of home-based palliative hospice care in Ontario (Klinger et al. 2013). The study found the average costs were approximately CAD$117.95 per patient day or a total of CAD$17,112.19 per patient over the 15-month study period. These findings are roughly equivalent to the Ontario Auditor General's reporting that the average per day palliative care costs in the last month of a patient's life is under CAD$100/day for home-based palliative care. Alternatively, the average costs of other palliative services were CAD$1,100 per day in an acute-care hospital bed, CAD$630 to $770 per day in a bed in a palliative-care unit, and CAD$460 per day in a hospice bed. There is incongruence regarding these costs. A 2010 report estimated that it costs approximately CAD$4,700 per client annually to provide palliative care in the home as compared to CAD$19,000 for acute care annually. A piloted palliative home care service that ran in Ontario from 2000 to 2001 cost CAD$5,586 per patient for a year. From a system perspective, a 2013 study in Ontario projected that expanding in-home palliative care to those currently not receiving such services (approximately 45,000 people per year) can avoid CAD$191 million to CAD$385 million in health care costs. Shifting just 10% of patients at end of life from acute care to home care would save CAD$9 million a year.

A study of palliative care costs in the last 5 years of life among patients in Halifax, Montreal, Winnipeg, Edmonton, and Victoria found that the mean total cost of outpatient palliative care increased by 70% from the first to the last month of life, and the mean total cost of home care was 4.5 times higher during the last month of life compared to 5 months before death. While costs for transportation gradually increased, costs of prescription medications decreased from the fifth to the second last month of life, and costs of medical equipment increased from the fifth to the third month but then decreased from the third to the last month before death (Dumont et al. 2010).

Few Canadian studies have accessed the costs of home-based palliative care from a societal perspective, which considers third-party insurance payments, travelling expenses, caregiving time devoted to patients and missed time from work and leisure. Yu et al. investigated the differences in societal costs of end-of-life care associated with hospital and home deaths, and found that there was no significant differences in total societal costs; however, the higher hospitalization costs for hospital death patients were ultimately equivalent to the unpaid caregiver time and outpatients service costs for home death patients (Yu et al. 2015) Diving deeper into the distribution of societal costs, Dumont et al.'s study of resources utilization during the palliative phase of care in five regions in Canada found that the costs across inpatient hospital care stays, home care, and informal caregiving time were paid for 71.3% by the public health care system, 26.6% by the family, 1.6% by not-for-profit organizations, and 0.5% by other payers. The majority of costs supported by the family were attributable to caregiving time (66.3%), followed by out-of-pocket costs (17.0%), home medical equipment or aids (6.7%), and home care (4.4%) (Dumont et al. 2009).

Further investigating the source of these non-public system expenses, Chai et al. interviewed 169 caregivers of patients receiving home-based palliative care as well as abstracted data on health care utilization of patients. This study determined that the average monthly cost per patient for these services over the last 12 months of the patient's life was CAD$14,924 per patient (2011 Canadian dollars), which broke down into 77% unpaid caregiving cost (i.e., caregiver time lost from market labor and leisure) (CAD$11,334), 21% publicly financed health care costs (i.e., costs incurred by the public sector in the organization and delivery of home-based palliative care services) (CAD$3,211), 2% privately financed costs (i.e., out-of-pocket costs for expenditures on consultations with clinicians, travel expenses, private insurance plans supplementing public insurance) (CAD$379). The study also found that the magnitude of costs increased exponentially over the last 12 months of life. A previous study by the same group found that the mean monthly cost per patient for services over the last 12 months of life was CAD$24,549 (2008 Canadian dollars), which broke down into 70% unpaid caregiving cost ($17,184), 26% publicly financed health care costs (CAD$6,396), 4% privately financed costs (CAD$870) (Guerriere et al. 2010).

3.3 Cost Effectiveness of Home-Based Palliative Care (Australia)

A systematic review and meta-analysis of the impact of community specialist palliative care services found the evidence to be inconclusive regarding whether the impact these services have on home deaths, symptoms, and costs. Importantly, none of the studies in this review found a significant effect in favor of an alternative intervention (Luckett et al. 2013). Kralik et al. compared home-based palliative care service utilization among patient with cancer and non-cancer conditions and found that patients with cancer were referred earlier, patients with non-cancer conditions were higher users of home-based palliative care services over a longer period of time (Kralik and Anderson 2008). An Australian home-based palliative care model was found to cost AUD$3,489 per patient, which was largely offset by lower mean inpatient care costs (AUD$2,450), resulting in a net incremental cost of AUD$1001 per patient (McCaffrey et al. 2013).

4 Highlighting of Organizations that Have Been Successful in Their Implementation of Outpatient Palliative Care

4.1 Johns Hopkins Medicine Palliative Care Program (Baltimore, USA)

Palliative care delivery at Johns Hopkins began at the Sidney Kimmel Comprehensive Cancer Centre (SKCCC) with outpatient palliative care, which was run primarily by pharmacy for cancer patients for three half days a week. Once two fulltime palliative care providers joined the hospital, physicians co-led the clinic with pharmacy, and the program also included access to a psychology nurse liaison, social workers (to address psychosocial issues and hospice referrals), and one chaplain. Often there were palliative care fellows staffing the clinic for half the year along with pharmacy residents and pharmacy students. The number of outpatient visits that were billed increased from 200 to over 1000/year from 2011 to 2016.

In 2013, the program developed a half day clinic for non-oncology patients, including those with severe neurological disorders, mitochondrial diseases, chronic obstructive pulmonary disorder (COPD), pulmonary hypertension, and cirrhosis. Due to funding, this clinic for non-oncology patients is only provided by a palliative care physician and an additional palliative care fellow for half the year. The program consults with all patients prior to left ventricular assist device (LVAD) and heart transplant, and periodically sees patients with pulmonary hypertension, heart failure, and liver disease in embedded clinics with the respective teams. Across inpatient and outpatient services, the program uses the modified

Memorial Symptom Assessment Scale Condensed (MSAS-C) for symptom assessments, spiritual, psycho-social assessments, as well as engages in prognosis evaluation after speaking with specialists. Over half of the patients in the program are primarily referred to receive symptom management; the remaining patients primarily are referred for either goals of care discussions and/or evaluation for hospice.

We have recently estimated the total impact of the palliative care program on the health center, and 2016 activity should save the institution nearly five million dollars (Isenberg et al. 2017) (Fig. 2).

With the increased acceptance of palliative care at Johns Hopkins Medicine among providers, coupled with increased institutional buy-in and more and more accountable care organizations, the program is in the process of developing home-based palliative care with an already established geriatric home-based care program, JHome. This multiprogram collaboration involves stakeholders from home care, geriatrics, pharmacy,

Financial impact	Cases/year projected 2016	Financial impact per case	Contribution ($/year)	5 year total contribution
IP PCU margin (1)			$100,000	$500,000
IP PCU cost $1595 savings/transfer (2)	154	$1,595	$245,630	$1,228,150
PC IP consult cost savings per case, $2,374 for patients discharged alive (3)	1355	$2,374	$3,216,770	$16,083,850
PC IP consult cost savings per case, $6,871 for decedents, 11% died (4)	167	$6,871	$1,147,457	$5,737,285
JHFAU vetted savings			***$4,709,857***	***$23,549,285***
Early PC OP consult cost savings per case. $5198/case – if seen 3 months before death compared to near death	297	$5,198	$245,630	$34,355,000
Hospice referrals cost savings per case, $4348/case; assumes half of the actual savings of $8697 in the last year[i]	800	$4,348	$3,478,400	$17,392,000
Professional fees, 50% collection rate			$500,000	$2,500,000
Improvement in HCAHPS (2% of Medicare reimbursement in 2017).			?	
Increased ICU bed availability leading to revenue			?	
Reduction in 30 day readmissions			?	
Goodwill; impact on disparities ; charitable contributions			?	
Total impact			**$13,643,744**	**$101,345,570**

PC palliative care; IP inpatient; PCU palliative care unit; JHFAU Johns Hopkins Fiscal Analysis Unit; HCAHPS Hospital Consumer Assessment of Healthcare Providers and Systems

Fig. 2 Financial impact of the palliative care program on the health system, projected to 2016

business development, and the hospital's financial analysis unit.

The outpatient program has encountered some challenges, in particular approximately 25% of outpatient visits are no shows. To address this issue, one of the program's administrative assistants calls patients 2 days before scheduled visits to confirm attendance. This process has decreased no show rates by approximately 25%. The program sees over 1000 patients/year with 468 unique medical record number visits, which are either new visits and/or patients who have not been seen in a year. They have half day clinics for patients with cancer 3 days per week and a half day clinic for patients who have non-cancer diagnoses. Outpatient palliative care program accounts for 14% of the total program work Relative Value Units (wRVUs). The program expects each provider to meet wRVU goals and to cover at least half their salaries and benefits, with the hospital absorbing the rest.

It is critical to bill and collect appropriately for professional fees or the program will not succeed. We show two "Levels of Care" billed by two practitioners who saw patients of similar severity. Provider one – based on chart review and time spent with the patient – is not billing enough to cover his/her salary. Note that provider B documented her time consuming, difficult medical decision-making visit in subsequent visits with the 99233 code (Fig. 3a, b).

The Harry J. Duffey Family endowed the Palliative Care Program at the cancer center, which has now spread across all disciplines. There is an endowed annual lecture on "Hope" and an endowed professorship in Neuromodulation with emphasis on Scrambler Therapy (Majithia et al. 2016). A memorial service is held yearly at the cancer center, and one for all the patients who have died on the Osler Medical Service. Scholarly activities have included the updating of the national clinical practice guidelines in

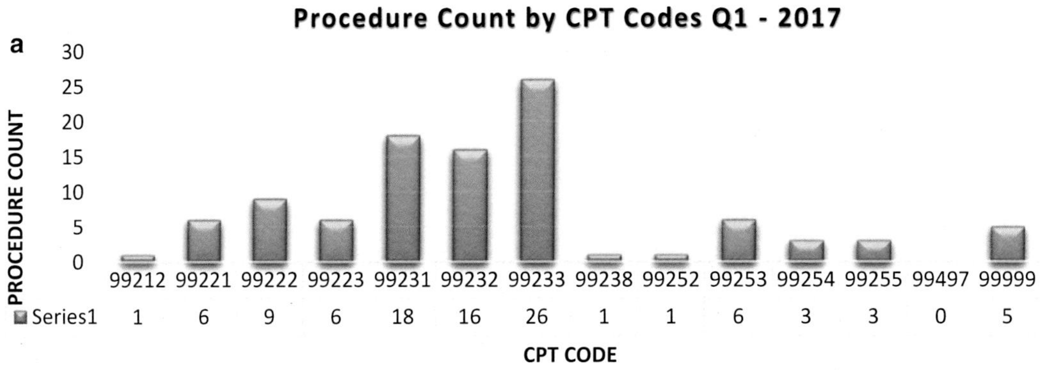

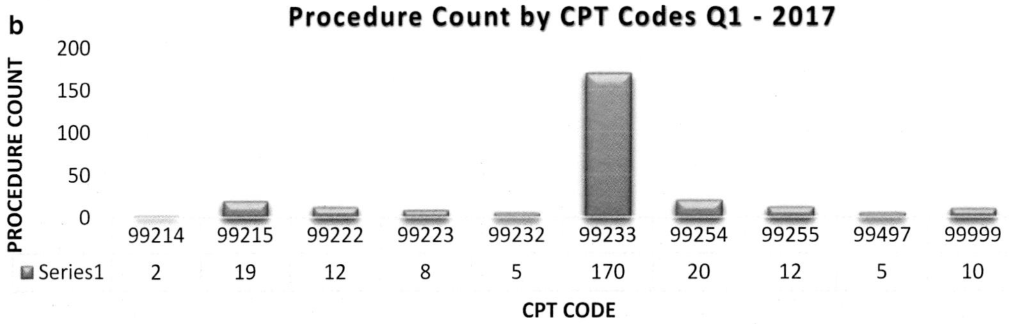

Fig. 3 (**a**) Different billing codes from two providers who gave the same service. (**b**) Different billing codes representative of the actual work performed

palliative care (Ferrell et al. 2017; Levy et al. 2016); communication in the neonatal intensive care unit; neuromodulation for relief of pain from cancer, HIV, post-mastectomy syndrome; integration of palliative care with hospitalist work; and one widely accepted play ("Life Support") presented locally and at the national meeting.

4.2 The Symptom Management Service at the Helen Diller Family Comprehensive Cancer Center, UCSF (San Francisco, CA)

The Symptom Management Service (SMS) is the clinic-based palliative care program at UCSF's comprehensive cancer center. The SMS provides comanagement with the oncology teams. The majority of referrals are for pain and depression. Approximately, 60% of patients in the SMS have metastatic disease. The SMS was launched in 2005 in Genito-Urinary Oncology with a single half-day clinic staffed by a palliative care physicians and social worker. In 2008, the SMS was available to patients throughout the cancer center. Currently, the SMS has grown to offer 25 half-day clinics weekly across both cancer center campuses. In 2017, the SMS had 605 new patients and 1,436 follow up visits. The program includes physicians (1.9 FTE total across 7 physicians), a nurse practitioner (1.0 FTE), a nurse (1.0 FTE), a program coordinator (1.0 FTE), a practice manager (0.5 FTE), and a chaplain (0.2 FTE). Among SMS staff, physicians are supported from clinical billing revenue. All other staff are supported by the medical center. Social workers are shared with the cancer center programs, as are psychologists and nutritionists. The SMS trains palliative care fellows, oncology fellows, medical residents, medical students, nursing students, and pharmacy residents. SMS clinics are primarily stand-alone but with an expanding number if embedded clinics, including in Breast Oncology and Gastrointestinal Oncology.

The SMS primarily has served patients with solid tumors (the top referring programs are Breast, GI, and GU oncology) but is currently expanding with 2 half-days embedded in the Bone Marrow Transplant Clinic (at yet a third UCSF campus). The SMS program includes annual memorial services at two cancer center campuses, a video legacy project for patients, cancer center awards to leading faculty and staff, and a campus-wide lecture series. The SMS oversees inpatient palliative care services at the affiliated cancer hospital. At UCSF, in addition to outpatient palliative care for cancer patients provided by the SMS, inpatient palliative care is available at the main university hospital; there is a home-based palliative care service for UCSF patients in San Francisco county, and an outpatient palliative care clinic for non-cancer patients will be launching soon.

SMS research has demonstrated improved clinical outcomes in nearly all symptoms assessed and persistence of benefit over more than 80 days (Bischoff et al. 2013). Patients have similar improvement regardless of gender, age, ethnicity, disease stage, disease progression, and concurrent oncologic treatments. In another study, clinician and financial outcomes were explored among UCSF patients who died of cancer. Patients who received palliative care early (in the SMS, prior to 90 days before death) had improved end-of-life outcomes, health care utilization, and total costs compared to patients who received palliative care late (within 90 days of death, primarily from inpatient palliative care consultation).

4.3 Temmy Latner Centre for Palliative Care at Sinai Health System (Toronto, Canada)

The Temmy Latner Centre for Palliative Care (TLCPC) is a department in Sinai Health System (Toronto) that began in 1989, initially providing both hospital and home-based care with a team comprised of one physician, a clinical nurse specialist, social worker, and two chaplains. Co-founded by Dr. Larry Librach and Dr. Frank Ferris, the program is the first and largest organized home palliative care program in Ontario (Temmy Latner Centre for Palliative Care 2015).

As of 2015, the program has 21 physicians on staff (17 in the Home-Care program and 6 in the In-Hospital Care Program), 2 full-time equivalent (FTE) coordinators, and 3.8 FTE staff (Seow et al. 2013). The program receives referrals from physicians across the Greater Toronto Area. As of 2017, the program includes: a home-based palliative care program serving residents of the Greater Toronto Area, a 32-bed inpatient palliative care unit, and inpatient consultation services within the Sinai Health System. The home-based care program partners with community agencies (i.e., Community Care Access Centres) to provide multidisciplinary palliative care in the home, and there is a physician available to patients 24 h a day, 7 days a week. In addition to the care it provides, the clinicians in the program assist with education providers at Mount Sinai Hospital, as well as providing training in palliative care to all medical students and many postgraduate medical trainees in many specialties at the University of Toronto.

Seow et al. evaluated the effectiveness of the home-based palliative care program comparing 676 patients who received home-based care from TLCPC from April 2009–March 2011, to a comparison group of patients matched on demographics and primary diagnoses. The study found that compared to the control group, TLCPC patients had a 30% (relative risk = 0.70) lower risk of being in the hospital in the last 2 weeks of life, a 35% (RR = 0.66) lower risk of dying in the hospital, a 53% (RR = 0.47) lower risk of visiting an Emergency Department in the last 2 weeks of life, and a three times (RR = 3.02) greater risk of dying someplace outside of the hospital (Seow et al. 2013) A study of patients in this program found that the average monthly cost for these services over the last 12 months of the patient's life was CAD$14,924 per patient (2011 Canadian dollars), which broke down into 77% unpaid caregiving cost (i.e., caregiver time lost from market labor and leisure) (CAD$11,334), 21% publicly financed health care costs (i.e., costs incurred by the public sector in the organization and delivery of home-based palliative care services) (CAD$3,211), 2% privately financed costs (i.e., out-of-pocket costs for expenditures on consultations with clinicians, travel expenses, private insurance plans supplementing public insurance) (CAD$379) (Chai et al. 2014).

4.4 Outpatient Specialist Palliative Care Clinic, Scarborough, North Yorkshire, England

The specialist palliative care clinic in Scarborough via Scarborough General Hospital (SGH) serves a population of about 220,000 across a mixed urban-rural setting. This program is associated with Hull York Medical School and is in partnership with Saint Catherine's Hospice. The hospice is an independent charity and gets 70% of its funds from the community donors. The rest is provided by the NHS. Patients have access to lymphedema clinic, complementary therapy, and those in the area have access to bereavement services. They have a community specialist palliative care nurse advisory service including a neurology palliative nurse specialist. In addition, they provide an out of hours phone advice service for patients and relatives and non-palliative care health care professionals which also acts as a liaison point for those at home who may need a medical visit from the GP out of hours service. Patients do not need to be otherwise known to the hospice to be registered for this service. They have an active education center which seeks to upskill non-palliative care clinicians who do the bulk of generalist palliative care, including running 2-day advanced communication skills courses. Palliative care providers are employed by the hospice and NHS Trust and work together as one team across all the settings – hospital, community, and hospice. This ensures continuity of care in all settings. There is excellent integration with oncology, cardiology, movement disorder clinic, neurology, and respiratory medicine. The group uses a needs-based model rather than a prognosis-based model in all aspects of the service. In the UK, the term end-of-life indicates someone with a prognosis of 6–12 months.

5 Blueprint of How to Make Outpatient Palliative Care Sustainable and Replicable

From our clinical experiences, the following are key tips that can help to create and/or enhance outpatient and home-based palliative care delivery: 1. Train your team in standardized care that includes goals of care discussions. This means to acknowledge barriers to engaging in these conversations, convince all providers to engage in Advance Care Planning (ACP) such that the difficult discussions are had, and add communication prompts (e.g., communication checklist or even a temporary tattoo (Leong et al. 2016)). The prompts can be built into your electronic medical record system. Use systematic way to assess systems such as a spiritual distress scale, a symptom assessment scale like the Edmonton Symptom Assessment Scale (ESAS). Train all providers in how to complete (and then measure, for program impact) other possible outcomes like the Physician Orders for Life Sustaining Treatment (POLST) completion, hospice referrals, and readmissions.

Second, obtain buy-in from leadership and administrators by asking them what matters most and measuring your impact on it. One qualitative study interviewed clinical and operations leaders at local, regional, and national levels in the US Veterans Health Administration (VHA) to gauge organizational factors that were potentially influencing the adoption of outpatient care in chronic illness. Participants perceived outpatient palliative care as a lower priority for them because there are not sufficient performance measures to gauge improvement nor incentivize update of palliative care. Participants expressed that their buy-in would be increased if were demonstrated to them that the costs of the program offset health service utilization costs, and that issues regarding staffing and space requirements were being sufficiently addressed. Participants were also concerned that palliative care be done as complimentary to other forms of care, to ensure that clinicians did not feel threatened by the palliative care team; building clinician trust and buy-in is perceived as integral, as well as clarifying the roles and responsibilities of outpatient palliative care and primary/specialty care for disease management in advanced chronic illness (Bekelman et al. 2016).

Third, do not be isolated; interface with the larger organization. It is important to align the patient-centered symptom management goals of outpatient and home-based palliative care with the organization's financial interests, as it may enable more budgetary, political, or operational support (Cassel et al. 2015). Promote the program to providers in the institution to help increase referrals to the program. To do so, it is important to build relationships with providers, as well as educate providers about palliative care processes (e.g., what is involved, how to refer).

Fourth, make the referral and consult process as easy as possible. Make sure the process is as streamlined as possible. Remember to ALWAYS send a letter to the referring doctor to close the loop. It usually takes 3 min in EPIC or Cerner. When interacting to a patient's other providers in the organization, engage in conversations about prognosis – make sure you obtain permission to discuss prognosis from the involved surgeon or oncologist, as well as the patient.

Fifth, consider with whom to partner. Existing inpatient programs may be convinced to enhance outpatient palliative care programs through the consideration that they help to prevent over-utilization of the costliest health care services, which typically get provided at end-of-life. These programs also help to prevent readmissions and 30-day mortality admissions, which many hospitals in the USA and elsewhere are penalized for in-payment models. The business case is often the easiest to make! Other potential partners include: local meals on wheels program, hospital bed supplier, and personal support worker (i.e., home health aides, community health worker) agencies.

Sixth, make sure your own team is interdisciplinary as that is where much of the evidence of beneficial impact lies, not with individual palliative care providers (Ferrell et al. 2016). At the team level, give team members feedback and performance reviews based on evidence like

Fig. 3 above; budget time and finances for travel; monitor team burnout; and facilitate team building exercises (e.g., the group at Hopkins has a bi-monthly palliative care movie night. As you see more complex and difficult patients, develop strategies for dealing with complex patients. Some hints include the following (Text Box 1).

Text Box 1: Dealing with Difficult Families or Patients

- Build rapport – ask about joys (e.g., family)
- Address symptoms first – always the easy place to start
- Set expectations
- Figure out their goal
- Involvement with case management, social workers, and other supportive staff
- Notes – show data as to why you are making a recommendation
- Discuss coping strategies
- If family/caregiver is present, ask how they are coping too
- See regularly – monthly
- Email between visits
- Collaborate with specialists about care

Billing, income, and costs are crucial to long-term institutional support. Go after professional fees as appropriate, and in the USA, use the new Advance Care Planning codes which encourage physicians to document and bill for ACP discussions. Remember, though that while savings are system wide and might accrue to the ICUs, neurology, and home care, the costs are localized and usually come from one cost center. Plug in to national/regional groups like Center to Advance Palliative Care (CAPC) for knowledge sharing and collaborations. Use the Center to Advance Palliative Care (CAPC) office and home-based program design toolkits. They provide all the information and tools you need to launch office and home-based palliative care programs.

Bull et al. synthesized and identified five key barriers to outpatient palliative care (Bull et al. 2012). While these five are specific to the USA, many of them translate to other settings.

1. Large scale organizational challenges may hinder services delivery (e.g., differences in provider subspecialization, operational challenges, and lack of sufficient palliative care-trained providers to deliver services).
2. Limited funding to cover the costs of outpatient palliative care. For example, in the USA, Medicare covers palliative care for people with clear terminal diagnoses but not for people with chronic conditions. In Canada, reimbursements for home-based visits do not adequately compensate for the time that providers may spend visiting with patients in their home and travelling to the homes.
3. There is a lack of a gold-standard business model for outpatient palliative care, which means that each organization offering the services must create a business case for senior leadership to justify the incorporation of the program.
4. The fragmentation of care across settings (i.e., from inpatient to outpatient care) can result in difficult coordinating outpatient palliative care post-discharge. Further, as patients with palliative care needs often have multiple providers, it becomes challenges for outpatient palliative care to coordinate services and reduce redundancies with more acute care specialists.
5. There is a shortage of palliative care-trained physicians, nurse practitioners, and other health professionals, which results in few providers able to deliver outpatient or home-based services, let alone inpatient services.

To aid success, consider process changes that can help to reduce financial losses that may impede the success of programs. For example, Bull et al.'s use of Quality Assessment and Performance Improvement Cycles allowed them to identify challenges and inefficiencies in the Four Season's palliative care outpatient programs, develop strategies to overcome various barriers, institute said strategies and ultimately decrease financial losses by 40% (Kamal et al. 2011a, b) (Text Box 2).

Text Box 2: Ways to Improve Efficiency and the Bottom Line

- Do daily or weekly rounds for home-based patients (via teleconference) as needed to trouble-shoot
- Standardize the palliative care visit combining best practice components of care, identified by the National Quality Forum
  - For scheduling, 1 h for new patients, half hour for follow-ups
  - Keep an additional slot open for urgent appointments to avoid emergency rooms visits.
- Standardize data collection using established, validated data collection tools, and regularly aggregate and analyze the data. Bull and colleagues developed the Quality Data Collection Tool (QDACT), in partnership with colleagues at Duke University Medical Center. Use templates, Smart Phrases, and anything else that makes you more efficient.
- Increase referrals to palliative care by reaching out to providers across the health care system and other facilities
- Engage in several initiatives to increase referrals from palliative care to hospice (e.g., using quality metrics to track referrals, educating providers about referral process)
- Mentor providers to hone skills in palliative care delivery
- Introduce incentives to increase provider productivity and satisfaction (e.g., use of a nonfinancial bonus, extra paid time off, for providers who meet performance targets)
- Work to build a culture of accountability with regular performance reviews and sharing of team success
- Increase workforce to reduce provider strain and burnout
- Ensure that coding and billing are accurate by checking the billing, and engaging in education sessions

Text Box 2: Ways to Improve Efficiency and the Bottom Line (continued)

- Ensure that leadership time is best spent, and introduce administrators to perform administrative tasks, so that providers can focus on clinical work
- Clarify job expectations for providers and try to offload some of their non-clinical work to administrative staff

6 Conclusion

Community-based palliative care has become the focus of palliative care's growth and opportunity. Twelve of the largest randomized control trials on palliative care are community-based and result in equal or greater survival, positive satisfaction from patients and caregivers, and equal or less cost. Surprisingly, sometimes the business case is the easiest to make (Cassel et al. 2015). With health care financing that embraces value-based programs such as shared savings, bundled payments, global budget revenues, community-based palliative care shows great promise and may be part of the solution to provide better care for patients at a cost we can afford.

References

Alesi ER, Fletcher D, Muir C, Beveridge R, Smith TJ. Palliative care and oncology partnerships in real practice. Oncology (Williston Park). 2011;25(13):1287–90, 1292–3.

Bekelman DB, Rabin BA, Nowels CT, Sahay A, Heidenreich PA, Fischer SM, Main DS. Barriers and facilitators to scaling up outpatient palliative care. J Palliat Med. 2016;19:456–9.

Bell CL, Somogyi-Zalud E, Masaki KH. Methodological review: measured and reported congruence between preferred and actual place of death. Palliat Med. 2009;23:482–90.

Bischoff K, Weinberg V, Rabow MW. Palliative and oncologic co-management: symptom management for outpatients with cancer. Support Care Cancer. 2013;21(11):3031–7. https://doi.org/10.1007/s00520-013-1838-z. Epub 2013 Jun 21.

Bookbinder M, Glajchen M, McHugh M, Higgins P, Budis J, Solomon N, Homel P, Cassin C, Portenoy RK. Nurse practitioner-based models of specialist palliative care at home: sustainability and evaluation of feasibility. J Pain Symptom Manag. 2011;41:25–34.

Brian Cassel J, Kerr KM, McClish DK, Skoro N, Johnson S, Wanke C, Hoefer D. Effect of a home-based palliative care program on healthcare use and costs. J Am Geriatr Soc. 2016;64:2288–95.

Brumley R, Enguidanos S, Jamison P. Increased satisfaction with care and lower costs: results of a randomized trial of in-home palliative care. J Am Geriatr Soc. 2007;55:993–1000.

Bull JH, Whitten E, Morris J, Hooper RN, Wheeler JL, Kamal A, Abernethy AP. Demonstration of a sustainable community-based model of care across the palliative care continuum. J Pain Symptom Manag. 2012;44:797–809.

Cassel JB, Kerr KM, Kalman NS, Smith TJ. The business case for palliative care: translating research into program development in the US. J Pain Symptom Manag. 2015;50:741–9.

Chai H, Guerriere DN, Zagorski B, Coyte PC. The magnitude, share and determinants of unpaid care costs for home-based palliative care service provision in Toronto, Canada. Health Soc Care Community. 2014; 22:30–9.

Cohen J, Houttekier D, Onwuteaka-Philipsen B, Miccinesi G, Addington-Hall J, Kaasa S, Bilsen J, Deliens L. Which patients with cancer die at home? A study of six European countries using death certificate data. J Clin Oncol. 2010;28:2267–73.

Davis MP, Temel JS, Balboni T, Glare P. A review of the trials which examine early integration of outpatient and home palliative care for patients with serious illnesses. Ann Palliat Med. 2015;4:99–121.

Dumont S, Jacobs P, Fassbender K, Anderson D, Turcotte V, Harel F. Costs associated with resource utilization during the palliative phase of care: a Canadian perspective. Palliat Med. 2009;23:708–17.

Dumont S, Jacobs P, Turcotte V, Anderson D, Harel F. The trajectory of palliative care costs over the last 5 months of life: a Canadian longitudinal study. Palliat Med. 2010;24:630–40.

Dumont S, Jacobs P, Turcotte V, Turcotte S, Johnston G. Palliative care costs in Canada: a descriptive comparison of studies of urban and rural patients near end of life. Palliat Med. 2015;29:908–17.

Ferrell BR TJ, Temin S, Alesi ER, Balboni TA, Basch E, Firn J, Paice JA, Peppercorn JM, Phillips T, Strasser F, Zimmermann C, Smith TJ. The integration of palliative care into standard oncology care: American Society of Clinical Oncology Clinical Practice Guideline update. J Clin Oncol. 2016. ePub ahead of print.

Ferrell BR, Temel JS, Temin S, Alesi ER, Balboni TA, Basch EM, Firn JI, Paice JA, Peppercorn JM, Phillips T, Stovall EL, Zimmermann C, Smith TJ. Integration of palliative care into standard oncology care: American Society of Clinical Oncology Clinical Practice Guideline update. J Clin Oncol. 2017;35(1):96–112. Epub 2016 Oct 28. Review. PMID: 28034065.

Gagnon B, Nadeau L, Scott S, Dumont S, MacDonald N, Aubin M, Mayo N. The Association Between Home Palliative Care Services and Quality of End-of-Life Care Indicators in the Province of Québec. J Pain Symptom Manage. 2015;50(1):48–58. https://doi.org/10.1016/j.jpainsymman.2014.12.012.

Gardiner C, Brereton L, Frey R, Wilkinson-Meyers L, Gott M. Exploring the financial impact of caring for family members receiving palliative and end-of-life care: a systematic review of the literature. Palliat Med. 2014;28:375–90.

Gomes B, Calanzani N, Higginson I. Reversal of the British trends in place of death: time series analysis 2004–2010. Palliat Med. 2012;26:102–7.

Gomes B, Calanzani N, Gysels M, Hall S, Higginson IJ. Heterogeneity and changes in preferences for dying at home: a systematic review. BMC Palliat Care. 2013a;12:7.

Gomes B, Calanzani N, Curiale V, McCrone P, Higginson IJ. Effectiveness and cost-effectiveness of home palliative care services for adults with advanced illness and their caregivers. Cochrane Database of Systematic Reviews. 2013b; Issue 6, pp 13–33. Art. No.: CD007760. https://doi.org/10.1002/14651858.CD007760.pub2.

Guerriere DN, Zagorski B, Fassbender K, Masucci L, Librach L, Coyte PC. Cost variations in ambulatory and home-based palliative care. Palliat Med. 2010;24:523–32.

Higginson IJ, Sen-Gupta GJ. Place of care in advanced cancer: a qualitative systematic literature review of patient preferences. J Palliat Med. 2000;3:287–300.

Hoek PD, Schers HJ, Bronkhorst EM, Vissers KCP, Hasselaar JGJ. The effect of weekly specialist palliative care teleconsultations in patients with advanced cancer -a randomized clinical trial. BMC Med. 2017;15(1):119. https://doi.org/10.1186/s12916-017-0866-9.

Isenberg SR, Lu C, McQuade J, Chan KKW, Gill N, Cardamone M, Torto D, Langbaum T, Razzak R, Smith TJ. Impact of a new palliative care program on health system finances: an analysis of the Palliative Care Program Inpatient Unit and Consultations at Johns Hopkins Medical Institutions. J Oncol Pract. 2017;13(5):e421–30. https://doi.org/10.1200/JOP.2016.014860. Epub 2017 Feb 28. PMID: 28245147.

Jang RW, Krzyzanowska MK, Zimmermann C, Taback N, Alibhai SM. Palliative care and the aggressiveness of end-of-life care in patients with advanced pancreatic cancer. J Natl Cancer Inst. 2015;107(3). https://doi.org/10.1093/jnci/dju424. Print 2015 Mar. pii: dju424.

Kamal AH, Bull J, Stinson C, Blue D, Smith R, Hooper R, Kelly M, Kinsella J, Philbrick M, Gblokpor A, et al. Collecting data on quality is feasible in community-based palliative care. J Pain Symptom Manag. 2011a;42:663–7.

Kamal AH, Currow DC, Ritchie C, Bull J, Wheeler JL, Abernethy AP. The value of data collection within a palliative care program. Curr Oncol Rep. 2011b; 13:308–15.

Kerr CW, Donohue KA, Tangeman JC, Serehali AM, Knodel SM, Grant PC, Luczkiewicz DL, Mylotte K, Marien MJ. Cost savings and enhanced hospice enrollment with a home-based palliative care program implemented as a hospice–private payer partnership. J Palliat Med. 2014;17:1328–35.

Kerr K, Cassel JB, Rabow MW, et al., for California Health Care Foundation. Uneven terrain: mapping palliative care need and supply in California. 2015. www.chcf.org/publications/2015/02/palliative-care-data. Last accessed 30 Oct 2017.

Klinger CA, Howell D, Marshall D, Zakus D, Brazil K, Deber RB. Resource utilization and cost analyses of home-based palliative care service provision: the Niagara West End-of-Life Shared-Care Project. Palliat Med. 2013;27:115–22.

Kralik D, Anderson B. Differences in home-based palliative care service utilisation of people with cancer and non-cancer conditions. J Clin Nurs. 2008;17:429–35.

Leong M, Shah M, Smith TJ. How to avoid late chemotherapy. J Oncol Pract. 2016;12(12):1208–10. Epub 2016 Sep 30.

Levy M, Smith T, Alvarez-Perez A, Back A, Baker JN, Beck AC, Block S, Dalal S, Dans M, Fitch TR, Kapo J, Kutner JS, Kvale E, Misra S, Mitchell W, Portman DG, Sauer TM, Spiegel D, Sutton L, Szmuilowicz E, Taylor RM, Temel J, Tickoo R, Urba SG, Weinstein E, Zachariah F, Bergman MA, Scavone JL. Palliative care version 1.2016. J Natl Compr Cancer Netw. 2016;14(1):82–113. PMID: 26733557.

Luckett T, Davidson PM, Lam L, Phillips J, Currow DC, Agar M. Do community specialist palliative care services that provide home nursing increase rates of home death for people with life-limiting illnesses? A systematic review and meta-analysis of comparative studies. J Pain Symptom Manag. 2013;45:279–97.

Lustbader D, Mudra M, Romano C, Lukoski E, Chang A, Mittelberger J, Scherr T, Cooper D. The impact of a home-based palliative care program in an accountable care organization. J Palliat Med. 2017;20:23–8.

Majithia N, Smith TJ, Coyne PJ, Abdi S, Pachman DR, Lachance D, Shelerud R, Cheville A, Basford JR, Farley D, O'Neill C, Ruddy KJ, Sparadeo F, Beutler A, Loprinzi CL. Scrambler therapy for the management of chronic pain. Support Care Cancer. 2016;24(6):2807–14. https://doi.org/10.1007/s00520-016-3177-3. Epub 2016 Apr 4.

McCaffrey N, Agar M, Harlum J, Karnon J, Currow D, Eckermann S. Is home-based palliative care cost-effective? An economic evaluation of the Palliative Care Extended Packages at Home (PEACH) pilot. BMJ Support Palliat Care. 2013;3:431–5.

Muir JC, Daly F, Davis MS, Weinberg R, Heintz JS, Paivanas TA, Beveridge R. Integrating palliative care into the outpatient, private practice oncology setting. J Pain Symptom Manag. 2010;40(1):126–35. https://doi.org/10.1016/j.jpainsymman.2009.12.017. PMID: 20619215.

Muir JC, Scheffey C, Young HM, Vilches AO, Davis MS, Connor SR. Opioid prescribing practices before and after initiation of palliative care in outpatients. J Pain Symptom Manag. 2013;45(6):1107–11. https://doi.org/10.1016/j.jpainsymman.2012.06.006. Epub 2012 Sep 25. PMID: 23017605.

Obermeyer Z, Makar M, Abujaber S, Dominici F, Block S, Cutler DM. Association between the Medicare hospice benefit and health care utilization and costs for patients with poor-prognosis cancer. JAMA. 2014;312(18): 1888–96. https://doi.org/10.1001/jama.2014.14950.

Pouliot K, Weisse CS, Pratt DS, DiSorbo P. First-year analysis of a new, home-based palliative care program offered jointly by a community hospital and local visiting nurse service. Am J Hosp Palliat Care. 2017;34(2): 166–172. https://doi.org/10.1177/1049909115617139.

Rabow MW, Smith AK, Braun JL, Weissman DE. Outpatient palliative care practices. Arch Intern Med. 2010;170(7): 654–5. https://doi.org/10.1001/archinternmed.2010.56. PMID: 20386012.

Rabow M, Kvale E, Barbour L, Cassel JB, Cohen S, Jackson V, Luhrs C, Nguyen V, Rinaldi S, Stevens D, et al. Moving upstream: a review of the evidence of the impact of outpatient palliative care. J Palliat Med. 2013;16:1540–9.

Sarmento VP, Gysels M, Higginson IJ, Gomes B. Home palliative care works: but how? A meta-ethnography of the experiences of patients and family caregivers. BMJ Support Palliat Care. 2017. https://doi.org/10.1136/bmjspcare-2016-001141.

Scheffey C, Kestenbaum MG, Wachterman MW, Connor SR, Fine PG, Davis MS, Muir JC. Clinic-based outpatient palliative care before hospice is associated with longer hospice length of service. J Pain Symptom Manag. 2014;48(4):532–9. https://doi.org/10.1016/j.jpainsymman.2013.10.017. Epub 2014 Mar 27. PMID: 24680626.

Scibetta C, Kerr K, Mcguire J3, Rabow MW. The costs of waiting: implications of the timing of palliative care consultation among a cohort of decedents at a comprehensive cancer center. J Palliat Med. 2016;19(1):69–75. https://doi.org/10.1089/jpm.2015.0119. Epub 2015 Nov 30.

Seow H, Brazil K, Barbera L, Sussman J, Pereira J, Marshall D, Husain A, Austin P. The effectiveness of palliative care expert-consult teams. Toronto: Focus on the Temmy Latner Centre for Palliative Care (TLCPC) Team; 2013.

Statistics. NCfH: Health, United States, 2010: with special feature on death and dying. CDC.gov; 2010.

Sun Z, Laporte A, Guerriere DN, Coyte PC. Utilisation of home-based physician, nurse and personal support worker services within a palliative care programme in Ontario, Canada: trends over 2005–2015. Health Soc Care Community. 2017;25:1127–38.

Temmy Latner Centre for Palliative Care. History of the Temmy Latner Centre for Palliative Care. In: Sinai Health System (ed) 2015. http://www.tlcpc.org/tlcpc/history. Accessed May 30, 2018.

Teno JM, Gozalo PL, Bynum JP, Leland NE, Miller SC, Morden NE, Scupp T, Goodman DC, Mor V. Change in end-of-life care for Medicare beneficiaries: site of death, place of care, and health care transitions in 2000, 2005, and 2009. JAMA. 2013;309:470–7.

Wilson I, Carter AE, Berg KM. Improving the self-report of HIV antiretroviral medication adherence: is the glass half full or half empty. Curr HIV/AIDS Rep. 2009; 6:177–86.

Yu M, Guerriere DN, Coyte PC. Societal costs of home and hospital end-of-life care for palliative care patients in Ontario, Canada. Health Soc Care Community. 2015; 23:605–18.

Serious Illness and Out-of-Pocket Spending

101

Yolanda W. H. Penders and Aline de Vleminck

Contents

Abstract

The last years of life are one of the most costly periods in terms of formal healthcare provision, often attributed to a high amount of critical care, hospital admissions, and care home stays. Some of these costs are borne directly by the patient and their family carers: out-of-pocket costs. Out-of-pockets costs include insurance premiums, deductibles, and all costs for services not covered by health insurance or government-funded healthcare. Specifically for the last phase of life, research has

Y. W. H. Penders (✉)
Epidemiology, Biostatistics and Prevention Institute, University of Zürich, Zürich, Switzerland
e-mail: yolanda.penders@uzh.ch

A. de Vleminck
End-of-life care research group, Department of Family Medicine and Chronic Care, Vrije Universiteit Brussel, Jette, Belgium
e-mail: aline.de.vleminck@vub.ac.be

R. D. MacLeod, L. Van den Block (eds.), *Textbook of Palliative Care*,
https://doi.org/10.1007/978-3-319-77740-5_104

focused on insurer costs rather than out-of-pocket costs. The ability to design policy solutions is contingent on understanding the total societal costs, including both formal and out-of-pocket costs. While both the likelihood of out-of-pocket costs and the amount differ across healthcare systems and countries, they can have potentially serious consequences for patients and families, from refusing treatment to bankruptcy.

In this chapter, we discuss the distribution of costs in different health care systems and how different types of health care systems can have an effect on out-of-pocket costs. Next, we discuss how certain diseases (such as cancer or Alzheimer's disease) or vulnerable groups (people with a low income) may be particularly associated with higher out-of-pocket costs. Last, we review the impact of palliative care on out-of-pocket costs. We show how specialized palliative care can have a positive but limited impact on out-of-pocket costs and cannot on its own alleviate all out-of-pocket costs associated with serious illness.

1 Introduction

Being ill can be expensive. Even in systems where healthcare is accessible to and affordable for all, the consequences of serious illness can have far-reaching financial implications. In this chapter, we will examine the out-of-pocket costs that people with a serious illness or in the last phase of life may expect; how these costs are related to health care system and diagnosis; what the impact of these costs is on patients and families; and how specialized palliative care and the aging population may impact out-of-pocket costs.

2 What Are the Costs Associated with Serious Illness?

When considering the costs of healthcare, our first thought is often the direct costs of care: costs of treatment and medication, devices and supports such as wheelchairs, labor costs of healthcare professionals, and care in an institutional setting such as a nursing home. Serious illness, whether it is chronic or acute, often requires a great deal of care throughout the disease trajectory and particularly in the last phase of life. Indeed, much of the high cost of end-of-life care lies in the high amount of critical care, hospital admissions, and stays in a long-term care facility that people at the end of life require (Emanuel et al. 2002; Polder et al. 2006; Fassbender et al. 2009; Langton et al. 2014).

Beyond these direct costs of care, however, is a layer of secondary costs not quite so visible: opportunity costs in the healthcare system – the time and money spent on one patient cannot be spent on another – as well as lost income and economic activity on the part of the patient. There is also an impact on informal carers, whose caregiving activities are unpaid labor for the benefit of the patient. Informal carers may lose part of their income as a result of both the expenses of caring for the patient and time off from work that may be required. Caregivers also may be in more need of physical or mental healthcare themselves as a result of their caregiving activity. Finally, there are funeral costs that occur after death, as well as potential continued costs for next of kin associated with complex grief.

Thus, total costs can be divided into costs borne by the government or health insurance companies, so-called formal costs, and costs borne directly by the patient and their family carers that are not reimbursed through health insurance, so-called out-of-pocket costs. Out-of-pocket costs include insurance premiums, deductibles, plus all costs for services not covered by health insurance or government-funded healthcare – including many of the indirect costs mentioned above. Taken together, the sum total of all costs associated with serious illness and end-of-life care is referred to as the societal costs. Depending on the healthcare system and personal situation of the patient, out-of-pocket costs can be negligible or a reason for financial ruin. The financial burden of terminal illness can in this way contribute to the stress and psychological burden of patients and their families.

Given the complexity of the costs associated with terminal illness and end-of-life care, quantifying these costs is not an easy task. Most research in this area focuses on formal costs, which are easier to measure through governmental and insurance records. It is this type of study that is often cited to support claims that palliative care can be more cost-effective than regular care. The impact of palliative care on out-of-pocket cost can often only be determined indirectly. A 2014 systematic review found that the main focus of studies investigating the costs of palliative care was on formal or direct costs, with little focus on informal or out-of-pocket costs (Smith et al. 2014).

3 Distribution of Costs in Different Healthcare Systems

It is practically impossible to compare the proportion of formal coverage and out-of-pocket spending between healthcare systems in a straightforward manner. Apart from the complexity of measuring costs of care mentioned previously, such a comparison must also take into account things like insurance premiums and means-tested pricing or reimbursement schemes. However, there are certain patterns distinguishable in costs based on the type of healthcare system used in different countries. A classic division of healthcare systems is in the following four groups:

3.1 Beveridge Model

In countries employing the Beveridge model of healthcare, so named after William Beveridge who designed Britain's National Health Service, all healthcare is provided and financed by the government without out-of-pocket payments. This system may also be called a "single payer national health service model" (not to be confused with national health insurance/single payer models, where all residents of a country have mandatory health insurance). Examples of such countries are the United Kingdom and Denmark. People living in a country that employs the Beveridge model never pay out-of-pocket for care, unless they choose private treatment that is not covered by the government (e.g., elective plastic surgery or alternative medicine). Whereas costs to patients are minimized, in actual practice, patients in countries employing the Beveridge model often experience long wait times for medical services as budgeted resources rarely meet the population's actual needs. For example, in the UK, while the NHS has established a general maximum waiting time of 18 weeks for a nonurgent referral, this target had not been met since 2016 (Care Quality Commission 2018). In addition, the indirect costs of care, such as loss of income by the patient and informal carers, are not necessarily covered in such a system.

3.2 The Bismarck Model

The Bismarck model, named after Prussian chancellor Otto von Bismarck, is based on three principles: (1) The government is responsible for universal access to healthcare, (2) health policy is implemented by the smallest political and administrative units in society, and (3) elected officials negotiate the terms of medical care and reflect the interest of different medical professions. Health insurance in a Bismarck model is financed through payroll taxes and all residents are required to have health insurance. Insurance providers cannot refuse clients. This system may also be called a "nonprofit sickness fund" system or a "social insurance model." Examples of such countries are Germany, Switzerland, and Japan. While clinics and hospitals in the Bismarck model may be private and for-profit, the government enforces strict financial control, reducing the costs per capita.

3.3 The National Health Insurance/Single Payer Model

In countries that use a single payer model, medical care is privately run but paid for by a government-run insurance program that all residents pay into. Examples of such countries are Canada and South Korea. The NHI system can be seen as a combination of the Beveridge (because government-paid) and Bismarck (because privately run) models. The government can decide which treatments and forms of care they will pay for. Like the Beveridge model, a downside of this system is the potentially long waiting lists.

3.4 Out-of-Pocket Model

In some countries, there is no formal healthcare system. All healthcare is paid for by the patients, sometimes with intervention from nongovernmental organizations, and no systematic insurance or reimbursement scheme exists. This system may also be called a "market-driven system." Many low-income countries fall in this category. In such countries, all costs are carried by the patient and care can quickly become unaffordable. People may not seek medical attention until very late in the disease trajectory, at which point curative or life-prolonging treatments may no longer be an option and intensive care is needed. Care for the dying outside the formal healthcare system may be dependent largely on next-of-kin or religious or charity organizations.

3.5 Other

Finally, there are countries that use none of these healthcare systems, while other countries use a combination of systems. The United States of America, one of the most expensive healthcare system in the world costing more than 17% of GDP, employs a combination of all four models for different groups of the population (Institute of Medicine and National Research Council 2013). Another example of a healthcare system that is not easily classified is the Russian system, which is an NHS system on paper (i.e., free to all), but also requires compulsory medical insurance, and there is open and sometimes hostile competition between state-run and private healthcare services.

An overview of the impact of each system on out-of-pocket costs is given in Table 1.

From this classification, it would appear obvious that out-of-pocket costs are higher in some models than in other – with the Beveridge model at the bottom and the pure out-of-pocket system at the top. While this general hierarchy holds, even in a Beveridge model out-of-pocket costs can be a reality. Data from the World Health Organization Global Health Expenditure Database showed that in 2015, household out-of-pocket payments for healthcare were US$644 per capita in the UK. This is the average and does not reflect only those patients with a serious illness or in the last phase of life. A system which relies strongly on out-of-pocket costs runs the risk of catastrophic health expenditure in a large number of households, meaning that the financial situation in these households is one serious illness away from financial ruin (McIntyre et al. 2006). Apart from making healthcare inaccessible to a segment of the population, this causes financial insecurity among people at risk for serious illnesses and generally does not have a good impact on the economy (Xu et al. 2003).

The above classification is much-used and widely known, but it does not provide full information on the organization of a healthcare system nor on the financial burden to patients. The amount of out-of-pocket costs is not necessarily equal in countries that employ the same healthcare system. Furthermore, such general information does not necessarily tell us about the costs associated with serious illness or care in the last phase of life, which may include types of care that are less likely to be reimbursed such as specialist palliative care and care in long-term care facilities. Additionally, health insurance premiums may be higher in some countries than in others, which in itself is a type of out-of-pocket cost.

Additional information relevant to care in the case of serious illness may be found in other classifications. One such classification is the ANCIEN typology of long-term care developed as part of the ENEPRI project (Kraus et al. 2010). The ENEPRI project classified long-term care systems in European countries using two approaches, one focused on system characteristics and one focused on the use and financing of care. For the latter, they ascertained among other things how much is spent on long-term care, which portion of spending is private, and how much support is available for informal caregivers. This classification therefore takes both formal and out-of-pocket costs into account.

Table 1 Healthcare systems and out-of-pocket costs

System	Exemplary countries	Advantages	Disadvantages	Effect on out-of-pocket costs
Beveridge model	United Kingdom, Denmark, Hong Kong	Accessibility of care for all	Long waiting lists; government decides which treatments should be reimbursed	Low; all or almost all direct and supportive care is free at the point of delivery. Private alternatives that incur costs may exist
Bismarck model	Germany, Japan	Accessibility of care for all; collective negotiating power of government decreases formal costs	Economic incentives may push overtreatment and -medication	Moderate; most care is reimbursed through insurance, but additional expenses may be necessary
National Health Insurance model	Canada, South Korea	Accessibility of care for all; collective negotiating power of government decreases formal costs	Government decides which treatments should be reimbursed	Moderate; most care is reimbursed through insurance, but additional expenses may be necessary
Out-of-pocket model	Kenya, Thailand	Low formal costs	Inaccessibility of care to people of lower socio-economic strata	High; in principle all costs are paid for out-of-pocket
United States model	United States	Advanced equipment and treatment more readily available than in other systems	High insurance premiums; inaccessibility of care to uninsured people; high formal costs	Variable; heavily dependent on type of insurance and insurance provider

1. EU Cluster 1

   In countries in this cluster, many people rely on or expect to rely on formal long-term care in the last phase of life and most long-term care facilities are publicly funded. However, reliance on informal care remains important; for that reason, support for informal caregiving is high. Public spending on long-term care is low. This cluster includes Belgium, Germany, Slovakia, and the Czech Republic.
2. EU Cluster 2

   Systems in this cluster are characterized by high public spending and low private funding. As in cluster 1, many people expect to use formal long-term care at some point. While support for informal caregiving is high in cluster 2 as well, use of informal caregiving is low, possibly due to highly funded and well-developed formal long-term care options. This cluster includes Sweden, the Netherlands, and Denmark and may be termed the "Scandinavian model."
3. EU Cluster 3

   Long-term care systems in this cluster have fewer publicly funded long-term care facilities and formal long-term care is more likely to be privatized. These systems are further characterized by moderate public spending, high private funding, and a moderate use of formal care. Use of informal care is high, as is support for the use of informal care. This cluster includes Finland, France, Austria, England, and Spain.
4. EU Cluster 4

   The differences between clusters 3 and 4 are mainly in the support for informal care, which is low in cluster 4 even though usage of informal care is high. Like cluster 3, long-term care systems in this cluster are characterized by low public spending, high private funding, and low use of formal care. This cluster includes Italy and Hungary.

The impact of these systems on out-of-pocket costs is shown in Table 2. This typology of long-term care systems suggests that in clusters 3 and 4, out-of-pocket spending for long-term care will be higher as there are few publicly funded options. This may be problematic in particular for countries in cluster 4, where informal care alternatives are also badly supported. Note, however, that a use of formal over informal care is not in itself

Table 2 Long-term care typologies from the EU project ANCIEN and out-of-pocket costs

System	Exemplary countries	Advantages	Disadvantages	Effect on out-of-pocket costs
Cluster 1: High use of formal care, low spending	Belgium, Germany	Strong support for informal care	Low support for formal long-term care; strong reliance on informal care	Moderate; high out-of-pocket spending for formal long-term care, but good support for informal care
Cluster 2: High use of formal care, high spending	Sweden, the Netherlands	Strong support for both formal and informal long-term care	High formal costs	Low; public funding for formal long-term care is high and use of informal care is low
Cluster 3: Moderate use of formal care, moderate spending	Finland, Austria	Strong support for informal care; long-term care is often privatized	High out-of-pocket costs for formal long-term care; strong reliance on informal care	Moderate; high out-of-pocket spending for privatized formal care, but good support for informal care
Cluster 4: Low use of formal care, low spending	Italy, Hungary	Long-term care is often centered in the community; low formal costs	Little support for informal care, even though reliance on informal care is strong	High; out-of-pocket costs for formal long-term care are high and support for informal care low

problematic, as long as adequate support – both financial and psychological – is available for informal carers. Preferences for formal or informal care differ per country and should not be taken as absolutes (European Commission 2007).

Neither the overall healthcare system classification nor the EU ANCIEN typology of long-term care can explain all differences between countries in out-of-pocket costs for care in the context of serious illness or the last phase of life. One study that did investigate out-of-pocket costs in the last year of life in 13 European countries found substantial differences in the percentage of people who had any out-of-pocket costs for care (between 26% of decedents in Spain and 96% in Sweden), the amount these people had to pay on average (between 2% (Netherlands) and 25% (Czech Republic) of median household income), and the relative contribution of different types of healthcare to out-of-pocket costs (Penders et al. 2017). These differences did not conform to any recognizable typology of healthcare systems, but were likely a result of a combination of factors. Nevertheless, healthcare system characteristics can help us to make general predictions about the likelihood of high or low out-of-pocket costs for care.

There is currently no clear picture on how formal costs and out-of-pocket costs relate to each other in most healthcare systems. Most studies investigate either one or the other; a cursory review of the literature turned up only one study investigating both (Kotlarz et al. 2009). There are two intuitive answers regarding the relation between out-of-pocket costs and insurer costs. The first is that particular aspects of healthcare, for example, medication, that have low out-of-pocket costs must therefore have (relatively) high insurer costs and vice versa. The second is that low out-of-pocket costs are related to low insurer costs and high out-of-pocket costs are linked to high insurer costs, because some types of care are just expensive and the burden is shared. Neither view is currently supported by evidence, except for the aforementioned study which showed that for certain chronic illnesses, such as osteoarthritis, both out-of-pocket and insurer costs are high.

4 Differences in Out-of-Pocket Costs Between Diagnoses

Regardless of which proportion of costs is paid out of pocket, a person's diagnosis can influence the costs they can be expected to have at the end of life. Certain serious illnesses may require more care than others or have more treatment options available. For example, a person with dementia is more likely to require care in a long-term care facility, whereas a person with cancer is more likely to require expensive treatments. Also, depending on the healthcare system, certain types of care required for different illnesses may be more or less expensive.

Two diagnoses with particularly high out-of-pocket costs across the board are cancer and dementia, though for different reasons. Research has found that the biggest contribution to care of cancer patients in the last 6 months of life were hospital stays (up to an average of US$20,559 in the last month of life) and hospice use, which accounted for 36% of costs in the last month of life (Chastek et al. 2012). Within people with cancer in the USA, those who use chemotherapy have a more than 50% increase in out-of-pocket costs for care, and even more if they used chemotherapy in the last 30 days of life (Bao et al. 2017). Even among insured Americans, almost half reported significant or catastrophic (subjective) financial burden and even more reduced spending on food and clothing to pay for treatment (Zafar et al. 2013). The informal caregivers of people with cancer can also expect significant costs, both in terms of money and time: a study in Ireland found that the approximate average out-of-pocket costs for informal carers of people with colorectal cancer was €4476 (including travel), on top of €25,365 of time costs, i.e., the worth of the hours spent on caregiving tasks if the carers were paid the average hourly wage in Ireland (Hanly et al. 2013). As the estimated survival time for many forms of cancer goes up, cancer is becoming more of a chronic illness in some cases, with all the additional costs this implies: more months of medication costs, longer periods of time spent on informal caregiving, and a higher chance for informal caregivers to drop out of the labor market.

For people with dementia, research in the USA showed that while their formal expenditures over the last 5 years of life were the same as for people without dementia, the average societal costs were more than $100,000 higher for those with dementia than those who died of cancer, with out-of-pocket spending for people with dementia representing 32% of wealth measured 5 years before death compared with 11% for people without dementia (Kelley et al. 2015). Meanwhile in Europe, secondary and institutional care – including care by specialist physicians, hospital care, care in a long-term care facility and hospice care – were shown to be the largest contributors to out-of-pocket costs in nine out of 13 countries studied, constituting up to 76% of out-of-pocket costs in the last year of life (Penders et al. 2017). This was primarily attributable to care in long-term care facilities, and having difficulties with activities of daily life (independently of being chronically ill), two things people with dementia in particular may be confronted with. Especially in countries in ANCIEN clusters 3 and 4, stays in long-term care facilities may be extremely burdensome.

This is not to say that other diagnoses are necessarily cheap, especially in different healthcare contexts. In China, although the government has a policy to provide free healthcare to people with tuberculosis, the average out-of-pocket cost for tuberculosis was 11% of the median annual household income (Pan et al. 2013). In India, the out-of-pocket costs for kidney transplantations start at 386% of median household income and rise to 634%, essentially making treatment for kidney failure inaccessible to the majority of the population (Ramachandran and Jha 2013). On the other hand, advanced cancer treatments may be less available in these countries, so the costs of cancer may be relatively low compared to the USA. In countries with a lower average life expectancy (e.g., 68 years in India vs. 81 in the EU-28), a dementia trajectory or chronic illness trajectory may be considerably shorter and the total out-of-pocket costs therefore lower. Which disease groups or population groups are at risk for higher out-of-pocket costs therefore depends on both the treatment options and availability of care, burden of illness, and healthcare context.

5 The Impact of Out-of-Pocket Costs on Patients, Families, and Quality of Life

A study in 13 European countries showed that out-of-pocket costs in the last year of life have been found to be up to a quarter of median household income (Penders et al. 2017). And in countries with a pure out-of-pocket system, any serious illness carries with it the risk of financial ruin. High out-of-pocket costs, the full extent of which is often only known after death, can put patients and families for impossible choices: do we start or continue this treatment or not? Patients, but especially next-of-kin may be willing to spend "whatever it takes" on prolonging the life of their relative, to their own detriment and often without a clear view of what the benefits of certain treatments are – or indeed, if there realistically are any benefit. However, especially for chronic treatments – for instance, certain medication – the financial burden will eventually catch up. Higher out-of-pocket spending has been associated with non-adherence to treatments and higher rates of therapy discontinuation in the USA and elsewhere (Hennessy et al. 2016; Dusetzina et al. 2014). Older people in particular are vulnerable to negative effects of high out-of-pocket costs and sometimes cite high costs as a reason not to initiate or adhere to treatment or care, potentially decreasing quality of life in the final stage of life (Soumerai et al. 2006; Chao et al. 2008; Neugut et al. 2011). Older people often do not want to feel like they are a burden on their family, and high out-of-pocket costs may be one way they perceive this burden.

The financial burden of care can indeed weigh heavily on the shoulders of family carers: Hudson (2003), for example, reported that a quarter of his sample of family carers had stopped work or taken part-time work in order to care for dying family members at home. Soothill et al. (2003) in their survey of 200 carers noted that 44% retired to care for dying family members. This can reduce the capacity of households to deal with financial costs associated with long-term care. A study conducted in Italy found that a one-fourth of families of cancer patients have to use all their savings to pay for care at the end of life and around 45% have difficulties in managing their regular employment (Rossi et al. 2007).

Financial stress and a low income level are linked to a higher perceived burden and a more frequent exhibition of depressive symptoms amongst informal carers (Papastavrou et al. 2007; Andrén and Elmståhl 2007). Since most older people do not want to be a burden on their family, this may further dissuade them from engaging useful but expensive healthcare. Informal caregivers participate less in the labor market as a direct consequence of their caregiving activities, but also experience more physical problems and psychological distress. A meta-analysis of 176 studies found that caregiver depressive symptoms were associated with more physical health problems (Pinquart and Sörensen 2007). A study among female caregiving and noncaregiving twins found that caregiving was associated with lower mental health functioning, higher anxiety, higher perceived stress, and higher levels of depression and suggested that while both common genes and environment contributed to vulnerability to stress and consequently informal caregivers' functioning, caregiving lead to psychological distress even for those who were not particularly vulnerable to stress (Vitaliano et al. 2014). Another study found that up to 62% of family caregivers experience a high level of psychological distress, compared to 19% in the general population (Dumont et al. 2006).

There is also a disproportionate impact of out-of-pocket costs on people from lower socio-economic strata. Many people do not have the amount of savings recommended by financial advice bureaus, and these are mostly people from lower socio-economic strata. A bill of a few hundred dollars or euros can be disastrous for them where it would be inconvenient for most. Studies have shown that there are many differences in the use of healthcare by people from different socio-economic strata, as well as their health outcomes. For example, people from lower socio-economic strata are less likely to seek healthcare and may have less access to certain healthcare services (even with insurance) (Adamson et al. 2003; Allin et al. 2009). Additionally, there are gender disparities in the impact of out-of-pocket costs. Research has shown that most informal caregivers are women and that informal caregiving decreased women's participation in the labor market

(Viitanen 2005). As women may be relatively economically disadvantaged compared to men, their dropping out of the labor market can be particularly harmful.

In some cases, the financial burden of end-of-life care can be extremely high. The USA is a strong outlier in this respect, as a Western country where out-of-pocket costs make up a substantial proportion of healthcare costs. Studies have shown that in the USA, medical debts are the main reason for an increasing number of bankruptcies, up to 62% in 2007 (Himmelstein et al. 2009; Himmelstein et al. 2005). This does not just mean that families are left destitute: patients with cancer who filed for bankruptcy had almost twice as much risk of mortality as those who did not (Ramsey et al. 2016). The introduction of the Patient Protection and Affordable Care Act (ACA) in 2010 introduced out-of-pocket maximums, and the 2016 maximum was still a problematic 22% of the median annual personal income in the USA. This is still an improvement over the previous situation. Before the ACA, the average out-of-pocket expenditures for Medicare beneficiaries in the last 5 years of life exceeded total household assets for a quarter of decedents who were not survived by a spouse, and nonhousing assets for an additional 43% (Kelley et al. 2013). For those who were survived by a spouse, these figures were 10% and 24%, respectively, essentially leaving the widow or widower penniless. There are indications that the ACA has improved access and reduced financial burden for many patients, but it is not yet known how the situation will develop in the coming years (Dixon et al. 2017; Mahendraratnam et al. 2017).

Good support for family carers may partly alleviate the financial burden of care. Several countries, such as Belgium, France, and Germany, have policy measures in place that allow family carers to adapt their working patterns or take a leave of absence while retaining their employee rights (Maetens et al. 2017). While such regulations provide stability, financial compensation for informal caregiving occurs only in a limited number of countries.

6 The Impact of Specialist Palliative Care on Out-of-Pocket Costs

Many studies attempt to show that palliative care is cost effective, that is, not more expensive than regular (curative or life-prolonging) care. However, most evidence focusses only on formal costs and outcomes vary due to the diverse nature of palliative care initiatives. In a systematic review, it was found that specialist palliative care is most frequently found to be less costly relative to comparator groups with the difference being statistically significant in most cases when looking at formal costs (Smith et al. 2014). The same review found that, of the 46 included studies, only one focused on out-of-pocket costs – they found that there was no difference in the out-of-pocket costs of people who used hospice care in the USA and those who did not (Taylor Jr 2009). Another review on home-based palliative care services found that of 23 included studies six reported the cost-effectiveness of the tested programs, but evidence for cost-effectiveness was inconclusive (Gomes et al. 2009). Of these six, only one – a study from 1992 on home-based care for people with AIDS in northern Italy – provided a full economic evaluation using cost-utility ratios (Tramarin et al. 1992). A second study in the UK included both inpatient care and informal care in its cost-effectiveness analysis (Higginson et al. 2009). Both studies showed that home-based palliative care appeared to reduce costs, though the UK study showed no differences in costs to informal caregivers. Studies on the cost-effectiveness of hospital-based palliative care consultations show a fairly consistent impact on costs through lower (re-)hospitalization and intensive care unit admissions, but also do not take out-of-pocket costs into account (May et al. 2014, 2015). Likewise, hospice use in the USA has been shown to be cost-effective in terms of Medicare costs, but out-of-pocket costs were not studied (Kelley et al. 2013).

It is clear that although palliative care is less expensive than regular care in terms of formal costs, the impact on out-of-pocket costs is not studied sufficiently. Often out-of-pocket costs are not measured directly in costs research, though a few studies do exist. A Canadian study looked at the various costs incurred in the last year of life of patients who received care from a multi-disciplinary, home-based palliative care team. They found that while out-of-pocket expenditures in the last 12 months of life (in a single payer healthcare system) were only CA$379, the costs of formal care – the care provided by the home-care team as well as all other publicly funded medical costs – were almost 10 times as high. However, this was dwarfed by the unpaid caregiving costs – that is, the time dedicated to caregiving activities by families and friends, assigned a monetary value – which were more than CA$11,000 per month (Chai et al. 2014). With rising care needs as death approached, so did the monthly costs, with total costs in the last month of life averaging more than CA$30,000. Another study of the same palliative care service found that the societal costs were more than CA$34,000 per patient over the palliative trajectory (an average of 4 months).

What we can surmise from the available evidence is that while specialist palliative care can decrease out-of-pocket costs at the end of life, this is in no way guaranteed, and cost-effectiveness in terms of formal costs does not necessarily translate to a decrease in out-of-pocket costs. There are multiple reasons for this:

- Palliative care is often only available in the last phase of life, whereas out-of-pocket costs associated with serious illness are likely to occur earlier in the disease trajectory as well.
- Palliative care is often set up as an alternative to potentially overly aggressive hospital care or life-prolonging treatment. Its aim in these cases is not to provide support *in addition* to standard care.
- Many specialist palliative care initiatives are not community based and are thus not able to provide the type of support that is most likely to have an impact on the financial aspects of care.
- Palliative care often does not provide adequate support for family carers, both during the last phase of life and after death.
- The presence or absence of palliative care is unlikely to have an impact on certain parts of out-of-pocket costs no matter the way it is delivered, such as the missed labor market participation of both patient and family during the last phase of life.

While some of these reasons can be addressed – such as earlier initiation of specialist palliative care or better emotional support for family carers – others are almost impossible to change. It may therefore be wrong to assume that palliative care *should* have a large impact on out-of-pocket costs. However, full economic evaluations of specialist palliative care initiatives would do well to take the impact on informal and out-of-pocket costs into account.

7 Implications of Out-of-Pocket Costs for the Growing Population of Older People

Across the world, populations are aging. While many older people are able to maintain a good degree of independence, social engagement, and continued physical health, many do not – one study in the USA estimated that as few as 12% of people aged 65 and over achieve this ideal of "successful aging" (McLaughlin et al. 2010). Older people are likely to have severe or catastrophic disabilities and are at a higher risk of illnesses such as cancer and cardiovascular disease, and older people with dementia are likely to end up living and eventually dying in long-term care facilities (Reyniers et al. 2015; Gill et al. 2010). As such, an increase in the proportion of older people will have an impact on all aspects of healthcare, including chronic and long-term care, institutionalized care, and specialized end-of-life care.

First, as medical advances are made and life-prolonging treatments become more effective, certain types of care, like care for some forms of cancer, will become chronic care. Care will be provided for longer to patients with care needs that will increase, either steadily or in jolts, as time goes on. This will drive up the costs of both formal and informal care. It is unlikely in these cases that patients will be able to reliably provide income through work, so sustained medical costs may impose a significant financial burden if not adequately compensated. Long-term caregiving may also be especially burdensome for informal carers, both physically and psychologically. Informal caregiving over a number of years may also put informal carers at higher risk of losing their job than caregiving over a shorter period of time.

Second, an aging population puts more pressure on the long-term care system, whether that is based mostly on formal or informal care. The home setting is the preferred place of care of many older people (Wiles et al. 2011; Gott et al. 2004). Governments, healthcare organizations, and next-of-kin generally want to enable people to live at home for as long as possible. Even as demand rises, the number of beds in long-term care facilities in some countries has decreased (European Commission 2007). This means that an increasing number of older people living at home will have dementia, difficulties with multiple activities of daily living, and multimorbidity and that a larger number of informal caregivers will be affected. This will affect the presumed cost-effectiveness of encouraging people to stay at home longer: while care in a care home is expensive, it does not follow that home care is "cheap." People with difficulties with more than two activities of daily living are at risk for higher out-of-pocket costs (Penders et al. 2017), and chronically ill people and those with multimorbidities use a large portion of healthcare, financially speaking, regardless of setting (Aldridge and Kelley 2015). Older people living at home are also more likely to be hospitalized than older people living in a long-term care facility, which increases care costs. A study in the Netherlands found that the average societal costs of healthcare for hospitalized older people were €30,000 per year, with almost one third of that being informal healthcare costs between hospital discharge and 12-month follow-up (Asmus-Szepesi et al. 2014). Particularly older patients with a high risk score at the time of hospital admission (i.e., those who were most frail and had most physical and mental limitations) were likely to incur high costs, with informal care costs almost twice as high as the lowest risk group and formal costs (excluding the original hospitalization) more than twice as high. Furthermore, a prospective cohort study in the Netherlands found that when a person with dementia was admitted to a long-term care facility during the course of the study, the psychological distress of informal caregivers improved (Borsje et al. 2016). By promoting informal care in the home setting as an alternative for long-term care facilities, a larger number of informal carers is at risk of physical and psychological health issues. These issues may contribute to decreased labor market participation and loss of income and may place an additional burden on the healthcare system.

Not only are care homes one of the, if not the, most expensive types of care for care receivers in European countries; they are also the type of care that it is most likely people have to pay out-of-pocket for. This is a worrying combination. As the population of Europe ages, more older people will spend their final phase of life in a care or nursing home (Houttekier et al. 2011; Gomes and Higginson 2008). Private funding of long-term care facilities is usually unaffordable for residents, with average long-term care expenditures accounting for 60% to 80% of disposable income (OECD 2005). Means-tested contributions to long-term care, where those with a higher income or more wealth pay more and those with a lower income are subsidized such as in the Netherlands and the UK, may seem to be a solution to this problem, but in practice has been shown to also have an adverse impact on the accessibility of care for people of a low socioeconomic status (Comas-Herrera et al. 2010). Keeping (or making) care in long-term care facilities affordable for people from all backgrounds and socioeconomic statuses will be necessary to ensure the growing population of older people will be able to access appropriate care.

Unfortunately, the total costs of long-term care facilities and remaining at home are very difficult to compare. A fair comparison should not only include all the costs that were already mentioned in this chapter, but also expenses such as rent and food which are included in a long-term care facility but are always out-of-pocket in the home setting. Without a detailed comparison, it is unknown if care in a long-term care facility would still be so (relatively) expensive once food, rent, and assorted costs of living are included in the equation. On the other hand, people who move to a long-term care facility are more likely to have a severe care burden, complex multimorbidities, and dementia. If they remain at home instead, additional home care would be required which would drive up the costs of living at home. However, at least one study showed that in most countries, at least half of people who received home care did not have to pay for it out of pocket, suggesting there are systems in place to avoid the financial burden of home care falling solely on the care receivers' shoulders (Penders et al. 2017). If this is the case, policy makers should ensure these systems are robust enough to also provide for an influx of people with high care burden who would otherwise have lived in long-term care facilities.

8 Conclusion and Summary

The costs of end-of-life care are complex and sometimes hard to quantify. Out-of-pocket costs relating to care in the last phase of life affect most patients and their next-of-kin. To determine the burden of out-of-pocket costs on patients and their families in different healthcare systems, both direct and indirect costs must be taken into account. Financial stress can worsen health of both the patient and informal caregivers and in the worst case, can deter patients from seeking adequate and timely medical care. Cost-effectiveness studies of palliative care initiatives should study the total societal costs, including both formal and out-of-pocket costs.

References

Adamson J, Ben-Shlomo Y, Chaturvedi N, Donovan J. Ethnicity, socio-economic position and gender – do they affect reported health – care seeking behaviour? Soc Sci Med. 2003;57(5):895–904.

Aldridge MD, Kelley AS. The myth regarding the high cost of end-of-life care. Am J Public Health. 2015; 105(12):2411–5.

Allin S, Masseria C, Mossialos E. Measuring socioeconomic differences in use of health care services by wealth versus by income. Am J Public Health. 2009;99(10):1849–55.

Andrén S, Elmståhl S. Relationships between income, subjective health and caregiver burden in caregivers of people with dementia in group living care: a cross-sectional community-based study. Int J Nurs Stud. 2007;44(3):435–46.

Asmus-Szepesi KJE, Koopmanschap MA, Flinterman LE, TJ Bakker, Mackenbach JP, Steyerberg EW. Formal and informal care costs of hospitalized older people at risk of poor functioning: a prospective cohort study. Arch Gerontol Geriatr. 2014;59(2):382–92.

Bao Y, Maciejewski RC, Garrido MM, Shah MA, Maciejewski PK, Prigerson HG. Chemotherapy use, end-of-life care, and costs of care among patients diagnosed with stage IV pancreatic cancer. J Pain Symptom Manag. 2017;12:335. https://doi.org/10.1016/j.jpainsymman.

Borsje P, Hems MA, Lucassen PL, Bor H, Koopmans RR, Pot AM. Psychological distress in informal caregivers of patients with dementia in primary care: course and determinants. Fam Pract. 2016;33(4):374–81. https://doi.org/10.1093/fampra/cmw009.

Care Quality Commission. The state of healthcare and adult social care in England 2016/17. Presented to Parliament pursuant to section 83(4)(a) of the Health and Social Care Act 2008. 2018; Available from https://www.gov.uk/government/publications. ISBN: 978-1-5286-0051-4.

Chai H, Guerriere DN, Zagorski B, Coyte PC. The magnitude, share and determinants of unpaid care costs for home-based palliative care service provision in Toronto, Canada. *Health & social care in the community*. 2014;22(1):30–9.

Chao L-W, Pagán JA, Soldo BJ. End-of-life medical treatment choices: do survival chances and out-of-pocket costs matter? Med Decis Mak. 2008;28(4):511–23.

Chastek BB, Harley C, Kallich J, Newcomer L, Paoli CJ, Teitelbaum AH. Healthcare costs for patients with cancer at the end of life. J Oncol Pract. 2012;8(6s): 75–80.

Comas-Herrera A, King D, Malley J, Pickard L, Wittenberg R. The long-term care system for the elderly in England. s.l. ENEPRI research report no. 74; 2010.

Dixon MS, Cole AL, Dusetzina SB. Out-of-pocket spending under the affordable care act for patients with cancer. Cancer J. 2017;23(3):175–80.

Dumont S, Turgeon J, Allard P, Gagnon P, Charbonneau C, Vézina L. Caring for a loved one with advanced cancer: determinants of psychological distress in family caregivers. J of Pall Med. 2006;9(4):912–21.

Dusetzina SB, Winn AN, Abel GA, Huskamp HA, Keating NL. Cost sharing and adherence to tyrosine kinase inhibitors for patients with chronic myeloid leukemia. J Clin Oncol. 2014;32(4):306–11.

Emanuel EJ, Ash A, Yu W, Gazelle G, Levinsky NG, Saynina O, et al. Managed care, hospice use, site of death, and medical expenditures in the last year of life. Arch Intern Med. 2002;162(15):1722–8.

European Commission. Health and long-term care in the European Union, Special eurobarometer. Brussels: European Commission; 2007.

Fassbender K, Fainsinger RL, Carson M, Finegan BA. Cost trajectories at the end of life: the Canadian experience. J Pain Symptom Manag. 2009;38(1): 75–80.

Gill TM, Gahbauer EA, Han L, Allore HG. Trajectories of disability in the last year of life. N Engl J Med. 2010;362:1173–80.

Gomes B, Higginson IJ. Where people die (1974—2030): past trends, future projections and implications for care. Palliat Med. 2008;22(1):33–41.

Gomes B, Calanzani N, Curiale V, McCrone P, Higginson IJ. Effectiveness and cost-effectiveness of home palliative care services for adults with advanced illness and their caregivers. Cochrane Database Syst Rev. 2009;6: CD007760.

Gott M, Seymour J, Bellamy G, Clark D, Ahmedzai S. Older people's views about home as a place of care at the end of life. Palliat Med. 2004;18(5):460–7.

Hanly P, Céilleachair AÓ, Skally M, O'Leary E, Kapur K, Fitzpatrick P, Staines A, Sharp L. How much does it cost to care for survivors of colorectal cancer? Caregiver's time, travel and out-of-pocket costs. Support Care Cancer. 2013;21(9):2583–92.

Hennessy D, Sanmartin C, Ronksley P, Weaver R, Campbell D, Manns B, Tonelli M, Hemmelgarn B. Out-of-pocket spending on drugs and pharmaceutical products and cost-related prescription non-adherence among Canadians with chronic disease. Health Rep. 2016;27(6):3.

Higginson IJ, McCrone P, Hart SR, Burman R, Silber E, Edmonds PM. Is short-term palliative care cost-effective in multiple sclerosis? A randomized phase II trial. J Pain Symptom Manag. 2009;38(6):816–26.

Himmelstein DU, Warren E, Thorne D, Woolhandler S. Illness and injury as contributors to bankruptcy. Health Aff (Millwood). (February 2, 2005); [Web exclusive] content.healthaffairs.org/cgi/reprint/hlthaff.w5.63v1.

Himmelstein DU, Thorne D, Warren E, Woolhandler S. Medical bankruptcy in the United States, 2007: results of a national study. Am J Med. 2009;122(8):741–6.

Houttekier D, Cohen J, Surkyn J, Deliens L. Study of recent and future trends in place of death in Belgium using death certificate data: a shift from hospitals to care homes. BMC Public Health 2011;11(1):1.

Hudson P. Home-based support for palliative care families: challenges and recommendations. Med J Aust. 2003; 179(6):S35–7.

Institute of Medicine and National Research Council. US health in international perspective: shorter lives, poorer health. Washington, DC: The National Academies Press; 2013. https://doi.org/10.17226/13497.

Kelley AS, McGarry K, Fahle S, Marshall SM, Du Q, Skinner JS. Out-of-pocket spending in the last five years of life. J Gen Intern Med. 2013;28(2):304–9.

Kelley AS, McGarry K, Gorges R, Skinner JS. The burden of healthcare costs for patients with dementia in the last 5 years of life. Ann Intern Med. 2015;163(10):729–36.

Kotlarz H, Gunnarsson CL, Fang H, Rizzo JA. Insurer and out-of-pocket costs of osteoarthritis in the US: evidence from national survey data. Arthritis Rheum. 2009; 60(12):3546–53.

Kraus M, Riedel M, Mot E, Willemé P, Röhrling G, Czypionka T. A typology of long-term care systems in Europe. ENEPRI Research Report No. 91; 2010.

Langton JM, Blanch B, Drew AK, Haas M, Ingham JM, Pearson S-A. Retrospective studies of end-of-life resource utilization and costs in cancer care using health administrative data: a systematic review. Palliat Med. 2014;27

Maetens A, Beernaert K, Deliens L, Aubry R, Radbruch L, Cohen J. Policy measures to support palliative care at home: a cross-country case comparison in three European countries. J Pain Symptom Manag. 2017; 54(4):523–9.

Mahendraratnam N, Dusetzina SB, Farley JF. Prescription drug utilization and reimbursement increased following state Medicaid expansion in 2014. J Manag Care Special Pharm. 2017;23(3):355–63.

May P, Normand C, Morrison RS. Economic impact of hospital inpatient palliative care consultation: review of current evidence and directions for future research. J Palliative Med. 2014;17(9):1054–63.

May P, Garrido MM, Cassel JB, Kelley AS, Meier DE, Normand C, Smith TJ, Stefanis L, Morrison RS. Prospective cohort study of hospital palliative care teams for inpatients with advanced cancer: earlier consultation is associated with larger cost-saving effect. J Clin Oncol. 2015;33(25):2745.

McLaughlin SJ, Connell CM, Heeringa SG, Li LW, Roberts KS. Successful aging in the United States: prevalence estimates from a National Sample of older adults. J Gerontol B Psychol Sci Soc Sci. 2010;65B(2): 216–26.

McIntyre D, Thiede M, Dahlgren G, Whitehead M. What are the economic consequences for households of illness and of paying for health care in low-and middle-income country contexts?. Soc Sci Med. 2006;62(4): 858–65.

Neugut AI, Subar M, Wilde ET, et al. Association between prescription co-payment amount and compliance with adjuvant hormal therapy in women with early-stage breast cancer. J Clin Oncol. 2011;29(10):2534–42.

Organisation for Economic Co-Operation and Development. Long-term care for older people. Paris: OECD; 2005.

Pan HQ, Bele S, Feng Y, Qiu SS, Lü JQ, Tang SW, Shen HB, Wang JM, Zhu LM. Analysis of the economic burden of diagnosis and treatment of tuberculosis patients in rural China. Int J Tuberc Lung Dis. 2013; 17(12):1575–80.

Papastavrou E, Kalokerinou A, Papacostas SS, Tsangari H, Sourtzi P. Caring for a relative with dementia: family caregiver burden. J Adv Nurs. 2007;58(5):446–57.

Penders YWH, Rietjens J, Albers G, Croezen S, Van den Block L. Differences in out-of-pocket costs of healthcare in the last year of life of older people in 13 European countries. Palliat Med. 2017;31(1):42–52.

Pinquart M, Sörensen S. Correlates of physical health of informal caregivers: a meta-analysis. J Gerontol Ser B. 2007;62(2):P126–37.

Polder JJ, Barendregt JJ, Van Oers H. Healthcare costs in the last year of life – the Dutch experience. Soc Sci Med. 2006;63(7):1720–31.

Pyenson B, Connor S, Fitch K, Kinzbrunner B. Medicare cost in matched hospice and non-hospice cohorts. J Pain Symp Manage. 2004;28(3):200–10.

Ramachandran R, Jha V. Kidney transplantation is associated with catastrophic out of pocket expenditure in India. PLoS One. 2013;8(7):e67812.

Ramsey SD, Bansal A, Fedorenko CR, Blough DK, Overstreet KA, Shankaran V, Newcomb P. Financial insolvency as a risk factor for early mortality among patients with cancer. J Clin Oncol. 2016;34(9):980.

Reyniers T, Deliens L, Pasman HR, Morin L, Addington-Hall J, Frova L, Cardenas-Turanzas M, Onwuteaka-Philipsen B, Naylor W, Ruiz-Ramos M, Wilson DM. International variation in place of death of older people who died from dementia in 14 European and non-European countries. J Am Med Dir Assoc. 2015;16(2):165–71.

Rossi PG, Beccaro M, Miccinese G, et al. Dying of cancer in Italy: impact on family and caregiver. The Italian survey of dying of Cancer. J Epidemiol Community Health. 2007;61:547–54.

Smith S, Brick A, O'Hara S, Normand C. Evidence on the cost and cost-effectiveness of palliative care: a literature review. Palliat Med. 2014;28(2):130–50. https://doi.org/10.1177/0269216313493466.

Soothill K, Morris SM, Harman JC, et al. Informal carers of cancer patients: what are their unet psychosocial needs? Health Soc Care Commun. 2003;9(6):464–75.

Soumerai SB, Pierre-Jacques M, Zhang F, et al. Cost-related medication nonadherence among elderly and disabled Medicare beneficiaries. Arch Intern Med. 2006;166:1829–35.

Taylor DH, Ostermann J, Van Houtven CH, Tulsky JA, Steinhauser K. What length of hospice use maximizes reduction in medical expenditures near death in the US Medicare program?. Soc Sci Med. 2007;65(7):1466–78.

Taylor DH Jr. The effect of hospice on Medicare and informal care costs: the U.S. experience. J Pain Symptom Manag. 2009;38:110–4.

Tramarin A, Milocchi F, Tolley K, Vaglia A, Marcolini F, Manfrin V, de Lalla F. An economic evaluation of home-care assistance for AIDS patients: a pilot study in a town in northern Italy. AIDS (London, England). 1992 Nov;6(11):1377–83.

Viitanen TK. Informal elderly care and female labour force participation across Europe, ENEPRI Research Report No.13. Brussels: European Network of Economic Policy Research Institutes; 2005.

Vitaliano PP, Strachan E, Dansie E, Goldberg J, Buchwald D. Does caregiving cause psychological distress? The case for familial and genetic vulnerabilities in female twins. Ann Behav Med. 2014;47(2):198–207.

Wiles JL, Leibing A, Guberman N, Reeve J, Allen RE. The meaning of "ageing in place" to older people. Gerontolgist. 2011;52(3):357–66. https://doi.org/10.1093/geront/gnr098.

Xu K, Evans DB, Kawabata K, Zeramdini R, Klavus J, Murray CJ. Household catastrophic health expenditure: a multicountry analysis. The Lancet. 2003;362(9378):111–7.

Zafar SY, Peppercorn JM, Schrag D, Taylor DH, Goetzinger AM, Zhong X, Abernethy AP. The financial toxicity of cancer treatment: a pilot study assessing out-of-pocket expenses and the insured cancer patient's experience. The Oncologist. 2013;18(4):381–90.

Index

R. D. MacLeod, L. Van den Block (eds.), *Textbook of Palliative Care*,
https://doi.org/10.1007/978-3-319-77740-5

C

G

I

J

K

L

O

Q

T

U

V